Tumors of the Uterine Corpus and Gestational Trophoblastic Diseases

AFIP Atlas of Tumor Pathology

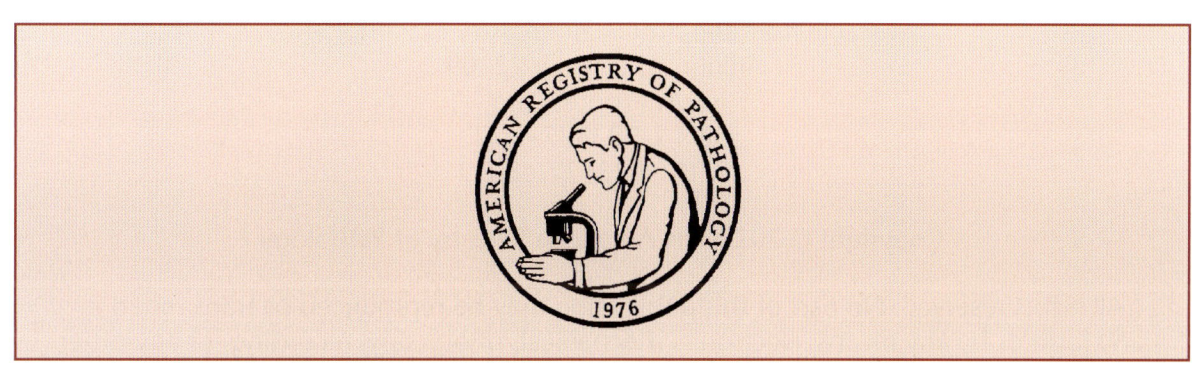

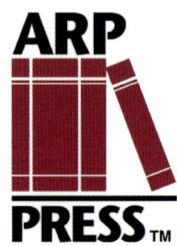

ARP PRESS

Arlington, Virginia

Senior Director of Publications: Mirlinda Q. Caton
Production Editor: Dian S. Thomas
Technical Editor and Subscription Manager: Magdalena C. Silva
Copy Editor: Audrey Kahn
Editorial Assistant: Elizabeth Tomlinson

Available from the American Registry of Pathology
Arlington, Virginia 22209
www.arppress.org
ISBN 1-933477-48-2
978-1-933477-48-0

Copyright © 2020 The American Registry of Pathology

All rights reserved. No part of this publication may be reproduced or transmitted in any form or by any means: electronic, mechanical, photocopy, recording, or any other information storage and retrieval system without the written permission of the publisher.

Printed in Korea

AFIP ATLAS OF TUMOR PATHOLOGY

Fourth Series
Fascicle 30

TUMORS OF THE UTERINE CORPUS AND GESTATIONAL TROPHOBLASTIC DISEASES

by

Esther Oliva, MD
Pathologist, Massachusetts General Hospital
Professor of Pathology, Harvard Medical School
Boston, Massachusetts

David C. Wilbur, MD
Pathologist, Massachusetts General Hospital
Professor of Pathology, Harvard Medical School
Boston, Massachusetts

Neil J. Sebire, MBBS, BClinSci MD, FRCPath FRCOG
Professor of Pathology, Great Ormond Street Hospital and Institute of Child Health (UCL)
Consultant Pathologist to the Trophoblastic Disease Unit, Charing Cross Hospital
London, United Kingdom

Robert A. Soslow, MD
Attending Pathologist, Memorial Hospital
Member, Memorial Sloan Kettering Cancer Center
Professor of Pathology and Laboratory Medicine, Weill Cornell Medicine
New York, New York

Published by
American Registry of Pathology
Arlington, Virginia
2020

AFIP ATLAS OF TUMOR PATHOLOGY

EDITOR
Steven G. Silverberg, MD
Department of Pathology
University of Maryland School of Medicine
Baltimore, Maryland

ASSOCIATE EDITOR
Ronald A. DeLellis, MD
Warren Alpert Medical School
of Brown University
Providence, Rhode Island

ASSOCIATE EDITOR
Leslie H. Sobin, MD
Armed Forces Institute of Pathology
Washington, DC

EDITORIAL ADVISORY BOARD

Jorge Albores-Saavedra, MD	Médica Sur Clinic and Foundation Mexico City, Mexico
William J. Frable, MD	Virginia Commonwealth University Richmond, Virginia
Kim R. Geisinger, MD	Wake Forest University School of Medicine Winston-Salem, North Carolina
Leonard B. Kahn, MD	Long Island Jewish Medical Center New Hyde Park, New York
Donald West King, MD	National Library of Medicine Bethesda, Maryland
James Linder, MD	University of Nebraska Medical Center Omaha, Nebraska
Virginia A. LiVolsi, MD	University of Pennsylvania Medical Center Philadelphia, Pennsylvania
Elizabeth A. Montgomery, MD	Johns Hopkins University School of Medicine Baltimore, Maryland
Juan Rosai, MD	Istituto Nazionale Tumori Milan, Italy
Mark H. Stoler, MD	University of Virginia Health System Charlottesville, Virginia
William D. Travis, MD	Memorial Sloan Kettering Cancer Center New York, New York
Mark R. Wick, MD	University of Virginia Medical Center Charlottesville, Virginia

Manuscript reviewed by:
Marisa Nucci, MD
Pei Hui, MD

EDITORS' NOTE

The Atlas of Tumor Pathology has a long and distinguished history. It was first conceived at a cancer research meeting held in St. Louis in September 1947, as an attempt to standardize the nomenclature of neoplastic diseases. The first series was sponsored by the National Academy of Sciences-National Research Council. The organization of this formidable effort was entrusted to the Subcommittee on Oncology of the Committee on Pathology, and Dr. Arthur Purdy Stout was the first editor-in-chief. Many of the illustrations were provided by the Medical Illustration Service of the Armed Forces Institute of Pathology (AFIP), the type was set by the Government Printing Office, and the final printing was done at the Armed Forces Institute of Pathology. The American Registry of Pathology (ARP) purchased the Fascicles from the Government Printing Office and sold them virtually at cost. Over a period of 20 years, approximately 15,000 copies each of nearly 40 Fascicles were produced. The worldwide impact of these publications over the years has largely surpassed the original goal. They quickly became among the most influential publications on tumor pathology, primarily because of their overall high quality, but also because their low cost made them easily accessible the world over to pathologists and other students of oncology.

Upon completion of the first series, the National Academy of Sciences-National Research Council handed further pursuit of the project over to the newly created Universities Associated for Research and Education in Pathology (UAREP). A second series was started, generously supported by grants from the AFIP, the National Cancer Institute, and the American Cancer Society. Dr. Harlan I. Firminger became the editor-in-chief and was succeeded by Dr. William H. Hartmann. The second series' Fascicles were produced as bound volumes instead of loose leaflets. They featured a more comprehensive coverage of the subjects, to the extent that the Fascicles could no longer be regarded as "atlases" but rather as monographs describing and illustrating in detail the tumors and tumor-like conditions of the various organs and systems.

Once the second series was completed, with a success that matched that of the first, ARP, UAREP, and AFIP decided to embark on a third series. Dr. Juan Rosai was appointed as editor-in-chief, and Dr. Leslie Sobin became associate editor. A distinguished Editorial Advisory Board was also convened, and these outstanding pathologists and educators played a major role in the success of this series, the first publication of which appeared in 1991 and the last (number 32) in 2003.

The same organizational framework applies to the current fourth series, but with UAREP and AFIP no longer functioning, ARP is now the responsible organization. New features include a hardbound cover and illustrations almost exclusively in color. There is also an increased emphasis on the cytopathologic (intraoperative, exfoliative, or fine needle aspiration) and molecular features that are important in diagnosis and prognosis. What does not change from the three previous series, however, is the goal of providing the practicing pathologist with thorough, concise, and up-to-date information on the nomenclature and classification; epidemiologic, clinical, and pathogenetic features; and, most importantly, guidance in the diagnosis of the tumors and tumorlike lesions of all major organ systems and body sites.

As in the third series, a continuous attempt is made to correlate, whenever possible, the nomenclature used in the Fascicles with that proposed by the World Health Organization's Classification of Tumors, as well as to ensure a consistency of style. Close cooperation between the various authors and their respective liaisons from the Editorial Board will continue to be emphasized in order to minimize unnecessary repetition and discrepancies in the text and illustrations.

Particular thanks are due to the members of the Editorial Advisory Board, the reviewers, the editorial and production staff, and the individual Fascicle authors for their ongoing efforts to ensure that this series is a worthy successor to the previous three.

Steven G. Silverberg, MD
Ronald A. DeLellis, MD
Leslie H. Sobin, MD

PREFACE AND ACKNOWLEDGMENTS

Since the publication of the Third Series Fascicle of the Uterine Corpus, molecular discoveries have deepened our understanding of epithelial, mesenchymal, and mixed müllerian tumors of the uterus, fueling a new and still evolving classification of the different categories of uterine neoplasms. For example, The Cancer Genomic Atlas of Endometrial Cancer has provided enormous insight to refine the classification of the different subtypes of endometrial carcinoma linked to important prognostic and therapeutic implications. At the same time, molecular findings have allowed for the discovery of familial syndromes associated with uterine corpus neoplasms, and identification of patients at increased risk for developing specific tumors, with the subsequent implementation of genetic counseling and appropriate treatment guidelines. Molecular underpinnings have also assisted in the development of new and potentially more predictive morphologic criteria for endometrial preoplasia, namely the endometrial intraepithelial neoplasia (EIN) system.

Another example of the impact of molecular findings in uterine tumors is represented by the breakthroughs in the classification of endometrial stromal tumors. Within the category of low-grade endometrial stromal sarcomas, we now recognize a myriad of morphologic variants, some of which may be seen in association with some high-grade endometrial stromal sarcomas. Although these morphologic variants often share immunohistochemical and molecular findings with typical endometrial stromal tumors, they were typically misdiagnosed in the past as other mesenchymal tumors, likely with secondary prognostic and therapeutic consequences. The spectrum of high-grade endometrial stromal sarcomas is broadening, each associated with specific morphologic, immunohistochemical and molecular characteristics that differ from undifferentiated uterine sarcoma, a tumor likely to disappear in future classifications. Furthermore, we are now able to recognize most of all these tumors based on morphology or with the utilization of immunohistochemistry as a surrogate of molecular signatures. In the field of gestational trophoblastic disease, major strides have been made in the identification of early complete hydatidiform mole with important treatment implications in the understanding and classification of hydatidiform moles with the addition of molecular genotyping into the working algorithm, and in the classification of trophoblastic tumors, with the recognition of epithelioid trophoblastic tumors, atypical placental site nodule, and mixed trophoblastic tumors as new entities.

In this Uterine Corpus Fascicle, we hope to offer the reader an objective as well as complete overview of the pathology of the uterine corpus accompanied by a vast number of high-quality illustrations, some of which have been provided by friends and colleagues from around the world. This "group" effort has helped improve the quality of this fascicle. It has been a long journey, but as coauthors we have enjoyed working together, and it has been a learning experience for all of us. Many individuals have also contributed in different ways to the fruition of this fascicle. We want to give special thanks to Drs. Dipti Sajed, Zehra Ordulu, Drucilla Roberts, and Robert H. Young. We also want to thank our support staff including Joanne Schiavo, Souad Mouni, Maya Dada, Steve Conley, and Michelle Lee, without whom this effort would not have been accomplished successfully.

We also wish to thank Drs. Steven Silverberg and Ronald DeLellis for inviting us to take on this project. In addition, we thank Dr. Pei Hui and Dr. Marisa Nucci for their helpful manuscript review and, finally, we wish to thank Mirlinda Caton and her team at the American Registry of Pathology for their tremendous support in completing this very important task.

Esther Oliva, MD
David C. Wilbur, MD
Neil J. Sebire, MD
Robert A. Soslow, MD

DEDICATIONS

Als meus pares, Pere i Mercè, per el vostre constant ajut al llarg de la meva carrera i vida lluny de casa i per ensenyar-me a mirar endavant sense tenir por als obstacles. Amb tota la meva estimació.

To the giants of gynecologic pathology, Dr. Jaime Prat, Dr. Robert H. Young, and Dr. Robert E. Scully who gave me the opportunity to learn and grow under their mentorship.

Esther Oliva

To my grandchildren, Crosby, Lucy, Gracie, Riley, James, and Genevieve, the most recent generation who remind me daily of the constancy, wonder, and delight to be found in the circle of life.

David C. Wilbur

To my husband, Michael Ogborn, for his unwavering support and encouragement.

To my dear departed parents, Arlene and Edwin Soslow, who imparted to me great curiosity and enthusiasm for education and teaching.

To my mentors, Dr. Richard Kempson and Dr. Michael Hendrickson, who kindled my passion for scientific discovery, taught me to always "put the patient first," and to interpret morphology within a relevant clinical context.

Robert A. Soslow

Permission to use copyrighted illustrations has been granted by:

Elsevier
Fertility and Sterility 1950;1:5. For figure 1-8.

Wolters Kluwer Health, Inc
American Journal of Surgical Pathology 2018;42:5-6. For figures 10-60 and 10-61.
International Journal of Gynecological Pathology 2010;29:513-22. For figure 2-15.
Lea & Febiger 1918:1263. For figure 1-6.

Springer
Nature 2012:25. For figure 1-1.

CONTENTS

1. Embryology, Anatomy, and Histology of the Uterine Corpus 1
   - Embryology 1
   - Anatomy 2
   - Histology 3
   - Endometrial Cytology 13
2. Non-Neoplastic Lesions 19
   - Endometrial Metaplasias 19
     - Endometrial Epithelial Metaplasias 19
       - Tubal (Ciliated) Metaplasia 19
       - Mucinous Metaplasia 21
       - Papillary (Lehman and Hart) Proliferations 24
       - Squamous Metaplasia 28
       - Papillary Syncytial Metaplasia 30
       - Eosinophilic Metaplasia 32
       - Hobnail and Clear Changes 33
       - Arias-Stella Reaction 33
       - Other Pregnancy/Hormonally Related Alterations 33
     - Endometrial Stromal Metaplasias 37
       - Smooth Muscle Metaplasia 37
       - Osseous Metaplasia 37
       - Cartilaginous and Fatty Metaplasia 38
       - Glial Tissue 38
       - Other Stromal Metaplasias 39
   - Inflammatory/Infectious Processes 40
     - Chronic Endometritis 40
     - Necrotizing Endometritis 43
     - Lymphoma-Like Lesions 43
     - Thermal Ablation 43
     - Chemotherapy and Radiation-Induced Changes 45
     - Viral Infections 46
     - Intrauterine Device (IUD)-Related Changes 46
     - Other Inflammatory Processes 46
   - Atypical Stromal Cells 49
   - Myxoid Change in the Endometrium/Myometrium 50
   - Adenomyosis 52
   - Blue Nevus 54
   - Other Processes 54

3. Endometrial Polyp 63
    Clinical Features 63
    Pathogenesis 63
    Gross Findings 63
    Microscopic Findings 64
    Differential Diagnosis 68
4. Endometrial Precancerous Neoplasia 75
    Epidemiology 75
    Clinical Features 76
    Gross Findings 76
    Molecular Genetic Findings 76
    Diagnostic Criteria 77
    Differential Diagnosis 82
5. Endometrioid Carcinoma and Related Carcinomas 89
    General Features and Epidemiology 89
    Clinical Features 91
    Gross Findings 91
    Microscopic Findings 91
        Architectural Features 91
        Cellular Features 93
        Stromal Features 99
        Treatment-Related Changes 101
    Grading 103
    Cytology of Endometrial Neoplasia 108
    Related Carcinomas 111
        Mucinous Carcinoma 111
        Ciliated Carcinoma 111
        Secretory Carcinoma 111
        Villoglandular Carcinoma 111
        Endometrioid Carcinoma Admixed with Other Elements ... 112
        Undifferentiated and Dedifferentiated Carcinoma 112
    Staging 119
        Myometrial Invasion 119
        Lymphovascular Invasion 124
        Cervical Involvement 125
        Synchronous Endometrioid Endometrial and Ovarian Carcinomas 128
        Lymph Node Metastases 129
    Immunohistochemical Findings 131
    Molecular Genetic Findings 133
    Differential Diagnosis 137
    Treatment and Prognosis 149

6. Serous Carcinoma 165
    General Features 165
    Clinical Features 165
    Gross Findings 166
    Microscopic Findings 166
    Precursors 173
    Immunohistochemical and Molecular Genetic Findings 174
    Differential Diagnosis 174
    Treatment and Prognosis 179

7. Clear Cell Carcinoma 187
    Definition 187
    General Features 187
    Clinical Features 187
    Gross Findings 187
    Microscopic Findings 188
        Architectural Findings 188
        Cytologic Findings 191
        Stromal Features 192
        Anaplastic or "Undifferentiated" Clear Cell Carcinoma 192
        Precursors 195
    Immunohistochemical Findings 195
    Molecular Genetic Findings 196
    Differential Diagnosis 197
    Treatment and Prognosis 202

8. Familial Cancer Syndromes 209
    Lynch Syndrome 209
        Definition 209
        General Features 209
        Pathophysiology and Genetics 209
        Screening and Diagnosis 210
        Gross Findings 212
        Microscopic Findings 212
        Immunohistochemical Findings 216
        Comprehensive Screening System 220
        Treatment and Prognosis 220
    Lynch-Like Syndrome 222
        Definition 222
        General Features and Epidemiology 222
        Pathophysiology and Genetics 222
    POLE and POLD1 Germline Mutations 223
    Cowden Syndrome 223

Hereditary Breast and Ovarian Cancer Syndromes (*BRCA* Syndromes) 224
Rare and Controversial Drivers of Endometrial Carcinoma 224
9. Endometrial Stromal Tumors 229
Endometrial Stromal Nodule and Endometrial Stromal Sarcoma 229
Definition 229
Clinical Features 229
Gross Findings 229
Microscopic Findings 231
Immunohistochemical Findings 244
Molecular Genetic Findings 247
Differential Diagnosis 250
Treatment and Prognosis 256
High-Grade Endometrial Stromal Sarcomas 258
Definition 258
YWHAE-FAM22 (*YWHAE-NUTM2*) High-Grade Endometrial Stromal Sarcoma 258
Clinical Features 258
Gross Findings 258
Microscopic Findings 258
Immunohistochemical and Molecular Genetic Findings 258
Differential Diagnosis 259
Treatment and Prognosis 262
ZC3H7B-BCOR High-Grade Endometrial Stromal Sarcoma 262
Clinical Features 262
Gross Findings 262
Microscopic Findings 263
Immunohistochemical and Molecular Genetic Findings 263
Differential Diagnosis 265
Treatment and Prognosis 267
High-Grade Endometrial Stromal Sarcoma in a Background of Low-Grade
Endometrial Stromal Sarcoma 267
Undifferentiated Uterine Sarcoma 268
Definition 268
Clinical Features 268
Gross Findings 268
Microscopic Findings 269
Immunohistochemical and Molecular Genetic Findings 269
Differential Diagnosis 269
Treatment and Prognosis 270
Uterine Tumors Resembling Ovarian Sex Cord Tumors 270
Definition 270
Clinical Features 270

Gross Findings 270
Microscopic Findings 270
Immunohistochemical Findings 271
Ultrastuctural Findings 274
Molecular Genetic Findings 274
Differential Diagnosis 276
Treatment and Prognosis 276

10. Smooth Muscle and Other Mesenchymal Tumors 289
    Leiomyoma and Variants 289
        Definition 289
        Epidemiology and General Features 289
        Clinical Features 290
        Gross Findings 291
        Microscopic Findings 295
            Leiomyoma with Bizarre Nuclei ("Symplastic" Leiomyoma) 297
            Fumarate Hydratase-Deficient 300
            Cellular Leiomyoma 301
            Mitotically Active Leiomyoma 302
            Leiomyoma with Hydropic (Including Diffuse and Perinodular) Change .. 304
            "Dissecting" Leiomyoma Including Cotyledonoid Leiomyoma 304
            Hemorrhagic Cellular "Apoplectic") Leiomyoma 306
            Drug-Related Changes in Leiomyoma 308
            Epithelioid Leiomyoma 309
            Myxoid Leiomyoma 310
            Leiomyoma with Heterologous Elements 310
            Diffuse Leiomyomatosis 311
            Parasitic Leiomyoma 311
            Diffuse Peritonal Leiomyomatosis 312
            Leiomyoma with Vascular Invasion 312
            Intravenous Leiomyomatosis 313
            Benign Metastasizing Leiomyoma 315
        Immunohistochemical Findings 315
        Molecular Genetic Findings 317
        Differential Diagnosis 319
        Treatment and Prognosis 323
    Leiomyosarcoma 324
        Definition 324
        Epidemiology and General Features 324
        Clinical Features 325
        Gross Findings 325
        Microscopic Findings 326

   Spindle 326
   Epithelioid 330
   Myxoid 331
   Dedifferentiated 333
   Other 333
  Immunohistochemical Findings 333
  Molecular Genetic Findings 334
  Differential Diagnosis 335
  Treatment and Prognosis 337
Smooth Muscle Tumors of Uncertain Malignant Potential (Atypical Leiomyoma) ... 339
Other Mesenchymal Tumors 340
  PEComa 340
   Definition 340
   Epidemiology and General Features 341
   Gross Findings 341
   Microscopic Findings 341
   Immunohistochemical Findings 345
   Differential Diagnosis 346
   Treatment and Prognosis 347
  Rhabdomyosarcoma 348
   Definition 348
   Clinical Features 348
   Gross Findings 348
   Microscopic Findings 348
   Immunohistochemical and Molecular Genetic Findings 348
   Differential Diagnosis 349
   Treatment and Prognosis 351
  Inflammatory Myofibroblastic Tumor 351
   Definition and General Features 351
   Clinical Features 351
   Gross Findings 351
   Microscopic Findings 351
   Immunohistochemical Findings 352
   Molecular Genetic Findings 352
   Ultrastructural Findings 354
   Differential Diagnosis 354
   Treatment and Prognosis 355
  Vascular Tumors 356
  Alveolar Soft Part Sarcoma 356
  Lipoma and Liposarcoma 358

		Solitary Fibrous Tumor	358
		Other Mesenchymal Tumors	359
11.	Mixed Epithelial-Stromal Tumors		383
	Carcinosarcoma		383
		Definition	383
		General Features	383
		Clinical Features	383
		Gross Findings	383
		Microscopic Findings	383
		Pathogenisis	389
		Immunohistochemical Findings	389
		Molecular Genetic Findings	390
		Differential Diagnosis	391
		Treatment and Prognosis	393
	Low-Grade Müllerian Adenosarcoma		394
		Definition	394
		General Features	394
		Clinical Features	394
		Gross Findings	394
		Microscopic Findings	395
		Immunohistochemical Findings	403
		Molecular Genetic Findings	405
		Differential Diagnosis	405
		Treatment and Prognosis	407
	Müllerian Adenofibroma		408
	Adenomyoma		408
		Definition	408
		Clinical Features	408
		Gross Findings	409
		Microscopic Findings	409
		Differential Diagnosis	409
		Treatment and Prognosis	411
	Atypical Polypoid Adenomyoma		411
		Definition	411
		Clinical Features	411
		Gross Findings	411
		Microscopic Findings	411
		Immunohistochemical and Molecular Genetic Findings	413
		Differential Diagnosis	414
		Treatment and Prognosis	414

12. Miscellaneous and Metastatic Malignancies ... 421
    Neuroendocrine Carcinomas ... 421
    Squamous Cell Carcinoma ... 423
    Mesonephric-Like Carcinoma ... 424
    Primitive Neuroectodermal Tumors ... 426
    Wilms Tumor ... 428
    Pure Germ Cell Tumors and Carcinomas with Germ Cell-Like Differentiation ... 429
        Yolk Sac Tumors ... 429
        Hepatoid Tumors ... 431
        Uterine Teratomas ... 431
        Nongestational Tumors with Trophoblastic Differentiation ... 431
    Sex Cord-Stromal Tumors ... 433
    Metastases and Direct Extension to Uterine Corpus from Adjacent Gynecologic
        Organs ... 433
        Primary Adnexal/Peritoneal Carcinomas ... 435
        Primary Cervical Carcinomas ... 435
    Metastases from Extragynecologic Sites ... 437
    Hematolymphoid Malignancies ... 438
13. Gestational Trophoblastic Diseases ... 445
    Normal Trophoblastic Development ... 446
        Trophoblast Stem Cells and Early Development ... 450
    Gestational Trophoblastic Diseases ... 452
        Staging ... 452
        Epidemiology ... 452
        Genetics ... 453
        Imprinting ... 454
        Familial Recurrent (Biparental) Hydatidiform Moles ... 455
        Genetic Testing of Hydatidiform Moles ... 455
        Genetic Features Influencing Outcome ... 456
        Genetic Testing of Gestational Trophoblastic Tumors ... 456
        Human Chorionic Gonadotrophin as a Biomarker of Gestational Trophoblastic
            Disease ... 457
        Gestational Trophoblastic Disease Subtypes ... 457
            Hydatidiform Moles ... 458
                Complete Hydatidiform Mole ... 459
                Partial Hydatidiform Mole ... 464
                Invasive Hydatidiform Mole ... 469
                Metastatic Molar Disease ... 470
                Ectopic Hydatidiform Mole ... 470
                Twin Pregnancy with Hydatidiform Mole ... 470
                Immunohistochemical Findings ... 471

  Differential Diagnosis 472
  Treatment and Prognosis. 475
Gestational Trophoblastic Tumors 476
 Choriocarcinoma 476
  Definition 476
  Clinical Features 476
  Gross Findings 477
  Microscopic Findings. 477
  Immunohistochemical and Molecular Genetic Findings 480
 Intermediate Trophoblastic Lesions 481
  Placental Site Trophoblastic Tumor 481
   Clinical Features. 482
   Gross Findings 482
   Microscopic Findings. 482
   Immunohistochemical and Molecular Genetic Findings 483
   Treatment and Prognosis. 484
  Epithelioid Trophoblastic Tumor 485
   Clinical Features. 485
   Gross Findings 485
   Microscopic Findings. 485
   Immunohistochemical Findings 488
   Molecular Genetic Findings. 488
   Treatment and Prognosis. 488
   Curettage Specimens of Trophoblastic Tissue 489
  Exaggerated Placental Site Reaction 489
  Placental-Site Nodule/Atypical Placental Site Nodule. 489
 Mixed Gestational Trophoplastic Tumors 490
 Nongestational Tumors with Trophoblastic Phenotype 492
Index 507

1 EMBRYOLOGY, ANATOMY, AND HISTOLOGY OF THE UTERINE CORPUS

EMBRYOLOGY

The paramesonephric (müllerian) ducts, originally described by Johannes Muller in 1830 (1), are the precursors of the fallopian tubes, uterine corpus, cervix, and upper vagina. They arise from mesoderm lateral to the mesonephric (wolffian) ducts formed in the 7th week of gestation. The paramesonephric ducts develop from thickenings and focal invaginations of the coelomic epithelium on the upper poles of the mesonephros. They course down the urogenital ridge to terminate at the primitive urogenital sinus.

Initial paramesonephric duct development is under the influence of the *Wnt* family of genes, particularly Wnt4, which promotes cell migration (2). In subsequent weeks the absence of "müllerian-inhibiting substance," a glycoprotein normally produced in the male testicular Sertoli cells in response to sex-determining region Y (SRY) protein, allows the paramesonephric ducts to develop, accompanied by the regression of the paired wolffian ducts (3).

The paramesonephric ducts grow caudally and laterally toward the urogenital ridges. At approximately 8 weeks, the lower portion of the combined paramesonephric ducts fuses with the ascending endoderm of the urogenital sinus at the sinus tubercle. Between 9 and 11 weeks of gestation, the lower medial portions of the paramesonephric ducts develop central lumens and complete their fusion to form the uterus and upper two thirds of the vagina, while the lateral portions remain hollow, funnel shaped, and open to the peritoneal cavity, becoming the fallopian tubes (fig. 1-1). The sinovaginal bulb forms the lower third of the vagina.

Within the uterus, the cervix becomes distinct from the corpus via an intervening constriction. The cervix constitutes about two thirds, and the corpus about one third of the structure at this stage. Reversal in size to a larger uterine corpus does not take place until the early teenage years. The upper end of the fused structure contains the precursor cells for the endometrium, myometrium, and uterine serosa, which begin their development at about 19 weeks of gestation. A midline septum normally persists in the developing uterus until about 20 weeks (fig. 1-2).

Between 20 weeks and birth, the uterine circumference grows by about three-fold and the width increases by about two-fold. During this

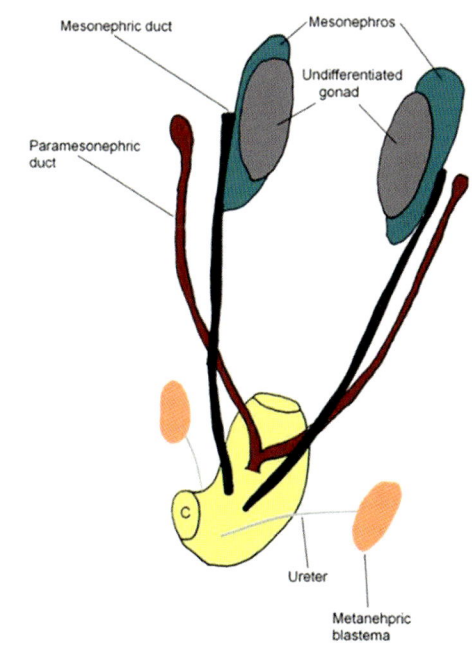

Figure 1-1

EMBRYONIC GENITOURINARY TRACT

This schematic shows the embryonic genitourinary tract between 6 and 8 weeks of gestation. (Figure 4b from Healey A. Embryology of the female reproductive tract. In: Mann GS, Blair JC, Garden AS, eds. Imaging of gynecologic disorders in infants and children, medical radiology. Diagnostic imaging. Berlin: Springer-Verlag; 2012:25.)

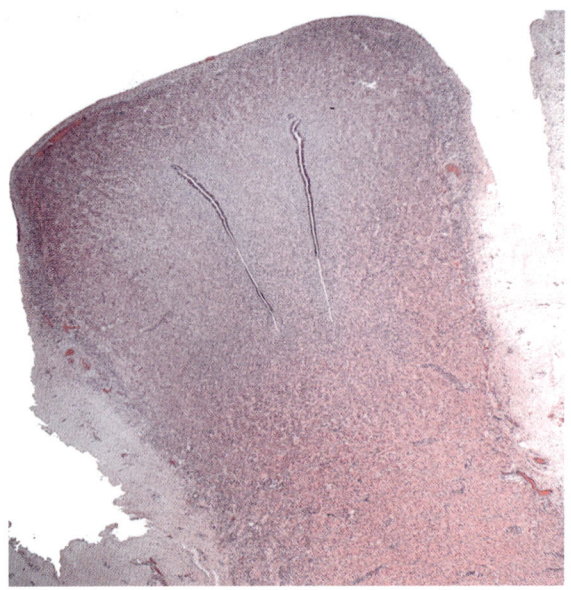

Figure 1-2

DEVELOPING UTERUS AT 20 WEEKS' GESTATION

The two uterine chambers and a divided septum are seen.

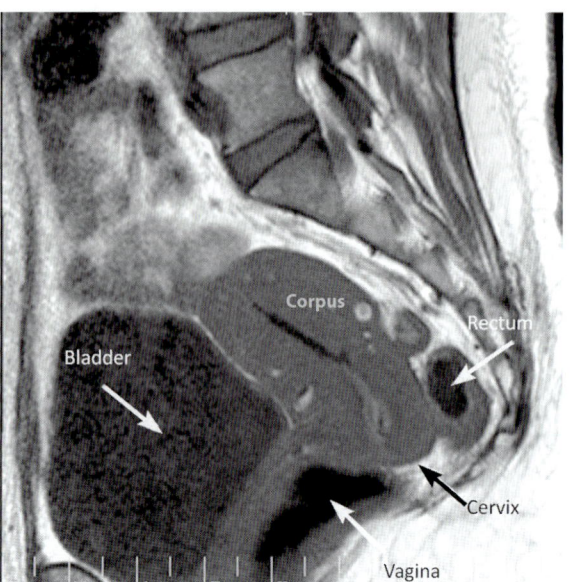

Figure 1-3

FEMALE GENITAL TRACT

In this sagittal magnetic resonance image (MRI) of the female genital tract, the relationship of the uterus to the bladder anteriorly and the rectum posteriorly is visualized. (Courtesy of Dr. S. F. Wilbur, Rochester, NY.)

time, the endometrium and the myometrium continue to differentiate and develop under regulation by the *Wnt* gene family. Wnt7a is expressed in luminal epithelium and Wnt5a is expressed in the mesenchymal elements (4). The endometrium changes from a simple columnar surface epithelium supported by an underlying fibroblastic stroma, to an invaginating, gland-forming epithelium extending toward the developing myometrium. At birth, the endometrium resembles an adult pattern of differentiation since it is still under maternal hormonal influence, but at about 1 month after maternal hormonal withdrawal, the endometrium reverts to an atrophic pattern until puberty.

A variety of developmental anomalies can occur during organogenesis, including septate uterus, which is caused by the lack of regression of the fused wall of the paramesonephric ducts; bicornuate uterus, caused by lack of fusion of the ducts; and unicornuate uterus, caused by duct regression or fusion failure (5).

ANATOMY

The uterine corpus is a thick-walled muscular structure located in the pelvis between the bladder on the anterior side and the rectum posteriorly (fig. 1-3). The nulliparous uterus measures about 75 mm in length, 50 mm in width across the fundus, and about 25 mm in thickness. It weighs between 40 and 100 g. Multiparous uteri are 20 to 30 percent larger and can be more than double the weight of nulliparous uteri (6).

The uterine corpus is a triangular structure, broadest at the fundus. The narrow area above the internal os is the isthmus (also known as the lower uterine segment), and the area of connection to the fallopian tubes corresponds to the cornua. The corpus is typically oriented at a right angle in relation to the vagina, pointed anteriorly, but this positioning can be variable as the uterus is mobile on its ligamentous suspension.

The anterior serosal surface is covered by peritoneum to a midlevel before being reflected back over the upper surface of the bladder (fig. 1-4). On the posterior surface, the peritoneal covering extends further inferiorly before reflecting back over the rectosigmoid colon. This difference in level of peritoneal covering allows for a distinction between anterior and posterior uterine surfaces in gross specimens (fig. 1-5). The location of the fallopian tubes also allows for orientation of specimens as they communicate

Embryology, Anatomy, and Histology of the Uterine Corpus

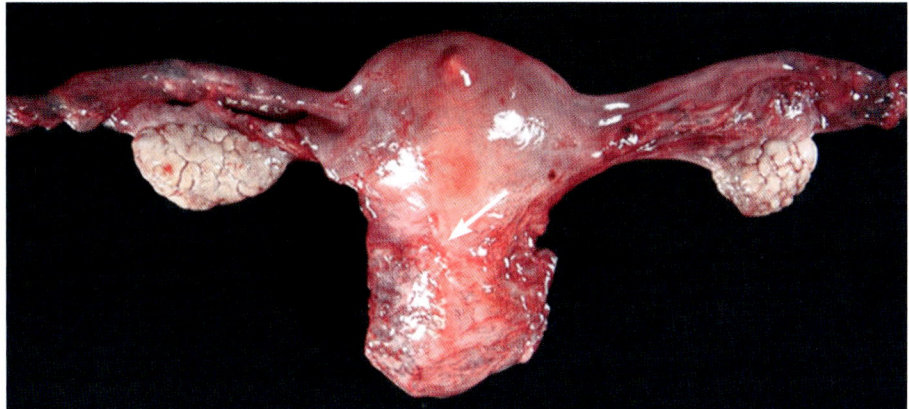

Figure 1-4

ANTERIOR VIEW OF THE UTERUS

The constriction demarcating the uterine corpus and cervix is clearly visible. The peritoneum extends only part of the way down the anterior surface since it reflects back over the surface of the bladder in this location (arrow).

Figure 1-5

LATERAL VIEW OF THE UTERUS

The peritoneal reflection is more caudally located on the posterior surface (single arrow) than on the anterior surface (double arrow). Orientation is also assisted by the posterior location of the fallopian tube stump, which is located behind the round ligament (triple arrow).

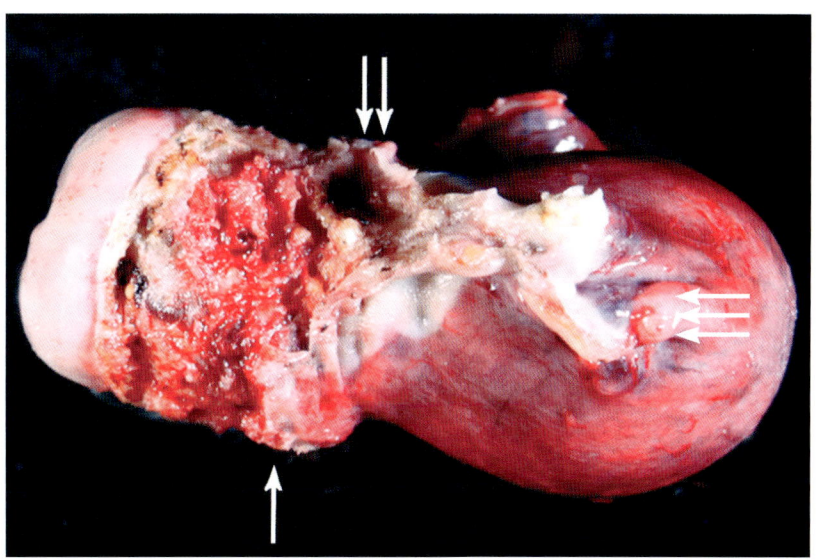

with the corpus posterior and caudally to the round ligaments. The anterior and posterior peritoneal coverings meet laterally to form the broad ligaments, which attach to the pelvic side wall. The broad and round ligaments suspend the uterus in its typical anteverted position.

The blood supply of the uterine corpus is predominantly derived from the uterine arteries, which branch from the internal iliac (hypogastric) arteries. The ovarian artery, which most commonly arises from the aorta, passes by the ovary and supplies the upper portions of the uterine corpus via anastomoses with the branches of the uterine artery (fig. 1-6). Branches of these arteries enter the serosa and course both radially and circumferentially (arcuate arteries) into the myometrium. The vessel density decreases at the myometrial-endometrial interface, which is significantly less vascularized. Endometrial vessels are supplied by myometrial radial arteries and end in the basal and spiral arterioles, the latter supplying the functional endometrial layers.

Uterine lymphatics are in close proximity to the arterial blood supply and drain via subserosal lymphatic plexuses to the pelvic and periaortic lymph nodes. A few lymphatics from the fundic area drain via the round ligament route to the superficial inguinal lymph nodes (7).

HISTOLOGY

The microscopic anatomy of the uterine corpus is divided into three layers: serosal surface, myometrium, and endometrium. The outer layer, or serosal surface (serosa), is composed of a single layer of mesothelium. The myometrium is the muscular layer and has three zones: the external zone, composed of longitudinal smooth

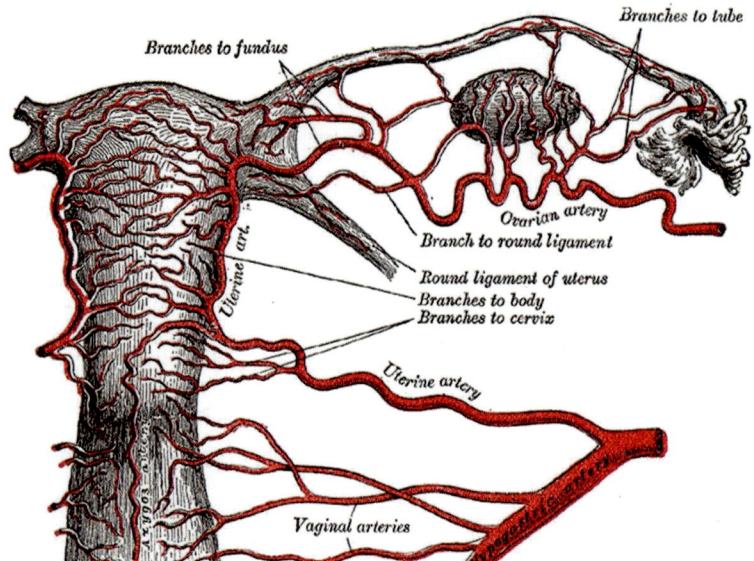

Figure 1-6

VASCULATURE OF THE UTERINE CORPUS

Blood supply is predominantly from the uterine arteries, which branch from the internal iliac arteries and from the ovarian arteries. The arterial blood enters via the uterine serosa, courses radially as the arcuate arteries, finally supplying the functional endometrium via the spiral arteries. (Fig. 1170 from Gray H. Anatomy of the human body, 20th ed. [revised and re-edited by Lewis W] Philadelphia: Lea & Febiger; 1918:1263.)

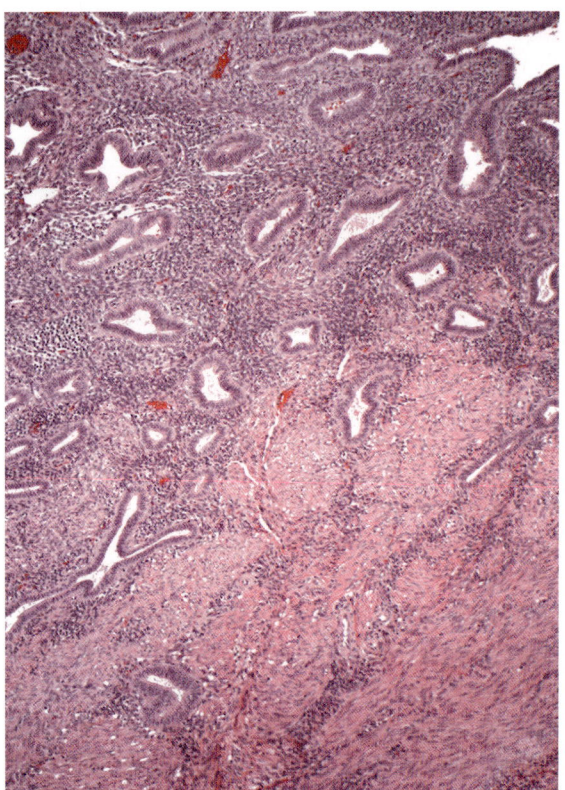

Figure 1-7

ENDOMETRIAL-MYOMETRIAL INTERFACE

Basal endometrium is present at the endometrial-myometrial interface. It consists of relatively small (non-cycling) glands lined by cuboidal/low columnar epithelial cells.

muscle fibers and containing the vascular and lymphatic plexuses; the middle zone, composed of interdigitating smooth muscle fibers; and the internal zone, containing circumferential smooth muscle fibers. The endometrial lining forms the third layer.

The endometrium is composed of surface epithelium and deep glands with surrounding endometrial stroma. The endometrial tissue is divided into a basal nonfunctioning layer and a superficial layer, the functionalis, which undergoes cyclical changes during the menstrual cycle. The basalis layer consists of small glands with cuboidal to low columnar epithelium showing little or no mitotic activity (fig. 1-7). The functionalis is further divided into the superficial portion, the compacta, which contains few glands and more stroma, and the deeper layer, the spongiosa, which contains more glands and less stromal tissue. The endometrial lining is most developed in the fundic regions and less in the lower uterine segment. In the latter area, endometrium histologically resembles the basalis. The endometrial epithelium in this area gradually merges with the endocervical epithelium and is much less responsive to the controlling ovarian hormones driving cellular changes in the fundic endometrial lining (7).

During the menstrual cycle, the endometrial functionalis layers undergo significant histologic changes. The length of the cycle is viewed,

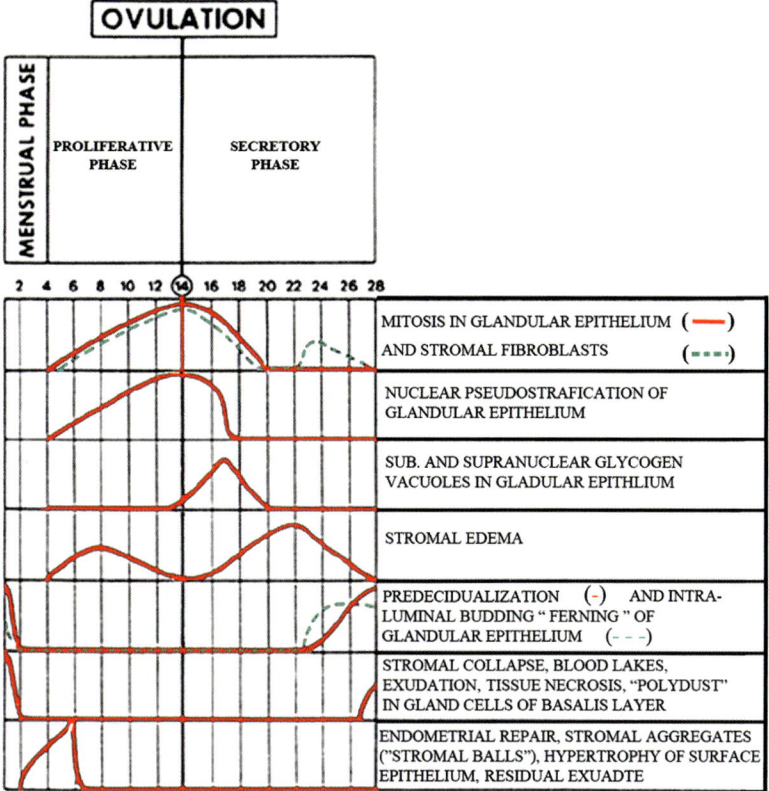

Figure 1-8

ENDOMETRIAL CYCLE AND DAILY MORPHOLOGIC CHARACTERISTICS

(Adapted from figure 1 from Noyes RW, Hartig AT, Rock J. Dating the endometrial biopsy. Fertil Steril 1950;1:5.)

by convention, as a 28-day event, although significant variability is noted clinically. Day 1 is considered to be the first day of the menses and day 14 represents the day of ovulation. The postmenses, preovulation portion of the cycle is referred to as the proliferative phase (days 4 to 14), and the postovulation portion of the cycle is referred to as the secretory phase (days 15 to 28). Histologic examination of the endometrium can identify functional issues related to infertility and irregular menstrual bleeding, such as anovulation and luteal phase defects (8). The useful features in endometrial dating and their temporal relationships are shown in figure 1-8 (7,9).

The proliferative phase of the menstrual cycle, under the influence of estrogenic stimulation, consists of growth and development of endometrial glands, stroma, and vasculature, resulting in an increased thickness of the endometrial compartment. As proliferation progresses, the columnar endometrial cells become pseudostratified, show mitotic activity, and increase in size; the glands, which begin as small, round, and uniform, become larger and more tortuous, oriented perpendicular to the surface (figs. 1-9, 1-10). The endometrial stroma also is mitotically active, increased in overall volume, and becomes edematous. During a normal proliferative phase, glands remain well spaced, have few outpouchings in gland structure, and exhibit no evidence of premature breakdown (apoptotic glandular or stromal debris). The presence of any of these features may signify an anovulatory cycle, with extreme changes termed disordered proliferative endometrium, which can be mistaken for nonatypical hyperplasia (discussed later) (fig. 1-11).

The secretory phase begins following ovulation. The estrogen-primed endometrial tissue, now under the influence of progesterone, changes its activity from proliferation and growth to differentiation. The first changes are gradual loss over several days of pseudostratification and mitotic activity. The production of cytoplasmic glycogen in subnuclear vacuoles is evident in the first few days, culminating in the classic day 17 appearance often referred to as a "picket-fence" when nearly all cells show subnuclear vacuoles (fig. 1-12). At day 18, vacuoles are present above and below the nuclei. As changes progress, the subnuclear vacuoles become predominantly

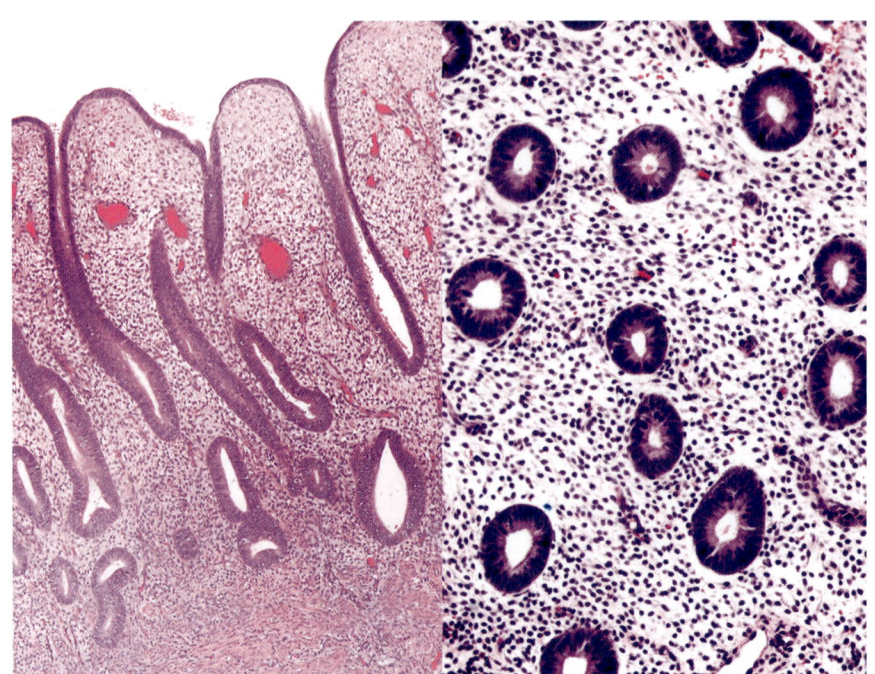

Figure 1-9

PROLIFERATIVE ENDOMETRIUM

Proliferative endometrium is composed of long tubular glands oriented from the surface to the base (left). In cross sectional view, the glands are small, round and evenly spaced (right).

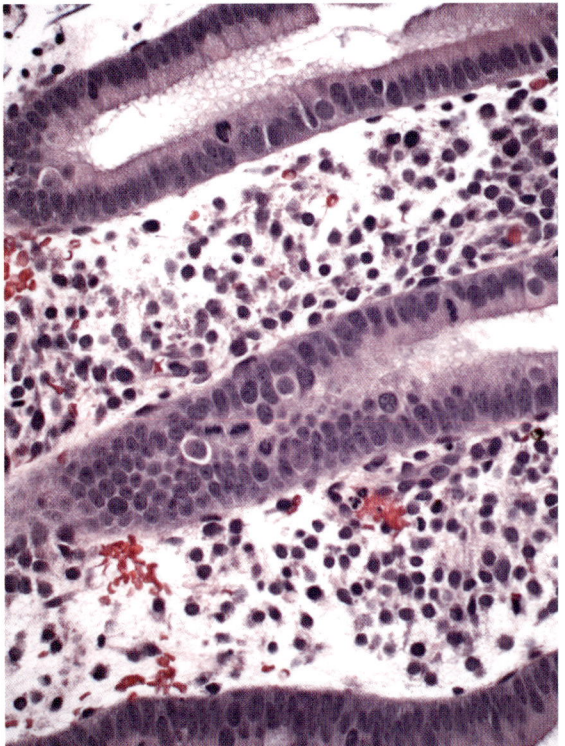
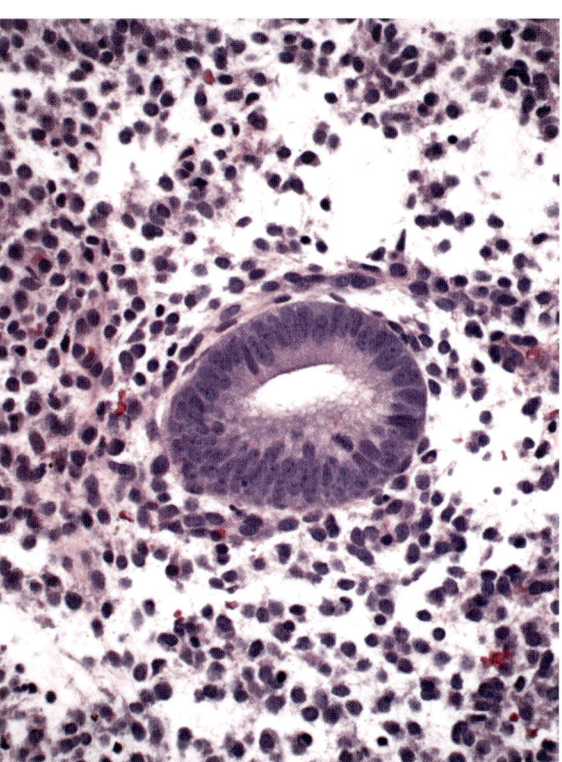

Figure 1-10

PROLIFERATIVE ENDOMETRIUM

Glands may have a long but straight tubular appearance (left). The epithelium is tall and nuclei are pseudostratified. Mitotic figures are evident. No cytoplasmic secretory product is noted (right).

Embryology, Anatomy, and Histology of the Uterine Corpus

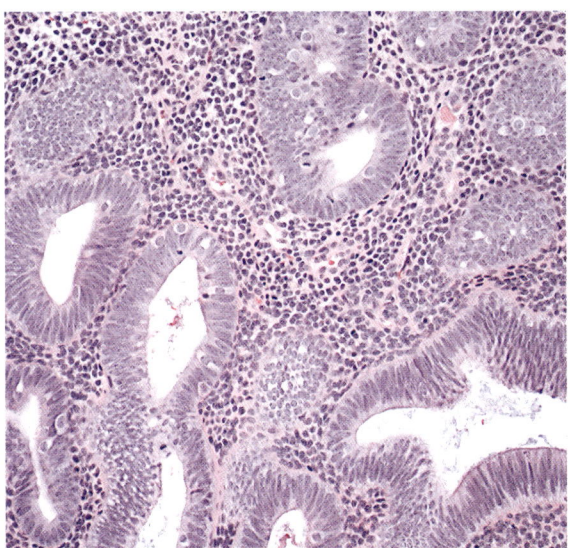 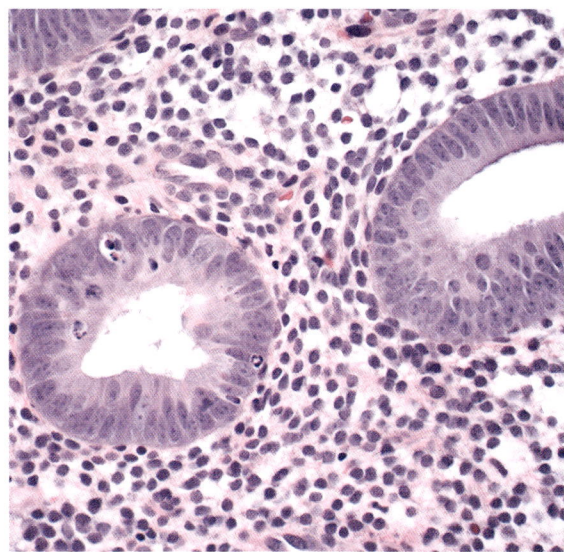

Figure 1-11

ALTERED PROLIFERATIVE ENDOMETRIUM

An ovulatory cycling leads to altered proliferative endometrium, with gland crowding and irregularity (left). Individual glands show evidence of breakdown or apoptosis, which can be seen in anovulatory cycles (right).

supranuclear and are secreted into the glandular lumens around day 20, leaving the nuclei in a basal position (fig. 1-13). Stromal edema becomes prominent at this stage.

In late stages of the secretory phase, the glands, having finished secreting, show regressive changes, with irregular contours, intraluminal secretion, some papillary tufting into the gland lumens, and eventually collapse (fig. 1-14). The glands maintain a similar appearance throughout the late secretory phase and hence are of little use in "dating" the endometrium. Fortunately, stromal changes take on characteristic temporal features that allow dating in this portion of the cycle. Coiling of the stromal arterioles becomes prominent within the edematous stroma at about day 23 and mitotic activity is detected in the perivascular stromal cells at this point (fig. 1-15). Predecidualization of the areas between the vessels follows, and then proceeds to involve the superficial portions of the stroma at about day 25. Predecidualized stromal cells contain abundant cytoplasm with enlarged nuclei and have an epithelioid appearance (fig. 1-16).

At days 26 to 28 (premenstrual phase), predecidual changes become prominent and diffuse, with infiltration by large granular lymphoid

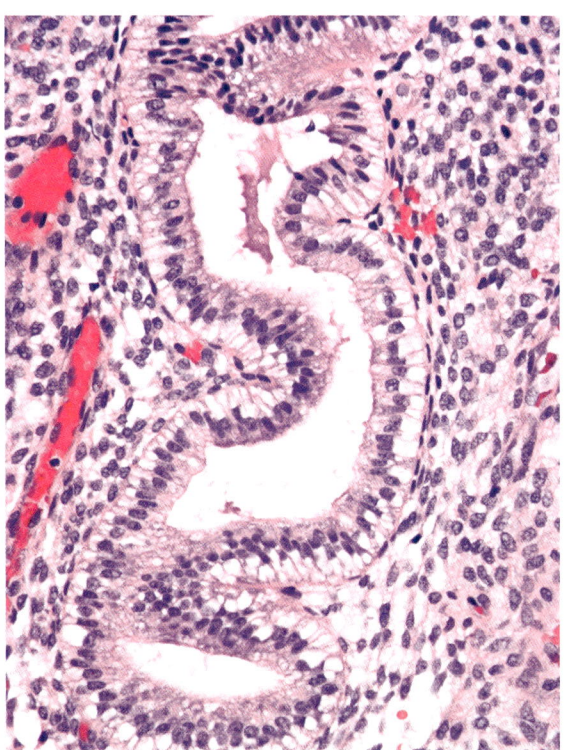

Figure 1-12

EARLY SECRETORY ENDOMETRIUM

At day 17, the classic "picket fence" appearance of subnuclear vacuoles is seen.

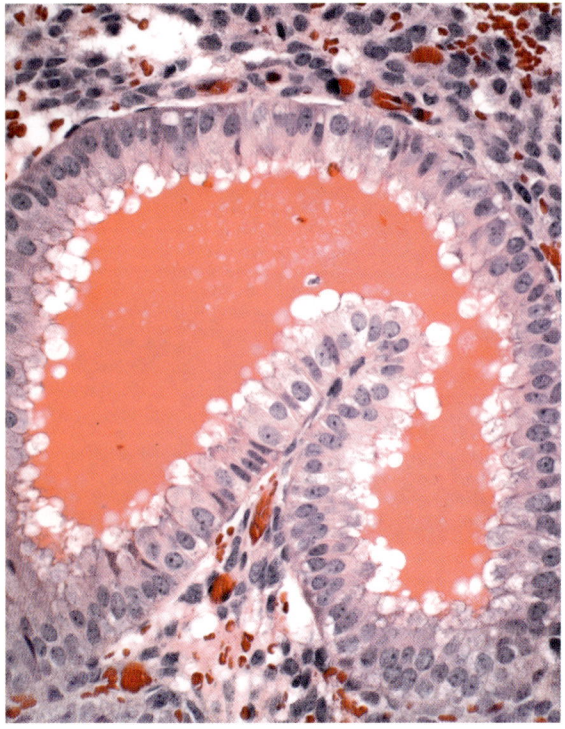

Figure 1-13

SECRETORY ENDOMETRIUM

By day 20, the vacuoles have moved to an apical position and secretion is present in the gland lumen.

cells, the "metrial" granulocytes. Infiltration by increasing numbers of granulocytes follows with stromal hemorrhage and some nuclear breakdown debris. The menstrual phase (days 1 to 4) follows, with large confluent areas of hemorrhage, fragments of degenerating endometrial glands and stroma showing apoptotic debris, and characteristic circular fragments of stromal condensation covered by degenerating endometrial epithelium ("exodus" ball formations commonly noted in postmenstrual cervical cytology specimens [see below under cytology]) (fig. 1-17). Some glands show excess cytoplasmic vacuolization during menses, referred to as "secretory recrudescence" (fig. 1-18). The presence of secretory glandular change may be helpful in differentiating the menstrual phase from extensive proliferative breakdown, and even from endometrial neoplasia, which can sometimes be misdiagnosed in curetted specimens from menstrual endometrium when plump epithelioid stromal cells predominate and can give a false impression of a high-grade carcinoma (fig. 1-19).

Dating of the endometrium is an important tool for patients with infertility or multiple spontaneous abortions. Lack of correlation of the dates of the clinical cycle and histologic

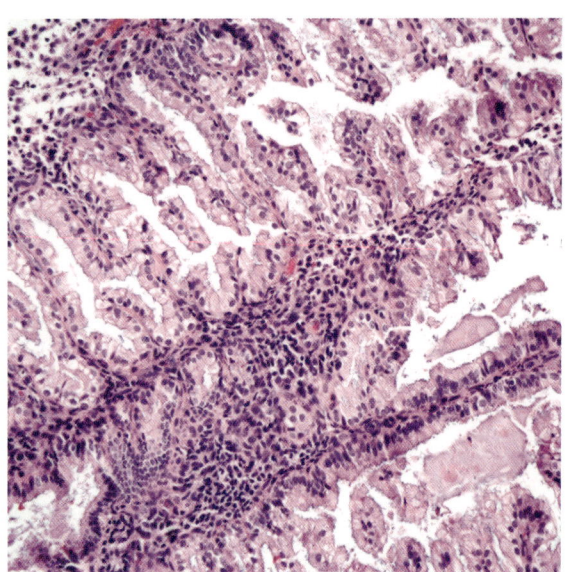 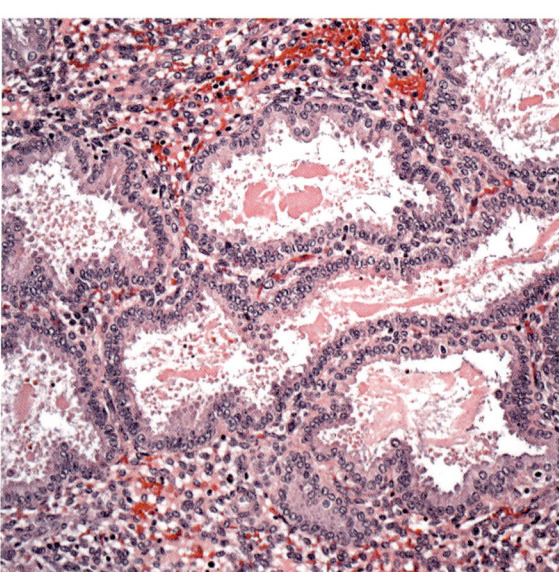

Figure 1-14

ADVANCED SECRETORY ENDOMETRIUM

By day 22, the secretory glands become more densely packed and tortuous (left). The secretion of the glands is exhausted, with no residual vacuoles (right). From this date going forward stromal changes are used to date the cycle.

dates can indicate hormonal imbalances. In dating endometrium under normal circumstances, the "leading edge" date, meaning the most advanced date indicated by histology, correlates best with the clinical date. Dyssynchronous patterns occur when the most advanced date and other areas within the biopsy show patterns that are more than 3 days apart. Other menstrual irregularities may show combinations of secretory and proliferative phase glands, discorrelations between secretory glands and stromal dates, and evidence of premature breakdown in clinically premenstrual specimens. As most of these presentations are not diagnostic of particular clinical entities, reporting the descriptive findings is generally recommended, which should prompt further clinical and laboratory investigations to determine the cause of the abnormality (8).

As a result of aging, infection, estrogen stimulation, or other reactive conditions, the endometrial epithelium may undergo a variety of benign metaplastic changes (10). The most common of these is tubal metaplasia, which consists of

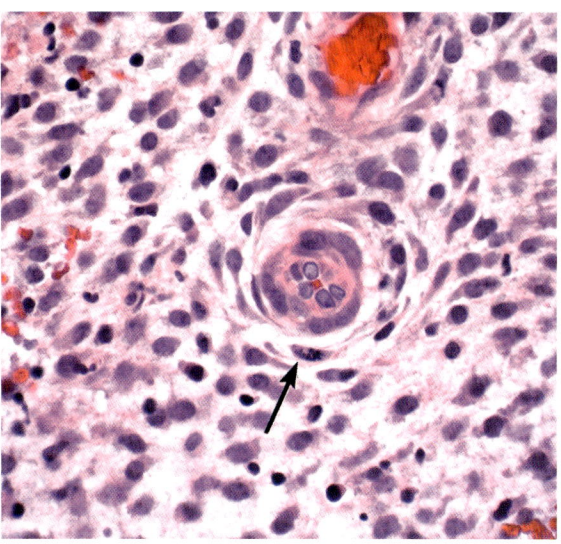

Figure 1-15

ADVANCED SECRETORY ENDOMETRIUM

A typical stromal feature of day 23 is the presence of mitotic figures in the cuffed spiral arteries (arrow).

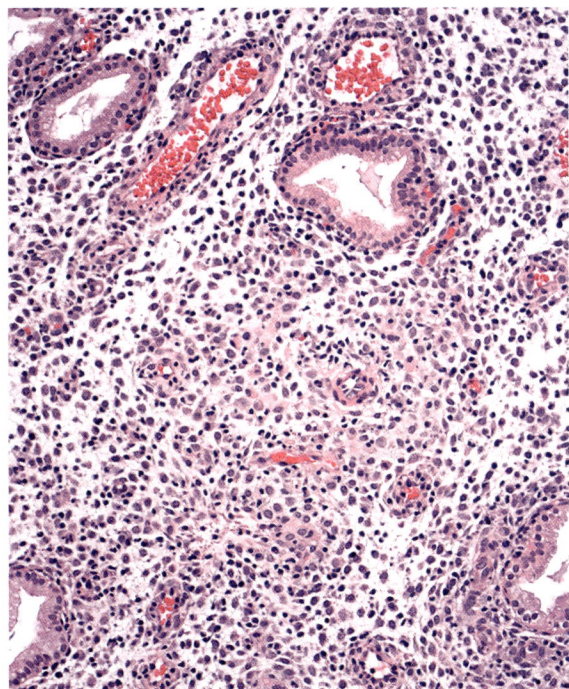 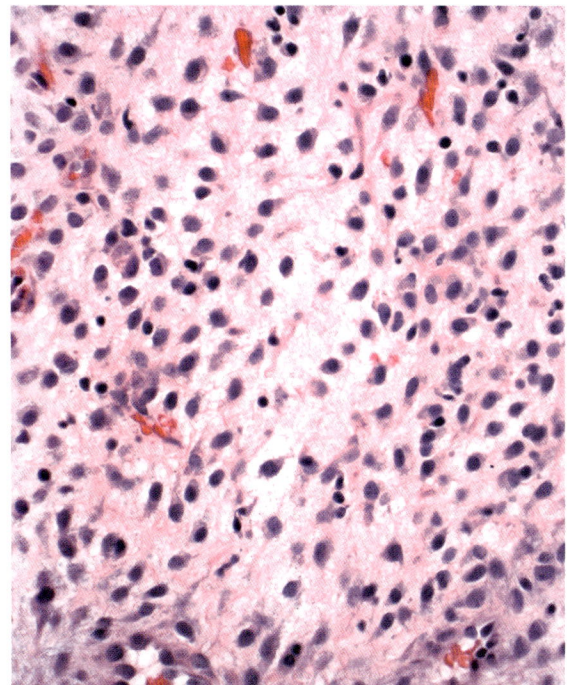

Figure 1-16

LATE SECRETORY ENDOMETRIUM

Secretory endometrium, at days 24 to 25, shows predecidualized stroma surrounding stromal arteries (left). Between day 24 and menses, the stromal cells show more abundant cytoplasm and the stroma is infiltrated by increasing numbers of inflammatory cells (right).

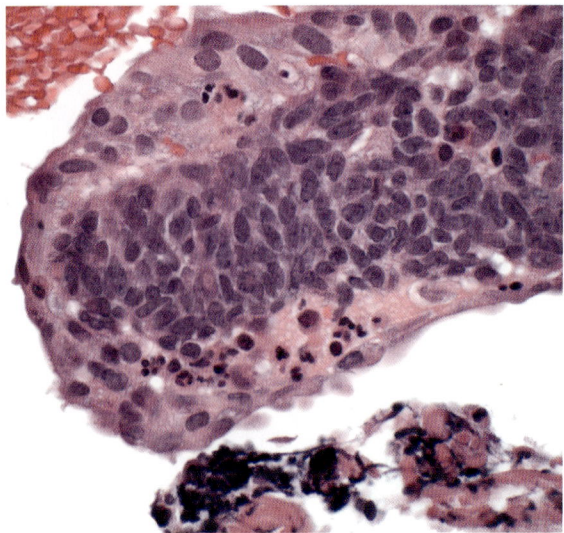

Figure 1-17

MENSTRUAL ENDOMETRIUM

At the time of menses, stromal breakdown beneath degenerating endometrial glands creates the classic "exodus" ball pattern, which can also be seen in Papanicolaou cytology specimens.

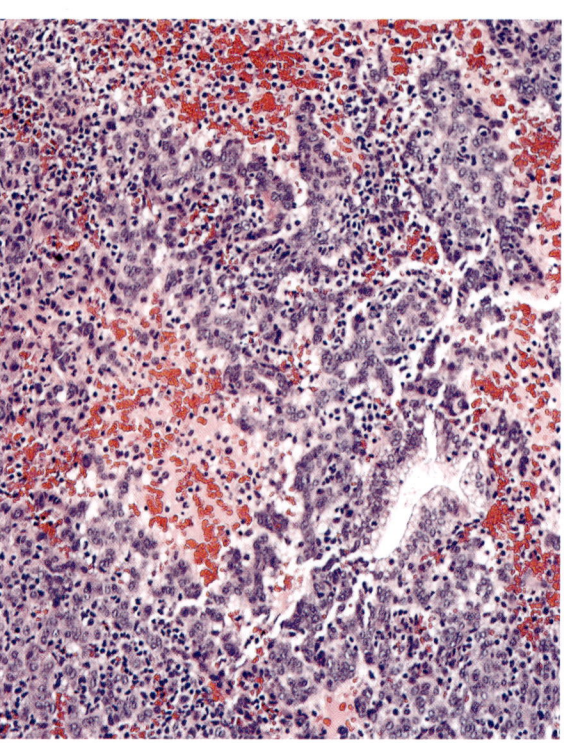

Figure 1-19

STROMA IN MENSTRUAL ENDOMETRIUM

Breakdown of stromal cells in menstrual endometrium can sometimes impart an epithelioid morphology, with large atypical nuclei and a trabecular pattern. This appearance can give a false impression of poorly differentiated carcinoma.

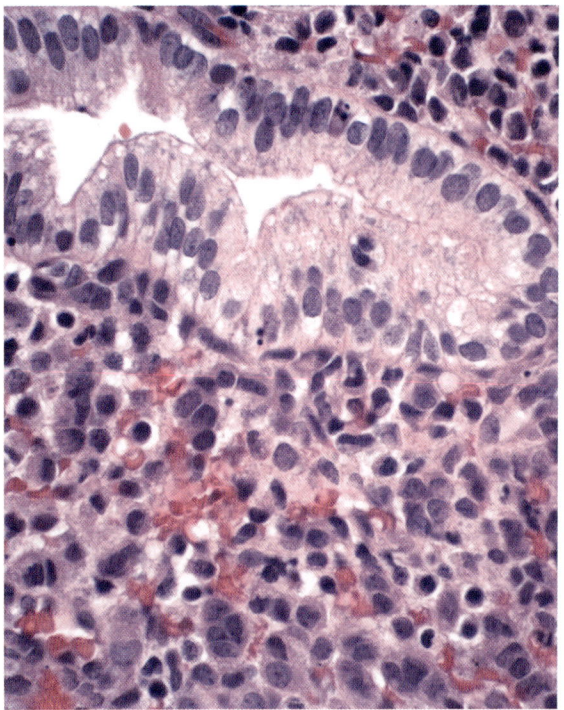

Figure 1-18

MENSTRUAL ENDOMETRIUM

The glands show cytoplasmic vacuolization "secretory recrudescence" as well as apoptoses.

an epithelial layer that appears identical to the lining of the fallopian tube. Tubal metaplasia includes the triad of ciliated, peg, and tall intercalated cells (fig. 1-20). Foci of tubal metaplasia are usually found in endometrial samples in women over the age of 30 years, and are therefore considered a normal transformative process of no clinical significance (see chapter 2).

Squamous metaplasia is generally associated with estrogenic stimulation. It consists of morules of benign squamous epithelium that fill the lumens of endometrial glands (fig. 1-21). Its presence should always prompt more thorough investigation for endometrial neoplasia since squamous metaplasia is also a common occurrence in endometrioid hyperplasia and carcinoma (see chapter 2).

Papillary or syncytial metaplasia consists of tufted, generally hobnail cells typically on the endometrial surface, that sometimes show complex architecture and nuclear atypia (fig. 1-22).

Embryology, Anatomy, and Histology of the Uterine Corpus

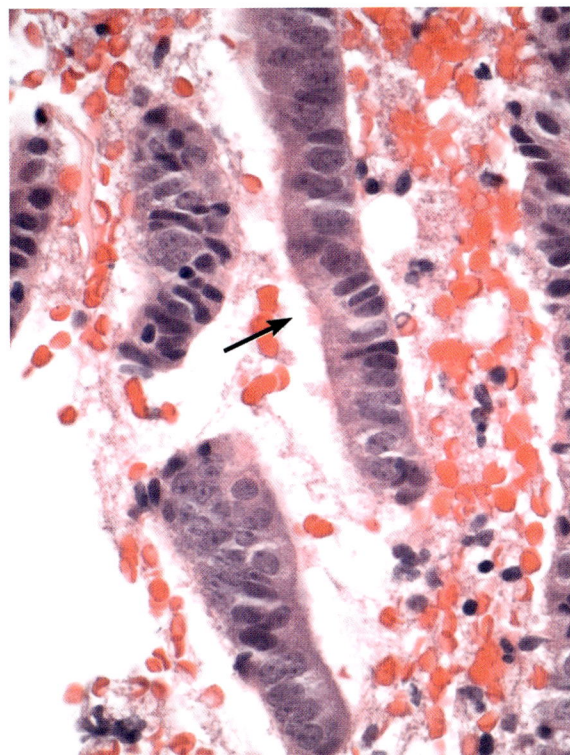

Figure 1-20

TUBAL METAPLASIA

Tubal metaplasia is common in late childbearing and perimenopausal women. In this illustration from a curetting, the normal endometrial lining is replaced by epithelium of fallopian tube-type with prominent ciliated apical borders (arrow).

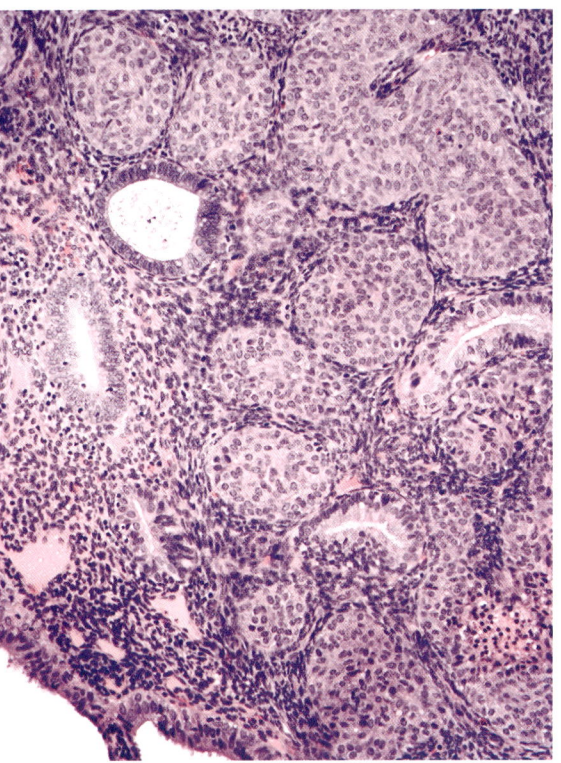

Figure 1-21

SQUAMOUS METAPLASIA

Squamous morules with banal cytologic features fill the endometrial glands.

This appearance may not represent a true metaplasia but a degenerative change, as it is typically noted in endometrium undergoing breakdown (menstrual or anovulatory changes) often in association with degenerated compact stroma.

The main entity in the differential diagnosis of papillary metaplasia is serous carcinoma, but the generally low nucleus to cytoplasmic ratios of the metaplastic cells and the lack of uniform nuclear atypia should prompt a benign interpretation. In small and fragmented biopsy samples, however, this distinction may be difficult and caution is advised (fig. 1-23) (11,12). In addition, cells can be immunoreactive for p53, which can lead to a false malignant interpretation. The use of a proliferation marker (e.g., Ki-67) should help with a proper interpretation since eosinophilic change shows little or no evidence of proliferation (fig. 1-24) (13) (see chapter 2).

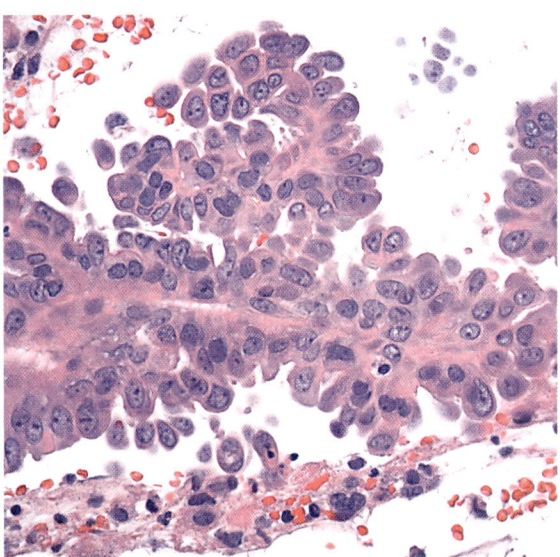

Figure 1-22

PAPILLARY METAPLASIA

Tufts of cells show reactive cytologic atypia. This is considered a degenerative phenomenon.

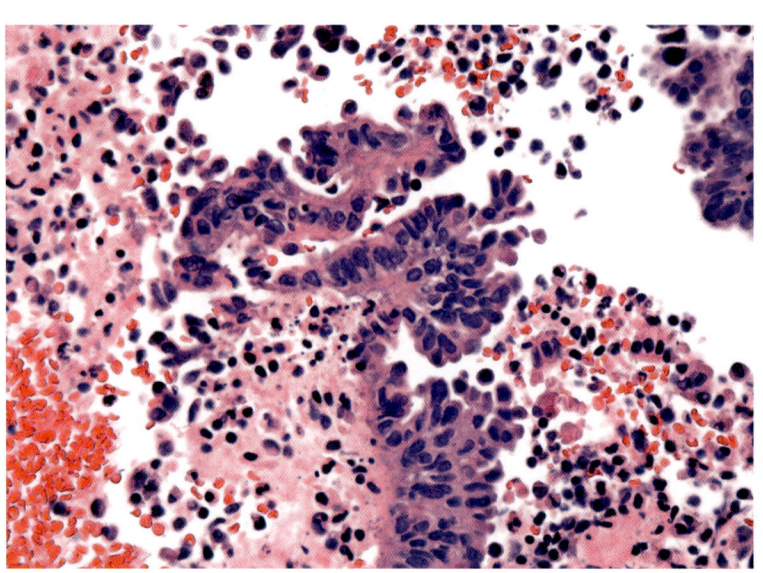

Figure 1-23
PAPILLARY METAPLASIA

Papillary metaplasia can undergo degenerative change with significant cytologic atypia. In small biopsies this appearance may suggest malignancy. The necrotic stroma is seen beneath the epithelium and the pyknotic epithelial nuclei have a dark "degenerative" appearance.

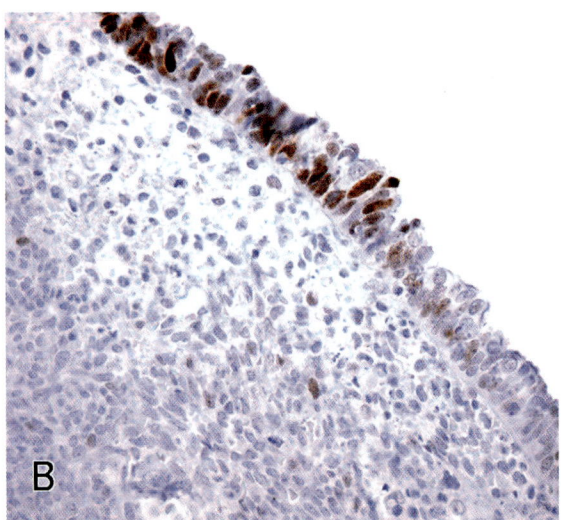

Figure 1-24
DEGENERATIVE CHANGES

Degenerative changes in the endometrial lining can simulate neoplasia (A). p53 immunohistochemistry may be positive, and if used alone, can lead to a malignant diagnosis (B). The use of a proliferation marker such as Ki-67 shows a low index and helps to label these atypical features as benign degenerative changes (C).

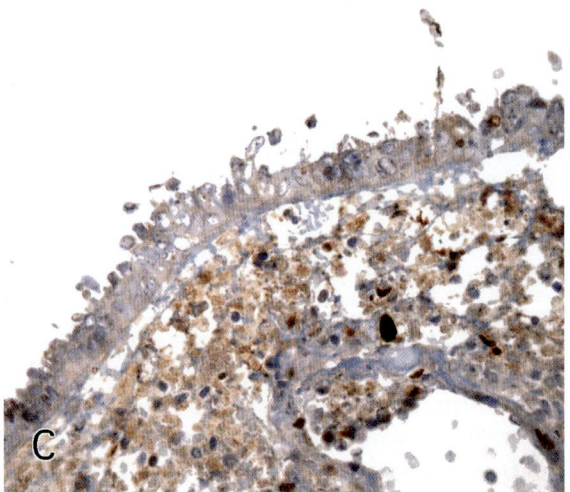

Embryology, Anatomy, and Histology of the Uterine Corpus

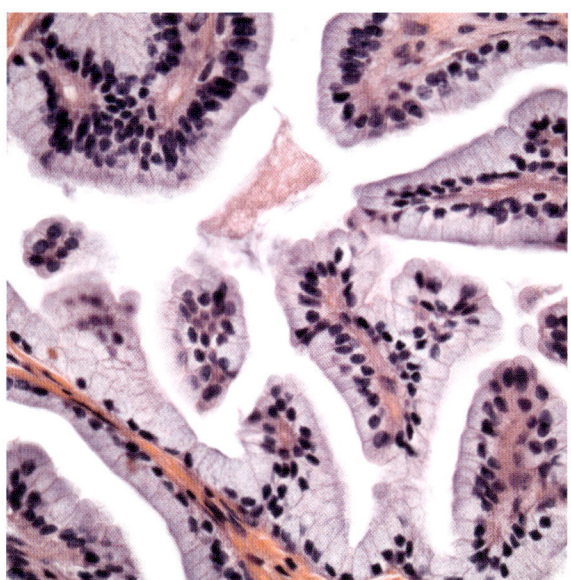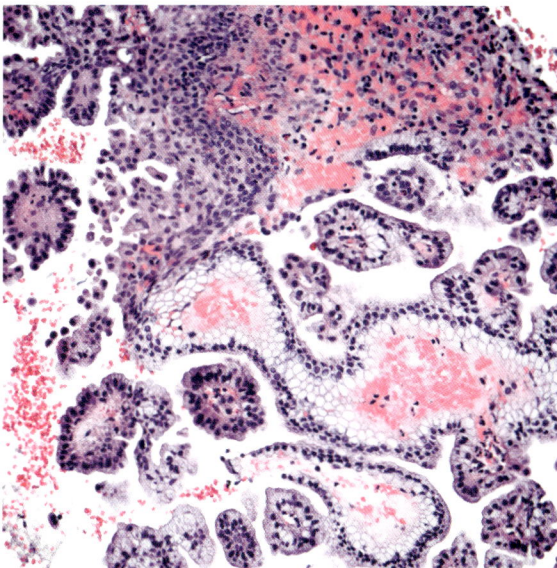

Figure 1-25

MUCINOUS METAPLASIA

The normal endometrial cells are replaced by columnar cells with bland nuclear features showing abundant mucin contents (left). Mucinous metaplasia can often be present in association with other metaplastic changes, in this case with papillary tufting (right).

Mucinous metaplasia consists of epithelium with prominent mucinous cytoplasm (fig. 1-25). Data suggest that this form of metaplasia could be a precursor lesion to mucinous adenocarcinoma (10) (see chapter 2).

Many patients receive progestational agents for contraception, suppression of bleeding, and treatment of hyperplasia. Progestational hormones affect the endometrium in a characteristic way, including atrophy of the endometrial glands and diffuse stromal decidualization (fig. 1-26). The appearance is reminiscent of the stroma associated with gestational endometrium (see below), but the finding of gland atrophy sets this pattern apart from hypersecretion seen with pregnancy.

Following implantation of a fertilized ovum, the endometrium shows the characteristic changes referred to as gestational endometrium. The glands show intraluminal epithelial projections ("ferning") and evidence of intraluminal secretions. Stromal edema is more prominent and stromal vessels become congested. The predecidual reaction is pronounced but devoid of inflammatory cells (fig. 1-27). Similar changes are seen with nongestational events such as persistent corpus luteum or corpus luteum cyst, and hence, evidence of pregnancy in the first few weeks is dependent on the identification of fetal tissue. After about 4 weeks, the gestational endometrial appearance becomes distinctive, with hypersecretory glandular changes that show exaggerated nuclear size and variability, and clear or eosinophilic cytoplasm, which can lead to the Arias-Stella reaction (fig. 1-28).

Following menopause and its associated withdrawal of hormonal support, the endometrium becomes inactive or atrophic. In the former circumstance, endometrial glands remain proliferative-like, showing pseudostratified architecture but with no evidence of active proliferation in the form of mitoses (fig. 1-29). Over time, the endometrial epithelium becomes cuboidal, often with associated cystic glandular change (cystic atrophy) (fig. 1-30).

ENDOMETRIAL CYTOLOGY

The cytology of the endometrium is dependent on the method of sampling. In cervical cytology specimens, the most common scenario by which endometrial cells appear is via exfoliation. In normal cycling women, exfoliated endometrial cells are present during and after

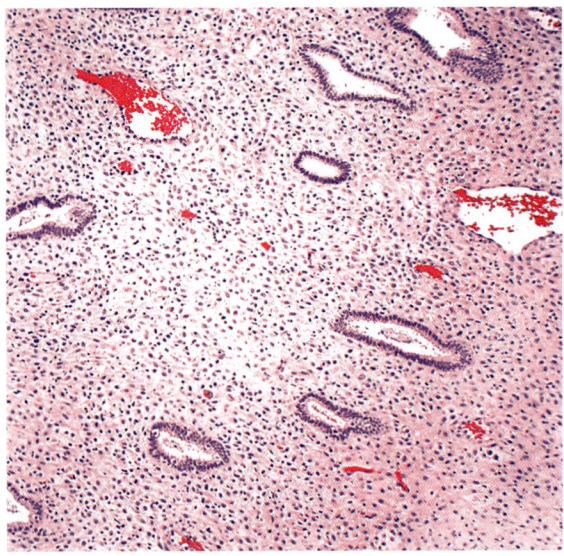

Figure 1-26

PROGESTATIONAL HORMONE EFFECT

The stroma undergoes marked pseudodecidualization and the glands become atrophic.

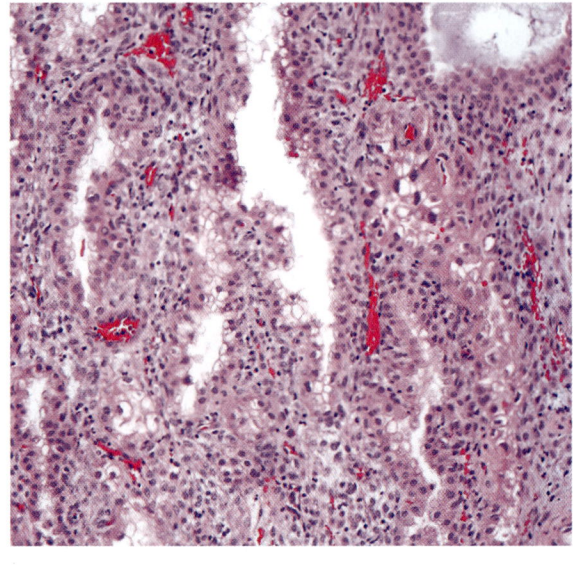

Figure 1-27

DECIDUAL STROMAL CHANGE IN PREGNANCY

Successful implantation leads to marked decidual stromal change, similar to progestational hormone effect. In contrast to the latter, gestational endometrial glands show complex proliferation.

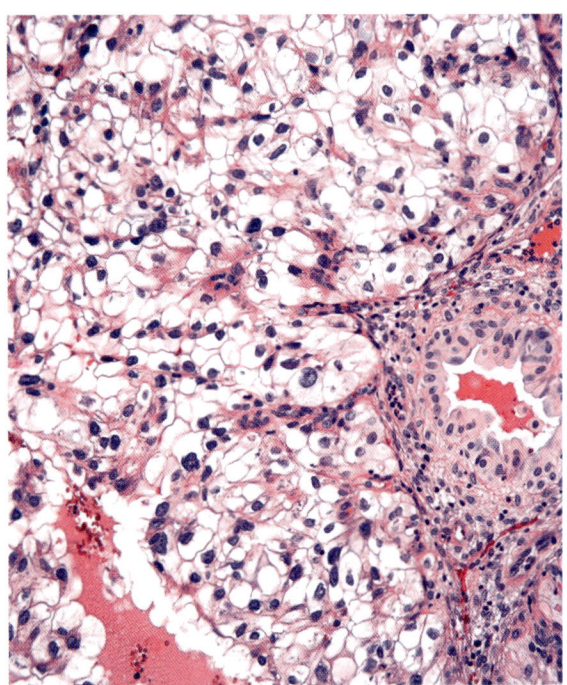
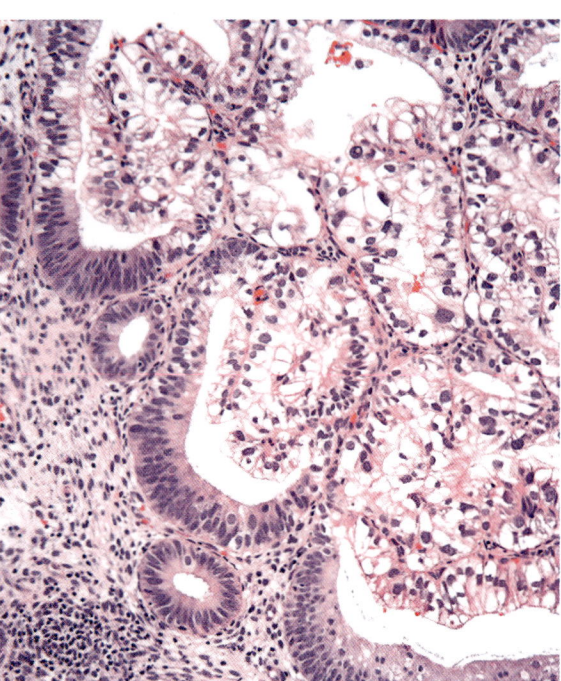

Figure 1-28

ARIAS-STELLA REACTION

The hypersecretory glandular epithelium shows nuclear atypia including pleomorphic forms (left). Some nuclei show degenerative change. The cytoplasm is abundant and may show clearing, causing concern for clear cell carcinoma. There is often transition to normal appearing endometrial lining within glands (right).

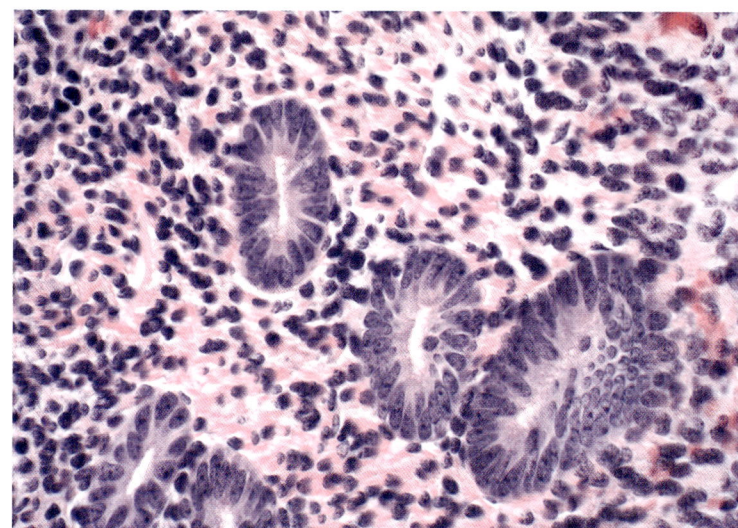

Figure 1-29
PERIMENOPAUSAL OR EARLY POSTMENOPAUSAL ENDOMETRIUM
Endometrial glands become inactive but can still show some degree of pseudostratification of nuclei ("inactive" endometrium).

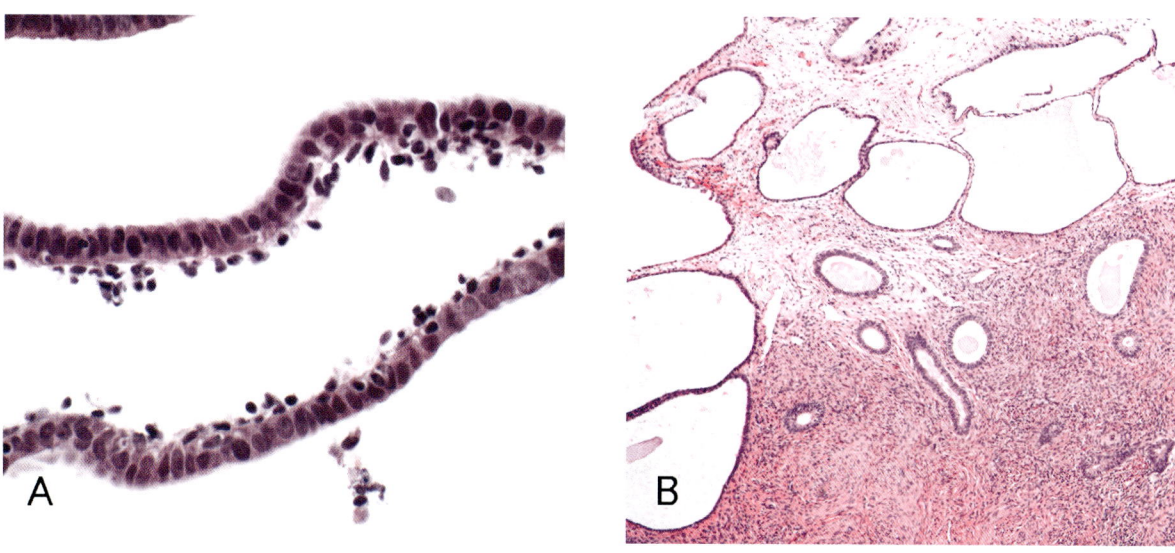

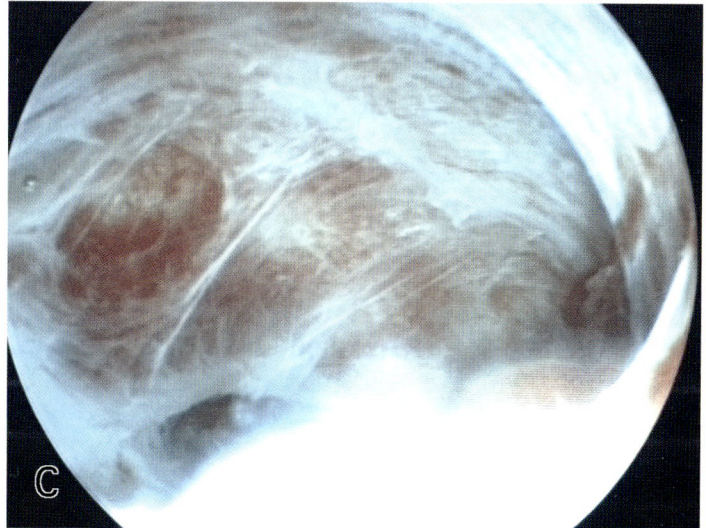

Figure 1-30
POSTMENOPAUSAL ENDOMETRIUM
In curettage specimens, endometrium is often found as strips of cuboidal epithelium with attached spindled stromal cells. This appearance is referred to as "atrophic" endometrium (A). Intact atrophic endometrium often shows prominent cystic change (B). Hysteroscopy appearance of endometrial atrophy (C).

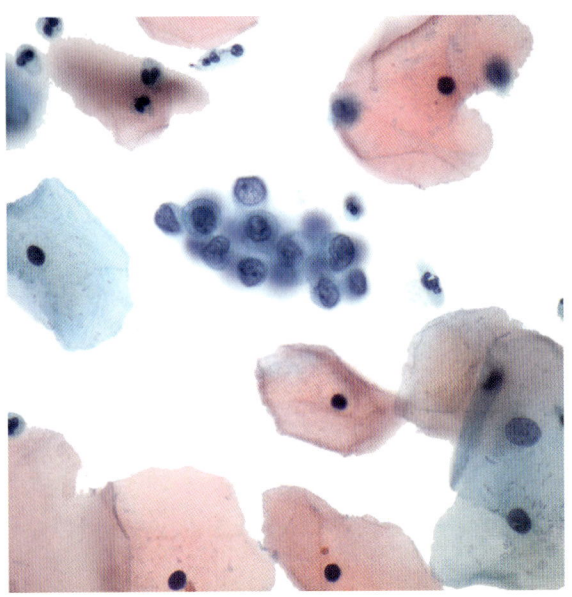

Figure 1-31

SHED ENDOMETRIAL CELLS

Shed endometrial cells are small and cuboidal. They can be present as individual cells or as small groups of cells.

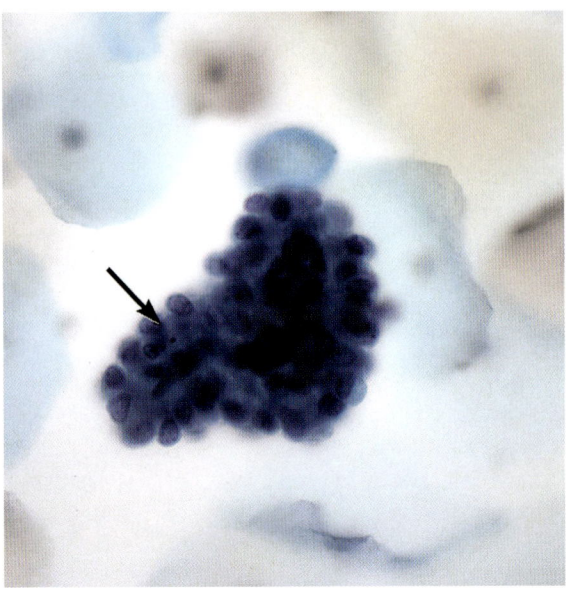

Figure 1-32

SHED ENDOMETRIAL CELLS

Endometrial cells shed from the surface of the endometrium form three-dimensional balls of small cells. No columnar features are seen in distinction to directly sampled endometrium. Degenerative granules (apoptotic debris) can be seen within the group (arrow).

the menses, generally up until day 12. During menses, small and large three-dimensional aggregates of endometrial glandular and stromal cells are present in a background of blood, consistent with the breakdown phase of the cycle (fig. 1-31). Individual endometrial glandular cells may also be present.

The normal exfoliated endometrial glandular cell is small, with a nucleus about the same size as the nucleus of an intermediate squamous cell. The nuclei are typically hyperchromatic and have an indented configuration. They show granular chromatin, an appearance that is consistent with the degenerative nature of the exfoliated cell. The cytoplasm is scant, with occasional degenerative vacuoles. In three-dimensional groups, there may be significant karyorrhectic/apoptotic debris and nuclear enlargement, also consistent with the degenerative process (fig. 1-32).

Reactive changes may be accentuated in liquid-based cytology specimens, most likely due to rapid fixation and preservation (fig. 1-33). In such cases, enlarged nuclei with nucleoli may be present. Knowledge of the menstrual dates, the presence of stromal breakdown, and cytoplasm showing large "degenerative" vacuoles, differentiate these groups from atypical endometrial cells, which otherwise may suggest a neoplastic process.

In days 6 to 10, a particular cytologic pattern referred to as exodus shows three-dimensional balls of endometrial stromal cells surfaced by endometrial glandular cells (fig. 1-34).

In cases where endocervical sampling devices reach the lower uterine segment, typical in patients with prior cervical excisions, endometrial cells can be sampled directly. In such a scenario, the architectural features of normal endometrium may be present in cytologic samples. These include intact endometrial glands and stromal fragments (figs. 1-35, 1-36). In contrast to the three-dimensional clusters present in exfoliative samples, directly sampled endometrial glands show pseudostratified layering of nuclei with retention of tubular structures and two-dimensional sheets of columnar cells. These groups can mimic the pseudostratified architecture of endocervical neoplasia. Endometrial nuclei, however, are much smaller and lack the cytologic atypia present in endocervical adenocarcinoma in situ. In addition, a background of endometrial

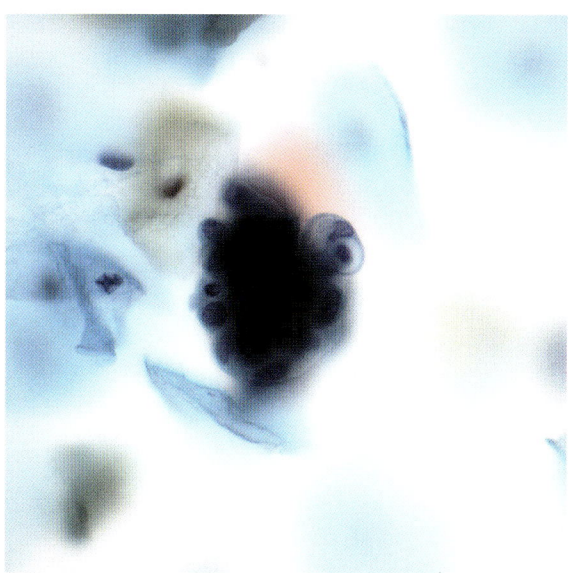

Figure 1-33
SHED ENDOMETRIAL CELLS
Degenerative changes, such as vacuolization and nuclear pleomorphism, are common in shed endometrial cells.

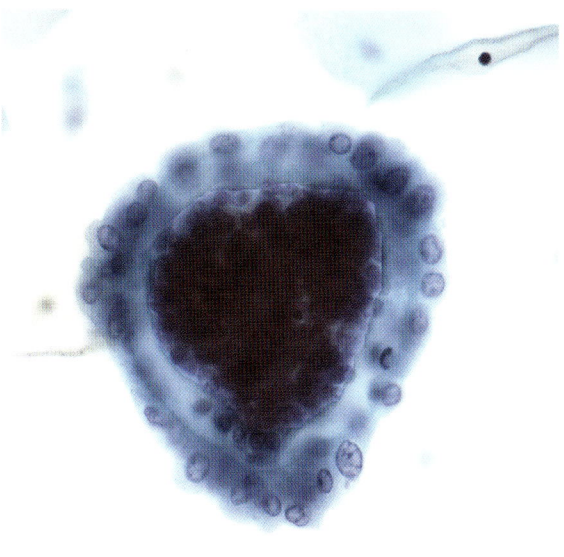

Figure 1-34
EXODUS PATTERN
This three-dimensional structure commonly found in cervical cytology specimens following the menstrual period consists of a central core of stromal cells and an outer rim of endometrial glandular cells. Compare this illustration to the same structure noted in the biopsy specimen of menstrual endometrium in figure 1-17.

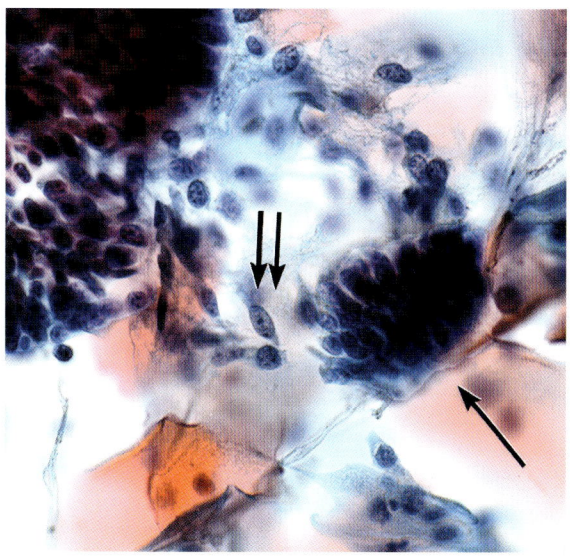

Figure 1-35
DIRECTLY SAMPLED ENDOMETRIUM
Direct sampling of the endometrium yields epithelial cells which appear in their in situ configuration as pseudostratified strips (arrow). The background often contains individual spindled endometrial stromal cells (double arrow).

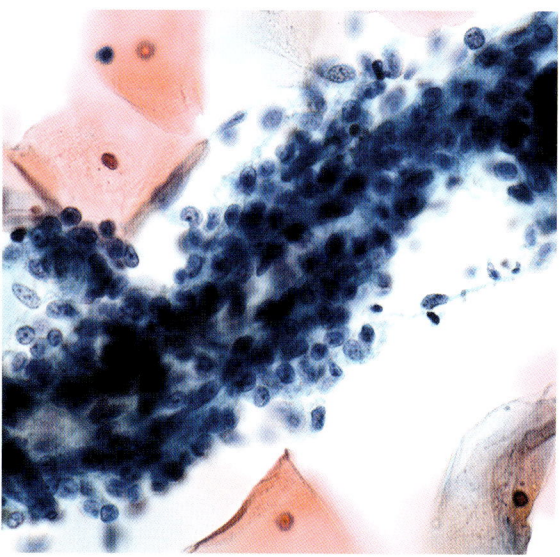

Figure 1-36
DIRECTLY SAMPLED ENDOMETRIUM
Large fragments of spindled endometrial stromal cells are seen. The spindled cells are attached to the surface of a stromal vessel.

stromal fragments and individual spindled stromal cells attached to the surface of the tubular groups helps in the differential diagnosis.

The presence of exfoliated endometrial cells in postmenopausal women can be concerning because of an association that was noted with concurrent endometrial neoplasia (hyperplasia and adenocarcinoma). Studies before 2001 showed that this association was as high as 17 percent. Because of this association, the second edition of the Bethesda System (2001) (15) recommended reporting benign endometrial cells in all women over the age of 40 years. In the following decade, reporting became more prevalent and the predictive value fell dramatically to a 3 percent association with endometrial neoplasia. In the 3rd edition of the Bethesda System (2015) (14), the reporting age was raised to 45 years, and concurrent American Society for Colposcopy and Cervical Pathology (ASCCP) management guidelines recommended an endometrial biopsy only if the patient was clinically postmenopausal (16). Hopefully, these changes will improve the predictive value of this common finding.

REFERENCES

1. Muller J. Bildungsgeschichte der Genitalien aus anatomischen Untersuchungen an Embryonen des Menschen und der Thiere nebst einem Anhang über die chirurgische Behandlung der Hypospadia. 1830; Dusseldorf: Arnz.
2. Prunskaite-Hyyrylainen R, Skovorodkin I, Xu Q, Miinalainen I, Shan J, Vainio SJ. Wnt4 coordinates directional cell migration and extension of the mullerian duct essential for ontogenesis of the female reproductive tract. Hum Mol Genet 2016;25:1059-73.
3. Healey A. Embryology of the female reproductive tract. In: Mann GS, Blair JC, Garden AS, eds. Imaging of gynecologic disorders in infants and children. Berlin: Springer-Verlag; 2012:21-30.
4. Miller C, Pavlova A, Sassoon DA. Differential expression patterns of Wnt genes in the murine female reproductive tract during development and the estrous cycle. Mech Dev 1998;76:91-9.
5. Jacquinet A, Millar D, Lehman A. Etiologies of uterine malformations. Am J Med Genet A 2016;170:2141-72.
6. McCluggage WG. Benign diseases of the endometrium. In: Kurman RJ, Ellison LH, Ronnett BM, eds. Blaustein's pathology of the female genital tract. New York: Springer; 2011:307-8.
7. Mutter GL, Ferenczy A. Anatomy and histology of the uterine corpus. In: Kurman RJ, eds. Blaustein's pathology of the female genital tract. New York: Springer-Verlag; 2002:383-406.
8. Mazur MT, Kurman RJ. Diagnosis of endometrial biopsies and curettings: a practical approach, 2nd ed. New York: Springer; 2005.
9. Noyes RW, Hertig AT, Rock J. Dating the endometrial biopsy. Am J Obstet Gynecol 1975;122:262-3.
10. Yoo SH, Park BH, Choi J, et al. Papillary mucinous metaplasia of the endometrium as a possible precursor of endometrial mucinous adenocarcinoma. Mod Pathol 2012;25:1496-507.
11. Nicolae A, Preda O, Nogales FF. Endometrial metaplasias and reactive changes: a spectrum of altered differentiation. J Clin Pathol 2011;64:97-106.
12. Zaman SS, Mazur MT. Endometrial papillary syncytial change. A nonspecific alteration associated with active breakdown. Am J Clin Pathol 1993;99:741-5.
13. McCluggage WG, McBride HA. Papillary syncytial metaplasia associated with endometrial breakdown exhibits an immunophenotype that overlaps with uterine serous carcinoma. Int J Gynecol Pathol 2012;31:206-10.
14. Cibas ES, Chelmow D, Waxman AG, Moriarty AT. Endometrial cells: the how and when of reporting. In: Nayar R, Wilbur DC, eds. The Bethesda System for reporting cervical cytology. Heidelberg: Springer; 2015:91-102.
15. Moriarty AT, Cibas ES. Endometrial cells: the how and why of reporting. In: Solomon D, Nayar R, eds. The Bethesda system for reporting cervical/vaginal cytologic diagnoses. New York: Springer; 2003.
16. Massad LS, Einstein MH, Huh WK, et al. 2012 updated consensus guidelines for the management of abnormal cervical cancer screening tests and cancer precursors. J Low Genit Tract Dis 2013;17(Suppl 1):S1-S27.

2 NON-NEOPLASTIC LESIONS

ENDOMETRIAL METAPLASIAS

Metaplastic changes may occur in the epithelium or stromal compartments (Table 2-1). They are most commonly epithelial, involve surface or endometrial glands, reflecting the plasticity of the müllerian epithelium. They may be seen in association with endometrial polyps, hyperestrogenic states including tamoxifen use, and in a variety of reactive processes, but in many cases such association is lacking. Most importantly, changes in epithelial metaplasias may suggest a malignant process or an association with neoplastic conditions, thus, it is important to be aware of the spectrum of their appearances and associations.

ENDOMETRIAL EPITHELIAL METAPLASIAS

Epithelial metaplasia is the replacement of endometrioid-type epithelium by other types of epithelium, most often of müllerian type. Frequently, more than one type of metaplasia is seen. Epithelial metaplasia typically represents an incidental finding in endometrial curettage or biopsy specimens performed for abnormal vaginal bleeding or discharge.

Tubal (Ciliated) Metaplasia

Tubal (ciliated) metaplasia is the most common type of metaplasia seen in normal proliferative endometrium, most frequently in the lower uterine segment and in endometrial polyps (1). In premenopausal and menopausal women, tubal metaplasia becomes more extensive with increasing anovulatory cycles due to higher estrogen levels. It is often associated with eosinophilic (oxyphilic) metaplasia. When fully developed, it is characterized by cells that are reminiscent of the fallopian tube lining: predominantly ciliated cells, with secretory cells and intercalated cells less commonly seen. The cells have columnar, eosinophilic, or sometimes, clear cytoplasm with terminal bars and luminal cilia, round vesicular nuclei and small but visible nucleoli (figs. 2-1, 2-2).

Glands involved by tubal metaplasia appear "thicker" than the surrounding unaffected endometrial glands due to nuclear pseudostratification. The glandular architecture may be complex, with closely spaced glands that may show cribriforming, particularly in polyps, an appearance suggestive of complex hyperplasia, especially if cilia are not prominent (fig. 2-3). Tubal metaplasia may be cytologically atypical and present in endometrial hyperplasia and less commonly, endometrioid carcinoma, thus, cytologic and architectural features should be evaluated in relation to these features in the surrounding glands (2).

The ciliated cells may have an increased nuclear to cytoplasmic ratio, enlarged nuclei, and prominent nucleoli ("atypical ciliated metaplasia") (fig. 2-4), resulting in concern for serous carcinoma, especially in curettage specimens. However, mitoses are typically scant, no apoptoses are noted, and cells maintain a

Table 2-1

ENDOMETRIAL METAPLASIAS

Epithelial
  Tubal
  Mucinous (endocervical, pyloric, intestinal)
  Papillary proliferations (simple, complex, diffuse)
  Squamous (morular, glycogenated)
  Papillary syncytial
  Eosinophilic
  Hobnail and clear
  Arias-Stella reaction
  Other pregnancy/hormonally related

Stromal
  Smooth muscle
  Osseous
  Cartilaginous and adipose
  Glial
  Other

Tumors of the Uterine Corpus and Gestational Trophoblastic Diseases

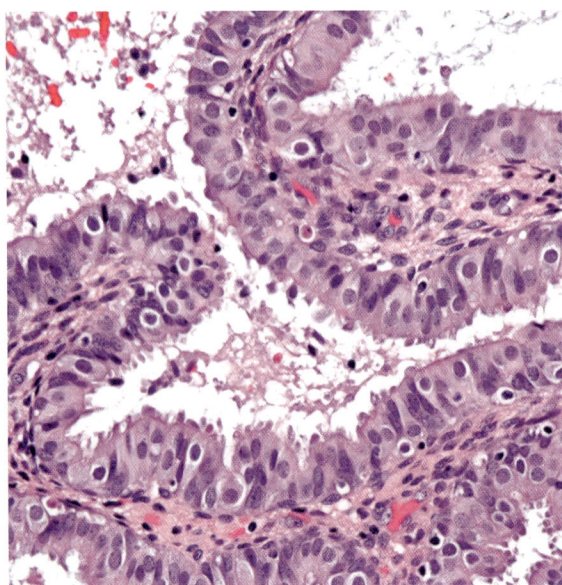

Figure 2-1

TUBAL METAPLASIA

Ciliated, secretory, and intercalated cells line endometrial glands. Ciliated cells have basally located nuclei, abundant eosinophilic cytoplasm, terminal bars, and cilia.

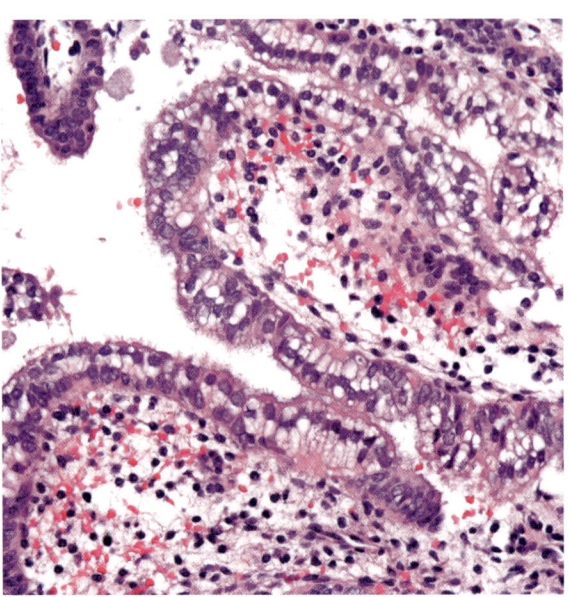

Figure 2-2

TUBAL METAPLASIA

Endometrial cells have clear subnuclear vacuoles as seen in early secretory phase but they also contain terminal cilia.

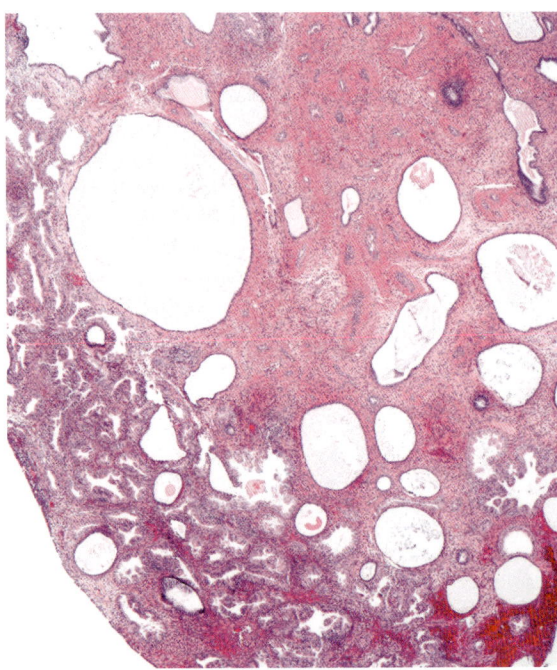

Figure 2-3

TUBAL METAPLASIA WITHIN AN ENDOMETRIAL POLYP

Tubal metaplasia often results in a "thicker" appearance to the endometrial glands that may secondarily impart a complex architecture simulating endometrial hyperplasia.

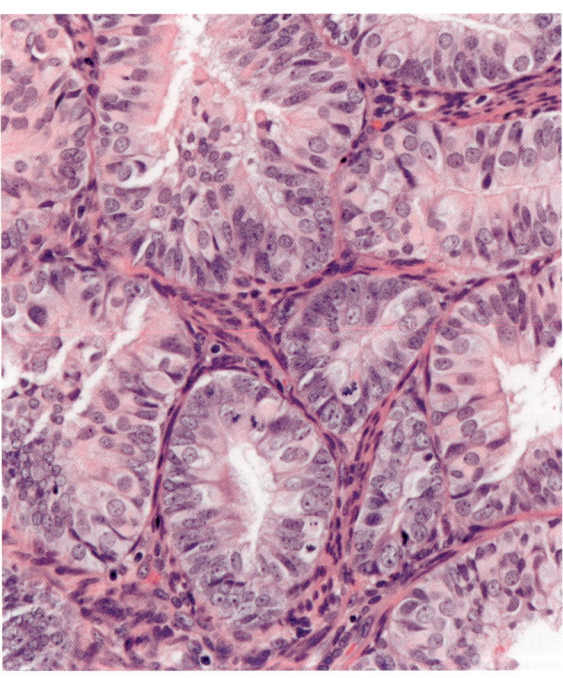

Figure 2-4

ATYPICAL TUBAL METAPLASIA

Cytologic atypia is present as enlarged rounded nuclei with vesicular chromatin, nucleoli, and mitoses.

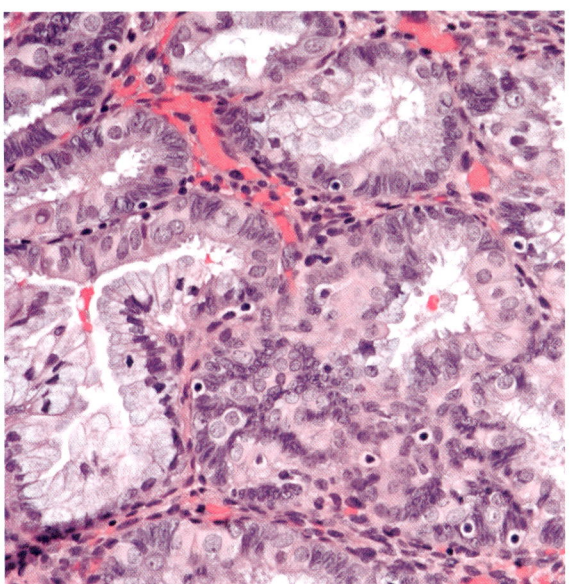 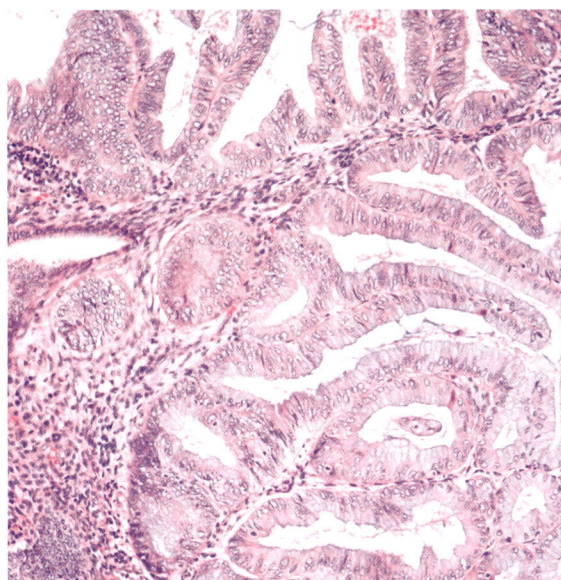

Figure 2-5

MUCINOUS METAPLASIA

Endocervical-type cells with small basally located nuclei and abundant columnar cytoplasm line simple endometrial glands located on the left (left). They are seen next to endometrial glands showing tubal metaplasia. Endometrioid carcinoma with mucinous metaplasia (right). There is complex architecture with back to back glands and villous growth in the absence of cytologic atypia.

cohesive appearance. They show a wild-type pattern of p53 staining, even when cytologically atypical, while Ki-67 expression is typically low (less than 5 percent), with only rare exceptions. Human telomerase reverse transcriptase staining is also negative, an immunoprofile that differs significantly from serous carcinoma (3). p16 staining is typically patchy positive (in contrast to diffuse and strong positivity in high-grade serous carcinoma) (4), and PAX2 and BCL2 are positive in secretory cells (1). Tubal metaplasia, including atypical forms, is not associated with an increased frequency of subsequent endometrial hyperplasia/carcinoma (3), although some investigators postulate that ciliated tubal metaplasia is likely a precursor of ciliated endometrioid-type carcinoma (1).

Mucinous Metaplasia

Mucinous (endocervical-type) metaplasia is uncommon (24 percent) when compared to tubal (58 percent), eosinophilic (48 percent), and squamous (34 percent) metaplasias as reported in a large comprehensive study (5). It is most often seen in postmenopausal patients or those in a hyperestrogenic state (6). Endometrial polyps, especially those that are tamoxifen related, may show mucinous metaplasia (7); this type of metaplasia represents the second most frequent type following tubal metaplasia in this setting in one study (8), indicating the close association of mucinous metaplasia and tamoxifen therapy.

Mucinous metaplasia of pyloric type involving the endometrium and other organs of the female genital tract may occur in patients with Peutz-Jeghers syndrome (9,10). Rarely, *intestinal-type metaplasia* may be seen in the endometrium (11).

Mucinous metaplasia is typically a focal finding in which cells with columnar to cuboidal cytoplasm are filled with mucin droplets and have basally located nuclei that may be small and hyperchromatic (compressed) or round and vesicular, similar to endocervical-type cells (fig 2-5, left). They may partially or completely replace the preexisting endometrial glandular lining, but complex architecture, except for rare tufting, or cytologic atypia should not be present (6,12). Frequently, mucinous metaplasia is associated with papillary, tubal, and eosinophilic metaplasia, imparting a variably complex appearance

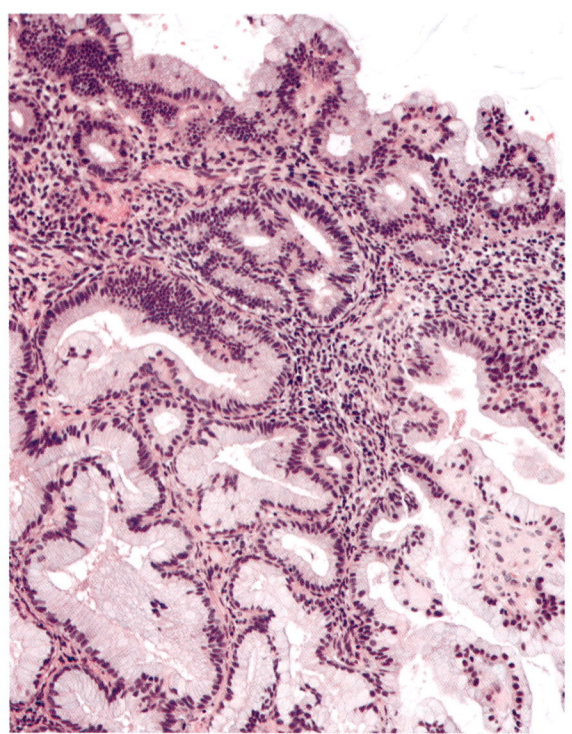

Figure 2-6

MUCINOUS METAPLASIA ASSOCIATED WITH FOCAL PAPILLARY ARCHITECTURE

Small papillae are lined by cells with abundant mucinous cytoplasm lacking cytologic atypia.

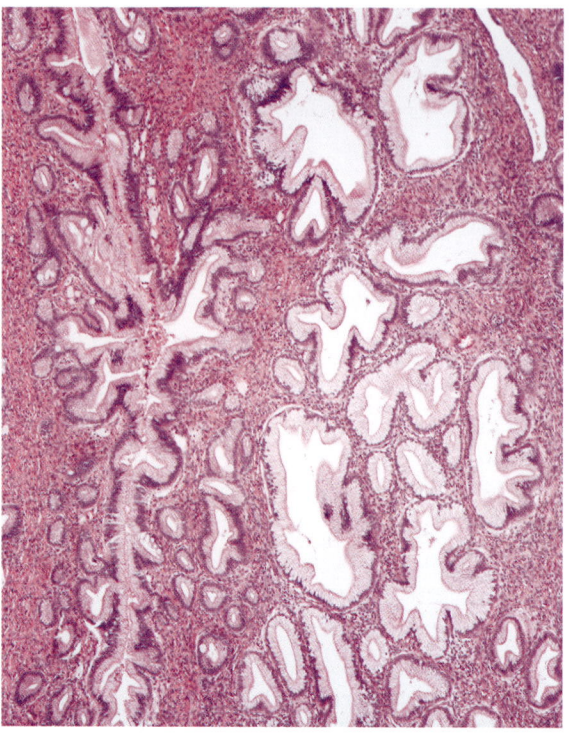

Figure 2-7

PYLORIC-TYPE MUCINOUS METAPLASIA

Most preexisting endometrial glands are replaced by mucinous cells with columnar, amphophilic cytoplasm reminiscent of gastric pyloric cells. One preserved gland is at top left. This patient had Peutz-Jeghers syndrome. (Courtesy of Dr. R. A. Soslow, New York, NY.)

(13). In such cases, the metaplastic changes are commonly, but not exclusively, present in a background of endometrial polyps in which either a simple or complex papillary architecture is noted (papillary proliferation of Lehman and Hart, discussed below) (fig. 2-6). Mucinous metaplasia shows low Ki-67 expression, focal p16 positivity, intact PTEN, ARID1A, and PAX2 expression, and wild-type p53 expression (14).

Mucinous metaplasia of the endometrium may be accompanied by mucinous metaplasia of the fallopian tube as well as multifocal mucinous neoplasia of the female genital tract (9,10,15), but in the latter, cells often have a pyloric-like appearance rather than resembling endocervical epithelium (fig. 2-7). This mucinous epithelium is positive for HIK1083 or MUC6 (10). Intestinal-type metaplasia may contain goblet as well as neuroendocrine cells (fig. 2-8), but it is rare and may be seen in association with intestinal metaplasia in the cervix. Cells have been reported to be CK7, CK20, CDX2, and villin positive while the neuroendocrine cells express chromogranin and p16 is negative (11,16).

The differential diagnosis of mucinous metaplasia includes mucinous carcinoma or endometrioid carcinoma with mucinous differentiation from the endometrium, atypical mucinous glandular proliferation, secondary involvement by mucinous carcinoma of the cervix, and less commonly, benign endocervical epithelium and metastatic carcinoma (exceedingly rare). Endometrial adenocarcinoma with mucinous differentiation is more common than pure mucinous carcinoma, but both typically show complex architecture, including back to back glands, cribriforming, and complex papillary/villous architecture (fig. 2-5, right). In a limited sample, complex architecture and associated abnormal (reactive) endometrial stroma should be carefully sought since nuclear atypia is frequently lacking in mucinous carcinoma and its precursors (6,17). Mucinous proliferations without confluent or cribriform architecture or cytologic atypia are classified by the most recent World Health Organization (WHO) classification as "atypical mucinous glandular proliferations" (18), and correspond to proliferations that are between metaplasia and carcinoma. In two studies, no morphologic feature was reliable to predict outcome (carcinoma versus non-neoplastic findings at hysterectomy) in patients with these lesions (12,19). As interobserver variability in the diagnosis of mucinous proliferations is high, it is difficult to ascertain which mucinous proliferation in a curettage/biopsy will be associated with mucinous carcinoma. To establish a diagnosis of mucinous metaplasia, no architectural complexity or cytologic atypia should be allowed (except if associated with papillary proliferations). Immunohistochemical stains are not helpful in this differential diagnosis, with the potential exception of KRAS. The finding of a *KRAS* mutation supports the diagnosis of atypical mucinous glandular proliferation/mucinous carcinoma (20).

Secondary endometrial involvement by usual endocervical carcinoma may disclose preservation of endometrial glandular architecture on low-power examination. However, at higher magnification, the glands are replaced by cells with markedly pseudostratified and hyperchromatic nuclei associated with frequent apical mitoses and apoptotic bodies. Also, usual-type endocervical adenocarcinomas are often depleted of mucin when compared to benign mucinous metaplasia. Although mucinous metaplasia may be focally positive for p16, the overall staining pattern contrasts with the strong and diffuse p16 positivity seen in usual-type endocervical carcinoma since it is human papillomavirus (HPV) related (21). If mucinous metaplasia is associated with papillary metaplasia, the cellular tufts of the latter are more frequently and intensively p16 positive but still do not show the diffuse staining seen in HPV-related adenocarcinomas. Progesterone receptor (PR) expression appears to decrease in mucinous metaplasia, nevertheless, it is positive (to some extent) in contrast to most endocervical carcinomas, which are typically negative, although exceptions occur (14).

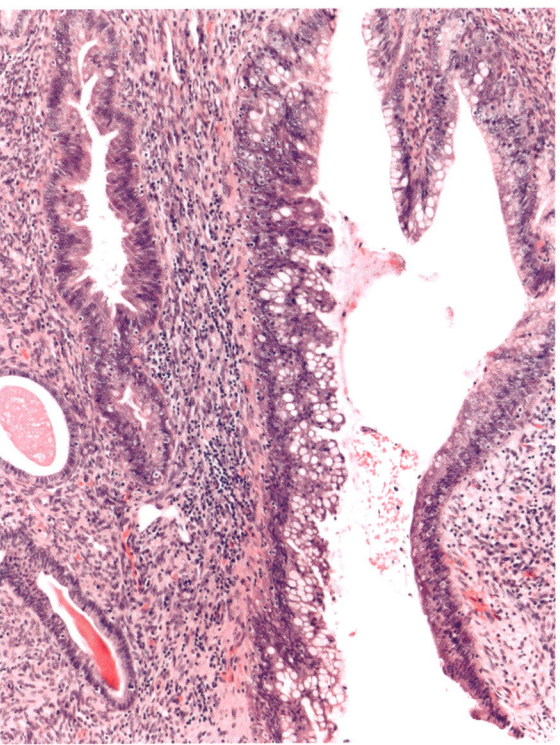

Figure 2-8

INTESTINAL-TYPE MUCINOUS METAPLASIA

The surface endometrium is lined by many goblet cells. (Courtesy of Dr. F. F. Nogales, Granada, Spain.)

Mucinous carcinoma of gastric type (adenoma malignum) can also partially or totally replace preexisting endometrial glands (fig. 2-9). Even though cytologic atypia may be minimal and mitotic activity absent in small samples, its morphologic appearance is different since neoplastic cells often have abundant, tall, eosinophilic or clear cytoplasm, an appearance similar to pyloric-type epithelium. p16 may be negative or focally positive (HPV unrelated) as may be seen in if mucinous metaplasia while PAX8 is often positive in both, thus, not helpful in this differential diagnosis (22). Estrogen receptor (ER) and PR expression favors mucinous metaplasia over gastric-type carcinoma, which is typically negative for these markers (23), while MUC6 favors a gastric-type carcinoma (22).

It may be very difficult to separate mucinous metaplasia from benign endocervix since the morphologic appearance of both is similar. In such cases, associated endometrial stroma,

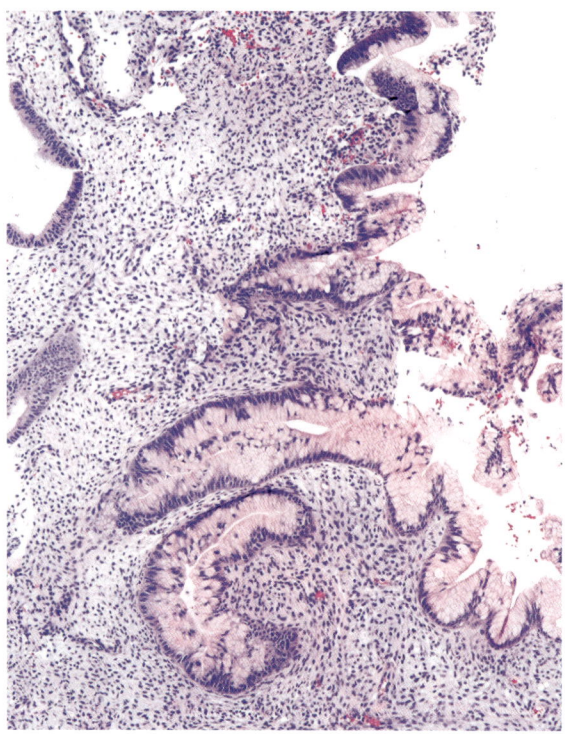

Figure 2-9

SECONDARY INVOLVEMENT BY CERVICAL "ADENOMA MALIGNUM"

The preexisting endometrial glands are replaced by tall epithelium with basally located but hyperchromatic and atypical nuclei and abundant pale cytoplasm.

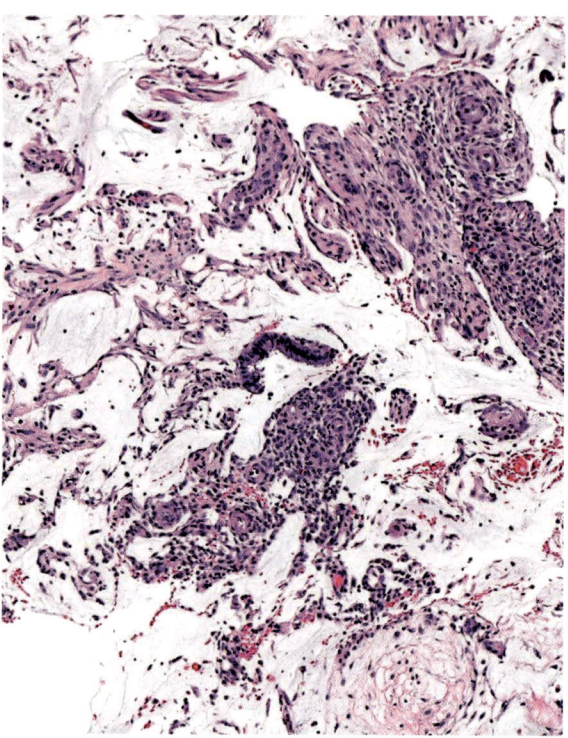

Figure 2-10

PSEUDOMYXOMA UTERI

Mucin dissects the endometrial stroma secondary to transtubal spread from a low-grade mucinous tumor of the appendix. The appearance is similar to that observed in pseudomyxoma peritonei. (Courtesy of Dr. P. N. Staats, Baltimore, MD.)

transition to endometrial-type epithelium, and where the sample was taken are helpful clues. The finding of reserve cells as a second layer under the mucinous epithelium points to an endocervical origin of the mucinous epithelium.

Rarely, low-grade appendiceal mucinous neoplasms associated with pseudomyxoma peritonei show endometrial involvement secondary to transtubal spread. Some of these patients present with mucinous discharge. Endometrial biopsies may show replacement of the endometrial epithelium by a low-grade mucinous neoplasm, which can be confused with mucinous intestinal metaplasia of the endometrium, since cells in this setting may be cytologically bland (fig. 2-10). A helpful clue to the diagnosis is an appearance similar to hyperplastic mucinous intestinal epithelium. Furthermore, there is typically extrauterine involvement of omentum, ovaries, and other organs (24,25).

Endometrial carcinomas with intestinal-type differentiation have been occasionally reported in the endometrium (26). The cells are CK20 and CDX2 positive, and often PAX8 negative, as occurs in intestinal metaplasia, but in contrast, there is abnormal architecture as well as cytologic atypia. Metastasis should be always excluded in this setting.

Endocervical mucinous metaplasia typically pursues a benign course when incidental, unassociated with architectural complexity or cytologic atypia, and the background endometrium is benign. A repeat curettage after 6 months of the initial diagnosis is advisable, especially if there is any degree of architectural abnormality (27).

Papillary (Lehman and Hart) Proliferations

Papillary proliferations are more often noted in postmenopausal women, but can be seen in younger women, typically with prolonged

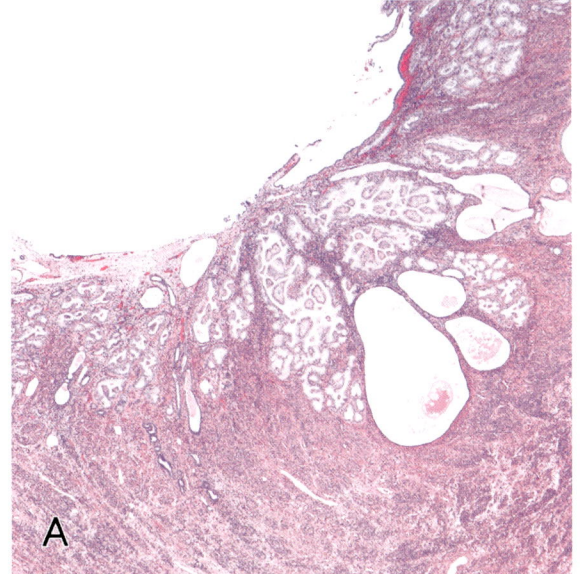

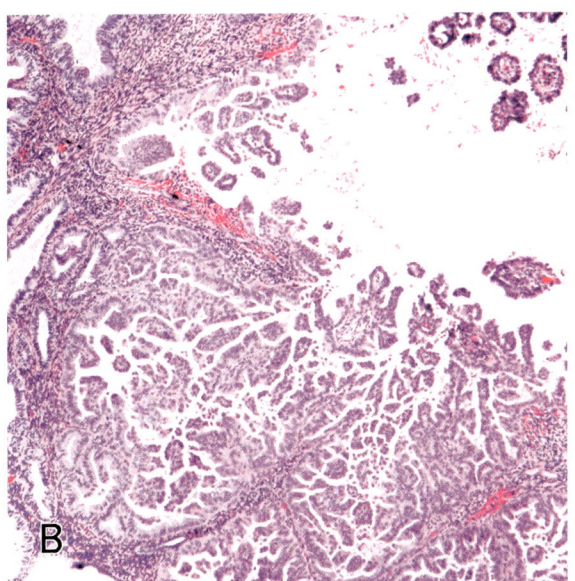
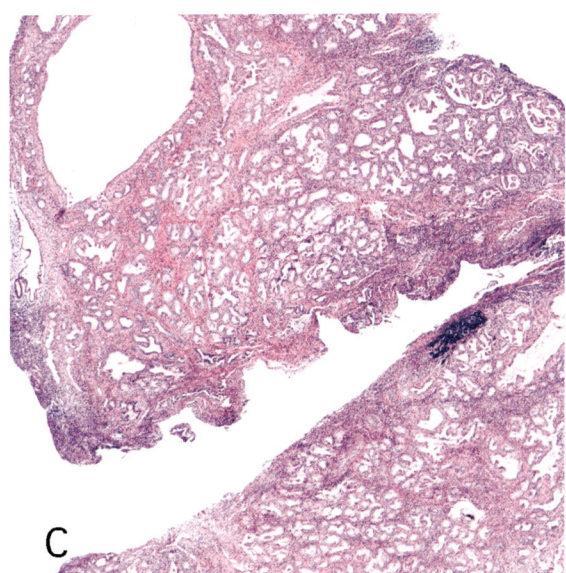

Figure 2-11

PAPILLARY (LEHMAN AND HART) PROLIFERATION

Nonpolypoid endometrium shows endometrial glands with simple intraluminal papillae and focal cystic gland dilation (A). Complex papillary architecture with secondary and tertiary branching within an endometrial polyp (not seen) (B). Diffuse involvement of endometrial polyp by intraluminal simple papillary growth (C).

hormonal drug intake and often associated with endometrial polyps (about 70 percent of cases), but can also be seen in nonpolypoid endometrium. They typically represent an incidental finding in curettings from women with abnormal vaginal bleeding (13,28). They tend to involve a small part of the endometrium but can be extensive.

Papillary proliferations are divided into simple and complex types based on the degree of complexity of the papillary growth. Simple architecture is defined by papillae having localized, short, predominantly nonbranching stalks, although occasional secondary or detached papillae are allowed (fig. 2-11A), while complex architecture shows either papillae with short or long stalks with frequent secondary or tertiary branching or diffuse and crowded intracystic papillae (fig. 2-11B) (28). Sometimes, changes may be extensive, with or without prominent branching of papillae and cellular budding (fig. 2-11C). The papillae have well-developed fibrovascular cores and may be slender or broad, with variable branching. The lining epithelium is one layer to multilayered, with or without prominent cell tufts, buds, and single detached cells (fig. 2-12). Metaplastic changes

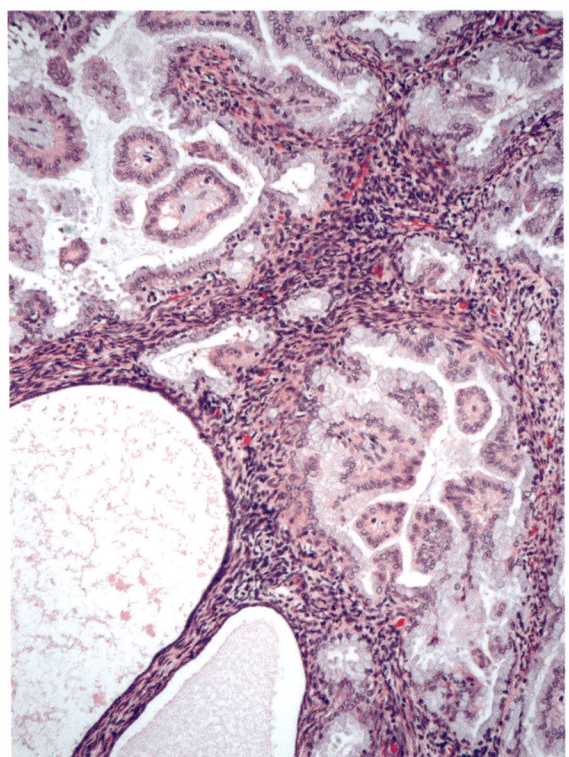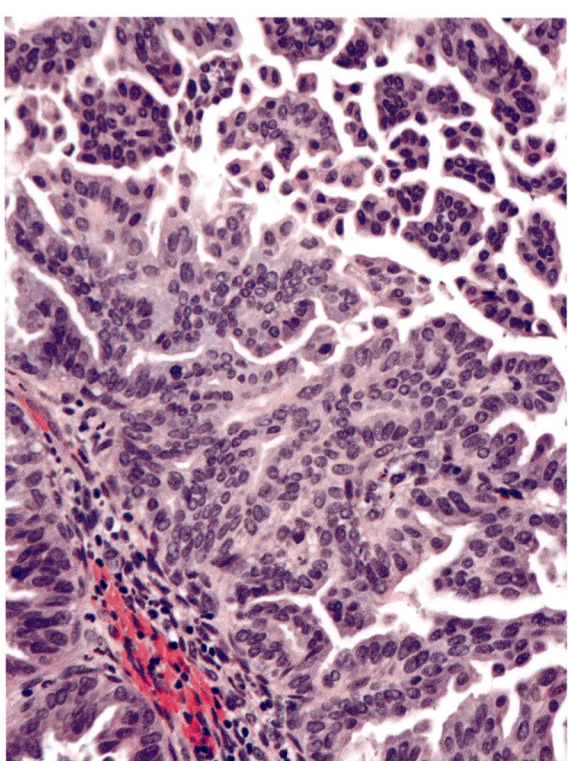

Figure 2-12

PAPILLARY (LEHMAN AND HART) PROLIFERATION

The endometrial glands have intraluminal simple but not branching papillae lined by banal mucinous epithelium (left). There is prominent branching with multilayered epithelium as well as cellular budding and cell tufts, minimal cytologic atypia but mitoses can be seen (right).

are seen in most cases (over 90 percent in the largest series [28]). Endocervical-type cuboidal to low-columnar lining is most common (seen in about 70 percent) (fig. 2-12, left), followed by eosinophilic (fig. 2-13), ciliated, and squamous metaplasia, and rarely hobnail metaplasia or surface syncytial change (13,28). In the two largest series, no goblet cells were identified (13,28). Nuclei are small and often oval and basally located. They may display small nucleoli but most importantly, no cytologic atypia is present, although scattered mitoses may be seen. When the architecture is complex, cytologic atypia is present, or changes are extensive (defined in one study [28] as presence of three or more foci within a specimen or involvement of over 50 percent of the endometrial polyp by either papillae with simple or complex architecture), the proliferation is regarded as atypical endometrial hyperplasia since it has been shown to be associated with endometrial neoplasia in a high percentage of follow-up hysterectomies (28,29).

Studies on the immunohistochemical profile of papillary proliferations are limited but typically not necessary for their diagnosis. They are ER and PR positive (although the latter shows reduced expression), with low Ki-67 (fig. 2-14, left), wild-type p53 expression (fig. 2-14, right), PTEN, and ARID-1A intact expression with either intact or reduced PAX2 expression. Papillary proliferations lined by mucinous epithelium may have intensively positive p16 cellular tufts (14,29,30).

The differential diagnosis of papillary proliferations includes endometrioid carcinoma and syncytial papillary change. The former may have a papillary architecture with villous or nonvillous papillae, or may have nonspecific papillae. Endometrioid carcinomas may also have mucinous metaplasia as mentioned above.

However, the architecture is typically complex, there is cytologic atypia, and often there are stromal changes that allow for the correct diagnosis in most instances even in limited material. Ki-67 is typically much lower in papillary proliferations than in carcinomas. Although *KRAS* mutations are not typically seen in mucinous metaplasia (14), they have been reported with high frequency in papillary mucinous metaplasia (12,14,20), thus, it is not helpful in the differential diagnosis with carcinoma. These findings have suggested that papillary mucinous metaplasia may represent a precursor of a subset of endometrioid carcinomas (12,14,20). Although papillary syncytial metaplasia is also seen in endometrial polyps and surface endometrium, in contrast to papillary proliferations, it is typically associated with stromal breakdown, lacks true papillae with fibrovascular cores, and often has prominent acute inflammatory inflammation associated with karyorrhectic nuclear debris (31).

Papillary proliferations are associated with a benign course when simple in architecture and limited (not diffuse) in amount. In this setting, the term "benign papillary proliferation of the endometrium" has been used. However, if the papillary proliferation is complex or extensive, even when simple in architecture, there is an

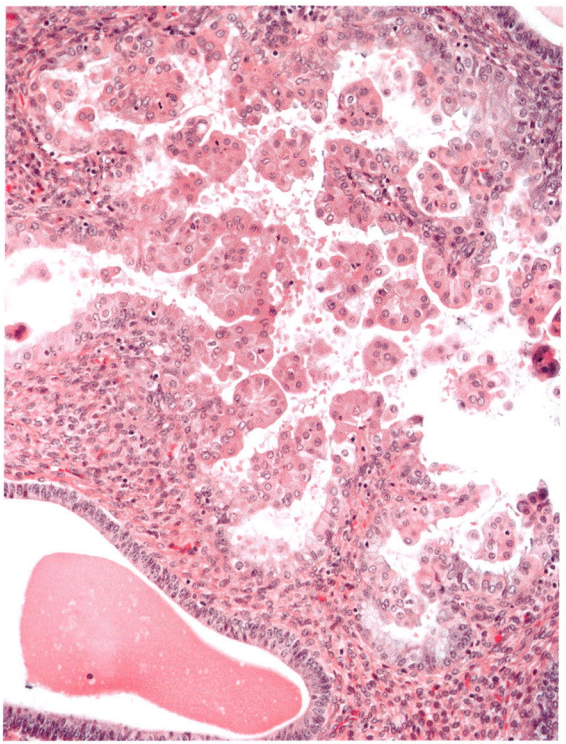

Figure 2-13

PAPILLARY (LEHMAN AND HART) PROLIFERATION

The papillae are lined by cells with striking oxyphilic change.

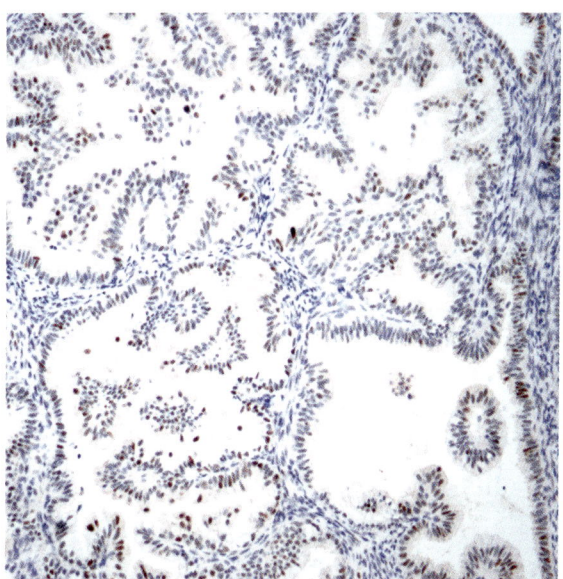

Figure 2-14

PAPILLARY (LEHMAN AND HART) PROLIFERATION

The cells display low Ki-67 expression (left) and wild-type p53 expression (right).

increased risk of associated endometrial neoplasia (atypical hyperplasia/carcinoma) and thus, should be termed "complex papillary hyperplasia" (28). As stated earlier, some authors postulate that papillary proliferations associated with mucinous metaplasia may be precursors of mucinous carcinoma, due to increased KRAS mutations in these cases (14,19).

Squamous Metaplasia

Squamous metaplasia is the third most common type of metaplasia within the endometrium, with a frequency of about 34 percent in one study (5). Squamous metaplasia is seen in premenopausal patients in association with polycystic ovarian disease or as an unusual response to estrogen or progesterone therapy or trauma (32). It has also been described after uterine embolization for leiomyomas and in association with chronic endometritis (32,33). In postmenopausal patients with a history of cervical stenosis, squamous metaplasia may be visible macroscopically when it is diffuse and keratinization is present; the result is whitish thickening of the endometrium, sometimes associated with small flecks (ichthyosis uteri). For the most part, however, this is an incidental finding in curettage or biopsy specimens.

Squamous metaplasia in the corpus can be present as *squamous morules (adenoacanthosis)* or conventional mature squamous metaplasia. On low-power microscopic examination, squamous morules (adenoacanthosis) are seen as free-floating small nodules or in association with endometrial glands, with replacement of one or several lumens by small and uniform cells with scant pink to purple cytoplasm and small, round, evenly spaced nuclei with inconspicuous nucleoli, some containing optically clear biotin-rich inclusions (34). There is absent or minimal (individual cell) keratinization, no visible intercellular bridges or cell membranes, and no mitoses. Central necrosis may be seen. Peripheral to the morules, one or more gland lumens may impart a complex (cribriform) appearance (fig. 2-15A,B). However, these are individual glandular units without neighboring gland crowding, cytologic atypia, or mitotic activity. Squamous morules may coalesce into broad sheets. Squamous morules are typically negative for epithelial membrane antigen (EMA) in contrast to glandular cells (35), but may be positive for some keratins. They often show strong β-catenin, CD10 and CDX2 expression (36) and can be ER-β positive, especially if they have abundant biotin-rich nuclear inclusions (37). They recently have been shown to express SATB2 (37a).

Mature (glycogenated) squamous metaplasia is characterized by sheets of polygonal pink cells with abundant eosinophilic to pale to vacuolated (clear) cytoplasm, small and vesicular central nuclei, small nucleoli, and no mitoses. Squamous differentiation is defined by the presence of visible cell membranes, intercellular bridges, and keratinization. It may be reparative and focal but, rarely, diffusely involves the endometrium (ichthyosis uteri) if secondary to cervical stenosis (fig. 2-15C). In the latter setting, it may also involve endometrial glands within adenomyosis. Mature squamous metaplasia is often p63, CD10, and ER positive with variable CDX2 expression and often display a low frequency of nuclear β-catenin positivity (36). The Ki-67 rate is very low in both squamous morules and mature squamous metaplasia (38).

In small samples, squamous morules should be distinguished from atypical polypoid adenomyoma, complex endometrial hyperplasia, and low-grade endometrioid carcinoma. The appearance of the squamous morules, including central necrosis, is identical in all instances. Four features should be evaluated given this differential diagnosis: amount and degree of architectural complexity of associated glands if present, cytologic atypia, and type of associated stroma. Squamous differentiation is uncommon in complex hyperplasia, but if present, typically has a morular appearance. In contrast, conventional mature squamous metaplasia is more common in endometrioid carcinomas (25 percent). In both instances (hyperplasia and carcinoma), there are abundant tissue fragments showing complex glandular architecture unassociated with morules, which still show cytologic atypia and mitotic activity (fig. 2-16, left). In carcinomas, the associated stroma may show marked inflammation indicative of endometrial stromal invasion, resulting in an appearance that differs from the resting endometrial stroma. The immunohistochemical profile of squamous morules in all these settings is identical, with CD10, nuclear CDX2, and β-catenin positivity

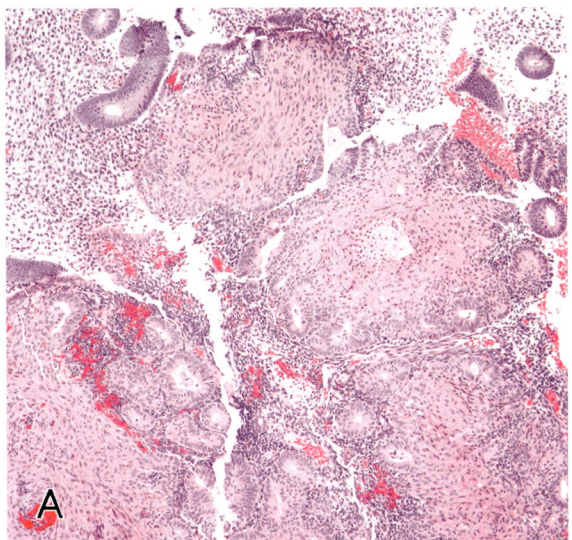
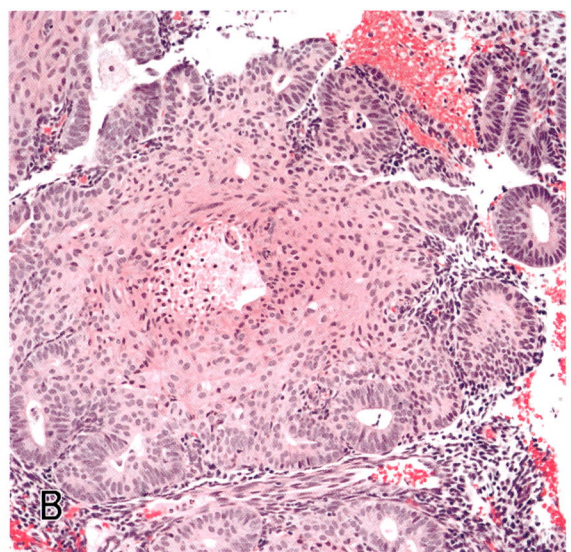
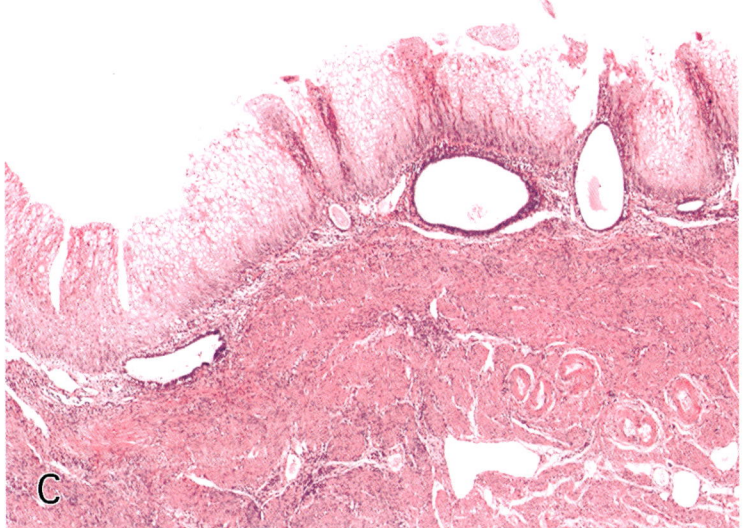

Figure 2-15

SQUAMOUS METAPLASIA

Squamous morules (adenoacanthosis) are seen as small nodules associated with normal-appearing endometrial glands, typically at the periphery. The cells have eosinophilic cytoplasm but the cell borders are difficult to identify. There is central necrosis (A). The associated endometrial glands have basally located nuclei and lack complex architecture (B). Mature glycogenated squamous replaces surface endometrium (Ichthyosis uteri) (C). (Modified from fig. 1A from Chew I, Post MD, Carinelli SG, et al. p16 expression in squamous and trophoblastic lesions of the upper female genital tract. Int J Gynecol Pathol 2010;29:513-22.)

and ER and p63 negativity (or only positive in most peripheral cells) (36,39,40) except one case reported where benign squamous morules were p63 positive (38). In atypical polypoid adenomyoma, there is muscular or fibromuscular stroma around the endometrial glands but no endometrial-type stroma. Thus, in curettage or biopsy specimens with squamous morules, it is important to evaluate the nonmorular accompanying endometrium. Furthermore, in atypical polypoid adenomyoma fragments are often part of a polypoid mass (41,42). β-catenin nuclear expression is also noted in atypical polypoid adenomyoma (43,44). Although the presence of isolated squamous morules has no clinical significance, surveillance is advised, especially if the sample is small and not representative of what is seen on hysteroscopy, as on occasion it may be the first manifestation of a premalignant or malignant process (45,46).

The differential diagnosis of mature squamous metaplasia includes endometrioid carcinoma with squamous differentiation, primary endometrial or cervical squamous cell carcinoma, and benign squamous epithelium from the cervix. Endometrioid carcinoma may show massive mature squamous differentiation in its original state or after medroxyprogesterone treatment (47) but atypical conventional endometrioid glands and malignant squamous epithelium are also seen in

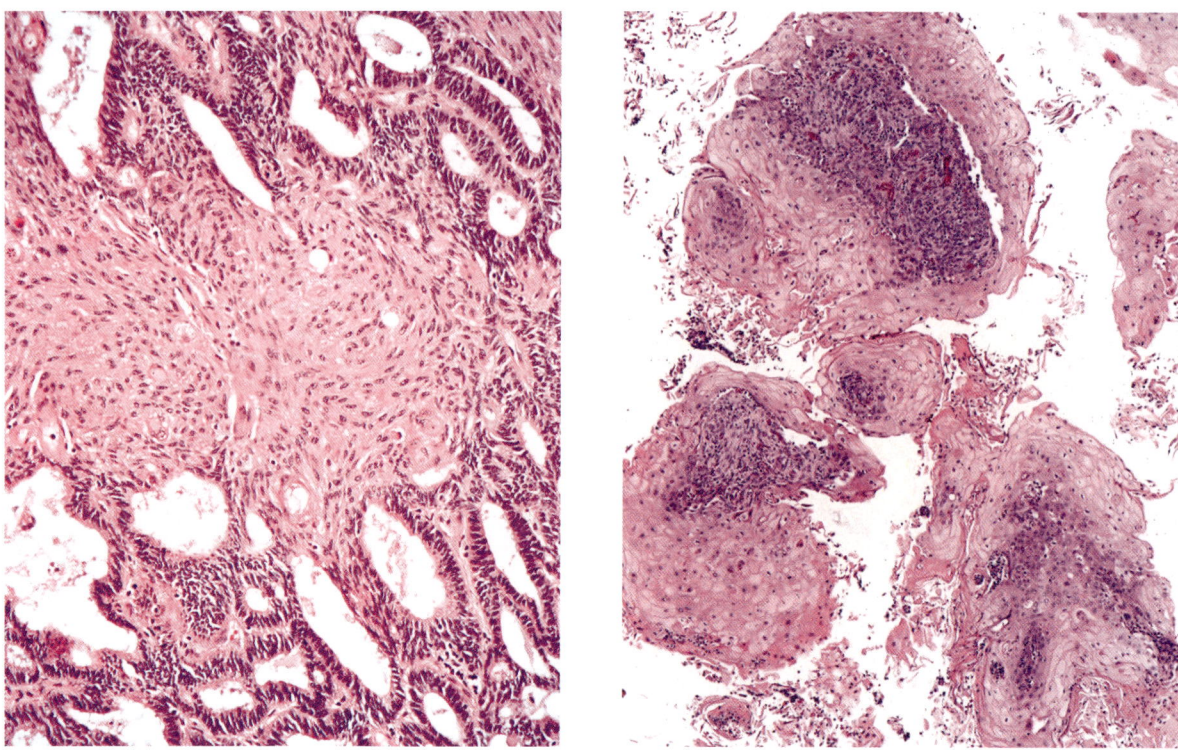

Figure 2-16

ENDOMETRIOID CARCINOMA WITH SQUAMOUS METAPLASIA

Squamous morules with bland cytologic features are seen in the background of a complex endometrioid glandular proliferation (left). Mature glycogenated squamous epithelium is a prominent component in some endometrioid carcinomas. Other areas display atypical endometrioid glands (right).

most (fig. 2-16, right). Primary squamous cell carcinoma of the endometrium is rare, typically seen in postmenopausal women. Although a mass is often suspected, sometimes examination may be difficult and some tumors may be highly differentiated. The finding of any abnormal architecture (i.e., papillarity) or any degree of cytologic atypia should suggest carcinoma (48–50). Extension of a cervical squamous cell carcinoma to the endometrium typically does not represent a diagnostic problem since cytologic atypia and mitotic activity are easy to identify and most are typically diffusely and strongly p16 positive as they are HPV related. On occasion, it may be difficult to distinguish mature squamous metaplasia from cervical squamous metaplastic epithelium. The latter is frequently associated with residual mucin droplets indicative of its origin. Immunostains are not helpful in this setting.

Papillary Syncytial Metaplasia

Stromal breakdown, whether or not a manifestation of menses, is often associated with *papillary syncytial metaplasia,* also termed *surface papillary syncytial change* or *eosinophilic syncytial change*. It is encountered in about 17 percent of curettage/biopsy specimens performed for abnormal uterine bleeding from women with a wide age range (5).

Papillary syncytial metaplasia is characterized by syncytial to papillary aggregates lacking fibrovascular cores, oriented in different planes, located on the endometrial surface and, less frequently, in superficial endometrial glands. The cells have variable amounts of eosinophilic cytoplasm, with rare vacuolization and indistinct cytoplasmic membranes ("syncytium"). Nuclei have a random orientation/distribution within the tufts, and they have small nucleoli and delicate chromatin. Below the syncytial

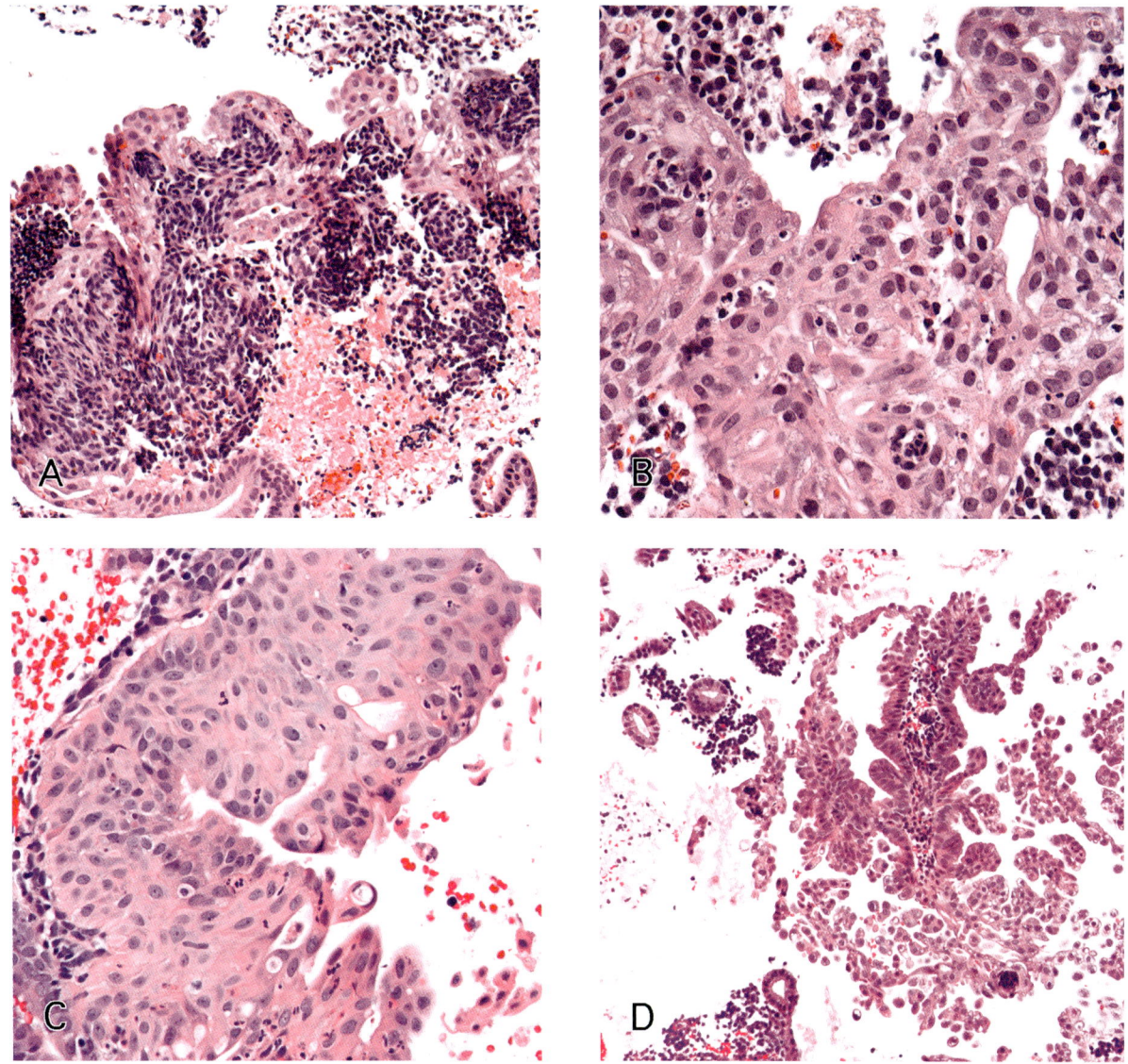

Figure 2-17

PAPILLARY SYNCYTIAL METAPLASIA

"Blue balls" of endometrial stroma, indicative of stromal breakdown, are associated with a syncytium of epithelial endometrial cells with eosinophilic cytoplasm and indistinct cell membranes that are piling up on top of each other due to the shrinking of underlying stroma (A). The nuclei are small with tiny nucleoli (B). Cells become larger, displaying some degree of cytologic atypia. They have enlarged nuclei and prominent nucleoli (C). If exuberant, with prominent budding of cells, serous carcinoma may be mimicked. Vacuolated cytoplasm and underlying stromal breakdown are seen (D).

tufts, the stroma is compacted and "blue," with nuclear debris (also noted in glandular epithelium), acute inflammation, and intravascular fibrin thrombi, as typically seen in stromal breakdown, facilitating the diagnosis (fig. 2-17A,B). In a number of cases, however, papillary syncytial metaplasia may show atypical features including hyperchromasia, some degree of pleomorphism, prominent nucleoli, and mitotic activity (fig. 2-17C) (51). In curettage specimens, these findings may raise the possibility of serous carcinoma (fig. 2-17D), especially if exuberant. Also, surface syncytial metaplasia has an immunohistochemical

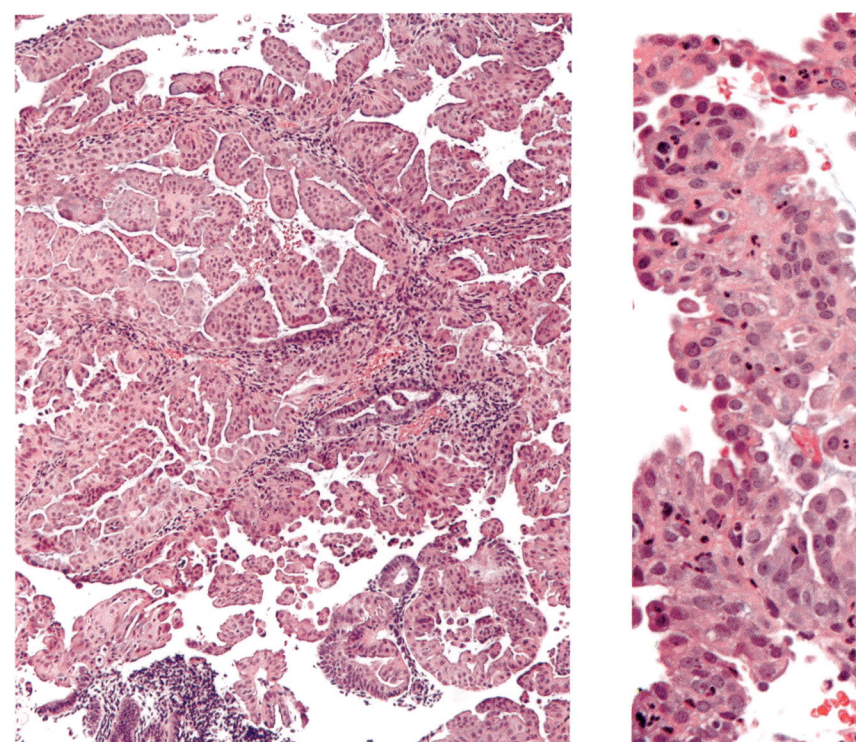

Figure 2-18

ENDOMETRIOID CARCINOMA WITH SURFACE SYNCYTIAL CHANGES

The associated glandular architecture is complex (left). Cytologic atypia and mitotic activity are present (right).

profile that overlaps to some extent with serous carcinoma, with decreased expression of ER and increased expression of p53 (although typically wild pattern) and diffuse p16 expression. Cyclin D1 is also overexpressed in papillary syncytial metaplasia (52). However, Ki-67 is always low (53–55) and typically there is a background of stromal breakdown.

Although surface syncytial metaplasia is seen in association with stromal breakdown in proliferative or secretory endometrium, endometrial hyperplasia and endometrioid carcinoma may show similar changes (fig. 2-18) (2,56). Thus, it is always important to evaluate the cytologic features of the proliferation as well as the nonpapillary or nonsyncytial endometrium. In contrast to endometrioid carcinomas, changes in papillary syncytial metaplasia are focal, true fibrovascular cores are lacking, and there is no overt cytologic atypia or mitotic activity. Some hypothesize that papillary syncytial metaplasia may represent early squamous metaplasia; nevertheless, it is accepted that this is a degenerative/regenerative change secondary to ischemia (31,51,57).

Eosinophilic Metaplasia

Endometrial cells sometimes display abundant eosinophilic cytoplasm, imparting an oncocytic or oxyphilic appearance, resulting in the terms "oncocytic" or "oxyphilic" metaplasia. This is often associated with tubal metaplasia. It can occur in non-neoplastic as well as neoplastic epithelium (2,5,58–60) and has been hypothesized to represent a reactive change to injury or an example of early mucinous metaplasia (fig. 2-13) (61). Cells display abundant eosinophilic cytoplasm, with round basally located nuclei and visible nucleoli. The overall appearance resembles that of ciliated metaplasia without the presence of cilia or the other cell types seen in tubal metaplasia. As it occurs with any type of metaplastic change, it is important to evaluate the cytologic and architectural features of the neighboring endometrial glands before making a diagnosis of eosinophilic metaplasia (5).

Hobnail and Clear Changes

Hobnail and clear changes are typically reactive changes that are present on the surface of the endometrium or in a polyp secondary to injury (a prior curettage or secondary to infarction). Hobnail change has also been described in about 25 percent of patients using the Mirena Coil (62). Hobnail cells have eosinophilic, clear, or vacuolated cytoplasm, often displaying hyperchromatic nuclei that are bulging into glandular lumens or surface endometrium (fig. 2-19). Typically, there is a transition to innocuous-appearing endometrial cells and no mitotic activity is noted. Even though examination at high-power magnification may raise concern for a clear cell or even serous carcinoma, especially in a curettage specimen, hobnail metaplasia is an incidental microscopic finding. Additionally, the stroma may be spindled, edematous, and inflamed in the setting of prior injury or ischemic changes in a polyp.

Clear cell change typically denotes hormonal alterations and may be seen in association with Arias-Stella reaction. Cells have clear cytoplasm due to abundant glycogen. They may form tufts and show pseudostratification. The nuclei typically have smudgy chromatin, and no mitotic activity is present. As with hobnail cells, clear change within endometrial glands may also cause concern for clear cell carcinoma. Importantly, this change represents a microscopic incidental finding (1,5).

Arias-Stella Reaction

In most instances, *Arias-Stella reaction* in the endometrium is easy to diagnose in the setting of pregnancy, puerperium, or oral contraceptive intake. However, when the history is not known or the reaction is seen in postmenopausal women (63), it may cause concern for neoplasia, most often clear cell carcinoma, especially in small samples. Worrisome features include abundant clear cytoplasm with hobnail nuclei, enlarged and hyperchromatic nuclei, rarely with nucleoli, and an exuberant "complex" appearance of the endometrial glands due hypersecretory change (fig. 2-20). Rarely, giant and bizarre nuclei of "monstrous type" may be seen either focally or diffusely within the endometrium (64). Glands affected by Arias-Stella reaction are ER positive but with less intensity than the noninvolved en-

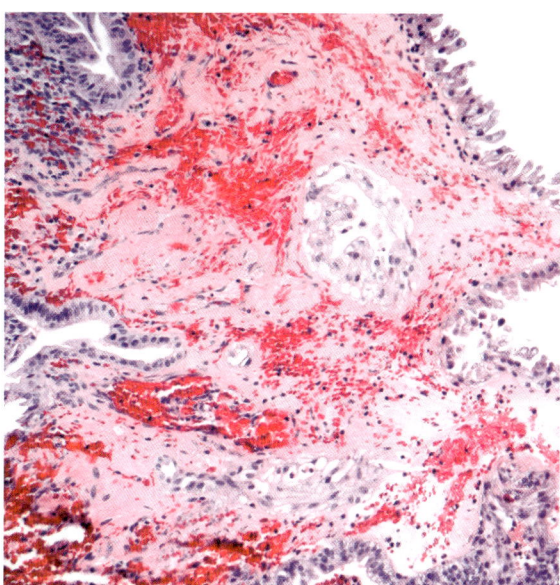

Figure 2-19

HOBNAIL METAPLASIA

Cells with eosinophilic and partially vacuolated cytoplasm and hobnailing nuclei are present on the surface of a partially infarcted endometrial polyp. The underlying stroma is hyalinized and hemorrhagic. Away from this area, the endometrial glands have a typical appearance.

dometrium, with lower or absent PR expression. There may be some degree of p53 positivity, but not aberrant expression (64,65).

The features that are helpful in this diagnosis include the low-power linear and parallel architecture of the glands which matches the normal preexisting endometrial architecture, sometimes partial gland involvement, degenerative nature of the nuclei, presence of nuclear pseudoinclusions, and absent mitotic activity (with rare exceptions since atypical Arias-Stella reaction may show occasional mitotic activity) (fig. 2-20) (66). Arias-Stella reaction shows low Ki-67 index (sometimes slightly elevated in pregnant women), in contrast to clear cell carcinoma, and p53 never displays strong and diffuse positivity (65) although clear cell carcinoma is only positive in about 30 of cases (67).

Other Pregnancy/ Hormonally Related Alterations

A myriad of changes are seen in the epithelial and stromal components of the endometrium in pregnant patients or those on progestational agents. Biotin-rich optically clear nuclei are a common finding in endometrial glands seen

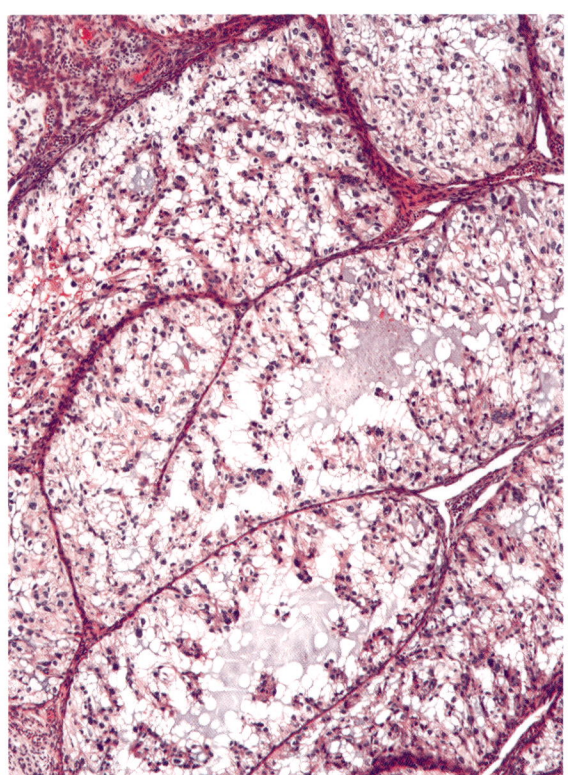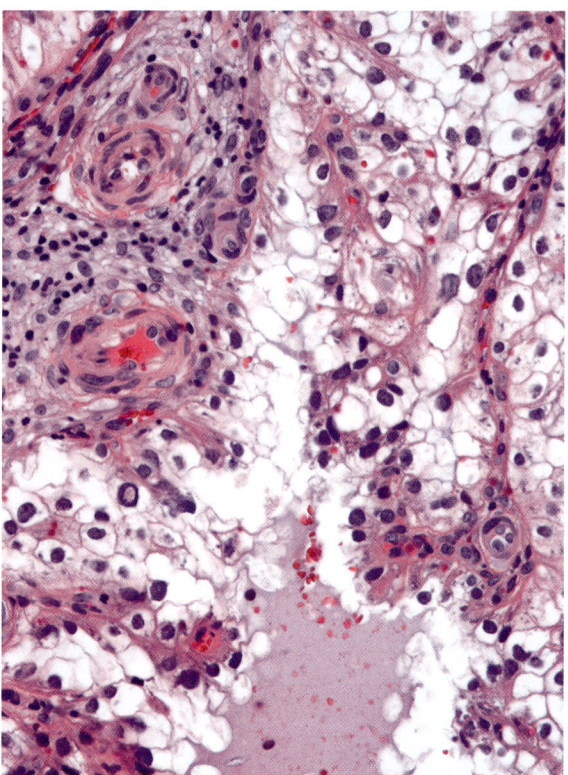

Figure 2-20

ARIAS-STELLA REACTION

Complex back-to-back appearance of the endometrial glands as well as abundant clear cytoplasm may cause concern for a neoplastic process (left). The cytologic features are bland, without prominent nucleoli and mitoses, but scattered smudgy nuclei and nuclear pseudoinclusions are seen (right).

during the second and third trimesters and puerperium, and are often seen in association with the Arias-Stella reaction (fig. 2-21, left) (68,69). Due to nuclear pseudoinclusions, nuclei immunostain for biotin with the peroxidase-antiperoxidase method. These intranuclear inclusions may be confused with herpes inclusions (69,70). Although decidua is typically seen in secretory phase endometrium or in patients on hormonal treatment and causes no diagnostic concerns, it may be seen in postmenopausal women and may have a polypoid appearance, associated necrosis, myxoid change, some degree of pleomorphism, and signet ring cells (fig. 2-21, right), these features suggesting a malignant process, including metastases (71). However, atypical areas merge with more typical decidual cells that have uniform nuclei with small nucleoli and no mitoses. Intracytoplasmic vacuoles are negative for mucicarmine, periodic acid–Schiff (PAS), and alcian blue and cells are keratin negative (72,73).

A wide variety of changes are seen in patients taking exogenous hormones, such as oral contraceptives, ovulation-induced therapy, hormonal replacement therapy, and antineoplastic hormonal therapy. Estrogen-only hormonal replacement is rarely administered in premenopausal women due to the high risk of developing endometrial hyperplasia and carcinoma, although the latter is typically low grade and low stage (74–76). If progesterone outweighs estrogen in an oral contraceptive, changes noted in the endometrium include stromal hyperplasia, decidual change, and glandular atrophy. However, if doses overall are small, glands are inactive with randomly distributed vacuoles and abortive secretions, with stromal edema or decidual change and thin blood vessels. The

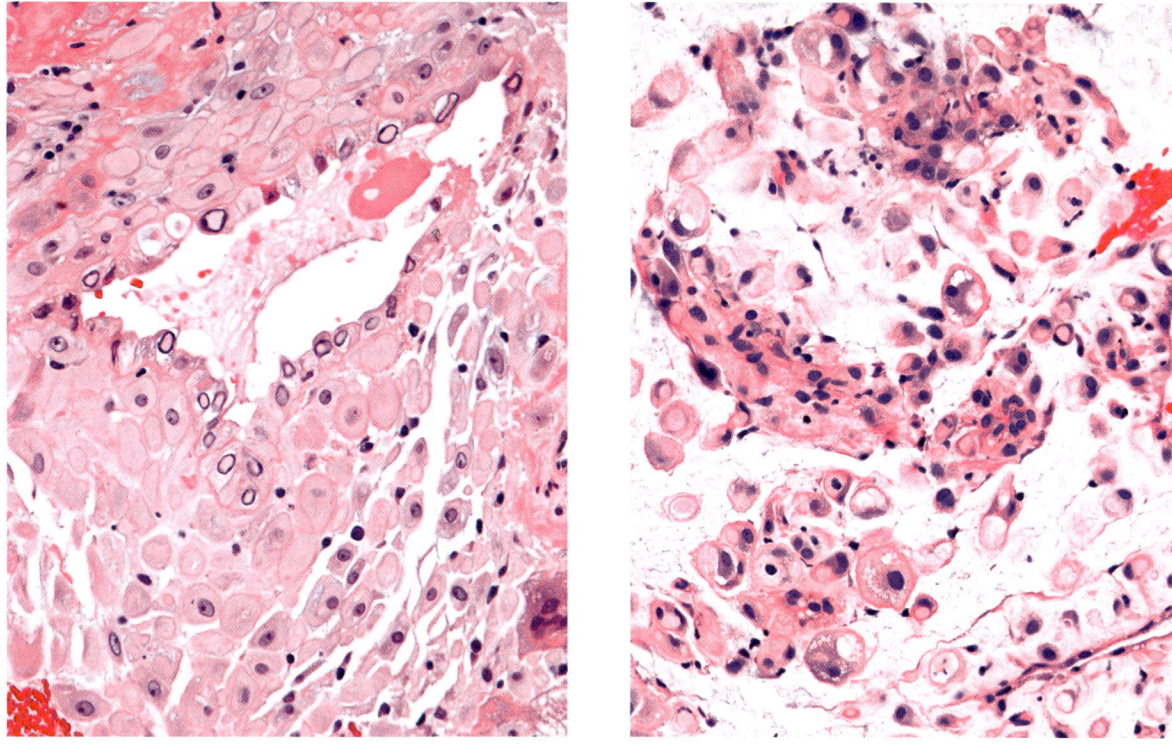

Figure 2-21

PREGNANCY OR HORMONALLY RELATED CHANGES

Biotin-rich optically clear nuclei within inactive endometrial glands and decidua (left). Decidua is associated with myxoid change and cytoplasmic vacuoles, mimicking signet ring cells (right).

endometrium of postmenopausal patients on hormone replacement therapy often shows mixed proliferative and secretory patterns, crowded endometrial glands, and endometrial metaplasias, including tubal, eosinophilic, mucinous, and papillary, which in aggregate may cause problems in interpretation. Patients with combined hormonal replacement therapies also often have endometrial polyps (77,78).

The purpose of progesterone for the treatment of endometrial hyperplasia or low-grade carcinoma is to stop glandular proliferation and induce gland maturation with secretory effect and stromal decidualization, although complex glandular architecture may persist (79). Progesterone may be administered for abnormal uterine bleeding, for contraception, or for endometriosis. In such instances, there is atrophy of the endometrial glands, which appear small and rounded, and lined by inactive cuboidal cells while the stroma is prominent due to pseudodecidual change and may be sprinkled with numerous lymphocytes (fig. 2-22A). In some instances, the stroma is expanded, displaying a polypoid appearance (decidual pseudopolyp) and may secondarily undergo extensive necrosis (fig. 2-22B). This tissue may be passed per vagina and cause concern for a malignant process, especially as hyperchromatic nuclei are striking and there may be associated myxoid change. However, high-power scrutiny shows ghosts of uniform polygonal cells (fig. 2-22C).

Progesterone receptor modulators (i.e., ulipristal acetate) used to treat leiomyomas and endometriosis as well as for contraception may produce a mass lesion (fig. 2-23, left) and impart a cystic appearance to the endometrial glands. These glands are lined by flat secretory-like endometrial cells with mitoses and apoptoses (simultaneous estrogen and progesterone effect), and if diffuse, may be confused with endometrial hyperplasia (fig. 2-23, right). Often, a prominent vascular component is also noted (80).

Figure 2-22
PREGNANCY OR HORMONALLY RELATED CHANGES

The striking polypoid appearance of the endometrium is due to extensive stromal pseudodecidualization (A). Pseudodecidualized polypoid stroma (decidual pseudopolyp) may undergo secondary necrosis. Cells may show hyperchromatic nuclei that may cause concern for malignancy if they pass through vagina (B). Most cells still have typical outlines of decidual cells (C).

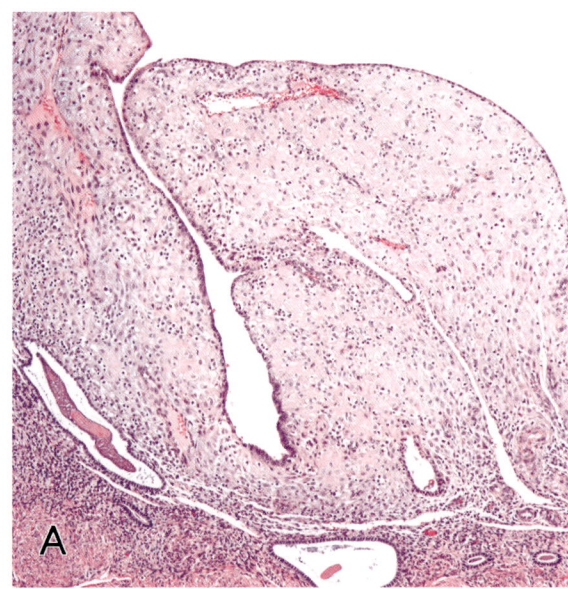

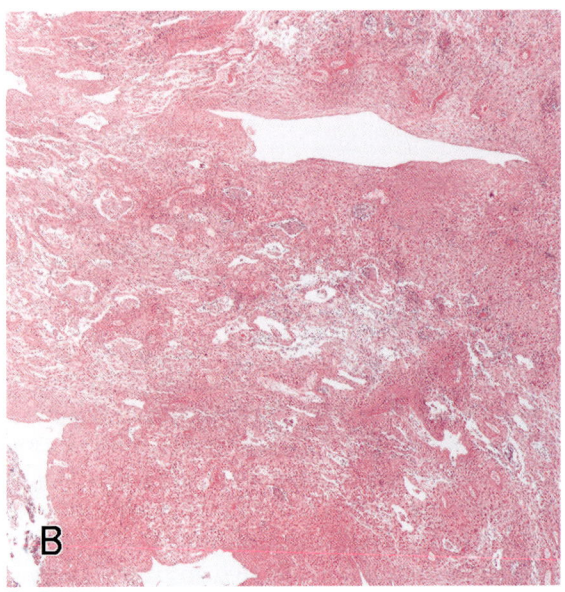

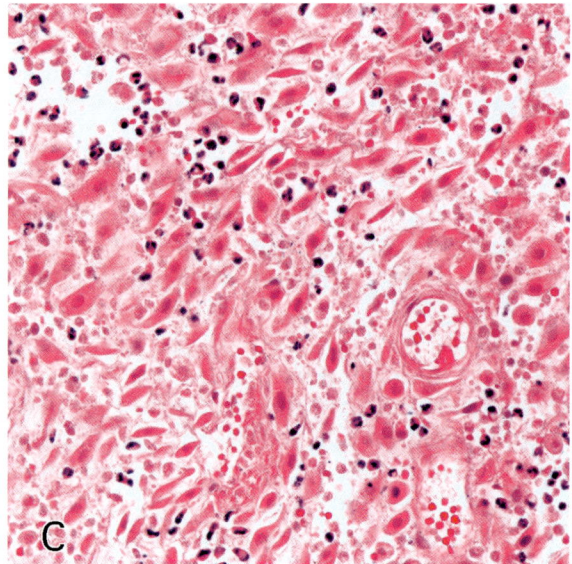

Gonadotropin-releasing hormone agonists used to reduce the size of large leiomyomas or cause iatrogenic endometrial suppression prior to ablation are associated with an inactive to atrophic appearance of the endometrium (81,82). Agents used to induce ovulation, if successful, show more advanced stromal maturation compared to the glandular elements (in biopsies often day 22 to 23 for stroma and 16 to 17 for glands). The glands tend to be smaller, less tortuous and with less secretions, and the pseudodecidual cells are smaller than expected with an overall decreased gland to stroma ratio (83).

Tamoxifen has a well-known antiestrogenic effect in breast cancer, but in the endometrium its effects range from antiestrogenic to weakly estrogenic depending on dose, duration of the treatment, and patient's hormonal status. Estrogenic changes affect not only the endometrium, but also the myometrium, with a consequent increase in size of the uterus (84–86). The most common alterations associated with tamoxifen are endometrial polyps, metaplasias (most commonly mucinous and squamous), hyperplasia, and carcinoma. However, most curettage specimens of patients on tamoxifen show an atrophic

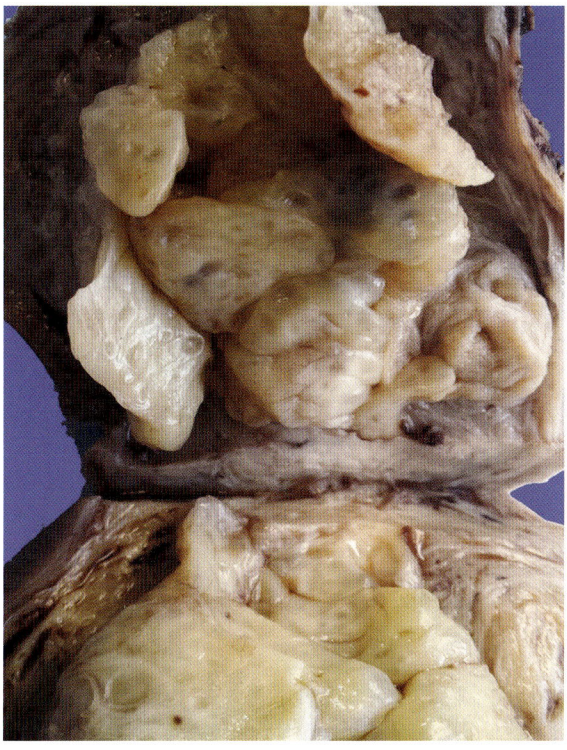 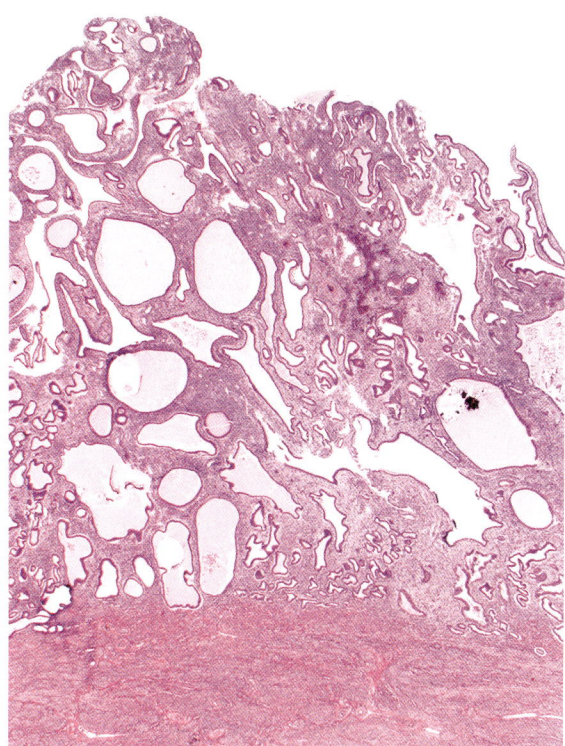

Figure 2-23

HORMONALLY RELATED CHANGES

Progesterone receptor modulators may cause a diffuse cystic change within the endometrium that grossly suggests a proliferative process (left). Strikingly dilated endometrial glands are seen microscopically (right). (Both figures courtesy of Dr. F. F. Nogales, Granada, Spain.)

endometrium. Endometrial polyps show endometrial glands oriented along their long axis as well as exuberant stroma that may protrude into the glands and periglandular stromal condensation, imparting a phyllodes-like morphology. Other changes include stromal fibrosis, myxoid change, and secondary infarction (7,8,87) (see chapter 3). p16 positivity in stromal cells does not separate tamoxifen-related from -unrelated polyps (88). Even though endometrioid carcinomas are more often seen in patients treated with tamoxifen (89), high-grade tumors, including serous and clear cell carcinoma and carcinosarcomas, have been reported (90–93) as well as müllerian adenosarcomas and leiomyosarcomas (94).

ENDOMETRIAL STROMAL METAPLASIAS

Smooth Muscle Metaplasia

Smooth muscle differentiation is likely the most common among stromal metaplasias. It is well known that endometrial polyps, even with an epithelioid morphology (95), atypical polypoid adenomyoma (42), and endometrial stromal tumors (96) show smooth muscle differentiation. Less frequently, foci of smooth muscle metaplasia are identified within the endometrium, similar to what is seen in endometriosis (97). Smooth muscle metaplasia is typically seen as small, short, intersecting fascicles of bland spindle cells with elongated nuclei and eosinophilic cytoplasm admixed with variable amounts of collagen, sometimes with a nodular configuration (fig. 2-24, left). It may represent the origin of submucosal leiomyomas.

Osseous Metaplasia

Osseous metaplasia is seen in the uterus as part of an endometrial carcinoma, malignant mixed müllerian tumor, and rarely, other tumors, but it is also an isolated finding in women of reproductive age who have a history of

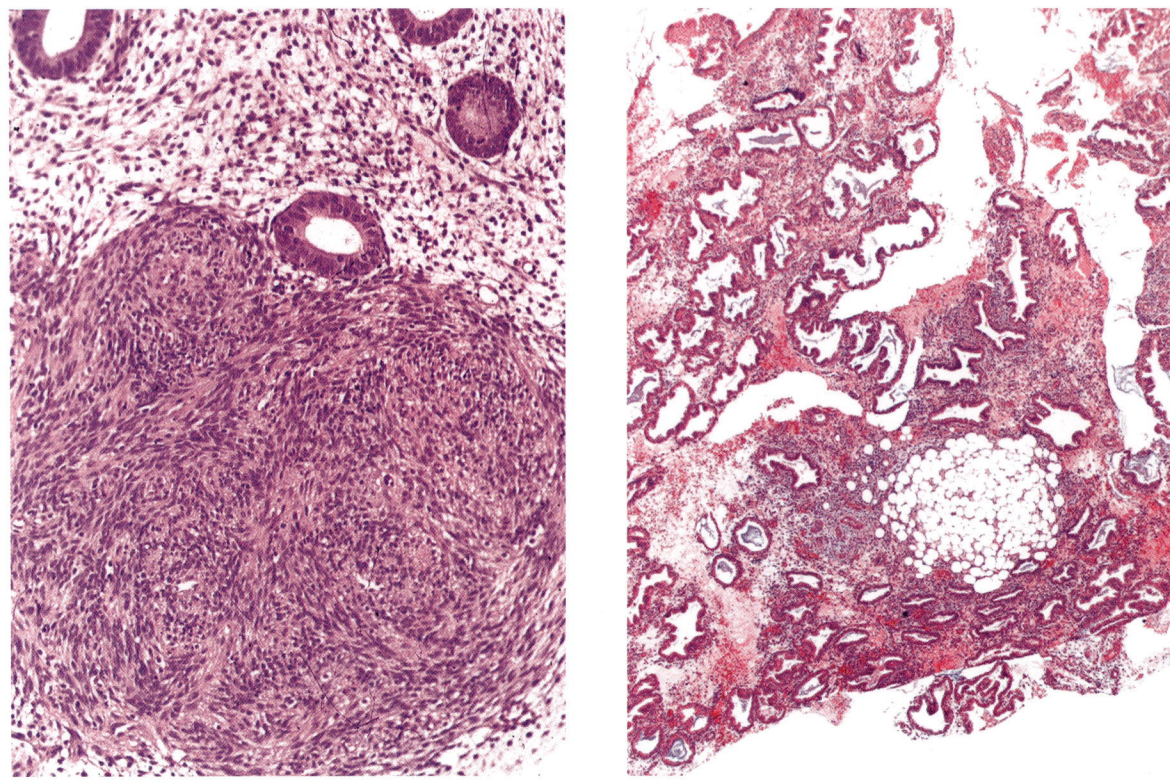

Figure 2-24

SMOOTH MUSCLE AND ADIPOSE METAPLASIA

Short whorling fascicles are composed of spindled cells with eosinophilic cytoplasm and fusiform nuclei (left). The fascicles form a well-defined nodule within the endometrial compartment. Mature adipocytes are noted between endometrial glands (right). (Courtesy of Dr. F. F. Nogales, Granada, Spain.)

prior gestation. In this scenario, it is postulated that the osseous metaplasia originates from retained embryonic contents, and less commonly, dystrophic calcification associated with chronic endometritis or metastatic calcification due to metabolic disorders (i.e., renal failure) (98,99). DNA studies have shown that both pathways exist (100,101). Bony spicules may be present within the discharged tissue and grossly, they are gray-white, sometimes disc-shaped fragments (102).

Cartilaginous and Fatty Metaplasia

Metaplastic cartilage is found rarely in the endometrium (103,104). It is thought to represent residual fetal tissue. *Fatty tissue* is rare in the endometrium (fig. 2-24, right) (105), but before making this diagnosis, two other possibilities should be strongly considered: uterine perforation, especially in the setting of pregnancy or in older women with a thin uterine wall, and pseudolipomatosis (106–108). The latter, which is more common and better characterized in the colon, is an artifactual microscopic change secondary to gaseous insufflation during hysteroscopy. The vacuoles vary in amount, distribution, and size (fig. 2-25), but they tend to be round or ovoid and unilocular. No peripheral nuclei are noted. They are S-100 protein negative (107,108).

Glial Tissue

Glial heterotopia is seen in the endometrium and cervix of reproductive age women, but it is a rare finding. Although different hypotheses explain its origin, currently, implantation from a prior pregnancy appears to be the most accepted, as a recent study reported an identical genetic profile, comparing implanted glial tissue presenting as a uterine polyp and fetal tissue from a prior abortion (109). Patients present with uterine bleeding, and an endometrial or cervical

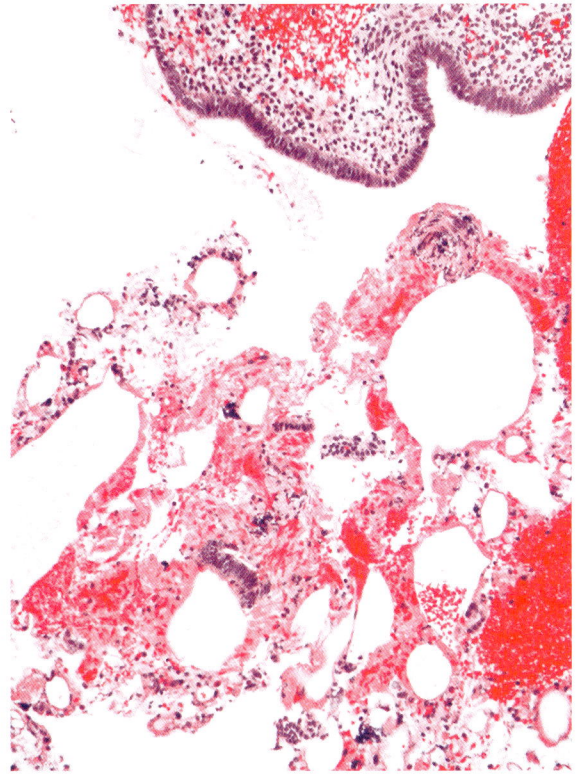

Figure 2-25

PSEUDOLIPOMATOSIS

Empty vacuoles have random size and distribution within the specimen. Peripheral nuclei are lacking.

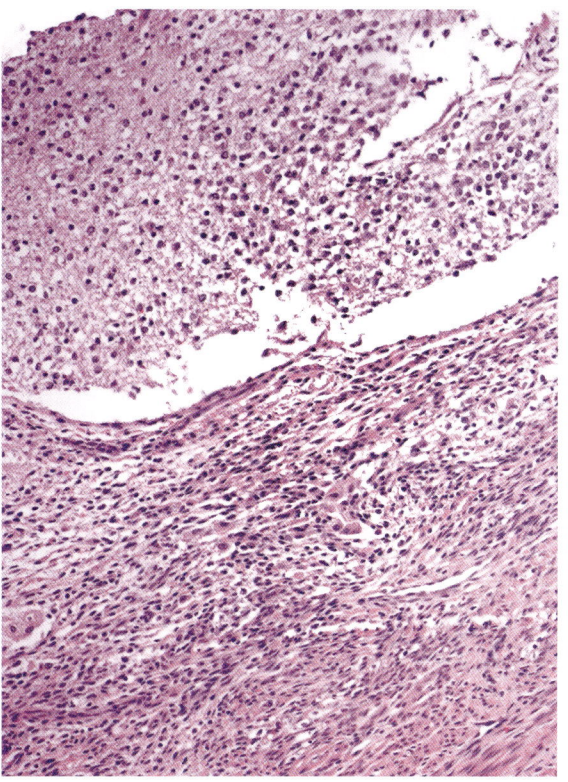

Figure 2-26

GLIAL TISSUE

Mature glial tissue composed of astrocytes in a fibrillary background is well demarcated from the surrounding endometrium. It likely represents remnants of a prior pregnancy.

polyp may be detected on exam (109–112). A history of prior abortion may be remote.

On microscopic examination, mature glial tissue, well demarcated from the surrounding endometrium, is composed of a homogeneous population of astrocytes, evenly distributed in a prominent fibrillary background (fig. 2-26). Rarely, neurons are seen. There may be an associated inflammatory response, mainly composed of lymphocytes. On occasion, cartilage, bone, and squamous epithelium are admixed with the glial tissue (113).

The differential diagnosis includes teratomas containing glial tissue, pure gliomas, or rare examples of endometrial adenocarcinoma or mixed müllerian tumors with glial differentiation. In all of these instances, a mass is noted, and on microscopic examination the glioma is a component of a primitive neuroectodermal tumor and is typically high grade (114,115). One reported exception is a polypoid tumor that filled the endometrial cavity of a 15-year-old girl; microscopic examination disclosed a low-grade fibrillary astrocytoma (116). Teratoma of the uterus is very rare when compared to its ovarian counterpart and typically shows an admixture of mature and fetal tissues in contrast to glial heterotopia (117).

Other Stromal Metaplasias

Extramedullary hematopoiesis is typically characterized by the production of granulocytic, erythrocytic, or megakaryocytic cells outside the bone marrow. The most common sites for extramedullary hematopoiesis are liver and spleen but it can be seen in any organ including the uterus. It may be an incidental finding within the endometrium or a leiomyoma (fig. 2-27) (118,119). In some cases, patients have hematologic disorders or less commonly, other neoplasms/conditions (120). It may form a mass

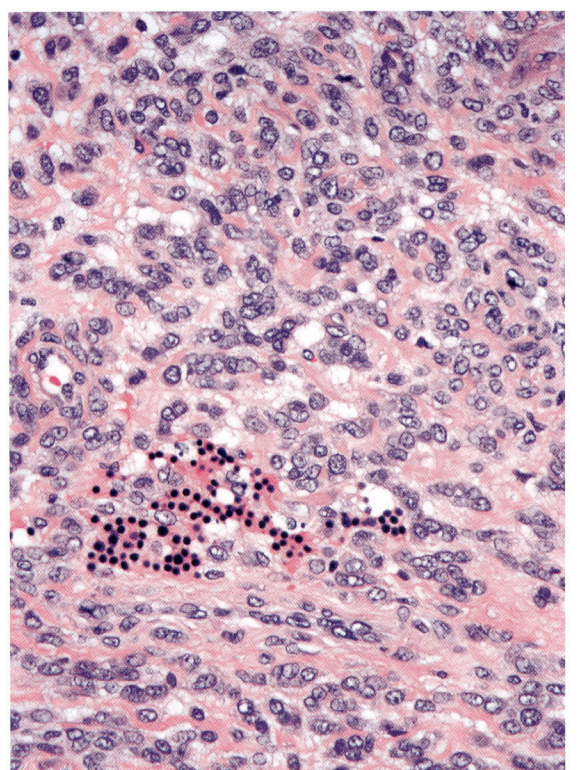 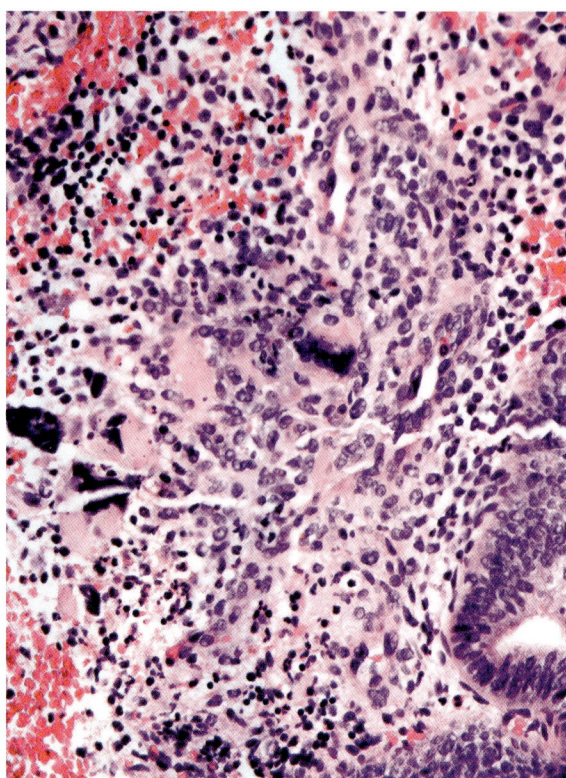

Figure 2-27

EXTRAMEDULLARY HEMATOPOIESIS

Erythrocytic precursors are present within a leiomyoma and typically represent an incidental finding (left). Megakaryocytes may be seen in the endometrium and due to the hyperchromatic nature of their multilobated nuclei, may cause concern for a malignant process (right).

lesion or may involve other organs within the gynecologic tract (118,121–123). The presence of extramedullary hematopoiesis should trigger further hematologic studies.

Stromal changes may occur secondary to levonorgestrel-releasing intrauterine devices. These include myxoid change, stromal hyalinization including hyaline nodules (fig. 2-28, left), calcification, and granulomatous reaction to amorphous eosinophilic material, likely necrotic decidualized stroma as well as synovial-like metaplasia (62,124–127). The latter is characterized by fibroblast-like stromal cells, often palisading, with a perpendicular orientation to the endometrial surface (fig. 2-28, right). Sometimes they form small nodules with the cells having a vimentin/CD68-positive and keratin-negative immunoprofile (127).

INFLAMMATORY/INFECTIOUS PROCESSES

Chronic Endometritis

Endometritis is divided into acute and chronic based on the predominant inflammatory component. *Acute endometritis* typically is associated with acute inflammation, including microabscesses that may secondarily destroy the underlaying epithelium. *Chronic endometritis* is often seen in the setting of recurrent pregnancy loss (including repeated implantation failure after in vitro fertilization), in women with an intrauterine device or pelvic inflammatory disease with secondary infertility, or in those with associated urinary tract infections. The most common pathologic organisms are *Neisseria gonorrhea, Chlamydia, Mycoplasma, Escherichia coli,* and *Streptococcus* (128–130).

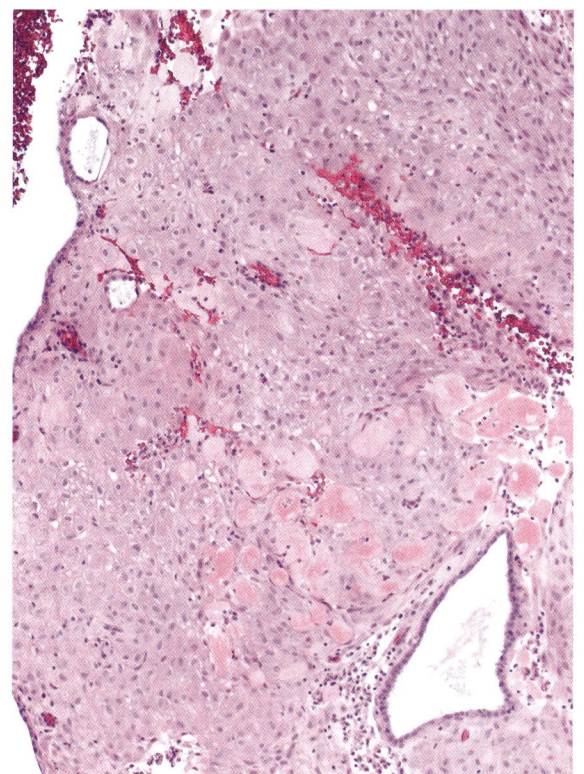 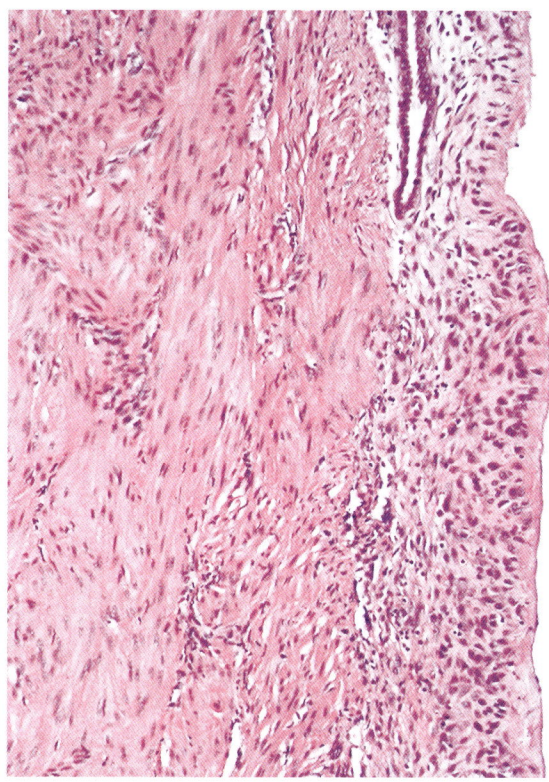

Figure 2-28

STROMAL CHANGES RELATED TO INTRAUTERINE DEVICES

Dense hyaline nodules are present in an extensively pseudodecidualized endometrial stroma with inactive endometrial glands (left). Synovial-like tissue composed of palisading fibroblast-like cells lines the endometrium of a patient with a levonorgestrel-releasing intrauterine device (right). (Courtesy of Dr. C. Stewart, Perth, Australia.)

Patients with clinically significant chronic endometritis often present with menorrhagia, menometrorrhagia, postmenopausal bleeding, or pelvic pain. To establish a diagnosis of chronic endometritis, plasma cells should be found within the endometrial stroma (fig. 2-29A). Plasma cells, sometimes abundant, are noted in the endometrium of asymptomatic patients and those with associated infection, but the diagnostic criteria for clinically significant chronic endometritis remains controversial. In florid examples, hysteroscopy may show multiple "micro" polyps, with small (less than 2 mm) vegetations which represent polypoid protrusions of the endometrium without a fibrovascular core, associated with prominent stromal edema (131).

At low-power magnification, the most characteristic feature is the spindle morphology of the endometrial stroma; other common features include altered/dysynchronous endometrial maturation, prominent edema, and hemorrhage. Reactive epithelial changes may be exuberant, including superficial eosinophilic change, acanthosis (32,132), and reactive-appearing nuclei with prominent nucleoli. Rarely, endometritis is associated with architectural abnormalities that suggest endometrial hyperplasia (fig. 2-29B).

The degree of stromal cell spindling correlates with the degree of plasma cell infiltration. In endometritis, plasma cells have been reported to reside near endometrial glands, surface endometrium, or lymphoid aggregates, but in recent studies a perivascular location has been noted to be most common (133). Other inflammatory cells are often present including lymphocytes, with or without germinal centers, eosinophils, and neutrophils but they are not diagnostic of chronic endometritis (fig. 2-29C). Stromal breakdown is commonly seen. Plasma cells may be difficult to identify or may be

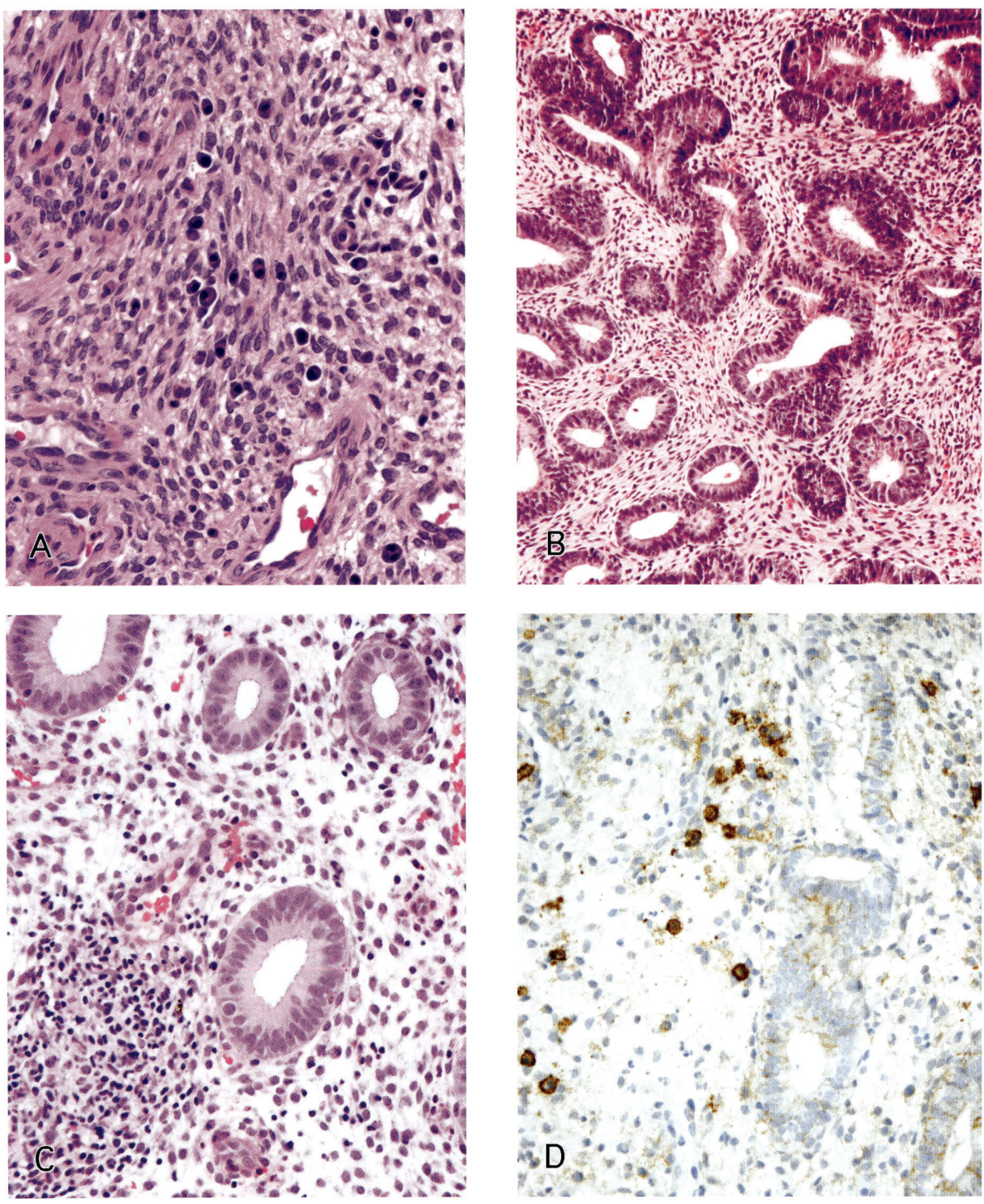

Figure 2-29

CHRONIC ENDOMETRITIS

Several plasma cells with typical morphology are noted (A). Endometrial glands are enlarged and have outpouches, raising the possibility of endometrial hyperplasia. Scrutiny of the stroma demonstrates plasma cells (B). Lymphocytes, which may form aggregates, as well as acute inflammatory cells are seen but are not diagnostic of chronic endometritis (C). CD138 highlights plasma cells in the background stroma (D).

confused with monocytoid stromal cells; thus histochemical (Giemsa) or immunohistochemical stains (CD138/syndecan-1) (fig. 2-29D) are used for differentiaton (134–136). Finding rare plasma cells with immunohistochemistry may have no clinical consequences, which questions the usefulness of these stains, particularly in asymptomatic patients.

Mimics of chronic endometritis include plasma cells overlying a leiomyoma, within an endometrial polyp, or in patients with anovulatory cycles (137). Basally located lymphocytes, on the other hand, may be seen in normal conditions and fluctuate during the endometrial cycle (138). If many plasma cells are noted, the possibility of overlooked endocervical tissue should be considered. Some studies have shown a good correlation between hysteroscopy, histologic diagnosis of chronic endometritis, and microbiologic results (130,131), but others have not found this correlation when asymptomatic patients are included (133,139).

Necrotizing Endometritis

Necrotizing endometritis is a rare form of endometritis characterized by periglandular lymphocytes (often predominating) and neutrophils that variably infiltrate glands, resulting in their expansion and partial or complete destruction, sometimes reminiscent of crypt abscesses in the colonic mucosa. Interestingly, no plasma cells are noted (140). Other findings include edema, spindling of the stromal cells, and focal reactive changes. Most patients, some under therapy with exogenous hormones, are premenopausal and present with vaginal bleeding. The etiology of this phenomenon is unclear. Diffuse necrotizing endometritis, even rarer than necrotizing endometritis, has been reported and may be related to the *Clostridium* family of anaerobic bacteria (141).

Lymphoma-Like Lesions

Acute and chronic inflammatory cells may be found in the endometrium, although typically less commonly than in the cervix. If abundant, they are often related to a prior procedure, intrauterine device, or chronic endometritis. If the inflammatory reaction is florid and contains large lymphoid cells (fig. 2-30, left), it may suggest lymphoma (most commonly a B-cell lymphoma) (fig. 2-30, right) (142). Patients may present with vaginal bleeding or a lesion may be found on radiologic examination (143,144).

Features that cause concern for a neoplasm include the presence of large lymphoid cells, including immunoblasts with brisk mitotic activity and abundant nuclear debris (fig. 2-30, left). These cells may form large, poorly defined aggregates lacking a mantle of mature lymphocytes (143,144). In contrast to lymphoma, the aggregates typically have a reactive appearance, with small lymphocytes, plasma cells, and neutrophils in a background of chronic endometritis. Although lymphoid cells may predominate, cells are not as monomorphic as seen in lymphoma, and immunohistochemistry shows a mixed infiltrate of B- and T-cells. Immunoglobulin heavy chain gene (*IGH*) rearrangement can be found in reactive lymphoma-like lesions, thus, these results should be correlated with the rest of immunohistochemical and morphologic findings (145).

An intravascular proliferation of reactive lymphoid blasts has been reported to mimic intravascular lymphoma in a polyp associated with a prominent chronic inflammatory infiltrate (146). The cells had brisk mitotic activity and a high MIB-1 index and raised suspicion for an angiocentric lymphoma. As occurs with other extravascular lymphoma-like lesions, it showed clonal rearrangement for *IGH*, but no evidence of lymphoma.

Thermal Ablation

Endometrial ablation is a common treatment modality, especially in premenopausal patients with dysfunctional uterine bleeding. The goal is to stop the bleeding by destroying the endometrium and superficial myometrium. The gross appearance may be initially alarming although it is quite characteristic, with a well-defined line where the thermal effect stops within the uterine wall (fig. 2-31, left).

The histologic changes depend on the interval between ablation and subsequent biopsy or hysterectomy. Within the first 3 months, the endometrium and superficial myometrium typically show ischemic necrosis (ghost cells can be seen) with associated fibrin deposition and, commonly, an exuberant foreign body giant granulomatous reaction (fig. 2-31, right). Variable acute inflammation is also seen. After 3 months, only the granulomatous foreign body

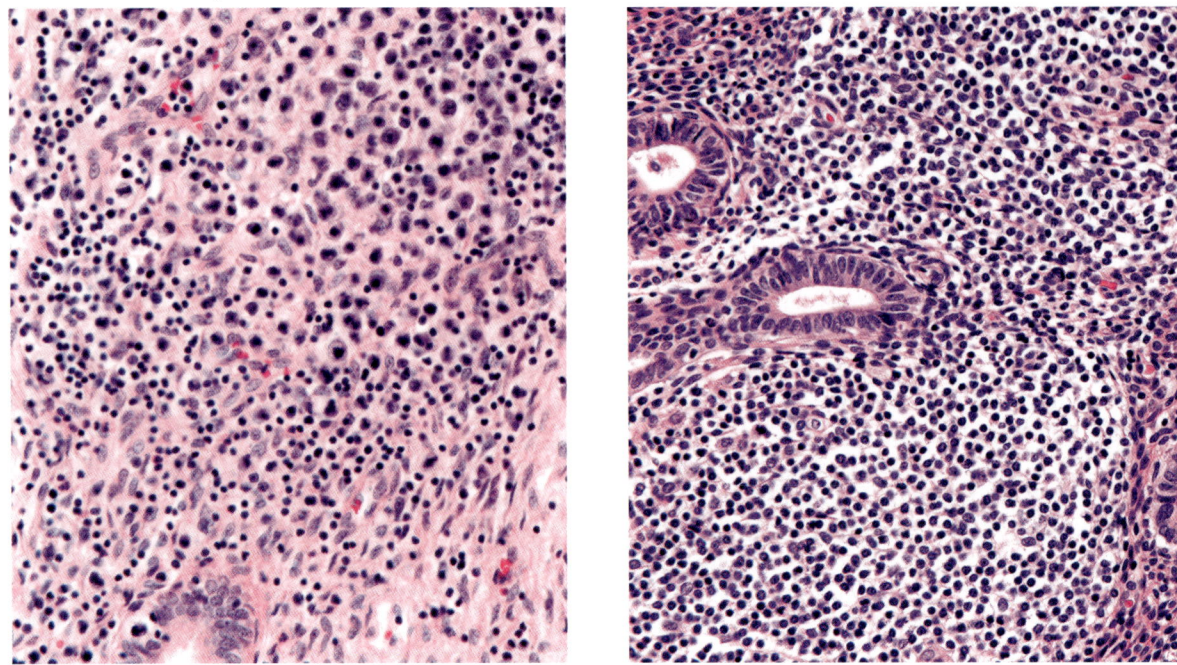

Figure 2-30

LYMPHOMA-LIKE LESION VERSUS LYMPHOMA

Although large cells (immunoblasts) are seen within the endometrium, they are admixed with small lymphocytes, plasma cells, and scattered granulocytes (left). B-cell lymphoma is composed of a monotonous population of small lymphocytes (right).

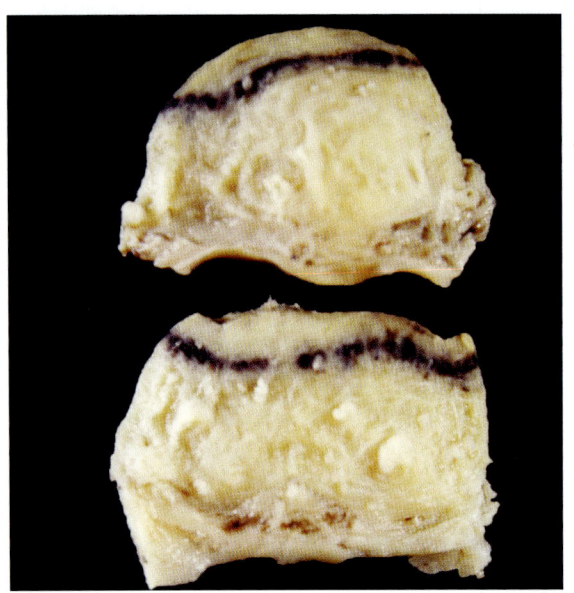 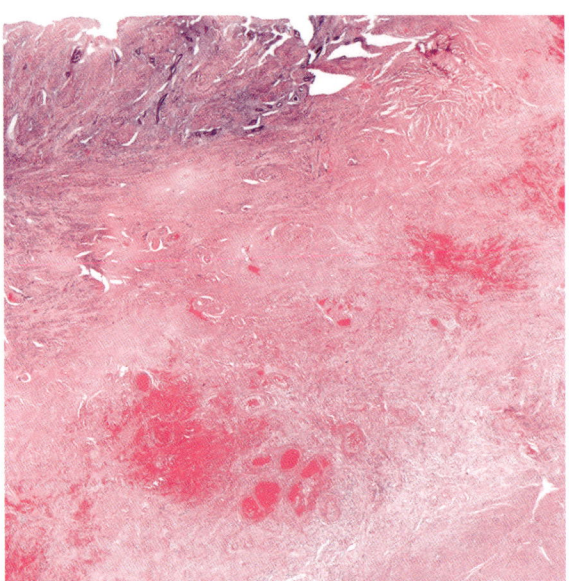

Figure 2-31

THERMAL ABLATION

Although grossly worrisome, a linear yellow band separated from the underlying myometrium by a dark line is characteristic (left). On microscopic examination, there is discrete but massive ischemic necrosis of the endometrium and superficial myometrium (right).

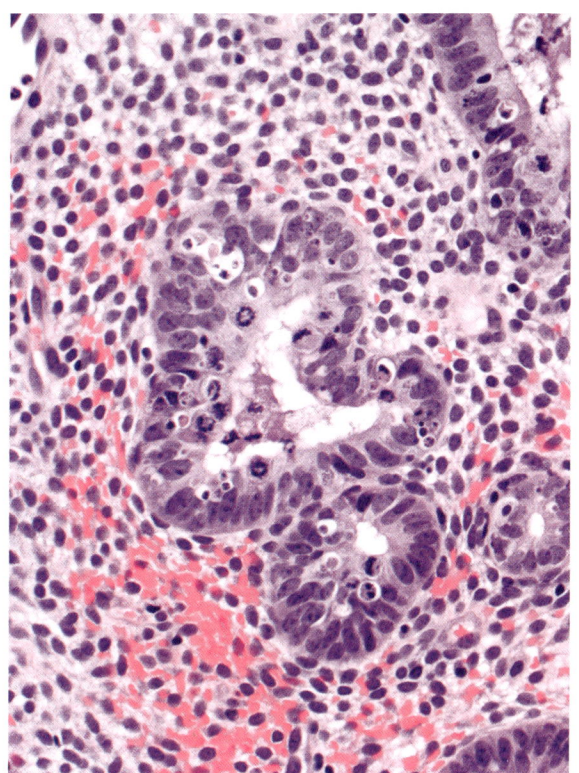 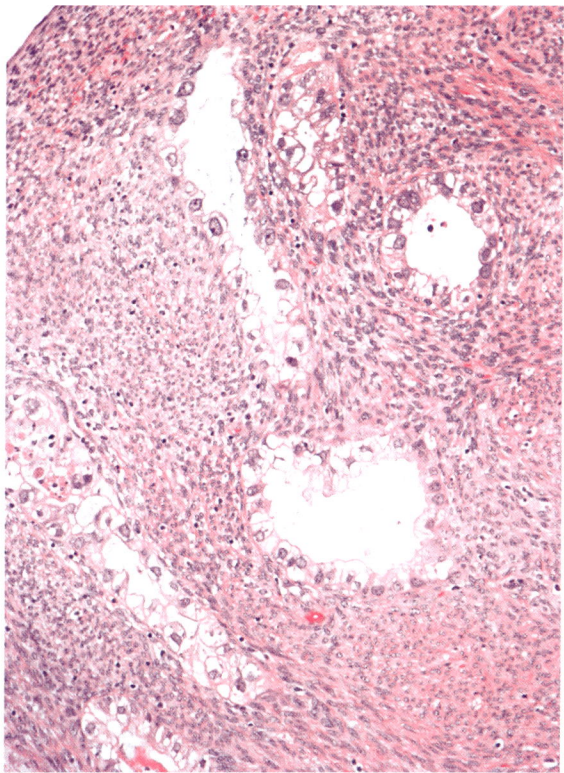

Figure 2-32

CHEMOTHERAPY AND RADIATION-INDUCED CHANGES

Brisk mitotic activity, with all divisions in metaphase, is characteristic of taxane effect in endometrial glands. Enlarged nuclei within endometrial glands may cause concern for serous carcinoma (left) (courtesy of Dr. M. F. Lerwill, Boston, MA). The smudgy texture of the chromatin and preserved nuclear to cytoplasmic ratio is typically seen in radiation effect (right).

giant cell reaction persists but over time, it is replaced by endometrial scarring, the endometrium represented by a single layer of flat to cuboidal cells directly against the myometrium. In some patients, the endometrium may be difficult or impossible to identify (147–150).

Chemotherapy and Radiation-Induced Changes

Chemotherapeutic agents cause a variety of cytologic changes within the endometrium, including cell enlargement and cytologic atypia with bizarre forms that may cause concern for a high-grade carcinoma, especially in curettage specimens of older patients. However, there is preservation of the nuclear to cytoplasmic ratio, abundant vacuolated cytoplasm, degenerative appearance of the chromatin, and low Ki-67 index (151).

Paclitaxel and other taxanes, commonly used in ovarian and breast cancer treatment, are specifically associated with brisk mitoses (all in metaphase) and apoptoses in otherwise unremarkable glands (fig. 2-32, left). This results from blocking cells at the G2/M phase of the cycle and inducing cell apoptoses by binding of taxanes to tubulin, which prevents normal depolymerization of microtubules within the mitotic spindle (152).

Radiation may cause changes within both compartments of the endometrium, but enlarged, irregular or hyperchromatic nuclei are typically the most obvious manifestation. There may also be clearing or vacuolization of the cytoplasm associated with hobnailing of the cells. When the history of prior radiation is not known, these changes suggest early serous carcinoma (intraepithelial carcinoma) since in both lesions, the glandular architecture is preserved. In contrast to serous carcinoma, the glandular cells of radiation change are cohesive, there is variation of nuclear shape and size,

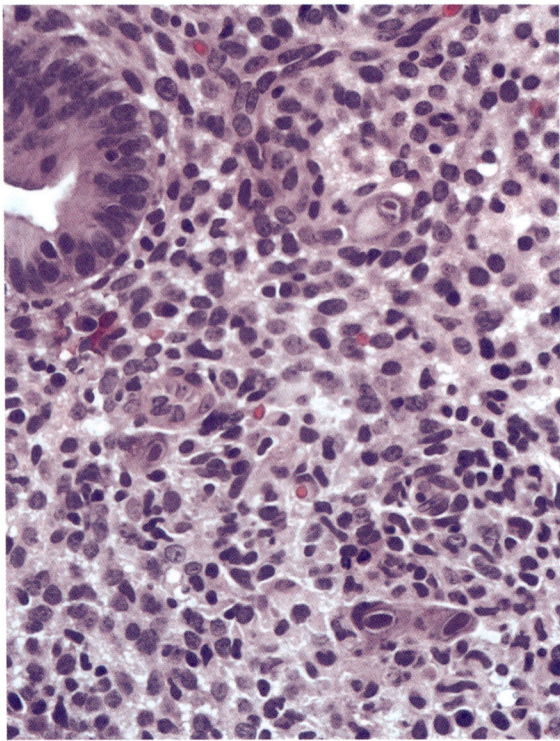

Figure 2-33

CYTOMEGALOVIRUS INFECTION

Several large intracellular inclusions characteristic of cytomegalovirus infection are present in a lymphoplasmacytic background.

from smudgy to innocuous (no homogenous hyperchromatism), and mitoses are absent (fig. 2-32, right). The finding of clear or hobnail cells may also raise concern for clear cell carcinoma, however, the typical patterns of that tumor are lacking as are the expected nuclear features and mitotic activity. Sometimes, the endometrial stromal cells show a reactive appearance with "plump" or multinucleated nuclei, hyalinization, and vascular changes.

Viral Infections

The most common viral infections in the uterus are *herpes* (153,154) and *cytomegalovirus* (155). Many affected patients are immunosuppressed (156). Patients may present with abdominal pain and foul-smelling vaginal discharge or generalized symptoms due to systemic dissemination.

The microscopic appearance of herpes endometritis includes acute inflammation and necrosis, while cytomegalovirus infection is often seen as chronic endometritis with abundant plasma cells, lymphocytes, and germinal centers or even granulomas (157). Both also display characteristic cytoplasmic and nuclear viral inclusions (fig. 2-33).

Intrauterine Device (IUD)-Related Changes

Patients with IUDs often have changes related to trauma and secondary inflammation, such as marked acute and chronic inflammation (endometritis with or without granulomas), reactive cytologic atypia, metaplasias, microcalcifications, and scarring. Changes are frequently seen in the areas close to the device but they may be extensive. *Actinomyces*, a gram-positive anaerobic bacteria, is seen in patients with long-standing IUD use. It causes a secondary ascending infection that results in tubo-ovarian abscesses (pelvic inflammatory disease) and can be lethal (158). *Actinomyces* organisms are seen in curettage specimens as granules with thin basophilic filaments radiating from a central granular eosinophilic core. They are typically Gram (Brown Hoppes stain) as well as Gomori methenamine silver positive (fig. 2-34) (159,160). They should be distinguished from pseudoactinomycotic granules which are also seen in patients with IUDs and are much more common. In contrast to *Actinomyces*, pseudoactinomycotic granules form club-like projections (pseudosulfur granules) without a dense central core and they are negative for Gram and silver stains; they are noninfectious structures. They are thought to represent an unusual response to a foreign body (Splendore-Hoeppli phenomenon) (fig. 2-35) (160,161). However, mixed granules have been reported (162).

In IUDs that release progestin (levonorgestrel), also known as a Mirena Coil, the endometrium has a characteristic appearance. Small inactive to atrophic glands have marked stromal pseudodecidualization hyaline nodule, myxoid change, and a sprinkling of granulated lymphocytes. Hobnail changes are also described in about 25 percent of patients using the Mirena Coil (62).

Other Inflammatory Processes

Mesothelial cells as well as histiocytes are found in curettage specimens. The latter may be conspicuous and form nodular aggregates. They are seen in patients with a wide range of ages. Abnormal vaginal bleeding is the most common

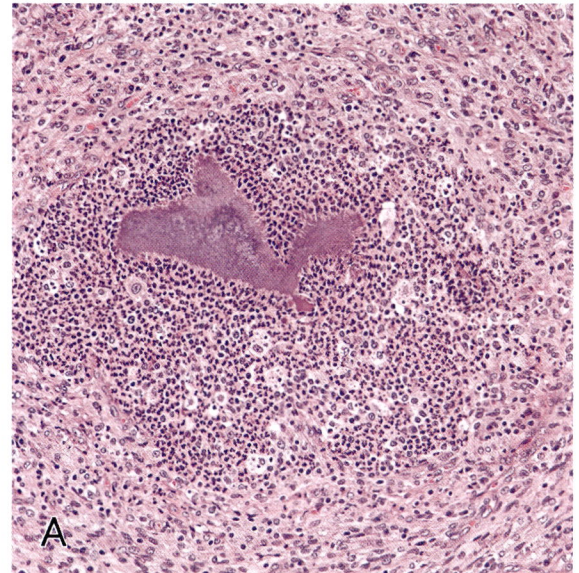

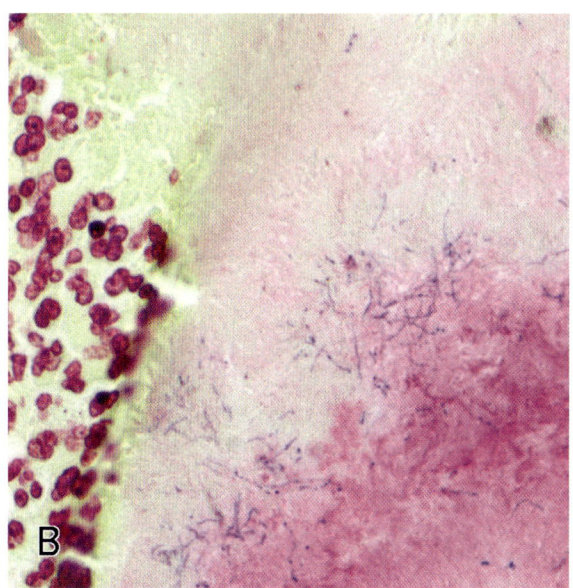
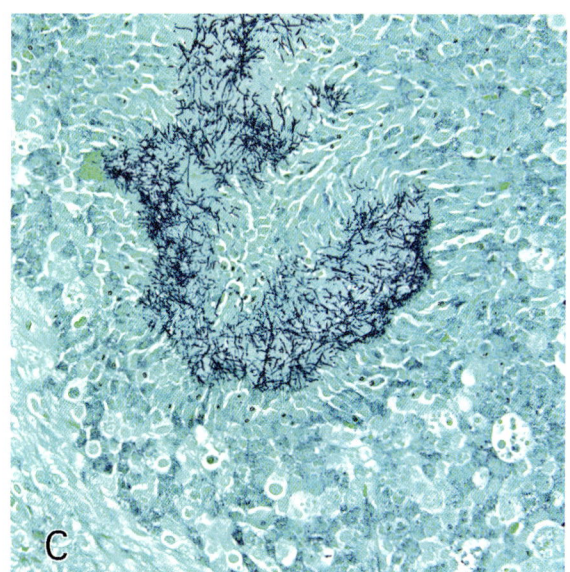

Figure 2-34

ACTINOMYCES INFECTION

Granules with thin radiating filaments are present within acute and chronic inflammation and are often seen in patients with IUDs. They are Brown and Hopes (B) and silver stain (C) positive.

presentation. The lesions are typically smaller than 1 cm, with cells at the periphery of the nodules having a less cohesive appearance than those in the center. The cells are typically uniform, with abundant, variably eosinophilic cytoplasm, reniform or grooved nuclei, tiny nucleoli, and lack mitotic activity (fig. 2-36). Some cells are large and display a plasmacytoid appearance, cytologic atypia, and a vacuole mimicking signet ring cells, and the nodules may have central necrosis, features that may be of concern. These histiocytes differ in morphology from those typically found in the abnormal endometrium of hyperplasia or carcinoma, which contain abundant vacuolated cytoplasm and tiny nuclei. They may be associated with mesothelial cells, eosinophils, and other inflammatory cells.

The differential diagnosis in these cases includes xanthogranulomatous endometritis, malakoplakia, and Langerhans cell histiocytosis. All these entities are rare; the former is often associated with a prominent chronic inflammatory infiltrate, while the others have specific histologic findings. A prior procedure resulting in injury may lead to these findings (163–165).

Figure 2-35

PSEUDOACTINOMYCOSIS

Club-like projections (pseudosulfur granules) are formed without a dense core (A). They are Brown and Hopes (B) and silver stain (C) negative.

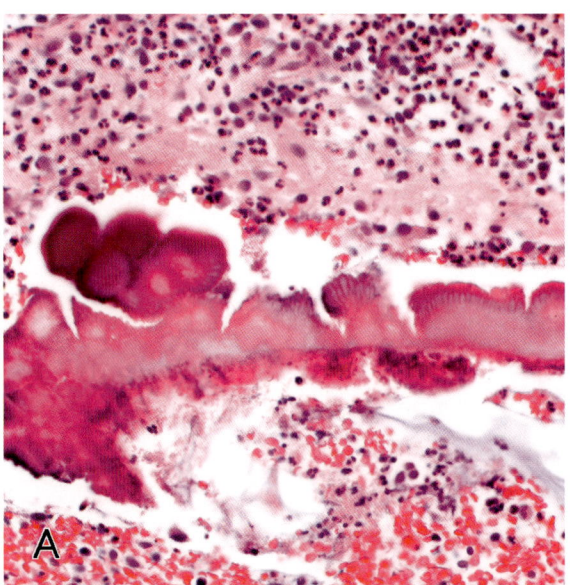

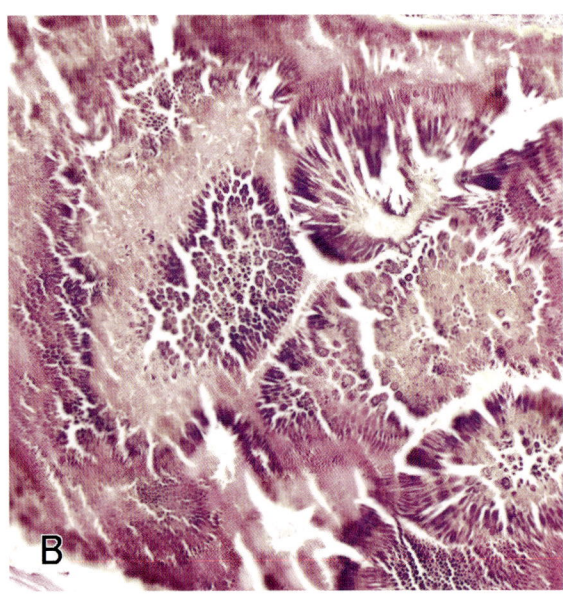

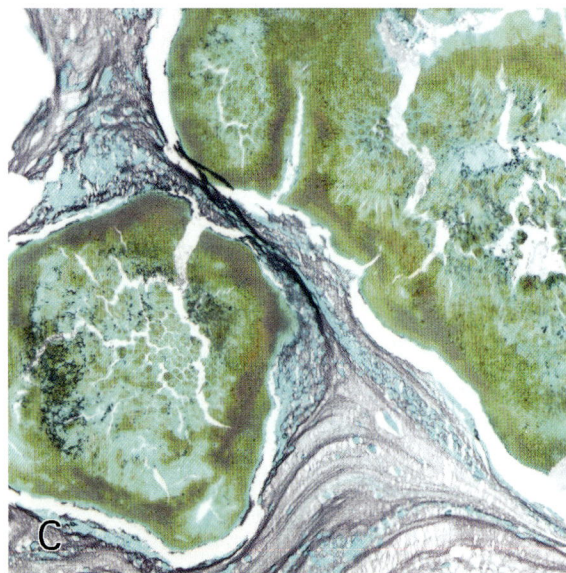

Malakoplakia in the endometrium typically affects postmenopausal women who present with abnormal bleeding. Rarely, it may produce a thickening or mass lesion (166). On microscopic examination, an exuberant diffuse histiocytic reaction without granulomas is observed. The histiocytes contain characteristic intracytoplasmic Michaelis-Gutmann bodies, a peculiar reaction to infection, and may be associated with lymphocytes (167,168).

Granulomas are seen occasionally within the endometrium as a manifestation of tuberculosis due to hematogenous spread. Patients often present with infertility (169,170). Granulomas are typically caseating. Confirmation is obtained with a Ziehl-Nielson stain for acid-fast bacteria or DNA polymerase chain reaction (PCR) (171). Granulomatous endometritis may be associated with *Enterobius vermicularis*, *Toxoplasma gondii*, and *cytomegalovirus* (172,173).

Sarcoidosis may also involve the endometrium, forming small, compact and noncaseating granulomas, typically in postmenopausal women. It is usually an incidental finding (174). Granulomas also occur after a procedure, due to the presence of a foreign body, or are idiopathic,

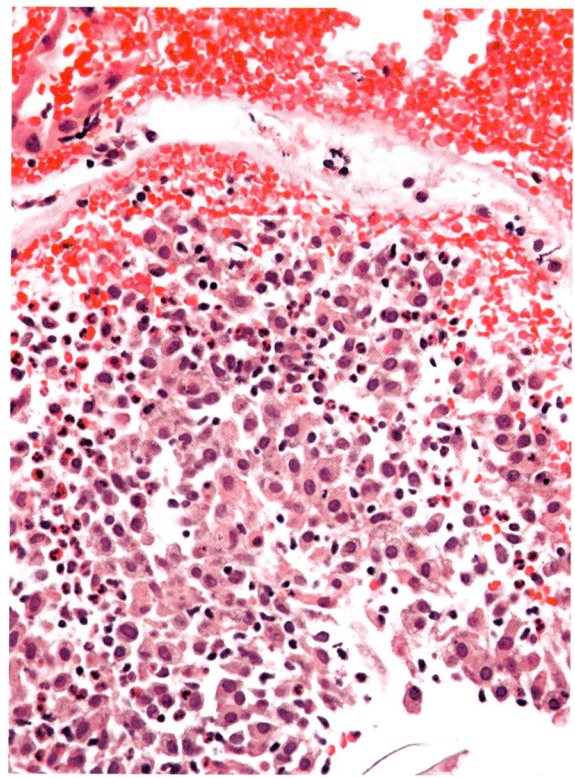

Figure 2-36

AGGREGATES OF HISTIOCYTES IN ENDOMETRIUM

Cells are uniform in appearance, and noncohesive.

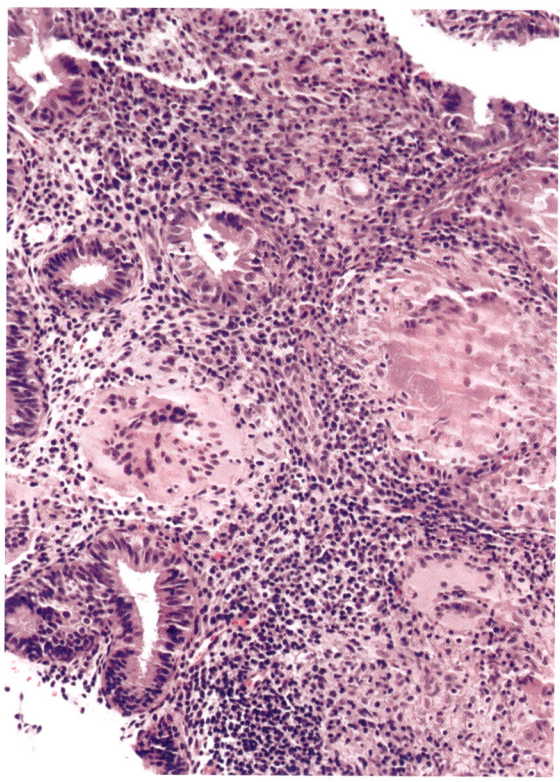

Figure 2-37

GRANULOMAS

Small granulomas with large multinucleated cells but lacking necrosis, are noted in the endometrium. They may be secondary to a prior procedure or idiopathic.

and thus, they are not necessarily indicative of infection or sarcoidosis (fig. 2-37) (175).

ATYPICAL STROMAL CELLS

Atypical stromal cells are occasionally seen in otherwise unremarkable endometrial polyps or in nonpolypoid endometrium (176,177). They are more common in the lower female genital tract, especially in fibroepithelial polyps from the vagina, vulva, and cervix (178).

Endometrial polyps with atypical stromal cells tend to occur in older women, often postmenopausal, when compared to usual endometrial polyps. Some patients have a history of hormonal intake and they present with abnormal vaginal bleeding. Atypical stromal cells are typically an incidental finding in specimens obtained for other reasons.

The atypical cells are distributed randomly within the stroma and, although they are occasionally seen as a linear band beneath the surface epithelium, they do not cluster around the endometrial glands. In most instances, their presence is focal, and less commonly, multifocal or diffuse (fig. 2-38). The cells may be polygonal, spindled, or stellate, and have enlarged, often hyperchromatic nuclei, sometimes with multinucleation. The chromatin pattern is often degenerative ("smudgy") without associated mitotic activity or cytologic atypia of the background stromal cells. Accompanying inflammatory cells are uncommon. The atypical stromal cells are positive for vimentin and estrogen, progesterone, and androgen receptors. Approximately one third express CD10 and half are desmin positive (177). Patients with these lesions have an uneventful outcome.

Problems occur in the differential diagnosis, especially in small samples, since the presence of atypical cells may suggest low-grade müllerian adenosarcoma, endometrial stromal

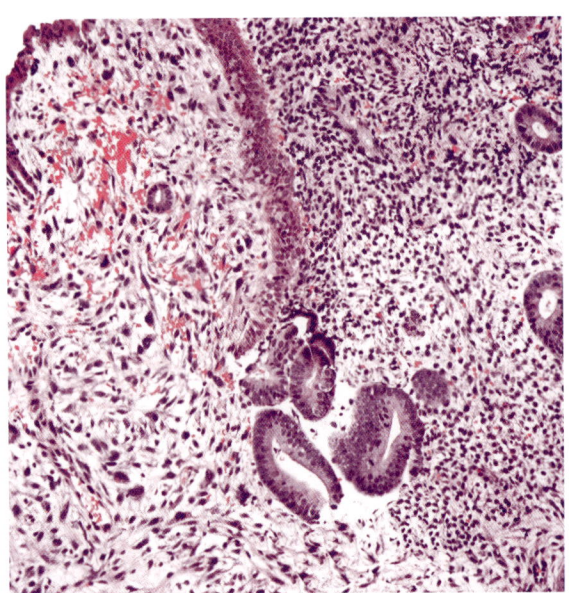 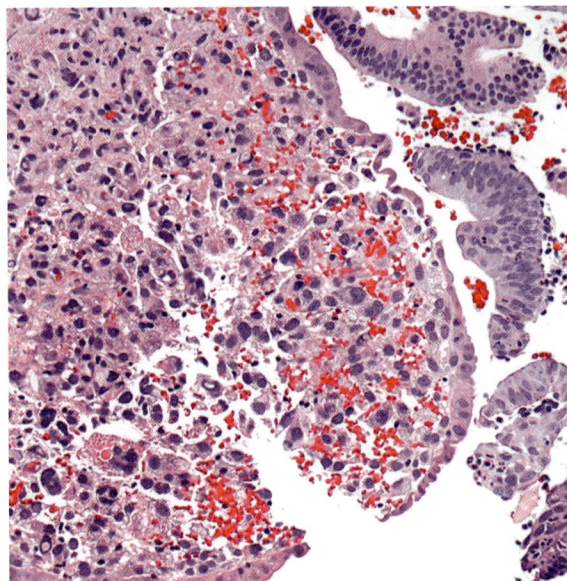

Figure 2-38

ATYPICAL STROMAL CELLS

Scattered enlarged stromal cells are present in a background of loose spindle stroma (left). Rarely, they form large aggregates, raising concern for a malignant neoplasm with a mesenchymal component (right).

tumor, smooth muscle tumor, or malignant mixed müllerian tumor. Low-grade müllerian adenosarcoma is characterized by condensation of stromal cells around the glands, the latter sometimes displaying a phyllodes-like architecture. At higher magnification, the stromal cells are atypical and show mitotic activity in most cases, but multinucleated and floret-like cells are not common (179). Highly atypical cells may be present if the stromal component is high grade or there is associated sarcomatous overgrowth; in such cases, the stromal cells are highly atypical (overtly sarcomatous) and associated with brisk mitotic activity. Rarely, endometrial stromal tumors (180) or smooth muscle tumors (either leiomyomas with bizarre nuclei or leiomyosarcoma) (181) show atypical "bizarre" cells. However, the background is highly cellular ("blue"), with small cells in stromal tumors, or fascicular with spindle cells in a smooth muscle tumor, both associated with some mitotic activity. One leiomyoma with bizarre nuclei and atypical stromal cells adjacent to the leiomyoma has been reported (182). A malignant mixed müllerian tumor is characterized by highly malignant epithelial and mesenchymal components. Even when only the mesenchymal component is available for review, it typically shows diffuse severe cytologic atypia, brisk mitotic activity, including atypical forms, associated with necrosis and hemorrhage, and heterologous elements (rhabdomyosarcoma or chondrosarcoma most common).

The etiology of the atypical stromal cells is unknown. They may be seen in endometrial polyps that undergo infarction, but in those cases, they tend to be near the area of infarction. In contrast to fibroepithelial polyps with atypical cells of the lower genital tract (often seen in pregnant woman or those taking oral contraceptives) such an association is not apparent in the endometrium (177). It has been postulated that atypical stromal cells are derived from multipotent mesenchymal cells with the capability to undergo smooth muscle or stromal differentiation (177).

MYXOID CHANGE IN THE ENDOMETRIUM/MYOMETRIUM

Interstitial expansion of the myometrium secondary to the deposition of acellular myxoid/mucin matrix can occur in patients with lupus erythematosus (myxoidosis) (183) or type I neurofibromatosis (184). It can also be of unknown etiology, although may be related to progestational effect (185). Patients are often suspected to have "enlarging" uterine leiomyomas and undergo hysterectomy.

On gross examination, the uterus may be large and the myometrial walls thickened without obvious lesions (if lupus related). On sectioning, the myometrium may have a "mucoid" appearance (in lupus) (183) or show no gross abnormalities.

Histologically, there is paucicellular myxoid material with focal, multifocal, or diffuse distribution within the myometrium. In lupus, the mucin often has a blue-gray flocculent quality and is associated with scant compressed collagen fibers, minimal inflammatory infiltrate (typically lymphocytes and plasma cells), and compressed small vessels (183). The endometrium, cervix, and serosa are typically spared. When not related to lupus, changes are focal or multifocal, and may involve the cervix. The myxoid areas can be well or poorly demarcated from the surrounding myometrium and contain widely separated bland fibroblasts as well as vessels and scattered entrapped smooth muscle cells, but no inflammatory infiltrate (fig. 2-39) (184,185). No cytologic atypia or mitotic activity has been reported.

In lupus-associated cases, the myxoid matrix stains for alcian blue, pH2.5 (without hyaluronidase) and colloidal iron (183). If lupus unrelated, cells within the myxoid areas are positive for CD10 and CD34 and rare cells are ER positive. Muscle markers, S-100 protein, and ALK1 are negative (184,185).

The differential diagnosis includes benign and, more commonly, malignant myxoid mesenchymal neoplasms, especially when only minimal material is procured. Smooth muscle tumors (186), endometrial stromal tumors (187), inflammatory myofibroblastic tumor (188,189), and less commonly, myxoma (190), myxoid liposarcoma (191), and nerve sheath tumors (192) are included in the differential diagnosis. Plexiform neurofibroma or malignant schwannoma are especially common in patients with neurofibromatosis (192). In all the above instances, there is a visible mass. In small samples, the finding of any degree of cellularity, cytologic atypia, or mitotic activity essentially rules out a benign myxoid change. When in doubt, lack of staining for muscle markers, ALK,

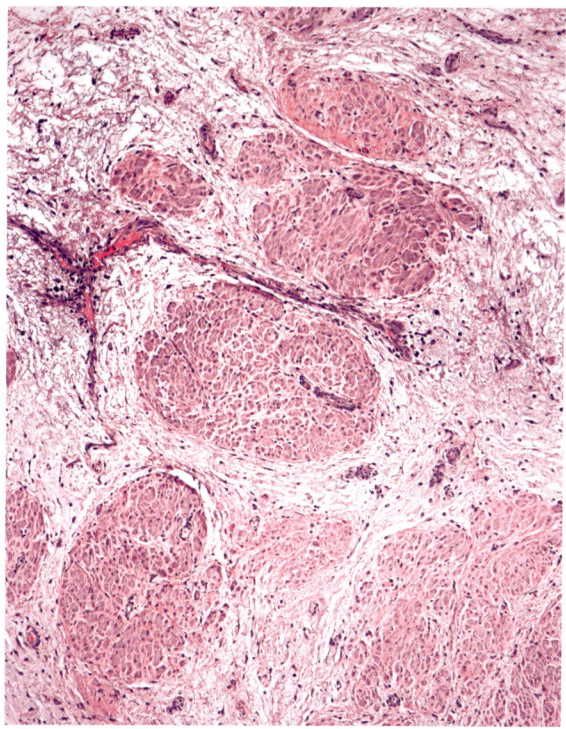

Figure 2-39

MYXOID CHANGE IN MYOMETRIUM

Paucicellular myxoid material is present within myometrial muscle bundles.

and S-100 protein helps to rule out smooth muscle tumors (although they often show patchy positivity), inflammatory myofibroblastic tumor, and malignant schwannoma. Endometrial stromal tumors, even when myxoid, tend to be more cellular than benign myxoid change and display arterioles and collagen bands of the type seen in areas of conventional endometrial stromal neoplasia. Immunohistochemical stains are not helpful in this differential diagnosis (187).

Pseudomyxoma endometrii may occur secondary to mucin deposition by a low-grade appendiceal mucinous neoplasm within the endometrium (25) and may mimic benign myxoid change or a myxoid neoplasm. The finding of free-floating mucinous epithelium is helpful. Furthermore, when there is involvement of the endometrium, other organs within the pelvis/peritoneum are also involved (24,25). Distinguishing myxoid matrix from mucin deposits is straightforward, since the latter is often associated with chronic inflammatory cells

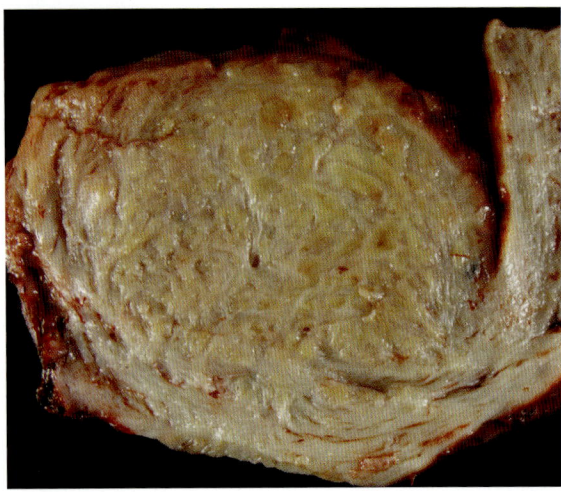 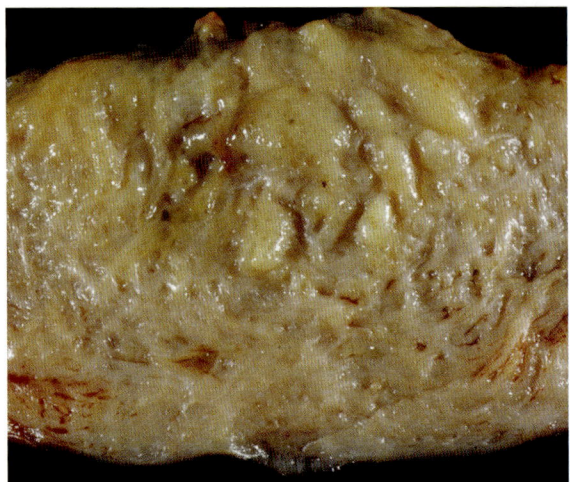

Figure 2-40

ADENOMYOSIS

A well-circumscribed intramyometrial mass may mimic a leiomyoma. The cut surface is strikingly trabeculated (left). Adenomyosis may diffusely affect the inner myometrium forming poorly defined small tan and soft nodules (right).

and macrophages and should be PAS positive. Recently, a gastrointestinal-type endometrial adenocarcinoma with focal "pseudomyxoma-type" invasion was reported; however, the mucin as occurs with secondary involvement by a low-grade appendiceal mucinous tumor was PAS positive and malignant tumor cells were present within the pools of mucin (193).

Rarely, focal myxoid change may be seen in the endometrium after a prior curettage. Typically, this should be an incidental finding but it may cause problems in the differential diagnosis in curettage specimens and may lead to overdiagnosis of a myxoid neoplasm. In such cases, clinical correlation is crucial.

ADENOMYOSIS

Adenomyosis is a non-neoplastic condition defined by the finding of endometrial stroma and glands (in variable admixtures) within the myometrium at least one medium-power field away from the endomyometrial junction (2 to 3 mm for a 10X objective). It has been postulated to occur due to abnormalities in the most superficial myometrial layers. Subendometrial smooth muscle hypertrophy, distortion of the normal architecture, and loss of inner myometrial function predispose to secondary infiltration of the myometrium by endometrial elements (194,195). Five to 70 percent of hysterectomy specimens have adenomyosis, depending on the strictness of the diagnostic criteria. It is mostly seen in late reproductive-aged women with nonspecific symptoms. Some investigators have found an increased incidence with parity and in postmenopausal breast cancer patients treated with tamoxifen (three to four times higher) (196,197).

The uterus may have a normal appearance, may show focal asymmetrical thickening, or may be diffusely enlarged. Rarely, adenomyosis is seen as an intramural mass that grossly mimics a leiomyoma (fig. 2-40, left). Typically, its abnormal appearance is a result of the neighboring smooth muscle hypertrophy. On sectioning, a prominent trabeculated surface may be noted, which corresponds to the hypertrophic smooth muscle surrounding adenomyosis. In the center of the hypertrophic muscle, small, reddish areas, occasionally with cyst formation, which correspond to the endometrial component, may be noted (fig. 2-40, right).

On microscopic examination, angulated islands of endometrial glands and stroma are seen within the myometrium (fig. 2-41A). The glands and stroma are typically inactive, but secretory changes, and in pregnancy or with exogenous hormones, decidual changes, may be seen (fig. 2-41B). Cystic glandular dilatation, epithelial metaplasias, and stromal fibrosis can occur

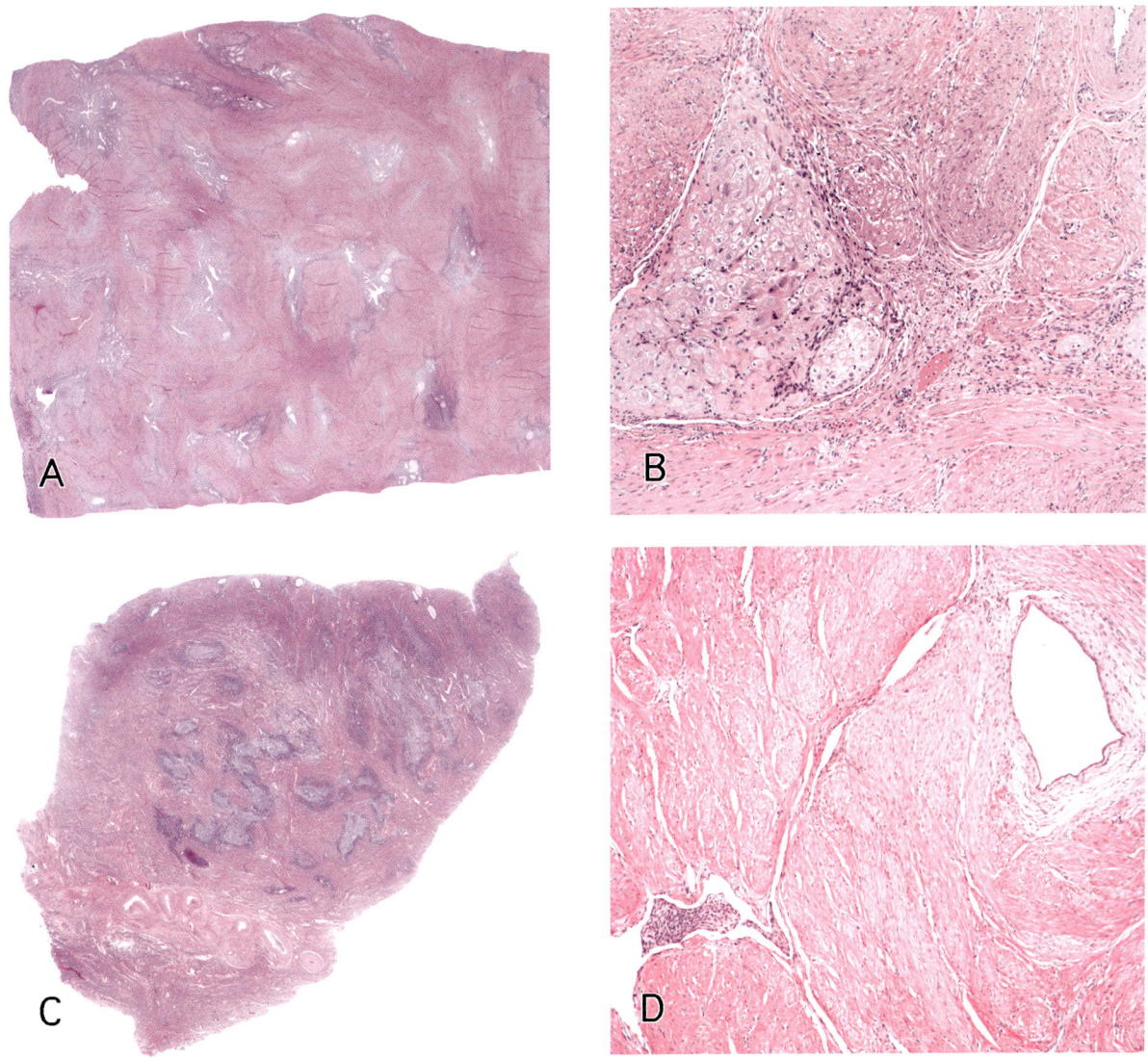

Figure 2-41

ADENOMYOSIS

Irregular and angulated islands of endometrial stroma, associated with variable numbers of endometrial glands, are present throughout the myometrium (A). Gland-poor adenomyosis replaced by decidua may mimic invasive squamous cell carcinoma (B). Gland-poor adenomyosis with blue islands of banal-appearing stromal cells unassociated with glands within the myometrium (C) or vessels (D) may be confused with an endometrial stromal sarcoma. Typical areas are seen nearby or in other sections.

(198). The surrounding hypertrophic myometrium typically forms ill-defined nodules.

Three features of adenomyosis may cause problems in the differential diagnosis: relative deficiency of stroma (i.e., gland-poor adenomyosis) (fig. 2-41C), location within vascular spaces (i.e., intravascular adenomyosis) (fig. 2-41D), and carcinoma or hyperplasia involving adenomyosis (199,200). Either of the first two findings may raise concern for a low-grade endometrial stromal sarcoma. However, in most cases, adenomyosis is an incidental finding in patients that have a hysterectomy performed for other reasons; it does not form a mass and conventional areas of adenomyosis are present nearby (199).

Adenomyosis may be secondarily involved by endometrial carcinoma, which should be distinguished from islands of myoinvasive carcinoma lacking an associated stromal response. To establish a definitive diagnosis of carcinoma within adenomyosis, foci of adenomyosis not involved by carcinoma are sought and a rim of benign endometrial stroma within that particular focus (201) is identified. The distinction is important as involvement of adenomyosis by an adenocarcinoma, even when deep in the myometrium, does not affect prognosis (202,203). CD10 is not helpful in this differential diagnosis as the stroma around neoplastic glands is also CD10 positive (204).

BLUE NEVUS

Blue nevus is a rare benign pigmented lesion in the female genital tract. It commonly involves the cervix and only occasionally is reported in the endometrium. Aggregates of cytologically bland pigmented spindle cells are present within the endometrial stroma and typically represent an incidental finding, even in a curettage specimen (205,206). It is postulated that melanocytes are derived from Schwann cells that may produce melanin at this site, or may be the result of abnormal migration of neural crest-derived cells during fetal development.

The differential diagnosis includes malignant melanoma, especially metastatic. Any other primary tumor containing melanin (primary malignant melanoma, carcinosarcoma, adenocarcinoma, PEComa, paraganglioma) (206) will be mass forming.

OTHER PROCESSES

Vasculitis of the female genital tract is rare; it is most often asymptomatic and isolated, occurring in the cervix. Panarteritis nodosa is frequently reported, followed by giant cell arteritis. These diseases can involve the uterus, fallopian tubes, and ovary (207) and usually involve one vessel rather than multiple vessels. Fibrinoid necrosis and inflammation are common findings that are associated with granulomatous inflammation in giant cell arteritis. Some of the affected patients also have polymyalgia rheumatica or temporal arteritis (208,209). Female genital tract involvement is only rarely associated with systemic vasculitis (207).

Ligneous endometritis is a rare inflammatory condition that affects all mucous membranes in patients with plasminogen deficiency. Involvement of the endometrium is rare in comparison to the cervix. Ligneous endometritis is characterized by fibrin deposition in the endometrium that may be associated with scattered acute and chronic inflammatory cells and multinucleated cells. Inflammation can be prominent if there is ulceration (210–212). Fibrin deposition in ligneous endometritis may mimic amyloidosis, but it does not stain with Congo red.

Amyloidosis involving the endometrium or myometrium is rare and patients typically present with menorrhagia or postmenopausal bleeding. It may occur in the setting of systemic amyloidosis, rheumatoid arthritis, or after renal transplant (213,214). It has been rarely reported in association with endometrial carcinoma (215).

REFERENCES

1. Nicolae A, Preda O, Nogales FF. Endometrial metaplasias and reactive changes: a spectrum of altered differentiation. J Clin Pathol 2011;64:97-106.
2. Kaku T, Silverberg SG, Tsukamoto N, et al. Association of endometrial epithelial metaplasias with endometrial carcinoma and hyperplasia in Japanese and American women. Int J Gynecol Pathol 1993;12:297-300.
3. Simon RA, Peng SL, Liu F, et al. Tubal metaplasia of the endometrium with cytologic atypia: analysis of p53, Ki-67, TERT, and long-term follow-up. Mod Pathol 2011;24:1254-61.
4. Horree N, Heintz AP, Sie-Go DM, van Diest PJ. p16 is consistently expressed in endometrial tubal metaplasia. Cell Oncol 2007;29:37-45.
5. Hendrickson MR, Kempson RL. Endometrial epithelial metaplasias: proliferations frequently misdiagnosed as adenocarcinoma. Report of 89 cases and proposed classification. Am J Surg Pathol 1980;4:525-42.
6. Nucci MR, Prasad CJ, Crum CP, Mutter GL. Mucinous endometrial epithelial proliferations: a morphologic spectrum of changes with diverse clinical significance. Mod Pathol 1999;12:1137-42.
7. Deligdisch L, Kalir T, Cohen CJ, de Latour M, Le Bouedec G, Penault-Llorca F. Endometrial histopathology in 700 patients treated with tamoxifen for breast cancer. Gynecol Oncol 2000;78:181-6.
8. Schlesinger C, Kamoi S, Ascher SM, Kendell M, Lage JM, Silverberg SG. Endometrial polyps: a comparison study of patients receiving tamoxifen with two control groups. Int J Gynecol Pathol 1998;17:302-11.
9. Mangili G, Taccagni G, Garavaglia E, Carnelli M, Montoli S. An unusual admixture of neoplastic and metaplastic lesions of the female genital tract in the Peutz-Jeghers syndrome. Gynecol Oncol 2004;92:337-42.
10. Mikami Y, Kiyokawa T, Sasajima Y, et al. Reappraisal of synchronous and multifocal mucinous lesions of the female genital tract: a close association with gastric metaplasia. Histopathology 2009;54:184-91.
11. Nicolae A, Goyenaga P, McCluggage WG, Preda O, Nogales FF. Endometrial intestinal metaplasia: a report of two cases, including one associated with cervical intestinal and pyloric metaplasia. Int J Gynecol Pathol 2011;30:492-6.
12. Alomari A, Abi-Raad R, Buza N, Hui P. Frequent KRAS mutation in complex mucinous epithelial lesions of the endometrium. Mod Pathol 2014;27:675-80.
13. Lehman MB, Hart WR. Simple and complex hyperplastic papillary proliferations of the endometrium: a clinicopathologic study of nine cases of apparently localized papillary lesions with fibrovascular stromal cores and epithelial metaplasia. Am J Surg Pathol 2001;25:1347-54.
14. Yoo SH, Park BH, Choi J, et al. Papillary mucinous metaplasia of the endometrium as a possible precursor of endometrial mucinous adenocarcinoma. Mod Pathol 2012;25:1496-507.
15. Anjarwalla S, Rollason TP, Rooney N, Hirschowitz L. Atypical mucinous metaplasia and intraepithelial neoplasia of the female genital tract—a case report and review of the literature. Int J Gynecol Cancer 2007;17:1147-50.
16. Wells M, Tiltman A. Intestinal metaplasia of the endometrium. Histopathology 1989;15:431-3.
17. Vang R, Tavassoli FA. Proliferative mucinous lesions of the endometrium: analysis of existing criteria for diagnosing carcinoma in biopsies and curettings. Int J Surg Pathol 2003;11:261-70.
18. Zaino R, Carinelli SG, Ellenson LH, et al. Epithelial tumours and precursors. In: Kurman R, Carcangiu ML, Herrington CS, Young RH, eds. Tumours of the uterine corpus. WHO classification of tumours of female reproductive organs. Lyon: IARC Press; 2014:125-35.
19. Rawish KR, Desouki MM, Fadare O. Atypical mucinous glandular proliferations in endometrial samplings: follow-up and other clinicopathological findings in 41 cases. Hum Pathol 2017;63:53-62.
20. He M, Jackson CL, Gubrod RB, et al. KRAS Mutations in mucinous lesions of the uterus. Am J Clin Pathol 2015;143:778-84.
21. Yemelyanova A, Vang R, Seidman JD, Gravitt PE, Ronnett BM. Endocervical adenocarcinomas with prominent endometrial or endomyometrial involvement simulating primary endometrial carcinomas: utility of HPV DNA detection and immunohistochemical expression of p16 and hormone receptors to confirm the cervical origin of the corpus tumor. Am J Surg Pathol 2009;33:914-24.
22. Carleton C, Hoang L, Sah S, et al. A detailed immunohistochemical analysis of a large series of cervical and vaginal gastric-type adenocarcinomas. Am J Surg Pathol 2016;40:636-44.
23. Mikami Y, McCluggage WG. Endocervical glandular lesions exhibiting gastric differentiation: an emerging spectrum of benign, premalignant, and malignant lesions. Adv Anat Pathol 2013;20:227-37.

24. McVeigh G, Shah V, Longacre TA, McCluggage WG. Endometrial involvement in pseudomyxoma peritonei secondary to low-grade appendiceal mucinous neoplasm: report of 2 cases. Int J Gynecol Pathol 2015;34:232-8.
25. Shaw KC, Kokh D, Ioffe OB, Staats PN. "Pseudomyxoma endometrii": endometrial deposition of acellular mucin from a low-grade appendiceal mucinous neoplasm as a rare mimic of myxoid uterine tumors. Int J Gynecol Pathol 2015;34:351-6.
26. Trippel M, Imboden S, Papadia A, et al. Intestinal differentiated mucinous adenocarcinoma of the endometrium with sporadic MSI high status: a case report. Diagn Pathol 2017;12:39.
27. Turashvili G, Childs T. Mucinous metaplasia of the endometrium: current concepts. Gynecol Oncol 2015;136:389-93.
28. Ip PP, Irving JA, McCluggage WG, Clement PB, Young RH. Papillary proliferation of the endometrium: a clinicopathologic study of 59 cases of simple and complex papillae without cytologic atypia. Am J Surg Pathol 2013;37:167-77.
29. Park CK, Yoon G, Cho YA, Kim HS. Clinicopathological and immunohistochemical characterization of papillary proliferation of the endometrium: a single institutional experience. Oncotarget 2016;7:39197-206.
30. Rekhi B, Menon S, Maheshwari A. Complex papillary hyperplasia of the endometrium: an uncommon case report with cytopathological features and diagnostic implications. Diagn Cytopathol 2015;43:163-8.
31. Shah SS, Mazur MT. Endometrial eosinophilic syncytial change related to breakdown: immunohistochemical evidence suggests a regressive process. Int J Gynecol Pathol 2008;27:534-8.
32. Crum CP, Richart RM, Fenoglio CM. Adenoacanthosis of endometrium: a clinicopathologic study in premenopausal women. Am J Surg Pathol 1981;5:15-20.
33. Amico P, Caltabiano R, Zizza G, Lanzafame S. About a case of diffuse endometrial squamous metaplasia after resectoscopic myomectomy: a potential diagnostic pitfall for gynecologists and pathologists. Appl Immunohistochem Mol Morphol 2010;18:392-5.
34. Gamachi A, Kashima K, Daa T, Nakatani Y, Tsujimoto M, Yokoyama S. Aberrant intranuclear localization of biotin, biotin-binding enzymes, and beta-catenin in pregnancy-related endometrium and morule-associated neoplastic lesions. Mod Pathol 2003;16:1124-31.
35. Chinen K, Kamiyama K, Kinjo T, et al. Morules in endometrial carcinoma and benign endometrial lesions differ from squamous differentiation tissue and are not infected with human papillomavirus. J Clin Pathol 2004;57:918-26.
36. Houghton O, Connolly LE, McCluggage WG. Morules in endometrioid proliferations of the uterus and ovary consistently express the intestinal transcription factor CDX2. Histopathology 2008;53:156-65.
37. Nakatani Y, Masudo K, Nozawa A, et al. Biotin-rich, optically clear nuclei express estrogen receptor-beta: tumors with morules may develop under the influence of estrogen and aberrant beta-catenin expression. Hum Pathol 2004;35:869-74.
37a. McCluggage WG, Van de Vijver K. SATB2 is consistently expressed in squamous morules associated with endometrioid proliferative lesions and in the stroma of atypical polypoid adenomyoma. Int J Gynecol Pathol 2018. [Epub ahead of print]
38. Terada T. Extensive squamous metaplasia (morules) of the otherwise normal endometrium: a case report with immunohistochemical studies. Int J Clin Exp Pathol 2013;6:543-5.
39. Blanco LZ Jr, Heagley DE, Lee JC, et al. Immunohistochemical characterization of squamous differentiation and morular metaplasia in uterine endometrioid adenocarcinoma. Int J Gynecol Pathol 2013;32:283-92.
40. Chiarelli S, Buritica C, Litta P, Ciani S, Guarch R, Nogales FF. An immunohistochemical study of morules in endometrioid lesions of the female genital tract: CD10 is a characteristic marker of morular metaplasia. Clin Cancer Res 2006;12(Pt 1):4251-6.
41. Mazur MT. Atypical polypoid adenomyomas of the endometrium. Am J Surg Pathol 1981;5:473-82.
42. Young RH, Treger T, Scully RE. Atypical polypoid adenomyoma of the uterus. A report of 27 cases. Am J Clin Pathol 1986;86:139-45.
43. Takahashi H, Yoshida T, Matsumoto T, et al. Frequent beta-catenin gene mutations in atypical polypoid adenomyoma of the uterus. Hum Pathol 2014;45:33-40.
44. Ota S, Catasus L, Matias-Guiu X, et al. Molecular pathology of atypical polypoid adenomyoma of the uterus. Hum Pathol 2003;34:784-8.
45. Lin MC, Lomo L, Baak JP, et al. Squamous morules are functionally inert elements of premalignant endometrial neoplasia. Mod Pathol 2009;22:167-74.
46. Litta P, Codroma A, D'Agostino G, Breda E. Morular endometrial metaplasia: review of the literature and proposal of the management. Eur J Gynaecol Oncol 2013;34:243-7.
47. Zaino RJ, Brady WE, Todd W, et al. Histologic effects of medroxyprogesterone acetate on endometrioid endometrial adenocarcinoma: a Gynecologic Oncology Group study. Int J Gynecol Pathol 2014;33:543-53.

48. Goodman A, Zukerberg LR, Rice LW, Fuller AF, Young RH, Scully RE. Squamous cell carcinoma of the endometrium: a report of eight cases and a review of the literature. Gynecol Oncol 1996;61:54-60.
49. Stockinger R, Sterlacci W, Neunteufel W, Boesl A, Spreitzer S, Offner F. Verrucous carcinoma of the endometrium: a rare and challenging diagnosis. Int J Gynecol Pathol 2014;33:298-301.
50. Bures N, Nelson G, Duan Q, Magliocco A, Demetrick D, Duggan MA. Primary squamous cell carcinoma of the endometrium: clinicopathologic and molecular characteristics. Int J Gynecol Pathol 2013;32:566-75.
51. Zaman SS, Mazur MT. Endometrial papillary syncytial change. A nonspecific alteration associated with active breakdown. Am J Clin Pathol 1993;99:741-5.
52. Ruhul Quddus M, Latkovich P, Castellani WJ, et al. Expression of cyclin D1 in normal, metaplastic, hyperplastic endometrium and endometrioid carcinoma suggests a role in endometrial carcinogenesis. Arch Pathol Lab Med 2002;126:459-63.
53. McCluggage WG, McBride HA. Papillary syncytial metaplasia associated with endometrial breakdown exhibits an immunophenotype that overlaps with uterine serous carcinoma. Int J Gynecol Pathol 2012;31:206-10.
54. Nicolae A, Preda O, Aneiros-Fernandez J, Palacios J, Biscuola M, Nogales FF. p16 INK4A positivity identifies endometrial surface papillary syncitial change as a regressive feature associated with desquamation. Histopathology 2011;58:483-6.
55. Haley SL, Malhotra RK, Qiu S, Eltorky ME. The immunohistochemical profile of atypical eosinophilic syncytial changes vs serous carcinoma. Ann Diagn Pathol 2011;15:402-6.
56. Jacques SM, Qureshi F, Lawrence WD. Surface epithelial changes in endometrial adenocarcinoma: diagnostic pitfalls in curettage specimens. Int J Gynecol Pathol 1995;14:191-7.
57. Gersell DJ. Endometrial papillary syncytial change. Another perspective. Am J Clin Pathol 1993;99:656-7.
58. Pitman MB, Young RH, Clement PB, Dickersin GR, Scully RE. Endometrioid carcinoma of the ovary and endometrium, oxyphilic cell type: a report of nine cases. Int J Gynecol Pathol 1994;13:290-301.
59. Fukuoka K, Hirokawa M, Shimizu M, et al. Oxyphilic cell variant of endometrioid adenocarcinoma. Pathol Int 1998;48:754-6.
60. Silver SA, Cheung AN, Tavassoli FA. Oncocytic metaplasia and carcinoma of the endometrium: an immunohistochemical and ultrastructural study. Int J Gynecol Pathol 1999;18:12-9.
61. Moritani S, Kushima R, Ichihara S, et al. Eosinophilic cell change of the endometrium: a possible relationship to mucinous differentiation. Mod Pathol 2005;18:1243-8.
62. Hejmadi RK, Chaudhri S, Ganesan R, Rollason TP. Morphologic changes in the endometrium associated with the use of the mirena coil: a retrospective study of 106 cases. Int J Surg Pathol 2007;15:148-54.
63. Huettner PC, Gersell DJ. Arias-Stella reaction in nonpregnant women: a clinicopathologic study of nine cases. Int J Gynecol Pathol 1994;13:241-7.
64. Arias-Stella J. The Arias-Stella reaction: facts and fancies four decades after. Adv Anat Pathol 2002;9:12-23.
65. Vang R, Barner R, Wheeler DT, Strauss BL. Immunohistochemical staining for Ki-67 and p53 helps distinguish endometrial Arias-Stella reaction from high-grade carcinoma, including clear cell carcinoma. Int J Gynecol Pathol 2004;23:223-33.
66. Arias-Stella J Jr, Arias-Velasquez A, Arias-Stella J. Normal and abnormal mitoses in the atypical endometrial change associated with chorionic tissue effect [corrected]. Am J Surg Pathol 1994;18:694-701.
67. DeLair DF, Burke KA, Selenica P, et al. The genetic landscape of endometrial clear cell carcinomas. J Pathol 2017;243:230-41.
68. Sakaki M, Hirokawa M, Sano T, et al. Ovarian endometriosis showing decidual change and Arias-Stella reaction with biotin-containing intranuclear inclusions. Acta Cytol 2003;47:321-4.
69. Mazur MT, Hendrickson MR, Kempson RL. Optically clear nuclei. An alteration of endometrial epithelium in the presence of trophoblast. Am J Surg Pathol 1983;7:415-23.
70. Yokoyama S, Kashima K, Inoue S, Daa T, Nakayama I, Moriuchi A. Biotin-containing intranuclear inclusions in endometrial glands during gestation and puerperium. Am J Clin Pathol 1993;99:13-7.
71. Jacques SM, Qureshi F, Ramirez NC, Lawrence WD. Unusual endometrial stromal cell changes mimicking metastatic carcinoma. Pathol Res Pract 1996;192:33-6.
72. Iezzoni JC, Mills SE. Nonneoplastic endometrial signet-ring cells. Vacuolated decidual cells and stromal histiocytes mimicking adenocarcinoma. Am J Clin Pathol 2001;115:249-55.
73. Clement PB, Scully RE. Idiopathic postmenopausal decidual reaction of the endometrium. A clinicopathologic analysis of four cases. Int J Gynecol Pathol 1988;7:152-61.
74. Shapiro S, Kelly JP, Rosenberg L, et al. Risk of localized and widespread endometrial cancer in relation to recent and discontinued use of conjugated estrogens. N Engl J Med 1985;313:969-72.

75. Brinton LA, Hoover RN. Estrogen replacement therapy and endometrial cancer risk: unresolved issues. The Endometrial Cancer Collaborative Group. Obstet Gynecol 1993;81:265-71.
76. Grady D, Gebretsadik T, Kerlikowske K, Ernster V, Petitti D. Hormone replacement therapy and endometrial cancer risk: a meta-analysis. Obstet Gynecol 1995;85:304-13.
77. Feeley KM, Wells M. Hormone replacement therapy and the endometrium. J Clin Pathol 2001;54:435-40.
78. Nand SL, Webster MA, Baber R, O'Connor V. Bleeding pattern and endometrial changes during continuous combined hormone replacement therapy. The Ogen/Provera Study Group. Obstet Gynecol 1998;91(Pt 1):678-84.
79. Gunderson CC, Dutta S, Fader AN, et al. Pathologic features associated with resolution of complex atypical hyperplasia and grade 1 endometrial adenocarcinoma after progestin therapy. Gynecol Oncol 2014;132:33-7.
80. Nogales FF, Crespo-Lora V, Cruz-Viruel N, Chamorro-Santos C, Bergeron C. Endometrial changes in surgical specimens of perimenopausal patients treated with ulipristal acetate for uterine leiomyomas. Int J Gynecol Pathol 2017. [Epub ahead of print]
81. Casper RF. Clinical uses of gonadotropin-releasing hormone analogues. CMAJ 1991;144:153-58.
82. Brooks PG, Serden SP, Davos I. Hormonal inhibition of the endometrium for resectoscopic endometrial ablation. Am J Obstet Gynecol 1991;164(Pt 1):1601-6; discussion 1606-8.
83. Benda JA. Clomiphene's effect on endometrium in infertility. Int J Gynecol Pathol 1992;11:273-82.
84. Ismail SM. Gynaecological effects of tamoxifen. J Clin Pathol 1999;52:83-8.
85. Seidman JD, Kurman RJ. Tamoxifen and the endometrium. Int J Gynecol Pathol 1999;18:293-6.
86. Cheng WF, Lin HH, Torng PL, Huang SC. Comparison of endometrial changes among symptomatic tamoxifen-treated and nontreated premenopausal and postmenopausal breast cancer patients. Gynecol Oncol 1997;66:233-7.
87. Kennedy MM, Baigrie CF, Manek S. Tamoxifen and the endometrium: review of 102 cases and comparison with HRT-related and non-HRT-related endometrial pathology. Int J Gynecol Pathol 1999;18:130-7.
88. Stewart CJ, Bharat C, Crook M. p16 immunoreactivity in endometrial stromal cells: stromal p16 expression characterises but is not specific for endometrial polyps. Pathology 2015;47:112-7.
89. Turbiner J, Moreno-Bueno G, Dahiya S, et al. Clinicopathological and molecular analysis of endometrial carcinoma associated with tamoxifen. Mod Pathol 2008;21:925-36.
90. Matsuo K, Ross MS, Bush SH, et al. Tumor characteristics and survival outcomes of women with tamoxifen-related uterine carcinosarcoma. Gynecol Oncol 2017;144:329-35.
91. Dallenbach-Hellweg G, Schmidt D, Hellberg P, et al. The endometrium in breast cancer patients on tamoxifen. Arch Gynecol Obstet 2000;263:170-7.
92. McCluggage WG, McManus DT, Lioe TF, Hill CM. Uterine carcinosarcoma in association with tamoxifen therapy. Br J Obstet Gynaecol 1997;104:748-50.
93. McCluggage WG, Sumathi VP, McManus DT. Uterine serous carcinoma and endometrial intraepithelial carcinoma arising in endometrial polyps: report of 5 cases, including 2 associated with tamoxifen therapy. Hum Pathol 2003;34:939-43.
94. Clement PB, Oliva E, Young RH. Mullerian adenosarcoma of the uterine corpus associated with tamoxifen therapy: a report of six cases and a review of tamoxifen-associated endometrial lesions. Int J Gynecol Pathol 1996;15:222-9.
95. Kenny SL, McCluggage WG. Adenomyomatous polyp of the endometrium with prominent epithelioid smooth muscle differentiation: report of two cases of a hitherto undescribed lesion. Int J Surg Pathol 2014;22:358-63.
96. Oliva E, Young RH, Amin MB, Clement PB. An immunohistochemical analysis of endometrial stromal and smooth muscle tumors of the uterus: a study of 54 cases emphasizing the importance of using a panel because of overlap in immunoreactivity for individual antibodies. Am J Surg Pathol 2002;26:403-12.
97. Scully RE. Smooth-muscle differentiation in genital tract disorders. Arch Pathol Lab Med 1981;105:505-7.
98. Perino A, Mangione D, Svelato A, et al. Chronic renal failure and endometrial osseous metaplasia: a hypothetical pathway. Acta Obstet Gynecol Scand 2013;92:118-9.
99. Kouakou F, Loue V, Kouame A, et al. Endometrial osseous metaplasia and infertility: a case report. Clin Exp Obstet Gynecol 2012;39:559-61.
100. Tulandi T, Al-Sunaidi M, Arseneau J, Tonin PN, Arcand SL. Calcified tissue of fetal origin in utero. Fertil Steril 2008;89:217-8.
101. Cayuela E, Perez-Medina T, Vilanova J, Alejo M, Canadas P. True osseous metaplasia of the endometrium: the bone is not from a fetus. Fertil Steril 2009;91:1293.
102. Garg D, Bekker G, Akselrod F, Narasimhulu DM. Endometrial osseous metaplasia: an unusual cause of infertility. BMJ Case Rep 2015;2015.
103. Podgornik F. [Metaplastic hyaline cartilage in endometrial tissue.] Ginekol Pol 1976;47:1191-2. [Polish]

104. Aabye R. Cartilage in the endometrium. Acta Obstet Gynecol Scand 1955;34:105-10.
105. Nogales FF, Pavcovich M, Medina MT, Palomino M. Fatty change in the endometrium. Histopathology 1992;20:362-3.
106. Deshmukh-Rane SA, Wu ML. Pseudolipomatosis affects specimens from endometrial biopsies. Am J Clin Pathol 2009;132:374-7.
107. Unger ZM, Gonzalez JL, Hanissian PD, Schned AR. Pseudolipomatosis in hysteroscopically resected tissues from the gynecologic tract: pathologic description and frequency. Am J Surg Pathol 2009;33:1187-90.
108. Heller A. Pseudolipomatosis in endometrial specimens does not represent uterine perforation. Int J Surg Pathol 2017;25:56-7.
109. Siddon A, Hui P. Glial heterotopia of the uterine cervix: DNA genotyping confirmation of its fetal origin. Int J Gynecol Pathol 2010;29:394-7.
110. Roca AN, Guajardo M, Estrada WJ. Glial polyp of the cervix and endometrium. Report of a case and review of the literature. Am J Clin Pathol 1980;73:718-20.
111. Calvert SM, Calvert RJ, Hjartardottir H, Beck I. Glial polyp: an unusual cause of post-coital bleeding. J Obstet Gynaecol 2000;20:205-6.
112. Russell P, de Costa C, Yeoh G. Fetal glial allograft in the endometrium: case report of a recurrent pseudo-tumor. Pathology 1993;25:247-9.
113. Gronroos M, Meurman L, Kahra K. Proliferating glia and other heterotopic tissues in the uterus: fetal homografts? Obstet Gynecol 1983;61:261-6.
114. Daya D, Lukka H, Clement PB. Primitive neuroectodermal tumors of the uterus: a report of four cases. Hum Pathol 1992;23:1120-9.
115. Chiang S, Snuderl M, Kojiro-Sanada S, et al. Primitive neuroectodermal tumors of the female genital tract: a morphologic, immunohistochemical, and molecular study of 19 cases. Am J Surg Pathol 2017;41:761-72.
116. Young RH, Kleinman GM, Scully RE. Glioma of the uterus. Report of a case with comments on histogenesis. Am J Surg Pathol 1981;5:695-9.
117. Stolnicu S, Szekely E, Molnar C, et al. Mature and immature solid teratomas involving uterine corpus, cervix, and ovary. Int J Gynecol Pathol 2017;36:222-7.
118. Creagh TM, Bain BJ, Evans DJ, Reid CD, Young RH, Flanagan AM. Endometrial extramedullary haemopoiesis. J Pathol 1995;176:99-104.
119. Cui X, Peker D, Greer HO, Conner MG, Novak L. Extramedullary hematopoiesis in uterine leiomyoma associated with numerous intravascular thrombi. Case Rep Pathol 2014;2014:957395.
120. Valeri RM, Ibrahim N, Sheaff MT. Extramedullary hematopoiesis in the endometrium. Int J Gynecol Pathol 2002;21:178-81.
121. Palatnik A, Narayan R, Walters M. Extramedullary hematopoiesis involving uterus, fallopian tubes, and ovaries, mimicking bilateral tuboovarian abscesses. Int J Gynecol Pathol 2012;31:584-7.
122. Gru AA, Hassan A, Pfeifer JD, Huettner PC. Uterine extramedullary hematopoiesis: what is the clinical significance? Int J Gynecol Pathol 2010;29:366-73.
123. Koch CA, Li CY, Mesa RA, Tefferi A. Nonhepatosplenic extramedullary hematopoiesis: associated diseases, pathology, clinical course, and treatment. Mayo Clin Proc 2003;78:1223-33.
124. Silverberg SG, Haukkamaa M, Arko H, Nilsson CG, Luukkainen T. Endometrial morphology during long-term use of levonorgestrel-releasing intrauterine devices. Int J Gynecol Pathol 1986;5:235-41.
125. Critchley HO, Wang H, Jones RL, et al. Morphological and functional features of endometrial decidualization following long-term intrauterine levonorgestrel delivery. Hum Reprod 1998;13:1218-24.
126. Phillips V, Graham CT, Manek S, McCluggage WG. The effects of the levonorgestrel intrauterine system (Mirena coil) on endometrial morphology. J Clin Pathol 2003;56:305-7.
127. Stewart CJ, Leake R. Endometrial synovial-like metaplasia associated with levonorgestrel-releasing intrauterine system. Int J Gynecol Pathol 2015;34:570-5.
128. Eckert LO, Thwin SS, Hillier SL, Kiviat NB, Eschenbach DA. The antimicrobial treatment of subacute endometritis: a proof of concept study. Am J Obstet Gynecol 2004;190:305-13.
129. Bouet PE, El Hachem H, Monceau E, Gariepy G, Kadoch IJ, Sylvestre C. Chronic endometritis in women with recurrent pregnancy loss and recurrent implantation failure: prevalence and role of office hysteroscopy and immunohistochemistry in diagnosis. Fertil Steril 2016;105:106-10.
130. Cicinelli E, De Ziegler D, Nicoletti R, et al. Chronic endometritis: correlation among hysteroscopic, histologic, and bacteriologic findings in a prospective trial with 2190 consecutive office hysteroscopies. Fertil Steril 2008;89:677-84.
131. Resta L, Palumbo M, Rossi R, Piscitelli D, Grazia Fiore M, Cicinelli E. Histology of micro polyps in chronic endometritis. Histopathology 2012;60:670-4.
132. Greenwood SM, Moran JJ. Chronic endometritis: morphologic and clinical observations. Obstet Gynecol 1981;58:176-84.
133. Smith M, Hagerty KA, Skipper B, Bocklage T. Chronic endometritis: a combined histopathologic and clinical review of cases from 2002 to 2007. Int J Gynecol Pathol 2010;29:44-50.

134. Adegboyega PA, Pei Y, McLarty J. Relationship between eosinophils and chronic endometritis. Hum Pathol 2010;41:33-7.
135. Bayer-Garner IB, Nickell JA, Korourian S. Routine syndecan-1 immunohistochemistry aids in the diagnosis of chronic endometritis. Arch Pathol Lab Med 2004;128:1000-3.
136. Bayer-Garner IB, Korourian S. Plasma cells in chronic endometritis are easily identified when stained with syndecan-1. Mod Pathol 2001;14:877-9.
137. Gilmore H, Fleischhacker D, Hecht JL. Diagnosis of chronic endometritis in biopsies with stromal breakdown. Hum Pathol 2007;38:581-4.
138. Kitaya K, Yasuo T. Aberrant expression of selectin E, CXCL1, and CXCL13 in chronic endometritis. Mod Pathol 2010;23:1136-46.
139. Pitsos M, Skurnick J, Heller D. Association of pathologic diagnoses with clinical findings in chronic endometritis. J Reprod Med 2009;54: 373-7.
140. Bennett AE, Rathore S, Rhatigan RM. Focal necrotizing endometritis: a clinicopathologic study of 15 cases. Int J Gynecol Pathol 1999;18:220-5.
141. Hale A, Kirby JE, Albrecht M. Fatal spontaneous clostridium bifermentans necrotizing endometritis: a case report and literature review of the pathogen. Open Forum Infect Dis 2016;6:1-4.
142. Bennett JA, Oliva E, Nardi V, Lindeman N, Ferry JA, Louissaint A Jr. Primary endometrial marginal zone lymphoma (MALT lymphoma): a unique clinicopathologic entity. Am J Surg Pathol 2016;40:1217-23.
143. Young RH, Harris NL, Scully RE. Lymphoma-like lesions of the lower female genital tract: a report of 16 cases. Int J Gynecol Pathol 1985;4:289-99.
144. Gaillot L, Allias F, Dubernard G, Berger F, Devouassoux-Shisheboran M. [Lymphoma-like lesions of the endometrium.] Ann Pathol 2008;28:504-7. [French]
145. Geyer JT, Ferry JA, Harris NL, Young RH, Longtine JA, Zukerberg LR. Florid reactive lymphoid hyperplasia of the lower female genital tract (lymphoma-like lesion): a benign condition that frequently harbors clonal immunoglobulin heavy chain gene rearrangements. Am J Surg Pathol 2010;34:161-8.
146. Bryant A, Lawton H, Al-Talib R, Wright DH, Theaker JM. Intravascular proliferation of reactive lymphoid blasts mimicking intravascular lymphoma—a diagnostic pitfall. Histopathology 2007;51:401-2.
147. Colgan TJ, Shah R, Leyland N. Post-hysteroscopic ablation reaction: a histopathologic study of the effects of electrosurgical ablation. Int J Gynecol Pathol 1999;18:325-31.
148. Ferryman SR, Stephens M, Gough D. Necrotising granulomatous endometritis following endometrial ablation therapy. Br J Obstet Gynaecol 1992;99:928-30.
149. McCulloch TA, Wagner B, Duffy S, Barik S, Smith JH. The pathology of hysterectomy specimens following trans-cervical resection of the endometrium. Histopathology 1995;27:541-7.
150. Tresserra F, Grases P, Ubeda A, Pascual MA, Grases PJ, Labastida R. Morphological changes in hysterectomies after endometrial ablation. Hum Reprod 1999;14:1473-7.
151. Kim EK, Yoon G, Kim HS. Chemotherapy-induced endometrial pathology: mimicry of malignancy and viral endometritis. Am J Transl Res 2016;8:2459-67.
152. Irving JA, McFarland DF, Stuart DS, Gilks CB. Mitotic arrest of endometrial epithelium after paclitaxel therapy for breast cancer. Int J Gynecol Pathol 2000;19:395-7.
153. McGill AL, Bavaro MF, You WB. Postpartum herpes simplex virus endometritis and disseminated infection in both mother and neonate. Obstet Gynecol 2012;120(Pt 2):471-3.
154. Mugo NR, Kiehlbauch J, Kiviat N, et al. Endometrial histopathology in patients with laparoscopic proven salpingitis and HIV-1 infection. Infect Dis Obstet Gynecol 2011;2011:407057.
155. Giraldo-Isaza MA, Jaspan D, Cohen AW. Postpartum endometritis caused by herpes and cytomegaloviruses. Obstet Gynecol 2011;117(Pt 2):466-7.
156. Brodman M, Deligdisch L. Cytomegalovirus endometritis in a patient with AIDS. Mt Sinai J Med 1986;53:673-5.
157. Frank TS, Himebaugh KS, Wilson MD. Granulomatous endometritis associated with histologically occult cytomegalovirus in a healthy patient. Am J Surg Pathol 1992;16:716-20.
158. Nakahira ES, Maximiano LF, Lima FR, Ussami EY. Abdominal and pelvic actinomycosis due to longstanding intrauterine device: a slow and devastating infection. Autops Case Rep 2017;7:43-7.
159. Pritt B, Mount SL, Cooper K, Blaszyk H. Pseudoactinomycotic radiate granules of the gynaecological tract: review of a diagnostic pitfall. J Clin Pathol 2006;59:17-20.
160. Kim YJ, Youm J, Kim JH, Jee BC. Actinomyces-like organisms in cervical smears: the association with intrauterine device and pelvic inflammatory diseases. Obstet Gynecol Sci 2014;57:393-6.
161. O'Brien PK, Roth-Moyo LA, Davis BA. Pseudosulfur granules associated with intrauterine contraceptive devices. Am J Clin Pathol 1981;75:822-5.
162. Boyle DP, McCluggage WG. Combined actinomycotic and pseudoactinomycotic radiate granules in the female genital tract: description of a series of cases. J Clin Pathol 2009;62:1123-6.

163. Kim KR, Lee YH, Ro JY. Nodular histiocytic hyperplasia of the endometrium. Int J Gynecol Pathol 2002;21:141-6.
164. Parkash V, Domfeh AB, Fadare O. Nodular histiocytic aggregates in the endometrium: a report of 7 cases. Int J Gynecol Pathol 2014;33:52-7.
165. Fukunaga M, Iwaki S. Nodular histiocytic hyperplasia of the endometrium. Arch Pathol Lab Med 2004;128:1032-4.
166. Wiltenburg W, Wouters MG, Uyterlinde AM, Sporken JM. [Malacoplakia of the female genital tract in a woman with postmenopausal bleeding.] Ned Tijdschr Geneeskd 2003;147:77-9. [Dutch]
167. Willen R, Stendahl U, Willen H, Trope. Malacoplakia of the cervix and corpus uteri: a light microscopic, electron microscopic, and X-ray microprobe analysis of a case. Int J Gynecol Pathol 1983;2:201-8.
168. Kawai K, Fukuda K, Tsuchiyama H. Malacoplakia of the endometrium. An unusual case studied by electron microscopy and a review of the literature. Acta Pathol Jpn 1988;38:531-40.
169. Sabadell J, Castellvi J, Baro F. Tuberculous endometritis presenting as postmenopausal bleeding. Int J Gynaecol Obstet 2007;96:203-4.
170. Mariara C, Koech A, Waweru P, Murage A. Endometrial tuberculosis compounding polycystic ovary syndrome in a subfertile woman: a case report. J Med Case Rep 2016;10:168.
171. Rivasi F, Curatola C, Garagnani L, Negri G. Detection of Mycobacterium tuberculosis DNA by polymerase chain reaction from paraffin samples of chronic granulomatous endometritis. Histopathology 2007;51:574-8.
172. al-Rufaie HK, Rix GH, Perez Clemente MP, al-Shawaf T. Pinworms and postmenopausal bleeding. J Clin Pathol 1998;51:401-2.
173. Hamid D, Baldauf JJ, Cuenin C, Ritter J. Treatment strategy for pelvic actinomycosis: case report and review of the literature. Eur J Obstet Gynecol Reprod Biol 2000;89:197-200.
174. Neumann G, Rasmussen KL, Olesen H. Premenopausal metrorrhagia as a symptom of sarcoidosis. Eur J Obstet Gynecol Reprod Biol 2002;104:171-3.
175. Smart PJ, Hetherington JF. Postoperative uterine granulomata following endometrial resection. Pathology 1995;27:209-11.
176. Lo Monaco M, Puzzo L, Brancato F, Torrisi A, Magro G. Endometrial atypical (bizarre) stromal cells: a potential diagnostic pitfall in biopsy. Pathol Res Pract 2004;200:625-7; discussion 629-30.
177. Tai LH, Tavassoli FA. Endometrial polyps with atypical (bizarre) stromal cells. Am J Surg Pathol 2002;26:505-9.
178. Nucci MR, Young RH, Fletcher CD. Cellular pseudosarcomatous fibroepithelial stromal polyps of the lower female genital tract: an underrecognized lesion often misdiagnosed as sarcoma. Am J Surg Pathol 2000;24:231-40.
179. Clement PB, Scully RE. Mullerian adenosarcoma of the uterus: a clinicopathologic analysis of 100 cases with a review of the literature. Hum Pathol 1990;21:363-81.
180. Baker PM, Moch H, Oliva E. Unusual morphologic features of endometrial stromal tumors: a report of 2 cases. Am J Surg Pathol 2005;29:1394-8.
181. Croce S, Young RH, Oliva E. Uterine leiomyomas with bizarre nuclei: a clinicopathologic study of 59 cases. Am J Surg Pathol 2014;38:1330-9.
182. Usubutun A, Karaman N, Ayhan A, Kucukali T. Atypical endometrial stromal cells related with a polypoid leiomyoma with bizarre nuclei: a case report. Int J Gynecol Pathol 2005;24:352-4.
183. Veras E, Junkins-Hopkins JM, Marinis S, Vang R. Myometrial myxoidosis: a report of 2 cases of a distinctive type of secondary myometrial hypertrophy in patients with lupus erythematosus. Int J Gynecol Pathol 2009;28:164-71.
184. Pugh A, McCluggage WG, Hirschowitz L. Multifocal uterine myxoid change: a newly recognized association with neurofibromatosis type 1. Int J Gynecol Pathol 2012;31:580-3.
185. McCluggage WG, Young RH. Myxoid change of the myometrium and cervical stroma: description of a hitherto unreported non-neoplastic phenomenon with discussion of myxoid uterine lesions. Int J Gynecol Pathol 2010;29:351-7.
186. Parra-Herran C, Schoolmeester JK, Yuan L, et al. Myxoid leiomyosarcoma of the uterus: a clinicopathologic analysis of 30 cases and review of the literature with reappraisal of its distinction from other uterine myxoid mesenchymal neoplasms. Am J Surg Pathol 2016;40:285-301.
187. Oliva E, Young RH, Clement PB, Scully RE. Myxoid and fibrous endometrial stromal tumors of the uterus: a report of 10 cases. Int J Gynecol Pathol 1999;18:310-9.
188. Parra-Herran C, Quick CM, Howitt BE, Dal Cin P, Quade BJ, Nucci MR. Inflammatory myofibroblastic tumor of the uterus: clinical and pathologic review of 10 cases including a subset with aggressive clinical course. Am J Surg Pathol 2015;39:157-68.
189. Bennett JA, Nardi V, Rouzbahman M, Morales-Oyarvide V, Nielsen GP, Oliva E. Inflammatory myofibroblastic tumor of the uterus: a clinicopathological, immunohistochemical, and molecular analysis of 13 cases highlighting their broad morphologic spectrum. Mod Pathol 2017;30:1489-503.

190. Barlow JF, Abu-Gazeleh S, Tam GE, et al. Myxoid tumor of the uterus and right atrial myxomas. S D J Med 1983;36:9-13.
191. McDonald AG, Dal Cin P, Ganguly A, et al. Liposarcoma arising in uterine lipoleiomyoma: a report of 3 cases and review of the literature. Am J Surg Pathol 2011;35:221-7.
192. Keel SB, Clement PB, Prat J, Young RH. Malignant schwannoma of the uterine cervix: a study of three cases. Int J Gynecol Pathol 1998;17:223-30.
193. Rubio A, Schuldt M, Guarch R, Laplaza Y, Giordano G, Nogales FF. Pseudomyxoma-type invasion in gastrointestinal adenocarcinomas of endometrium and cervix: a report of 2 cases. Int J Gynecol Pathol 2016;35:118-22.
194. Brosens JJ, Barker FG. Adenomyosis: time for a reappraisal. Lancet 1993;341:181-2.
195. Brosens I, Derwig I, Brosens J, Fusi L, Benagiano G, Pijnenborg R. The enigmatic uterine junctional zone: the missing link between reproductive disorders and major obstetrical disorders? Hum Reprod 2010;25:569-4.
196. Parazzini F, Vercellini P, Panazza S, Chatenoud L, Oldani S, Crosignani PG. Risk factors for adenomyosis. Hum Reprod 1997;12:1275-9.
197. Vercellini P, Parazzini F, Oldani S, Panazza S, Bramante T, Crosignani PG. Adenomyosis at hysterectomy: a study on frequency distribution and patient characteristics. Hum Reprod 1995;10:1160-62.
198. McCluggage WG, Desai V, Manek S. Tamoxifen-associated postmenopausal adenomyosis exhibits stromal fibrosis, glandular dilatation and epithelial metaplasias. Histopathology 2000;37:340-6.
199. Goldblum JR, Clement PB, Hart WR. Adenomyosis with sparse glands. A potential mimic of low-grade endometrial stromal sarcoma. Am J Clin Pathol 1995;103:218-23.
200. Meenakshi M, McCluggage WG. Vascular involvement in adenomyosis: report of a large series of a common phenomenon with observations on the pathogenesis of adenomyosis. Int J Gynecol Pathol 2010;29:117-21.
201. Cole AJ, Quick CM. Patterns of myoinvasion in endometrial adenocarcinoma: recognition and implications. Adv Anat Pathol 2013;20:141-7.
202. Mittal KR, Barwick KW. Diffusely infiltrating adenocarcinoma of the endometrium. A subtype with poor prognosis. Am J Surg Pathol 1988;12:754-8.
203. Ismiil N, Rasty G, Ghorab Z, et al. Adenomyosis involved by endometrial adenocarcinoma is a significant risk factor for deep myometrial invasion. Ann Diagnc Pathol 2007;11:252-7.
204. Toki T, Shimizu M, Takagi Y, Ashida T, Konishi I. CD10 is a marker for normal and neoplastic endometrial stromal cells. Int J Gynecol Pathol 2002;21:41-7.
205. Shintaku M, Tsuta K, Matsumoto T. Blue nevus of the endometrium. Int J Gynecol Pathol 2003;22:294-6.
206. Ishida M, Kagotani A, Yoshida K, Iwai M, Okabe H. Endometrioid adenocarcinoma concurrent with a blue nevus of the endometrium and uterine cervix: a case report. Oncol Lett 2013;6:1219-21.
207. Ganesan R, Ferryman SR, Meier L, Rollason TP. Vasculitis of the female genital tract with clinicopathologic correlation: a study of 46 cases with follow-up. Int J Gynecol Pathol 2000;19:258-65.
208. Bell DA, Mondschein M, Scully RE. Giant cell arteritis of the female genital tract. A report of three cases. Am J Surg Pathol 1986;10:696-701.
209. Buzzi A, Pezzica E, Crescini C, Sironi PL, Sonzogni A, Ziliani A. [Giant-cell arteritis of the female genital tract.] Minerva Ginecol 1993;45:425-8. [Italian]
210. Scurry J, Planner R, Fortune DW, Lee CS, Rode J. Ligneous (pseudomembranous) inflammation of the female genital tract. A report of two cases. J Reprod Med 1993;38:407-12.
211. Pantanowitz L, Fraser JL. Ligneous change of the female genital tract. Fertil Steril 2002;78:1123-4.
212. Taube ET, Frangini S, Caselitz J, et al. Ligneous cervicitis in a woman with plasminogen deficiency associated with an atypical form of microglandular hyperplasia: a case report and review of literature. Int J Gynecol Pathol 2013;32:329-34.
213. Winkler DD, Emery JA, Alan CB. Amyloidosis of the endometrium: an asymptomatic presentation. Obstet Gynecol 2004;104(Pt 2):1144-7.
214. Yue CC, Lampman JH, Park CH, Ballou SP. Secondary amyloidosis: diagnosis from an endometrial biopsy. Arthritis Rheum 1983;26:1295-6.
215. Kotru M, Chandra H, Singh N, Bhatia A. Localized amyloidosis in endometrioid carcinoma of the uterus: a rare association. Arch Gynecol Obstet 2007;276:383-4.

3 ENDOMETRIAL POLYP

An *endometrial polyp* is a benign growth of endometrial glands and stroma that protrudes above the endometrial surface. Endometrial polyps are covered by endometrioid epithelium. The endometrial glands may be uniformly or irregularly shaped and distributed within a stroma that can range from typical endometrial to a variety of other types (discussed below).

CLINICAL FEATURES

Endometrial polyps are common lesions, found in as many as 25 percent of women, typically in those over 40 years and postmenopausal. They are rare in premenarchal women. Endometrial polyps are often asymptomatic, but if large, can extend into and protrude through the cervical os, or undergo surface trauma. They may cause intermenstrual spotting/bleeding, menometrorrhagia, or postmenopausal bleeding. Polyps are also detected during infertility workups since they can be a contributing factor to the inability to conceive, likely due to mechanical interference.

Excisional curettage is generally adequate to treat polyp-related symptoms. Polyps commonly recur, however, as they are often incompletely removed during curettage or they regrow under continuing hormonal stimulation (1).

PATHOGENESIS

The pathogenesis of endometrial polyps is presumed to be an overgrowth of the endometrial basalis layer, probably (but not necessarily) resulting from estrogenic stimulation. Endometrial polyps do not predispose to endometrial neoplasia but can be mimics of neoplastic proliferations, particularly in fragmented specimens (discussed below). Polyps have been reported in patients taking tamoxifen for breast cancer, suggesting that endometrial polyps and neoplasia may share risk factors regardless of whether polyps are a true precursor to cancer (2). This concept is supported by the finding that about 25 percent of patients with endometrial carcinoma have accompanying endometrial polyp(s), similar to the background prevalence of endometrial polyps in the general population (1,3).

Among studies detailing the risk of endometrial carcinoma in the setting of polyps, two reported incidences of 3.5 (4) and 1.8 percent (5); the higher incidence study included patients that had received intracavitary radiation, a known risk factor for the development of endometrial cancer. Another study showed that 4.6 percent of polyps were associated with endometrial neoplasia (3.3 percent hyperplasia with atypia and 1.3 percent carcinoma) (6), while another showed only a slightly higher rate of carcinoma (3.2 percent), but a much higher rate of hyperplasia (11.3 percent), although the latter figure is likely too high, representing overdiagnosis of hyperplasia in the setting of a polyp (7). Yet, another study showed an 18 percent incidence of hyperplasia in endometrial polyps (7 percent atypical) with the number being even higher in postmenopausal women (21 percent; 12 percent atypical hyperplasia), again most likely representing overdiagnosis (8).

GROSS FINDINGS

On gross examination, endometrial polyps can be pedunculated or broad-based (fig. 3-1), with variable size. If large, they can fill the entire uterine cavity and be easily identified on radiologic exam (fig. 3-2). A large study of over 1,000 polyps found the size to range from 0.3 to 12.0 cm, with a mean slightly above 2 cm (9).

Endometrial polyps are found in any location within the uterine corpus or the lower uterine segment. In the latter location, they can protrude from the external os and be clinically misinterpreted as being of endocervical origin. Endometrial polyps are multiple in about 20 percent of cases. They typically display a smooth

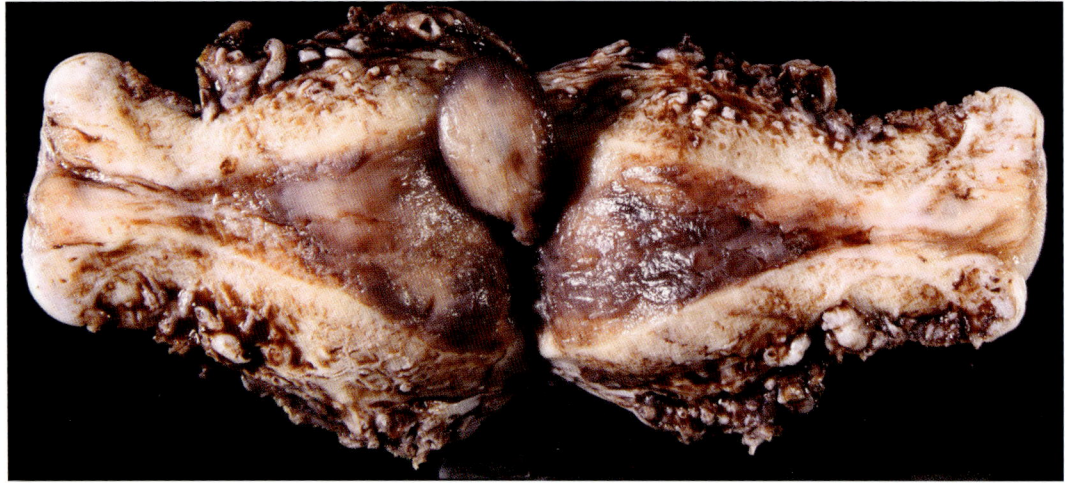

Figure 3-1

ENDOMETRIAL POLYP

Gross illustration of an endometrial polyp with the base in the apex of the uterine corpus. The tip of the polyp is hemorrhagic, which may lead to the common presenting symptom of abnormal uterine bleeding.

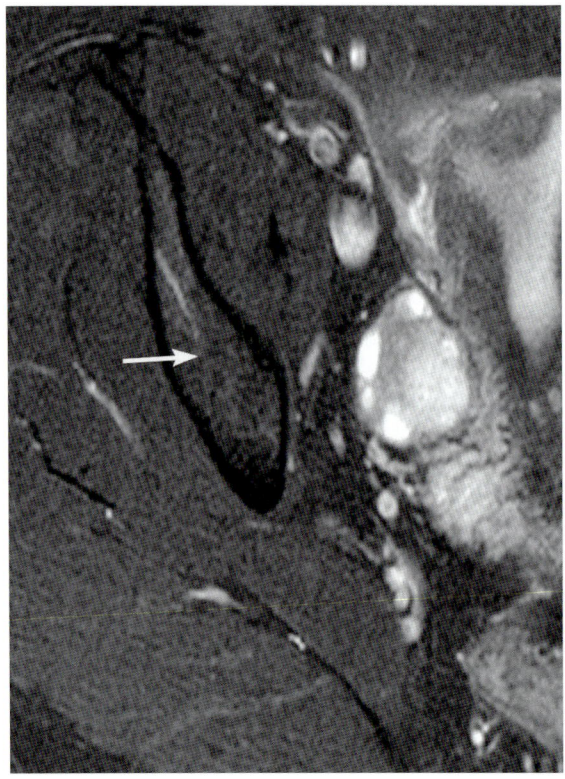

Figure 3-2

ENDOMETRIAL POLYP

Magnetic resonance imaging (MRI) of an endometrial polyp filling the uterine cavity (arrow). (Courtesy of Dr. S. F. Wilbur, Rochester, NY.)

tan surface, but red-brown granular areas may be seen secondary to erosion/trauma.

MICROSCOPIC FINDINGS

Microscopically, since endometrial polyps correspond to a three-dimensional structure, they are lined on three sides by endometrioid epithelium, which is typically derived from the basalis portion of the endometrium (fig. 3-3, left). The endometrial glands most commonly have a non-functioning inactive basalis, are proliferative type, or show a combination of these patterns (fig. 3-3, right). Mild secretory changes may be present, but it is unusual to see normally cycling secretory endometrium in polyps since they do not typically follow the normal endometrial cycle. In most cases, the endometrial glands are irregularly distributed within the polyp and have variable sizes and shapes, including outpouchings, angulation, and cystic change (fig. 3-4). The presence of cystic change should not be misdiagnosed as non-atypical hyperplasia within an endometrial polyp.

The stroma of the polyp is often abundant and composed of inactive endometrial stromal cells imparting a "compact" blue appearance, but may be hypocellular due to collagenization or fibrosis (fig. 3-5). The stroma can occasionally show smooth muscle differentiation (adenomyomatous polyp [10]), and rarely large,

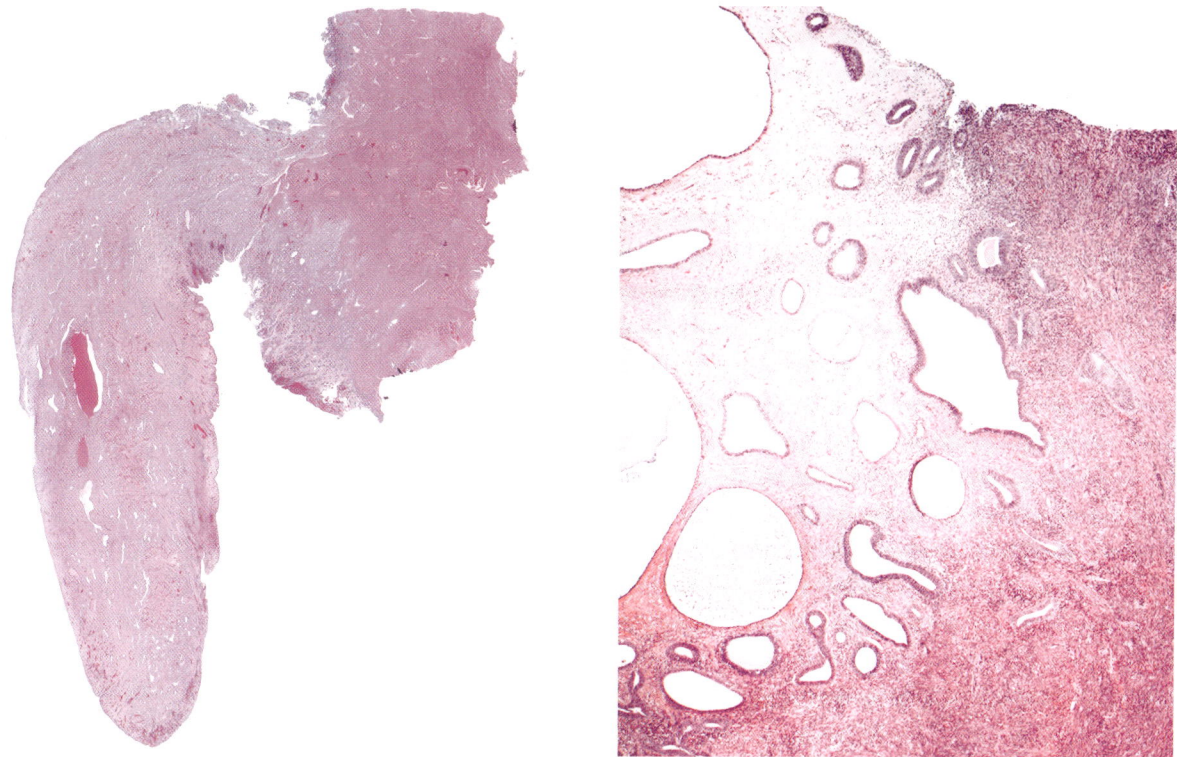

Figure 3-3

ENDOMETRIAL POLYP

Endometrial polyps form a three-dimensional structure arising from the basalis (left). A clear distinction is seen between the basalis and the collagenized polyp with prominent cystic glands (right).

atypical spindled or epithelioid stromal cells that are degenerative/reactive (fig. 3-6) (11). Histiocytes and inflammatory cells are often noted within the stroma, most frequently lymphocytes and plasma cells. In a patient with an endometrial polyp, the finding of plasma cells does not indicate the presence of chronic endometritis. It may be challenging in a curettage specimen to determine which fragments belong to the polyp and thus, in the presence of a definitive polyp, the diagnosis of chronic endometritis should be avoided. Intact polyps have prominent plexuses of thick-walled "feeder" vessels at the base or in the pedunculated stalk (fig. 3-7), a feature of significant diagnostic importance in fragmented specimens.

A variety of histologic patterns are seen in endometrial polyps, which has led in the past to their classification as hyperplastic, atrophic, or functional. Due to significant overlap in their appearance, this classification is not generally used in clinical practice, but may serve as an "exercise" to identify types of differentiation that may enter the differential diagnosis of non-polyp mimics in challenging specimens. For instance, the hyperplastic-type endometrial polyp shows more crowded endometrioid glands and more irregular pseudostratified cells within the glands than typical proliferative endometrial glands. This appearance needs to be distinguished from endometrial hyperplasia/endometrial intraepithelial neoplasia (EIN) (see chapter 4). Endometrial hyperplasia/EIN can involve an endometrial polyp, making a correct interpretation even more challenging. Atrophic polyps contain glands with low cuboidal epithelium and cystically dilated glands. Functional polyps, much less common than hyperplastic or atrophic polyps, show evidence of hormonal responsiveness and can, therefore, show either proliferative or, less commonly, secretory changes within the glands. Atrophic and functional

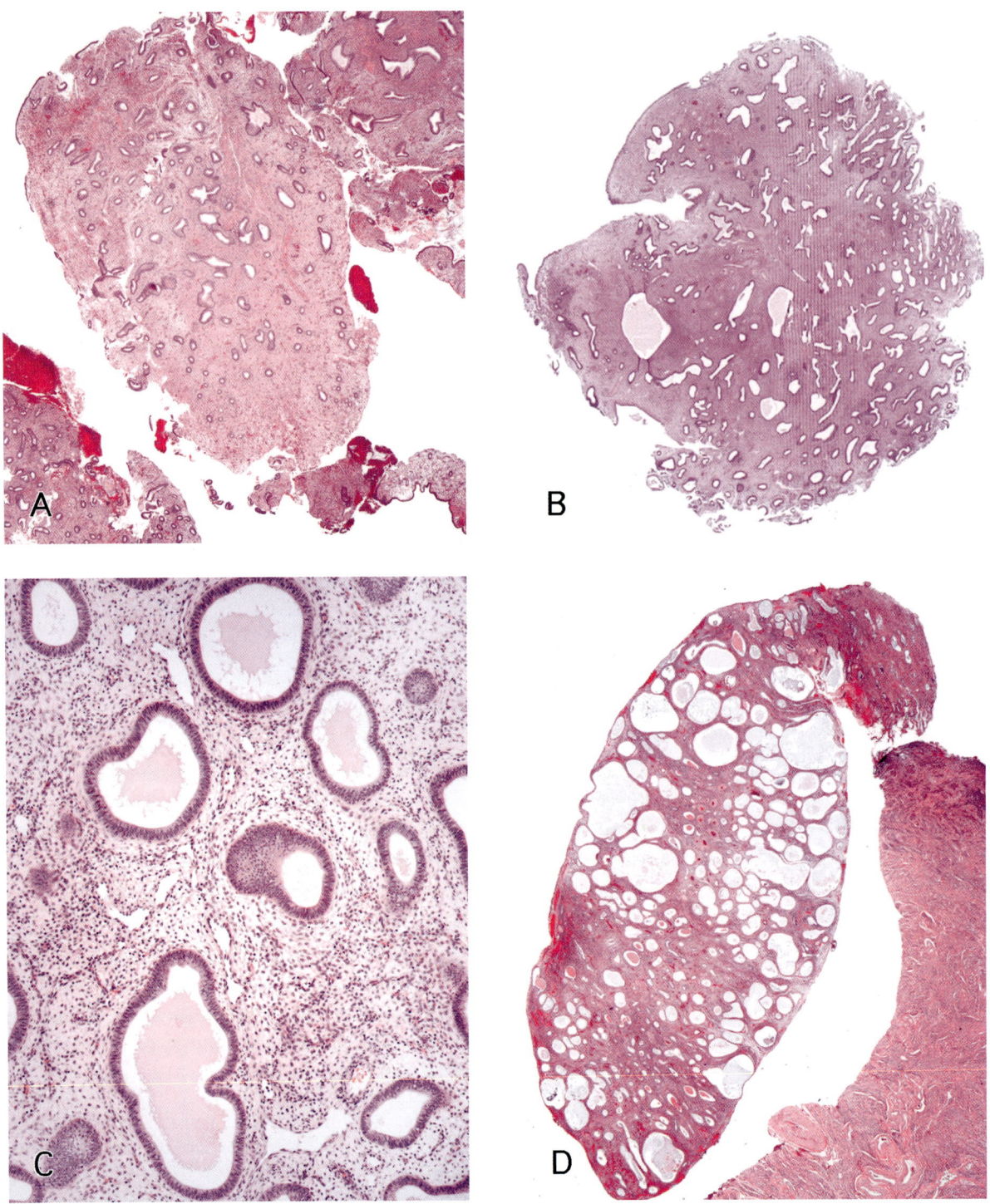

Figure 3-4

ENDOMETRIAL POLYP

The typical endometrial polyps, shown at low (A,B), and high (C) magnifications, display a disorganized arrangement of proliferative-type glands with some cystic change and a mild degree of gland irregularity. The latter contrasts with the more uniform small glands of the adjacent normal proliferative endometrium (A). Polyps may show prominent cystic change in the glands (D).

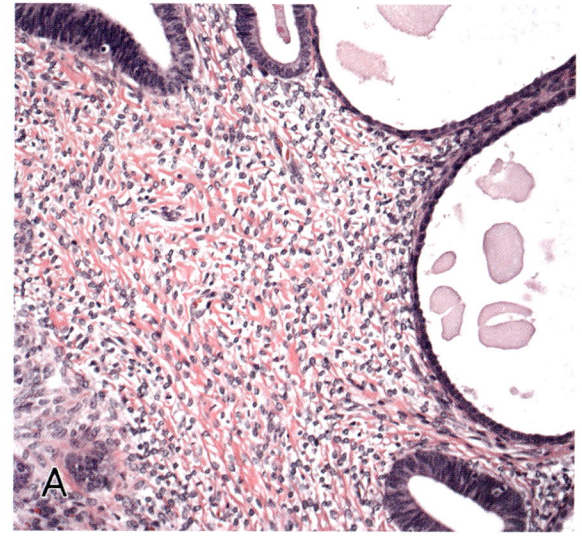
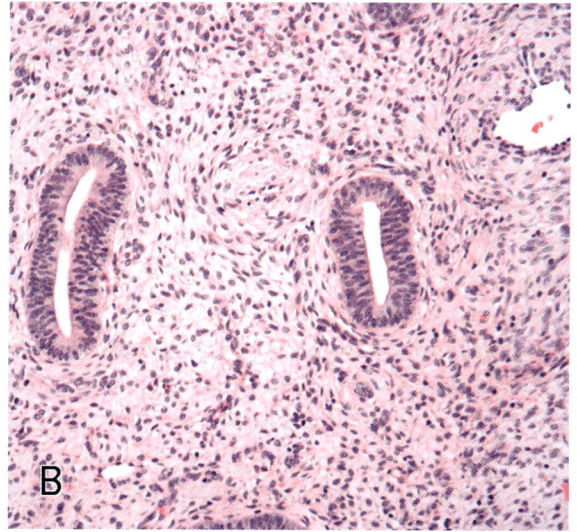
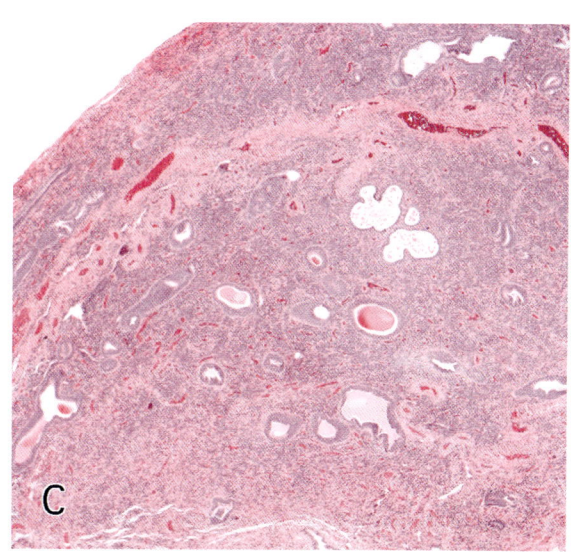

Figure 3-5

ENDOMETRIAL POLYP

Endometrial polyps can have typical endometrial stroma, however, areas of collagenization can be present either focally or extensively (A–C).

Figure 3-6

ATYPICAL STROMAL CELLS

Endometrial polyps can show atypical stromal cells with enlarged, irregular, and hyperchromatic nuclei. Although these cells may simulate sarcomatous change, they are reactive/degenerative in nature. Smudged chromatin and multinucleation are clues to the reactive nature of the cells.

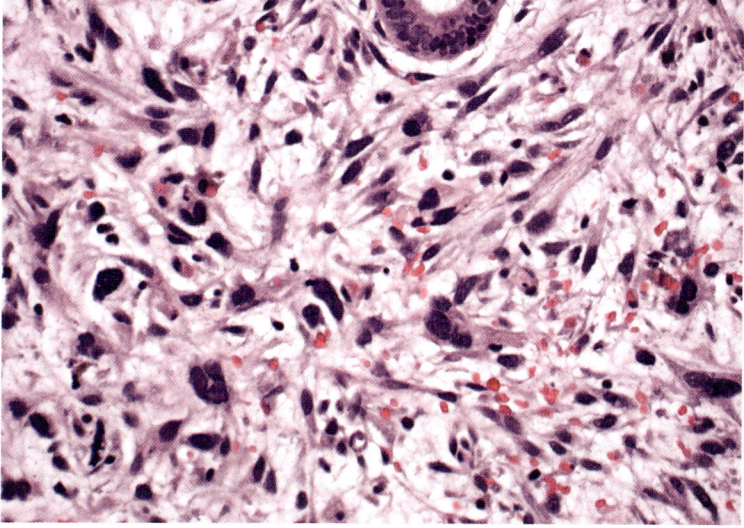

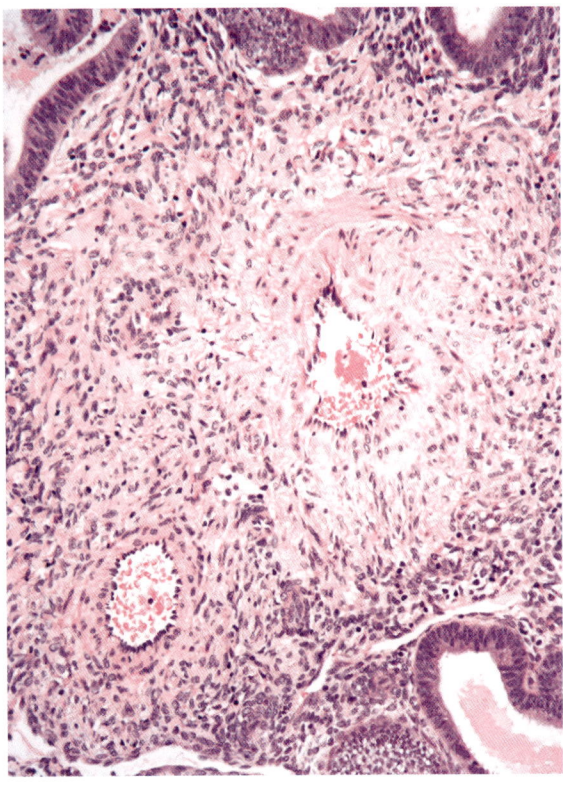

Figure 3-7

THICK-WALLED BLOOD VESSELS IN ENDOMETRIAL POLYP

A vascular plexus of thick-walled vessels is often found at the base of an endometrial polyp and can be a helpful clue to this diagnosis in curetted samples.

endometrial polyps usually do not cause problems in differential diagnosis (12).

A variety of metaplastic changes can be present in endometrial polyps, particularly when they undergo surface trauma or infarction. Tubal, squamous, papillary, and mucinous metaplasias, and eosinophilic degenerative or hobnail changes can involve small or large segments of the polyp epithelium and often they coexist (fig. 3-8).

The so-called Lehman-Hart polyp or papillary proliferation of Lehman and Hart, shows exuberant but variable architecturally complex papillary tufts of cytologically bland metaplastic epithelium (any type but most commonly mucinous) with fibrovascular cores within the surface or glands of an endometrial polyp. This metaplastic change frequently involves a significant proportion of the polyp (fig. 3-8B) (13,14). If simple and limited in amount, these changes typically are associated with an uneventful outcome. When architecturally complex, they can be difficult to differentiate from atypical hyperplasia, particularly in fragmented curettage specimens. When complex or extensive, they have been shown to be associated with (about 15 percent) concurrent endometrial hyperplasia or low-grade endometrial adenocarcinoma and thus, they should be regarded as analogous to atypical hyperplasia, and the term "complex papillary hyperplasia" is advised to alert the clinician (14) (see chapter 2).

Although endometrial polyps in patients with breast cancer treated with tamoxifen do not have pathognomonic histologic features, they are frequently large and more often associated with stromal fibrosis and mucinous metaplasia. Some investigators have also described staghorn glands and stromal condensation around the glands in patients taking tamoxifen (fig. 3-9). As patients with tamoxifen are at higher risk for the development of endometrial hyperplasia/carcinoma and may have metastatic breast carcinoma, it is important to closely evaluate endometrial polyps in this setting in order to exclude these diagnoses (15–18). If the metastatic breast carcinoma is of lobular type, it may be a subtle morphologic finding in the polyp stroma (19). If the diagnosis of hyperplasia is made in polyps whether associated or not with tamoxifen therapy (especially in a curettage specimen), it is important to evaluate the nonpolypoid endometrium as hyperplasia may not be limited to the endometrial polyp. The finding of non-polyp areas of hyperplasia suggests more aggressive patient treatment.

DIFFERENTIAL DIAGNOSIS

Endometrial polyps may focally display a morphology that suggests a low-grade müllerian adenosarcoma. Concerning histologic features include focal abnormal "phyllodes-like" architecture of the endometrial glands (most common), focal periglandular stromal condensation and increased mitoses which may be seen in isolation or combined. This group represented less than 0.02 percent of all endometrial polyps at one institution (20). Follow-up in these patients is usually uneventful but they are typically young and thus, overtreatment should be avoided.

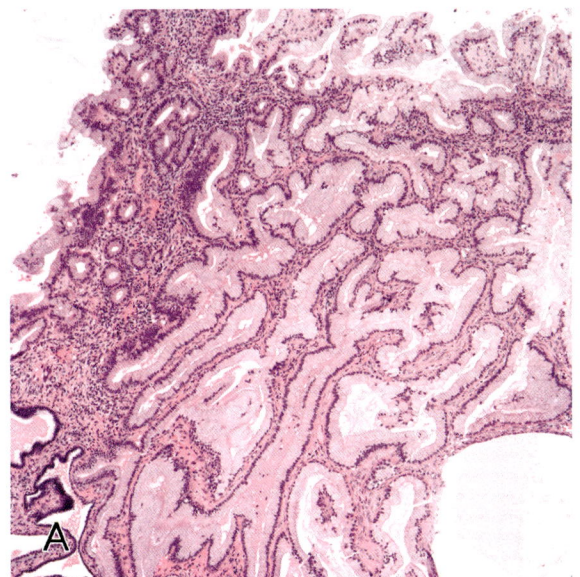

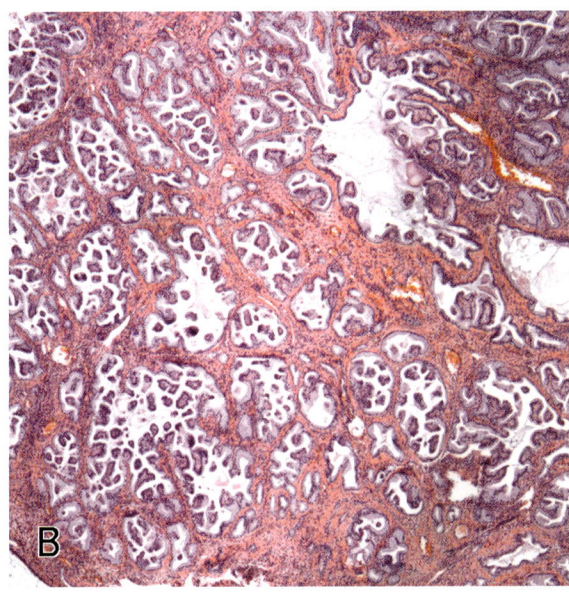

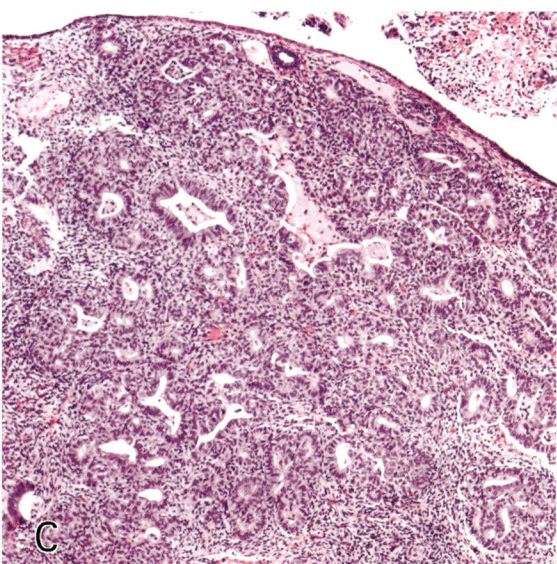

Figure 3-8
MUCINOUS METAPLASIA

Mucinous metaplasia within a polyp is common and may cause concern for carcinoma (A). Papillary proliferation of Lehman and Hart occurs often in polyps and shows extensive metaplastic changes with prominent tufted epithelium. This variant can cause concern for endometrial neoplasia, particularly in fragmented specimens due to the complex architecture. When markedly crowded, it is best to treat such proliferations as potentially neoplastic due to the high association (up to 15%) with endometrial hyperplasia/cancer (B). Tubal metaplasia can also impart a busy appearance to the endometrial glands and be overdiagnosed as hyperplasia (C).

As noted above, true endometrial neoplasia (hyperplasia/EIN), and serous and clear cell carcinomas are occasionally present in endometrial polyps (fig. 3-10). These neoplasms can diffusely involve the polyp or may represent very small foci. Even small malignant tumors involving polyps should, in most cases, be treated similarly to their counterparts found in the native endometrial tissue. Importantly, the finding of a malignancy in a polyp does not mean that the nonpolypoid endometrium is uninvolved.

Young women with a diagnosis of atypical endometrial hyperplasia/EIN or endometrioid carcinoma confined to a polyp can be treated conservatively in order to preserve fertility, provided there has been a thorough examination of the endometrial lining via curettage. In older patients, even small foci of high-grade intraepithelial carcinoma (serous) in a polyp may prompt hysterectomy and full staging (20). Patients with only a minor focus of high-grade carcinoma in an otherwise atrophic curetted polyp have been shown to have advanced disease on hysterectomy (21,22).

Atypical polypoid adenomyoma (APA) may have a gross appearance similar to an

Tumors of the Uterine Corpus and Gestational Trophoblastic Diseases

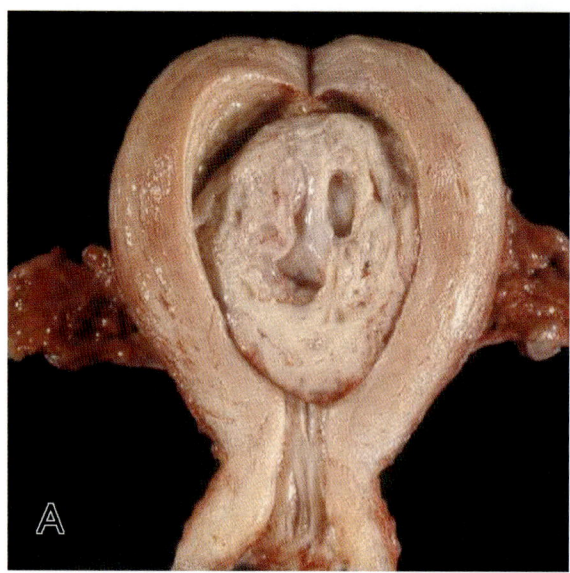

Figure 3-9

TAMOXIFEN-RELATED POLYP

A large polyp (A) is characterized by a heavily collagenized stroma (B,C), and fills the endometrial cavity. (Courtesy of Dr. X. Matias-Guiu, Barcelona, Spain.)

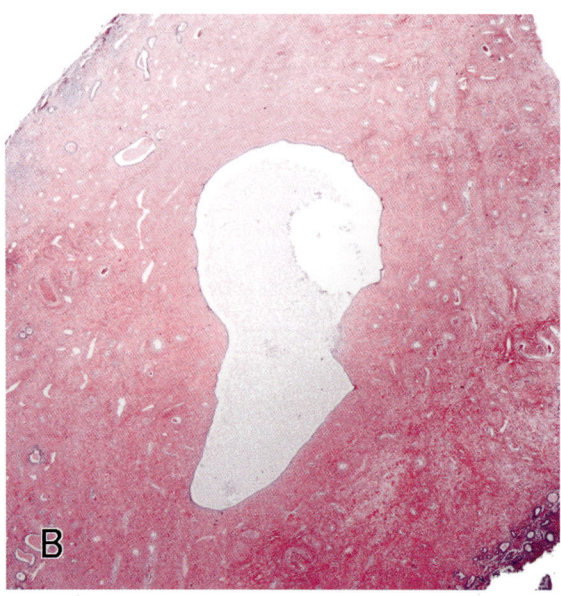

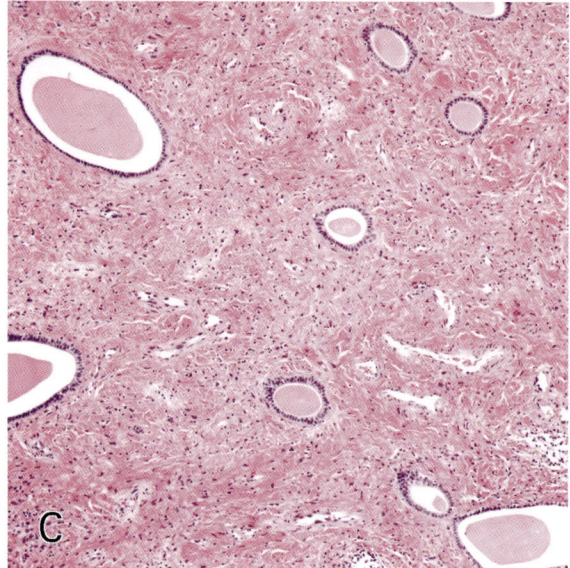

endometrial polyp and thus may enter into the differential diagnosis. It is found in reproductive or perimenopausal women with a mean age of 39 years (23). It shares risk factors with endometrial neoplasia, including estrogen stimulation, nulliparous status, obesity, and Turner syndrome. Conservative management is generally recommended. On microscopic examination, the major diagnostic consideration is not an endometrial polyp but low-grade endometrioid carcinoma, particularly in fragmented specimens. In contrast to typical endometrial polyp, APA more commonly involves the lower uterine segment. Like typical endometrial polyp, APA also presents with abnormal bleeding but in contrast to the latter, consists of haphazardly arranged atypical endometrioid glands within a cellular smooth muscle stroma. The endometrioid glands show prominent pseudostratification, enlarged nuclei, prominent nucleoli, and mitotic activity. The cytoplasm is abundant and eosinophilic. These cellular features are similar to those seen in atypical endometrial hyperplasia; however, although the glands may be packed, there is a characteristic lobular architecture. A common and helpful feature is

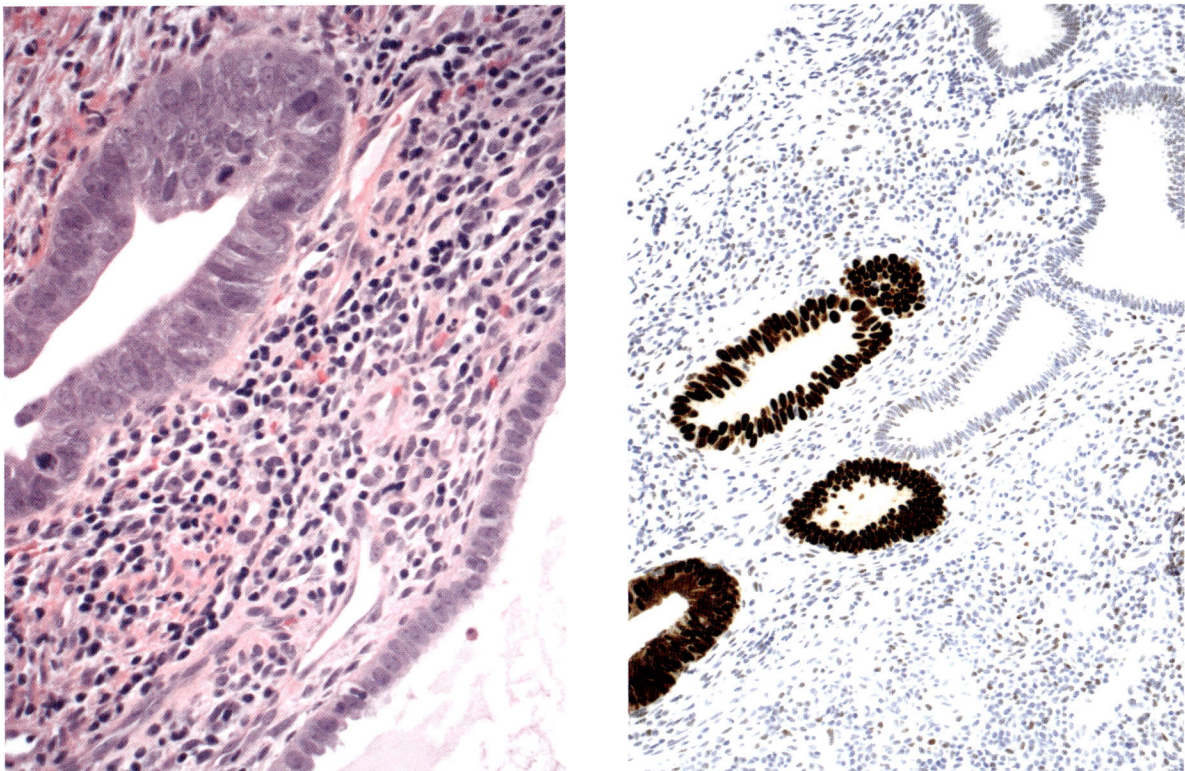

Figure 3-10

SEROUS CARCINOMA IN ENDOMETRIAL POLYP

Serous carcinoma is identified in otherwise benign-appearing endometrial polyp. The neoplastic glands can be focal or diffuse and often are innocuous-appearing at low magnification. The typical appearance of serous carcinoma is shown (left) in comparison to the normal benign glands. The serous carcinoma cells are tall, with marked atypia and frequent mitotic activity. p53 clearly delineates normal from neoplastic glands (right).

the presence of squamous morules within the gland lumens, sometimes with central necrosis, which can expand the glands, leading to a cribriform appearance. The stromal smooth muscle is arranged in short interlacing fascicles as opposed to the long muscle bundles present in normal myometrial tissue, and can be mitotically active (fig. 3-11). In contrast, smooth muscle in endometrial polyps tends to be located in the stalk and it is much less prominent. The low-power lobular architecture, presence of smooth muscle around groups of endometrial glands, squamous morule formation, and lack of gland crowding and architectural complexity are keys to a correct interpretation. Nevertheless, APA, as occurs in endometrial polyps, may be associated with malignancy, typically endometrioid carcinoma (23).

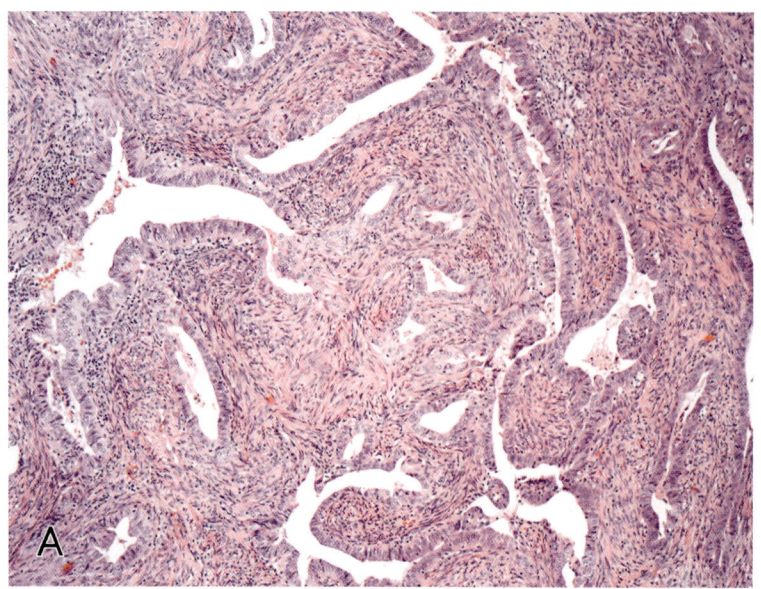
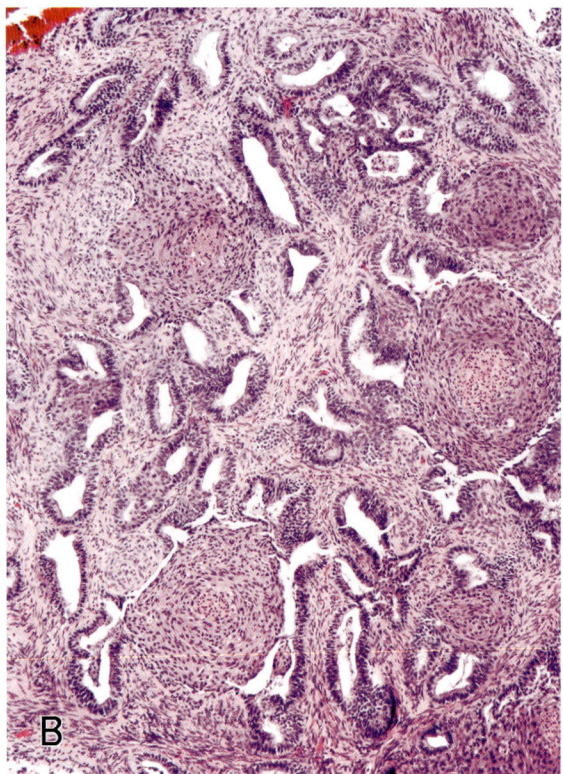
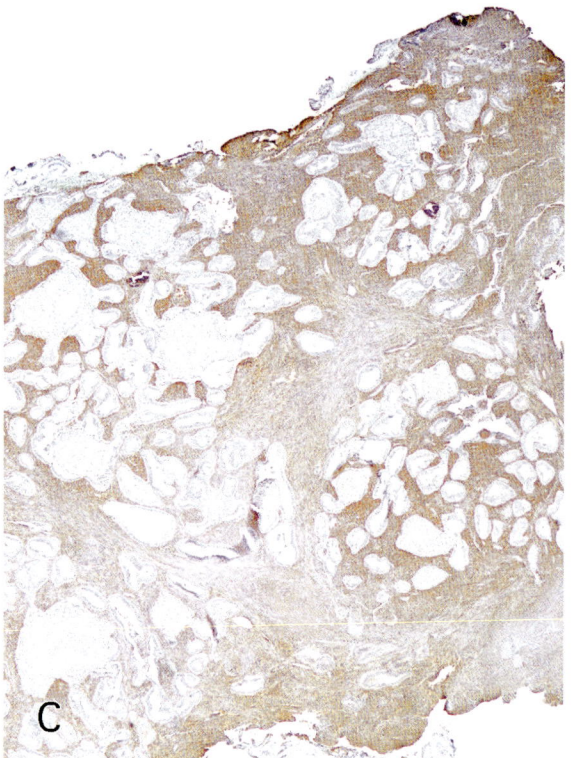

Figure 3-11

ATYPICAL POLYPOID ADENOMYOMA

Atypical polypoid adenomyoma may have a gross appearance similar to an endometrial polyp. However, it is composed of short interlacing fascicles of smooth muscle that separate endometrial glands (A). A classic feature is the benign morular squamous metaplasia that fills and expands the endometrial glands (B). Actin highlights the smooth muscle stroma as well as a vague nodular architecture (C).

REFERENCES

1. Lieng M, Istre O, and Qvigstad E. Treatment of endometrial polyps: a systematic review. Acta Obstet Gynecol Scand 2010; 89:992-1002.
2. Kalampokas T, Sofoudis C, Anastasopoulos C, et al. Effect of tamoxifen on postmenopausal endometrium. Eur J Gynaecol Oncol 2013;34:325-8.
3. Van Bogaert LJ. Clinicopathologic findings in endometrial polyps. Obstet Gynecol 1988;71:771-3.
4. Salm R. The incidence and significance of early carcinomas in endometrial polyps. J Pathol 1972;108: 47-53.
5. Martin-Ondarza C, Gil-Moreno A, Torres-Cuesta L, et al. Endometrial cancer in polyps: a clinical study of 27 cases. Eur J Gynaecol Oncol 2005;26: 55-8.
6. Elfayomy AK, Soliman BS. Risk factors associated with the malignant changes of symptomatic and asymptomatic endometrial polyps in premenopausal women. J Obstet Gynaecol India 2015;65:186-92.
7. Bakour SH, Khan KS, Gupta JK. The risk of premalignant and malignant pathology in endometrial polyps. Acta Obstet Gynecol Scand 2000;79:317-20.
8. Rahimi S, Marani C, Renzi C, Natale ME, Giovannini P, Zeloni R. Endometrial polyps and the risk of atypical hyperplasia on biopsies of unremarkable endometrium: a study on 694 patients with benign endometrial polyps. Int J Gynecol Pathol 2009;28:522-8.
9. Peterson WF, Novak ER. Endometrial polyps Obstet Gynecol 1956;8:40-9.
10. Strickland KC, Quade BJ, Nucci MR, Howitt BE. The clinicopathologic and immunohistochemical features of adenomyomatous polyps. Mod Pathol 2016;29,312A(Supplement 2).
11. Lo Monaco M, Puzzo L, Brancato F, Torrisi A, Magro G. Endometrial atypical (bizarre) stromal cells: a potential diagnostic pitfall in biopsy. Pathol Res Pract 2004;200:625-7; discussion 629-30.
12. Sherman ME, Mazur MT, Kurman RJ. Benign diseases of the endometrium. In: Kurman RJ, ed. Blaustein's Pathology of the female genital tract. New York: Springer; 2002:448-51.
13. Lehman MB, Hart WR. Simple and complex hyperplastic papillary proliferations of the endometrium: a clinicopathologic study of nine cases of apparently localized papillary lesions with fibrovascular stromal cores and epithelial metaplasia. Am J Surg Pathol 2001;25:1347-54.
14. Ip PP, Irving JA, McCluggage WG, Clement PB, Young RH. Papillary proliferation of the endometrium: a clinicopathologic study of 59 cases of simple and complex papillae without cytologic atypia. Am J Surg Pathol 2013;37:167-77.
15. Schlesinger C, Kamoi S, Ascher SM, Kendell M, Lage JM, Silverberg SG. Endometrial polyps: a comparison study of patients receiving tamoxifen with two control groups. Int J Gynecol Pathol 1998;17: 302-11.
16. Kennedy MM, Baigrie CF, Manek S. Tamoxifen and the endometrium: review of 102 cases and comparison with HRT-related and non-HRT-related endometrial pathology. Int J Gynecol Pathol 1999;18:130-7.
17. Nuovo MA, Nuovo GJ, McCaffrey RM, Levine RU, Barron B, Winkler B. Endometrial polyps in postmenopausal patients receiving tamoxifen. Int J Gynecol Pathol 1989;8:125-31.
18. Deligdisch L, Kalir T, Cohen CJ, de Latour M, Le Bouedec G, Penault-Llorca F. Endometrial histopathology in 700 patients treated with tamoxifen for breast cancer. Gynecol Oncol 2000;78:181-6.
19. Houghton JP, Ioffe OB, Silverberg SG, McGrady B, McCluggage WG. Metastatic breast lobular carcinoma involving tamoxifen-associated endometrial polyps: report of two cases and review of tamoxifen-associated polypoid uterine lesions. Mod Pathol 2003;16:395-8.
20. Howitt BE, Quade BJ, Nucci MR. Uterine polyps with features overlapping with those of Mullerian adenosarcoma: a clinicopathologic analysis of 29 cases emphasizing their likely benign nature. Am J Surg Pathol 2015;39:116-26.
21. Wheeler DT, Bell KA, Kurman RJ, Sherman ME. Minimal uterine serous carcinoma: diagnosis and clinicopathologic correlation. Am J Surg Pathol 2000;24:797-806.
22. Sherman ME, Bitterman P, Rosenshein NB, Delgado G, Kurman RJ. Uterine serous carcinoma. A morphologically diverse neoplasm with unifying clinicopathologic features. Am J Surg Pathol 1992;16:600-10.
23. Longacre TA, Chung MH, Rouse RV, Hendrickson MR. Atypical polypoid adenomyofibromas (atypical polypoid adenomyomas) of the uterus. A clinicopathologic study of 55 cases. Am J Surg Pathol 1996;20:1-20.

4 ENDOMETRIAL PRECANCEROUS NEOPLASIA

The term *endometrial hyperplasia* has over the years been applied to a heterogeneous group of lesions that have included both true precursors of endometrioid-type endometrial carcinoma and benign proliferations having some histologic features that mimic a true neoplastic process. In 1985, Kurman et al. (1) in a seminal study subdivided endometrial hyperplasia into two categories based on the presence of cytologic atypia. The authors found that the presence of cytologic atypia within endometrial hyperplasia was highly predictive of progression to or concurrent endometrial adenocarcinoma. The architectural pattern (simple versus complex) was thought to show additional risk, with "complex/atypical" lesions showing the highest rates of association with endometrioid carcinoma. Additional work, however, has shown that interobserver reproducibility in the assessment of what constitutes "cytologic atypia" and "architectural complexity" have been poor (2–4). The most recent World Health Organization (WHO)/International Society of Gynecological Pathologists (ISGYP) terminology (2014) continues to recognize cytologic atypia as a strong prognostic factor, but has eliminated architecture (simple versus complex) from its lexicon, leaving a binary system of nonatypical and atypical hyperplasia (5).

More recently, and in parallel to the hyperplasia classification noted above, another system, the endometrial intraepithelial neoplasia (EIN) concept, has been put forth. Studies using this designation have been shown to be more accurate than the classic hyperplasia classification in predicting which lesions progress to or have concurrent carcinoma (6,7). Although EIN has a conceptual basis tied to the molecular biology of endometrial cancer, as with the endometrial hyperplasia system, EIN utilizes histologic criteria alone to arrive at a diagnosis. The 2014 WHO terminology recognizes this parallel system as a correlate to atypical hyperplasia, although it has been shown that a small percentage of EIN lesions would, by histologic criteria, fall into the non-atypical hyperplasia category (8). Interestingly, lesions classified as EIN have been shown to capture carcinoma in the non-atypical hyperplasia category, indicative of the potential heightened importance of EIN criteria. As each system has clinical relevance and synergistic use, both are now accepted and are presented below.

EPIDEMIOLOGY

The diagnosis of endometrial hyperplasia/EIN is purely morphologic which has been shown to have poor interobserver reproducibility. Hence, historic data about prevalence and risk of cancer can be unreliable. However, the link between the endometrial hyperplasia/EIN/cancer spectrum and unopposed estrogen stimulation is robust. The use of exogenous estrogen as well as increased levels of endogenous estrogen associated with obesity, nulliparity, diabetes, and polycystic ovary disease have all been shown to be risk factors for endometrial neoplasia (9). As expected, significant declines in the incidence of all neoplastic categories were noted following the discontinuance of unopposed estrogen therapy in the mid 1970s. Rates have increased in recent years, most likely as a result of the obesity epidemic and its concomitant association with increased systemic estrogen levels (10,11).

The incidence of nonatypical hyperplasia is highest in women in the mid-50s compared to those of the mid-60s for both atypical hyperplasia/EIN and endometrioid carcinoma (the latter is rare below 30 years of age). In large population studies, most patients diagnosed with hyperplasia have nonatypical hyperplasia (as many as 85 percent) with the remainder having atypical hyperplasia (12,13). Compiled data shows important differences in prognosis between the two categories. Up to 80 percent of patients with atypical hyperplasia may already have carcinoma at the time the "hyperplasia" is

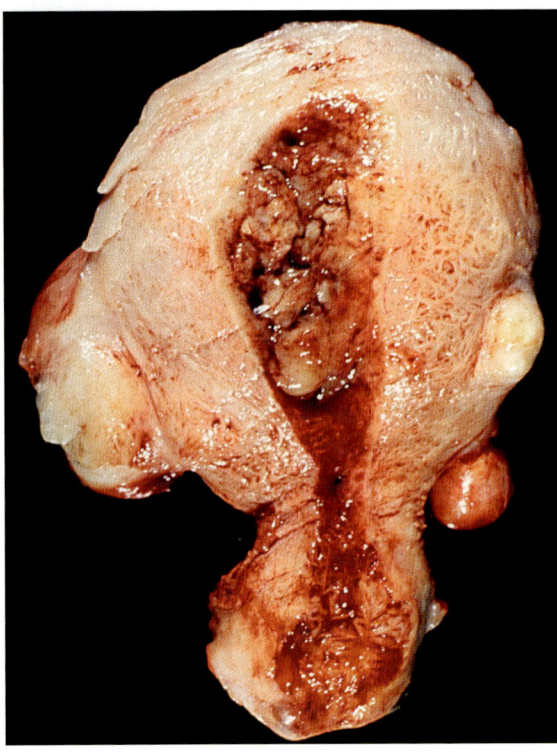

Figure 4-1

ENDOMETRIAL HYPERPLASIA IN A HYSTERECTOMY SPECIMEN

Endometrial precancers can show no obvious gross abnormality or they may present with a thickened endometrial lining. In this example, the endometrium is thickened with knobby surface projections.

diagnosed, or will progress to carcinoma within a 20-year follow-up period, as originally noted by Kurman (14). In contrast, only a small (1 to 3 percent) percentage of nonatypical hyperplasias evolve to carcinoma (1,13). Similar findings have been reported with EIN studies (15). As many as 15 percent of patients with EIN have concurrent carcinoma and 35 percent had persistent EIN on subsequent biopsy (8,16,17).

CLINICAL FEATURES

Endometrial hyperplasia/EIN usually presents as abnormal uterine bleeding at either premenopausal or postmenopausal age. The finding of benign endometrial cells in Papanicolaou tests from postmenopausal women was associated with a 12 percent rate of hyperplasia on follow-up in earlier studies (pre-2001). Because of this association, the 2nd edition of the Bethesda cervical cytology reporting system recommended reporting this finding in women over 40 years of age (18). Increased reporting of benign endometrial cells in Papanicolaou tests ensued, with a substantial drop in the positive predictive value of endometrial biopsies. The incidence of associated hyperplasia/cancer dropped to about 2 percent, with most cases showing that the endometrial cells were likely due to anovulation or normal menstrual flow in cycling women. This considerable loss of predictive value led the 3rd edition of the Bethesda reporting terminology to revise its recommendations, increasing the reportable age for benign-appearing endometrial cells in cervical cytology specimens to 45 years, with the caveat that this is applied only in postmenopausal women or when the menstrual status is not known. This change in the age threshold is expected to return the predictive value to higher levels (19).

Cervical cytology specimens containing "atypical" endometrial cells have a higher correlation with hyperplasia and carcinoma, although in most such instances, patients already have clinically apparent bleeding (20). Ultrasound of the uterine corpus for endometrial thickening in women having abnormal uterine bleeding has shown no significant predictive value for hyperplasia or carcinoma, however, measuring the endometrial "stripe" by ultrasonography (heterogeneity or cystic changes) does correlate with a higher risk of endometrial hyperplasia or carcinoma in all women regardless of bleeding history (21).

GROSS FINDINGS

Hyperplastic endometrium may be associated with no gross findings or a diffuse or polypoid thickening of the endometrial lining (fig. 4-1). In biopsy or curettage specimens there may be more voluminous amounts of tissue in the submitted sample, with larger tissue fragments than would be expected, especially in postmenopausal patients where scant tissue is the norm.

MOLECULAR GENETIC FINDINGS

The molecular alterations associated with endometrial hyperplasia/EIN overlap with those observed in endometrial adenocarcinoma, although they are typically encountered at a lower frequency. These include microsatellite instability, PAX2 inactivation, and mutations in PTEN, *PIK3CA*, *K-RAS*, and *CTNNB1* (22–25). *PTEN* mutations have been found in 15 to 55 percent of endometrial hyperplasias, with and without cytologic atypia, suggesting that PTEN loss represents an early event in endometrial carcinogenesis. A similar frequency of PTEN loss has been noted in EIN and proliferative endometrium (49 percent normal versus 44 percent EIN), significantly lower when compared to carcinomas (68 percent). In contrast, a similar prevalence of PAX2 loss has been shown in EIN and carcinoma (71 percent versus 77 percent loss), significantly higher than that observed in normal proliferative endometrium (36 percent) (26). Overall, however, coincident loss of PAX2 and PTEN expression is more common in precancers and carcinomas.

PTEN and *K-RAS* mutations occur in lesions with microsatellite instability typically involving MLH1, secondary to MLH1 promoter hypermethylation, a late event within the spectrum of hyperplasia/EIN/carcinoma (23,27). In contrast to *PTEN* mutations, *PIK3CA* mutations are associated with endometrial carcinoma but are uncommon in endometrial hyperplasia. They are frequently mutually exclusive with *PTEN* mutations (28). CTNN1 mutations are commonly seen in endometrial hyperplasia associated with squamous morular metaplasia and are not associated with other abnormalities (29).

Endometrial hyperplasia/EIN has a greater risk of association with genetic syndromes, particularly in younger women having Cowden and Lynch syndromes (30–32). Molecular evidence supports the clonal expansion of individual glands forming a premalignant lesion, challenging the long-held assumption that endometrial precancers exist as a continuum of diffuse and progressive disease.

DIAGNOSTIC CRITERIA

According to the WHO 2014 classification, hyperplasia, both nonatypical and atypical, is an exaggerated proliferation of glands, with an increase in gland to stroma ratio as compared to normal proliferative endometrium. The architectural patterns are highly variable but have in common back to back gland crowding with little intervening stroma, abnormal gland distribution, and irregular individual gland complexity showing branching, outpouchings, papillae, and cystic change (fig. 4-2). In nonatypical proliferations, the dividing line between hyperplasia and "disordered proliferative endometrium," a consequence of anovulatory cycling, can be difficult if not arbitrary (discussed below). Nonatypical hyperplasia shows nuclear features that are similar to those seen in cycling proliferative endometrium (fig. 4-3). Atypical hyperplasia shows gland crowding and an architecture similar to that described for nonatypical hyperplasia (fig. 4-4). However, aberrant nuclear changes, including enlargement, hyperchromasia, coarsely granular chromatin, pleomorphism, loss of polarity, large nucleoli, and mitotic activity are present (fig. 4-5). Unfortunately, evaluation of nuclear atypia is poorly reproducible, leading to significant overlap between the two categories. Zaino et al. (2) noted the poor reproducibility of atypical hyperplasia in a study in which a panel of pathologists rescored biopsies carrying a referral diagnosis of "atypical hyperplasia." They confirmed this diagnosis in only 38 percent of cases, with a kappa statistic showing poor reproducibility. In another study, Allison et al. (3) obtained similar results when a group of pathologists were asked to classify a random set of endometrial biopsies using the 1994 WHO system. Cytologic atypia, the best predictor of outcome in the WHO schema, was the feature leading to the most disagreement. These studies reflect the subjective nature of histologic assessment of premalignant endometrial lesions and help to partially explain the subsequent pursuit of more reliable diagnostic criteria to predict the risk/presence of endometrial cancer (Table 4-1).

Based on objective molecular data, Mutter et al. (7,33,34) sought to identify morphologic correlates of genetically-defined, clinically high-risk endometrial lesions to better subclassify endometrial proliferations as EIN, carcinoma, or mimics. An initial objective computer-assisted morphometric analysis informed the development of specific histologic criteria for EIN that could be applied in routine pathology practice. As in the hyperplasia system, the proposed EIN criteria also combined architecture and cytology, but with arguably less ambiguous definitions. The area of glands exceeds that of the stroma (stroma volume less than 55 percent), the cytology of the endometrial glands with crowding differs

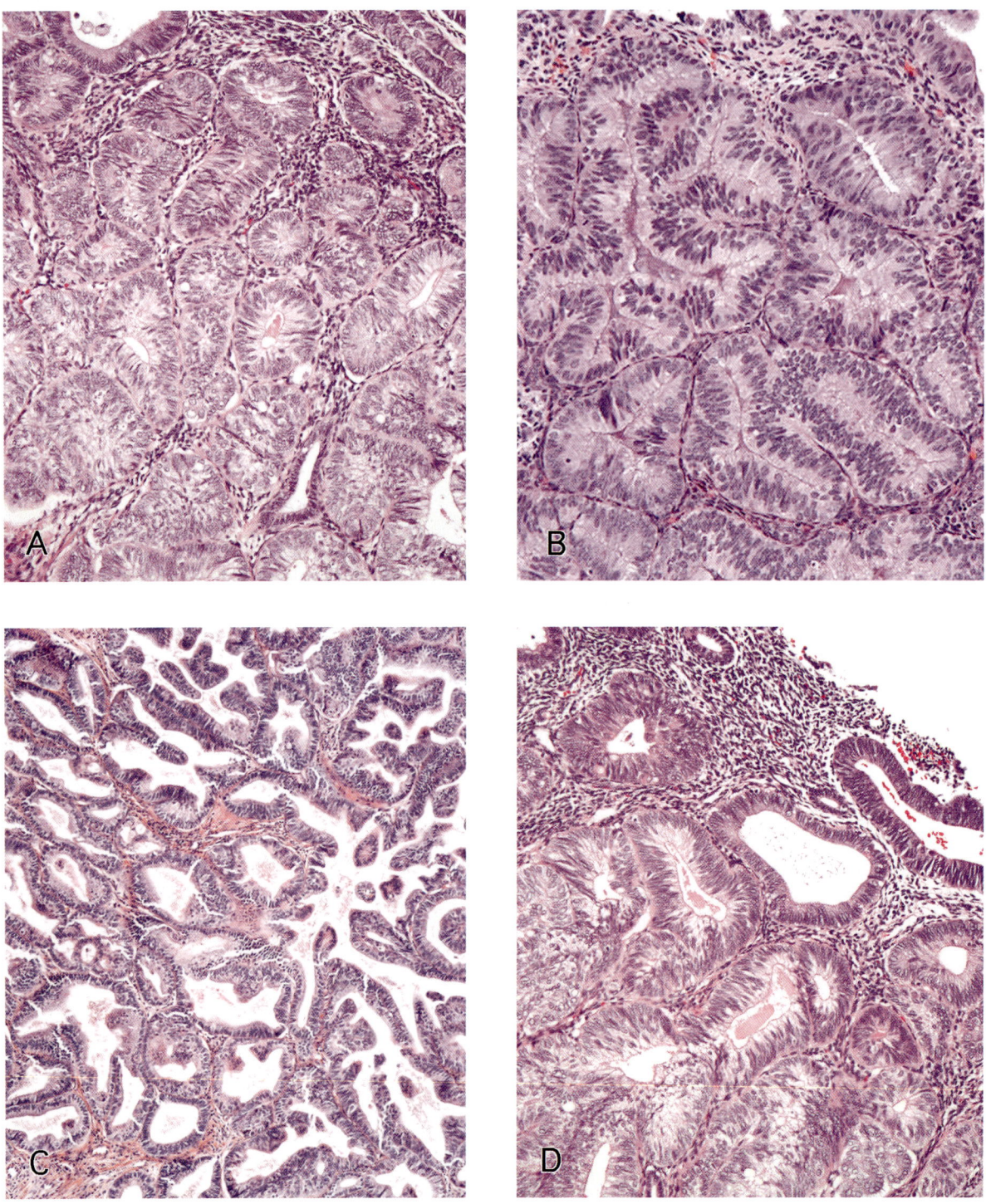

Figure 4-2

NONATYPICAL HYPERPLASIA

The glands show crowding, contour irregularities with outpouchings (A), gland branching (B), and papillae (C). The appearance of the glands is distinctly different from the background endometrial glands, which show less cytoplasm, less columnar cytoplasm, and less gland irregularity (D). The latter criterion is a necessary feature for the diagnosis of endometrial intraepithelial neoplasia (EIN). In all examples, the nuclear characteristics resemble those of normal proliferative endometrium.

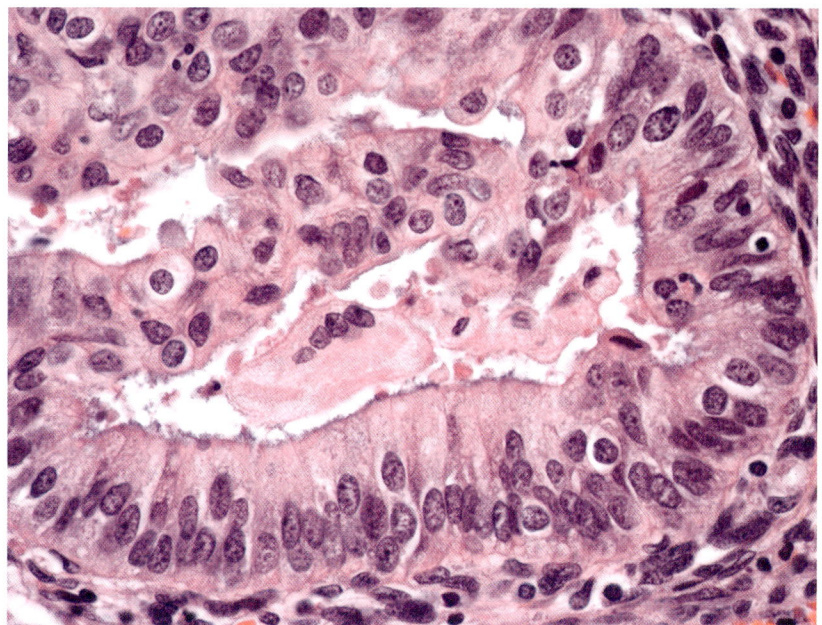

Figure 4-3

NONATYPICAL HYPERPLASIA

The cytologic features of nonatypical hyperplasia resemble those of normal cycling proliferative endometrium with uniform, oval to elongated nuclei.

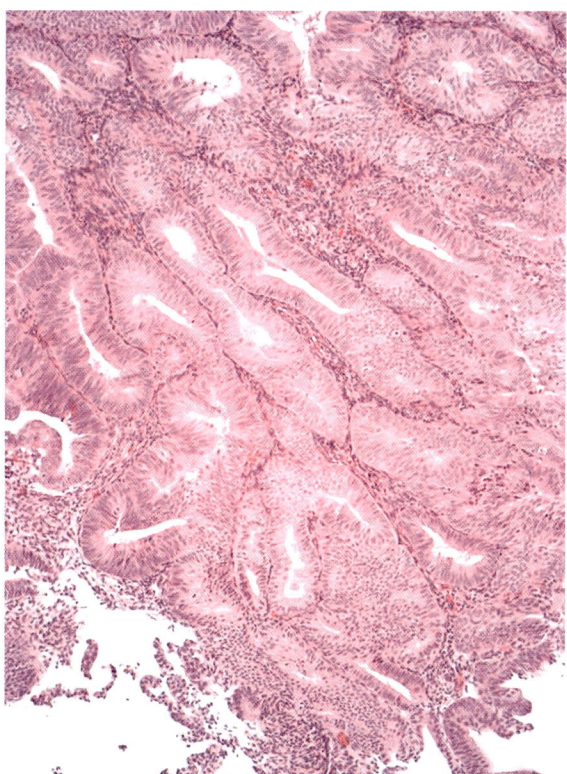 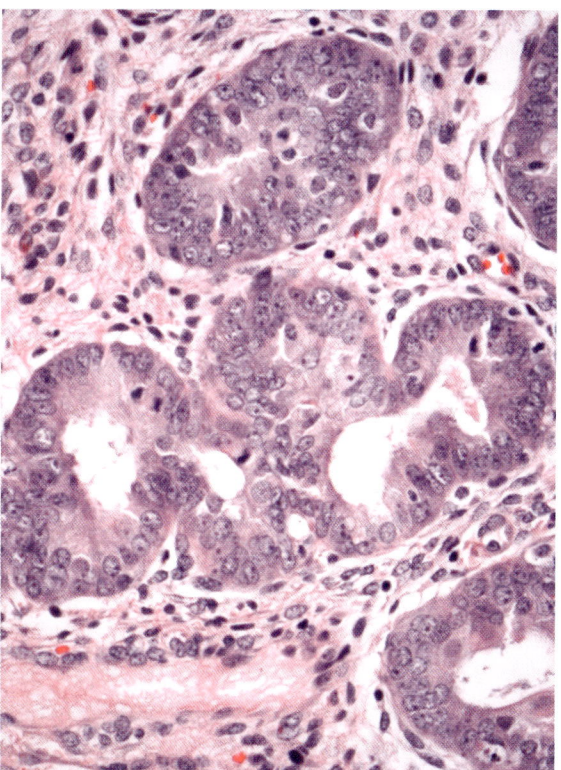

Figure 4-4

ATYPICAL HYPERPLASIA

The architectural configuration of the glands is similar to that of nonatypical hyperplasia with crowding and contour irregularity (left). At intermediate magnification, nuclear pseudostratification and frequent mitoses suggest atypical hyperplasia (right).

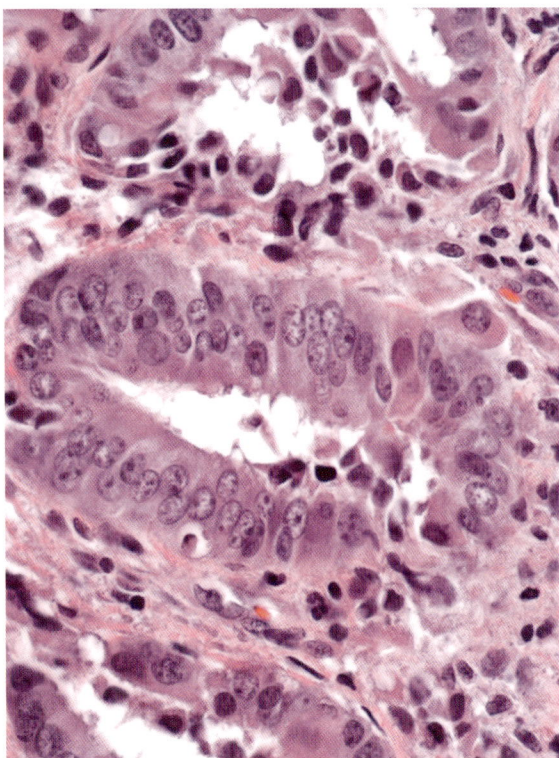

Figure 4-5

ATYPICAL HYPERPLASIA

The cytologic features of atypical hyperplasia resemble those of well-differentiated adenocarcinoma: nuclear size and shape variation, disorganization, prominent nucleoli, and hyperchromatic granular chromatin. Mitoses are more frequent than in nonatypical hyperplasia.

Table 4-1

CRITERIA FOR THE DIAGNOSIS OF ENDOMETRIAL PRECANCEROUS LESIONS

Nonatypical Hyperplasia
Exaggerated proliferation of endometrial glands
Variable architecture but may have some or all of the following features:
  irregular gland distribution
  gland complexity
  irregular individual glands—outpouching, branching, papillae, cystic dilatation
Increased gland to stroma ratio
Nuclear features similar to normal cycling proliferative endometrial glands

Atypical Hyperplasia
Exaggerated proliferation of endometrial glands
Variable architecture but may have some or all of the following features:
  irregular gland distribution
  gland complexity
  irregular individual glands—outpouching, branching, papillae, cystic dilatation
Increased gland to stroma ratio
Atypical nuclear features:
  enlargement
  pleomorphism (irregularity)
  prominent nucleoli
  hyperchromasia with coarse chromatin
  increased number of mitoses

Endometrial Intraepithelial Neoplasia (EIN)
Increased gland to stroma ratio (area occupied by glands exceeds that occupied by stroma)
Maximal linear dimension of crowded gland area exceeds 1mm
Cytology of crowded glands differs from background (nonaffected) endometrial glands
Benign (e.g., disordered proliferative endometrium, endometrial polyp) and malignant (e.g., endometrial carcinoma) entities are excluded

from the background endometrium, the maximum linear dimension of the crowded gland focus is at least 1 mm, and mimics (disordered proliferative endometrium, endometrial polyp, metaplasias) and endometrial cancer need to be excluded (figs. 4-6, 4-7). In a study reclassifying biopsies previously diagnosed by the WHO system using these EIN criteria, Hecht et al. (8) showed high interobserver (unanimous agreement on 75 percent of cases) and intraobserver reproducibility. A more recent international study demonstrated that, after self-training with published EIN guidelines, 79 percent of diagnoses made by 20 practicing pathologists were concordant with expert subspecialty diagnoses, showing moderate interobserver reproducibility for the diagnosis of EIN (35).

The performance of the EIN system is encouraging given the potential for improvement in reproducibility among pathologists and the relative ease with which the criteria may be learned and applied. In a direct comparison of the WHO and EIN criteria, the two do seem to fare similarly. Lacey et al. (15) evaluated the same original cases using the hyperplasia and EIN criteria independently and showed that the progression to carcinoma was comparable using both criteria. One salient difference seems to be relevant since it underscores the importance of diagnostic categories for clinical management. EIN criteria identify a minority of cases having cancer that would have been classified as nonatypical hyperplasia. The potential higher sensitivity of an EIN

Endometrial Precancerous Neoplasia

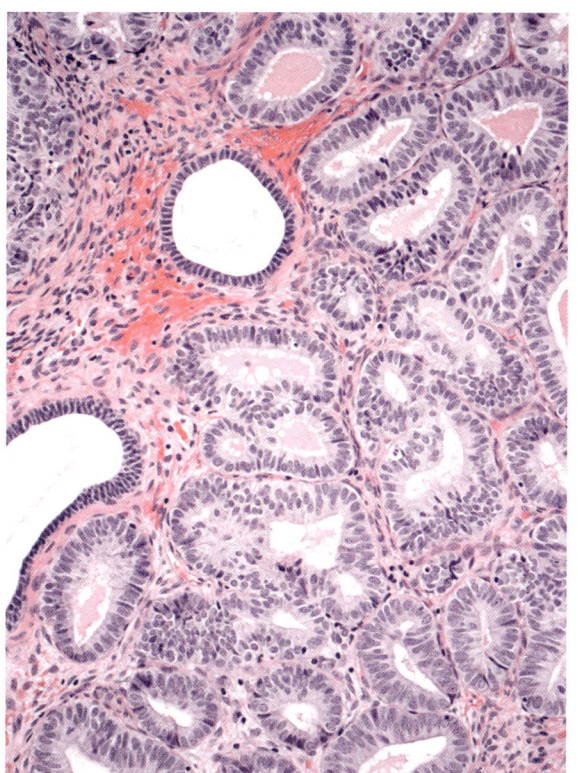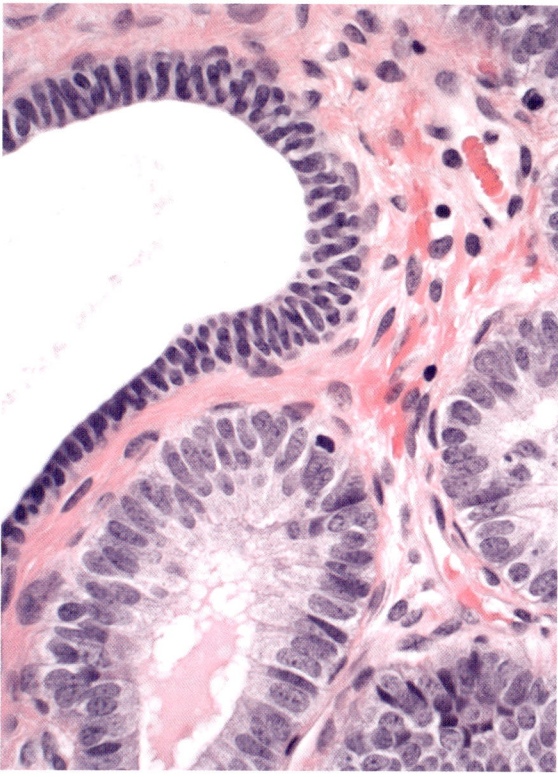

Figure 4-6

ENDOMETRIAL INTRAEPITHELIAL NEOPLASIA

Endometrial intraepithelial neoplasia criteria add the presence of background endometrium that is different than the glands of the putative precancerous lesion. The background cystically dilated glands show less height and cytoplasm than the precancerous glands at low (left) and high (right) magnification.

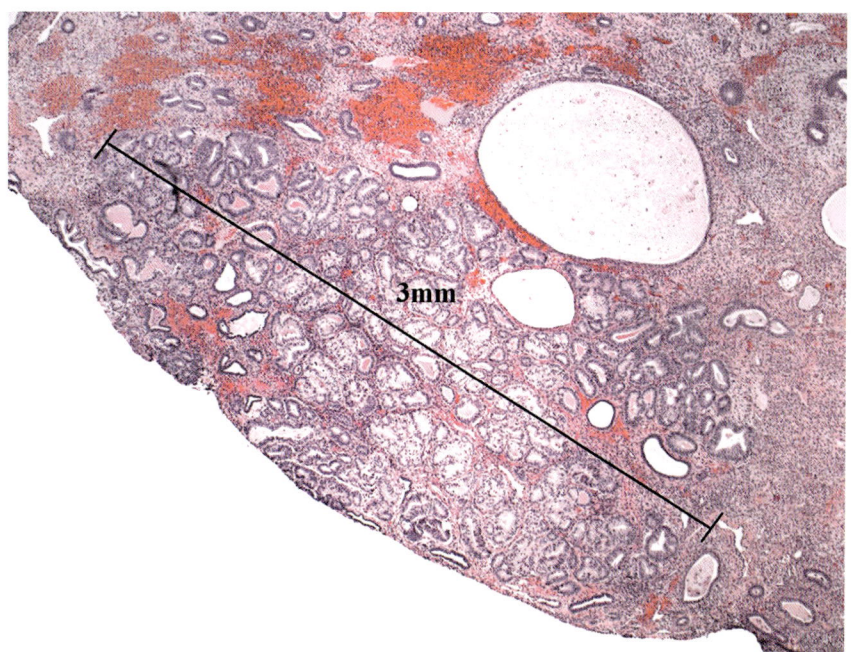

Figure 4-7

ENDOMETRIAL INTRAEPITHELIAL NEOPLASIA

The size of the crowded glandular area must be greater than 1 mm to qualify for a designation of EIN. In this example, the abnormal glandular proliferation measures 3 mm in greatest linear dimension.

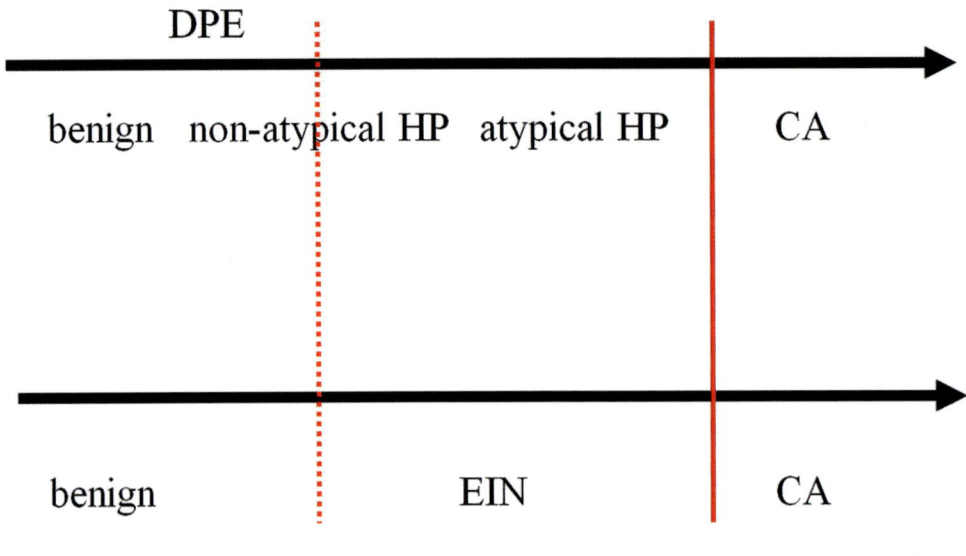

Figure 4-8

CONCEPTUAL VIEW OF ENDOMETRIAL PRECANCER TERMINOLOGY

This schematic shows the sequence from normal to cancer on two lines: the upper represents the nonatypical/atypical hyperplasia continuum and the bottom represents the EIN continuum. The approximate location of disordered proliferative endometrium (DPE) on the morphologic spectrum is shown. DPE overlaps with nonatypical hyperplasia. The solid red line on the right forms the "hard" distinction of precancer from cancer in both systems. The dotted line on the left shows the much more subjective distinction of benign from precancer. The EIN criteria are more predictive of true precancer since they better discriminate DPE from precancer.

diagnosis, with associated higher specificity for a malignant outcome demonstrated in several studies, indicates that use of the EIN criteria may be better at excluding cancer (7,36). As a recent Committee Opinion by the American College of Obstetrics and Gynecology suggests, the EIN schema may be slightly better at establishing criteria for distinguishing pathologic entities that should be managed differently (37). The EIN criterion of assessing the differences between the cytologic appearance of the putative lesion and the background benign endometrium appears to add sensitivity in facilitating an accurate and clinically relevant assessment.

Nevertheless, despite the appeal of the EIN system, the hyperplasia system continues to be the most widely used among pathologists, with its well-recognized, albeit somewhat subjective, criteria, and its greater acceptance/understanding among clinicians. From a practical standpoint, incorporating the useful points of both systems may be of most benefit in deciding which lesions are truly at risk of harboring cancer and which can be managed conservatively, particularly on the lower end of the disordered proliferative endometrium (DPE)/non-atypical hyperplasia morphologic spectrum (fig. 4-8).

DIFFERENTIAL DIAGNOSIS

The most common and problematic issue in endometrial neoplasia interpretation is distinguishing endometrial hyperplasia from a benign process, including even normal proliferative or secretory endometrium, in fragmented curettage specimens. In 100 consecutive cases referred with a diagnosis of hyperplasia, Winkler et al. (38), downgraded 16 to some variant of normal endometrium. Exuberant proliferative appearance, particularly in fragmented biopsy specimens in which the stroma may collapse or be broken apart, can lead to an artifactually crowded pattern of endometrial glands, with telescoped glands showing double lumens. In patients having prior curettage specimens, endometrial tissue may show significant reactive nuclear changes potentially leading to an impression of cytologic atypia, which can overlap with the findings in atypical hyperplasia.

Secretory endometrium, with its normal endometrial thickening, is abundant in a biopsy or curettage specimens and can lead to a concern that an endometrial neoplasia is present. In non-neoplastic secretory specimens, a homogeneous and delicate gross appearance of the endometrium is appreciated. Microscopic examination may show abundant crowded glands, leading to an overinterpretation of hyperplasia. Recognition of the secretory nature of the crowded glands is critical since "secretory hyperplasia," or true endometrial hyperplasia with diffuse secretory change, is extremely rare and thought to be secondary to ovulation occurring in a neoplastic endometrium, resulting in extreme crowding and disorganization (fig. 4-9) (39). The uniformity of glands in a linear orientation and parallel array and lack of cytologic atypia allow an appropriate benign interpretation.

In special circumstances, physiologic changes due to persistent estrogenic stimulation, or anovulatory proliferative patterns, can lead to mild glandular crowding, and when of long duration, the crowding can be more pronounced and the glands can become irregular. These patterns are frequently misinterpreted as non-atypical endometrial hyperplasia, but should be classified as DPE.

Distinction of DPE from endometrial hyperplasia/EIN requires careful examination of the distribution and uniformity of the "abnormal" glands. Glands from neoplastic lesions have a different morphologic appearance than the background glands and these areas of dissimilarity may be focal (more than 1 mm) or diffuse. In contrast, non-neoplastic processes show glandular uniformity across the specimen, with a similar appearance to the background non-crowded/noncomplex endometrial glands. In addition, anovulatory patterns typically show evidence of gland or stromal breakdown (40).

When evaluating endometrial samples with changes suggesting hyperplasia but on the "low end" of the spectrum where DPE and nonatypical hyperplasia are the major considerations in the differential diagnosis, the criteria in the EIN scheme should be applied. If the proliferation does not meet the criteria for EIN, it is unlikely to represent a significant risk for endometrial adenocarcinoma, and can be classified "down" (see fig. 4-8).

Endometrial metaplasias can histologically suggest endometrial neoplasia, particularly if only

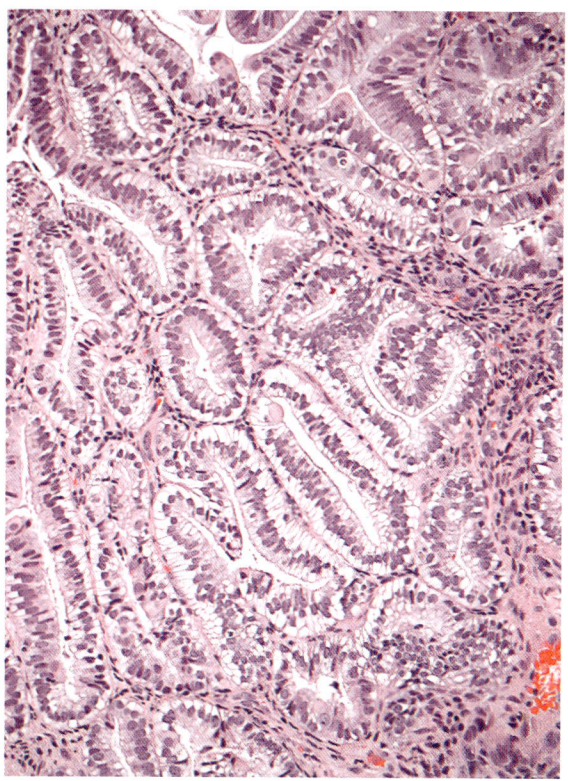

Figure 4-9

SECRETORY HYPERPLASIA

Secretory hyperplasia is a rare entity indicative of ovulation in a preexisting hyperplastic endometrium. Based on the nuclear characteristics, this example would be considered nonatypical hyperplasia.

small fragments of tissue are obtained in a curetted or biopsy specimen. Endometrial metaplasias can show solid growth, architectural complexity with crowded glands, and some degree of nuclear atypia. Although in most instances this distinction is straightforward, one important exception is the presence of complex patterns, which should be classified cautiously with recommendation for follow-up as they may be associated with endometrial cancers, especially if the process is extensive (fig. 4-10). In particular, complex mucinous metaplasia/proliferations are associated with malignancy-related mutations and with underlying carcinoma in a small number of cases (fig. 4-10) (41).

Endometrial polyp is often misdiagnosed as endometrial hyperplasia. In one study, most samples erroneously classified as endometrial hyperplasia were reclassified as endometrial

Figure 4-10
COMPLEX PAPILLARY METAPLASIA

Complex papillary metaplasia can be difficult to discriminate from hyperplasia/EIN. Glands are crowded but show a distinct metaplastic appearance, with abundant mucinous/eosinophilic cytoplasm, with or without vacuolated and ciliated cells. Metaplasias are often associated with reactive/inflammatory processes such as chronic endometritis (A). Ki-67 shows a lower proliferative index when compared to hyperplasia/EIN (B). Mucinous metaplasia should be interpreted with caution when showing complex architecture and tufting. Such changes should prompt careful follow up (C).

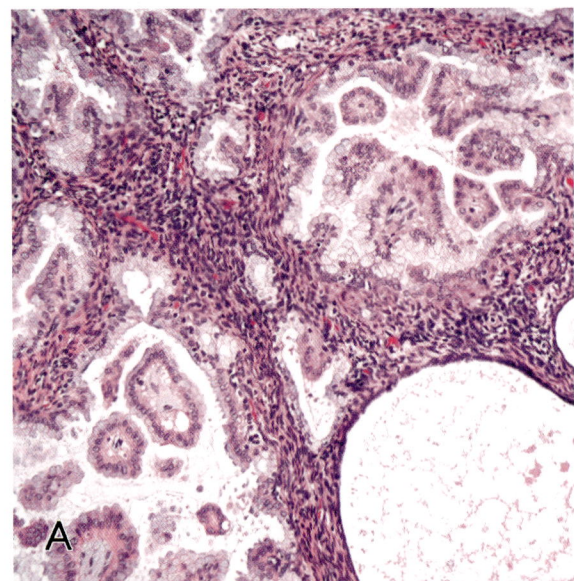

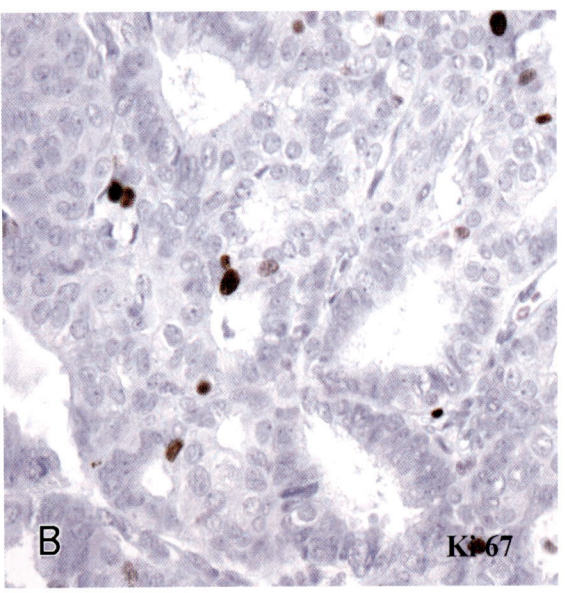

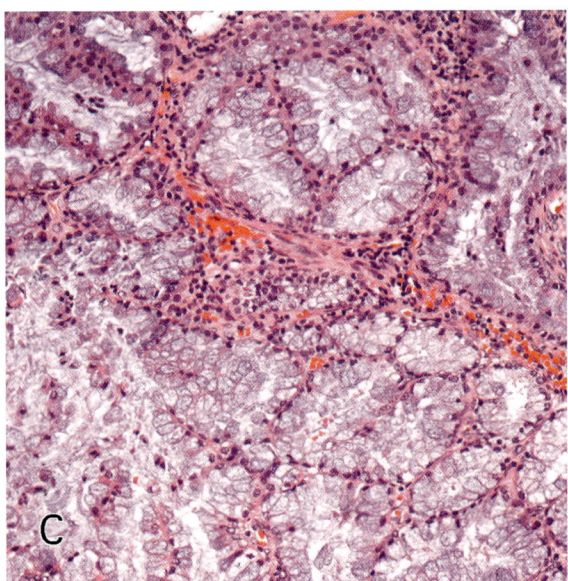

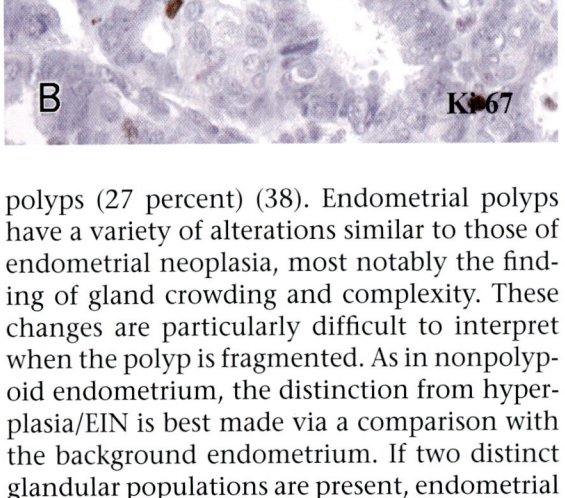

polyps (27 percent) (38). Endometrial polyps have a variety of alterations similar to those of endometrial neoplasia, most notably the finding of gland crowding and complexity. These changes are particularly difficult to interpret when the polyp is fragmented. As in nonpolypoid endometrium, the distinction from hyperplasia/EIN is best made via a comparison with the background endometrium. If two distinct glandular populations are present, endometrial hyperplasia/EIN should be a strong consideration. If the abnormal glands can be seen overgrowing benign-appearing glands, it is most likely that the polyp contains a neoplastic focus (fig. 4-11). Classic stromal features described in endometrial polyps, including vascular plexuses and dense collagenized stroma, also help establish a correct interpretation.

It may be difficult to differentiate endometrial hyperplasia/EIN and well-differentiated endometrial adenocarcinoma. As described for endometrial carcinoma, the presence of back to back glands without intervening stroma, complex cribriform glands showing fusion, and extended gland lumens leads to a diagnosis of endometrial carcinoma (42). These architectural

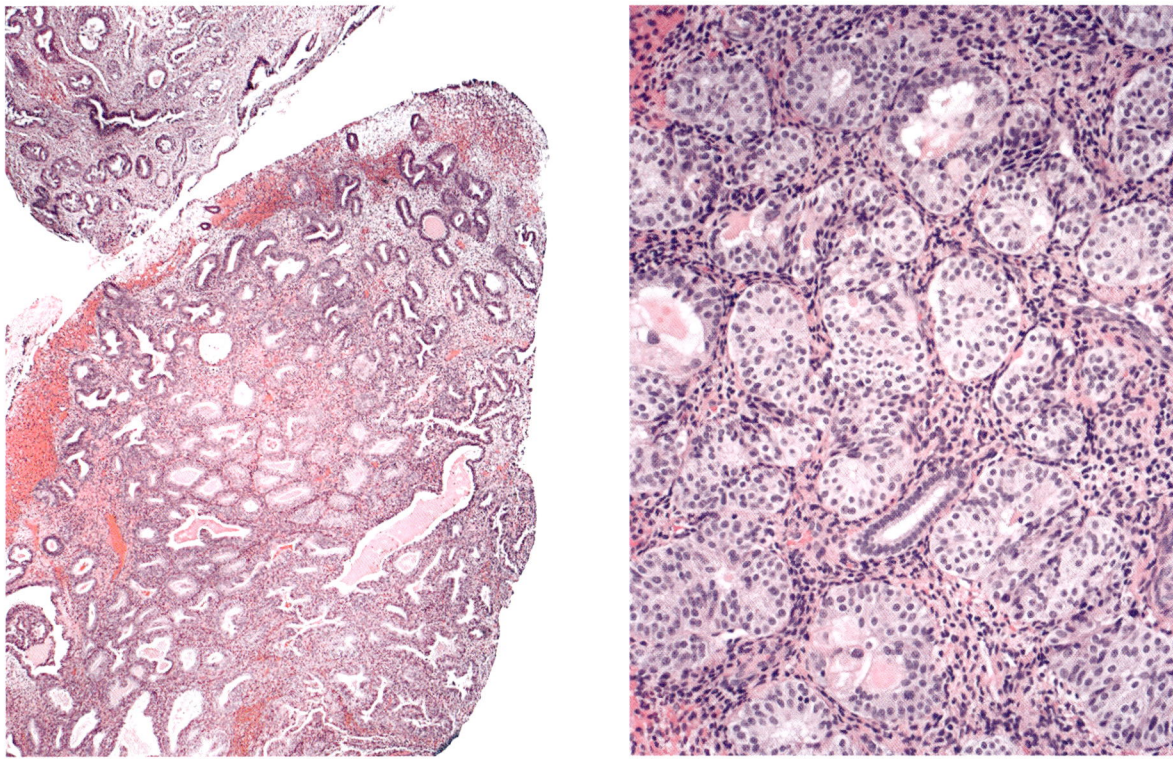

Figure 4-11

HYPERPLASIA/EIN IN POLYPS

Application of the hyperplasia/EIN criteria in endometrial polyps can be difficult as they often show crowded benign glands. In this example, benign glands are morphologically distinct from the surrounding hyperplastic crowded glands, allowing for a designation as hyperplasia/EIN (left: low magnification; right: high magnification).

features are important to identify even if they involve only small areas of the specimen. Proliferations with features of carcinoma involving an area as little as 2.1 mm have been associated with myoinvasive carcinoma (43). Epithelial features such as pseudostratification and cytologic atypia are of less value in this differential diagnosis as both atypical hyperplasia/EIN and well-differentiated endometrial adenocarcinoma can show such changes (42).

REFERENCES

1. Kurman RJ, Kaminski PF, Norris HJ. The behavior of endometrial hyperplasia. A long-term study of "untreated" hyperplasia in 170 patients. Cancer 1985;56:403-12.
2. Zaino RJ, Kauderer J, Trimble CL, et al. Reproducibility of the diagnosis of atypical endometrial hyperplasia: a Gynecologic Oncology Group study. Cancer 2006;106:804-11.
3. Allison KH, Reed SD, Voigt LF, Jordan CD, Newton KM, Garcia RL. Diagnosing endometrial hyperplasia: why is it so difficult to agree? Am J Surg Pathol 2008;32:691-8.
4. Ordi J, Bergeron C, Hardisson D, et al. Reproducibility of current classifications of endometrial endometrioid glandular proliferations: further evidence supporting a simplified classification. Histopathology 2014;64:284-92.
5. Zaino R, Carinelli SG, Ellenson LH, et al. Epithelial tumours and precursors. In: Kurman RJ, Carcanjiu ML, Herrington CS, Young RH, eds. WHO classification of tumours of the female reproductive organs. Lyon: IARC Press; 2014:125-6.
6. Baak JP, Nauta JJ, Wisse-Brekelmans EC, Bezemer PD. Architectural and nuclear morphometrical features together are more important prognosticators in endometrial hyperplasias than nuclear morphometrical features alone. J Pathol 1988;154:335-41.
7. Mutter GL. Endometrial intraepithelial neoplasia (EIN): will it bring order to chaos? The Endometrial Collaborative Group. Gynecol Oncol 2000;76:287-90.
8. Hecht JL, Ince TA, Baak JP, Baker HE, Ogden MW, Mutter GL. Prediction of endometrial carcinoma by subjective endometrial intraepithelial neoplasia diagnosis. Mod Pathol 2005;18:324-30.
9. Parazzini F, La Vecchia C, Bocciolone L, Franceschi S. The epidemiology of endometrial cancer. Gynecol Oncol 1991;41:1-16.
10. Grady D, Gebretsadik T, Kerlikowske K, Ernster V, Petitti D. Hormone replacement therapy and endometrial cancer risk: a meta-analysis. Obstet Gynecol 1995;85:304-13.
11. Epplein M, Reed SD, Voigt LF, Newton KM, Holt VL, Weiss NS. Risk of complex and atypical endometrial hyperplasia in relation to anthropometric measures and reproductive history. Am J Epidemiol 2008;168:563-70; discussion: 571-6.
12. Lacey JV Jr, Chia VM, Rush BB, et al. Incidence rates of endometrial hyperplasia, endometrial cancer and hysterectomy from 1980 to 2003 within a large prepaid health plan. Int J Cancer 2012;131:1921-9.
13. Reed SD, Newton KM, Clinton WL, et al. Incidence of endometrial hyperplasia. Am J Obstet Gynecol 2009;200:678.e1-6.
14. Trimble CL, Kauderer J, Zaino R, et al. Concurrent endometrial carcinoma in women with a biopsy diagnosis of atypical endometrial hyperplasia: a Gynecologic Oncology Group study. Cancer 2006;106:812-9.
15. Lacey JV Jr, Mutter GL, Nucci MR, et al. Risk of subsequent endometrial carcinoma associated with endometrial intraepithelial neoplasia classification of endometrial biopsies. Cancer 2008;113:2073-81.
16. Kane SE, Hecht JL. Endometrial intraepithelial neoplasia terminology in practice: 4-year experience at a single institution. Int J Gynecol Pathol 2012;31:160-5.
17. Semere LG, Ko E, Johnson NR, et al. Endometrial intraepithelial neoplasia: clinical correlates and outcomes. Obstet Gynecol 2011;118:21-8.
18. Moriarty AT, Cibas ES. Endometrial cells: the how and why of reporting. In: Solomon D, Nayar R, eds. The Bethesda System for reporting cervical/vaginal cytologic diagnoses. New York: Springer; 2003.
19. Cibas ES, Chelmow D, Waxman AG, Moriarty AT. Endometrial cells: the how and when of reporting. In: Nayar R, Wilbur DC, eds. The Bethesda System for reporting cervical cytology. Heidelberg: Springer Press; 2015:91-102.
20. Gomez-Fernandez CR, Ganjei-Azar P, Behshid K, Averette HE, Nadji M. Normal endometrial cells in Papanicolaou smears: prevalence in women with and without endometrial disease. Obstet Gynecol 2000;96:874-8.
21. Kim MJ, Kim JJ, Kim SM. Endometrial evaluation with transvaginal ultrasonography for the screening of endometrial hyperplasia or cancer in premenopausal and perimenopausal women. Obstet Gynecol Sci 2016;59:192-200.
22. Prat J, Gallardo A, Cuatrecasas M, Catasus L. Endometrial carcinoma: pathology and genetics. Pathology 2007;39:72-87.
23. Matias-Guiu X, Catasus L, Bussaglia E, et al. Molecular pathology of endometrial hyperplasia and carcinoma. Hum Pathol 2001;32:569-77.
24. Suhaimi SS, Ab Mutalib NS, Jamal R. Understanding molecular landscape of endometrial cancer through next generation sequencing: what we have learned so far? Front Pharmacol 2016;7:409.
25. Joshi A, Ellenson LH. PI3K/PTEN/AKT genetic mouse models of endometrial carcinoma. Adv exp Med Biol 2017;943:261-73.

26. Monte NM, Webster KA, Neuberg D, Dressler GR, Mutter GL. Joint loss of PAX2 and PTEN expression in endometrial precancers and cancer. Cancer Res 2010;70:6225-32.
27. Kanaya T, Kyo S, Sakaguchi J, et al. Association of mismatch repair deficiency with PTEN frameshift mutations in endometrial cancers and the precursors in a Japanese population. Am J Clin Pathol 2005;124:89-96.
28. Hayes MP, Wang H, Espinal-Witter R, et al. PIK-3CA and PTEN mutations in uterine endometrioid carcinoma and complex atypical hyperplasia. Clin Cancer Res 2006;12(Pt 1):5932-5.
29. Brachtel EF, Sanchez-Estevez C, Moreno-Bueno G, Prat J, Palacios J, Oliva E. Distinct molecular alterations in complex endometrial hyperplasia (CEH) with and without immature squamous metaplasia (squamous morules). Am J Surg Pathol 2005;29:1322-9.
30. Huang M, Djordjevic B, Yates MS, et al. Molecular pathogenesis of endometrial cancers in patients with Lynch syndrome. Cancer 2013;119:3027-33.
31. Stambolic V, Tsao MS, Macpherson D, Suzuki A, Chapman WB, Mak TW. High incidence of breast and endometrial neoplasia resembling human Cowden syndrome in pten+/- mice. Cancer Res 2000;60:3605-11.
32. Bartosch C, Pires-Luis AS, Meireles C, et al. Pathologic findings in prophylactic and non-prophylactic hysterectomy specimens of patients with Lynch syndrome. Am J Surg Pathol 2016;40:1177-91.
33. Mutter GL. Histopathology of genetically defined endometrial precancers. Int J Gynecol Pathol 2000;19:301-9.
34. Mutter GL, Baak JP, Crum CP, Richart RM, Ferenczy A, Faquin WC. Endometrial precancer diagnosis by histopathology, clonal analysis, and computerized morphometry. J Pathol 2000;190:462-9.
35. Usubutun A, Mutter GL, Saglam A, et al. Reproducibility of endometrial intraepithelial neoplasia diagnosis is good, but influenced by the diagnostic style of pathologists. Mod Pathol 2012;25:877-84.
36. Yang YF, Liao YY, Peng NF, Li LQ, Xie SR, Wang RB. Prediction of coexistent carcinomas risks by subjective EIN diagnosis and comparison with WHO classification in endometrial hyperplasias. Pathol Res Pract 2012;208:708-12.
37. The American College of Obstetricians and Gynecologists Committee Opinion no. 631. Endometrial intraepithelial neoplasia. Obstet Gynecol 2015;125:1272-8.
38. Winkler B, Alvarez S, Richart RM, Crum CP. Pitfalls in the diagnosis of endometrial neoplasia. Obstet Gynecol 1984;64:185-94.
39. Truskinovsky AM, Lifschitz-Mercer B, Czernobilsky B. Hyperplasia and carcinoma in secretory endometrium: a diagnostic challenge. Int J Gynecol Pathol 2014;33:107-13.
40. Mazur MT, Kurman RJ. Dysfunctional Uterine bleeding. In: Mazur MT, Kurman RJ. Diagnosis of endometrial biopsies and curettings. A practical approach. New York: Springer: 1995:101-3.
41. McKenney JK, Longacre TA. Low-grade endometrial adenocarcinoma: a diagnostic algorithm for distinguishing atypical endometrial hyperplasia and other benign (and malignant) mimics. Adv Anat Pathol 2009;16:1-22.
42. Yoo SH, Park BH, Choi J, et al. Papillary mucinous metaplasia of the endometrium as a possible precursor of endometrial mucinous adenocarcinoma. Mod Pathol 2012;25:1496-507.
43. Kurman RJ, Norris HJ. Evaluation of criteria for distinguishing atypical endometrial hyperplasia from well-differentiated carcinoma. Cancer 1982;49:2547-59.

5 ENDOMETRIOID CARCINOMA AND RELATED CARCINOMAS

Definition. *Endometrioid carcinomas* are carcinomas showing endometrioid differentiation defined by the presence, at least focally, of glands reminiscent of proliferative endometrium lined by columnar cells with ovoid or elongated nuclei, intermediate or low nuclear to cytoplasmic (N/C) ratio, and no severe cytologic atypia (fig. 5-1). Some tumors lacking the above features may show squamous differentiation or combinations of mucinous and tubal differentiation (figs. 5-2, 5-3).

GENERAL FEATURES AND EPIDEMIOLOGY

It was estimated that 621,612 women were diagnosed with endometrial carcinoma in the United States in 2012 and approximately 55,000 new cases were diagnosed in 2015 (25.1 per 1,000,000 women per year), representing 3.3 percent of all new cancers (1). Approximately 10,170 women in the United States died from endometrial carcinoma in 2015, representing 1.7 percent of all cancer deaths; approximately 82 percent of patients survived their disease. Rates for newly diagnosed endometrial cancer and cancer death have not changed significantly over the past 10 years. A closer look at the data reveals that the incidence of endometrial carcinoma in Caucasian patients decreased significantly from 1975 to 1990 and then leveled off, while the

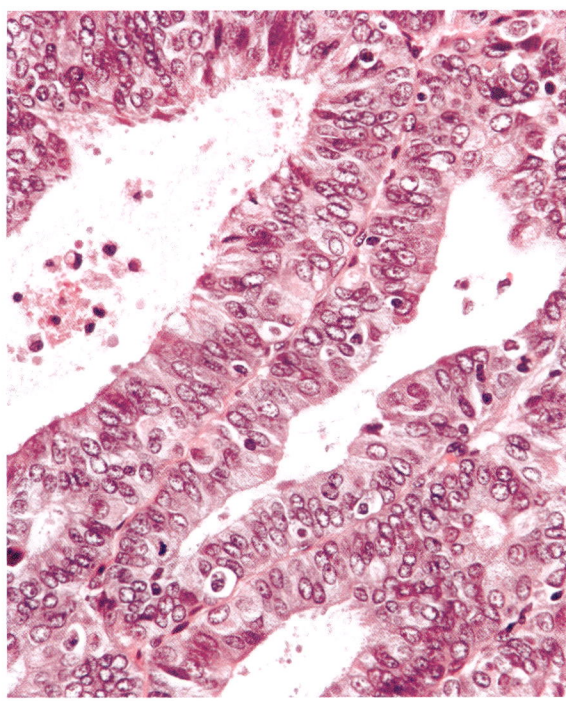

Figure 5-1

LOW-GRADE ENDOMETRIOID CARCINOMA

Glands are lined by columnar cells with eosinophilic cytoplasm and pseudostratified, low-grade oval nuclei.

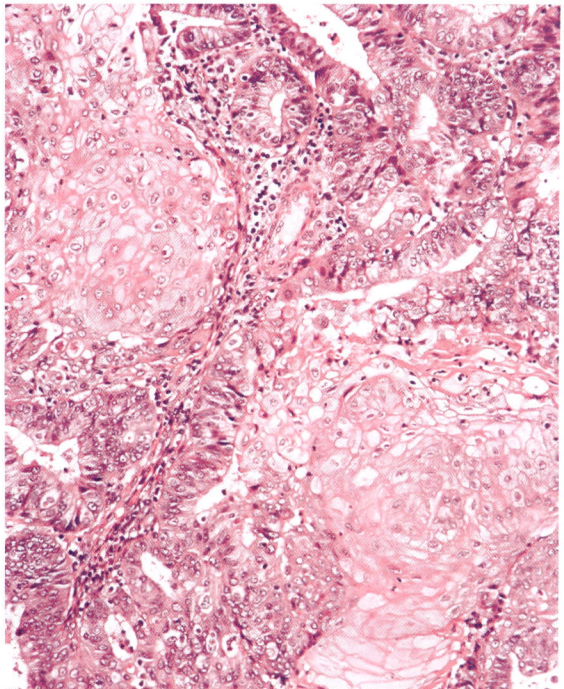

Figure 5-2

LOW-GRADE ENDOMETRIOID CARCINOMA

Squamous differentiation, a confirmatory feature of endometrioid carcinoma, is seen.

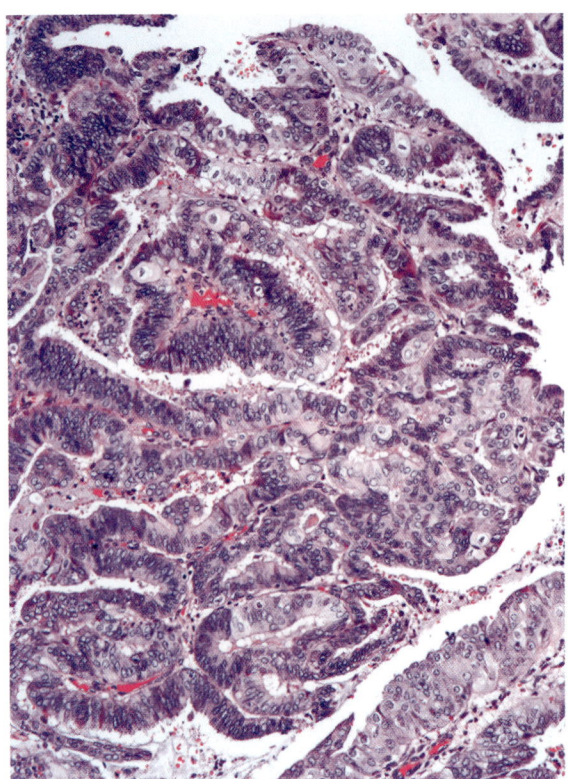 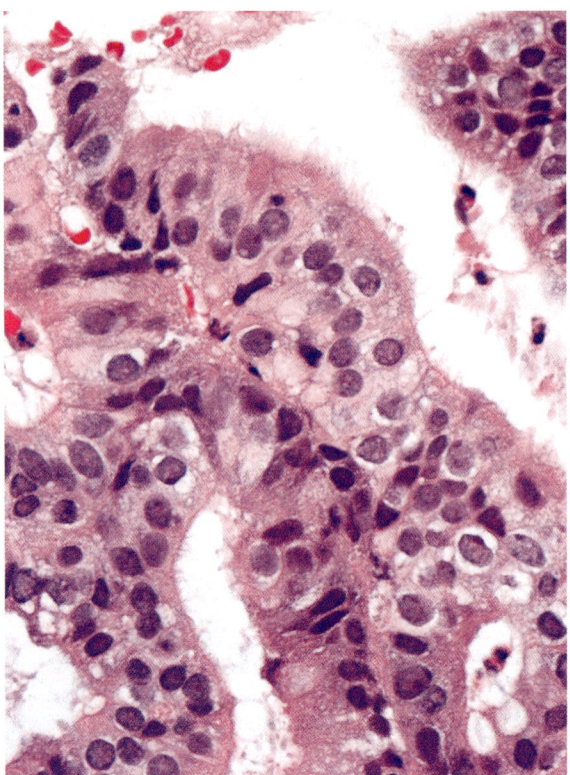

Figure 5-3

ENDOMETRIOID CARCINOMA

Cells showing tubal differentiation have lighter eosinophilic cytoplasm compared to conventional endometrioid cells and contain a terminal bar with cilia (left). The nuclei lack appreciable cytologic atypia (right).

incidence in African-American women was stable until about 1990, when it began to increase.

Endometrial carcinoma is most frequently diagnosed in women between 55 and 64 (median, 62) years in the United States; the median age at death is approximately 70 years (1). The incidence of endometrial carcinoma is equal among races, with slightly lower rates in Asian, Pacific Islander, Native American, and Hispanic women compared to Caucasian and African-American women. Death rates among patients of African descent double that of patients from other ethnic backgrounds. This important difference may be due to an increased risk for developing serous carcinoma (2–8), comorbid conditions, and lack of appropriate care (9), as well as other factors not yet understood.

Features typically regarded as risk factors in endometrial cancer are most pertinent to the International Federation of Gynecology and Obstetrics (FIGO) grades 1 and 2 endometrioid carcinomas (previously referred to as "type I endometrial carcinoma") (10). These include: unopposed estrogen (11,12), obesity (13,14), late menopause (after age 52 years), menometrorrhagia, Stein-Leventhal syndrome (including infertility, anovulatory menses, hirsutism and other endocrine abnormalities), family history of multiple cancers, personal history of breast or rectal cancer, infertility or nulliparity, adult-type granulosa cell tumor, hypertension, and diabetes mellitus (13,15). Tamoxifen is also thought by many to increase the risk of developing endometrioid (16–22) and serous carcinomas (23,24).

Although most endometrioid carcinomas display the characteristics of "type I endometrial carcinoma" as described by Bokhman (25), these tumors are highly heterogeneous. A subset of FIGO grade 3 endometrioid carcinomas has more in common with "type II endometrial carcinoma" from a clinicopathologic perspective (26). When Brinton et al. (10) compared the epidemiological risk factors of endometrioid carcinomas and serous, clear cell, carcinosarcoma, and "mixed epithelial" carcinomas (i.e., "type II"), they found more similarities between FIGO grade 3 endometrioid carcinomas and "type II carcinomas" than between FIGO grade 3 endometrioid carcinomas and low-grade endometrioid carcinomas (10). This study also documented significant heterogeneity within the "type 2" category of carcinomas, calling into question the validity of categorizing endometrial carcinomas in this way.

The most common hereditary cancer syndrome linked to endometrial carcinoma is Lynch syndrome. It has been estimated that between 2 and 6 percent of endometrial carcinomas are Lynch syndrome related (discussed in chapter 8).

CLINICAL FEATURES

Most patients with endometrioid carcinoma present with vaginal bleeding. Rarely, they have signs or symptoms secondary to extra-uterine disease, such as lymphadenopathy or pulmonary or bone lesions. Occasionally, carcinomas are an incidental finding in biopsies performed for a thickened endometrial stripe on sonography (usually performed in patients on tamoxifen therapy), during surgery for an ovarian tumor (commonly adult granulosa cell tumor or a synchronous ovarian endometrioid carcinoma), or at prophylactic surgery in patients with known Lynch syndrome.

In-office endometrial biopsy is the most frequent diagnostic sampling modality, but dilatation and curettage should be considered when the biopsy yields minimal diagnostic tissue, the patient desires a fertility-sparing therapeutic approach (27), and the differential diagnosis includes endocervical adenocarcinoma. A cone biopsy may be performed in the latter scenario if curettage, imaging, and immunohistochemistry cannot discern the origin. Approximately 70 percent of patients present with tumor confined to the uterus, 20 percent have regional lymph node or adnexal metastases, and a small number have distant (abdominal, visceral, and supradiaphragmatic) metastases or are unstaged (1). Rates of distant metastases at presentation increase with age (over 10 percent of patients over 75 years).

GROSS FINDINGS

The uterus is often enlarged. The tumor is typically centered in the corpus (fig. 5-4) but may arise in the lower uterine segment. There is usually a single, dominant exophytic mass, but some endometrioid carcinomas display multiple nodules, are deeply invasive without an obvious mass, or produce a variably thickened endometrium. Some tumors are found within an endometrial polyp. They typically have a shaggy and ulcerated surface and a soft grey-white cut section surface (fig. 5-5). Occasionally, no tumor is grossly seen after the initial diagnostic biopsy or curettage (28).

Assessment of size may be important in the intraoperative setting as some gynecologic oncologists base the decision to perform lymphadenectomy, at least in part, on that feature (29). It is crucial to assess the depth of myometrial invasion. When serially sectioning into the myometrium, distinguishing a myometrial invasive carcinoma from adenomyosis may be challenging. Adenomyosis typically has a trabeculated/nodular appearance whereas invasive carcinoma displays a more homogeneous appearance and is firmer on palpation. It is also important to grossly evaluate the status of the uterine serosa, cervix, and adnexa for staging purposes.

MICROSCOPIC FINDINGS

Endometrioid adenocarcinomas have a wide range of architectural, cytologic (cytoplasmic and nuclear), and stromal features. However, any tumor should show, at least focally, glands reminiscent of proliferative endometrium lined by columnar cells containing ovoid or elongated, slightly pseudostratified nuclei, with an intermediate or low N/C ratio, without severe cytologic atypia (fig. 5-1). In the absence of such features, the tumor should show squamous differentiation or combinations of mucinous and tubal differentiation (figs. 5-2, 5-3). These features, taken together, are referred to as "confirmatory endometrioid features."

Architectural Features

The glandular and papillary components of endometrioid carcinoma are varied and should always be evaluated in the context of the nuclear and cytoplasmic features of the tumor. Glandular complexity includes closely packed tubular glands

Figure 5-4
ENDOMETRIOID CARCINOMA

A multinodular, exophytic tumor involves most of the endometrial cavity (A). A large, hemorrhagic endometrial mass shows extensive ulceration and myometrial invasion on cross section. The mass is yellow, with an exophytic component (B). Dedifferentiated endometrial carcinoma occupies the entire endometrial cavity (C). (Courtesy of Dr. C. Tornos, Stony Brook, NY.)

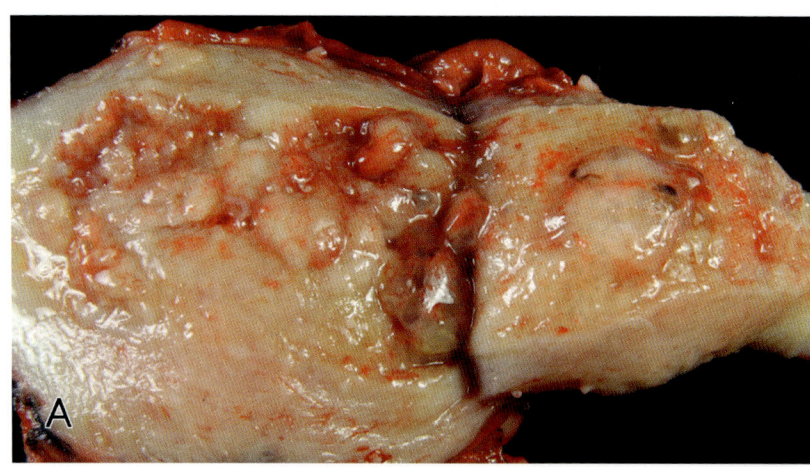

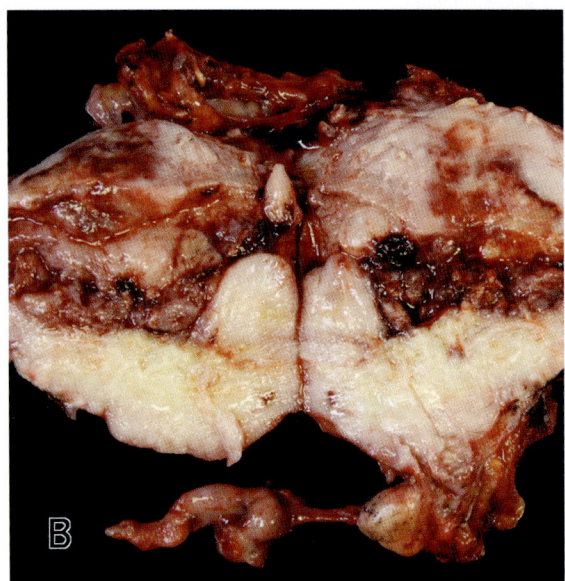

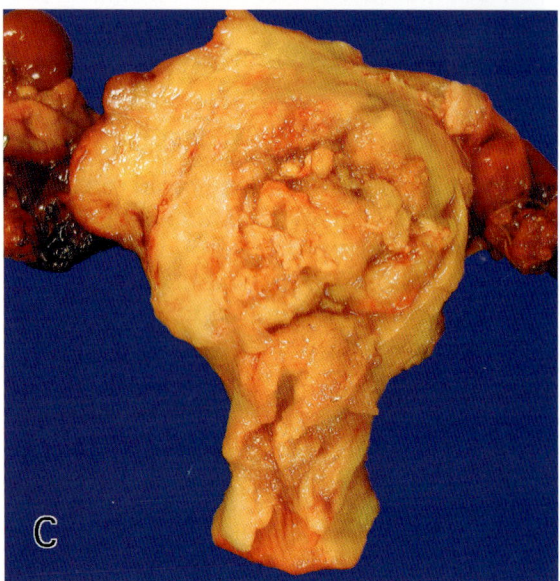

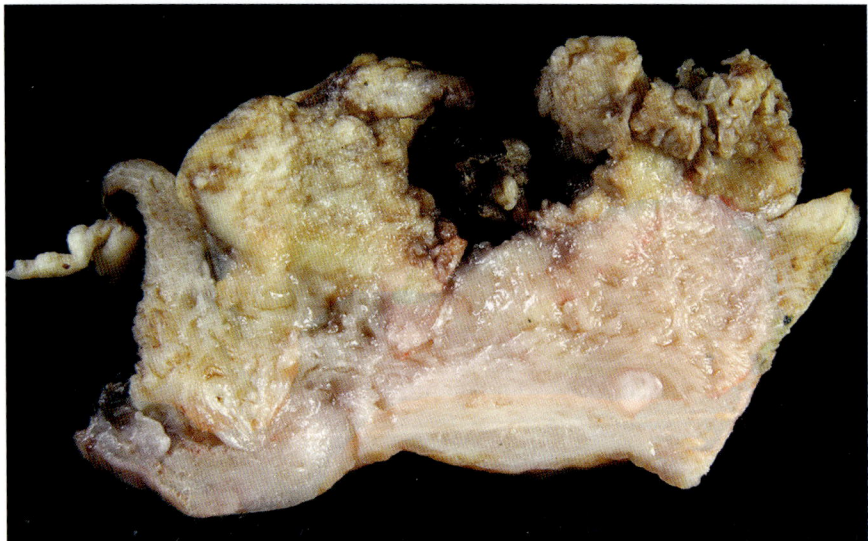

Figure 5-5
ENDOMETRIOID ADENOCARCINOMA INVADING MYOMETRIUM

Cross section displays irregular contoured extension of the tumor into myometrium.

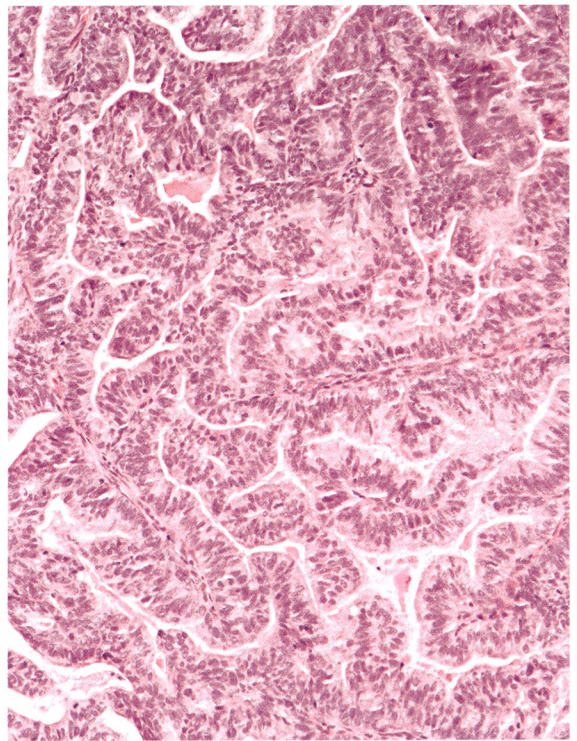

Figure 5-6

ENDOMETRIOID ADENOCARCINOMA WITH LABYRINTHINE ARCHITECTURE

"Wandering lumens" uninterrupted by endometrial stroma.

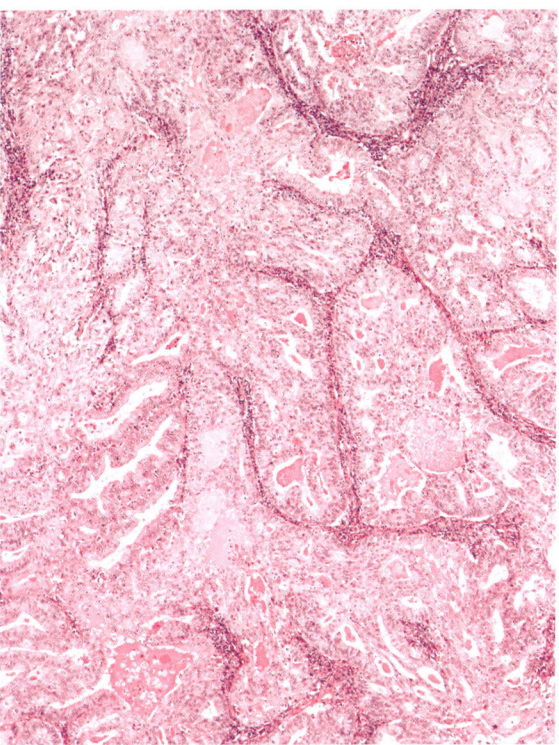

Figure 5-7

ENDOMETRIOID ADENOCARCINOMA WITH MACROGLANDULAR ARCHITECTURE

Large glands have extensive intraglandular cribriform structures.

lacking intervening stroma; fused glands, which sometimes result in a labyrinthine appearance (fig. 5-6); and large glands, "macroglands," with cribriform architecture and micropapillae (fig. 5-7). Gland lumens may contain eosinophilic secretions or mucin and some show necrosis similar to that seen in colonic carcinomas.

Papillary architecture ranges from nondescript papillae to "small nonvillous papillae" (30), in which single cells or small tight clusters of cells with abundant eosinophilic cytoplasm protrude into glandular lumens (fig. 5-8), to villous papillae (fig. 5-9), with long, thin and finger-like papillae with or without branching (villoglandular) or transitional cell-like morphology (fig. 5-10). Since both serous and clear cell carcinomas typically feature papillary architecture, it is crucial to scrutinize the nuclear features in these papillary areas to avoid diagnostic misclassification. Some tumors display trabecular and corded arrangements, sometimes mimicking the growth of adult granulosa or Sertoli cell tumors of the ovary (sex cord-like or corded morphology) (fig. 5-11) (31–34).

When a solid architecture is present, it seamlessly emerges from the glandular and papillary components (fig. 5-12). The solid component often shows a nested or trabecular architecture of cohesive cells. A patternless growth (lacking epithelial differentiation) is uncommon and should suggest undifferentiated carcinoma. Solid areas may display cells with a spindle morphology (fig. 5-13), which may be mitotically active, but lack overt nuclear pleomorphism. These tumors are currently diagnosed as low-grade endometrioid carcinomas.

Cellular Features

Cytoplasmic. The typical glands or papillae of low-grade endometrioid adenocarcinoma are lined by columnar cells with variable amounts of pale to deeply eosinophilic cytoplasm (fig. 5-1).

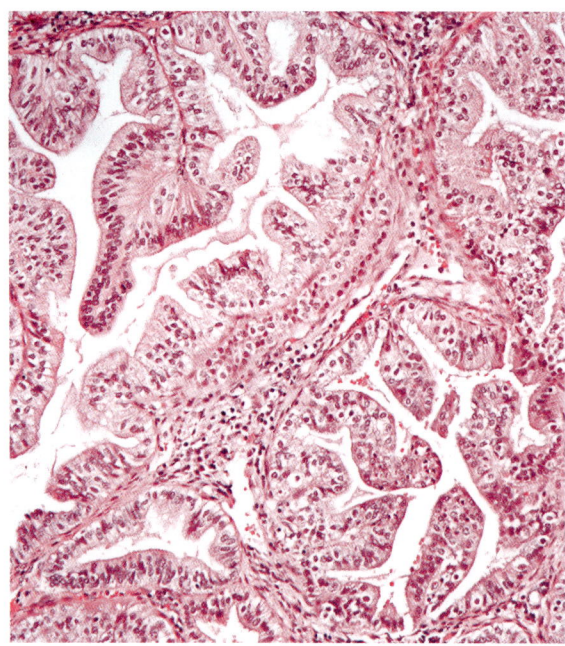 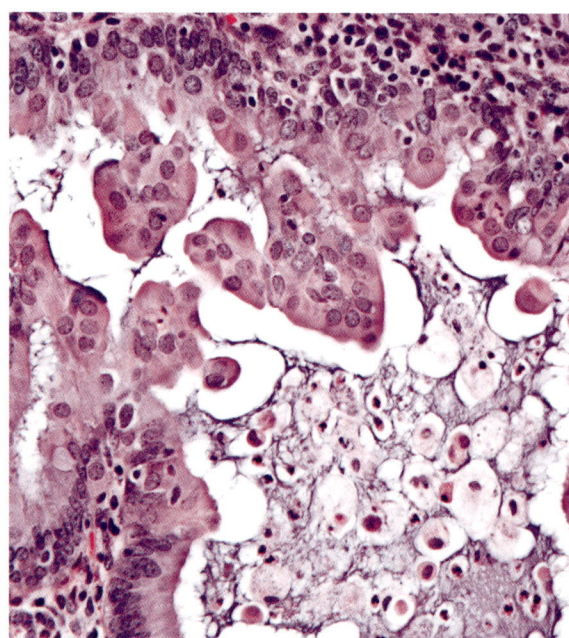

Figure 5-8

ENDOMETRIOID ADENOCARCINOMA WITH PAPILLAE

Nonspecific papillary architecture (left) and "small nonvillous papillae" (right) are seen. The latter designation refers to clusters of eosinophilic cells lacking atypia that project into glandular lumens. The cytology differs from serous carcinoma and it is typically low grade.

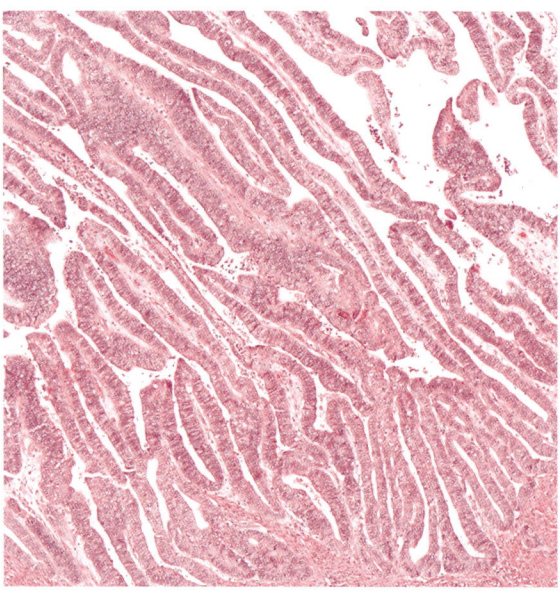 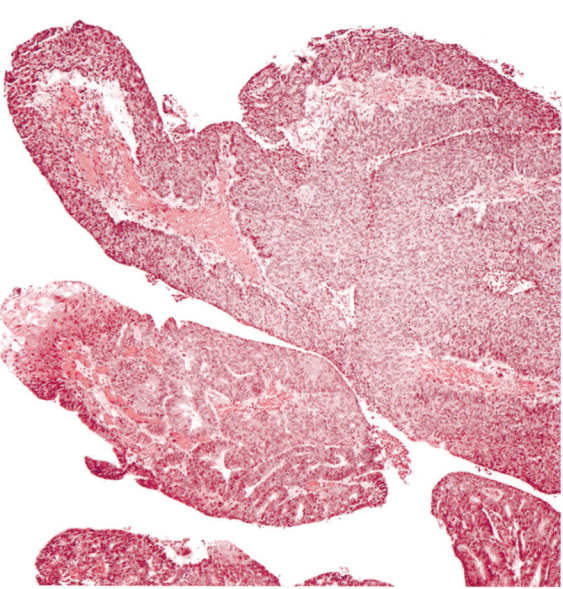

Figure 5-9

VILLOGLANDULAR ENDOMETRIOID ADENOCARCINOMA

The villiform papillae are long, thin, and "finger-like." The nuclear grade should be low to distinguish this subtype of endometrioid carcinoma from serous carcinoma.

Figure 5-10

ENDOMETRIOID ADENOCARCINOMA WITH TRANSITIONAL CELL CARCINOMA-LIKE ARCHITECTURE

Broad papillae with multilayered epithelium superficially resemble some papillary urothelial carcinomas. Confirmatory low-grade endometrioid glands are shown.

Endometrioid Carcinoma and Related Carcinomas

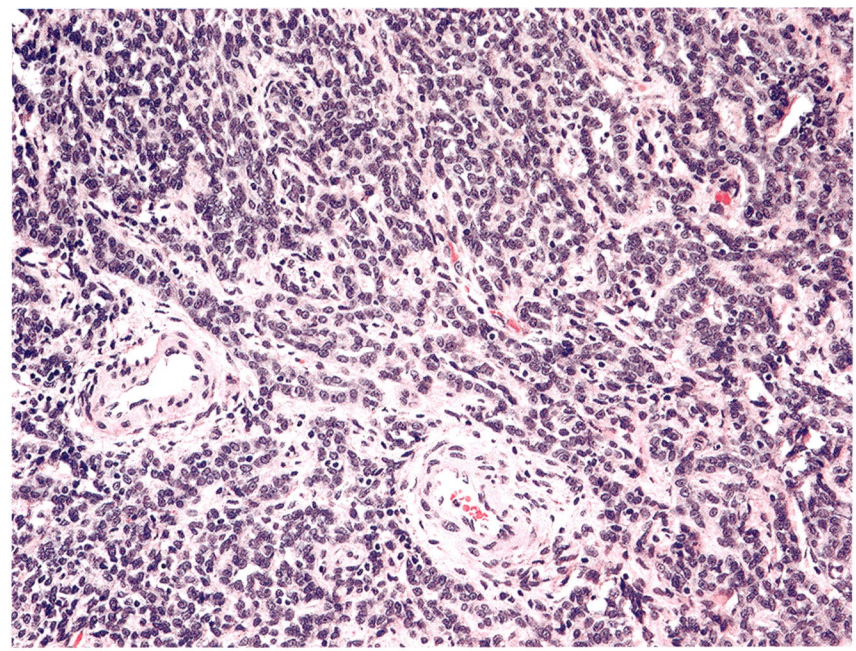

Figure 5-11

ENDOMETRIOID ADENOCARCINOMA WITH SEX CORD-LIKE PATTERN

This appearance is reminiscent of compressed Sertoli tubules or cords of granulosa cells.

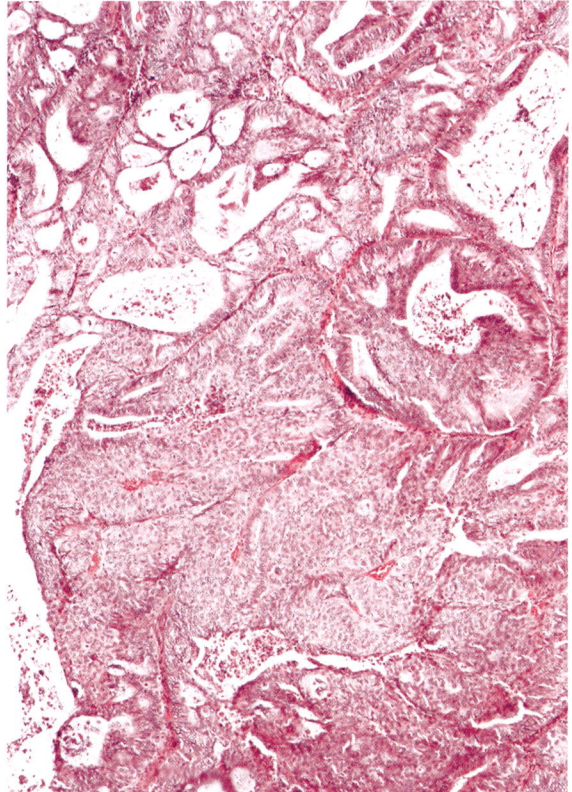
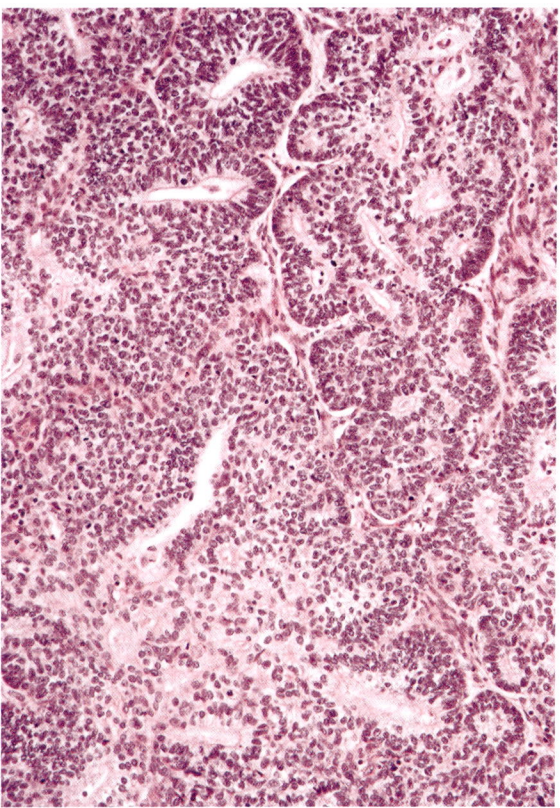

Figure 5-12

ENDOMETRIOID ADENOCARCINOMA

Seamless transition from glandular to solid architecture (left and right) is seen. If the latter represents less than 50 percent of the tumor it is classified as grade 2.

Figure 5-13
ENDOMETRIOID CARCINOMA WITH SPINDLE CELLS
Well-differentiated endometrioid glands "merge" with low-grade spindle cells set in a hyaline matrix (A). Endometrioid glands transition to narrow, spindly cords (B). Squamous metaplastic epithelium may also transition to spindle cells (C).

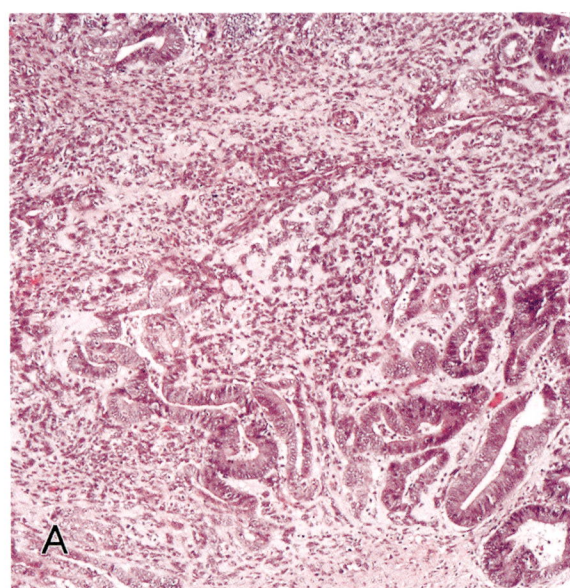

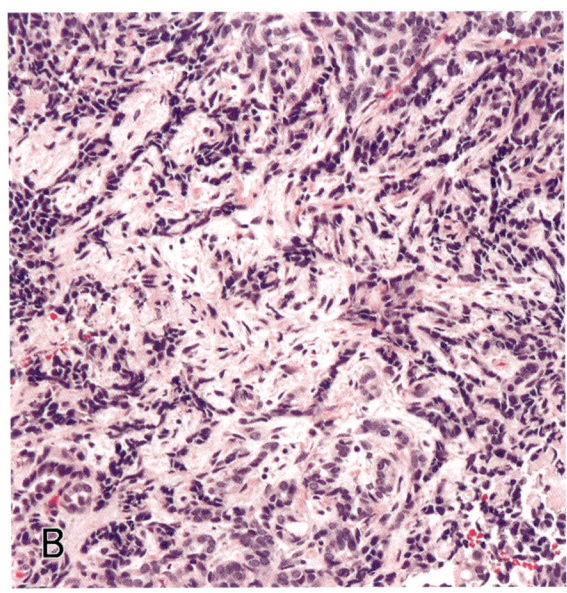

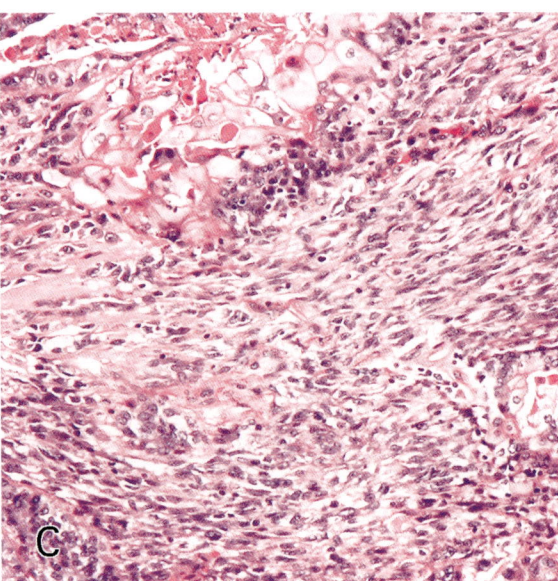

They often exhibit squamous differentiation, which manifests as round, syncytial aggregates of nonkeratinizing squamous cells that may have central necrosis (squamous morules) (fig. 5-14), solid nests of nonkeratinizing squamous cells (fig. 5-15), or keratinizing squamous cells with intercellular bridges with or without extracellular keratin pearls (fig. 5-16). Squamous cells as well as glandular cells may display cytoplasmic clearing. Endometrioid cells with clear cytoplasm may contain subnuclear and supranuclear vacuoles resembling secretory endometrium or show nonspecific cytoplasmic clearing (fig. 5-17).

Tubal differentiation with cilia and an apical bar (often randomly distributed but may be extensive) (fig. 5-3) and mucinous differentiation resembling non-neoplastic endocervical cells (fig. 5-18) are common. The latter occasionally displays a "microglandular hyperplasia-like" architecture (fig. 5-18C) (35,36). Microglandular hyperplasia-like endometrioid carcinoma is characterized by back-to-back microacinar glands lined by mucinous epithelium, often admixed with acute inflammatory cells, which resembles microglandular hyperplasia of the endocervix. It has recently been reported that mucinous differentiation in the presence of tumor-infiltrating lymphocytes is a feature of sporadically occurring microsatellite unstable endometrioid carcinomas (37).

Spindle cells with scant to moderate eosinophilic cytoplasm either merge with glandular elements or are in continuity with squamous epithelium and, as mentioned earlier, have low-grade cytologic features (31). Surface papillary syncytial change (syncytium of cells with randomly oriented nuclei) (38) and oxyphilic metaplasia (39–41) are uncommon and goblet cell and argyrophil metaplasias are rare (42,43).

Nuclear. The major problems in assessment of nuclear grade in endometrioid carcinomas are related to what constitutes severe cytologic atypia and the amount of which is sufficient to move a FIGO grade 1 to grade 2 or a FIGO grade 2 to grade 3 tumor. In order to upgrade a tumor, there is general consensus that a substantial number of tumor cells should demonstrate severe cytologic atypia in the form of marked nuclear enlargement, with or without pleomorphism,

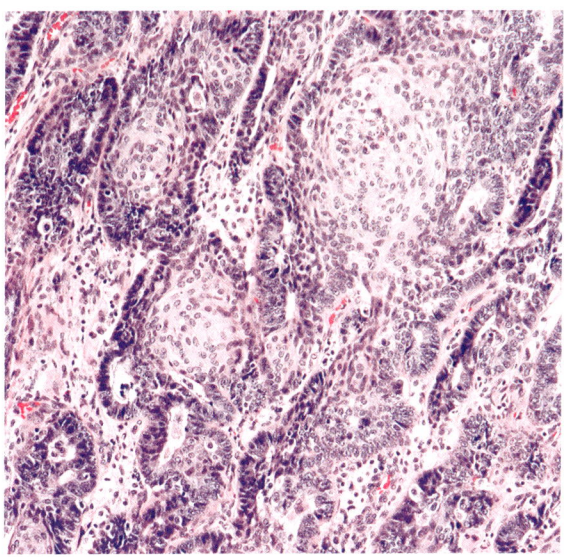

Figure 5-14

ENDOMETRIOID ADENOCARCINOMA WITH SQUAMOUS MORULES

There are round aggregates of nonkeratinizing squamous differentiation.

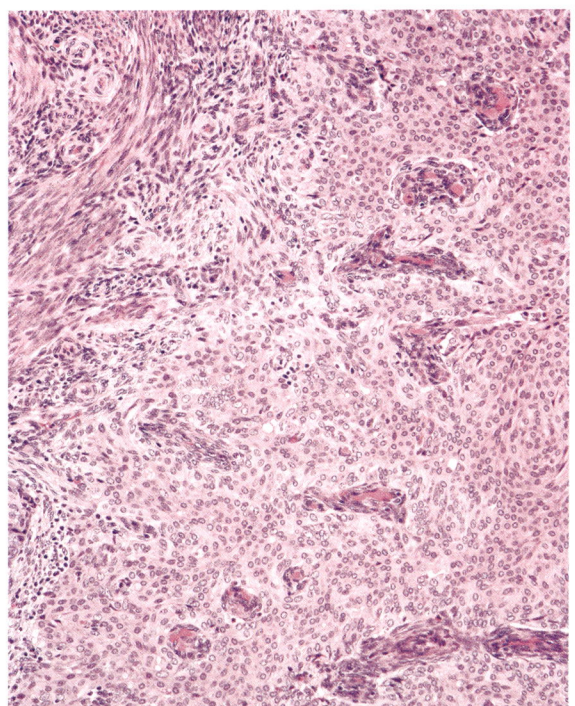 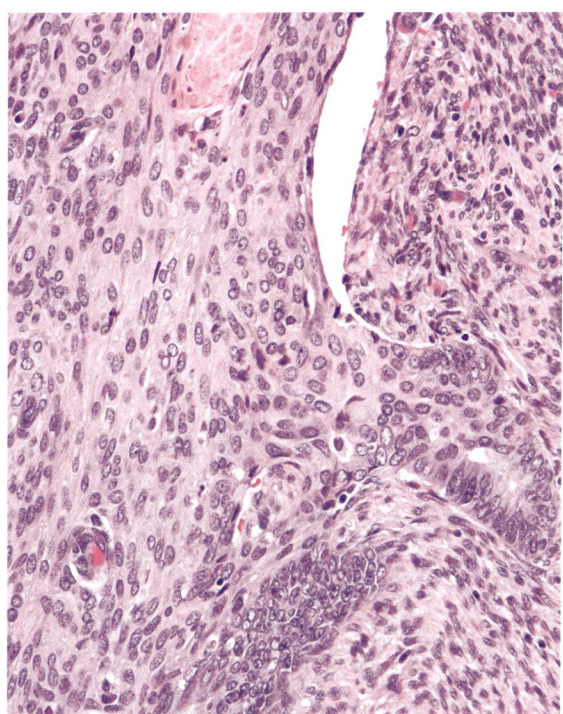

Figure 5-15

ENDOMETRIOID ADENOCARCINOMA WITH NONKERATINIZING SQUAMOUS DIFFERENTIATION

"Streaming" is a characteristic feature of some endometrioid carcinomas with squamous metaplasia. Note bland cytologic appearance.

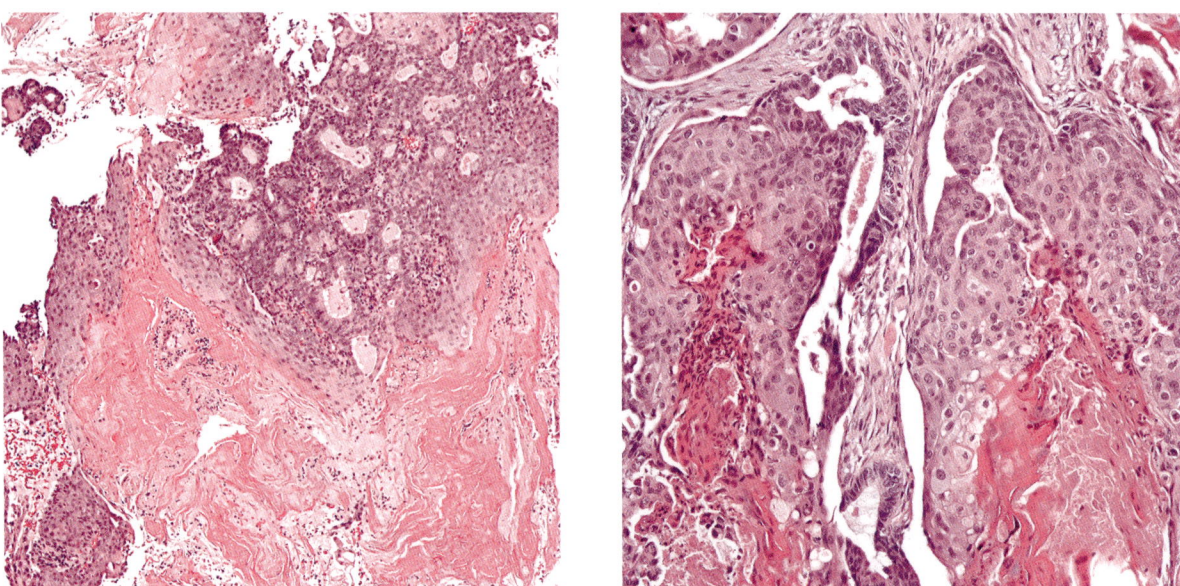

Figure 5-16

ENDOMETRIOID ADENOCARCINOMA WITH KERATINIZING SQUAMOUS DIFFERENTIATION
Abundant keratin is seen.

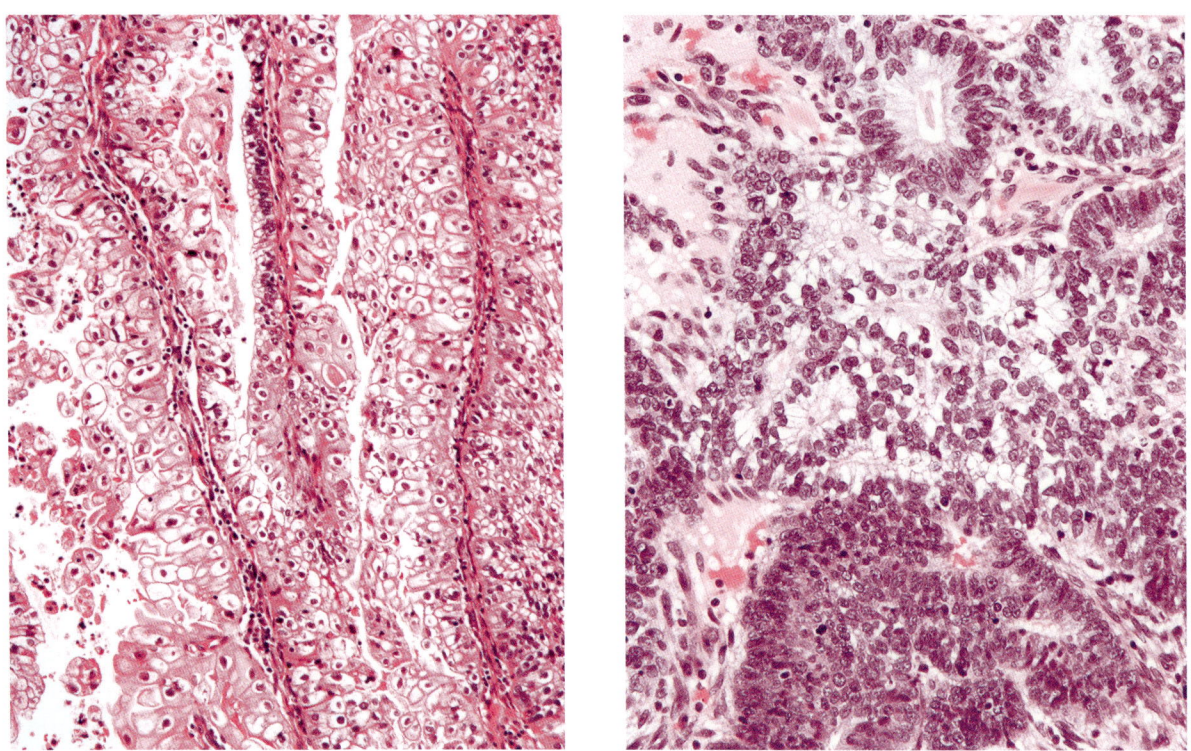

Figure 5-17

ENDOMETRIOID ADENOCARCINOMA WITH CLEAR CELLS
Glycogenated squamous differentiation (left) and secretory-like change within the endometrioid epithelium (right) display clear cytoplasm.

Endometrioid Carcinoma and Related Carcinomas

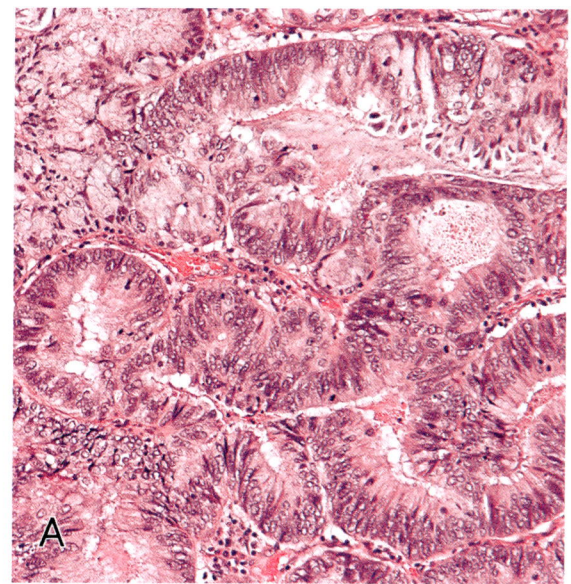

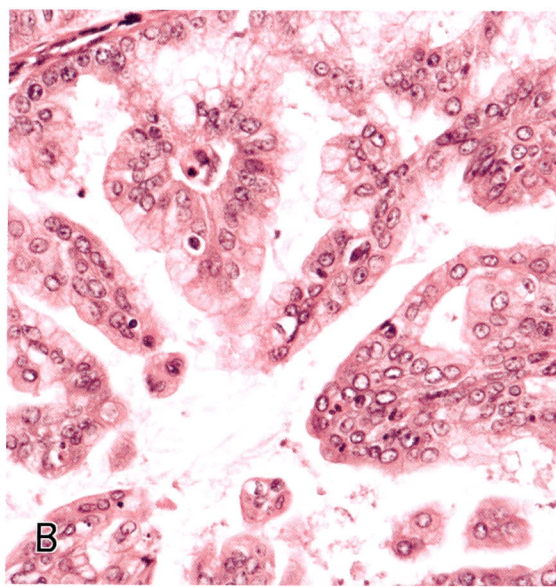

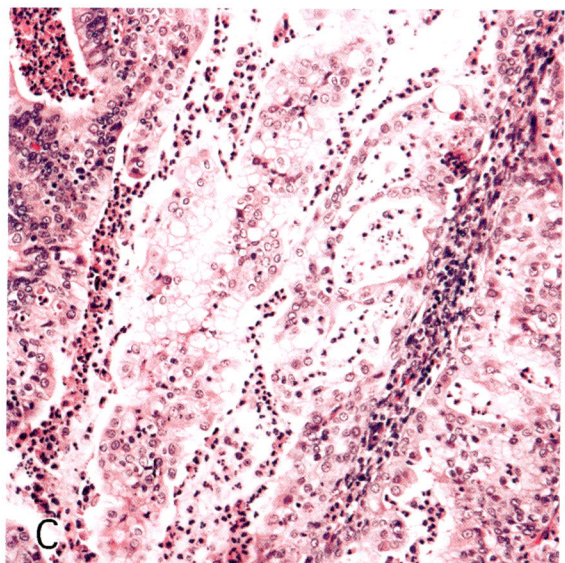

Figure 5-18

ENDOMETRIOID ADENOCARCINOMA WITH MUCINOUS DIFFERENTIATION

FIGO grade 1 endometrioid adenocarcinoma with a component of bland-appearing cells with intracytoplasmic mucin (A). Low-grade endometrioid carcinoma with occasional mucinous metaplastic cells arranged in intraglandular papillae and micropapillae (B). Microglandular hyperplasia-like endometrioid carcinoma. Although this tumor shares with microglandular hyperplasia the finding of microglands, mucinous differentiation, and neutrophilic infiltration, this example contains endometrioid glandular neoplasia at left, including both mucinous and tubal differentiation (C).

irregular nuclear outlines, coarse chromatin, and prominent nucleoli, but a standardized system does not exist (44). It might be helpful to assign nuclear grade based on the Nottingham breast carcinoma grading formulation (fig. 5-19) (45). The squamous epithelium, in most instances, displays bland nuclear features, but may be overtly malignant in rare instances.

Stromal Features

Alterations may exist in the endometrial stroma surrounding endometrioid carcinomas. These include a subtle myofibroblastic or fibroblastic reaction often associated with inflammatory cells (fig. 5-20) (46,47), a prominent lymphocytic infiltrate within the stroma, and the presence of stromal foam cells, often in aggregates (fig. 5-21). In some endometrioid carcinomas, the stroma may be hyalinized (fig. 5-22) or transition to osteoid or overt bony metaplasia (fig. 5-23) (31), which should not be misconstrued as malignant heterologous elements. The latter stromal changes are more frequently noted in endometrioid carcinomas with sex cord-like, corded, or spindled growth (fig. 5-13), particularly when squamous differentiation is also present. Endometrioid

Figure 5-19

ENDOMETRIOID ADENOCARCINOMA: NUCLEAR GRADING

Grade 1 nuclei are typically uniform in size and lack overt chromatin abnormalities (A). Grade 2 nuclei are larger and have chromatin abnormalities in contrast to grade 1, but lack overt pleomorphism (B). Grade 3 nuclei show marked nuclear variation in size, shape, and chromatin quality (C).

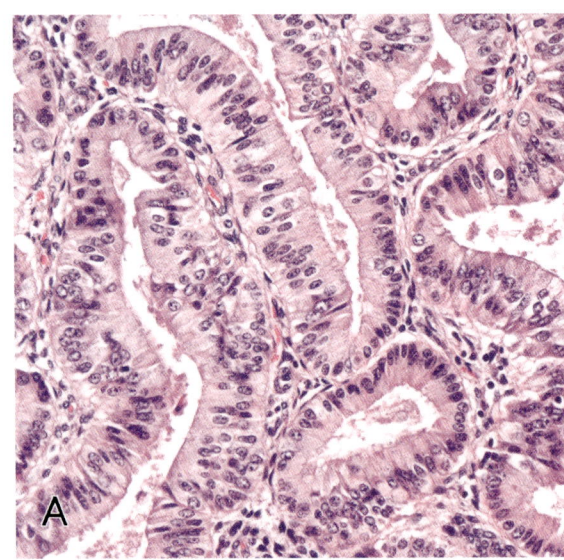

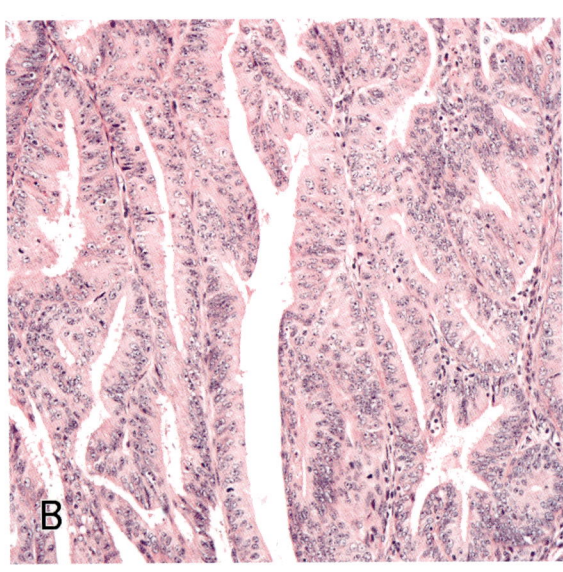

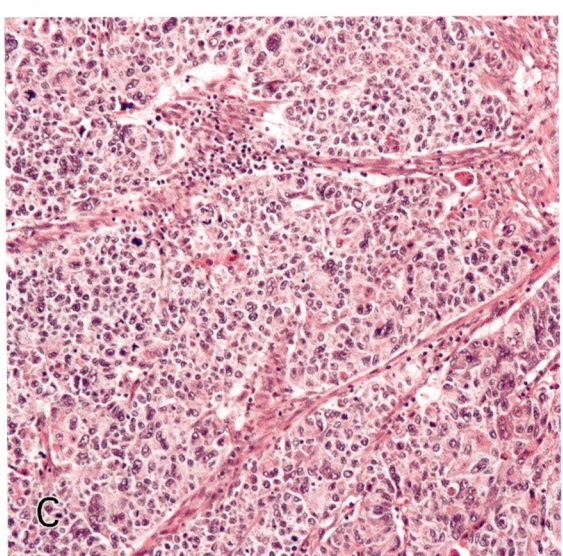

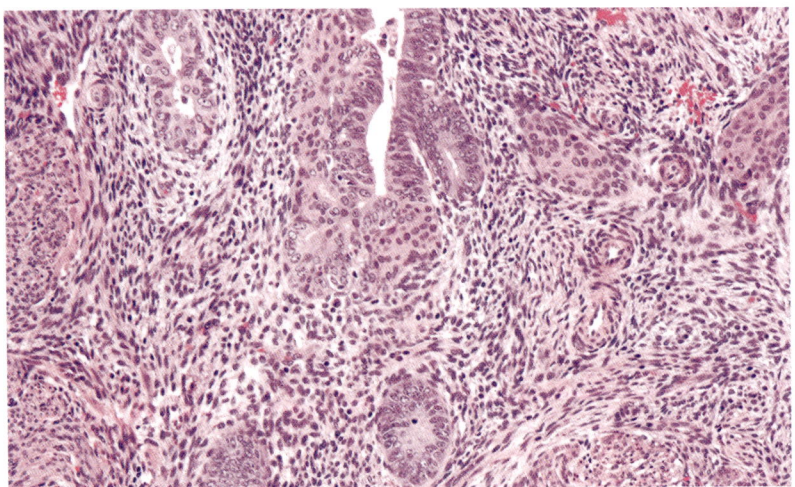

Figure 5-20

ENDOMETRIOID ADENOCARCINOMA WITH "ALTERED ENDOMETRIAL STROMA"

Subtle fibromyxoid stroma surrounds neoplastic glands.

carcinomas with extensive lymphovascular invasion may be associated, paradoxically, with psammoma bodies within or near the lymphovascular spaces (fig. 5-24) (48).

Treatment-Related Changes

Progestational therapy is used as an alternative to surgery in selected patients with low-grade endometrioid carcinoma. Tumors may partially or totally regress and follow-up biopsies, especially in young patients, may only show inactive or secretory endometrium in a background of pseudodecidualized stroma, without residual glandular confluence or significant nuclear atypia (fig. 5-25) (49,50). An exception to the latter is Arias-Stella change (fig. 5-26), where nuclear atypia may manifest as enlarged, ovoid or round nuclei with irregular outlines and a granular, vesicular, or "smudgy" appearance of the chromatin.

There is a wide range of histologic changes associated with a suboptimal, partial response of hyperplasia and carcinoma to progestins (51–54). Glands show reduced nuclear stratification, the N/C ratio decreases as nuclear size decreases and cells gain cytoplasm, and nucleoli disappear. These findings result from extensive

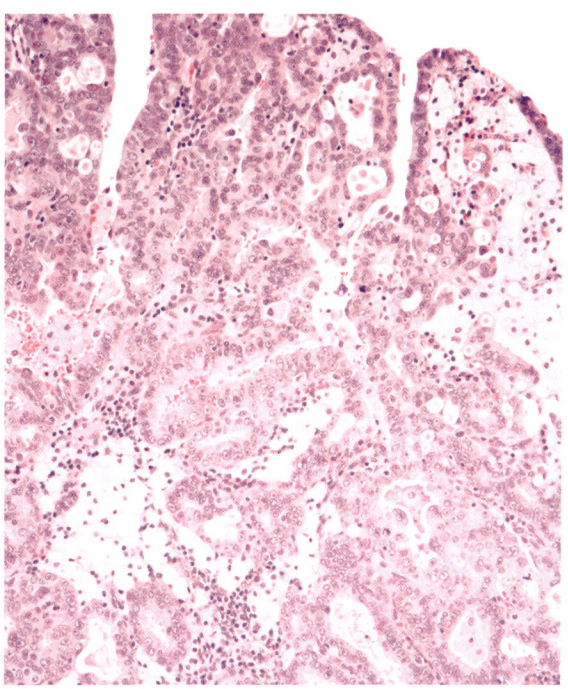

Figure 5-21

ENDOMETRIOID ADENOCARCINOMA WITH AGGREGATES OF STROMAL FOAM CELLS

In a curettage specimen, this finding helps localize the neoplastic process to the endometrium.

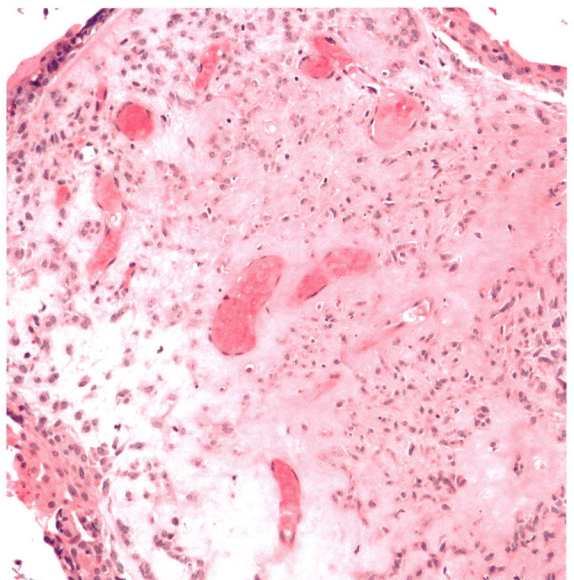
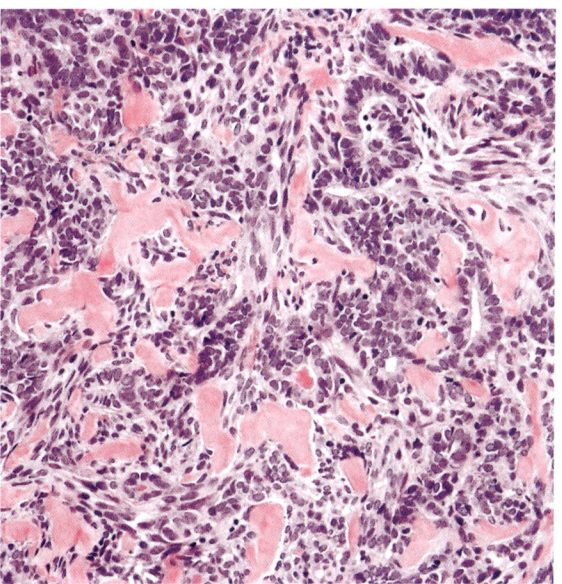

Figure 5-22

ENDOMETRIOID ADENOCARCINOMA WITH STROMAL HYALINIZATION

This appearance is typically seen in corded and hyalinized endometrioid carcinomas (left). Obvious glandular differentiation makes the diagnosis straightforward, but in some cases, careful search for such features (focally present in right), is necessary.

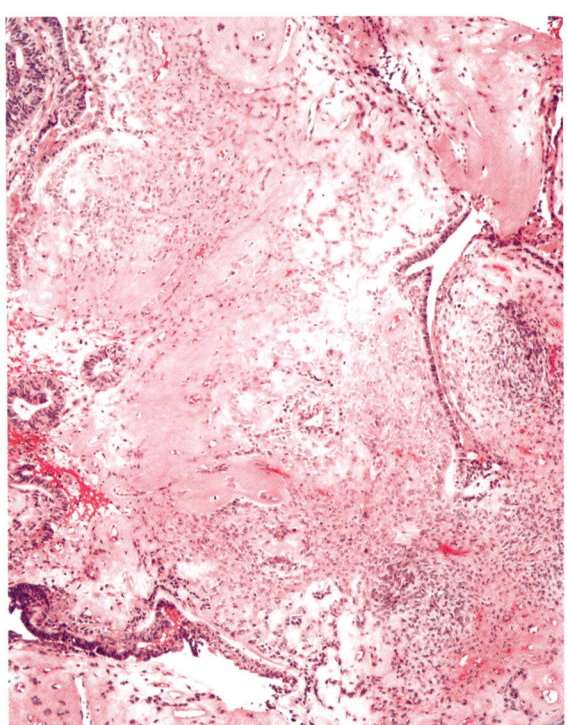 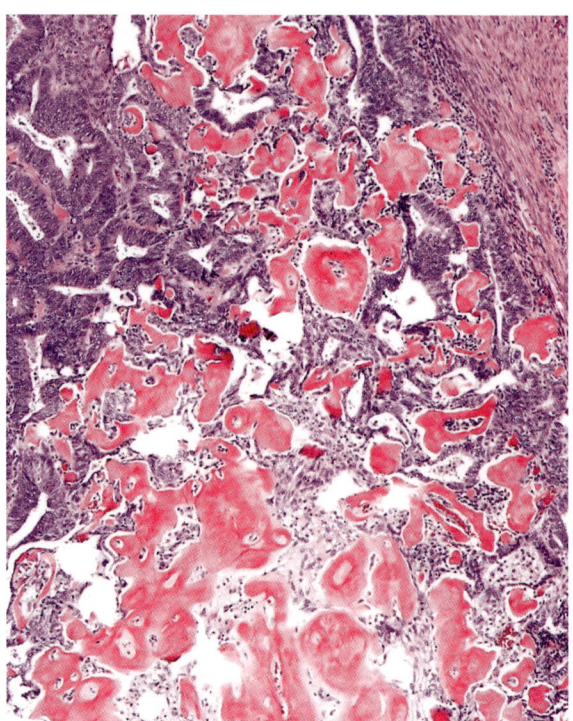

Figure 5-23

ENDOMETRIOID ADENOCARCINOMA WITH FEATURES SUGGESTING HETEROLOGOUS DIFFERENTIATION

Chondromyxoid and sclerotic stroma resembles osteoid (left) and mature osteoid is noted in some tumors (right). These findings are not diagnostic of carcinosarcoma.

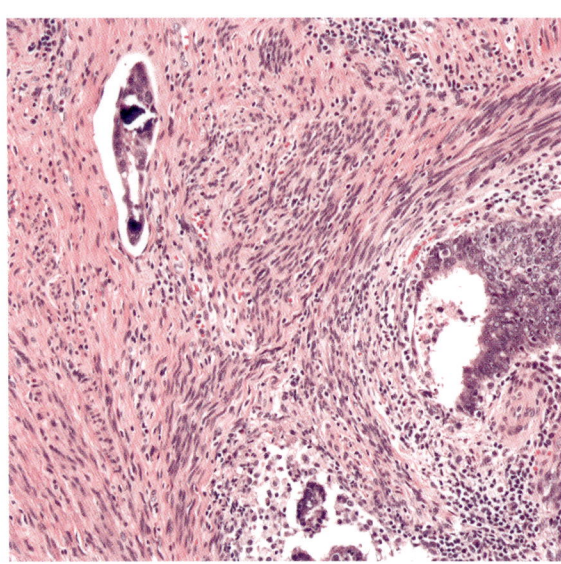 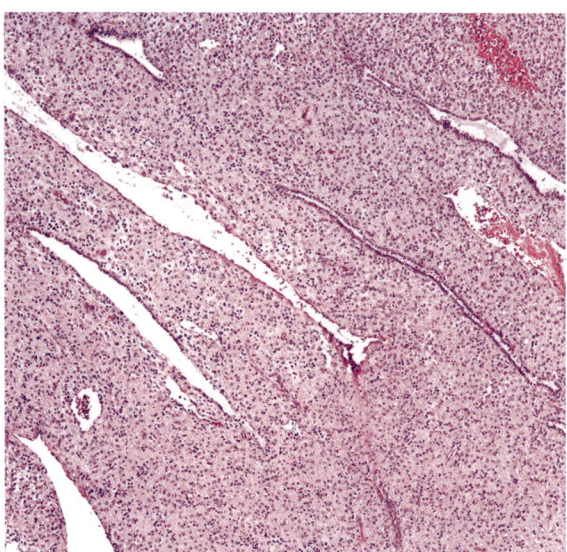

Figure 5-24

ENDOMETRIOID ADENOCARCINOMA WITH A PSAMMOMA BODY

This rare finding is associated with aggressive lymphovascular invasion.

Figure 5-25

ENDOMETRIOID ADENOCARCINOMA WITH COMPLETE RESPONSE TO PROGESTATIONAL THERAPY

Atrophic endometrium sits on pseudodecidualized stroma.

metaplastic changes, including secretory and eosinophilic and, less frequently, squamous and mucinous. These changes may complicate the overall interpretation of the biopsy; however, focal glandular crowding, cribriforming, or papillary growth allows recognition of residual hyperplasia or carcinoma. In one study, features predictive of treatment failure included glandular crowding and presence of prominent nucleoli (54).

The terminology used in these scenarios is not uniform among pathologists, but some investigators have proposed the following: "progestin-treated hyperplasia" for residual closely spaced or back-to-back glands lacking nuclear atypia, "progestin-treated atypical hyperplasia" for residual closely spaced back-to-back glands with nuclear atypia (fig. 5-27), and "progestin-treated carcinoma" for residual confluent glandular or papillary architecture, usually with nuclear atypia (54). In practice, it may be difficult to distinguish among these categories and in such instances it is usually sufficient to describe the lesion and compare its appearance and extent to that in preceding biopsies. The descriptive term "residual low-grade endometrioid neoplasia with treatment effect" may be used for such cases. Key information to convey to the gynecologist includes whether complete response has been achieved, and if not, the degree of response as compared to the previous biopsy(ies).

GRADING

FIGO Grading System. Endometrioid, mucinous, secretory, villoglandular, and ciliated carcinomas should be graded using this system (55); FIGO grading should not be used when endometrioid, mucinous, or ciliated differentiation cannot be established. All other tumor types are typically high grade (i.e., serous and clear cell carcinomas). A grading scheme proposed by Gilks et al. (56) can be used if the tumor type is uncertain (discussed below).

FIGO grade 1 (well-differentiated) endometrioid carcinoma displays a complex glandular or papillary architecture, but lacks a significant solid component (less than 5 percent solid nonsquamous elements). The nuclear grade can be 1 or 2 on a scale of 1 to 3 (fig. 28). FIGO grade 2 (moderately differentiated) endometrioid

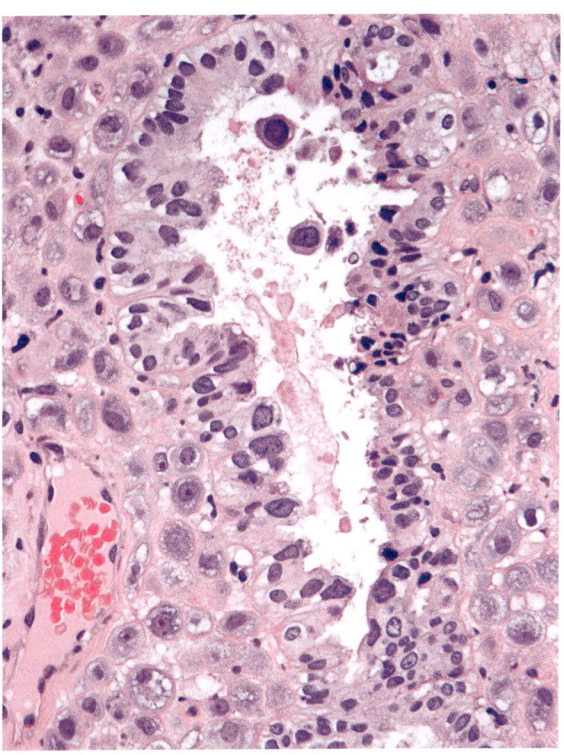

Figure 5-26

ARIAS-STELLA PHENOMENON IN A TREATED ENDOMETRIOID CARCINOMA

This patient, previously diagnosed with FIGO grade 1 endometrioid carcinoma, experienced complete resolution of disease with progestational therapy. Hobnail cells with degenerative nuclear features are found in a gland set in pseudodecidualized stroma.

carcinoma shows glandular and/or papillary architecture with solid nonsquamous elements representing 5 percent or more but 50 percent or less of the tumor (fig. 5-28). The glandular and papillary components must meet the criteria for endometrioid differentiation.

What constitutes solid nonsquamous architecture is often subjective. Many pathologists accept confluent tumor nests with barely perceptible microacini as evidence of solid architecture (fig. 5-29). Solid areas of squamous differentiation should be not counted when grade is assigned, which is easy when squamous differentiation is keratinizing. However, distinguishing solid nonsquamous elements from nonkeratinizing squamous differentiation may be difficult or impossible. Pathologists may base the grade on the appearance of the nuclei

Figure 5-27

ENDOMETRIOID NEOPLASIA WITH PROGESTIN EFFECT

Atypical hyperplasia shows residual complex architecture and prominent eosinophilic metaplastic change (A,B). Cribriform architecture and prominent nucleoli are diagnostic of residual adenocarcinoma. Eosinophilic, mucinous, and tubal metaplasia are also seen (C).

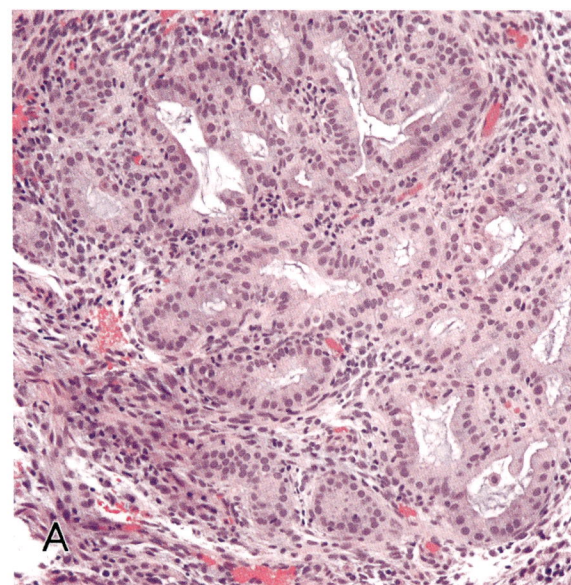
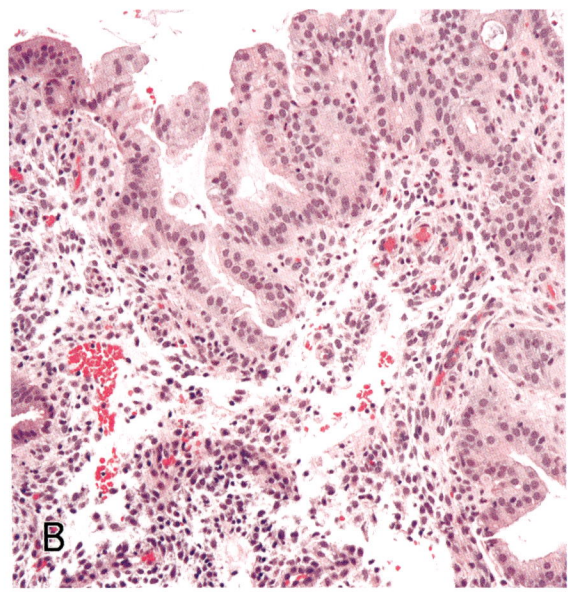
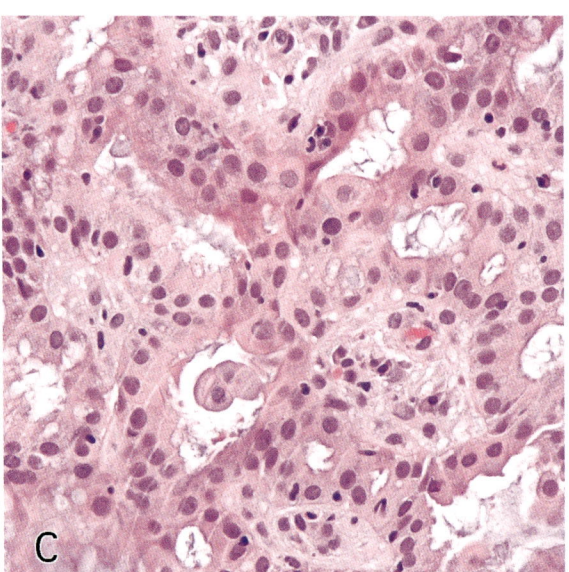

in the solid areas. If they appear similar to the nuclei of the gland-forming components, they are accepted as evidence of solid nonsquamous tumor (fig. 5-30).

Some FIGO grade 2 endometrioid carcinomas may contain a significant component of grade 3 nuclei (severely atypical) (fig. 5-31) (44). In this case, the tumor must still have an endometrioid morphology and no evidence of serous or clear cell carcinoma.

FIGO grade 3 (poorly differentiated) endometrioid carcinoma has a predominantly solid (over 50 percent) nonsquamous architecture (fig. 5-32). Some nonendometrioid carcinomas show extensive solid architecture; therefore, this finding in isolation does not classify an endometrial tumor as FIGO grade 3 endometrioid carcinoma. Low-grade endometrioid glandular or papillary architecture or squamous differentiation must be present at least focally. Although squamous differentiation is not considered in the FIGO grading algorithm, some endometrioid carcinomas contain cytologically malignant-appearing squamous epithelium within an otherwise gland-forming endometrioid carcinoma (fig. 5-33). Such tumors were

Endometrioid Carcinoma and Related Carcinomas

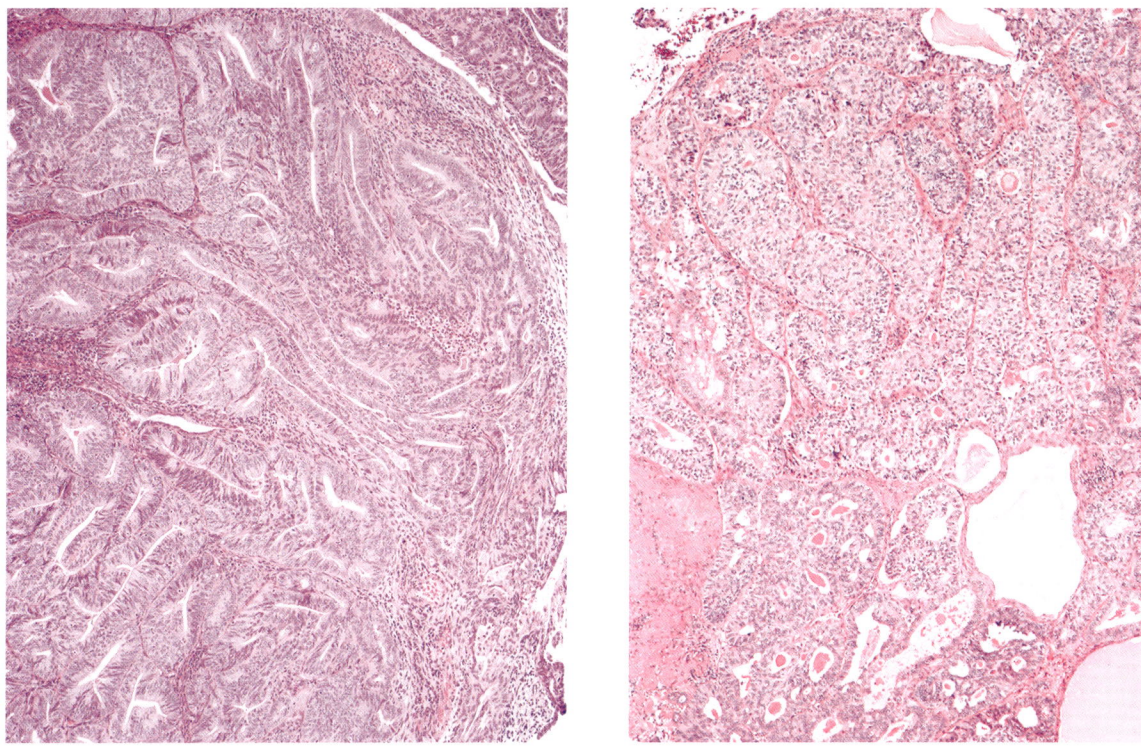

Figure 5-28

LOW-GRADE ENDOMETRIOID ADENOCARCINOMA

FIGO grade 1 (left) and FIGO grade 2 (right) endometrioid adenocarcinomas. In contrast to grade 1 tumors, grade 2 carcinomas contain solid, nonsquamous elements in 5 percent or more and less than 50 percent of the tumor. The transition from glandular to solid areas is typically seamless.

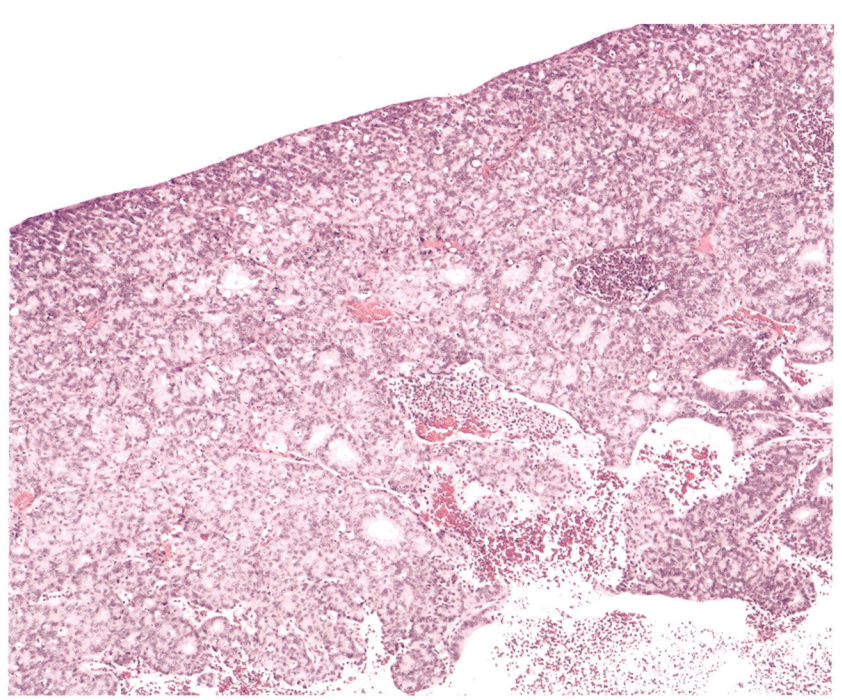

Figure 5-29

"SOLID ARCHITECTURE" REPRESENTED BY BACK-TO-BACK MICROACINI

Even though tiny glandular lumens are present, most pathologists consider this appearance to represent solid architecture for the purposes of FIGO grading.

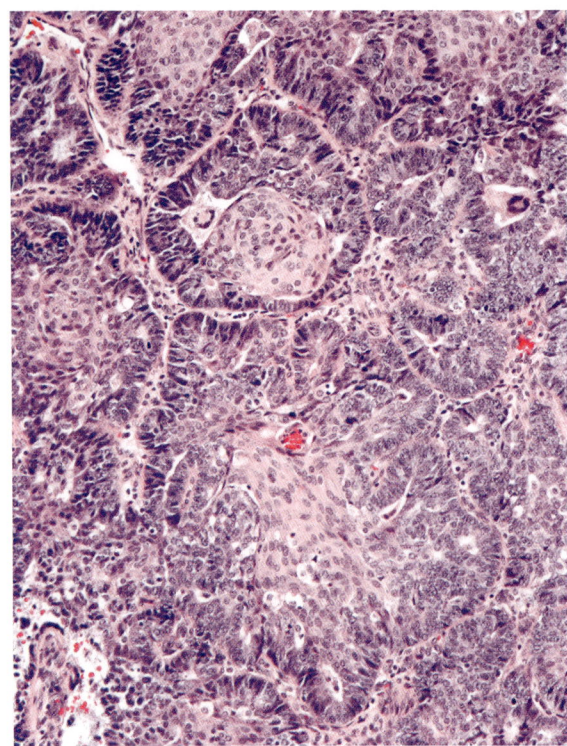

Figure 5-30

ENDOMETRIOID ADENOCARCINOMA WITH SOLID ARCHITECTURE DUE TO SQUAMOUS MORULES

This is a FIGO grade 1 endometrioid adenocarcinoma. Squamous morules should not be considered evidence of solid architecture for grading purposes.

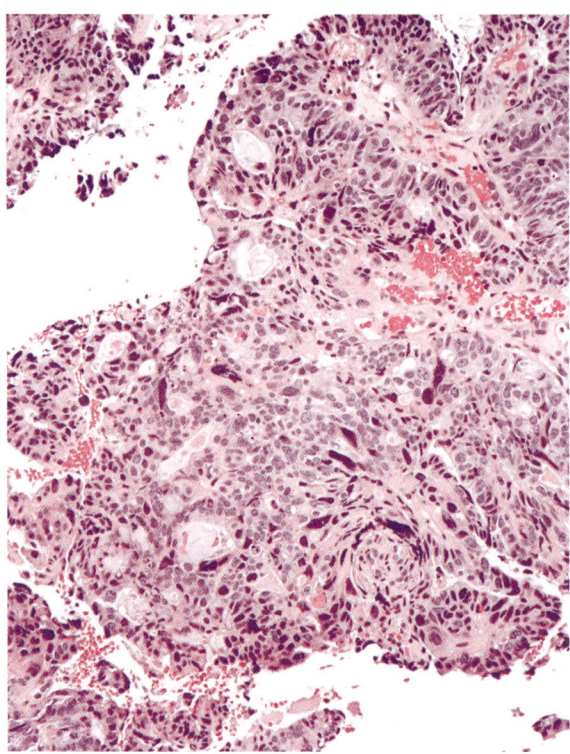

Figure 5-31

ENDOMETRIOID ADENOCARCINOMA WITH SEVERE CYTOLOGIC ATYPIA

Severe nuclear atypia is an indication to upgrade the tumor.

previously regarded as "adenosquamous carcinoma" and are considered by most pathologists to represent FIGO grade 3 carcinomas.

On occasion, a FIGO grade 3 endometrioid carcinoma exhibits the architectural features of a FIGO grade 2 tumor, but in addition have a significant component of grade 3 nuclei (44). As discussed earlier, serous or clear cell carcinoma should be excluded when this combination of features is present.

Non-FIGO Grading Systems. There has been recent interest in exploring binary schemes to replace the traditional FIGO grading criteria (57,58), as most binary grading schemes have superior interobserver diagnostic agreement compared to a three-tiered grading scheme. Several binary grading scheme proposals have shown that endometrioid adenocarcinoma can be readily divided into two main prognostic groups, low- and high-risk, based on a number of features associated with increased tumor aggressiveness, with estimation of solid growth being a good foundation for grade assessment. Understanding the clinical impact of adopting any binary grading system is complicated by variations in patient management and absence of widely accepted consensus on indications for extensive surgical staging in patients with a preoperative diagnosis of low-grade endometrioid carcinoma.

The binary grading scheme proposed by Lax et al. (59) stratified patients into three distinctive prognostic groups. Patients with low-grade endometrioid carcinoma, FIGO stages 1A and 1B (FIGO 1988), had the best prognosis; patients with low-grade endometrioid carcinoma, FIGO stages 1C and higher, and high-grade endometrioid carcinoma, FIGO stages 1B and 1C, had intermediate outcomes; and patients with high-grade carcinoma with extrauterine disease

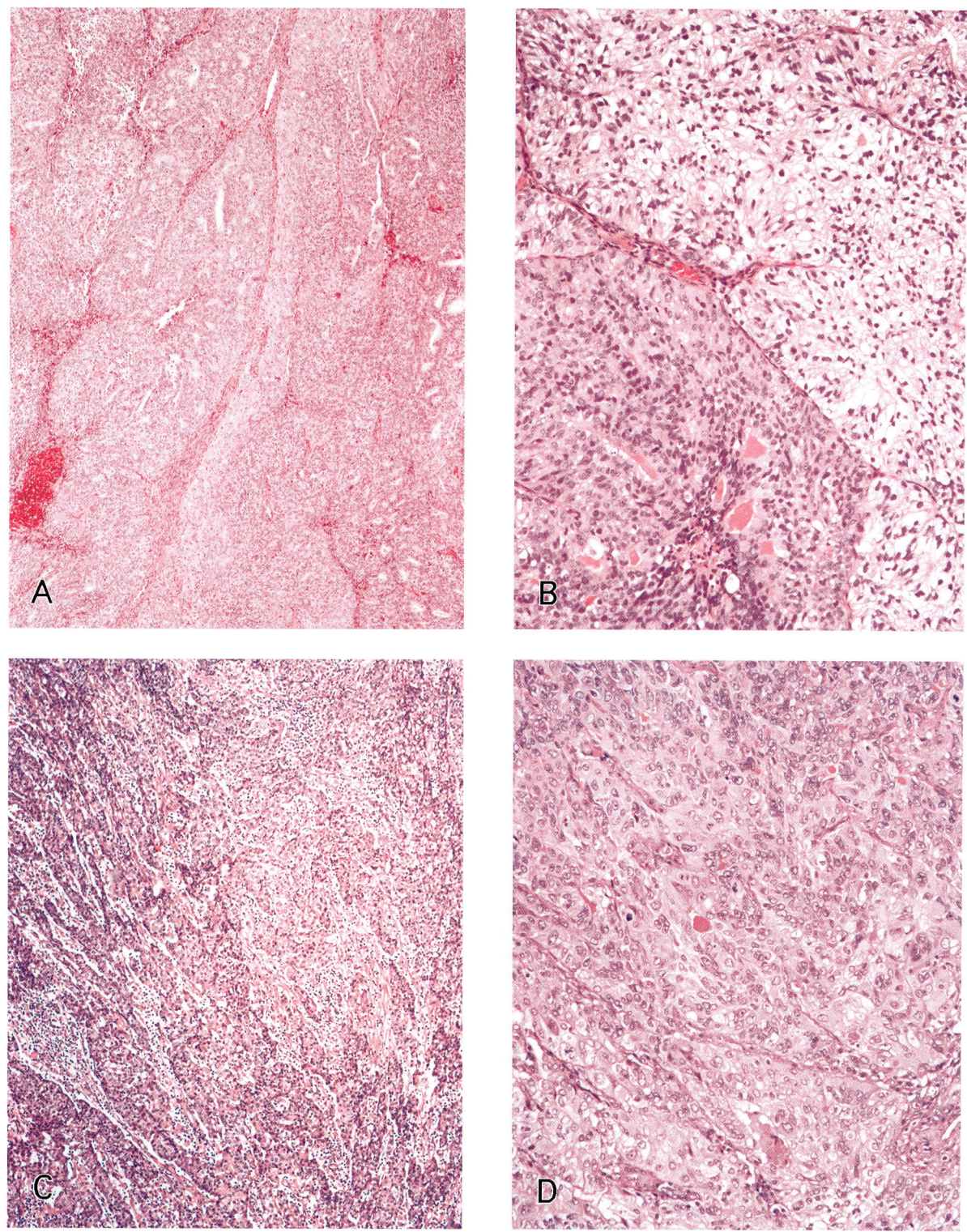

Figure 5-32
GRADE 3 ENDOMETRIOID ADENOCARCINOMA
Predominantly or exclusively solid architecture is present.

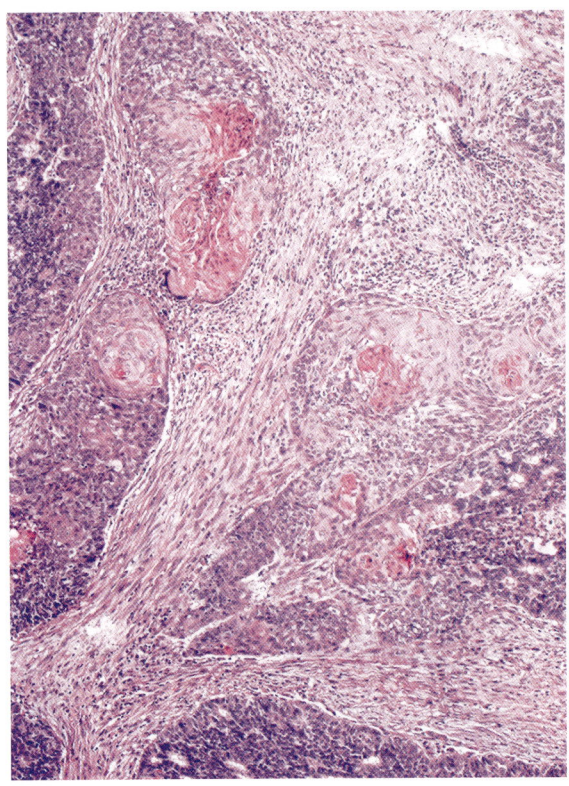

Figure 5-33

GRADE 3 ENDOMETRIOID ADENOCARCINOMA

There is a malignant-appearing squamous component.

The third binary grading scheme collapses FIGO grades into low-grade and high-grade. Classification and regression tree (CART) statistical analysis of 1,544 endometrioid carcinomas from a single institution demonstrated that after tumor stage, division into high-grade (FIGO grade 3) and low-grade (FIGO grades 1 and 2) was the second most informative prognostic parameter (60). This study also demonstrated that while FIGO grade 1 tumors had a significantly lower rate of lymph node metastases than FIGO grade 2 tumors overall (6.6 versus 11.6 percent; p=0.003), differences disappeared when adjusted for depth of myometrial invasion. These results indicate that a binary system based on the known FIGO grading system, collapsing grades 1 and 2 into a low-grade category, is a feasible alternative to the three-tiered FIGO grading when the patient undergoes staging surgery. Distinction between FIGO grade 1 and grade 2 endometrioid carcinomas retains value in biopsy and curettage specimens when the decision to perform staging surgery is based in part on tumor grade.

CYTOLOGY OF ENDOMETRIAL NEOPLASIA

Papanicolaou tests are not considered an effective screening method for endometrial neoplasia because of a lack of sensitivity. Reports of malignant endometrial cells present in Pap tests from patients with carcinoma range from 18 to 50 percent (61–63). If atypical endometrial cells and age over 40 years are added to the equation, the predictive value increases to as high as 77 percent (61,63). The cells of endometrial hyperplasia and carcinoma can be identified with good reliability when present.

In the 2014 Bethesda terminology (64), abnormal endometrial cells are classified into two categories: atypical endometrial cells and endometrial adenocarcinoma. Unlike atypical endocervical cells, which are further classified into "not otherwise specified" and "favor neoplasia" subcategories, this type of distinction between endometrial atypias has been shown to be less reproducible and less reliable, primarily due to cellular degeneration in shed endometrial cells and benign mimics. Atypical endometrial cells can be seen in association with benign endometrial polyp, chronic endometritis, intrauterine device, and endometrial neoplasia. Reports show that after finding atypical endometrial cells, 15

had the worst clinical outcomes. A tumor was classified as high-grade when at least two of the following three criteria were present: more than 50 percent solid architecture (without distinction between squamous and nonsquamous), diffusely infiltrative pattern of myometrial invasion, and tumor cell necrosis. Interobserver and intraobserver agreement was superior compared to the FIGO system. This binary grading scheme is applicable only to endometrioid carcinomas diagnosed in hysterectomy specimens.

The binary grading scheme proposed by Gilks et al. (56) separates clinically low-grade and high-grade tumors irrespective of tumor histotype and can therefore be used when the histotype is uncertain. A tumor is classified as high-grade when at least two of the following three criteria are present: diffusely high nuclear grade, predominant papillary or solid architecture, and mitotic index of more than 5 mitoses per 10 high-power fields.

Endometrioid Carcinoma and Related Carcinomas

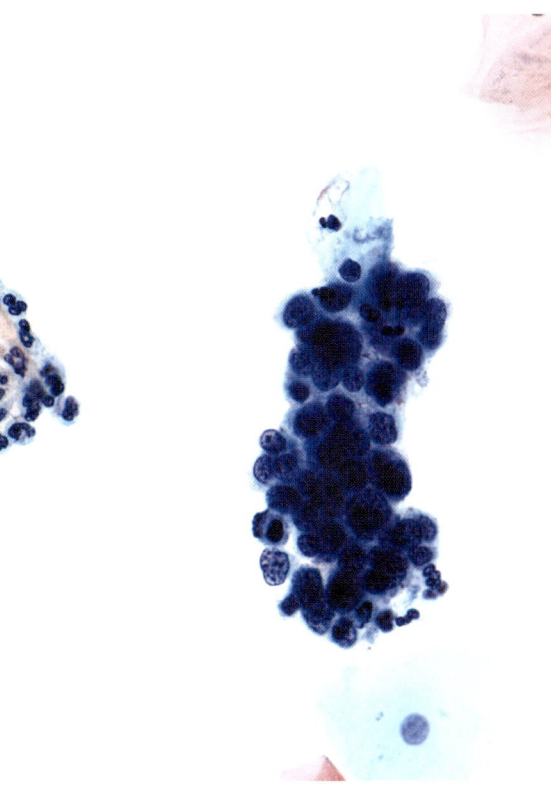

Figure 5-34

ATYPICAL ENDOMETRIAL CELLS

This group of cells is densely packed with a high N/C ratio, hyperchromasia, and coarse chromatin. The nuclei show mild enlargement compared to normal endometrial cells. Follow-up showed no evidence of endometrial neoplasia. The atypical features are attributable to degenerative changes in exfoliated endometrium due to menses.

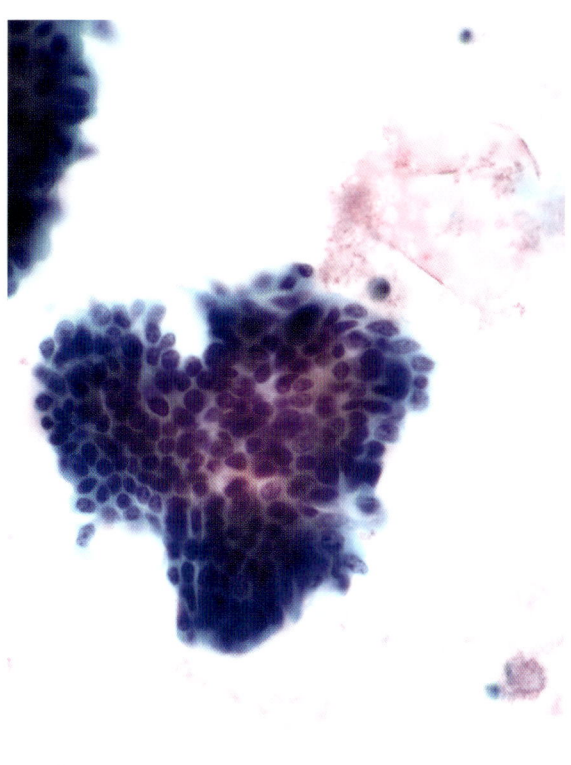

Figure 5-35

ATYPICAL ENDOMETRIAL CELLS

This large group of cells shows similar nuclear features to those present in figure 5-34. The background shows granular diathesis material ("watery" diathesis). Follow-up showed grade 1 endometrioid endometrial adenocarcinoma.

to 20 percent of patients have a carcinoma (6). The criteria for interpretation as atypical endometrial cells include cells occurring in small to medium-sized three-dimensional groups showing nuclei that are slightly enlarged as compared to normal endometrial cells, hyperchromatic cells, and cells having chromatin with heterogeneous granularity. Occasionally, small nucleoli are present. Cytoplasm is scant and may show vacuolization (figs. 5-34, 5-35) (64).

The diagnostic features of cells exfoliated from endometrioid carcinoma become progressively more recognizable as the tumor grade increases. Grade 1 tumors only show mild nuclear changes and are interpreted only as "atypical." When cells from higher-grade carcinomas are present, the nuclear size proportionally increases, as does nuclear pleomorphism (both in size and shape). Nuclei are hyperchromatic, with coarse irregular chromatin showing cleared areas, and with nucleolar prominence proportionate to grade. Cytoplasm is scant, with a resultant high N/C ratio (fig. 5-36). The background of the slide may show a "watery" or finely granular diathesis. Vacuolated cells filled with neutrophils are commonly present in endometrial carcinomas but are not specific, as they can also be seen in degenerating epithelia, often in association with polyps (fig. 5-37). Tumor cells associated with high-grade serous carcinoma of the endometrium resemble their ovarian counterparts being very large with prominent macronucleoli, often in cohesive "tufted" three-dimensional groups (fig. 5-38) (64).

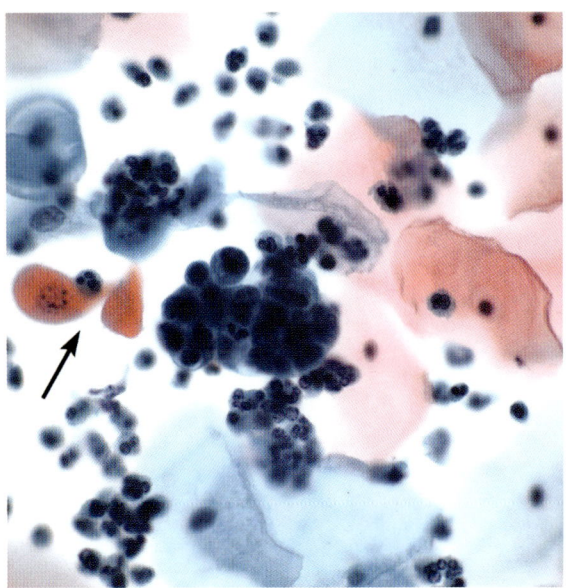 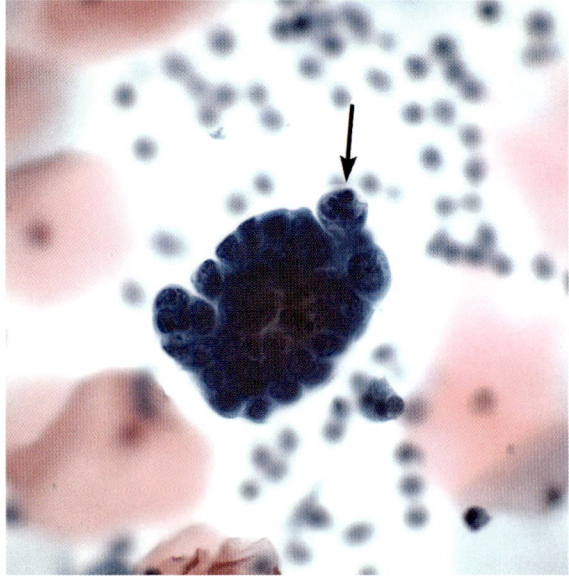

Figure 5-36

ENDOMETRIAL ADENOCARCINOMA

This three-dimensional group shows enlarged nuclei greater in size than those in figures 5-34 and 5-35. The nuclei are irregular, hyperchromatic, and show prominent nucleoli and coarse chromatin. Just below the group are two cells with squamous keratinization (arrow) derived from the squamous metaplasia commonly present in low-grade endometrioid adenocarcinoma (left). A higher-grade carcinoma has large and irregular nuclei. Neutrophils are present within the cell at the margin (arrow) (right).

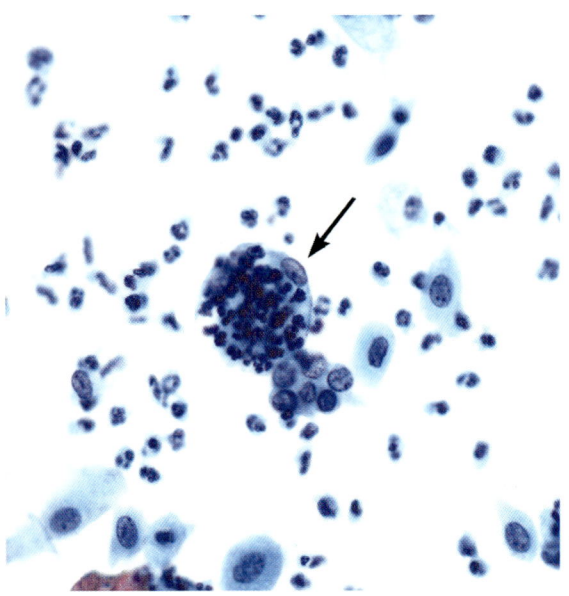 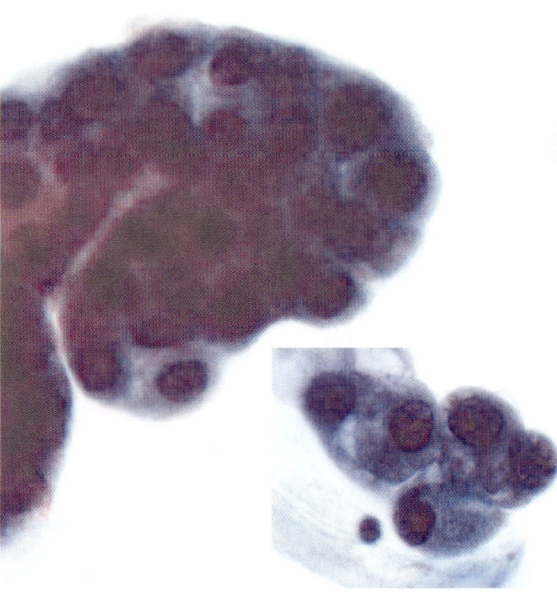

Figure 5-37

ENDOMETRIAL ADENOCARCINOMA

Isolated vacuolated cells containing neutrophils are common in endometrial adenocarcinoma (arrow), however, they are not specific since they are seen in other degenerating processes such as occur on the surface of polyps.

Figure 5-38

ENDOMETRIAL SEROUS CARCINOMA

Low magnification shows the tufted three-dimensional group often present in this carcinoma. At high magnification (inset), large nuclei with prominent nucleoli are noted.

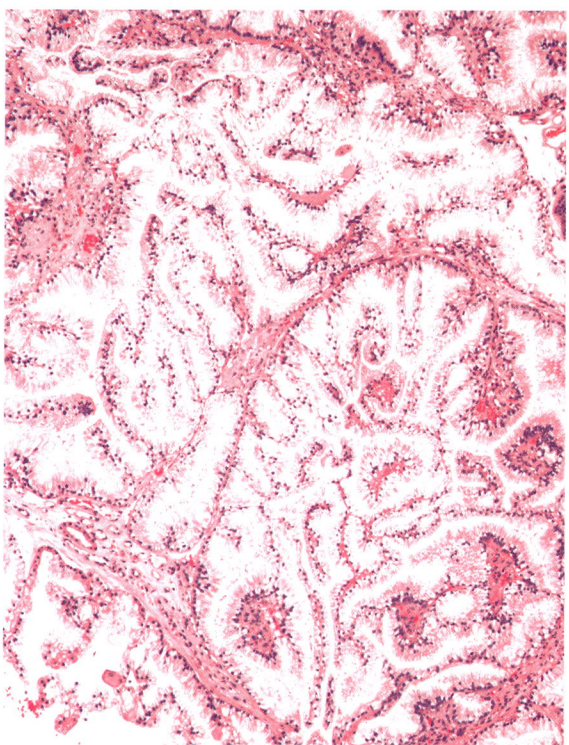

Figure 5-39

MUCINOUS CARCINOMA

The tumor cells have abundant mucin and are reminiscent of endocervical cells with bland nuclear features but complex architecture.

RELATED CARCINOMAS

Mucinous Carcinoma

Most *mucinous adenocarcinomas* resemble endometrioid carcinomas with mucinous differentiation (65–67). It has been arbitrarily proposed that endometrioid carcinomas containing a major component of cells (more than 50 percent in 2014 World Health Organization classification) (68) with intracellular mucin be placed in the "mucinous carcinoma" category. The cells have an appearance reminiscent of endocervical cells. The finding of intraluminal mucin alone does not place a tumor in this category since this feature may be seen in other tumor types. The diagnosis of mucinous carcinoma should only be made in hysterectomy specimens, since typical endometrioid carcinomas often show mucinous metaplasia, especially on their surface (69).

Mucinous carcinomas display a variably complex glandular or papillary architecture, sometimes with cystically dilated glands (fig. 5-39). Solid growth is uncommon. Some tumors resemble microglandular hyperplasia of endocervix (see fig. 5-18C) (35,36,70) or even minimal deviation adenocarcinoma, mucinous type, of the cervix (67). Abundant extracellular mucin and acute inflammatory infiltrates may be seen (67). Oxyphilic cells may be admixed with mucinous cells and, rarely, goblet or argentaffin cells. Most mucinous carcinomas have low-grade nuclear features, thus the diagnosis, especially in biopsy or curettage specimens, is based on architectural complexity (71).

These tumors tend to have indolent behavior, as they are often confined to the endometrium. The prognosis is similar to that reported for endometrioid carcinomas matched for grade and stage (72).

Ciliated Carcinoma

Ciliated carcinomas are rare. They have an overall appearance identical to conventional endometrioid carcinomas, with glands predominantly lined by ciliated cells (see fig. 5-3). In some cases, gland lumens are tiny and impart a "solid" low-power appearance. They tend to be indolent tumors, especially as the nuclear grade is usually low (73).

Secretory Carcinoma

A variant of endometrioid carcinoma, *secretory carcinoma* displays a significant component of cells with glycogen-rich supranuclear and/or subnuclear cytoplasmic vacuoles imparting an appearance similar to secretory phase endometrium (see fig. 5-17) (74–76). It is rarely seen in its pure form (less than 2 percent), but is more often encountered as a minor component of an otherwise conventional endometrioid carcinoma. This morphology may be seen in patients on hormonal therapy or related to the finding of a corpus luteum in the ovary, but in most cases these associations are lacking. The adjacent uninvolved endometrium may have a mid- or late-secretory appearance.

Villoglandular Carcinoma

Villoglandular carcinomas are composed predominantly of long and thin (finger-like) papillae (figs. 5-9, 5-40) (77–79), often admixed with a minor component of endometrioid glands. A villoglandular component is seen in 10 to 15 percent of endometrioid carcinomas but this morphology is rarely seen in pure form. The papillae are lined by columnar "endometrioid-type" cells with low nuclear grade. Squamous differentiation may be present. Although villoglandular architecture is more common in the surface compartment of the tumor, it may also be noted in the myoinvasive component.

Villoglandular carcinomas tend to be indolent when they have low nuclear grade, and there is limited or no myometrial invasion, paralleling the behavior of conventional endometrioid carcinomas. Some data indicate that myometrial invasive villoglandular carcinomas may pursue an aggressive course.

Endometrioid Carcinoma Admixed with Other Elements

Endometrioid carcinomas can be admixed with the following elements: small and large cell neuroendocrine carcinomas (80–82), central- and peripheral-type primitive neuroectodermal tumors (83–85), trophoblastic and germ cell tumors (86–88), and Wilms tumor (89–91) (see chapter 12).

Undifferentiated and Dedifferentiated Carcinoma

Undifferentiated carcinoma is defined as a malignant epithelial neoplasm with no recognizable differentiation on morphologic grounds. This diagnosis should be made only after excluding other entities in the differential diagnosis. It occurs over a wide age range (median, 55 years), with 45 percent of patients being over 50 years (92). They mainly present with vaginal bleeding, and only a minority with abdominal pain. Most tumors are centered in the uterine corpus, but a significant minority arises in the lower uterine segment. Extrauterine disease is seen in 40 to 60 percent of patients at presentation (92,93).

The macroscopic features of undifferentiated and dedifferentiated (described below) carcinomas are not well described in the literature. Based on anecdotal experience, these tumors do not have distinguishing gross characteristics, although they have a tendency to be large and necrotic (see fig. 5-4C).

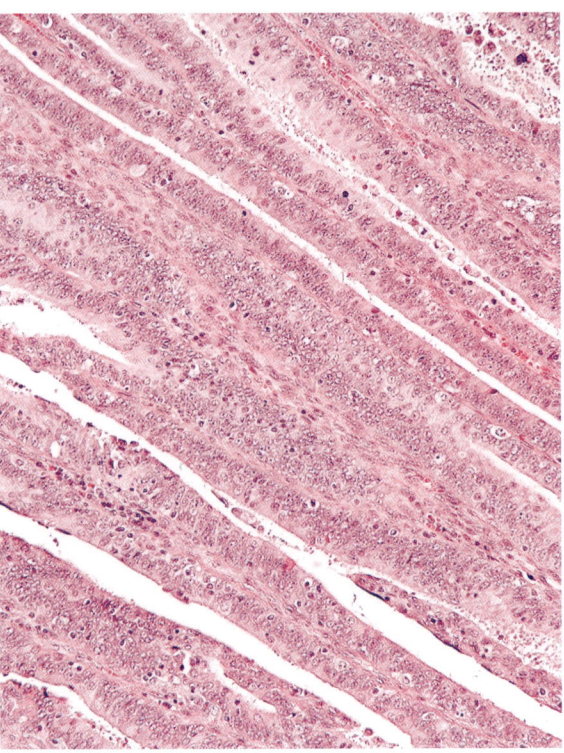

Figure 5-40

VILLOGLANDULAR ENDOMETRIOID ADENOCARCINOMA

This carcinoma has villoglandular features and nuclear grade 2. The presence of a higher nuclear grade should suggest serous carcinoma.

Morphologically, there are at least two general types of undifferentiated carcinoma (94): *monomorphic undifferentiated carcinoma* and *pleomorphic undifferentiated carcinoma*. Monomorphic undifferentiated carcinoma is composed of noncohesive medium to large sized cells arranged in sheets without any obvious nested or trabecular architecture (fig. 5-41). The low-power appearance frequently overlaps with that of lymphoma, plasmacytoma, high-grade endometrial stromal sarcoma, and small cell carcinoma as gland formation is lacking. If poorly fixed, smaller cells may be noted. Although some degree of nuclear size variability is seen within a tumor, overt pleomorphism is absent, with only rare exceptions in which pleomorphic nuclei are found focally (fig. 5-42). Chromatin may be condensed and a dark or small nucleolus may be present. The mitotic activity is typically brisk (over 25 mitoses per 10 high-power fields). Approximately one-quarter of tumors have rhabdoid cells with

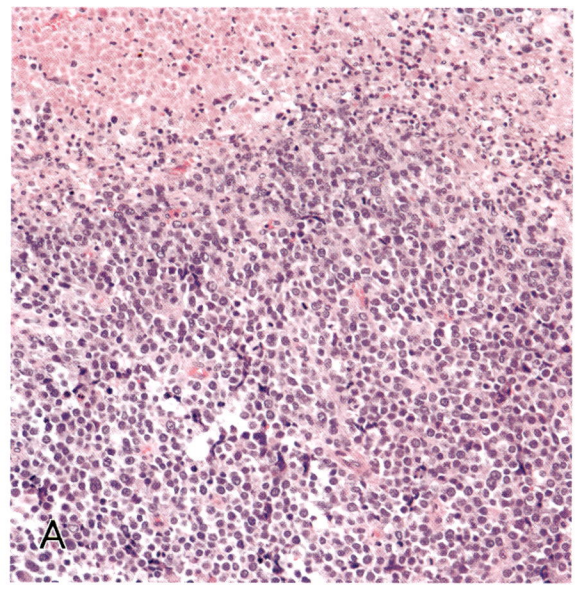

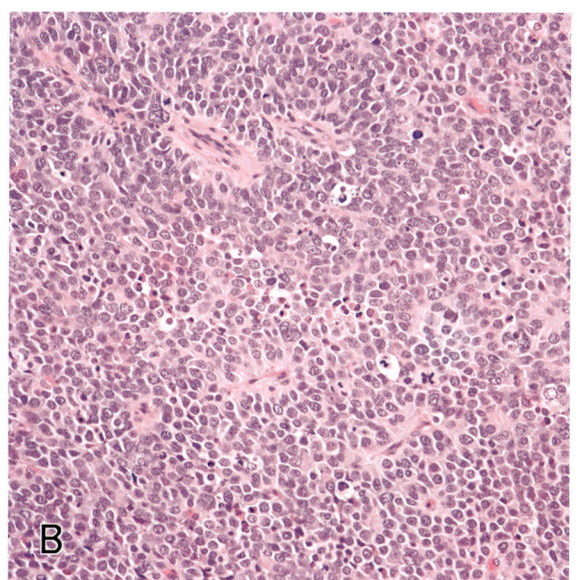
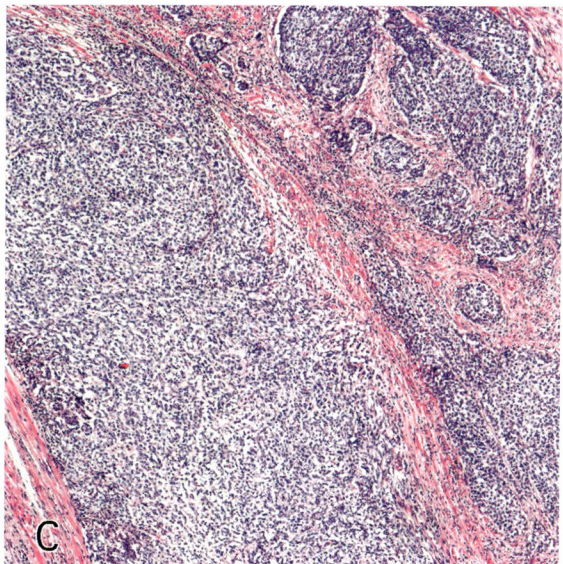

Figure 5-41

UNDIFFERENTIATED ENDOMETRIAL CARCINOMA

Tumor cells are monotonous and dyshesive without nests, trabeculae, or glands. Necrosis is common (A). There is a similarity to lymphoma and small cell carcinoma. Tumor cells grow in sheets (B), and typically show destructive myometrial invasion (C).

abundant globoid pink cytoplasm and a displaced vesicular nucleus with large nucleolus, imparting a plasmacytoid appearance (fig. 5-43). Although associated stroma is generally inapparent, some tumors, particularly those with rhabdoid cells, display a myxoid matrix (fig. 5-44). Tumor-infiltrating lymphocytes are common (92), and if prominent, the morphologic appearance may resemble a lymphoepithelial-like carcinoma of cervix or nasopharynx (fig. 5-45). Abrupt keratinization, seen as keratin pearls, is rare (fig. 5-46).

A component of FIGO grade 1 or 2 endometrioid carcinoma is seen juxtaposed to the undifferentiated carcinoma in about 40 percent of tumors (95) (fig. 5-47). These tumors are designated as *dedifferentiated carcinoma* or mixed *differentiated and undifferentiated carcinoma*. As the differentiated endometrioid and undifferentiated components are usually found in the most superficial and deeper aspects the tumor, respectively, a diagnosis of FIGO grade 1 endometrioid carcinoma may be rendered in the curettage specimen and a diagnosis of undifferentiated carcinoma may be made at hysterectomy, or a diagnosis of FIGO grade 1 endometrioid carcinoma at hysterectomy and that of

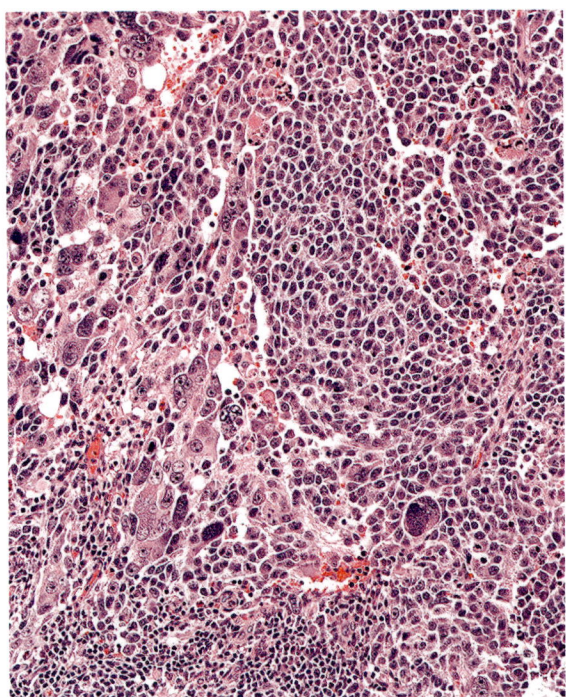

Figure 5-42

UNDIFFERENTIATED ENDOMETRIAL CARCINOMA

Pleomorphic nuclei are seen focally in a background of monomorphic nuclei.

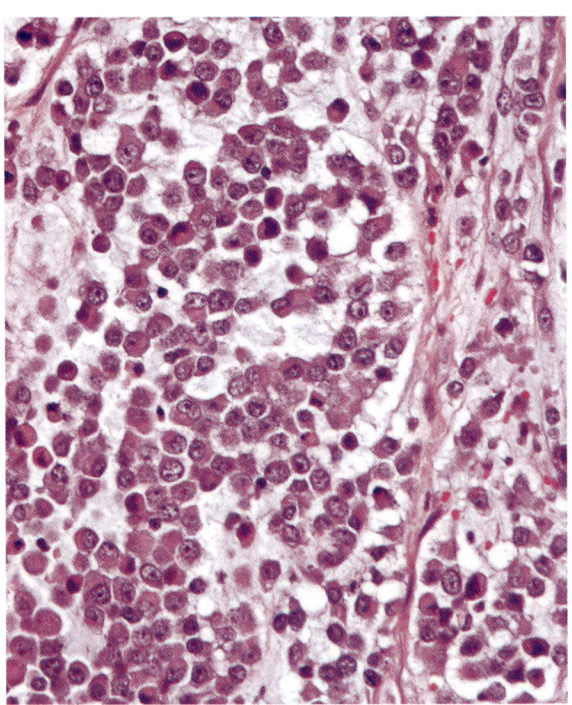

Figure 5-43

UNDIFFERENTIATED ENDOMETRIAL CARCINOMA

Rhabdoid tumor cells are floating in a myxoid matrix.

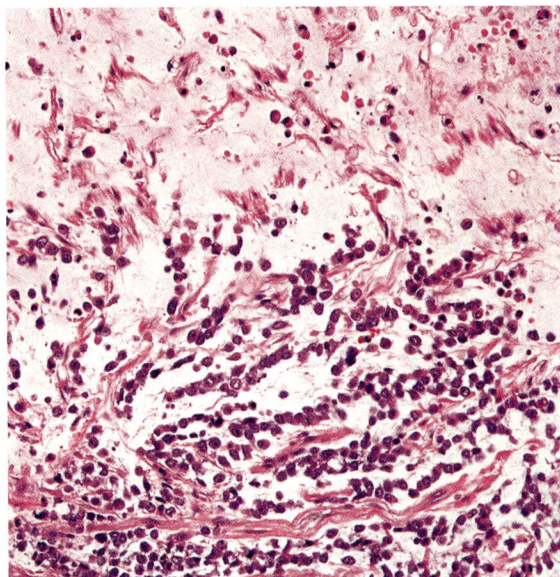

Figure 5-44

UNDIFFERENTIATED ENDOMETRIAL CARCINOMA

Prominent myxoid matrix is seen.

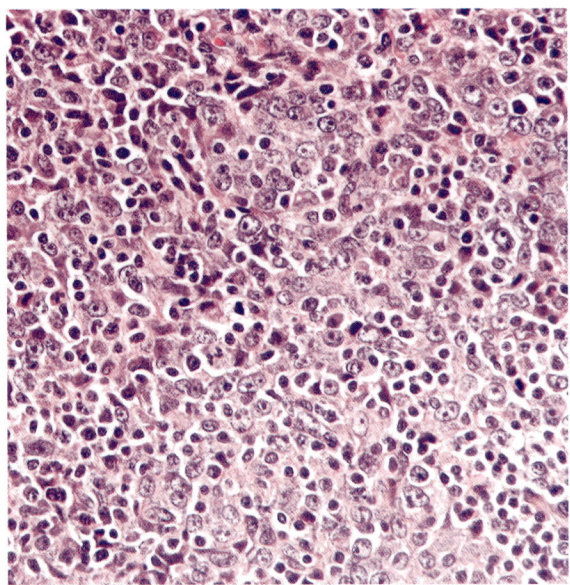

Figure 5-45

UNDIFFERENTIATED ENDOMETRIAL CARCINOMA

The dense tumor-infiltrating lymphocytes impart an appearance similar to that seen in a lymphoepithelioma-like carcinoma. This tumor lacked expression of MLH1 and PMS2.

undifferentiated carcinoma in a metastatic site. Rarely, a FIGO grade 3 carcinoma is juxtaposed to an undifferentiated carcinoma (fig. 5-48) and in that scenario it is still reasonable to diagnose these tumors as mixed undifferentiated and grade 3 endometrioid carcinoma.

Rarely, undifferentiated carcinoma can have a spindled morphology (fig. 5-49). Most of these neoplasms have been diagnosed as carcinosarcomas, but they diverge from the characteristic carcinosarcoma, which typically features a high-grade carcinoma (most often with serous or hybrid morphology) and a high-grade mesenchymal component (see chapter 11). Another rare combination is that of low-grade endometrioid carcinoma with both monomorphic and pleomorphic undifferentiated components, or even low-grade endometrioid carcinoma with pleomorphic undifferentiated components lacking overtly sarcomatoid features. Since there is no consensus or published criteria on diagnostic terminology, tumors with the aforementioned features may be diagnosed as dedifferentiated

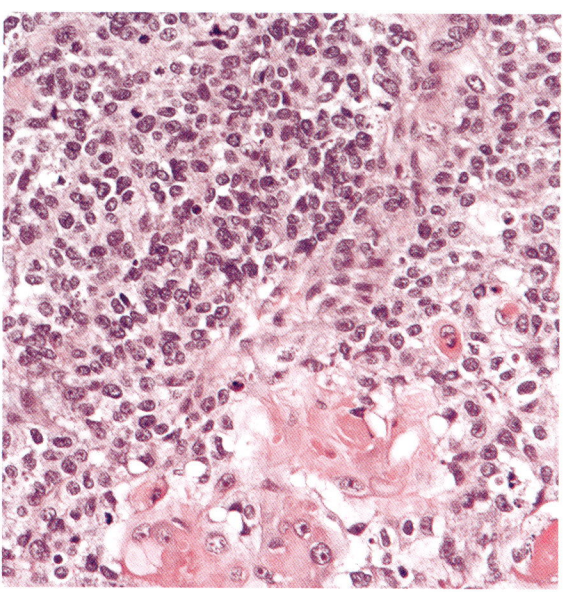

Figure 5-46

UNDIFFERENTIATED ENDOMETRIAL CARCINOMA WITH ABRUPT KERATINIZATION

This is the only type of epithelial differentiation allowable in undifferentiated carcinoma.

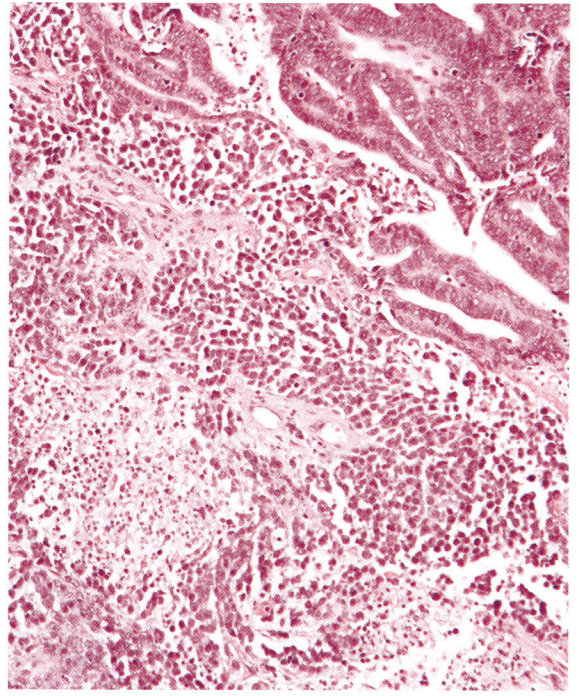
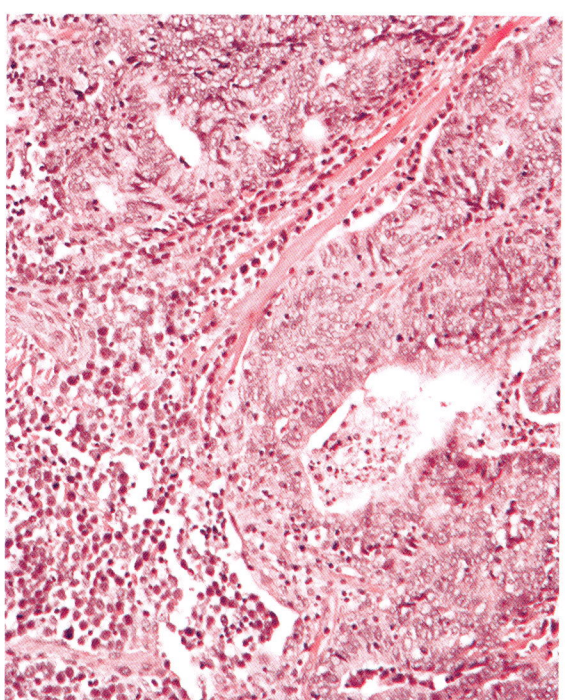

Figure 5-47

DEDIFFERENTIATED ENDOMETRIAL CARCINOMA (MIXED WELL-DIFFERENTIATED ENDOMETRIOID AND UNDIFFERENTIATED CARCINOMA)

A FIGO grade 1 endometrioid carcinoma is juxtaposed to an undifferentiated carcinoma.

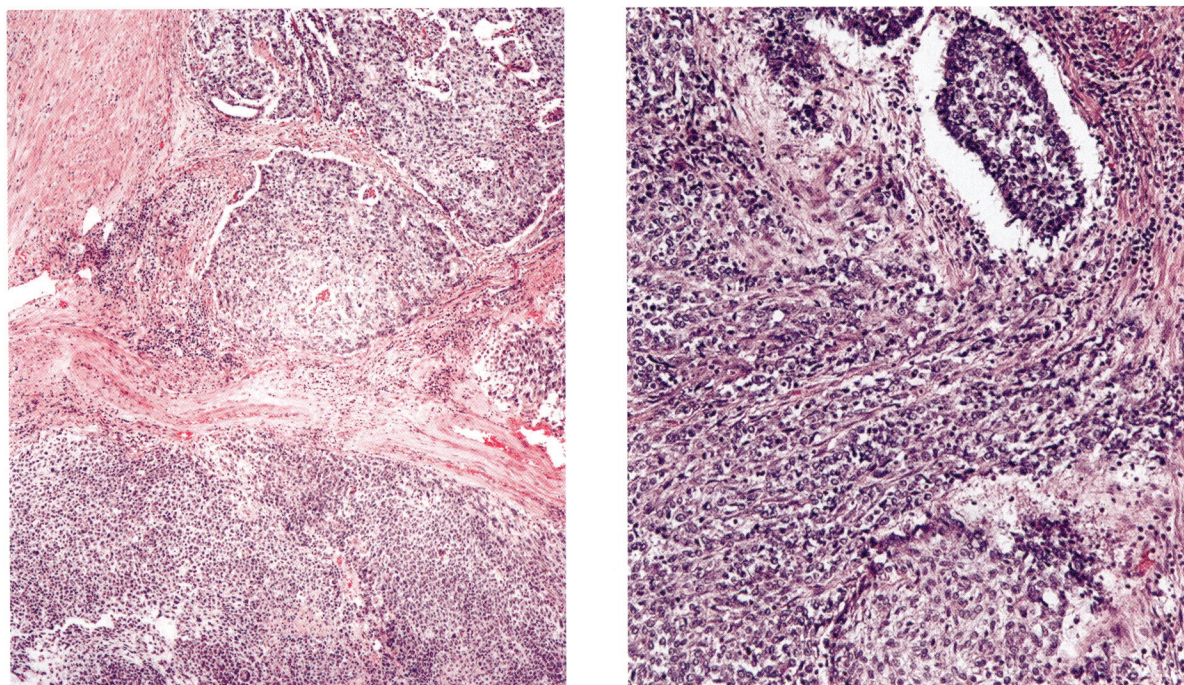

Figure 5-48

DEDIFFERENTIATED ENDOMETRIAL CARCINOMA (MIXED POORLY DIFFERENTIATED ENDOMETRIOID AND UNDIFFERENTIATED CARCINOMA)

The nested and cohesive appearance of FIGO grade 3 endometrioid carcinoma contrasts with the dyshesive appearance of the undifferentiated carcinoma.

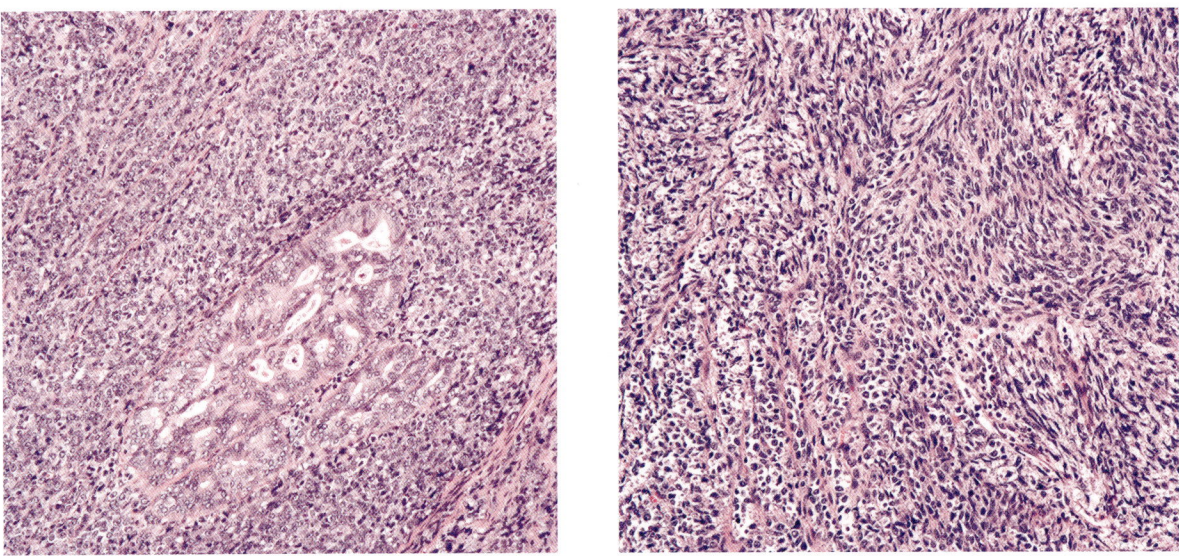

Figure 5-49

DEDIFFERENTIATED ENDOMETRIAL CARCINOMA WITH SPINDLE CELLS

Spindling is barely perceptible in the left figure, but is well developed in the right. These tumors might be diagnosed as carcinosarcoma, but their appearance and expected immunophenotype and genotype differ significantly from most carcinosarcomas, which are typically characterized by high-grade or pleomorphic epithelial and mesenchymal elements.

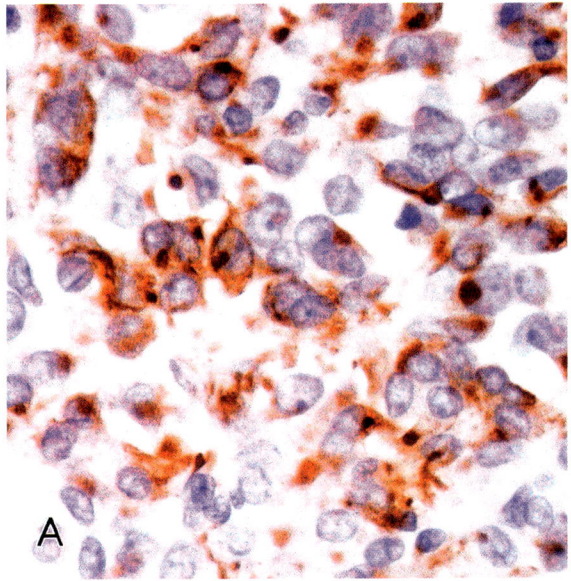

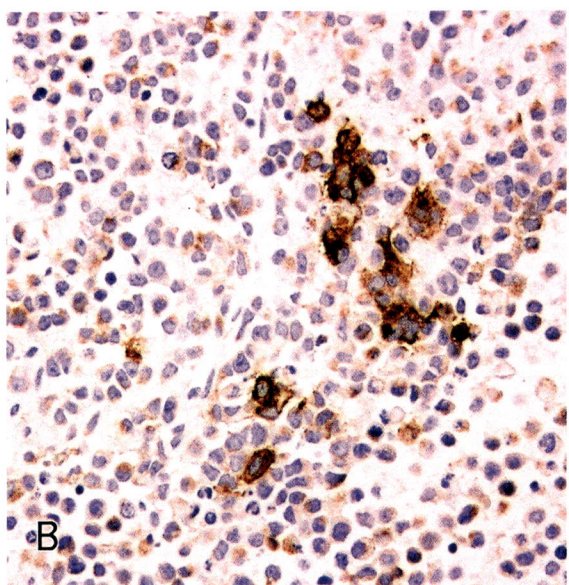

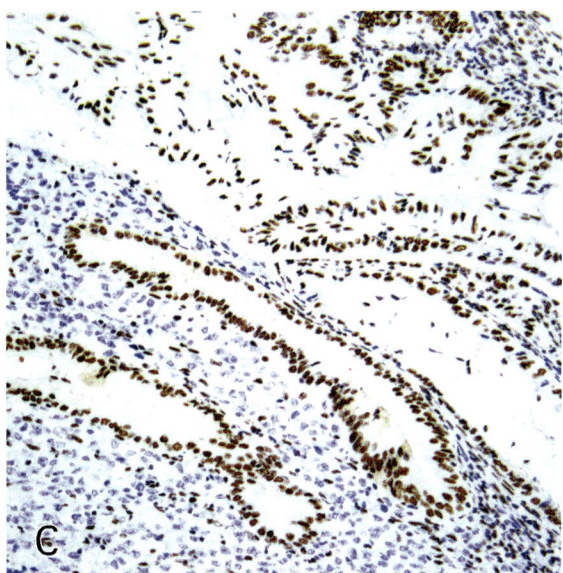

Figure 5-50

UNDIFFERENTIATED ENDOMETRIAL CARCINOMA: IMMUNOPHENOTYPE

Focal expression of CK18 (A), EMA (B), and loss of expression of BRG-1 (C) is seen in the undifferentiated component, the latter preserved in the endometrioid component. *SMARCA-4* mutation may be involved in the process of dedifferentiation.

carcinoma, endometrioid carcinoma with tumor giant cells (see following), or carcinosarcoma.

Undifferentiated carcinomas, monomorphic type, are divided into two subcategories based on molecular findings: 1) with chromatin remodeling abnormalities and microsatellite instability (more common); 2) with *Tp53* mutation and microsatellite stability (less common) (96). The former displays evidence of epithelial differentiation with epithelial membrane antigen (EMA) (93) and CK18 labeling in only a minority of tumor cells (fig. 5-50) (92). Rarely, they harbor *POLE* exonuclease domain mutations (97). Diffuse pancytokeratin and PAX8 expression are lacking and estrogen receptor (ER) and progesterone receptor (PR) are typically negative. Tumor cells express vimentin and may be positive for CD138. No or limited E-cadherin labeling is seen (96,98). Chromogranin and synaptophysin may be positive, but typically in a minority of tumor cells (93).

The most common evidence of chromatin remodeling abnormalities involves loss of expression of BRG-1, due to mutations in *SMARCA4*, along with frequent loss of expression of SMARCA2 (96). Another important pathway involves loss of expression of BAF250a/ARID1A,

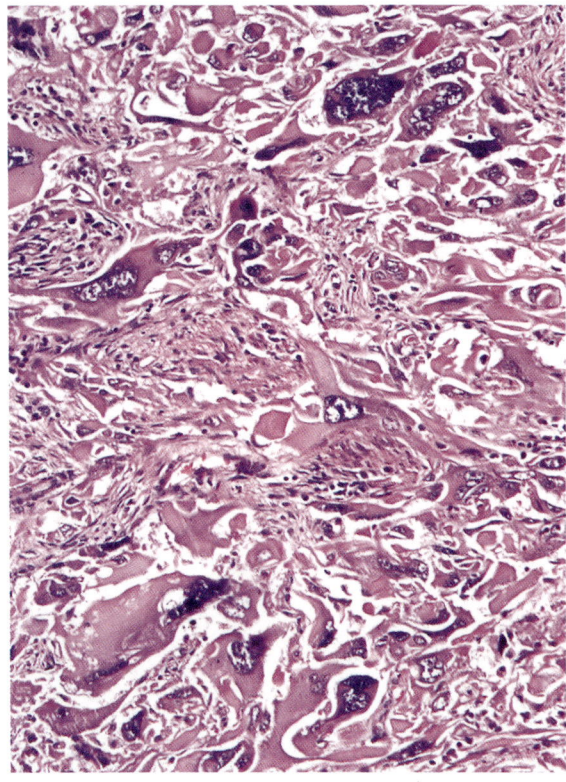

Figure 5-51

GIANT CELL CARCINOMA OF ENDOMETRIUM

This tumor type resembles giant cell/pleomorphic/sarcomatoid carcinomas of pancreas and lung. Although it may exist in pure form, it is more likely to be found associated with endometrioid or serous carcinoma.

due to mutations in *ARID1A*, along with loss of expression of ARID1B and mutations in *ARID1B* (99). Rarely, loss of expression of BAF47/INI-1, due to mutations in *SMARCB1*, has been reported (96). Approximately half to three quarters of these tumors are microsatellite unstable (92,96), mostly due to *hMLH1* promoter methylation. Occasional DNA mismatch repair (MMR) germline mutations diagnostic of Lynch syndrome have been reported (100). The second group of monomorphic undifferentiated carcinomas with *Tp53* mutation tends to show substantially more labeling with pancytokeratins, EMA, PAX8, ER, and PR, compared to tumors with chromatin remodeling abnormalities and microsatellite instability, as well as aberrant p53 staining (81,96).

Undifferentiated carcinomas are part of a family of carcinomas that are thought to arise via epithelial to mesenchymal transition (EMT), a process by which epithelial cells lose polarity and intercellular adhesion, while acquiring properties of mesenchymal cells. In uterine tumors, EMT typically involves upregulation of the micro-RNA-200 series, with consequent upregulation of established EMT-related proteins such as ZEB-1, SNAIL, and TWIST, and downregulation of E-cadherin (98). The emergence of an undifferentiated component is possibly due to acquisition of an *SMARCA4* (96) or *ARID1B* mutation (99), leading to loss of expression in the undifferentiated component in a majority of such tumors.

A small number of endometrial carcinomas containing tumor giant cells have been reported as giant cell carcinoma of endometrium (pleomorphic undifferentiated carcinoma) (101,102). The tumor giant cells are usually keratin negative and lack resemblance to any differentiated endometrial carcinoma. The appearance is reminiscent of giant cell carcinomas found in the lung and pancreas (fig. 5-51). In most cases, the giant cell component is admixed with a differentiated endometrial carcinoma, most commonly an endometrioid carcinoma.

Clinically, approximately two-thirds of patients with undifferentiated/dedifferentiated carcinomas have pelvic and para-aortic lymph node metastases, and less frequently, have vaginal, visceral, and abdominal dissemination. An infrequent, but alarming finding is explosive lymphadenopathy simulating lymphoma (92). Extrauterine disease at presentation is an ominous finding. Between 55 percent and 95 percent of patients have persistent disease or have died of disease at follow-up (92,93). Patients with undifferentiated or dedifferentiated carcinoma have a poorer clinical outcome than those with FIGO grade 3 endometrioid carcinoma (93). Small series have suggested that the clinical outcome is similar to that of high-grade neuroendocrine carcinomas (103) and carcinosarcomas (104).

Patients with *SMARCA4*- or *SMARCB1*-mutated tumors (including those with loss of expression of the corresponding protein by immunohistochemistry) can be enrolled in therapeutic trials of EZH2 inhibitors thought to induce synthetic lethality (105). Patients with DNA MMR-deficient undifferentiated or dedifferentiated carcinomas may also benefit from immunomodulatory therapies (106). These therapies are thought to be effective in patients whose tumors are microsatellite unstable, carry a high mutational load, and contain numerous tumor-infiltrating lymphocytes, all characteristics that are frequently encountered in these tumors. DNA MMR deficient tumors, as well as those harboring *POLE* exonuclease domain mutations, may be prognostically favorable (107).

STAGING

Table 5-1 shows the current FIGO staging scheme (2009) for endometrial carcinoma (108,109), which differs from the 1988 classification. The main differences between the two classifications are: combining prior stage 1A (tumor confined to the endometrium) and stage IB (tumor infiltrating less than half of myometrium) as stage IA; dropping peritoneal washing status as part of staging; and disregarding endocervical mucosal involvement by tumor as stage II. However, this staging scheme is imperfect. It ignores definitions for staging adequacy (110) and significant clinical heterogeneity within each substage, and it does not account for mode of dissemination, suggesting that lymphovascular and peritoneal spread, direct extension, and implantation without invasion are clinically equivalent. Furthermore, it does not provide clear definitions for cervical stromal invasion; how to stage endometrial carcinoma with pelvic extension in the absence of or in addition to uterine serosal, parametrial, or adnexal involvement; what constitutes minimal parametrial involvement; and whether lymphovascular invasion in extrauterine sites qualifies as metastatic disease.

Myometrial Invasion

Determining the presence and depth of myometrial invasion can be challenging. A number of studies have reported discrepancy rates of approximately 30 percent among pathologists, with gynecologic pathologists reporting less myometrial invasion and smaller measurements (111–114). Figure 5-52 illustrates the methodology used to measure the depth of myometrial invasion in different settings, while Figure 5-53 demonstrates obvious examples of myometrial invasion. Overcalling the presence and depth of myometrial invasion is thought to be secondary to several factors including inherent irregular endomyometrial junction, inapparent or metaplastic endometrial stroma around the tumor, and measuring tumor thickness instead of depth of invasion. The location of the endomyometrial junction must be sought or at least estimated to avoid measuring tumor thickness, especially in exophytic tumors (fig. 5-54). A less common mistake is to underestimate the depth of myometrial invasion due to unfamiliarity with certain patterns of invasion, such as the microcystic elongated and fragmented (MELF) and adenoma malignum-like, discussed below.

Most uteri have an irregular endomyometrial junction. The endomyometrial interface can be appreciated at low-power magnification and recognized as intact when its contour is smooth and/or undulating ("valleys"), endometrial stroma and/or benign endometrial glands are present at the myometrial interface, and a stromal (desmoplasia or inflammation) response is absent. Adherence to these rules avoids misclassifying endometrium-confined tumors as showing the rather uncommonly encountered "pushing pattern" of invasion, in which a stromal response is present.

The same rules apply to the distinction of adenomyosis colonized by adenocarcinoma from adenocarcinoma that has invaded myometrium. Altered or myoid metaplastic endometrial stroma may resemble myometrium and therefore lead to the mistaken impression of myometrial invasion. At high-power magnification, myoid metaplastic endometrial stroma reveals seamless transition to typical-appearing endometrial

Table 5-1

INTERNATIONAL FEDERATION OF GYNECOLOGY AND OBSTETRICS (FIGO) 2009 STAGING OF ENDOMETRIAL CARCINOMA AND CARCINOSARCOMA

IA:	Tumor confined to the uterus; no or < ½ myometrial invasion
IB:	Tumor confined to the uterus; ½ or more myometrial invasion
II:	Cervical stromal invasion, but not beyond uterus
IIIA:	Tumor invades serosa or adnexa
IIIB:	Vaginal and/or parametrial involvement
IIIC1:	Pelvic lymph node involvement
IIIC2:	Para-aortic lymph node involvement
IVA:	Tumor invasion of bladder and/or bowel mucosa
IVB:	Distant metastases including abdominal and/or inguinal lymph nodes metastases

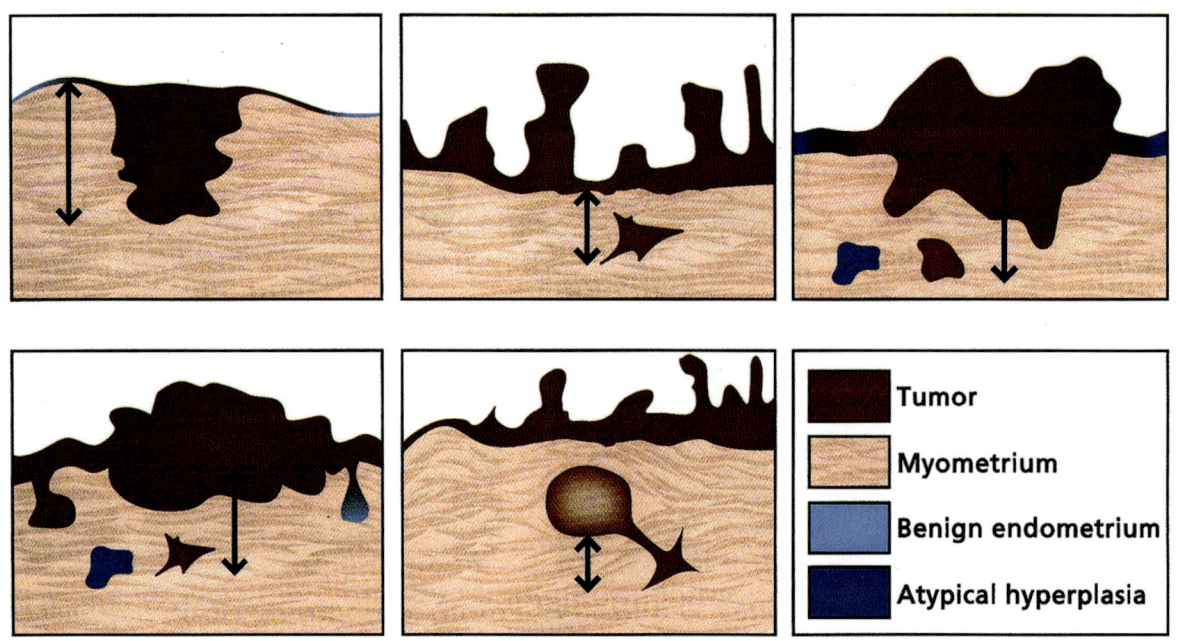

Figure 5-52

MYOMETRIAL INVASION

Diagram illustrating method for measuring depth of myometrial invasion. (Diagram 7.1 Soslow RA, Longacre TA. Uterine pathology. Cambridge illustrated surgical pathology. Cambridge University Press; 2012:139).

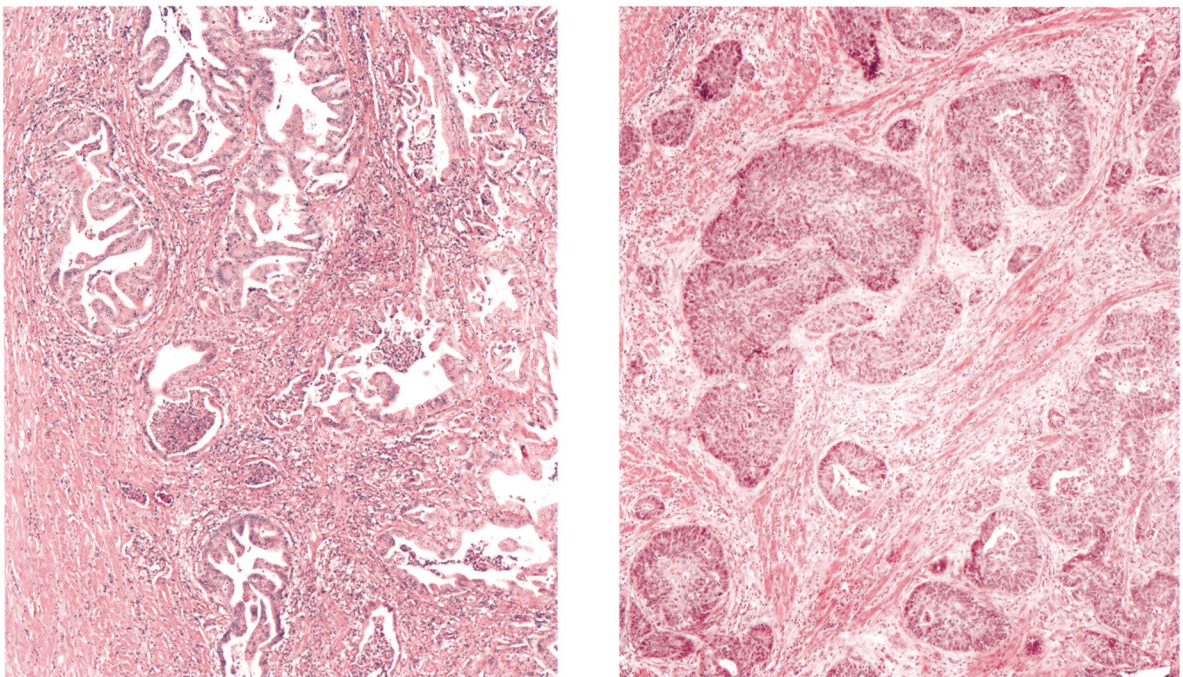

Figure 5-53

MYOMETRIAL INVASION

Irregularly contoured glands and nests of tumor are present in myometrium with a desmoplastic response.

stroma (fig. 5-55). The appearance of this stroma, including spiral arterioles, provides a contrast between the fibrillary nature of altered stroma and the well-organized bundles of myometrial smooth muscle. Within the foci of adenomyosis involved by carcinoma, it is helpful to look for rare benign glands often present at the periphery ("sentinel glands"). When there is difficulty distinguishing between adenomyosis colonized by carcinoma and invasive carcinoma, it is important to evaluate for the presence of adenomyosis elsewhere in the myometrium. If conventional adenomyosis is not found, the presence of myoinvasive carcinoma is favored. CD10 immunostaining may not be helpful, as metaplastic endometrial stroma may show only weak reactivity; furthermore, some myoinvasive carcinomas have a peripheral rim of attenuated spindle cells that are CD10 positive (115).

Another issue related to carcinoma involving adenomyosis is how to measure carcinoma invading from adenomyosis, an issue that is, unfortunately, not addressed in the FIGO staging scheme. One approach to this problem is to report the depth of myometrial invasion by measuring the distance between the invasive focus and the adjacent area of adenomyosis (fig. 5-56) (111).

The MELF (microcystic, elongated, and fragmented) pattern of invasion (116–123) is detected at low-power magnification due to its associated myxoinflammatory response within the myometrium (fig. 5-57). The neoplastic glands may be difficult to recognize as they can be obscured by the striking acute inflammation, sometimes forming microabscesses. Not infrequently, foci of MELF invasion are seen at the leading edge of the carcinoma and sometimes deeper in the myometrium, and discontinuous from that invasive front or adjacent to adenomyosis colonized by carcinoma. When multiple patterns of invasion are noted, the MELF pattern typically represents the deepest extent of invasion, thus, close scrutiny of the myometrium should be performed in order to exclude deepest invasion, which may change the FIGO stage. The invasive cells frequently differ in appearance when compared to the more superficially situated adenocarcinoma component. MELF cells often have a "squamoid" or eosinophilic, elongated/attenuated or histiocytic appearance with low N/C ratios and tiny to absent nucleoli.

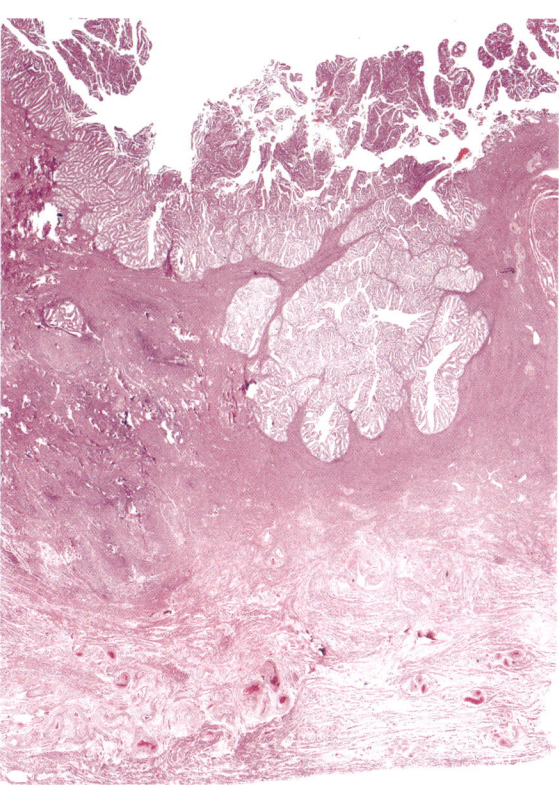

Figure 5-54

EXOPHYTIC ADENOCARCINOMA

There is a highly irregular endomyometrial junction, but no myometrial invasion. A rounded contour is seen at the endomyometrial junction, with subtle surrounding muscular hyperplasia and superficially placed adenomyosis.

It is sometimes difficult to distinguish MELF invasion from lymphovascular invasion in the myometrium as the attenuated cytoplasm of the invasive tumor cells can resemble endothelium (fig. 5-57). Endothelial markers, such as FLI-1, podoplanin, and CD31 may be helpful in this distinction.

MELF invasion is statistically associated with lymphovascular invasion and metastases to regional lymph nodes, but it is not a prognostic indicator independent of stage (116,119–123). MELF invasion is an example of epithelial to mesenchymal transition present at the invasive front of endometrial carcinomas, with consequent loss of epithelial cell adhesion molecules such as E-cadherin (52,117,118) and this pattern appears to be over-represented in tumors with mucinous and papillary morphology (124) as well as with defective MLH1 expression (125).

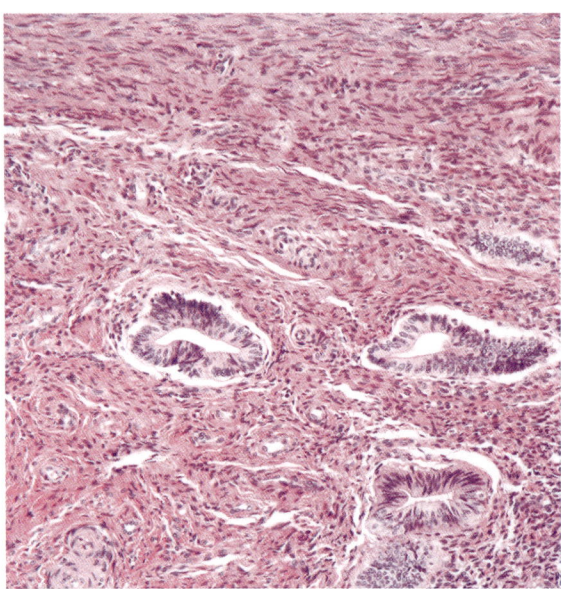 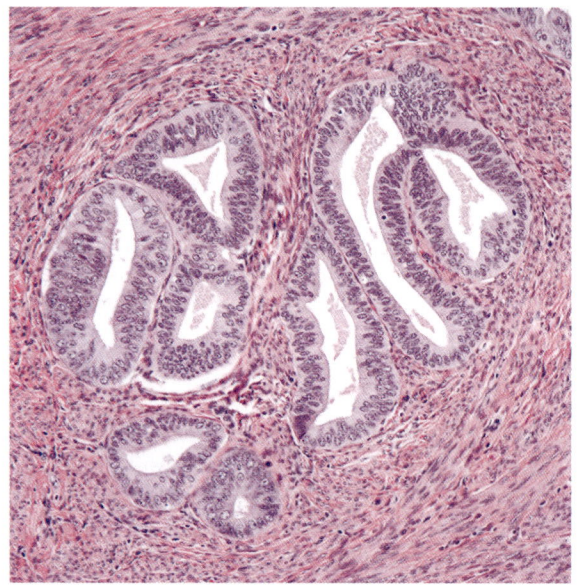

Figure 5-55

METAPLASTIC ENDOMETRIAL STROMA IN ADENOMYOSIS MIMICS MYOMETRIAL INVASION

Benign glands of adenomyosis are invested in endometrial stroma with a myofibroblastic appearance (left). This appearance is occasionally confused with myometrium, leading to an inaccurate diagnosis of myometrial-invasive adenocarcinoma. Myofibroblastic endometrial stroma shows fibrillary appearance and retention of spiral-like arterioles. Hyperplasia in adenomyosis with myofibroblastic stroma is surrounded by circumferential, hyperplastic myometrium (right).

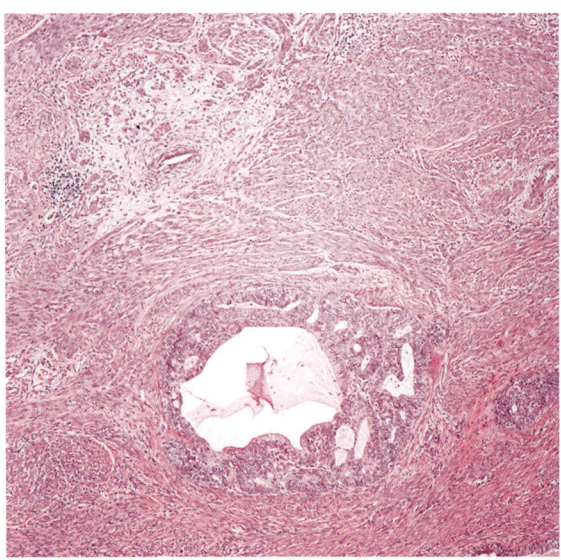

Figure 5-56

MYOINVASION ADJACENT TO ADENOMYOSIS

Invasion is indicated at top by the irregularly shaped patch of myxoinflammatory reaction and the small, attenuated gland within. If this is the only focus of myometrial invasion, the depth of invasion can be measured from the adenomyosis to the invasive focus.

The adenoma malignum-like invasion pattern displays well-formed endometrioid glands haphazardly distributed throughout the myometrium without an obvious stromal response (fig. 5-58) (120,126), a feature shared with minimal deviation adenocarcinoma of the endocervix; however, despite a similar name, these two entities are otherwise completely unrelated. The adenoma malignum-like pattern of invasion is distinguished from adenomyosis by the presence of a chaotic arrangement of neoplastic glands, which contrasts with the low-power appearance of clustered endometrial glands and endometrial stroma characteristic of adenomyosis. The adenoma malignum-like pattern of invasion is probably prognostically similar to conventional myometrial invasion patterns but experience is limited.

Another pattern of myometrial invasion that features nests of well-differentiated glands invading myometrium is the "adenomyosis-like" (120) pattern of invasion (fig. 5-59). This is characterized by clusters of large glands forming irregular islands that may contain

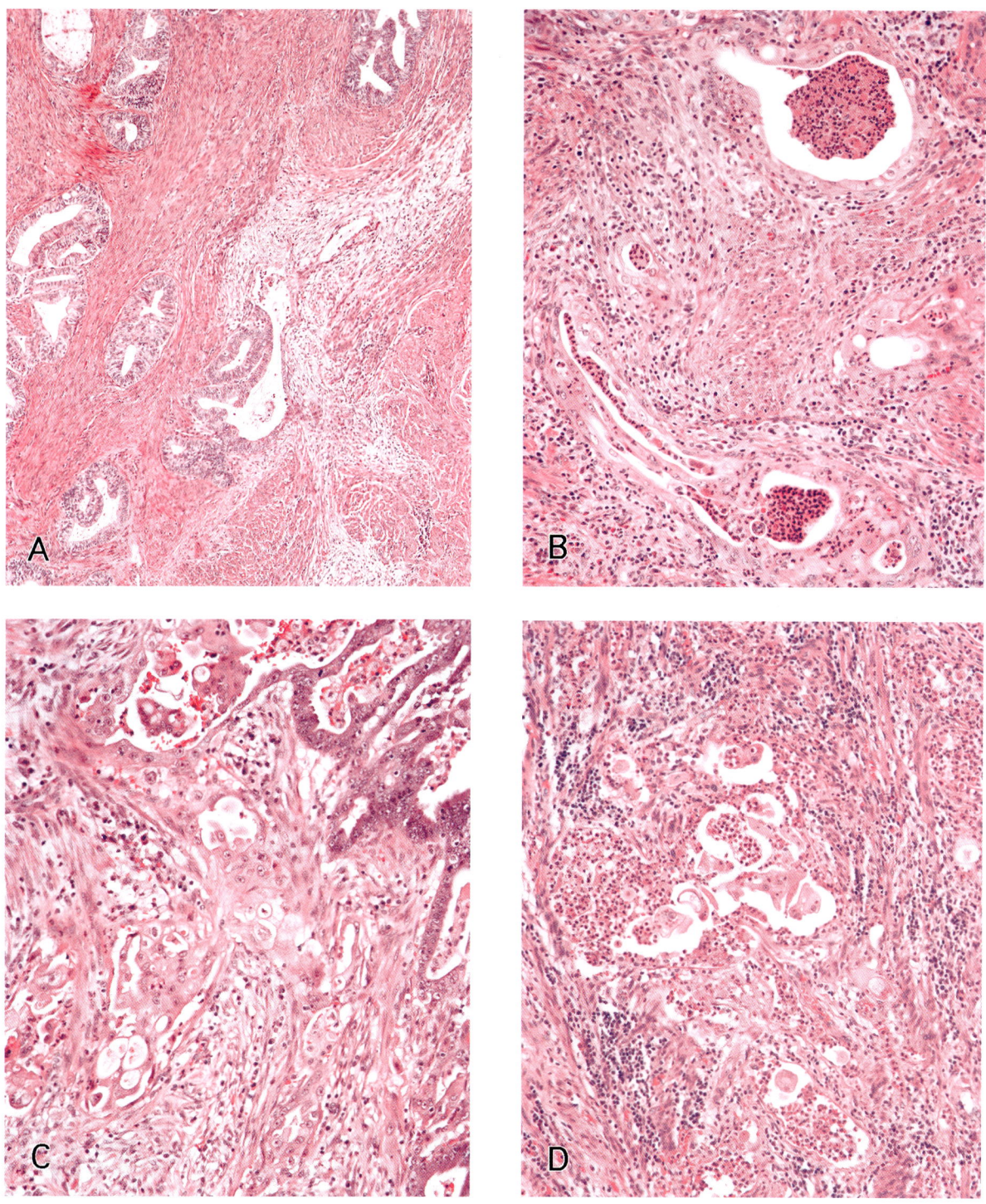

Figure 5-57

MICROCYSTIC ELONGATED AND FRAGMENTED (MELF) PATTERN OF MYOINVASION

At low power, irregular patches of myxoinflammatory infiltrate in the myometrium are the first clue to the diagnosis (A). The classic high-power appearance of MELF includes elongated microcysts, fragmented glands, and intraluminal microabscesses (B). Squamoid metaplastic changes are common (C). The epithelial fragmentation in this pattern of invasion may resemble lymphovascular invasion (D).

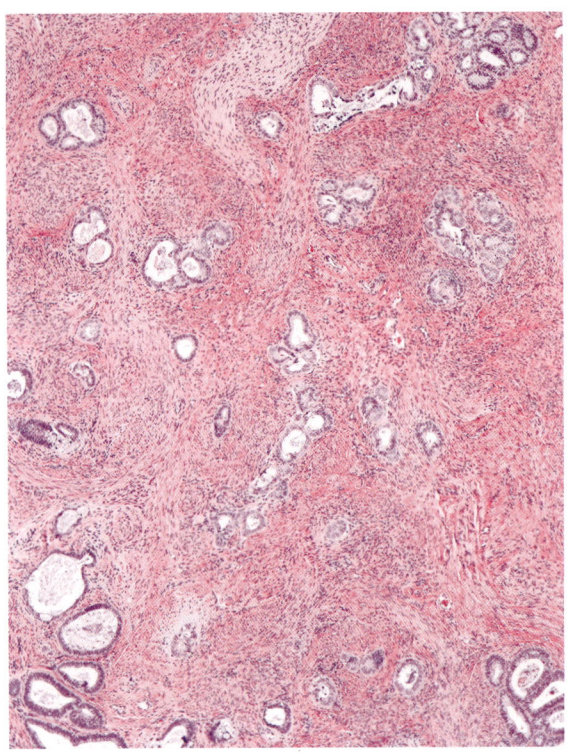 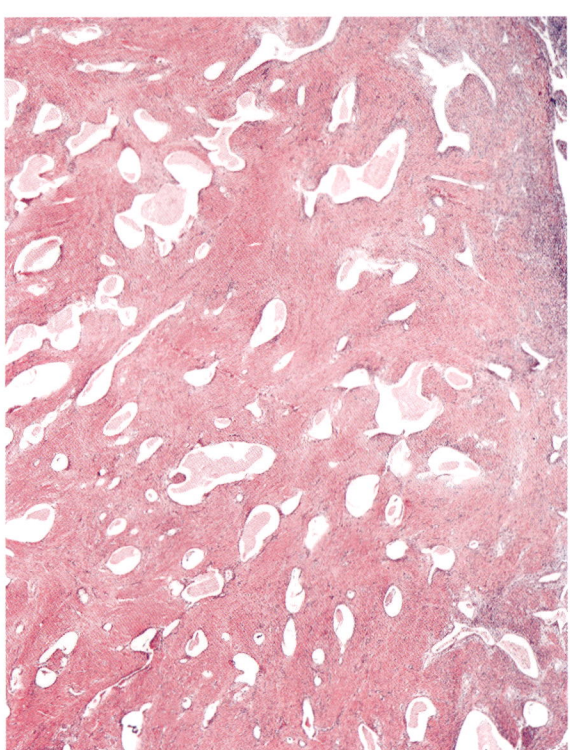

Figure 5-58

ADENOMA MALIGNUM-LIKE PATTERN OF MYOINVASION

Well-differentiated glands are haphazardly distributed throughout the myometrium without an obvious stromal response.

villous papillae. It differs from adenomyosis by the lack of benign glands and associated endometrial stroma. It shows irregular borders and a variable stromal response, particularly when MELF-pattern invasion is also present. Some cases represent the invasive portion of a villoglandular carcinoma.

The poorly described "pushing pattern" of invasion should only be reported as a form of myometrial invasion when there is an associated stromal response (fig. 5-60). This pattern is overdiagnosed when the endometrium is expanded and replaced by adenocarcinoma in the presence of an irregular endomyometrial junction.

Lymphovascular Invasion

Both the presence and extent of lymphovascular invasion (fig. 5-61) are prognostically important in endometrioid and related carcinomas (127–130). Lymphovascular invasion should be assessed at the advancing edge of the tumor. Foci suspicious for lymphovascular invasion should not be interpreted as "positive" when a tumor embolus is found within the carcinoma.

A challenging differential diagnosis involves the distinction of lymphovascular invasion from artifactual tissue displacement into myometrial vessels (fig. 5-62), spaces not lined by endothelium, fallopian tube lumens, and peritoneal washings. This phenomenon is encountered more commonly in laparoscopic and robotic procedures than with open, or traditional, operative approaches (131–135). Although artifactual tumor displacement was initially thought to be the result of tumor disruption during uterine manipulation, it is currently believed that the operative procedure leads to the formation of friable tumor fragments that can be dragged through the tissue during prosection. Formalin fixation for several hours before prosection has been reported to minimize the occurrence of these artifacts (132). Clues to the correct diagnosis include the presence of neoplastic and non-neoplastic endometrium and endometrial

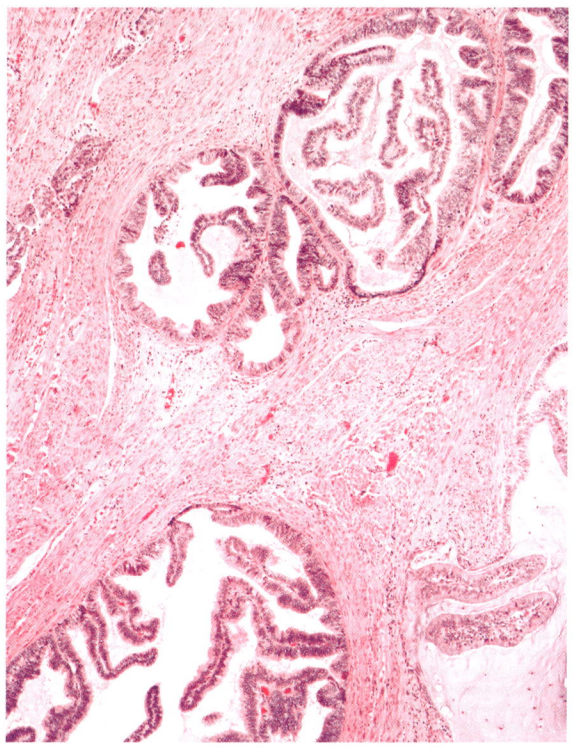

Figure 5-59

ADENOMYOSIS-LIKE PATTERN OF MYOINVASION

Groups of round glands with internal architectural complexity (a villoglandular pattern seen here) invade myometrium without an obvious stromal response. This pattern of myoinvasion lacks associated endometrial stroma. Lymphovascular invasion is shown at the top.

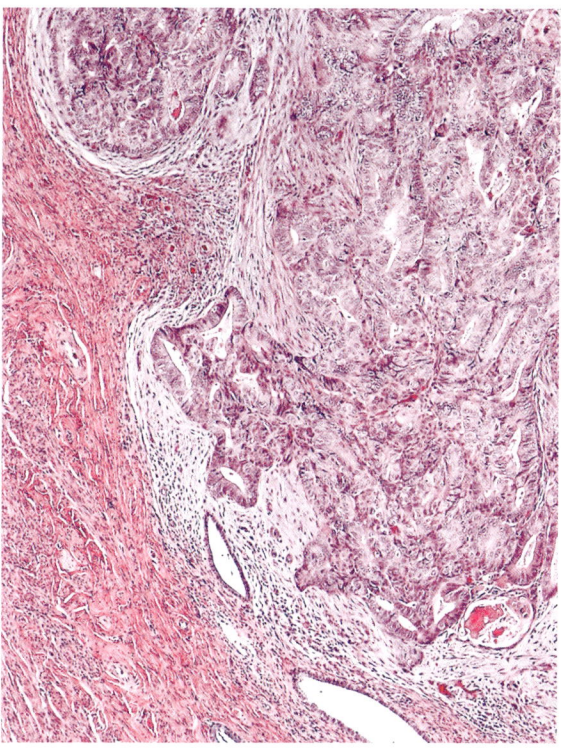

Figure 5-60

PUSHING PATTERN OF MYOINVASION

The endometrioid carcinoma invades the stroma of the lower uterine segment, displaying an irregular contour and a stromal reaction, both of which are required to diagnose invasion in this context.

stroma, often crushed and distorted, in vessels (lymphatics, capillaries, veins, and arteries) and nonendothelial-lined spaces of varying sizes, both close to the tumor and distantly. It is occasionally impossible to confidently diagnose lymphovascular invasion in the presence of displaced tumor within vessels, emphasizing the importance of formalin fixation before serially sectioning the endomyometrium.

Cervical Involvement

A reproducible diagnosis of cervical stromal invasion is complicated by the absence of anatomic boundaries, or definitions thereof, that separate cervix from the lower uterine segment and secondary involvement of endocervical glands from cervical stroma (fig. 5-63) (135,136). A confident diagnosis of cervical stromal involvement is made only when the neoplastic focus is bounded proximally and distally by normal endocervical glands. Tumors at the junction between endocervix and lower uterine segment cannot be convincingly regarded as cervical involvement when the tumor is juxtaposed against endocervical tissue only distally. Unequivocal stromal invasion can only be recognized when the invasive focus underlies normal ectocervix or endocervical glands or a stromal reaction is present (figs. 5-64, 5-65).

It is important to accurately distinguish embryologic (mesonephric) remnants and endocervical hyperplasias from endometrioid adenocarcinomas secondarily involving cervical stroma with an adenoma malignum-like invasion pattern (137). Since some endometrioid carcinomas of the corpus or lower uterine segment have a paradoxically highly differentiated appearance in the cervical stroma (i.e., adenoma

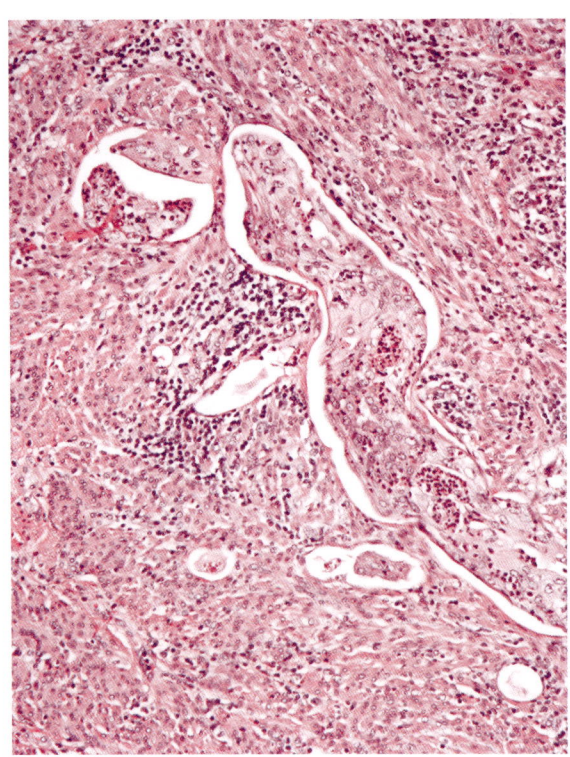 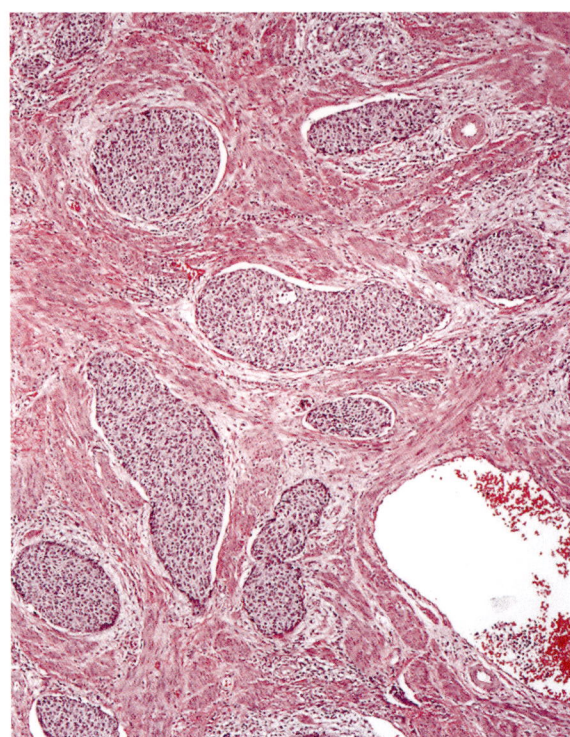

Figure 5-61

LYMPHOVASCULAR INVASION

Classic appearance (left). Extensive intravascular tumor emboli could be mistaken for myometrial invasion. Retraction around some of the emboli reveals an endothelial lining. The depth of lymphovascular invasion should not be reported as the depth of myometrial invasion (right).

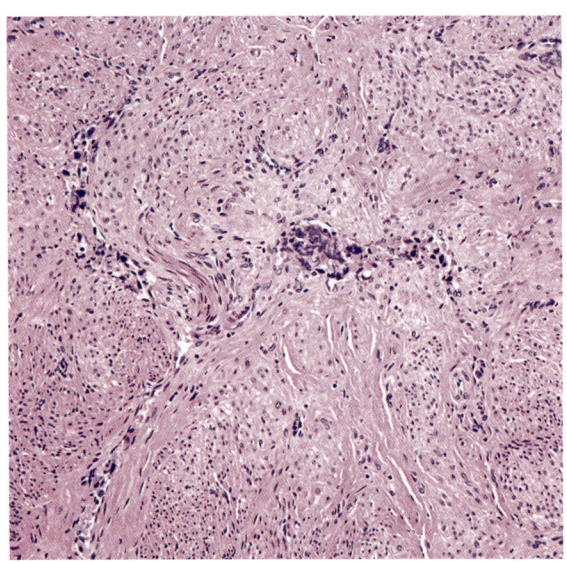 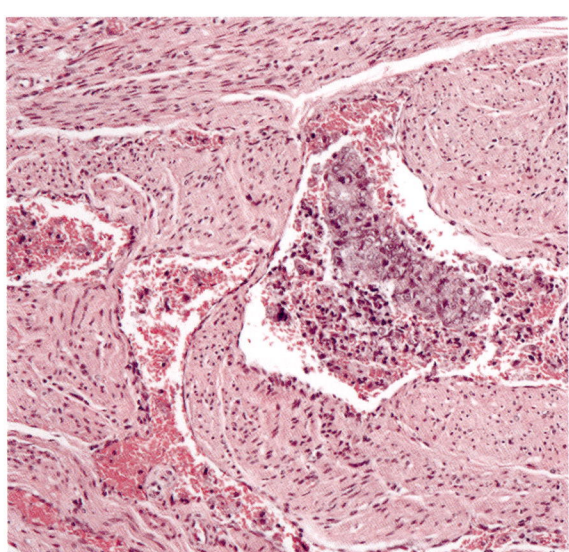

Figure 5-62

ARTIFACTUAL TISSUE DISPLACEMENT MIMICKING LYMPHOVASCULAR INVASION

Note the dyshesive, crushed, and often degenerative appearance of the tumor within vessels but also with cleft-like spaces.

Endometrioid Carcinoma and Related Carcinomas

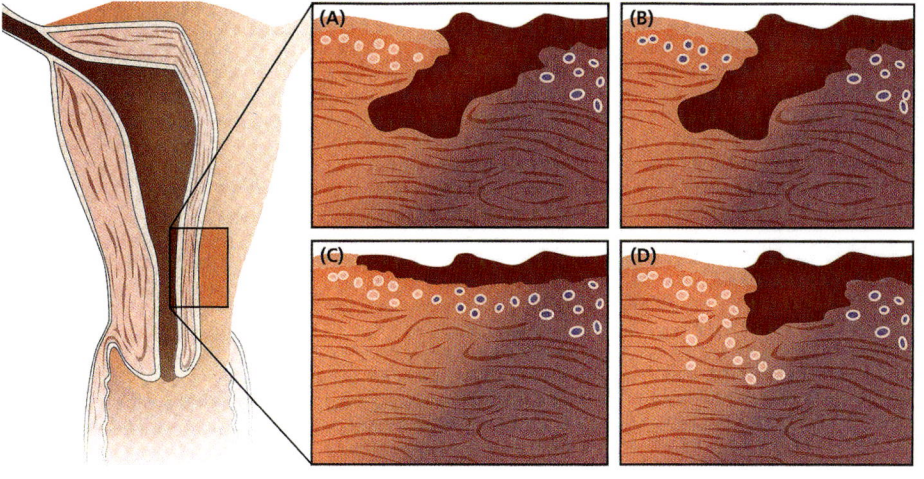

Figure 5-63

CERVICAL STROMAL INVASION

Diagram illustrating method for assessing presence of cervical stromal invasion. (Diagram 7.2 Soslow RA, Longacre TA. Uterine pathology. Cambridge illustrated surgical pathology. Cambridge University Press; 2012: 143).

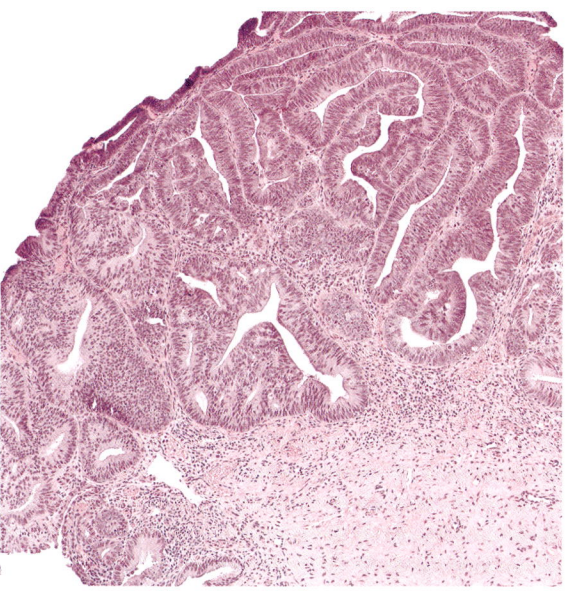

Figure 5-64

ENDOCERVICAL MUCOSAL COLONIZATION BY ENDOMETRIOID ADENOCARCINOMA

The endocervical mucosa is replaced by well-differentiated endometrioid adenocarcinoma, but no confluent growth suggestive of stromal invasion is seen.

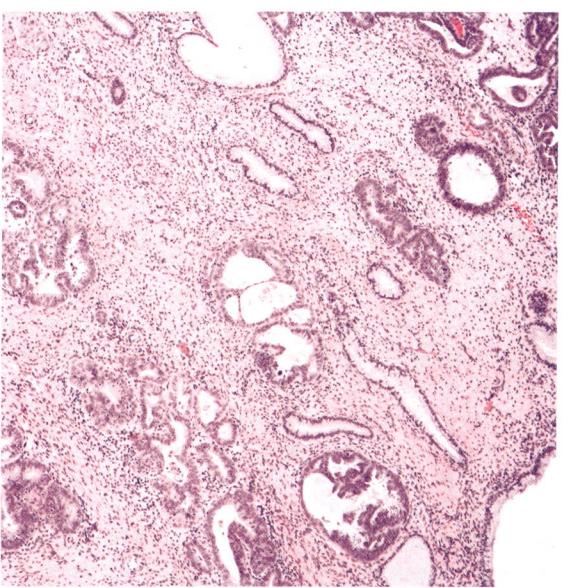

Figure 5-65

CERVICAL STROMAL INVASION BY ENDOMETRIOID CARCINOMA

Infiltrative adenocarcinoma located in between non-neoplastic endocervical glands.

malignum-like), identification of a transition between carcinoma in the lower uterine segment and cervix by extensive sectioning is important. A high threshold is needed to diagnose small or equivocal foci of cervical stromal invasion, as there are some data that suggest cervical stromal invasion alone is not independently associated with clinical outcome (135,138). Cervical stromal invasion tends to coexist with other factors known to influence poor outcome, such as deep myometrial invasion, high cytologic grade, and lymphovascular invasion.

Rare endometrioid adenocarcinomas preferentially invade the cervical stroma rather than myometrium; thus, the predominant location of the invasion does not necessarily inform the tumor type or primary site (137). Similarly, rare endocervical adenocarcinomas colonize the lower uterine segment and endometrium (139)

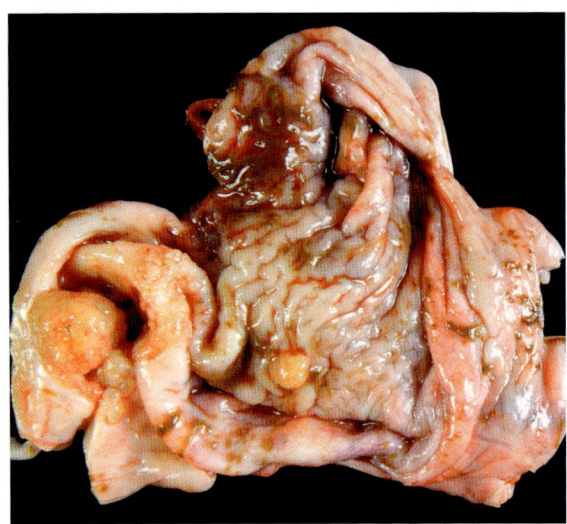 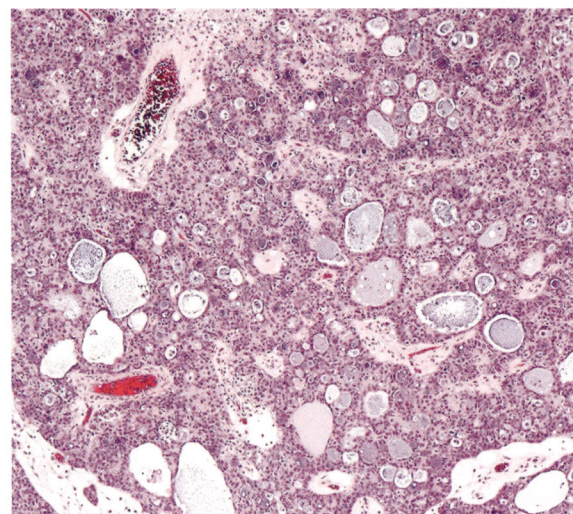

Figure 5-66

SYNCHRONOUS OVARIAN ENDOMETRIOID ADENOCARCINOMA

Most synchronous adenocarcinomas in the ovary arise in an endometriotic cyst (left) and are endometrioid (right).

and may preferentially invade myometrium but not the cervical wall. The distinction between an endocervical adenocarcinoma preferentially involving corpus and an endometrioid adenocarcinoma predominantly involving cervix may require the use of immunohistochemistry.

Synchronous Endometrioid Endometrial and Ovarian Carcinomas

The coexistence of endometrioid tumors involving endometrium and ovary presents difficulties for stage assignment, prognostication, and therapy. Synchronous adenocarcinomas of ovary and endometrium should be staged separately and each site is usually assigned FIGO stage I. Clinicopathologic studies support favorable outcomes in affected patients although not as favorable as in patients with only one stage I carcinoma (140–143). When an endometrial carcinoma metastasizes to the ovary, on the other hand, it is regarded as FIGO stage IIIA.

The guidelines that separate synchronous from metastatic tumors are meant to segregate tumors into two clinically meaningful categories: indolent if synchronous or potentially aggressive if metastatic. These guidelines were developed based on histologic findings but several investigators have reported clonal relationships between "synchronous" endometrial and ovarian carcinomas (144–148). Although most synchronous tumors represent metastases from a genotypic perspective, there is no clinical evidence that shared clonality in this context is associated with aggressive clinical behavior.

There are two prototypes of synchronous endometrial and ovarian carcinomas. The most common scenario occurs in young patients with paradoxically histologically similar tumors in both sites and a unilateral ovarian tumor (fig. 5-66) (140,142,149–152). Most of these tumors occur sporadically, although some are diagnosed in the setting of Lynch syndrome (153). The ovarian tumor is typically large, and associated with endometriosis or a borderline tumor (Table 5-2). Typical patterns of metastatic endometrial carcinoma, on the other hand, include bilateral ovarian involvement, size less than 10 cm, surface involvement, and a nodular growth with preservation of ovarian stroma between nodules (Table 5-3).

Less commonly, synchronous carcinomas are of different types (fig. 5-67). They are found more frequently in Lynch syndrome patients, particularly when either pure or mixed clear cell carcinoma is present in either site (100,154). These tumors are not clonally related (147) and thus, they represent synchronous tumors both from clinical and genotypic perspectives. Tables

5-2 and 5-3 present guidelines rather than diagnostic criteria for such scenarios as in many cases, it is difficult to distinguish metastases from synchronous tumors with certainty. It is important in such scenarios to inform the gynecologist that a precise diagnosis cannot be made with certainty.

Lymph Node Metastases

Metastatic endometrial carcinoma in lymph nodes is usually easy to recognize. Metastases from tumors with a MELF pattern of invasion can be overlooked as they are represented by only single cells and small clusters of

Table 5-2
GUIDELINES FOR RECOGNIZING SYNCHRONOUS ENDOMETRIAL AND OVARIAN CARCINOMAS WITH SIMILAR HISTOLOGY[a]

Endometrium
  Low-grade endometrioid carcinoma, no or superficial myometrial invasion and no lymphovascular invasion

Ovary
  Low-grade endometrioid carcinoma
  Associated endometriosis, müllerian borderline tumor
  Expansile invasion
  Large, unilateral tumor
  Patient <50 years

[a]Adapted from Soslow RA. Practical issues related to uterine pathology: staging, frozen section, artifacts, and Lynch syndrome. Mod Pathol 2016;29(Suppl 1):S59-77.

Table 5-3
GUIDELINES FOR RECOGNIZING METASTATIC ENDOMETRIOID CARCINOMA OF ENDOMETRIUM TO OVARY[a]

Bilateral ovarian involvement

Small ovaries (<10 cm)

Multinodular configuration

Surface involvement

No associated endometriosis or müllerian borderline tumor

Destructive stromal invasion

[a]Adapted from Soslow RA. Practical issues related to uterine pathology: staging, frozen section, artifacts, and Lynch syndrome. Mod Pathol 2016;29(Suppl 1):S59-77.

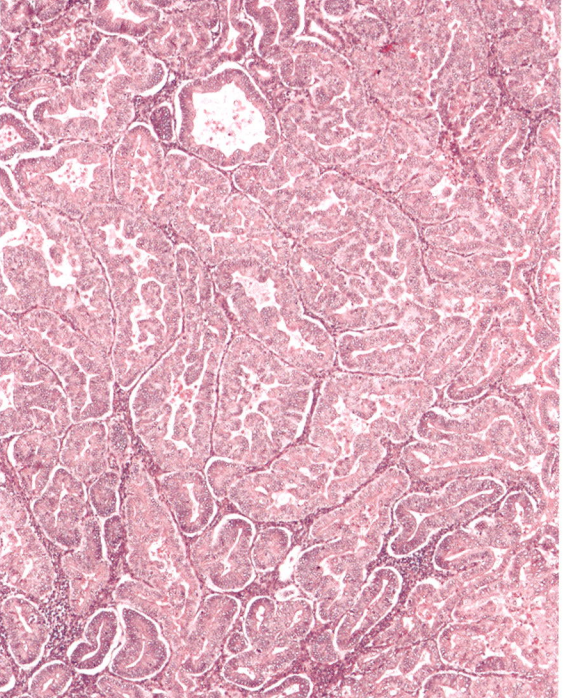
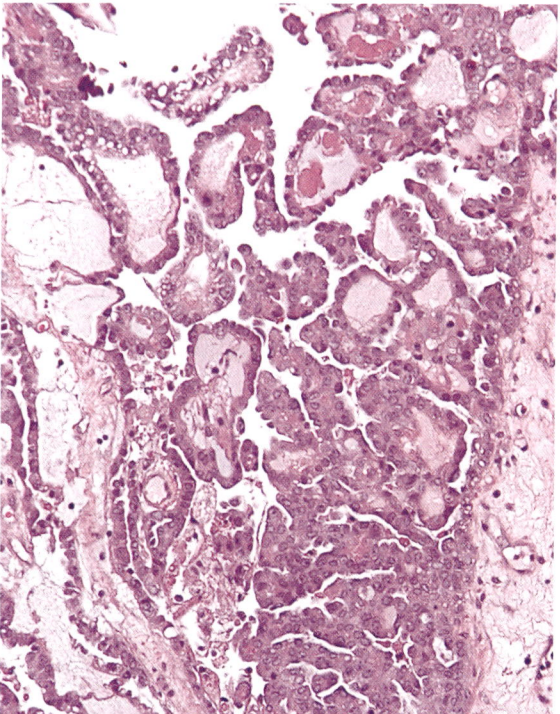

Figure 5-67

SYNCHRONOUS OVARIAN AND ENDOMETRIAL CARCINOMA OF DIFFERING HISTOTYPES
Endometrioid adenocarcinoma of endometrium (left) with synchronous clear cell carcinoma of ovary (right).

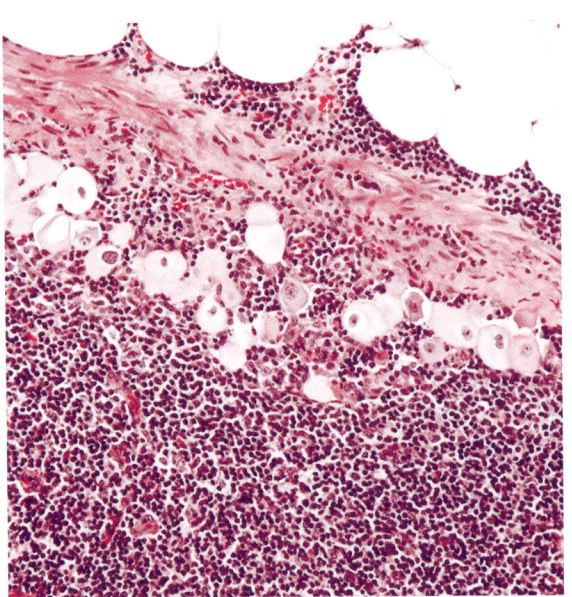 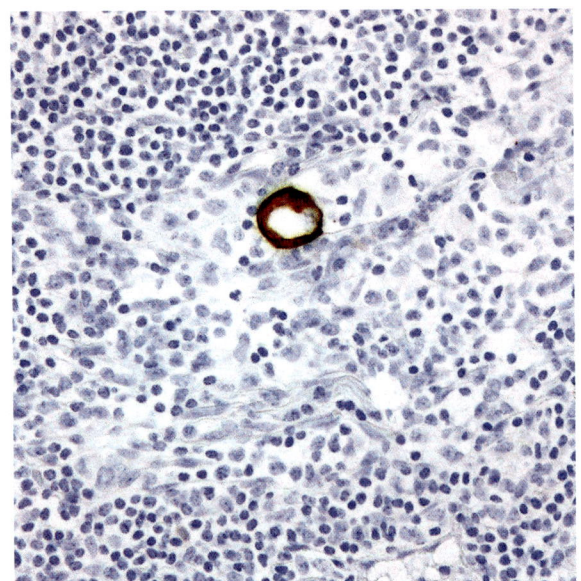

Figure 5-68

METASTATIC ENDOMETRIOID CARCINOMA TO LYMPH NODE

Subtle histiocyte-like tumor cells in lymph node sinuses are often seen in tumors with a MELF pattern of invasion (left). Pancytokeratin stain (AE1/AE3) marks an isolated tumor cell within a sentinel pelvic lymph node (right).

histiocytoid-like or bland-appearing cells with dense eosinophilic cytoplasm (fig. 5-68) (155). The increasing use of cytokeratin immunohistochemistry for ultra-staging in sentinel lymph nodes makes recognition easier, but it presents problems for stage assignment and decision for adjuvant therapy.

Sentinel lymph node sampling is an emerging technique to replace lymph node sampling or full lymphadenectomy. Performing lymph node dissection for every patient with endometrial cancer has met considerable resistance due to comorbidities, such as lower extremity lymphedema (156), but also increased operative time, need for a gynecologic oncologist, number of blocks and slides generated, and overall high cost.

Patients undergoing sentinel lymph node mapping (157–161) are in most instances accurately staged (about 95 percent) without lymphadenectomy and can be spared the risk of lymphedema. Before the procedure, blue dye or tracer is injected into the lower uterine segment. Mapping at the time of surgery highlights the sentinel node(s), which will be removed. In addition, any enlarged lymph nodes and all blue dye/tracer-negative lymph nodes that are contralateral to the sentinel lymph nodes are also excised (158). Frozen section is not performed as lymph node stage is assigned by examining permanent sections of sentinel lymph nodes. Additional lymphadenectomy, either at the time of sentinel lymph node mapping or as part of a subsequent operative procedure, is unnecessary for stage assignment and is not therapeutic.

One of the most prevalent schemes for sentinel lymph node sectioning follows. The sentinel lymph nodes are breadloafed at 2-mm intervals and entirely submitted for microscopic examination. Two hematoxylin and eosin (H&E) slides and pancytokeratin-immunostained slides are prepared, separated by 50 microns. Unlike patients with breast cancer, these patients do not undergo a second surgery for completion of lymph node dissection if sentinel lymph node(s) is positive for carcinoma. Problems with implementation, however, involve challenges with accurate mapping in patients with high body mass index (BMI) and when the surgeon has insufficient experience with the procedure.

From the pathology perspective, problems occur when undue reliance is placed upon the use of cytokeratin immunohistochemical stains to detect low-volume metastases. Ultra-staging

Table 5-4
DISCRIMINATORY IMMUNOMARKERS WITH KNOWN PERFORMANCE CHARACTERISTICS IN ENDOMETRIAL CARCINOMAS

Marker	Standardization	References for Standardization and Reproducibility
p53	Aberrant expression in SC/CS>CC>EMC[a] Diagnostically useful in proper context Independent association with outcome	26, 168, 272–174, 278–285
p16	Aberrant expression in SC/CS>CC>EMC (mostly high-grade)	168, 280, 281, 283
Her2/neu	Overexpression in SC>CC; see Table 6 Possible therapeutic target	130, 286–289
ER/PR	Expression in EMC>SC Expression associated with low stage Therapeutic target	130, 168, 285, 290–292
PTEN	Loss of expression in EMC>CC>SC Diagnostically useful in proper context Pathway therapeutic target	170, 293–296
β-catenin (CTNNB1)	Aberrant expression in ~20% of EMC Potential association with adverse outcome	274, 297, 298
HNF-1β	Expression in CC>EMC>SC Diagnostically useful in proper context	299–303
DNA MMR proteins	Loss of expression in UC>EMC>CC>SC Lynch syndrome screening Diagnostically useful in proper context Possible therapeutic importance	100, 154, 304, 305

[a]SC = serous carcinoma; CS = carcinosarcoma; CC = clear cell carcinoma; EMC = endometrioid carcinoma; UC = undifferentiated carcinoma.

with cytokeratin immunohistochemistry has revealed a number of endometrial carcinomas with low-volume nodal disease, including single keratin-positive cells, isolated tumor cells, and micrometastases, using the definitions from breast pathology (157–162). Although pathologists and gynecologists may consider these scenarios to represent FIGO stage IIIC, some caution is warranted. Most patients in whom isolated tumor cells are found in lymph nodes have clinical stage I, FIGO grade 1 endometrioid adenocarcinoma with or without MELF pattern of invasion, which in the absence of isolated tumor cells would be considered low- or, at most, intermediate-risk disease. The College of American Pathologists now categorizes isolated tumor cells as N0(i+) and indicates that the finding is of uncertain significance. Considering these patients to have FIGO stage IIIC carcinomas may contaminate a category where adjuvant therapy constitutes standard of care. It is, therefore, considered controversial by some pathologists to use ultra-staging to identify low-volume metastases. Recent studies (163,164) have shown that patients with isolated tumor cells or micrometastases in lymph nodes have significantly better survival rates than those with macrometastases. However, at least in one study, many patients opted to be treated with chemotherapy and radiotherapy, thus making it impossible to know whether patients with N0(i+) endometrial carcinoma would benefit from adjuvant therapy.

IMMUNOHISTOCHEMICAL FINDINGS

A detailed list of antibodies that can be used as diagnostic adjuncts and as putative prognostic markers in endometrioid and related carcinomas is provided in Tables 5-4 to 5-6. Most endometrioid carcinomas coexpress PAX8 (165), pancytokeratins, and CK7 (166,167), but the expression may be weak or absent in poorly differentiated carcinomas. Vimentin is almost universally present, at least focally, and typically expressed in a "basolateral pattern" (fig. 5-69) (168). Most tumors also express cell surface glycoproteins, such as BerEP4, B72.3, MOC31, and CA125, as well as

Table 5-5
POSSIBLE ENDOMETRIAL CARCINOMA DISCRIMINATORY MARKERS

Marker	Significance (Reference)	Drawback
TFF-3 (Trefoil factor 3)	Preferentially expressed in EMC[a] (306)	Limited data
Mesothelin	Expression associated with SC (282)	Limited data
Folate binding protein	Expression associated with SC (307)	Limited data
BRCA1	Loss of expression in SC subset (308, 309)	Uncertain whether this can be assessed in unselected sections represented in a TMA
WT1	Preferential expression in CS>SC>EMC (310)	Typically positive in adnexal SC
IMP-3 (insulin-like growth factor II mRNA-binding protein)	Preferentially expressed in SC (306)	Unclear whether discriminatory power superior to p53 or p16; expression is not restricted to SC (311)
E-cadherin	Epithelial-mesenchymal transition marker Loss of expression in UC>CS/SC>EMC (98)	Only limited studies included UCs

[a]EMC = endometrioid carcinoma; SC = serous carcinoma; CS = carcinosarcoma; CC = clear cell carcinoma; UC = undifferentiated carcinoma; TMA = tissue microarray.

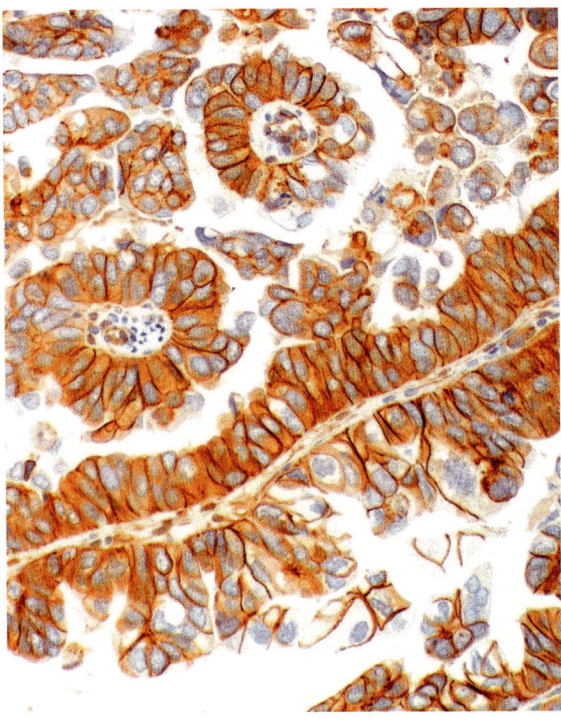

Figure 5-69

VIMENTIN-POSITIVE ENDOMETRIOID ADENOCARCINOMA

Vimentin shows a basolateral pattern of staining in tumor cells.

EMA. Endometrioid carcinomas usually express ER and PR, but the percentage of positive tumor cells tends to decrease with increasing grade. Approximately 10 percent of low-grade endometrioid carcinomas and as many as 40 percent of FIGO grade 3 carcinomas are negative for ER and PR (168). Some carcinomas with extensive secretory change may display attenuated PR staining.

Loss of expression of PTEN is found in at least half of tumors (169,170), while ARID1A and DNA MMR protein loss or microsatellite instability is documented in approximately 25 percent (fig. 5-70) (169). Loss of ARID1a expression is more prevalent in high-grade than low-grade endometrioid carcinomas (171).

Among all endometrioid and related carcinomas, undifferentiated and dedifferentiated carcinomas are most likely to be MMR deficient (92,96) (see chapter 8). p53 shows aberrant expression (overexpression more frequently than absence of expression) in 10 to 20 percent of tumors (fig. 5-71), almost always FIGO grade 3 (172). The overall estimate of aberrant p53 expression in this group is about 20 percent, but reported rates range from 2.5 to 69.0 percent (26,56,172–177). p16 typically shows patchy expression in endometrioid carcinomas, although diffuse, strong expression can be encountered, especially in FIGO grade 3 carcinomas, similar to p53 (168). Endometrioid carcinomas with mucinous differentiation may show cytoplasmic labeling with monoclonal antibodies against carcinoembryonic antigen (mCEA) and CDX2, but more than weak and focal CK20 staining is typically absent (178).

Table 5-6
ENDOMETRIAL CARCINOMA MARKERS WITH POSSIBLE PROGNOSTIC VALUE

Marker	Significance (Reference)	Drawback
L1CAM	Prognostically significant cell adhesion molecule (312)	Uncertain how to interpret the stain
CD163	Macrophage marker Expression associated with deeply myometrial invasive tumors, increased microvessel density, lymph node metastasis (313)	Suggest evaluating evasive tumor edge
HIF 1A (hypoxia-inducible factor 1α subunit)	Expression associated with deeply myometrial invasive tumors, increased microvessel density (313)	Limited data
ZEB1	Marker of epithelial-mesenchymal transition Expressed in aggressive endometrial carcinoma, particularly CS[a] and UC (98, 286)	Limited data
Syndecan-1 (CD138)	Adhesion molecule Stromal expression, along with MMP-9, associated with poor prognosis (314)	Limited data
MMP2, 9 (matrix metalloproteinases)	Expression associated with lymphatic invasion and, possibly, prognosis (314)	Limited data Uncertain whether this can be assessed in unselected sections represented in a TMA
S100A4	Calcium binding protein Expression associated with high grade and high stage (315)	Limited data
Annexin-A2	Receptor/binding protein for proteases (cathepsin B, plasminogen and tissue plasminogen activator) and extracellular matrix proteins (type 1 collagen and tenascin C) involved in tumor invasion and metastasis May predict recurrence	
DNA MMR proteins	Defective MMR may be associated with chemo- and/or radio-responsiveness (275)	

[a]CS = carcinosarcoma; UC = undifferentiated carcinoma; TMA = tissue microarray; MMR = mismatch repair.

The immunophenotype of foci of keratinizing squamous differentiation and squamous morules (fig. 5-72) may differ from that of the glandular component. In a recent study, PAX8 was negative in 8 percent of foci of keratinizing squamous differentiation and 27 percent of squamous morules. ER and PR expression was found in only approximately 40 percent of foci of keratinizing squamous differentiation and 10 percent of nonkeratinizing squamous differentiation, a much lower rate than seen in the glandular elements of low-grade endometrioid adenocarcinomas. p16 was patchy positive in 82 percent of foci of keratinizing squamous differentiation and 88 percent of nonkeratinizing squamous differentiation (179) but p16 may show diffuse expression in these areas (180). p63 is predominantly positive in foci of keratinizing squamous differentiation but not morular differentiation (71 percent). The latter may also be strongly CD10 and CDX2 positive and show nuclear beta-catenin expression (181).

MOLECULAR GENETIC FINDINGS

Listed in decreasing order of prevalence are the most commonly dysregulated somatic genes in endometrioid carcinoma: *PTEN* (inactivating mutation), *PIK3CA* (activating mutation), *ARID1A* (inactivating mutation), *hMLH1* (promoter methylation), *KRAS* (including complex mucinous proliferations and carcinomas) (182), *CTNNB1*, *Tp53* (inactivating mutation), *polymerase E* ([*POLE*]; inactivating mutation), and *hMSH2* and *hMSH6* (inactivating mutations).

Recent work from the Cancer Genome Atlas (TCGA) indicates that there are four genomic classes of endometrioid carcinomas, each with a

Figure 5-70

ENDOMETRIOID ADENOCARCINOMA

ARID1A with geographic expression loss at right (A), PTEN loss (B), and MLH1 loss (C) in endometrioid adenocarcinoma. These abnormalities are seen most commonly in endometrioid carcinoma, less commonly in clear cell carcinoma, but not in serous carcinoma. Positive internal controls are seen throughout.

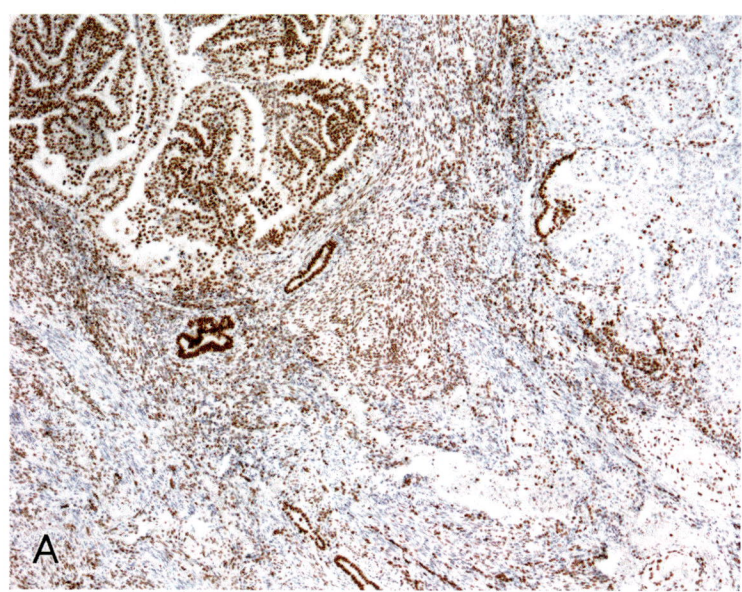

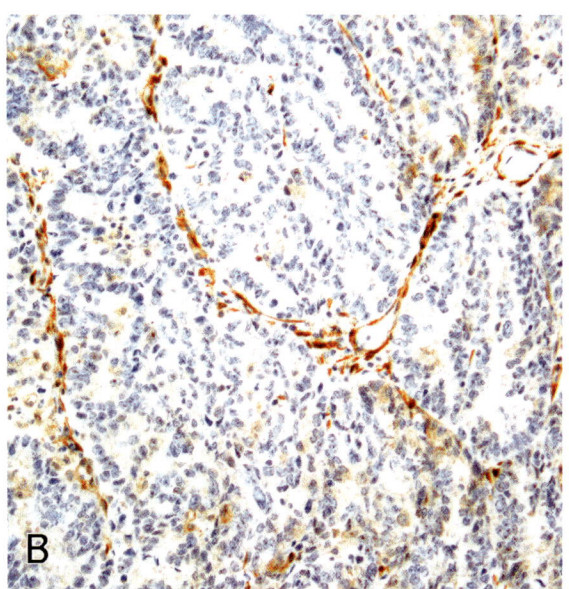

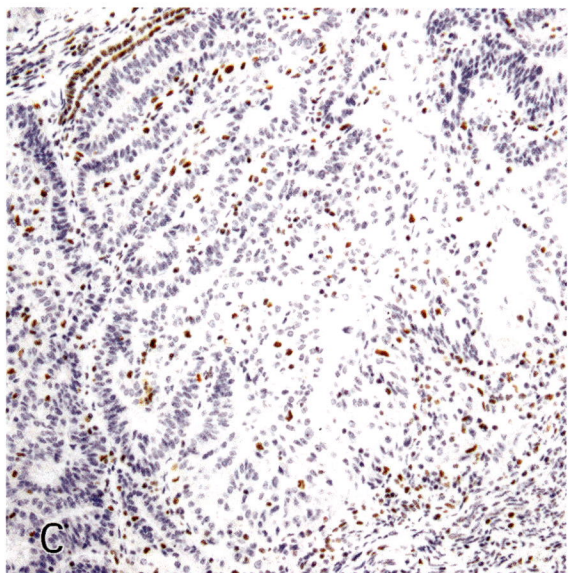

different mutational profile (183), which can be used to stratify these tumors into distinctive epidemiologic, morphologic, prognostic, and therapeutically predictive categories (184,185). The most prevalent group is the "copy number-low" (CN-L), which comprises most FIGO grades 1 and 2 carcinomas. These tumors are similar to the "type I" endometrial carcinomas defined originally by Bokhman (25). Their definition rests on the absence of large numbers of genomic amplifications and deletions, microsatellite instability, and *POLE* exonuclease domain hotspot mutations. There exists a good deal of morphologic, immunophenotypic, and genomic diversity within this group. Amplification at chromosome 1q is prognostically unfavorable (183) as is *CTNNB1* (β-catenin) mutation (186).

The next most prevalent group is the microsatellite instability-high (MSI-H), with most tumors showing methylation of the *hMLH1* promoter. This group is defined by the presence of MSI-H and "hypermutation" in the absence of *POLE* exonuclease domain hotspot mutations. This group comprises tumors ranging from FIGO 1 to 3 endometrioid carcinomas. These tumors have more mutations than the CN-L

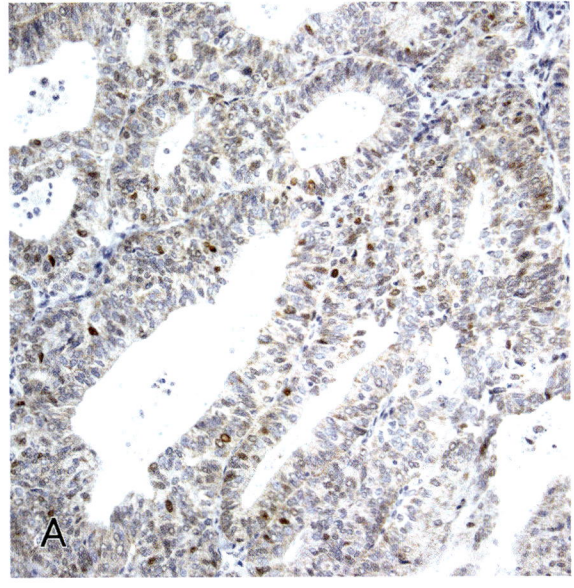
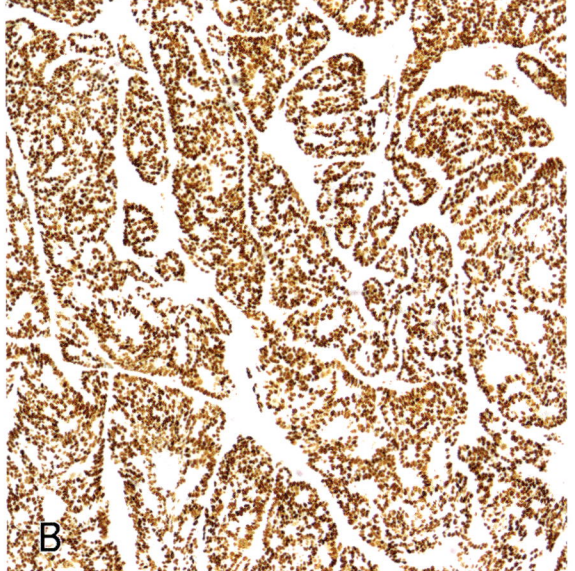
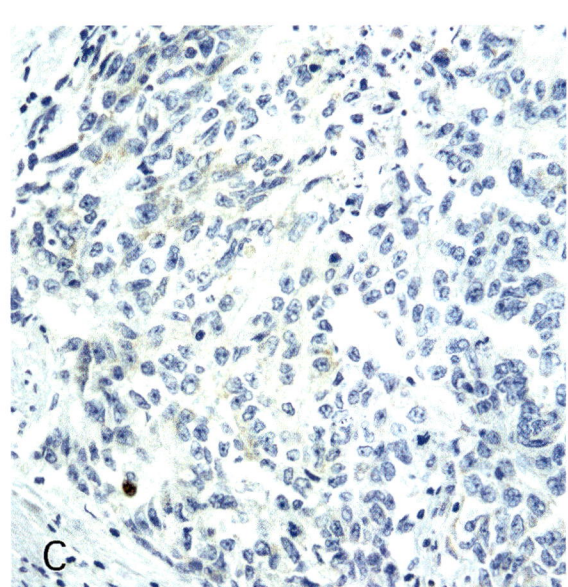

Figure 5-71

P53 IMMUNOHISTOCHEMISTRY IN ENDOMETRIOID ADENOCARCINOMA

Normal/wild type expression (A); overexpression (aberrant) (B); null pattern (aberrant) (C). A positive internal control is seen in C.

group (expressed as mutations per megabase and referred to as "hypermutated"), including *ARID1A*, *PTEN*, *PIK3CA*, and others.

The next two groups contain comparable numbers of endometrioid carcinomas: *POLE* and CN-H (or "serous-like"). Hotspot mutations in the exonuclease domain of *POLE* are mostly associated with FIGO grade 2 and 3 endometrioid carcinomas, with some being histologically similar to mixed endometrioid and serous carcinoma. These tumors have the highest numbers of mutations (expressed as mutations per megabase and referred to as "ultramutated"), including but not limited to *PTEN*, *PIK3CA*, *ARID1A*, *Tp53*, and *hMSH6*.

The serous-like group comprises about 20 percent of FIGO grade 3 endometrioid carcinomas. It is defined by the presence of large numbers of genomic amplifications and deletions, but a low number of mutations per megabase. Nearly all have *Tp53* mutations and may have *PTEN*, *PIK3CA*, or *ARID1A* mutations.

Each genomic group of endometrial endometrioid carcinomas has a typical morphologic

Figure 5-72

IMMUNOPHENOTYPE OF SQUAMOUS MORULES

Aberrant expression of beta-catenin (A); p16 (B); and CDX2 (C). The immunophenotype of squamous morules usually differs from that of gland-forming portions of the tumor and should, therefore, not be used to characterize the immunophenotype of the carcinoma.

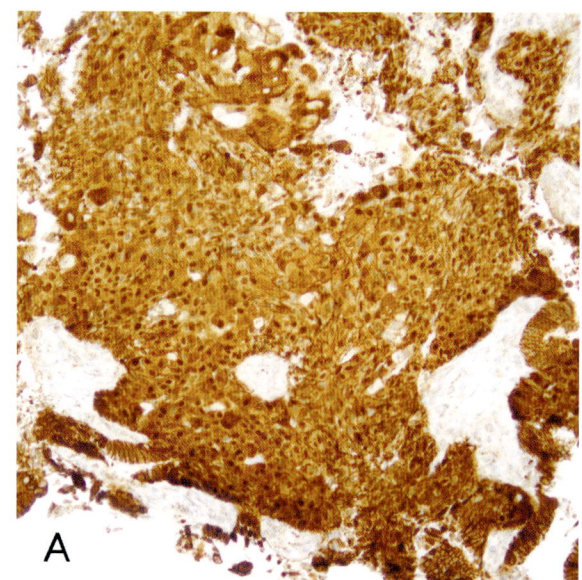

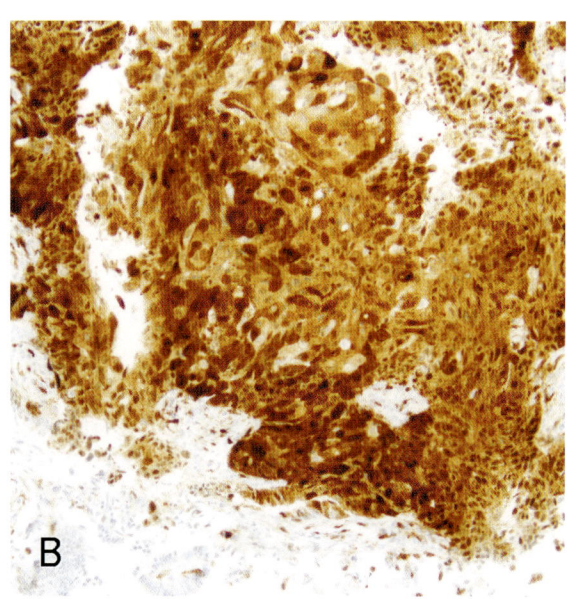

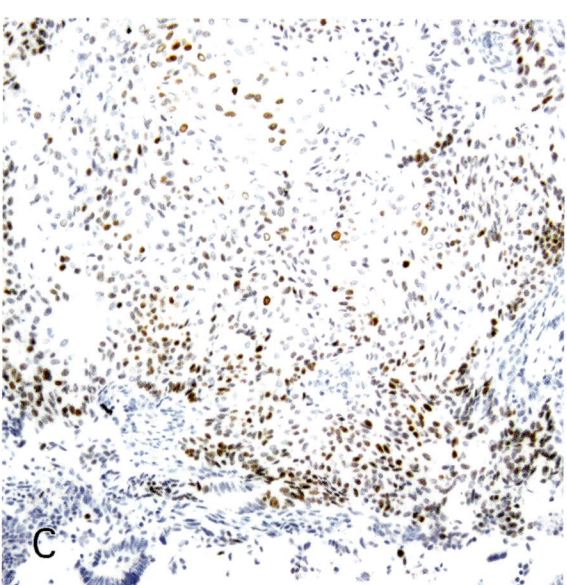

appearance, including peritumoral lymphocytes, tumor-infiltrating lymphocytes, and intratumoral heterogeneity in the *POLE* (fig. 5-73) (187,188), and MSI-H groups (fig. 5-74) (154,189), and diffuse high nuclear grade in the serous-like group (190). These histologic features, however, are not thought to be sufficiently robust for genomic group assignment.

A problem that is not adequately addressed with a histology-only approach is the existence of morphologically ambiguous tumors that reside in the *POLE*, MSI-H, and serous-like categories (but not the CN-L category) (fig. 5-75) (191,192) and the fact that many *POLE* endometrioid carcinomas have components or subclones that are histologically similar to serous carcinomas (fig. 5-73, right) (187). The TCGA dataset and similar datasets have been used to extract surrogate markers to classify endometrial cancers into one of the four genomic categories, and then validated the classifier in an independent set of cases (figs. 5-76, 5-77) (184,185). This classifier included MMR and p53 immunohistochemistry and sequencing of *POLE* exonuclease domains. Some authors refer to this simplified TCGA-based classification as the "PROMISE

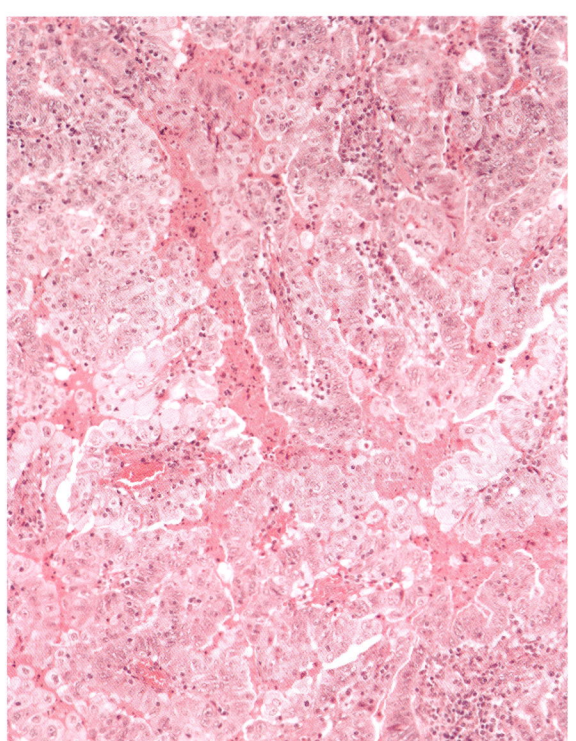 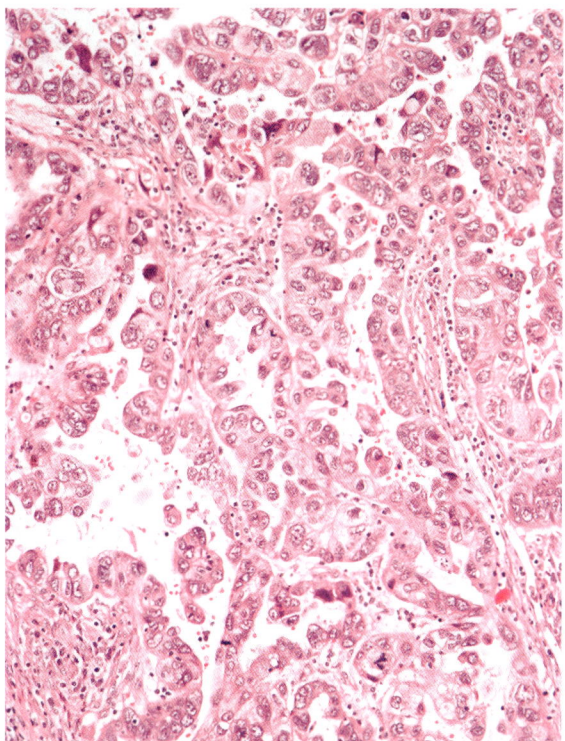

Figure 5-73

POLYMERASE EPSILON (*POLE*)-MUTATED ENDOMETRIOID ADENOCARCINOMA

Cytoplasmic eosinophilia and lymphoid aggregates are seen (left). A component of an otherwise typical endometrioid carcinoma mimics the appearance of serous carcinoma, although the nuclear to cytoplasmic ratio is marginally lower than in most serous carcinomas and contains tumor-infiltrating lymphocytes (right).

classifier" (proactive molecular risk classification tool for endometrial cancers) (184).

DIFFERENTIAL DIAGNOSIS

Atypical Hyperplasia/Endometrioid Intraepithelial Neoplasia (EIN). FIGO grade 1 endometrioid carcinoma is distinguished from atypical hyperplasia/EIN by its nuclear and architectural features (46,193). Any of the following architectural patterns is diagnostic of adenocarcinoma rather than atypical hyperplasia/EIN: closely packed tubular glands lacking intervening stroma, fused glands, a labyrinthine appearance, large glands containing cribriform architecture or micropapillae, and extensive papillary architecture (fig. 5-78). Some examples of atypical and nonatypical hyperplasia are effaced by extensive squamous differentiation, which may give the false impression of an architecturally complex lesion diagnostic of adenocarcinoma. A general rule of thumb is to ignore the squamous areas and concentrate instead on the architecture and nuclear features of glandular elements. Carcinoma in this context should only be diagnosed when unequivocal glandular confluence or appreciable nuclear atypia is present. Some pathologists use a size or volume criterion, in addition to appraisal of nuclear and architectural features, to distinguish atypical hyperplasia/EIN and adenocarcinoma (46,193).

Several quantitative guidelines have been proposed to establish a diagnosis of adenocarcinoma in a background of atypical hyperplasia/EIN. Kurman and Norris (46) proposed that the finding of a confluent glandular pattern, extensive papillary pattern, or replacement of stroma by masses of squamous epithelium in an area more than 2 mm (half of low-power field) qualified for carcinoma. Others establish the diagnosis of adenocarcinoma in this context only when the focus in question is estimated to constitute more than 30 percent of the lesion

Figure 5-74
MICROSATELLITE-UNSTABLE ENDOMETRIOID ADENOCARCINOMA

Tumor-infiltrating lymphocytes (A) and intratumoral heterogeneity (B,C). Although the prototype of intratumoral heterogeneity is dedifferentiated carcinoma, other types of heterogeneity can be encountered, particularly the combination of well- and poorly differentiated endometrioid carcinoma found side-by-side.

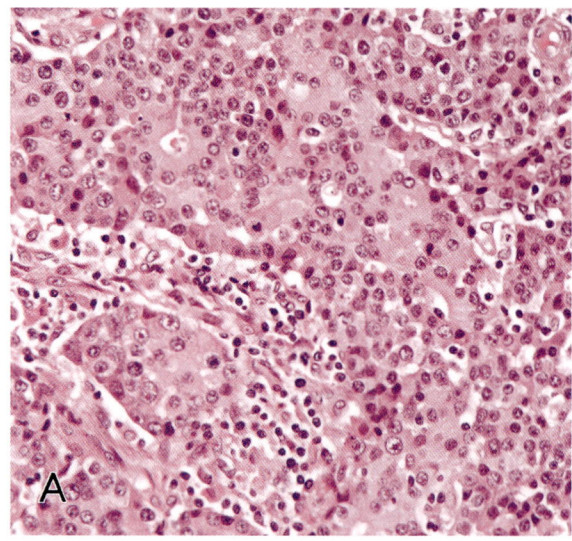

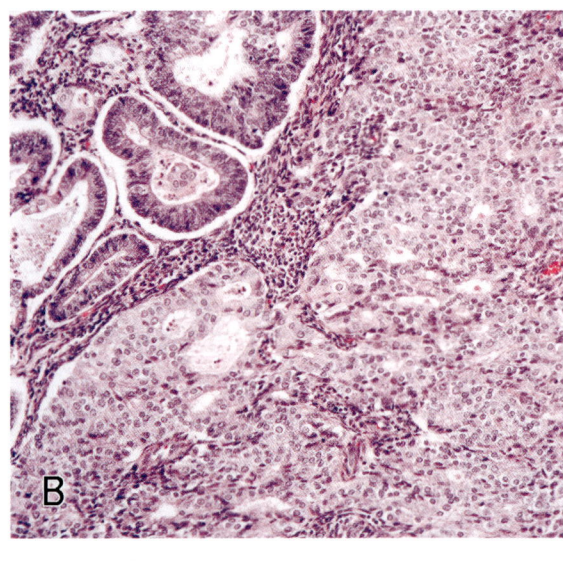

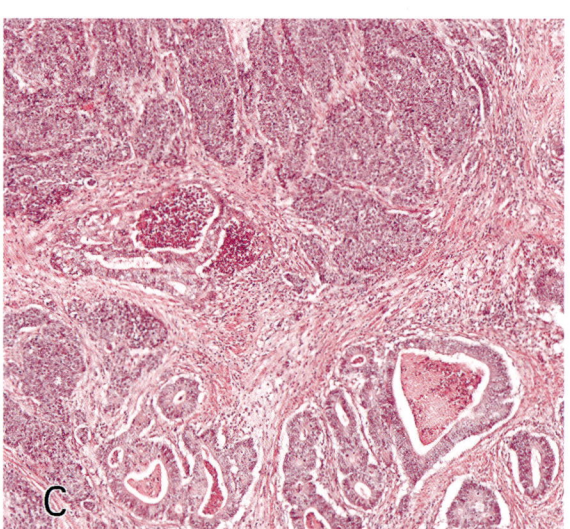

Figure 5-75
MORPHOLOGICALLY AMBIGUOUS ENDOMETRIAL CARCINOMA

This adenocarcinoma contains cells with eosinophilic cytoplasm lining tubular glands (suggestive of endometrioid carcinoma), monomorphic nuclei with prominent nucleoli (suggestive of clear cell carcinoma [oxyphilic clear cell carcinoma in this case]), and irregular luminal contours with highly atypical nuclei (suggestive of serous carcinoma).

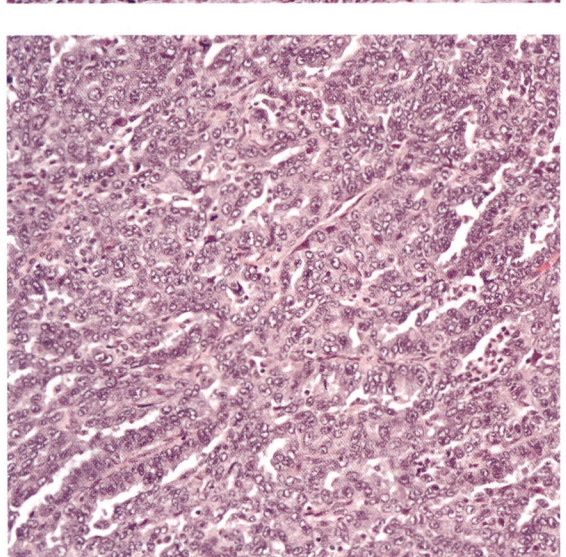

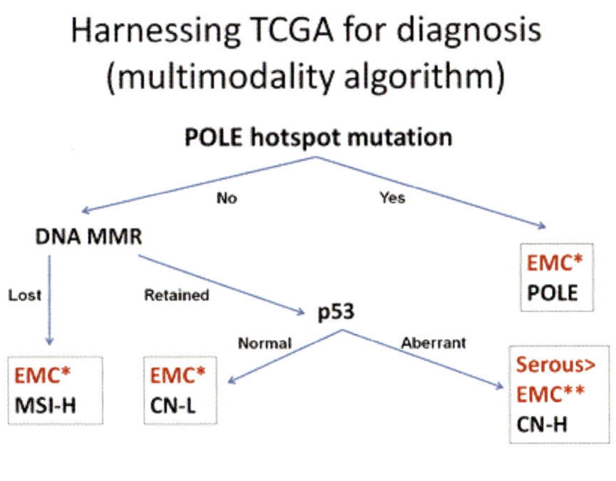

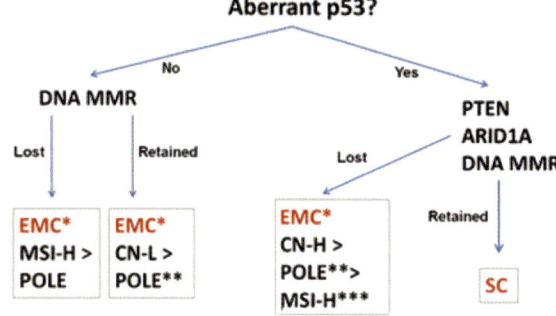

Figure 5-76

SIMPLIFIED TCGA CLASSIFIER

EMC: endometrioid carcinoma; MSI-H: microsatellite instability high; CN-L: copy number low (type I EMC); POLE: polymerase E hotspot mutant tumor; CN-H: copy number high (serous or serous-like endometrial carcinoma).

*EMC: it may also be applicable to clear cell carcinomas. Most tumors can be separated with review of H&E slides. **EMC: this assay does not distinguish CN-H G3 endometrioid carcinoma from serous carcinoma or CN-H clear cell carcinoma from serous carcinoma.

For laboratories that cannot perform *POLE* mutational analysis, an alternative method, although less precise, has been proposed, using immunohistochemistry (fig. 5-77). However, this algorithm may be as problematic as the simplified TCGA classifier because most laboratories have not optimized PTEN or ARID1A antibodies for routine diagnostic use.

Figure 5-77

ALTERNATIVE CLASSIFIER LACKING *POLE* MUTATIONAL ANALYSIS

EMC: endometrioid carcinoma; MSI-H: microsatellite instability high; CN-L: copy number low (type I EMC); POLE: polymerase E hotspot mutant tumor; CN-H: copy number high (serous or serous-like endometrial carcinoma).

EMC*: this may also be applicable to clear cell carcinomas. Most tumors can be separated with review of H&E slides. **POLE hotspot mutant endometrioid carcinoma in this context should be favored if tumor shows striking intratumoral heterogeneity or geographic outgrowth of a component simulating serous carcinoma and/or dense peritumoral and tumor-infiltrating lymphocytes. ***POLE hotspot mutant tumors may appear histologically similar to MSI-H endometrioid carcinoma. It can be difficult or impossible to distinguish tumors with both *POLE* and *Tp53* mutations from CN-H tumors in this algorithm.

(193). These cut-offs were suggested due to low rates of concurrent adenocarcinoma when foci resembling carcinoma are limited in size or volume in follow-up hysterectomy specimens. Despite these data, most pathologists would diagnose lesions with the above characteristics as "focal adenocarcinoma in a background of atypical hyperplasia/EIN" or "atypical hyperplasia/EIN bordering on adenocarcinoma."

Atypical Polypoid Adenomyoma (APA). This tumor resembles complex hyperplasia, with or without nuclear atypia, set in a polyp with myoid or myofibromatous stroma (193,194). This lesion characteristically occurs in women between 38 and 42 years, is typically centered in the lower uterine segment, and has a lobulated low-power architecture. If the lesion is fragmented, the appearance may be concerning for myometrial invasive endometrioid carcinoma, particularly when the glands are architecturally complex. In order to avoid this diagnostic pitfall, a diagnosis of myometrial invasive carcinoma should not be made in polypectomy, biopsy, or curettage specimens. As occurs with hyperplasia, APA can display a range of architectural complexity and nuclear atypia that approaches or resembles FIGO grade 1 endometrioid carcinoma (195). Given that most affected patients are young and the lesion is confined to a polyp, there is only minimal risk of concurrent myometrial invasive carcinoma or progression to myometrial invasive carcinoma. Therefore, excision of the polyp with endometrial curettage and hormonal therapy should be the treatment of choice.

Endocervical Adenocarcinoma. One of the most frequent differential diagnoses concerns FIGO grade 1 or 2 endometrioid carcinoma versus human papillomavirus (HPV)-associated (usual) endocervical adenocarcinoma. The diagnosis is usually straightforward in hysterectomy specimens, but it can be problematic in biopsy

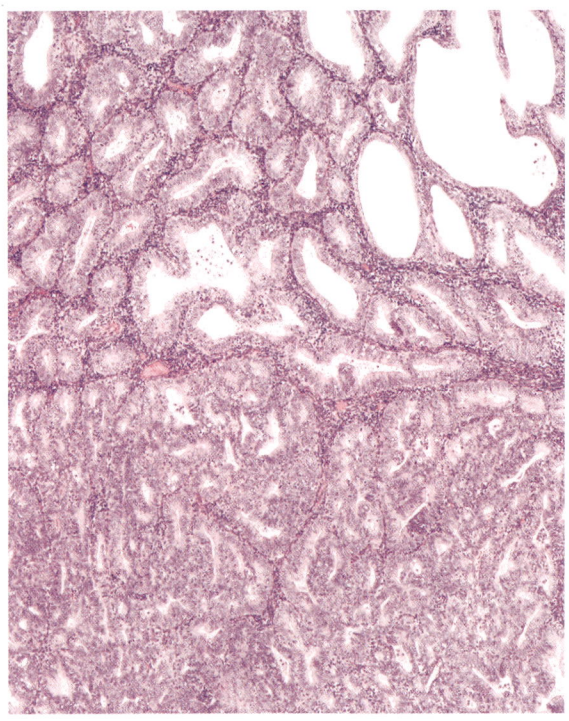

Figure 5-78

DISTINCTION BETWEEN ATYPICAL HYPERPLASIA AND ADENOCARCINOMA

Atypical hyperplasia retains interglandular stroma whereas adenocarcinoma shows back-to-back glands without intervening stroma.

and curettage specimens when the tumor is histologically high-grade, is endocervical but not HPV-associated, or is MSI-H. When doubt exists about the origin of the tumor even after applying immunohistochemistry, it is best to convey this information to the clinician so that clinical imaging or a cone biopsy can be performed. Even at hysterectomy, the diagnosis can be complicated by the presence of preferential cervical involvement by endometrioid carcinoma (137) or by extension of endocervical adenocarcinoma to the lower uterine segment or corpus (139).

HPV-associated endocervical adenocarcinoma mostly occurs in premenopausal and perimenopausal women, particularly in those with an established precursor such as high-grade squamous intraepithelial lesion (HSIL) or adenocarcinoma in situ (AIS). The presence of stromal foam cells, associated endometrial hyperplasia, or squamous differentiation within the neoplastic glands favors an endometrial endometrioid carcinoma. HPV-associated endocervical adenocarcinomas, in contrast to most glandular or papillary low-grade endometrioid carcinomas, show cells with more pseudostratified, elongated and darkly stained nuclei that are fairly uniform from cell to cell (fig. 5-79A). Low-grade endometrioid carcinomas, on the other hand, frequently contain an admixture of different cell types (endometrioid, squamous, mucinous, ciliated) with oval nuclei lacking condensed chromatin. A helpful differentiating feature in HPV-associated endocervical adenocarcinoma is the finding of conspicuous mitotic activity at the luminal/apical aspect of the cells in conjunction with basal karyorrhexis.

HPV-associated endocervical adenocarcinomas typically show diffuse and strong p16 overexpression and label with high-risk HPV in situ hybridization probes. They tend to be negative or only weakly positive for ER, PR (more reliably negative), and vimentin in contrast to low-grade endometrioid carcinomas (fig. 5-79B). Mucinous carcinomas of endometrium may show cytoplasmic CEA staining and MSI-H endometrioid carcinomas may be weakly positive or negative for ER and PR, complicating this differential diagnosis. MSI-H endometrioid carcinoma shows loss of expression of at least one DNA MMR protein (MLH1, PMS2, MSH2, and MSH6), unlike endocervical adenocarcinoma (196). Low-grade endometrioid carcinomas, as discussed previously, may display many p16 positive cells, but the staining is usually in a mosaic pattern rather than a uniform/diffuse pattern. Some high-grade endometrioid and clear cell carcinomas, and all serous carcinomas, however, show diffuse p16 overexpression (168). In this setting, it may be helpful to perform in situ hybridization for high-risk HPV. A positive signal indicates HPV infection and, indirectly, a diagnosis of HPV-associated endocervical adenocarcinoma. Fewer than 5 percent of HPV-associated endocervical adenocarcinomas show aberrant p53 staining (197), unlike many examples of high-grade endometrioid and clear cell carcinomas and nearly all serous carcinomas.

It is important to remain aware of the uncommon HPV-negative endocervical carcinomas. With the exception of frequent WT1 expression in adnexal serous carcinomas, clear cell and serous

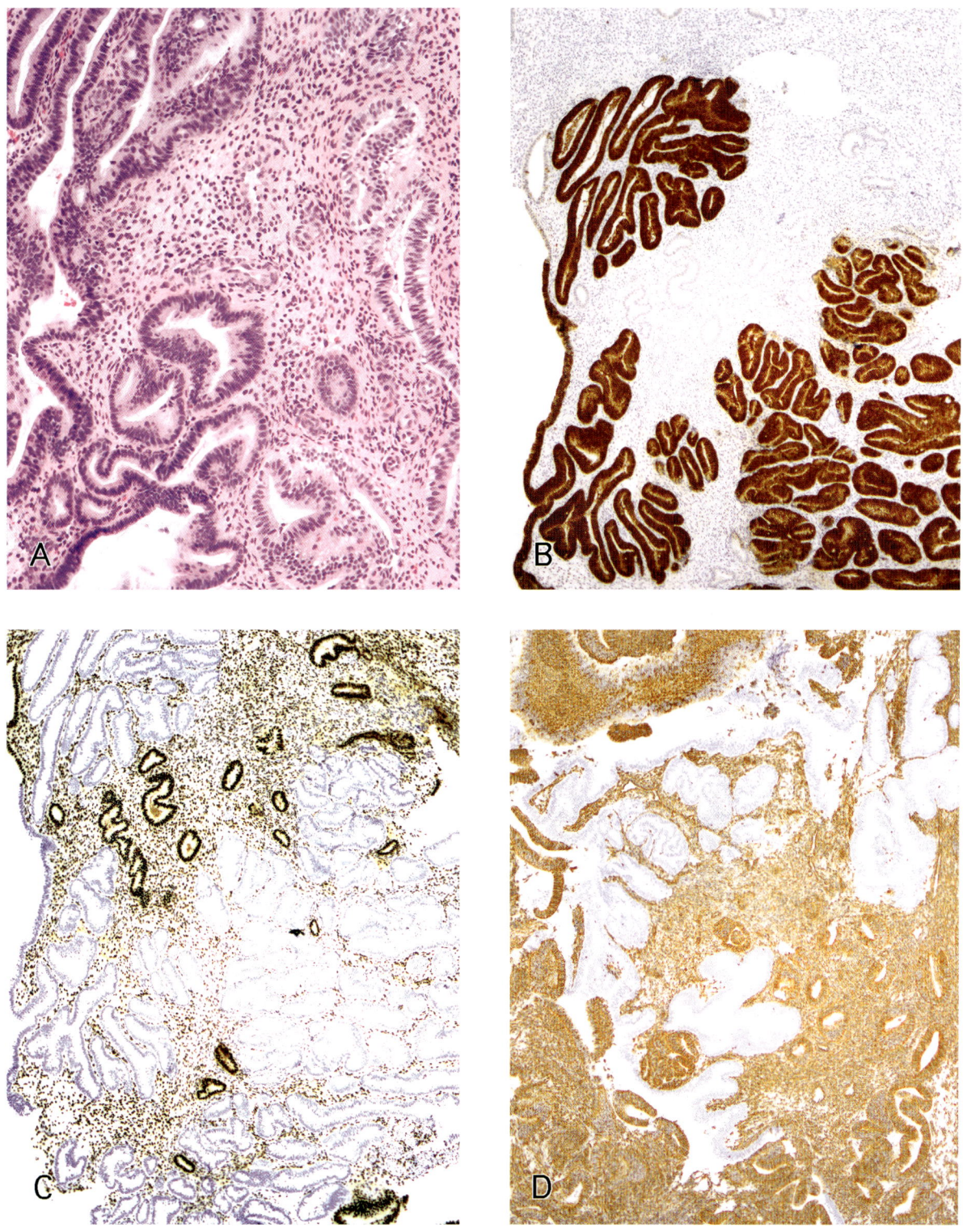

Figure 5-79
ENDOCERVICAL ADENOCARCINOMA COLONIZING LOWER UTERINE SEGMENT
Hyperchromatic nuclei and apical mitoses (A). The tumor is p16 positive (B), and PR (C) and vimentin negative (D).

carcinomas have the same morphology and more or less the same immunophenotype regardless of site of origin, thus, immunohistochemistry should not be used in the differential diagnosis. Serous carcinomas of the cervix are rare and before making such a diagnosis, the existence of a uterine, fallopian tube, ovarian, or peritoneal primary should be excluded.

Mesonephric carcinoma (cervix) and mesonephric-like carcinoma (endometrium) are also rare but display a wide range of morphologies and may simulate several types of carcinoma, including endometrioid carcinomas, particularly when ductal differentiation is present. A hysterectomy specimen usually provides sufficient material to enable recognition of the characteristically variable architectural patterns of cervical mesonephric carcinoma and its precursors, mesonephric remnants and hyperplasia (198,199). Useful immunohistochemical markers that may facilitate recognition of this tumor include GATA-3, reportedly positive in most mesonephric carcinomas although with variable staining intensity (200,201), and TTF-1, positive in a significant minority of mesonephric carcinomas and mesonephric-like carcinomas (202,203). In contrast, most endometrioid carcinomas are GATA-3 negative and only occasionally express TTF-1. Mesonephric carcinomas are usually ER/PR negative and known to variably express calretinin and CD10 (204,205). The latter two markers are also frequently expressed in endometrioid carcinomas (203) (see chapter 12).

Gastric-type adenocarcinoma of endocervix (GAS), including minimal deviation adenocarcinoma of mucinous type (206), may show histologic overlap with mucinous carcinoma of endometrium. Furthermore, imaging studies may localize this tumor to the upper endocervix or lower uterine segment, complicating interpretation. When encountered, lobular endocervical hyperplasia, severe nuclear atypia, and intestinal-type goblet cells suggest GAS over mucinous carcinoma of endometrium. GAS lacks ER/PR expression and may overexpress p53. Most show HNF-1β expression and many express carbonic anhydrase IX (207).

Microglandular Hyperplasia of Endocervix. Occasionally, endometrioid adenocarcinoma with mucinous differentiation resembles microglandular hyperplasia of endocervix, particularly in biopsy and curettage material (35,36,208). As most patients with microglandular hyperplasia are premenopausal or have been treated with progestins, and most patients with carcinoma of endometrium are postmenopausal, the patient's age and medication history are used as part of the initial diagnostic strategy. Nevertheless, some studies have reported microglandular hyperplasia in postmenopausal women and in those with no associated history of progestin therapy (209,210).

Morphologically, microglandular hyperplasia typically lacks nuclear atypia and mitotic activity, while frequently displaying a two-cell population consisting of reserve or basal cells and columnar secretory cells. Typical examples also show subnuclear and supranuclear cytoplasmic vacuoles (fig. 5-80). Both proliferations express ER and PR and Ki-67 is not helpful in this differential diagnosis. The benefit of vimentin staining in this differential diagnosis has recently been questioned (211,212). p16 labeling tends to be paradoxically elevated, but not diffuse, in endometrioid adenocarcinomas with mucinous differentiation, which contrasts with little or no p16 labeling in most cases of microglandular hyperplasia (213). A recent study concluded that a p16-positive/PAX2-negative phenotype favors a diagnosis of microglandular hyperplasia-like adenocarcinoma over microglandular hyperplasia (212). *K-ras* mutations are not identified in microglandular hyperplasia in contrast to 60 percent of endometrioid carcinomas with microglandular-like features (212a). p63 labeling of reserve or basal cells in microglandular hyperplasia (unpublished observations) can be used diagnostically if the clinical and morphologic features are confounding.

Endometrial Serous Carcinoma. This type of uterine carcinoma is diagnosed in the presence of diffuse, severe nuclear atypia when the morphologic features of endometrioid or clear cell carcinomas are lacking (190). In contrast to most endometrioid carcinomas, tumor cells are low columnar or polyhedral, and exhibit cellular stratification (as opposed to pseudostratification), tumor cell budding and detachment leading to irregular luminal borders and slit-like spaces, and a high N/C ratio. Serous carcinoma should be favored over endometrioid carcinoma, even when there is a

Endometrioid Carcinoma and Related Carcinomas

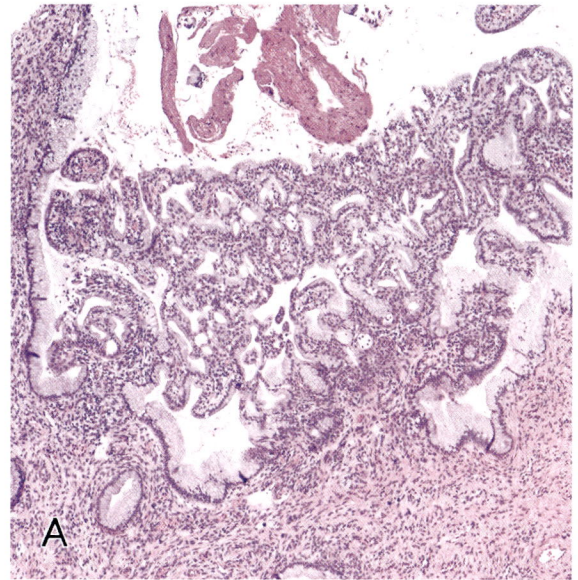
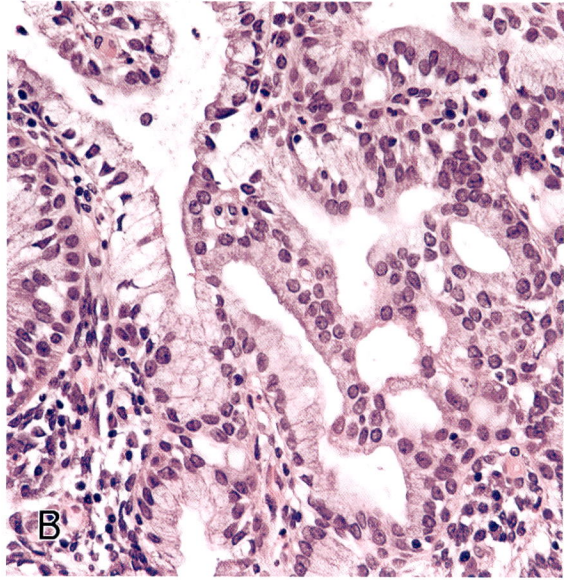
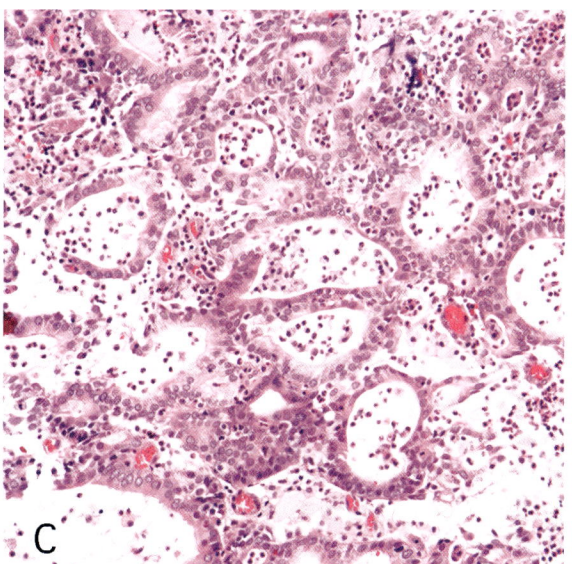

Figure 5-80

MICROGLANDULAR HYPERPLASIA OF ENDOCERVIX VERSUS MICROGLANDULAR HYPERPLASIA-LIKE ADENOCARCINOMA OF ENDOMETRIUM

Typical examples of microglandular hyperplasia (A,B). In biopsy or curettage, where anatomic landmarks are unclear, microglandular hyperplasia is the favored diagnosis in the presence of a reserve cell layer underlying mucinous epithelium (best seen at left in B) and absence of nuclear atypia and mitotic activity. Microglandular hyperplasia-like endometrioid adenocarcinoma (C) is more commonly encountered in postmenopausal patients.

predominant solid architecture, in the presence of diffusely distributed high-grade nuclei with striking pleomorphism and absence of endometrioid features (190). Early serous carcinoma may be "intraepithelial," colonizing preexisting surface endometrium or atrophic glands within the endometrium or an endometrial polyp. In contrast to well-developed serous carcinoma, it may be difficult to recognize as neoplastic on scanning magnification. The only indication of early serous carcinoma, referred to as endometrial intraepithelial carcinoma (EIC) or serous intraepithelial carcinoma (the preferred term, as it minimizes confusion with EIN) may be subtle cellular and nuclear enlargement, increased N/C ratio, and increased mitotic activity, particularly in the presence of a linear, well-delimited proliferation of tall blue cells on the endometrial surface or replacing atrophic glands. Aberrant p53 (diffuse and strong or absent) labeling and an elevated proliferative index with Ki-67 confirm this diagnosis. Gland forming endometrioid lesions only rarely display this immunophenotype. Loss of expression of ARID1A, PTEN, or one of the DNA MMR markers supports a diagnosis of endometrioid carcinoma, even when the p53 staining pattern is aberrant. Some *POLE*-mutated carcinomas mimic the appearance of serous carcinomas to a significant degree (see fig. 5-73).

Differentiating serous carcinoma from FIGO grade 3 endometrioid carcinoma with aberrant p53 staining can be challenging, as evidenced by poor rates of interobserver diagnostic concordance. The presence of focal low-grade endometrioid glandular components or squamous differentiation favors interpretation as endometrioid, but this is still subject to diagnostic discordance in some cases (214). Furthermore, tumors with an endometrioid genotype (i.e., CN-H with *p53* mutation along with *PTEN*, *PIK3CA*, or *ARID1A* mutation) may be histologically ambiguous (215), making distinction between serous-like/CN-H FIGO grade 3 endometrioid carcinoma and serous carcinoma difficult or impossible in routine clinical practice. Despite overall unfavorable clinical outcomes in the CN-H/serous-like genomic group, distinction between CN-H/serous-like FIGO grade 3 endometrioid carcinomas and serous carcinomas remain important as there is preliminary evidence that the former metastasize to the peritoneum less frequently than serous carcinoma and have lower rates of extrauterine disease at presentation (192). These findings suggest that efforts to accurately histotype endometrial carcinomas should continue.

Detailed analysis of *Tp53*-mutated FIGO grade 3 endometrioid carcinomas indicates that only *Tp53* mutation in the setting of CN-H places FIGO grade 3 endometrioid carcinomas in a high-risk clinical category. Some *Tp53* mutations found in the POLE and MSI-H categories involve portions of the *Tp53* gene that are not mutated in serous carcinomas (216) and, since some *Tp53* mutations in *POLE* and MSI-H carcinomas affect epitopes that do not lead to impaired degradation of p53 protein or truncation, there is imperfect correlation between *Tp53* mutation and aberrant p53 staining in these groups of tumors. Nevertheless, when faced with a FIGO grade 3 endometrioid carcinoma with aberrant p53 staining, the odds are in favor of a CN-H/serous-like tumor with a poor prognosis rather than a *POLE*-mutated or MSI-H carcinoma (184) (see below). A panel of markers or sequencing should be used to distinguish among the various genomic subtypes of endometrial carcinoma.

Clear Cell Carcinoma. Finding clear cytoplasm or hobnail cells is not diagnostic of clear cell carcinoma, since these features are also seen in endometrioid and serous carcinomas (217,218). A diagnosis of clear cell carcinoma should only be rendered in the presence of the definitional architectural and cytologic features. Clear cell carcinoma is typically characterized by an admixture of tubules, cysts, papillae, and much less commonly, a solid growth of tumor cells. The cysts vary in size and papillae tend to be small and rounded, frequently with myxoid stroma or a hyaline matrix, in contrast to most endometrioid carcinomas. Clear cells are seen in endometrioid carcinomas, within the glands or in areas of squamous differentiation, but cells do not contain large, round nuclei with prominent nucleoli or architectural patterns of clear cell carcinoma. Cellular stratification and columnar cells with nuclear pseudostratification are also not characteristic of clear cell carcinoma.

In contrast to most endometrioid carcinomas, clear cell carcinomas typically express strong hepatocyte nuclear factor-1 beta (HNF-1β), and napsin A, and are negative for ER and PR, with only occasional exceptions. Focal to moderate expression of HNF-1β and, to a lesser extent, napsin A can be encountered in some endometrioid carcinomas with clear cells (219–224). Aberrant p53 expression and p16 overexpression are not diagnostically helpful since both endometrioid and clear cell carcinomas may display these abnormalities (225–228).

Mixed Epithelial Carcinomas with an Endometrioid Component. This term has been used for two types of tumor: a carcinoma containing at least two distinct histologic components and a histologically ambiguous tumor (see figs. 5-73, 5-75) that displays overlapping features of at least two histotypes (i.e., "can't distinguish endometrioid or serous"). The most recent WHO classification stipulates that, in the former scenario, a "type II" endometrial carcinoma histotype must be present and the least prevalent component should represent at least 5 percent of the tumor. This excludes histologically ambiguous tumors from this category (187,215,229,230).

Despite the morphologic requirement for distinctive histotypes, a recent study indicates that, with only occasional exceptions, mixed epithelial carcinomas represent one tumor clone with divergent subclones. One study of "mixed endometrioid and serous carcinomas" (188) reported shared mutations in the "serous" and "endometrioid" components in 9 of 11 cases. Six tumors shared *Tp53* mutations and/or diffusely aberrant p53 staining in each component, without mutations typical of endometrioid carcinomas, indicating that these tumors should be considered serous carcinomas with glandular and papillary architecture. Three tumors were DNA MMR-deficient or *POLE* mutated with an endometrioid genotype, supporting a diagnosis of endometrioid carcinoma with intratumoral heterogeneity. The remaining 2 tumors showed different mutations in the two components, one being DNA MMR deficient. Thus, only 2 of 11 tumors fulfilled the criteria for "mixed endometrioid and serous carcinoma." Furthermore, only two reports of mixed endometrioid and low-grade serous carcinoma exist in the literature (229,231).

As for morphologically ambiguous endometrial carcinomas, a recent study reported aberrant p53 staining in all 13 tumors studied, 3 having "endometrioid-type" mutations, such as *PTEN* or *PIK3CA* (229). As these cases were ascertained by searching specifically for "mixed endometrioid and serous carcinomas," data appear to be enriched for p53 abnormalities in morphologically ambiguous carcinomas. Another recent study indicates that both MSI-H and *POLE*-mutated endometrioid carcinomas, neither of which typically displays aberrant p53 staining, can also display overlapping features of endometrioid and serous carcinoma (214).

When presented with a "mixed carcinoma" or a morphologically ambiguous endometrial carcinoma, the rarity of "mixed carcinoma" should be recognized, and p53 and DNA MMR immunohistochemistry and, if available, *POLE* mutational analysis performed (fig. 5-77).

Undifferentiated Carcinoma. Monomorphic undifferentiated endometrial carcinoma should be distinguished from endometrioid carcinoma with solid architecture (figs. 5-41, 5-46, 5-48). Unlike the cells of endometrioid carcinoma, tumor cells in undifferentiated carcinoma are noncohesive and arranged in monotonous sheets, infiltrate as single cells and large, poorly formed aggregates, or are distributed haphazardly in a myxoid stroma. Poorly fixed specimens are problematic and cannot be analyzed in some instances, even with the use of immunohistochemistry, as some tumors exist in a grey zone between the two entities. Absence of diffuse positivity for pancytokeratins, limited EMA and CK18 expression, limited or no expression of E-cadherin, loss of BRG-1 or INI-1 staining, and no expression of ER, PR, and PAX8 favor a diagnosis of undifferentiated carcinoma over grade 3 endometrioid carcinoma.

Other tumors in the differential diagnosis of undifferentiated carcinoma include serous carcinoma with a solid architecture (diffuse PAX8 and keratin expression), small and large cell neuroendocrine carcinoma (extensive chromogranin or synaptophysin expression), and rhabdomyosarcoma (desmin and myogenin expression). They can be identified by careful morphologic evaluation and the use of a limited panel of immunohistochemical stains. Since there can be a gradient of neuroendocrine expression from undifferentiated carcinoma to small cell neuroendocrine carcinoma, morphology should take precedence. Undifferentiated carcinomas seldom display nuclear molding, streaming, and crush artifact, which are characteristic of small cell carcinoma.

The distinction of undifferentiated carcinoma from lymphoma and plasmacytoma may be problematic as many undifferentiated carcinomas express CD138, like plasmacytoma, some display weak expression of lymphoid markers by flow cytometry, and others have oligoclonal lymphoid infiltrates. Aside from CD138, which is a nonspecific marker, undifferentiated carcinomas do not express lymphoid markers and do not show convincing evidence of B-cell clonality.

Undifferentiated carcinoma with monomorphic cells may also resemble high-grade endometrial stromal sarcoma. In contrast to the former, high-grade endometrial stromal sarcoma does not usually display dyshesive cells or contain rhabdoid or multinucleated cells. They may invade the myometrium with a pushing or tongue-like pattern, and most are centered in the myometrium, whereas undifferentiated carcinomas typically have a destructive pattern of invasion and are centered in the endometrium. The best characterized type of high-grade endometrial stromal sarcoma has a nested architecture, delicate vasculature, +/- a low-grade fibromyxoid component. It typically shows strong and diffuse cyclin D1 (232), BCOR, and c-KIT (233) expression, markers that are not frequently positive in undifferentiated carcinoma, with the exception of cyclin D1 (234). In these cases, claudin 4 may be useful in the differential diagnosis as it is reportedly positive in undifferentiated carcinoma but not sarcoma (235). The cyclin D1-positive variant of high-grade endometrial stromal sarcoma also features a characteristic recurrent translocation, t(10;17) (236). Although only present in 50 to 75 percent of tumors, the presence of DNA MMR deficiency favors an undifferentiated carcinoma.

Dedifferentiated Endometrial Carcinoma (Mixed Endometrioid and Undifferentiated Carcinoma.) The same morphologic and immunohistochemical criteria discussed for distinguishing undifferentiated carcinoma from grade 3 endometrioid carcinoma apply when evaluating the solid component of these mixed tumors, so as not to misdiagnose them as FIGO grade 2 or 3 endometrioid carcinoma.

The differential diagnosis of dedifferentiated carcinomas also includes mullerian adenosarcoma with stromal overgrowth and carcinosarcoma when the undifferentiated component is pleomorphic. With rare exceptions, mullerian adenosarcoma does not feature an adenocarcinoma in the epithelial compartment, and even with stromal overgrowth still has typical areas of adenocarcinoma facilitating the differential diagnosis. With rare exceptions, carcinosarcoma should only be diagnosed in the presence of histologically high-grade epithelial and mesenchymal elements (68). The epithelial component of a typical dedifferentiated carcinoma is FIGO grade 1 or 2 endometrioid carcinoma and thus fails to meet criteria for carcinosarcoma. Diagnosing a mixed endometrioid and undifferentiated carcinoma when the differentiated component is FIGO grade 3 can be problematic, however. In these cases, the small round blue cell component of the tumor should be carefully examined and studied with immunohistochemistry if necessary. Other tumors in this differential diagnosis include melanoma, lymphoma, plasmacytoma, rhabdomyosarcoma, and pleomorphic undifferentiated or pleomorphic heterologous uterine sarcoma (when malignant cartilage or osteoid is encountered). Differentiating pleomorphic undifferentiated carcinoma and sarcoma can be difficult and in some cases impossible. Carcinoma is favored when the tumor is centered in or appears to have arisen from the endometrium, when epithelial differentiation can be ascertained with at least focal expression of EMA or CK18, or when the tumor is DNA MMR deficient. Pleomorphic heterologous uterine sarcoma should be diagnosed when malignant heterologous elements are present. Since undifferentiated carcinomas may have myxoid matrix, which may resemble chondroid matrix, malignant chondrocytes should be identified before diagnosing a pleomorphic heterologous uterine sarcoma.

Squamous Cell Carcinoma. Occasionally, a curettage specimen contains only tumor fragments with squamous elements. If there is no clinical history or evidence of a cervical carcinoma precursor and no clinically appreciable cervical tumor, the possibility of endometrioid carcinoma with extensive squamous differentiation should be considered (fig. 5-81). Lack of p16 block-like expression, negative in situ hybridization for high-risk HPV, and expression of adenocarcinoma-associated glycoproteins B72.3 or BerEP4 in metaplastic areas help support a diagnosis of endometrioid carcinoma with extensive squamous differentiation.

Although there are some reports of HPV-associated squamous cell carcinoma of endometrium, most studies do not support this association (237–241). The small number of tumors studied with p16 indicate that, with only rare exceptions (237), diffuse p16 staining is not found in squamous carcinomas of the corpus (180,238).

Rare primary squamous cell carcinomas of endometrium have been reported (fig. 5-82). But before establishing this diagnosis, an endometrioid carcinoma with extensive squamous differentiation should be excluded (180,242,243). These tumors may be associated with ichthyosis uteri or extensive squamous metaplasia of endometrium (180,244–247).

Small Cell Neuroendocrine Carcinoma. At low-power magnification, small cell carcinoma may resemble high-grade endometrioid carcinoma because of solid/trabecular or nested architecture (see chapter 12). Furthermore, it may be admixed with an endometrioid component, and in that scenario, dedifferentiated carcinoma may be suggested (248). The diagnosis of small

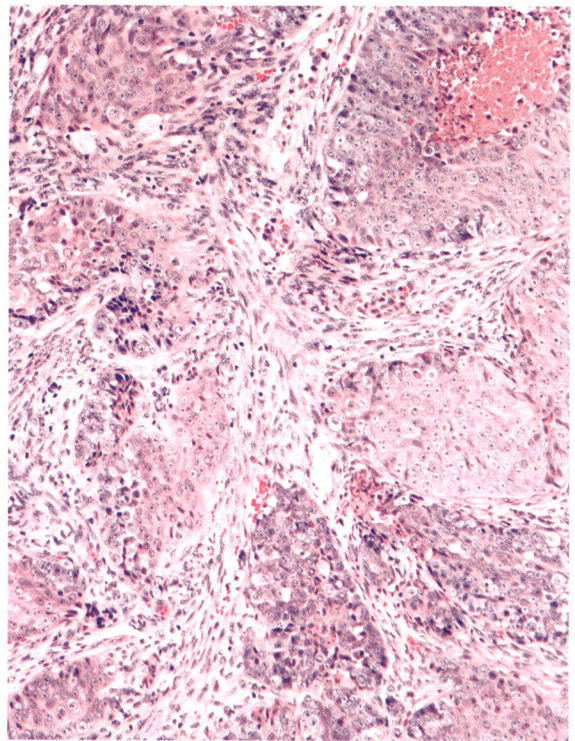

Figure 5-81

ENDOMETRIOID ADENOCARCINOMA MIMICKING SQUAMOUS CELL CARCINOMA

The primary differential diagnosis here is between endometrioid adenocarcinoma and cervical squamous carcinoma, as primary squamous cell carcinoma of the corpus is rare. A clue to the correct diagnosis is the very eosinophilic/squamous metaplastic appearance of the epithelium without keratinization or basaloid features. The diagnosis is usually apparent in a hysterectomy specimen, but can be difficult in a curetting, where immunohistochemistry and high-risk human papillomavirus (HPV) in situ hybridization can be performed as ancillary diagnostic tests.

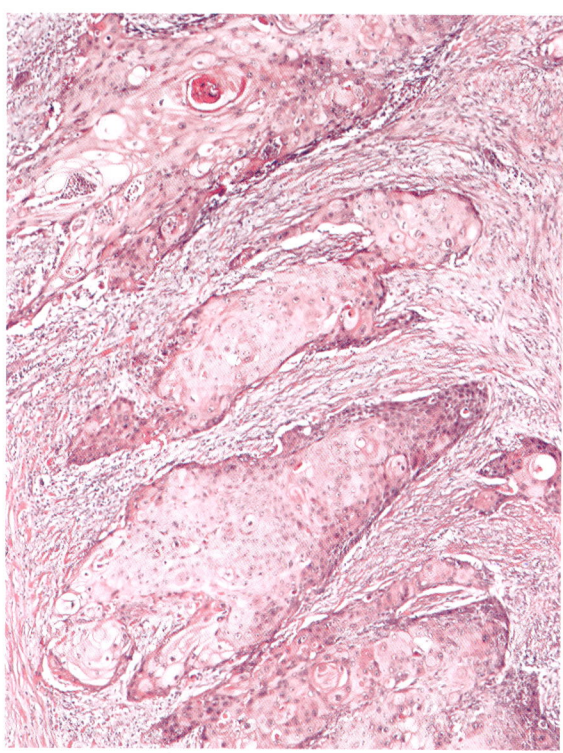

Figure 5-82

SQUAMOUS CELL CARCINOMA OF UTERINE CORPUS

This tumor is distinguished from endometrioid adenocarcinoma with squamous differentiation by extensive sampling that fails to reveal endometrioid glandular differentiation. The possibility of a cervical primary squamous cell carcinoma should always be excluded.

cell carcinoma should be suspected when the characteristic nuclear features, namely the "salt and pepper" chromatin with nuclear molding, streaming, and crush artifact, are present. If needed, expression of neuroendocrine markers, along with some keratin expression, should facilitate the diagnosis. However, neuroendocrine markers and cytokeratin expression may not be extensive in small cell carcinoma and may be attenuated or absent, particularly in small samples. On the other hand, endometrioid carcinomas may show neuroendocrine differentiation, thus the diagnosis relies on morphologic findings. If a diagnosis of small cell carcinoma can be established, a cervical origin should be ruled out first. Imaging and HPV analysis can be used in this setting.

Uterine Tumor Resembling Ovarian Sex Cord Tumor (UTROSCT). This is a rare uterine mesenchymal tumor showing extensive sex cord-like differentiation (32). In biopsy, curettage, and polypectomy specimens particularly, the tumor may have a mixed acinar, trabecular, or solid appearance that mimics FIGO grade 2 endometrioid carcinoma or the solid pattern of FIGO grade 3 endometrioid carcinoma. On gross examination, most of these tumors are well circumscribed, yellow to tan, and uniform in appearance, which often is in contrast with the appearance of endometrioid carcinoma. Although UTROSCTs are often keratin positive, they tend to be EMA negative. They frequently coexpress smooth muscle actin, with or without desmin and caldesmon, as well as inhibin, melan A, calretinin, WT1, and sometimes FOXL2 and CD10 (83,249). Thus, they are described as polyphenotypic, but some of these markers, including calretinin and CD10, may also be seen in endometrioid carcinomas.

Carcinoma with Yolk Sac Differentiation. This rare tumor, when presenting in adulthood, can be mixed with endometrioid carcinoma (164). The appearance is similar or identical to pure yolk sac tumor and SALL4 and glypican-3, are positive, while EMA and CK7 are negative in most cases.

Hepatoid Carcinoma. This rare neoplasm can be mixed with endometrioid carcinoma and may simulate solid endometrioid carcinoma with oxyphilic features (250,251). Trabecular or solid architecture with eosinophilic cells should suggest this diagnostic possibility. The presence of canalicular bile confirms the diagnosis, although this is a rare finding. These cells express hepar-1, alpha-fetoprotein (AFP), arginase, SALL4, and glypican-3, while EMA and CK7 are negative.

Wilms Tumor. Adult extrarenal Wilms tumor may resemble endometrioid carcinoma with tubular and spindle cell features. A triphasic appearance, consisting of simple tubules, glomeruloid structures, immature mesenchyme, and blastema, should establish the diagnosis, sometimes with associated rhabdomyoblastic differentiation (252–254). WT1 is positive, although this marker is not specific.

Primitive Neuroectodermal Tumor (PNET). The most common type of PNET, although rare, is central-type, lacking the *EWS* translocation (208,254). Only rare examples of peripheral PNET (i.e., Ewing sarcoma) have been described in the uterus (83,255). Central-type PNETs may resemble medulloblastoma, ependymoblastoma, or neuroblastoma. In small samples, the rosettes that are so characteristic of these tumors may mimic endometrioid tubules. Furthermore, endometrioid carcinoma may be seen in association with PNET. Central-type PNETs express synaptophysin, neurofilament, or GFAP, typically without pancytokeratin expression. Peripheral-type PNET only rarely enters in the differential diagnosis with endometrioid carcinoma, although it can resemble monomorphic undifferentiated carcinoma. The presence of an *EWS* translocation should be sought to confirm a diagnosis of peripheral-type PNET.

Non-Neoplastic Entities. Eosinophilic and hobnail metaplasia, Arias-Stella reaction, reparative and reactive changes, and radiation atypia may enter the differential diagnosis with endometrioid carcinoma because of cytoplasmic or nuclear features that depart from those of cycling or atrophic endometrium. In most instances, however, these non-neoplastic lesions lack the architectural complexity and cytologic features that characterize carcinoma. Reparative lesions, in particular, are often present in a background of loose inflamed stroma that in some cases corresponds to a previous biopsy site or intrauterine device-associated endometritis, but in this setting the most common problem is with clear cell or serous carcinoma. Papillary syncytial metaplasia is easy to recognize when closely associated with degenerating balls of endometrial stroma and fibrin, but its streaming appearance may suggest carcinoma when the stromal balls are scarce. Evidence of glandular and stromal breakdown elsewhere, which is supportive of papillary syncytial metaplasia, is usually present.

A range of papillary proliferations may be seen within the endometrium that fall short of a diagnosis of adenocarcinoma. Papillae that characterize carcinoma are: 1) villous (long, finger-like and frequently branched); 2) nonvillous but extensively branched; or 3) nonvillous with secondary architectural complexity, such as superimposed cribriform structures, and show notable nuclear atypia. Papillae lacking these features are referred to as "simple papillae" and their presence is not diagnostic of carcinoma. Such papillae are found on the surface of endometrial polyp(s) or nonpolypoid endometrium in older women, and they are benign if found focally, and cells lack nuclear atypia (256).

Mucinous proliferations without complex architecture are typically benign, however, in biopsy specimens, architecture may be difficult to evaluate and distinction from carcinoma may be exceedingly difficult. When benign-appearing mucin-rich cells are present singly or forming small tufts within normal preexisting endometrial glands or surface the likelihood of associated carcinoma is likely nonexistent. However, if any degree of architectural complexity is noted, the risk of coexistent adenocarcinoma can increase up to 65 percent (71,256a).

Metastatic Adenocarcinoma. Lobular carcinoma, colorectal adenocarcinoma (257–259), and drop metastases from fallopian tube, ovary, or peritoneum are the most frequently encountered metastases to the endometrium. Of these, only colorectal adenocarcinoma may cause confusion with endometrioid carcinoma owing to gland formation including complex architecture and pseudostratified nuclei. In contrast to most endometrioid carcinomas, the nuclei of metastatic colorectal adenocarcinomas are hyperchromatic, with obvious atypia along with a higher mitotic index when compared to the low-grade architecture. They often feature dirty necrosis and garland architecture. Many colorectal adenocarcinomas also contain variable numbers of goblet cells, which are present only exceptionally in endometrial carcinomas. CK7, CK20, PAX8, and SATB2 help in this differential diagnosis.

TREATMENT AND PROGNOSIS

FIGO stage and grade, patient age, performance status, and medical comorbidities are the most robust prognostic determinants of endometrioid carcinomas. In a classification and regression tree (CART) statistical analysis of prognostic determinants in endometrial cancer, one group reported that FIGO stage I (low stage) versus stages II to IV (high stage) was the most powerful prognostic discriminator (60). Among high-stage tumors, FIGO grades 1 and 2 (low-grade) clustered separately from the FIGO grade 3 (high-grade) carcinomas and among low-stage tumors, patients over 68 years had worse clinical outcomes than younger patients.

An endometrial carcinoma nomogram, a tool that predicts an individual patient's prognosis based on statistically robust discriminators, is used in some tertiary centers (260). The most important factors are FIGO stage and grade and patient age; only little weight is given to histologic subtype in the nomogram. A multivariate analysis of a limited sample of endometrial carcinomas also identified TCGA group assignment, but not histotype, as prognostically important (184).

Most patients with low-stage and low-grade endometrioid carcinoma have a good prognosis, but some have recurrences. Vaginal recurrences can often be salvaged, but extravaginal recurrences are typically responsible for adverse outcomes. Risk factors for extravaginal recurrences include deep myoinvasion, large size, tumor cell necrosis, lymphovascular invasion (particularly when present deeper than the invasive tumor front), lower uterine segment involvement, cervical involvement, and aneuploidy (121,261–264).

FIGO staging unfortunately ignores significant clinical heterogeneity within each substage and staging adequacy. For example, a 70-year-old patient with serous carcinoma who has undergone a hysterectomy, without peritoneal or lymph node staging and with 40 percent myometrial invasion (FIGO stage I), has an estimated 5-year survival rate of 66 percent; the same patient with FIGO grade 1 endometrioid carcinoma, 30 negative lymph nodes, and no myometrial invasion (FIGO stage I) has an estimated 5-year survival rate of 97 percent. Some investigators have proposed subclassification of FIGO stage I endometrial carcinomas to account for tumor type and grade, as well as staging adequacy (60). This scheme yields significantly more predictive information than either the FIGO 1988 or FIGO 2009 systems, as patients with uterus-confined unstaged nonendometrioid or FIGO grade 3 carcinomas have the worst prognosis and patients with well-staged FIGO grade 1 endometrioid carcinomas have the best outcome. There is, unfortunately, no consensus about what constitutes an adequate extent of lymph node dissection for accurate surgical staging.

The NCCN guidelines (265) used in the United States stratifies patients with endometrioid carcinoma based on surgical stage, grade, and depth of myometrial invasion primarily, with secondary stratification based on patient age, lymphovascular invasion, and tumor size. The guidelines state that "pelvic lymph node dissection…continues to be an important part of the surgical staging," thereby implying that lymph node sampling (not dissection) is suboptimal for adequate staging. Sentinel lymph node mapping is suggested as an alternative to full lymph node dissection in selected patients. The guidelines also call for collection of peritoneal washings even though this parameter is no longer used in the FIGO or AJCC staging schemes (214,265).

The decision tree starts with the assignment of patients into operable and inoperable categories, with consideration for fertility-sparing therapeutic approaches. Patients with inoperable endometrioid carcinoma are managed with a progestin-coated intrauterine device if the tumor is localized, pelvic radiation therapy for regional disease, and a combination of chemotherapy and pelvic radiation for systemic disease if the patient does not have associated comorbidities (266).

Patients with atypical hyperplasia/endometrial intraepithelial neoplasia (EIN) and low-grade endometrioid carcinoma (mostly FIGO grade 1 carcinoma) are candidates for fertility-sparing therapy if they are fertile, pelvic magnetic resonance imaging (MRI) is negative for myometrial invasion, progestin therapy (delivered systemically or by intrauterine device) is tolerated, and the patient is motivated to undergo close surveillance with endometrial biopsy at 3-month intervals. Such patients are typically counseled about the benefits and risks of this nonstandard protocol and are encouraged to become pregnant as soon as possible following resolution of hyperplasia or carcinoma and then undergo hysterectomy to prevent recurrence (51–54). Approximately 70 percent of patients have a complete response to therapy and, of those, 80 percent become pregnant. The median time to regression is about 6 months and most patients respond to progestational therapy within 9 months. Treatment of nonresponders is not standardized, although most gynecologists encourage hysterectomy. Approximately 40 percent of patients whose tumors initially regressed experience recurrence (267). Patients not desiring further fertility and postmenopausal patients who are deemed to have "operable" disease should undergo total hysterectomy and salpingo-oophorectomy using open, laparoscopic, or robotic techniques. Radical or modified radical hysterectomy can be considered if there is clinical evidence of cervical involvement while supracervical hysterectomy should be avoided.

Many prognostic and predictive immunomarkers have also been reported, but with the exception of aberrant p53 expression, correlated with tumor grade and TCGA subtype assignment, most have either not been validated as prognostically powerful in large studies or are dependent on other established prognostic variables (Tables 5-4–5-6). An example is IMP 3 (insulin-like growth factor II mRNA-binding protein), which tends to be expressed in tumors with aberrant p53 expression. Of lesser importance are the histologic subtype, depth of myometrial invasion, and presence of lymphovascular invasion, although it is likely that the latter two variables lose prognostic significance when accurate stage is taken into account.

There is vibrant clinical interest in TCGA group assignment for diagnostic, prognostic, and, eventually, therapeutic purposes. As mentioned previously, immunohistochemical study with DNA MMR markers and p53, along with *POLE* mutational analysis, can replicate TCGA group assignment (184), which is referred to as "PROMISE classifier" by one group (proactive molecular risk classification tool for endometrial cancers). A multivariate analysis confirmed independent associations between PROMISE and clinical outcome, but no such associations were found for histologic subtype.

Independent associations between the European Society for Medical Oncology (ESMO) clinical risk groups (268) and clinical outcomes were also reported. ESMO stratifies FIGO stage I endometrial carcinoma into three categories: low-risk, stage IA (grade 1 or 2 endometrioid); intermediate risk, FIGO stage IA (grade 3 endometrioid) or stage IB (grade 1 or 2 endometrioid); and high-risk, stage IB (grade 3 endometrioid) or any nonendometrioid carcinoma. Clinical risk group and PROMISE classifiers are generally concordant. *POLE* mutational analysis verifies low clinical risk (183,187,188,269–274), even with a deeply invasive high-grade carcinoma, while aberrant p53 staining in the absence of DNA MMR abnormalities and *POLE* mutation verifies the presence of an aggressive serous or serous-like adenocarcinoma (183,184,274). DNA MMR immunohistochemical testing is used for Lynch syndrome triage and, in selected cases, as a diagnostic adjunct. Additionally, there is accumulating evidence that MMR status also conveys information about therapeutic responsiveness, with MMR-deficient tumors having a superior response to adjuvant therapy (275). This multimodality classification is aspirational because assays are not available in most pathology laboratories.

Among patients with stages I and II carcinomas, adjuvant therapy is not necessarily needed for FIGO grade 1, stage IA carcinoma. Adjuvant therapy ranges from vaginal brachytherapy for increasing degrees of myometrial invasion and tumor grade, to vaginal brachytherapy with or without pelvic radiation therapy, and with or without chemotherapy for deeply invasive, high-grade carcinomas. Many gynecologic oncologists withhold pelvic radiation therapy if a proper lymph node dissection is performed. Adjuvant chemotherapy is used for stages IIIA-IVB and radiation is used in addition in many centers (266,276). Typical chemotherapeutic agents used in this setting are carboplatin and taxol. The 5-year survival rates for patients with endometrioid carcinoma reported in the SEER database (1) are: 97 percent for stage I patients under 50 (young patients) and 95 percent for stage I patients 50 years and older; 82 percent for young patients with adnexal or regional lymph node metastases and 66 percent for older patients; and 29 percent for young patients and 15 percent for older patients with distant disease.

Approximately 20 percent of patients experience recurrence. Pelvic and nodal recurrences after a diagnosis of FIGO grade 3 endometrioid carcinoma occur in approximately 50 percent; distant recurrences to lung or abdomen occur in about 50 percent, while liver, distant nodal, and peritoneal metastases occur in a few patients. Patients previously treated with radiation who experience a central pelvic recurrence without distant metastases may be offered pelvic exenteration. Recurrent endometrioid carcinoma, often MSI-H, is of higher grade than the primary in two thirds of cases, and frequently acquires clear cell change or mimics the appearance of clear cell carcinoma (231,277). Many of these grade-discordant metastases also show loss of PR expression.

REFERENCES

1. NIH National Cancer Institute: Surveillance Epidemiology, and End Results Program. Cancer Stat Facts. https://seer.cancer.gov/statfacts/html/corp.html
2. Randall TC, Armstrong K. Differences in treatment and outcome between African-American and white women with endometrial cancer. J Clin Oncol 2003;21:4200-6.
3. Sherman ME, Devesa SS. Analysis of racial differences in incidence, survival, and mortality for malignant tumors of the uterine corpus. Cancer 2003;98:176-86.
4. Cirisano FD Jr, Robboy SJ, Dodge RK, et al. The outcome of stage I-II clinically and surgically staged papillary serous and clear cell endometrial cancers when compared with endometrioid carcinoma. Gynecol Oncol 2000;77:55-65.
5. Santin AD, Bellone S, Siegel ER, et al. Racial differences in the overexpression of epidermal growth factor type II receptor (HER2/neu): a major prognostic indicator in uterine serous papillary cancer. Am J Obstet Gynecol 2005;192:813-8.
6. Ueda SM, Kapp DS, Cheung MK, et al. Trends in demographic and clinical characteristics in women diagnosed with corpus cancer and their potential impact on the increasing number of deaths. Am J Obstet Gynecol 2008;198:218.e1-6.
7. Wright JD, Fiorelli J, Schiff PB, et al. Racial disparities for uterine corpus tumors: changes in clinical characteristics and treatment over time. Cancer 2009;115:1276-85.
8. Smotkin D, Nevadunsky NS, Harris K, Einstein MH, Yu Y, Goldberg GL. Histopathologic differences account for racial disparity in uterine cancer survival. Gynecol Oncol 2012;127:616-9.
9. Ruterbusch JJ, Ali-Fehmi R, Olson SH, et al. The influence of comorbid conditions on racial disparities in endometrial cancer survival. Am J Obstet Gynecol 2014;211:627.e1-9.
10. Brinton LA, Felix AS, McMeekin DS, et al. Etiologic heterogeneity in endometrial cancer: evidence from a Gynecologic Oncology Group trial. Gynecol Oncol 2013;129:277-84.
11. Beral V, Banks E, Reeves G, Appleby P. Use of HRT and the subsequent risk of cancer. J Epidemiol Biostat 1999;4:191-210; discussion 210-5.
12. Pickar JH, Thorneycroft I, Whitehead M. Effects of hormone replacement therapy on the endometrium and lipid parameters: a review of randomized clinical trials, 1985 to 1995. Am J Obstet Gynecol 1998;178:1087-99.
13. Parazzini F, Franceschi S, La Vecchia C, Chatenoud L, De Cinto E. The epidemiology of female genital tract cancers. Int J Gynecol Cancer 1997;7:169-81.
14. Parazzini F, La Vecchia C, Bocciolone L, Franceschi S. The epidemiology of endometrial cancer. Gynecol Oncol 1991;41:1-16.

15. Brinton LA, Berman ML, Mortel R, et al. Reproductive, menstrual, and medical risk factors for endometrial cancer: results from a case-control study. Am J Obstet Gynecol 1992;167:1317-25.
16. Andersson M, Storm HH, Mouridsen HT. Incidence of new primary cancers after adjuvant tamoxifen therapy and radiotherapy for early breast cancer. J Natl Cancer Inst 1991;83:1013-7.
17. Cook LS, Weiss NS, Schwartz SM, et al. Population-based study of tamoxifen therapy and subsequent ovarian, endometrial, and breast cancers. J Natl Cancer Inst 1995;87:1359-64.
18. Fisher B, Costantino JP, Redmond CK, Fisher ER, Wickerham DL, Cronin WM. Endometrial cancer in tamoxifen-treated breast cancer patients: findings from the National Surgical Adjuvant Breast and Bowel Project (NSABP) B-14. J Natl Cancer Inst 1994;86:527-37.
19. Stewart HJ. The Scottish trial of adjuvant tamoxifen in nodenegative breast cancer. Scottish Cancer Trials Breast Group. J Natl Cancer Inst Monogr 1992;11:117-20.
20. Katase K, Sugiyama Y, Hasumi K, Yoshimoto M, Kasumi F. The incidence of subsequent endometrial carcinoma with tamoxifen use in patients with primary breast carcinoma. Cancer 1998;82:1698-703.
21. Ribeiro G, Swindell R. The Christie Hospital adjuvant tamoxifen trial. J Natl Cancer Inst Monogr 1992;11:121-5.
22. van Leeuwen FE, Benraadt J, Coebergh JW, et al. Risk of endometrial cancer after tamoxifen treatment of breast cancer. Lancet 1994;343:448-52.
23. Ferguson SE, Soslow RA, Amsterdam A, Barakat RR. Comparison of uterine malignancies that develop during and following tamoxifen therapy. Gynecol Oncol 2006;101:322-6.
24. Bland AE, Calingaert B, Secord AA, et al. Relationship between tamoxifen use and high risk endometrial cancer histologic types. Gynecol Oncol 2009;112:150-4.
25. Bokhman JV. Two pathogenetic types of endometrial carcinoma. Gynecol Oncol 1983;15:10-7.
26. Alvarez T, Miller E, Duska L, Oliva E. Molecular profile of grade 3 endometrioid endometrial carcinoma: is it a type I or type II endometrial carcinoma? Am J Surg Pathol. 2012;36:753-61.
27. Leitao MM Jr, Han G, Lee LX, et al. Complex atypical hyperplasia of the uterus: characteristics and prediction of underlying carcinoma risk. Am J Obstet Gynecol 2010;203:349 e1-6.
28. Ahmed QF, Gattoc L, Al-Wahab Z, et al. Vanishing endometrial cancer in hysterectomy specimens: a myth or a fact. Am J Surg Pathol 2015;39:221-6.
29. Mahdi H, Munkarah AR, Ali-Fehmi R, Woessner J, Shah SN, Moslemi-Kebria M. Tumor size is an independent predictor of lymph node metastasis and survival in early stage endometrioid endometrial cancer. Arch Gynecol Obstet 2015;292:183-90.
30. Murray SK, Young RH, Scully RE. Uterine endometrioid carcinoma with small nonvillous papillae: an analysis of 26 cases of a favorable-prognosis tumor to be distinguished from serous carcinoma. Int J Surg Pathol 2000;8:279-89.
31. Murray SK, Clement PB, Young RH. Endometrioid carcinomas of the uterine corpus with sex cord-like formations, hyalinization, and other unusual morphologic features: a report of 31 cases of a neoplasm that may be confused with carcinosarcoma and other uterine neoplasms. Am J Surg Pathol 2005;29:157-66.
32. Clement PB, Scully RE. Uterine tumors resembling ovarian sex-cord tumors. A clinicopathologic analysis of fourteen cases. Am J Clin Pathol 1976;66:512-25.
33. Eichhorn JH, Young RH, Clement PB. Sertoliform endometrial adenocarcinoma: a study of four cases. Int J Gynecol Pathol 1996;15:119-26.
34. Usadi RS, Bentley RC. Endometrioid carcinoma of the endometrium with sertoliform differentiation. Int J Gynecol Pathol 1995;14:360-4.
35. Young RH, Scully RE. Uterine carcinomas simulating microglandular hyperplasia. A report of six cases. Am J Surg Pathol 1992;16:1092-7.
36. Zaloudek C, Hayashi GM, Ryan IP, Powell CB, Miller TR. Microglandular adenocarcinoma of the endometrium: a form of mucinous adenocarcinoma that may be confused with microglandular hyperplasia of the cervix. Int J Gynecol Pathol 1997;16:52-9.
37. Sloan EA, Moskaluk CA, Mills AM. Mucinous differentiation with tumor infiltrating lymphocytes is a feature of sporadically methylated endometrial carcinomas. Int J Gynecol Pathol 2017;36:205-16.
38. Jacques SM, Qureshi F, Lawrence WD. Surface epithelial changes in endometrial adenocarcinoma: diagnostic pitfalls in curettage specimens. Int J Gynecol Pathol 1995;14:191-7.
39. Fukuoka K, Hirokawa M, Shimizu M, et al. Oxyphilic cell variant of endometrioid adenocarcinoma. Pathol Int 1998;48:754-6.
40. Pitman MB, Young RH, Clement PB, Dickersin GR, Scully RE. Endometrioid carcinoma of the ovary and endometrium, oxyphilic cell type: a report of nine cases. Int J Gynecol Pathol 1994;13:290-301.
41. Silver SA, Cheung AN, Tavassoli FA. Oncocytic metaplasia and carcinoma of the endometrium: an immunohistochemical and ultrastructural study. Int J Gynecol Pathol 1999;18:12-9.
42. Aguirre P, Scully RE, Wolfe HJ, DeLellis RA. Endometrial carcinoma with argyrophil cells: a histochemical and immunohistochemical analysis. Hum Pathol 1984;15:210-7.

98. Romero-Perez L, Lopez-Garcia MA, Diaz-Martin J, et al. ZEB1 overexpression associated with E-cadherin and microRNA-200 downregulation is characteristic of undifferentiated endometrial carcinoma. Mod Pathol 2013;26:1514-24.
99. Coatham M, Li X, Karnezis AN, et al. Concurrent ARID1A and ARID1B inactivation in endometrial and ovarian dedifferentiated carcinomas. Mod Pathol 2016;29:1586-93.
100. Garg K, Soslow RA. Lynch syndrome (hereditary non-polyposis colorectal cancer) and endometrial carcinoma. J Clin Pathol 2009;62:679-84.
101. Jones MA, Young RH, Scully RE. Endometrial carcinoma with a component of giant cell carcinoma. Int J Gynecol Pathol 1991;10:260-70.
102. Mulligan AM, Plotkin A, Rouzbahman M, Soslow RA, Gilks CB, Clarke BA. Endometrial giant cell carcinoma: a case series and review of the spectrum of endometrial neoplasms containing giant cells. Am J Surg Pathol 2010;34:1132-8.
103. Taraif SH, Deavers MT, Malpica A, Silva EG. The significance of neuroendocrine expression in undifferentiated carcinoma of the endometrium. Int J Gynecol Pathol 2009;28:142-7.
104. Schiavone M, Zivanovic O, Zhou Q, et al. Undifferentiated endometrial carcinomas: where do they fit in? Lab Invest 2015;96(Suppl 1):305A.
105. Morel D, Almouzni G, Soria JC, Postel-Vinay S. Targeting chromatin defects in selected solid tumors based on oncogene addiction, synthetic lethality and epigenetic antagonism. Ann Oncol 2017;28:254-69.
106. Eggink FA, Van Gool IC, Leary A, et al. Immunological profiling of molecularly classified high-risk endometrial cancers identifies POLE-mutant and microsatellite unstable carcinomas as candidates for checkpoint inhibition. Oncoimmunology 2017;6:e1264565.
107. Espinosa I, Lee CH, D'Angelo E, Palacios J, Prat J. Undifferentiated and dedifferentiated endometrial carcinomas with POLE exonuclease domain mutations have a favorable prognosis. Am J Surg Pathol 2017;41:1121-8.
108. Mutch DG. The new FIGO staging system for cancers of the vulva, cervix, endometrium, and sarcomas. Gynecol Oncol 2009;115:325-8.
109. Pecorelli S. Revised FIGO staging for carcinoma of the vulva, cervix, and endometrium. Int J Gynaecol Obstet 2009;105:103-4.
110. Zaino RJ, Kurman RJ, Diana KL, Morrow CP. Pathologic models to predict outcome for women with endometrial adenocarcinoma: the importance of the distinction between surgical stage and clinical stage—a Gynecologic Oncology Group study. Cancer 1996;77:1115-21.
111. Ali A, Black D, Soslow RA. Difficulties in assessing the depth of myometrial invasion in endometrial carcinoma. Int J Gynecol Pathol 2007;26:115-123.
112. Jacques SM, Qureshi F, Munkarah A, Lawrence WD. Interinstitutional surgical pathology review in gynecologic oncology: II. Endometrial cancer in hysterectomy specimens. Int J Gynecol Pathol 1998;17:42-5.
113. Kir G, Kir M, Cetiner H, Karateke A, Gurbuz A. Diagnostic problems on frozen section examination of myometrial invasion in patients with endometrial carcinoma with special emphasis on the pitfalls of deep adenomyosis with carcinomatous involvement. Eur J Gynaecol Oncol 2004;25:211-4.
114. Chafe S, Honore L, Pearcey R, Capstick V. An analysis of the impact of pathology review in gynecologic cancer. Int J Radiat Oncol Biol Phys 2000;48:1433-8.
115. Nascimento AF, Hirsch MS, Cviko A, Quade BJ, Nucci MR. The role of CD10 staining in distinguishing invasive endometrial adenocarcinoma from adenocarcinoma involving adenomyosis. Mod Pathol 2003;16:22-7.
116. Murray SK, Young RH, Scully RE. Unusual epithelial and stromal changes in myoinvasive endometrioid adenocarcinoma: a study of their frequency, associated diagnostic problems, and prognostic significance. Int J Gynecol Pathol 2003;22:324-33.
117. Stewart CJ, Little L. Immunophenotypic features of MELF pattern invasion in endometrial adenocarcinoma: evidence for epithelial mesenchymal transition. Histopathology 2009;55:91-101.
118. Stewart CJ, Brennan BA, Leung YC, Little L. MELF pattern invasion in endometrial carcinoma: association with low grade, myoinvasive endometrioid tumours, focal mucinous differentiation and vascular invasion. Pathology 2009;41:454-9.
119. Pavlakis K, Messini I, Vrekoussis T, et al. MELF invasion in endometrial cancer as a risk factor for lymph node metastasis. Histopathology 2011;58:966-73.
120. Quick CM, May T, Horowitz NS, Nucci MR. Low-grade, low-stage endometrioid endometrial adenocarcinoma: a clinicopathologic analysis of 324 cases focusing on frequency and pattern of myoinvasion. Int J Gynecol Pathol 2012;31:337-43.
121. Euscher E, Fox P, Bassett R, et al. The pattern of myometrial invasion as a predictor of lymph node metastasis or extrauterine disease in low-grade endometrial carcinoma. Am J Surg Pathol 2013;37:1728-36.
122. Han G, Lim D, Leitao MM Jr, Abu-Rustum NR, Soslow RA. Histological features associated with occult lymph node metastasis in FIGO clinical stage I, grade I endometrioid carcinoma. Histopathology 2014;64:389-98.

123. Hertel JD, Huettner PC, Pfeifer JD. Lymphovascular space invasion in microcystic elongated and fragmented (MELF)-pattern well-differentiated endometrioid adenocarcinoma is associated with a higher rate of lymph node metastasis. Int J Gynecol Pathol 2014;33:127-34.
124. Kihara A, Yoshida H, Watanabe R, et al. Clinicopathologic association and prognostic value of microcystic, elongated, and fragmented (MELF) pattern in endometrial endometrioid carcinoma. Am J Surg Pathol 2017;41:896-905.
125. Hussein YR, Garg K, Soslow RA, DeLair D. Endometrial carcinomas with DNA mismatch repair abnormalities: analysis of 75 cases. Mod Pathol 2013;26(Suppl 2):280A.
126. Longacre TA, Hendrickson MR. Diffusely infiltrative endometrial adenocarcinoma: an adenoma malignum pattern of myoinvasion. Am J Surg Pathol 1999;23:69-78.
127. Gal D, Recio FO, Zamurovic D, Tancer ML. Lymphvascular space involvement—a prognostic indicator in endometrial adenocarcinoma. Gynecol Oncol 1991;42:142-5.
128. Hanson MB, van Nagell JR Jr, Powell DE, et al. The prognostic significance of lymphvascular space invasion in stage I endometrial cancer. Cancer 1985;55:1753-7.
129. Ambros RA, Kurman RJ. Combined assessment of vascular and myometrial invasion as a model to predict prognosis in stage I endometrioid adenocarcinoma of the uterine corpus. Cancer 1992;69:1424-31.
130. Nofech-Mozes S, Ghorab Z, Ismiil N, et al. Endometrial endometrioid adenocarcinoma: a pathologic analysis of 827 consecutive cases. Am J Clin Pathol 2008;129:110-4.
131. Logani S, Herdman AV, Little JV, Moller KA. Vascular "pseudo invasion" in laparoscopic hysterectomy specimens: a diagnostic pitfall. Am J Surg Pathol 2008;32:560-5.
132. Kitahara S, Walsh C, Frumovitz M, Malpica A, Silva EG. Vascular pseudoinvasion in laparoscopic hysterectomy specimens for endometrial carcinoma: a grossing artifact? Am J Surg Pathol 2009;33:298-303.
133. Folkins AK, Nevadunsky NS, Saleemuddin A, et al. Evaluation of vascular space involvement in endometrial adenocarcinomas: laparoscopic vs abdominal hysterectomies. Mod Pathol 2010;23:1073-9.
134. Krizova A, Clarke BA, Bernardini MQ, et al. Histologic artifacts in abdominal, vaginal, laparoscopic, and robotic hysterectomy specimens: a blinded, retrospective review. Am J Surg Pathol 2011;35:115-26.
135. Zaino RJ, Abendroth C, Yemelyanova A, et al. Endocervical involvement in endometrial adenocarcinoma is not prognostically significant and the pathologic assessment of the pattern of involvement is not reproducible. Gynecol Oncol 2013;128:83-7.
136. McCluggage WG, Hirschowitz L, Wilson GE, Oliva E, Soslow RA, Zaino RJ. Significant variation in the assessment of cervical involvement in endometrial carcinoma: an interobserver variation study. Am J Surg Pathol 2011;35:289-94.
137. Tambouret R, Clement PB, Young RH. Endometrial endometrioid adenocarcinoma with a deceptive pattern of spread to the uterine cervix: a manifestation of stage IIb endometrial carcinoma liable to be misinterpreted as an independent carcinoma or a benign lesion. Am J Surg Pathol 2003;27:1080-8.
138. Orezzoli JP, Sioletic S, Olawaiye A, Oliva E, del Carmen MG. Stage II endometrioid adenocarcinoma of the endometrium: clinical implications of cervical stromal invasion. Gynecol Oncol 2009;113:316-23.
139. Reyes C, Murali R, Park KJ. Secondary involvement of the adnexa and uterine corpus by carcinomas of the uterine cervix: a detailed morphologic description. Int J Gynecol Pathol 2015;34:551-63.
140. Eifel P, Hendrickson M, Ross J, Ballon S, Martinez A, Kempson R. Simultaneous presentation of carcinoma involving the ovary and the uterine corpus. Cancer 1982;50:163-70.
141. Piura B, Glezerman M. Synchronous carcinomas of endometrium and ovary. Gynecol Oncol 1989;33:261-4.
142. Ulbright TM, Roth LM. Metastatic and independent cancers of the endometrium and ovary: a clinicopathologic study of 34 cases. Hum Pathol 1985;16:28-34.
143. Zaino R, Whitney C, Brady MF, DeGeest K, Burger RA, Buller RE. Simultaneously detected endometrial and ovarian carcinomas—a prospective clinicopathologic study of 74 cases: a gynecologic oncology group study. Gynecol Oncol 2001;83:355-62.
144. Guerra F, Girolimetti G, Perrone AM, et al. Mitochondrial DNA genotyping efficiently reveals clonality of synchronous endometrial and ovarian cancers. Mod Pathol 2014;27:1412-20.
145. Moreno-Bueno G, Gamallo C, Pérez-Gallego L, de Mora JC, Suárez A, Palacios J. Beta-catenin expression pattern, beta-catenin gene mutations, and microsatellite instability in endometrioid ovarian carcinomas and synchronous endometrial carcinomas. Diagn Mol Pathol 2001;10:116-22.
146. Kaneki E, Oda Y, Ohishi Y, et al. Frequent microsatellite instability in synchronous ovarian and endometrial adenocarcinoma and its usefulness for differential diagnosis. Hum Pathol 2004;35:1484-93.

43. Inoue M, Delellis RA, Scully RE. Immunohistochemical demonstration of chromogranin in endometrial carcinomas with argyrophil cells. Hum Pathol 1986;17:841-7.
44. Zaino RJ, Kurman RJ, Diana KL, Morrow CP. The utility of the revised International Federation of Gynecology and Obstetrics histologic grading of endometrial adenocarcinoma using a defined nuclear grading system: a Gynecologic Oncology Group study. Cancer 1995;75:81-6.
45. Elston CW, Ellis IO. Pathological prognostic factors in breast cancer. I. The value of histological grade in breast cancer: experience from a large study with long-term follow-up. Histopathology 1991;19;403-10.
46. Kurman RJ, Norris HJ. Evaluation of criteria for distinguishing atypical endometrial hyperplasia from well-differentiated carcinoma. Cancer 1982;49:2547-59.
47. Soslow RA, Chung MH, Rouse RV, Hendrickson MR, Longacre TA. Atypical polypoid adenomyofibroma (APA) versus well-differentiated endometrial carcinoma with prominent stromal matrix: an immunohistochemical study. Int J Gynecol Pathol 1996;15:209-16.
48. Parkash V, Carcangiu ML. Endometrioid endometrial adenocarcinoma with psammoma bodies. Am J Surg Pathol 1997;21:399-406.
49. Ramirez PT, Frumovitz M, Bodurka DC, Sun CC, Levenback C. Hormonal therapy for the management of grade 1 endometrial adenocarcinoma: a literature review. Gynecol Oncol 2004;95:133-8.
50. Randall TC, Kurman RJ. Progestin treatment of atypical hyperplasia and well-differentiated carcinoma of the endometrium in women under age 40. Obstet Gynecol 1997;90:434-40.
51. Gallos ID, Shehmar M, Thangaratinam S, Papapostolou TK, Coomarasamy A, Gupta JK. Oral progestogens vs levonorgestrel-releasing intrauterine system for endometrial hyperplasia: a systematic review and metaanalysis. Am J Obstet Gynecol 2010;203:547 e1-10.
52. Hahn HS, Yoon SG, Hong JS, et al. Conservative treatment with progestin and pregnancy outcomes in endometrial cancer. Int J Gynecol Cancer 2009;19:1068-73.
53. Reed SD, Voigt LF, Newton KM, et al. Progestin therapy of complex endometrial hyperplasia with and without atypia. Obstet Gynecol 2009;113:655-62.
54. Wheeler DT, Bristow RE, Kurman RJ. Histologic alterations in endometrial hyperplasia and well-differentiated carcinoma treated with progestins. Am J Surg Pathol 2007;31:988-98.
55. Announcements. FIGO stages-1988 revision. Gynecol Oncol 1989;35:125-7.
56. Alkushi A, Abdul-Rahman ZH, Lim P, et al. Description of a novel system for grading of endometrial carcinoma and comparison with existing grading systems. Am J Surg Pathol 2005;29:295-304.
57. Conlon N, Leitao MM Jr, Abu-Rustum NR, Soslow RA. Grading uterine endometrioid carcinoma: a proposal that binary is best. Am J Surg Pathol 2014;38:1583-7.
58. Guan H, Semaan A, Bandyopadhyay S, et al. Prognosis and reproducibility of new and existing binary grading systems for endometrial carcinoma compared to FIGO grading in hysterectomy specimens. Int J Gynecol Cancer 2011;21:654-60.
59. Lax SF, Kurman RJ, Pizer ES, Wu L, Ronnett BM. A binary architectural grading system for uterine endometrial endometrioid carcinoma has superior reproducibility compared with FIGO grading and identifies subsets of advance-stage tumors with favorable and unfavorable prognosis. Am J Surg Pathol 2000;24:1201-8.
60. Barlin JN, Soslow RA, Lutz M, et al. Redefining stage I endometrial cancer: incorporating histology, a binary grading system, myometrial invasion, and lymph node assessment. Int J Gynecol Cancer 2013;23:1620-8.
61. DuBeshter B, Warshal DP, Angel C, Dvoretsky PM, Lin JY, Raubertas RF. Endometrial carcinoma: the relevance of cervical cytology. Obstet Gynecol 1991;77:458-62.
62. Larson DM, Copeland LJ, Gallager HS, et al. Nature of cervical involvement in endometrial carcinoma. Cancer 1987;59:959-62.
63. Roelofsen T, Geels YP, Pijnenborg JM, et al. Cervical cytology in serous and endometrioid endometrial cancer. Int J Gynecol Pathol 2013;32:390-8.
64. Wilbur DC, Chhieng DC, Guidos B, Mody DR. Epithelial abnormalities: glandular. In: Nayar R, Wilbur DC, eds. The Bethesda system for reporting cervical cytoloty, 3rd ed. Cham: Springer; 2015:193-240.
65. Czernobilsky B, Katz Z, Lancet M, Gaton E. Endocervical-type epithelium in endometrial carcinoma: a report of 10 cases with emphasis on histochemical methods for differential diagnosis. Am J Surg Pathol 1980;4:481-9.
66. Tiltman AJ. Mucinous carcinoma of the endometrium. Obstet Gynecol 1980;55:244-7.
67. Fujiwara M, Longacre T. Low-grade mucinous adenocarcinoma of the uterine corpus: a rare and deceptively bland form of endometrial carcinoma. Am J Surg Pathol 2011;35:537-44.
68. Kurman RJ, Carcangiu ML, Herrington CS, Young RH. WHO classification of tumours of female reproductive organs, 4th ed. Lyon: IARC Press; 2014;6.
69. Clement PB, Young RH. Non-endometrioid carcinomas of the uterine corpus: a review of their pathology with emphasis on recent advances and problematic aspects. Adv Anat Pathol 2004;11:117-42.

70. Fukunaga M. Mucinous endometrial adenocarcinoma simulating microglandular hyperplasia of the cervix. Pathol Int 2000;50:541-5.
71. Nucci MR, Prasad CJ, Crum CP, Mutter GL. Mucinous endometrial epithelial proliferations: a morphologic spectrum of changes with diverse clinical significance. Mod Pathol 1999;12:1137-42.
72. Rauh-Hain JA, Vargas RJ, Clemmer J, et al. Mucinous adenocarcinoma of the endometrium compared with endometrioid endometrial cancer: a SEER analysis. Am J Clin Oncol 2016;39:43-8.
73. Hendrickson MR, Kempson RL. Ciliated carcinoma—a variant of endometrial adenocarcinoma: a report of 10 cases. Int J Gynecol Pathol 1983;2:1-12.
74. Kurman RJ, Scully RE. Clear cell carcinoma of the endometrium: an analysis of 21 cases. Cancer 1976;37:872-82.
75. Tobon H, Watkins GJ. Secretory adenocarcinoma of the endometrium. Int J Gynecol Pathol 1985;4:328-35.
76. Christopherman WM, Alberhasky RC, Connelly PJ. Carcinoma of the endometrium: I. A clinicopathologic study of clear-cell carcinoma and secretory carcinoma. Cancer 1982;49:1511-23.
77. Zaino RJ, Kurman RJ, Brunetto VL, et al. Villoglandular adenocarcinoma of the endometrium: A clinicopathologic study of 61 cases: a gynecologic oncology group study. Am J Surg Pathol 1998;22:1379-85.
78. Chen JL, Trost DC, Wilkinson EJ. Endometrial papillary adenocarcinomas: two clinicopathological types. Int J Gynecol Pathol 1985;4:279-88.
79. Hendrickson M, Ross J, Eifel P, Martinez A, Kempson R. Uterine papillary serous carcinoma: a highly malignant form of endometrial adenocarcinoma. Am J Surg Pathol 1982;6:93-108.
80. Huntsman DG, Clement PB, Gilks CB, Scully RE. Small-cell carcinoma of the endometrium. A clinicopathological study of sixteen cases. Am J Surg Pathol 1994;18:364-75.
81. Pocrnich CE, Ramalingam P, Euscher ED, Malpica A. Neuroendocrine carcinoma of the endometrium: a clinicopathologic study of 25 cases. Am J Surg Pathol 2016;40:577-86.
82. van Hoeven KH, Hudock JA, Woodruff JM, Suhrland MJ. Small cell neuroendocrine carcinoma of the endometrium. Int J Gynecol Pathol 1995;14:21-9.
83. Chiang S, Snuderl M, Kojiro-Sanada S, et al. Primitive neuroectodermal tumors of the female genital tract: a morphologic, immunohistochemical, and molecular study of 19 cases. Am J Surg Pathol 2017;41:761-72.
84. Daya D, Lukka H, Clement PB. Primitive neuroectodermal tumors of the uterus: a report of four cases. Hum Pathol 1992;23:1120-9.
85. Euscher ED, Deavers MT, Lopez-Terrada D, Lazar AJ, Silva EG, Malpica A. Uterine tumors with neuroectodermal differentiation: a series of 17 cases and review of the literature. Am J Surg Pathol 2008;32:219-28.
86. Ji M, Lu Y, Guo L, Feng F, Wan X, Xiang Y. Endometrial carcinoma with yolk sac tumor-like differentiation and elevated serum beta-hCG: a case report and literature review. Onco Targets Ther 2013;6:1515-22.
87. McNamee T, Damato S, McCluggage WG. Yolk sac tumours of the female genital tract in older adults derive commonly from somatic epithelial neoplasms: somatically derived yolk sac tumours. Histopathology 2016;69:739-51.
88. Shokeir MO, Noel SM, Clement PB. Malignant mullerian mixed tumor of the uterus with a prominent alpha-fetoprotein-producing component of yolk sac tumor. Mod Pathol 1996;9:647-51.
89. Bittencourt AL, Britto JF, Fonseca LE Jr. Wilms' tumor of the uterus: the first report of the literature. Cancer 1981;47:2496-9.
90. Garcia-Galvis OF, Stolnicu S, Muñoz E, Aneiros-Fernandez J, Alaggio R, Nogales FF. Adult extrarenal Wilms tumor of the uterus with teratoid features. Hum Pathol 2009;40:418-24.
91. McAlpine J, Azodi M, O'Malley D, et al. Extrarenal Wilms' tumor of the uterine corpus. Gynecol Oncol 2005;96:892-6.
92. Tafe LJ, Garg K, Chew I, Tornos C, Soslow RA. Endometrial and ovarian carcinomas with undifferentiated components: clinically aggressive and frequently underrecognized neoplasms. Mod Pathol 2010;23:781-9.
93. Altrabulsi B, Malpica A, Deavers MT, Bodurka DC, Broaddus R, Silva EG. Undifferentiated carcinoma of the endometrium. Am J Surg Pathol 2005;29:1316-21.
94. Abeler VM, Kjorstad KE, Nesland JM. Undifferentiated carcinoma of the endometrium. A histopathologic and clinical study of 31 cases. Cancer 1991;68:98-105.
95. Silva EG, Deavers MT, Bodurka DC, Malpica A. Association of low-grade endometrioid carcinoma of the uterus and ovary with undifferentiated carcinoma: a new type of dedifferentiated carcinoma? . Int J Gynecol Pathol 2006;25:52-8.
96. Hoang LN, Lee YS, Karnezis AN, et al. Immunophenotypic features of dedifferentiated endometrial carcinoma—insights from BRG1/INI1-deficient tumours. Histopathology 2016;69:560-9.
97. Rosa-Rosa JM, Leskela S, Cristobal-Lana E, et al. Molecular genetic heterogeneity in undifferentiated endometrial carcinomas. Mod Pathol 2016;29:1390-8.

147. Schultheis AM, Nq CK, De Filippo MR, et al. Massively parallel sequencing-based clonality analysis of synchronous endometrioid endometrial and ovarian carcinomas. J Natl Cancer Inst 2016;108:djv427.

148. Anglesio MS, Wang YK, Maassen M, et al. Synchronous endometrial and ovarian carcinomas: evidence of clonality. J Natl Cancer Inst 2016;108:djv428.

149. Zaino RJ, Unger ER, Whitney C. Synchronous carcinomas of the uterine corpus and ovary. Gynecol Oncol 1984;19:329-35.

150. Montoya F, Martin M, Schneider J, Matia JC, Rodriguez-Escudero FJ. Simultaneous appearance of ovarian and endometrial carcinoma: a therapeutic challenge. Eur J Gynaecol Oncol 1989;10:135-9.

151. Scully RE, Young RH, Clement PB. Tumors of the ovary, maldeveloped gonads, fallopian tube, and broad ligament. AFIP Atlas of Tumor Pathology, 3rd Series, Fascicle 23. Washington DC: American Registry of Pathology; 1998.

152. Soliman PT, Slomovitz BM, Broaddus RR, et al. Synchronous primary cancers of the endometrium and ovary: a single institution review of 84 cases. Gynecol Oncol 2004;94:456-62.

153. Aysal A, Karnezis A, Medhi I, Grenert JP, Zaloudek CJ, Rabban JT. Ovarian endometrioid adenocarcinoma: incidence and clinical significance of the morphologic and immunohistochemical markers of mismatch repair protein defects and tumor microsatellite instability. Am J Surg Pathol 2012;36:163-72.

154. Garg K, Leitao MM Jr, Kauff ND, et al. Selection of endometrial carcinomas for DNA mismatch repair protein immunohistochemistry using patient age and tumor morphology enhances detection of mismatch repair abnormalities. Am J Surg Pathol 2009;33:925-33.

155. McKenney JK, Kong CS, Longacre TA. Endometrial adenocarcinoma associated with subtle lymphvascular space invasion and lymph node metastasis: a histologic pattern mimicking intravascular and sinusoidal histiocytes. Int J Gynecol Pathol 2005;24:73-8.

156. Lu KH, Dinh M, Kohlmann W, et al. Gynecologic cancer as a "sentinel cancer" for women with hereditary nonpolyposis colorectal cancer syndrome. Obstet Gynecol 2005;105:569-74.

157. Barlin JN, Khoury-Collado F, Kim CH, et al. The importance of applying a sentinel lymph node mapping algorithm in endometrial cancer staging: beyond removal of blue nodes. Gynecol Oncol 2012;125:531-5.

158. Cibula D, Abu-Rustum NR, Dusek L, et al. Prognostic significance of low volume sentinel lymph node disease in early-stage cervical cancer. Gynecol Oncol 2012;124:496-501.

159. Frimer M, Khoury-Collado F, Murray MP, Barakat RR, Abu-Rustum NR. Micrometastasis of endometrial cancer to sentinel lymph nodes: is it an artifact of uterine manipulation? Gynecol Oncol 2010;119:496-9.

160. Khoury-Collado F, Murray MP, Hensley ML, et al. Sentinel lymph node mapping for endometrial cancer improves the detection of metastatic disease to regional lymph nodes. Gynecol Oncol 2011;122:251-4.

161. Kim CH, Soslow RA, Park KJ, et al. Pathologic ultrastaging improves micrometastasis detection in sentinel lymph nodes during endometrial cancer staging. Int J Gynecol Cancer 2013;23:964-70.

162. Abu-Rustum NR. Update on sentinel node mapping in uterine cancer: 10-year experience at Memorial Sloan-Kettering Cancer Center. J Obstet Gynaecol Res 2014;40:327-34.

163. Buda A, Crivellaro C, Elisei F, et al. Impact of indocyanine green (for sentinel lymph node mapping in early stage endometrial and cervical cancer: comparison with conventional radiotracer (99m)Tc and/or blue dye. Ann Surg Oncol 2016;23:2183-91.

164. Euscher ED, Lyons GR, Bassett RL, Silva E, Malpica A. Lymph node metastases in low grade endometrial carcinoma (LGEC): what matters? Lab Invest 2016;96(Suppl 1):282A-3A.

165. Ozcan A, Liles N, Coffey D, Shen SS, Truong LD. PAX2 and PAX8 expression in primary and metastatic müllerian epithelial tumors: a comprehensive comparison. Am J Surg Pathol 2011;35:1837-47.

166. Castrillon DH, Lee KR, Nucci MR. Distinction between endometrial and endocervical adenocarcinoma: an immunohistochemical study. Int J Gynecol Pathol 2002;21:4-10.

167. Wang NP, Zee S, Zarbo RJ, Bacchi CE, Gown AM. Coordinate expression of cytokeratins 7 and 20 defines unique subsets of carcinomas. Appl Immunohistochem 1996;3:99-107.

168. Reid-Nicholson M, Iyengar P, Hummer AJ, Linkov I, Asher M, Soslow RA. Immunophenotypic diversity of endometrial adenocarcinomas: implications for differential diagnosis. Mod Pathol 2006;19:1091-100.

169. Bosse T, ter Haar NT, Seeber LM, et al. Loss of ARID1A expression and its relationship with PI3K-Akt pathway alterations, TP53 and microsatellite instability in endometrial cancer. Mod Pathol 2013;26:1525-35.

170. Garg K, Broaddus RR, Soslow RA, Urbauer DL, Levine DA, Djordjevic B. Pathologic scoring of PTEN immunohistochemistry in endometrial carcinoma is highly reproducible. Int J Gynecol Pathol 2012;31:48-56.

171. Mao TL, Ardighieri L, Ayhan A, et al. Loss of ARID1A expression correlates with stages of tumor progression in uterine endometrioid carcinoma. Am J Surg Pathol 2013;37:1342-8.
172. Soslow RA, Shen PU, Chung MH, Isacson C. Distinctive p53 and mdm2 immunohistochemical expression profiles suggest different pathogenetic pathways in poorly differentiated endometrial carcinoma. Int J Gynecol Pathol 1998;17:129-34.
173. Egan JA, Ionescu MC, Eapen E, Jones JG, Marshall DS. Differential expression of WT1 and p53 in serous and endometrioid carcinomas of the endometrium. Int J Gynecol Pathol 2004;23:119-22.
174. Halperin R, Zehavi S, Habler L, Hadas E, Bukovsky I, Schneider D. Comparative immunohistochemical study of endometrioid and serous papillary carcinoma of endometrium. Eur J Gynaecol Oncol 2001;22:122-6.
175. Lax SF, Kendall B, Tashiro H, Slebos RJ, Hedrick L. The frequency of p53, K-ras mutations, and microsatellite instability differs in uterine endometrioid and serous carcinoma: evidence of distinct molecular genetic pathways. Cancer 2000;88:814-24.
176. Riethdorf L, Begemann C, Riethdorf S, Milde-Langosch K, Löning T. Comparison of benign and malignant endometrial lesions for their p53 state, using immunohistochemistry and temperature-gradient gel electrophoresis. Virchows Arch 1996;428:47-51.
177. Zannoni GF, Vellone VG, Arena V, et al. Does high-grade endometrioid carcinoma (grade 3 FIGO) belong to type I or type II endometrial cancer? A clinical-pathological and immunohistochemical study. Virchows Arch 2010;457:27-34.
178. Park KJ, Bramlage MP, Ellenson LH, Pirog EC. Immunoprofile of adenocarcinomas of the endometrium, endocervix, and ovary with mucinous differentiation. Appl Immunohistochem Mol Morphol 2009;17:8-11.
179. Blanco LZ Jr, Heagley DE, Lee JC, et al. Immunohistochemical characterization of squamous differentiation and morular metaplasia in uterine endometrioid adenocarcinoma. Int J Gynecol Pathol 2013;32:283-92.
180. Chew I, Post MD, Carinelli SG, et al. p16 expression in squamous and trophoblastic lesions of the upper female genital tract. Int J Gynecol Pathol 2010;29:513-22.
181. Houghton O, Connolly LE, McCluggage WG. Morules in endometrioid proliferations of the uterus and ovary consistently express the intestinal transcription factor CDX2. Histopathology 2008;53:156-65.
182. Alomari A, Abi-Raad R, Buza N, Hui P. Frequent KRAS mutation in complex mucinous epithelial lesions of the endometrium. Mod Pathol 2014;27:675-80.
183. Cancer Genome Atlas Research Network, Kandoth C, Schultz N, et al. Integrated genomic characterization of endometrial carcinoma. Nature 2013;497:67-73.
184. Talhouk A, McConechy MK, Leung S, et al. A clinically applicable molecular-based classification for endometrial cancers. Br J Cancer 2015;113:299-310.
185. Stelloo E, Bosse T, Nout RA, et al. Refining prognosis and identifying targetable pathways for high-risk endometrial cancer; a TransPORTEC initiative. Mod Pathol 2015;28:836-44.
186. Kurnit KC, Kim GN, Fellman BM, et al. CTNNB1 (beta-catenin) mutation identifies low grade, early stage endometrial cancer patients at increased risk of recurrence. Mod Pathol 2017;30:1032-41.
187. Hussein YR, Weigelt B, Levine DA, et al. Clinicopathological analysis of endometrial carcinomas harboring somatic POLE exonuclease domain mutations. Mod Pathol 2015;28:505-14.
188. Bakhsh S, Kinloch M, Hoang LN, et al. Histopathological features of endometrial carcinomas associated with POLE mutations: implications for decisions about adjuvant therapy. Histopathology 2016;68:916-24.
189. Shia J, Black D, Hummer AJ, Boyd J, Soslow RA. Routinely assessed morphological features correlate with microsatellite instability status in endometrial cancer. Hum Pathol 2008;39:116-25.
190. Hoang LN, McConechy MK, Köbel M, et al. Histotype-genotype correlation in 36 high-grade endometrial carcinomas. Am J Surg Pathol 2013;37:1421-32.
191. Bonora M, Wieckowski MR, Chinopoulos C, et al. Molecular mechanisms of cell death: central implication of ATP synthase in mitochondrial permeability transition. Oncogene 2015;34:1608.
192. Hussein YR, Broaddus R, Weigelt B, Levine DA, Soslow RA. The genomic heterogeneity of figo grade 3 endometrioid carcinoma impacts diagnostic accuracy and reproducibility. Int J Gynecol Pathol 2016;35:16-24.
193. Longacre TA, Chung MH, Jensen DN, Hendrickson MR. Proposed criteria for the diagnosis of well-differentiated endometrial carcinoma. A diagnostic test for myoinvasion. Am J Surg Pathol 1995;19:371-406.
194. Young RH, Treger T, Scully RE. Atypical polypoid adenomyoma of the uterus. A report of 27 cases. Am J Clin Pathol 1986;86:139-45.
195. Longacre TA, Chung MH, Rouse RV, Hendrickson MR. Atypical polypoid adenomyofibromas (atypical polypoid adenomyomas) of the uterus. A clinicopathologic study of 55 cases. Am J Surg Pathol 1996;20:1-20.

196. Mills AM, Liou S, Kong CS, Longacre TA. Are women with endocervical adenocarcinoma at risk for Lynch syndrome? Evaluation of 101 cases including unusual subtypes and lower uterine segment tumors. Int J Gynecol Pathol 2012;31:463-9.

197. Omori M, Hashi A, Kondo T, Katoh R, Hirata S. Dysregulation of CDK inhibitors and p53 in HPV-negative endocervical adenocarcinoma. Int J Gynecol Pathol 2015;34:196-203.

198. Clement PB, Young RH, Keh P, Ostor AG, Scully RE. Malignant mesonephric neoplasms of the uterine cervix. A report of eight cases, including four with a malignant spindle cell component. Am J Surg Pathol 1995;19:1158-71.

199. Ferry JA, Scully RE. Mesonephric remnants, hyperplasia, and neoplasia in the uterine cervix. A study of 49 cases. Am J Surg Pathol 1990;14:1100-11.

200. Howitt BE, Emori MM, Drapkin R, et al. GATA3 is a sensitive and specific marker of benign and malignant mesonephric lesions in the lower female genital tract. Am J Surg Pathol 2015;39:1411-9.

201. Roma AA, Goyal A, Yang B. Differential expression patterns of GATA3 in uterine mesonephric and nonmesonephric lesions. Int J Gynecol Pathol 2015;34:480-6.

202. Kenny SL MH, Jamison J, McCluggage WG. Mesonephric adenocarcinomas of the uterine cervix and corpus: HPV-negative neoplasms that are commonly PAX8, CA125, and HMGA2 positive and that may be immunoreactive with TTF1 and hepatocyte nuclear factor 1-beta. Am J Surg Pathol 2012;36:799-807.

203. McFarland M, Quick CM, McCluggage WG. Hormone receptor negative, TTF1 positive uterine and ovarian adenocarcinomas: report of a series of mesonephric-like adenocarcinomas. Histopathology 2016;68:1013-20.

204. McCluggage WG, Oliva E, Herrington CS, McBride H, Young RH. CD10 and calretinin staining of endocervical glandular lesions, endocervical stroma and endometrioid adenocarcinomas of the uterine corpus: CD10 positivity is characteristic of, but not specific for, mesonephric lesions and is not specific for endometrial stroma. Histopathology 2003;43:144-50.

205. Ordi J, Romagosa C, Tavassoli FA, et al. CD10 expression in epithelial tissues and tumors of the gynecologic tract: a useful marker in the diagnosis of mesonephric, trophoblastic, and clear cell tumors. Am J Surg Pathol 2003;27:178-86.

206. Kojima A, Mikami Y, Sudo T, et al. Gastric morphology and immunophenotype predict poor outcome in mucinous adenocarcinoma of the uterine cervix. Am J Surg Pathol 2007;31:664-72.

207. Carleton C, Hoang L, Sah S, et al. A detailed immunohistochemical analysis of a large series of cervical and vaginal gastric-type adenocarcinomas. Am J Surg Pathol 2016;40:636-44.

208. Fukunaga M, Nomura K, Endo Y, Ushigome S, Aizawa S. Carcinosarcoma of the uterus with extensive neuroectodermal differentiation. Histopathology 1996;29:565-70.

209. Greeley C, Schroeder S, Silverberg SG. Microglandular hyperplasia of the cervix: a true "pill" lesion? Int J Gynecol Pathol 1995;14:50-4.

210. Jones MW, Silverberg SG. Cervical adenocarcinoma in young women: possible relationship to microglandular hyperplasia and use of oral contraceptives. Obstet Gynecol 1989;73:984-9.

211. Qiu W, Mittal K. Comparison of morphologic and immunohistochemical features of cervical microglandular hyperplasia with low-grade mucinous adenocarcinoma of the endometrium. Int J Gynecol Pathol 2003;22:261-5.

212. Stewart CJ, Crook ML. PAX2 and cyclin D1 expression in the distinction between cervical microglandular hyperplasia and endometrial microglandular-like carcinoma: a comparison with p16, vimentin, and Ki67. Int J Gynecol Pathol 2015;34:90-100.

212a. Hong W, Abi-Raad R, Alomari AK, Hui P, Buza N. Diagnostic application of KRAS mutation testing in uterine microglandular proliferations. Hum Pathol 2015;46:1000-5.

213. Chekmareva M, Ellenson LH, Pirog EC. Immunohistochemical differences between mucinous and microglandular adenocarcinomas of the endometrium and benign endocervical epithelium. Int J Gynecol Pathol 2008;27:547-54.

214. Hussein YR BR, Weigelt B, Levine DA, Soslow RA. The genomic heterogeneity of FIGO grade 3 endometrioid carcinoma impacts diagnostic accuracy and reproducibility. Int J Gynecol Pathol 2016;35:16-24.

215. Soslow RA. Endometrial carcinomas with ambiguous features. Semin Diagn Pathol 2010;27:261-73.

216. Schultheis AM, Martelotto LG, De Filippo MR, et al. TP53 mutational spectrum in endometrioid and serous endometrial cancers. Int J Gynecol Pathol 2016:35:289-300.

217. Fadare O, Zheng W, Crispens MA, et al. Morphologic and other clinicopathologic features of endometrial clear cell carcinoma: a comprehensive analysis of 50 rigorously classified cases. Am J Surg Res 2013;3:70-95.

218. Silva EG, Young RH. Endometrioid neoplasms with clear cells: a report of 21 cases in which the alteration is not of typical secretory type. Am J Surg Pathol 2007;31:1203-8.

219. Fadare O, Desouki MM, Gwin K, et al. Frequent expression of napsin A in clear cell carcinoma of the endometrium: potential diagnostic utility. Am J Surg Pathol 2014;38:189-96.
220. Fadare O, Liang SX. Diagnostic utility of hepatocyte nuclear factor 1-beta immunoreactivity in endometrial carcinomas: lack of specificity for endometrial clear cell carcinoma. Appl Immunohistochem Mol Morphol 2012;20:580-7.
221. Han G, Soslow RA, Wethington S, et al. Endometrial carcinomas with clear cells: a study of a heterogeneous group of tumors including interobserver variability, mutation analysis, and immunohistochemistry with HNF-1beta. Int J Gynecol Pathol 2015;34:323-33.
222. Hoang LN, Han G, McConechy M, et al. Immunohistochemical characterization of prototypical endometrial clear cell carcinoma—diagnostic utility of HNF-1beta and oestrogen receptor. Histopathology 2014;64:585-96.
223. Iwamoto M, Nakatani Y, Fugo K, Kishimoto T, Kiyokawa T. Napsin A is frequently expressed in clear cell carcinoma of the ovary and endometrium. Hum Pathol 2015;46:957-62.
224. Lim D, Ip PP, Cheung AN, Kiyokawa T, Oliva E. Immunohistochemical comparison of ovarian and uterine endometrioid carcinoma, endometrioid carcinoma with clear cell change, and clear cell carcinoma. Am J Surg Pathol 2015;39:1061-9.
225. Arai T, Watanabe J, Kawaguchi M, et al. Clear cell adenocarcinoma of the endometrium is a biologically distinct entity from endometrioid adenocarcinoma. Int J Gynecol Cancer 2006;16:391-5.
226. DeLair DF, Burke KA, Selenica P, et al. The genetic landscape of endometrial clear cell carcinomas. J Pathol 2017;243:230-241.
227. Fadare O, Gwin K, Desouki MM, et al. The clinicopathologic significance of p53 and BAF-250a (ARID1A) expression in clear cell carcinoma of the endometrium. Mod Pathol 2013;26:1101-10.
228. Lax SF, Pizer ES, Ronnett BM, Kurman RJ. Clear cell carcinoma of the endometrium is characterized by a distinctive profile of p53, Ki-67, estrogen, and progesterone receptor expression. Hum Pathol 1998;29:551-8.
229. Espinosa I, D'Angelo E, Palacios J, Prat J. Mixed and ambiguous endometrial carcinomas: a heterogenous group of tumors with different clinicopathologic and molecular genetic features. Am J Surg Pathol 2016;40:972-81.
230. Soslow RA. High-grade endometrial carcinomas—strategies for typing. Histopathology 2013;62:89-110.
231. Soslow RA, Wethington SL, Cesari M, et al. Clinicopathologic analysis of matched primary and recurrent endometrial carcinoma. Am J Surg Pathol 2012;36:1771-81.
232. Lee CH, Ali RH, Rouzbahman M, et al. Cyclin D1 as a diagnostic immunomarker for endometrial stromal sarcoma with YWHAE-FAM22 rearrangement. Am J Surg Pathol 2012;36:1562-70.
233. Lee CH, Hoang LN, Yip S, et al. Frequent expression of KIT in endometrial stromal sarcoma with YWHAE genetic rearrangement. Mod Pathol 2014;27:751-7.
234. Shah VI, McCluggage WG. Cyclin D1 does not distinguish YWHAE-NUTM2 high-grade endometrial stromal sarcoma from undifferentiated endometrial carcinoma. Am J Surg Pathol 2015;39:722-4.
235. Schaefer IM, Agaimy A, Fletcher CD, Hornick JL. Claudin-4 expression distinguishes SWI/SNF complex-deficient undifferentiated carcinomas from sarcomas. Mod Pathol 2017;30:539-48.
236. Lee CH, Mariño-Enriquez A, Ou W, et al. The clinicopathologic features of YWHAE-FAM22 endometrial stromal sarcomas: a histologically high-grade and clinically aggressive tumor. Am J Surg Pathol 2012;36:641-53.
237. Giordano G, Azzoni C, D'Adda T, Merisio C. P16(INK4a) overexpression independent of Human Papilloma Virus (HPV) infection in rare subtypes of endometrial carcinomas. Pathol Res Pract 2003;199:533-8.
238. Horn LC, Richter CE, Einenkel J, Tannapfel A, Liebert UG, Leo C. p16, p14, p53, cyclin D1, and steroid hormone receptor expression and human papillomaviruses analysis in primary squamous cell carcinoma of the endometrium. Ann Diagn Pathol 2006;10:193-6.
239. Im DD, Shah KV, Rosenshein NB. Report of three new cases of squamous carcinoma of the endometrium with emphasis in the HPV status. Gynecol Oncol 1995;56:464-9.
240. Zidi YS, Bouraoui S, Atallah K, Kchir N, Haouet S. Primary in situ squamous cell carcinoma of the endometrium, with extensive squamous metaplasia and dysplasia. Gynecol Oncol 2003;88:444-6.
241. Yemelyanova A, Vang R, Seidman JD, Gravitt PE, Ronnett BM. Endocervical adenocarcinomas with prominent endometrial or endomyometrial involvement simulating primary endometrial carcinomas: utility of HPV DNA detection and immunohistochemical expression of p16 and hormone receptors to confirm the cervical origin of the corpus tumor. Am J Surg Pathol 2009;33:914-24.
242. Fluhman CF. Squamous epithelium in the endometrium in benign and malignant conditions. Surg Gynecol Obstet 1928;46:309-16.

243. Goodman A, Zukerberg LR, Rice LW, Fuller AF, Young RH, Scully RE. Squamous cell carcinoma of the endometrium: a report of eight cases and a review of the literature. Gynecol Oncol 1996;61:54-60.
244. Bewtra C, Xie QM, Hunter WJ, Jurgensen W. Ichthyosis uteri: a case report and review of the literature. Arch Pathol Lab Med 2005;129:e124-5.
245. Brown D Jr, Spjut HJ. Extensive squamous metaplasia of the endometrium (ichthyosis uteri). South Med J 1982;75:593-5.
246. Murhekar K, Majhi U, Sridevi V, Rajkumar T. Does "ichthyosis uteri" have malignant potential? A case report of squamous cell carcinoma of endometrium associated with extensive ichthyosis uteri. Diagn Pathol 2008;3:4.
247. Takeuchi K, Tsujino T, Yabuta M, Kitazawa S. A case of primary squamous cell carcinoma of the endometrium associated with extensive "ichthyosis uteri." Eur J Gynaecol Oncol 2012;33:552-4.
248. Pocrnich CE, Ramalingam P, Euscher ED, Malpica A. Neuroendocrine carcinoma of the endometrium: a clinicopathologic study of 25 cases. Am J Surg Pathol 2016;40:577-86.
249. de Leval L, Lim GS, Waltregny D, Oliva E. Diverse phenotypic profile of uterine tumors resembling ovarian sex cord tumors: an immunohistochemical study of 12 cases. Am J Surg Pathol 2010;34:1749-61.
250. Hoshida Y, Nagakawa T, Mano S, Taguchi K, Aozasa K. Hepatoid adenocarcinoma of the endometrium associated with alpha-fetoprotein production. Int J Gynecol Pathol 1996;15:266-9.
251. Shih A, Lui X, Silva AC, et al. Refined characterization of hepatoid differentiation in gynecologic tract neoplasms. Mod Pathol 2016;29(Suppl 2):309A.
252. Bittencourt AL, Britto JF, Fonseca LE Jr. Wilms' tumor of the uterus: the first report of the literature. Cancer 1981;47:2496-9.
253. McAlpine J, Azodi M, O'Malley D, et al. Extrarenal Wilms' tumor of the uterine corpus. Gynecol Oncol 2005;96:892-6.
254. García-Galvis OF, Stolnicu S, Muñoz E, Aneiros-Fernández J, Alaggio R, Nogales FF. Adult extrarenal Wilms tumor of the uterus with teratoid features. Hum Pathol 2009;40:418-24.
255. Yi T, Wang P, Lin L, Jiang W. Ewing's sarcoma/peripheral primitive neuroectodermal tumors of the uterus confirmed with fluorescence in situ hybridization in a 29-year-old Chinese female: a case report and published work review. J Obstet Gynaecol Res 2015;41:478-782.
256. Ip PP, Irving JA, McCluggage WG, Clement PB, Young RH. Papillary proliferation of the endometrium: a clinicopathologic study of 59 cases of simple and complex papillae without cytologic atypia. Am J Surg Pathol 2013;37:167-77.
256a. Vang R, Tavassoli FA. Proliferative mucinous lesions of the endometrium: analysis of existing criteria for diagnosing carcinoma in biopsies and curettings. Int J Surg Pathol 2003;11:261-70.
257. Kumar NB, Hart WR. Metastases to the uterine corpus from extragenital cancers. A clinicopathologic study of 63 cases. Cancer 1982;50:2163-9.
258. Kumar A, Schneider V. Metastases to the uterus from extrapelvic primary tumors. Int J Gynecol Pathol 1983;2:134-40.
259. Mazur MT, Hsueh S, Gersell DJ. Metastases to the female genital tract. Analysis of 325 cases. Cancer 1984;53:1978-84.
260. Polterauer S, Zhou Q, Grimm C, et al. External validation of a nomogram predicting overall survival of patients diagnosed with endometrial cancer. Gynecol Oncol 2012;125:526-30.
261. Abeler VM, Kjorstad KE, Berle E. Carcinoma of the endometrium in Norway: a histopathological and prognostic survey of a total population. Int J Gynecol Cancer 1992;2:9-22.
262. Pradhan M, Abeler VM, Danielsen HE, et al. Prognostic importance of DNA ploidy and DNA index in stage I and II endometrioid adenocarcinoma of the endometrium. Ann Oncol 2012;23:1178-84.
263. Proctor L, Pradhan M, Leung S, et al. Assessment of DNA ploidy in the ProMisE molecular subgroups of endometrial cancer. Gynecol Oncol 2017;146:596-602.
264. Roma AA, Rybicki LA, Barbuto D, et al. Risk factor analysis of recurrence in low-grade endometrial adenocarcinoma. Hum Pathol 2015;46:1529-39.
265. National Comprehensive Cancer Network, NNCC Clinical Practice Guidelines in Oncology (NCCN Guidelines®), Version 2.2016. Uterine Neoplasms 2016. https://www.universitycancercenters.com/wp-content/themes/uccenters-child/Pdf/NCCNUterine Neoplasms.pdf
266. SGO Clinical Practice Endometrial Cancer Working Group, Burke WM, Orr J, et al. Endometrial cancer: a review and current management strategies: part I. Gynecol Oncol 2014;134:385-92.
267. Aalders JG, Abeler V, Kolstad P. Recurrent adenocarcinoma of the endometrium: a clinical and histopathological study of 379 patients. Gynecol Oncol 1984;17:85-103.
268. Colombo N, Preti E, Landoni F, et al. Endometrial cancer: ESMO Clinical Practice Guidelines for diagnosis, treatment and follow-up. Ann Oncol 2013;24 (Suppl 6):vi33-8.

269. Billingsley CC, Cohn D, Mutch DG, Stephens JA, Suarez AA, Goodfellow PJ. Polymerase ε (POLE) mutations in endometrial cancer: clinical outcomes and implications for Lynch syndrome testing. Cancer 2015;121:386-94.
270. Billingsley CC, Cohn D, Mutch DG, Hade EM, Goodfellow PJ. Prognostic significance of POLE exonuclease domain mutations in high-grade endometrioid endometrial cancer on survival and recurrence: a subanalysis. Int J Gynecol Cancer 2016;26:933-8.
271. Church DN, Stelloo E, Nout RA, et al. Prognostic significance of POLE proofreading mutations in endometrial cancer. J Natl Cancer Inst 2014;107:402.
272. McConechy MK, Talhouk A, Leung S, et al. Endometrial carcinomas with POLE exonuclease domain mutations have a favorable prognosis. Clin Cancer Res 2016;22:2865-73.
273. Meng B, Hoang LN, McIntyre JB, et al. POLE exonuclease domain mutation predicts long progression-free survival in grade 3 endometrioid carcinoma of the endometrium. Gynecol Oncol 2014;134:15-9.
274. Stelloo E, Nout RA, Osse EM, et al. Improved risk assessment by integrating molecular and clinicopathological factors in early-stage endometrial cancer—combined analysis of PORTEC cohorts. Clin Cancer Res 2016;22:4315-24.
275. McMeekin DS, Tritchler DL, Cohn DE, et al. Clinicopathologic significance of mismatch repair defects in endometrial cancer: an NRG Oncology/Gynecologic Oncology Group study. J Clin Oncol 2016;34:3062-8.
276. SGO Clinical Practice Endometrial Cancer Working Group, Burke WM, Orr J, et al. Endometrial cancer: a review and current management strategies: part II. Gynecol Oncol 2014;134:393-402.
277. Rawish KR, Desouki Mm, Crispens MA, Fadare O. Conventional endometrioid adenocarcinomas of the endometrium recurring as clear cell tumors: comparative immunohistochemical analyses. Ann Diagn Pathol 2013;17:270-5.
278. Tashiro H, Isacson C, Levine R, Kurman RJ, Cho KR, Hedrick L. p53 gene mutations are common in uterine serous carcinoma and occur early in their pathogenesis. Am J Pathol 1997;150:177-85.
279. Ambros RA, Sheehan CE, Kallakury BV, et al. MDM2 and p53 protein expression in the histologic subtypes of endometrial carcinoma. Mod Pathol 1996;9:1165-9.
280. Chiesa-Vottero AG, Malpica A, Deavers MT, Broaddus R, Nuovo GJ, Silva EG. Immunohistochemical overexpression of p16 and p53 in uterine serous carcinoma and ovarian high-grade serous carcinoma. Int J Gynecol Pathol 2007;26:328-33.
281. Yemelyanova A, Ji H, Shih IeM, Wang TL, Wu LS, Ronnett BM. Utility of p16 expression for distinction of uterine serous carcinomas from endometrial endometrioid and endocervical adenocarcinomas: immunohistochemical analysis of 201 cases. Am J Surg Pathol 2009;33:1504-14.
282. Nofech-Mozes S, Khalifa MA, Ismiil N, et al. Immunophenotyping of serous carcinoma of the female genital tract. Mod Pathol 2008;21:1147-51.
283. Lax SF, Pizer ES, Ronnett BM, Kurman RJ. Clear cell carcinoma of the endometrium is characterized by a distinctive profile of p53, Ki-67, estrogen, and progesterone receptor expression. Hum Pathol 1998;29:551-8.
284. Alkushi A, Kobel M, Kalloger SE, Gilks CB. High-grade endometrial carcinoma: serous and grade 3 endometrioid carcinomas have different immunophenotypes and outcomes. Int J Gynecol Pathol 2010;29:343-50.
285. Darvishian F, Hummer AJ, Thaler HT, et al. Serous endometrial cancers that mimic endometrioid adenocarcinomas: a clinicopathologic and immunohistochemical study of a group of problematic cases. Am J Surg Pathol 2004;28:1568-78.
286. Singh M, Spoelstra NS, Jean A, et al. ZEB1 expression in type I vs type II endometrial cancers: a marker of aggressive disease. Mod Pathol 2008;21:912-21.
287. Singh P, Smith CL, Cheetham G, Dodd TJ, Davy ML. Serous carcinoma of the uterus-determination of HER-2/neu status using immunohistochemistry, chromogenic in situ hybridization, and quantitative polymerase chain reaction techniques: its significance and clinical correlation. Int J Gynecol Cancer 2008;18:1344-51.
288. Togami S, Sasajima Y, Oi T, et al. Clinicopathological and prognostic impact of human epidermal growth factor receptor type 2 (HER2) and hormone receptor expression in uterine papillary serous carcinoma. Cancer Sci 2012;103:926-32.
289. Santin AD, Bellone S, Van Stedum S, et al. Determination of HER2/neu status in uterine serous papillary carcinoma: comparative analysis of immunohistochemistry and fluorescence in situ hybridization. Gynecol Oncol 2005;98:24-30.
290. McConechy MK, Ding J, Cheang MC, et al. Use of mutation profiles to refine the classification of endometrial carcinomas. J Pathol 2012;228:20-30.
291. Arai T, Watanabe J, Kawaguchi M, et al. Clear cell adenocarcinoma of the endometrium is a biologically distinct entity from endometrioid adenocarcinoma. Int J Gynecol Cancer 2006;16:391-5.

292. Trovik J, Wik E, Werner HM, et al. Hormone receptor loss in endometrial carcinoma curettage predicts lymph node metastasis and poor outcome in prospective multicentre trial. Eur J Cancer 2013;49:3431-41.

293. Mutter GL, Lin MC, Fitzgerald JT, et al. Altered PTEN expression as a diagnostic marker for the earliest endometrial precancers. J Natl Cancer Inst 2000;92:924-30.

294. Lacey JV Jr, Mutter GL, Ronnett BM, et al. PTEN expression in endometrial biopsies as a marker of progression to endometrial carcinoma. Cancer Res 2008;68:6014-20.

295. Monte NM, Webster KA, Neuberg D, Dressler GR, Mutter GL. Joint loss of PAX2 and PTEN expression in endometrial precancers and cancer. Cancer Res 2010;70:6225-32.

296. Djordjevic B, Hennessy BT, Li J, et al. Clinical assessment of PTEN loss in endometrial carcinoma: immunohistochemistry outperforms gene sequencing. Mod Pathol 2012;25:699-708.

297. Schlosshauer PW, Ellenson LH, Soslow RA. Beta-catenin and E-cadherin expression patterns in high-grade endometrial carcinoma are associated with histological subtype. Mod Pathol 2002;15:1032-7.

298. Hayes MP, Douglas W, Ellenson LH. Molecular alterations of EGFR and PIK3CA in uterine serous carcinoma. Gynecol Oncol 2009;113:370-3.

299. Tsuchiya A, Sakamoto M, Yasuda J, et al. Expression profiling in ovarian clear cell carcinoma: identification of hepatocyte nuclear factor-1 beta as a molecular marker and a possible molecular target for therapy of ovarian clear cell carcinoma. Am J Pathol 2003;163:2503-12.

300. Kato N, Sasou S, Motoyama T. Expression of hepatocyte nuclear factor-1beta (HNF-1beta) in clear cell tumors and endometriosis of the ovary. Mod Pathol 2006;19:83-9.

301. Yamamoto S, Tsuda H, Aida S, Shimazaki H, Tamai S, Matsubara O. Immunohistochemical detection of hepatocyte nuclear factor 1beta in ovarian and endometrial clear-cell adenocarcinomas and nonneoplastic endometrium. Hum Pathol 2007;38:1074-80.

302. Köbel M, Kalloger SE, Carrick J, et al. A limited panel of immunomarkers can reliably distinguish between clear cell and high-grade serous carcinoma of the ovary. Am J Surg Pathol 2009;33:14-21.

303. Fadare O, Liang S. Diagnostic utility of hepatocyte nuclear factor 1-Beta immunoreactivity in endometrial carcinomas: lack of specificity for endometrial clear cell carcinoma. Appl Immunohistochem Mol Morphol 2012;20:580-7.

304. Broaddus RR, Lynch HT, Chen LM, et al. Pathologic features of endometrial carcinoma associated with HNPCC: a comparison with sporadic endometrial carcinoma. Cancer 2006;106:87-94.

305. Carcangiu ML, Radice P, Casalini P, Bertario L, Merola M, Sala P. Lynch syndrome--related endometrial carcinomas show a high frequency of nonendometrioid types and of high FIGO grade endometrioid types. Int J Surg Pathol 2010;18:21-6.

306. Mhawech-Fauceglia P, Yan L, Liu S, Pejovic T. ER+ /PR+ /TFF3+ /IMP3- immunoprofile distinguishes endometrioid from serous and clear cell carcinomas of the endometrium: a study of 401 cases. Histopathology 2013;62:976-85.

307. Dainty LA, Risinger JI, Morrison C, et al. Overexpression of folate binding protein and mesothelin are associated with uterine serous carcinoma. Gynecol Oncol 2007;105:563-70.

308. Garg K, Levine DA, Olvera N, et al. BRCA1 immunohistochemistry in a molecularly characterized cohort of ovarian high-grade serous carcinomas. Am J Surg Pathol 2013;37:138-46.

309. Hecht JL, Konstantinopoulos PA, Awtrey CS, Soslow RA. Immunohistochemical loss of BRCA1 protein in uterine serous carcinoma. Int J Gynecol Pathol 2014;33:282-7.

310. Dupont J, Wang X, Marshall DS, et al. Wilms tumor gene (WT1) and p53 expression in endometrial carcinomas: a study of 130 cases using a tissue microarray. Gynecol Oncol 2004;94:449-55.

311. Chen W, Husain A, Nelson GS, et al. Immunohistochemical profiling of endometrial serous carcinoma. Int J Gynecol Pathol 2017;36:128-39.

312. Zeimet AG, Reimer D, Huszar M, et al. L1CAM in early-stage type I endometrial cancer: results of a large multicenter evaluation. J Natl Cancer Inst 2013;105:1142-50.

313. Espinosa I, Jose Carnicer M, Catasus L, et al. Myometrial invasion and lymph node metastasis in endometrioid carcinomas: tumor-associated macrophages, microvessel density, and HIF1A have a crucial role. Am J Surg Pathol 2010;34:1708-14.

314. Oh JH, Kim JH, Ahn HJ, et al. Syndecan-1 enhances the endometrial cancer invasion by modulating matrix metalloproteinase-9 expression through nuclear factor kappaB. Gynecol Oncol 2009;114:509-15.

315. Xie R, Schlumbrecht MP, Shipley GL, Xie S, Bassett RL Jr, Broaddus RR. S100A4 mediates endometrial cancer invasion and is a target of TGF-beta1 signaling. Lab Invest 2009;89:937-47.

6 SEROUS CARCINOMA

Serous carcinoma of the endometrium is a high-grade, clinically aggressive malignancy that resembles high-grade serous carcinoma of the ovary, fallopian tube, and peritoneum (1-4). These tumors typically harbor a somatic *TP53* mutation and have numerous chromosomal amplifications and deletions (5).

GENERAL FEATURES

Serous carcinoma constitutes up to 10 percent of endometrial carcinomas and almost always occurs in a sporadic setting. In contrast to patients with endometrioid or clear cell carcinoma, those with serous carcinoma are more frequently African-American; 15 to 30 percent in some studies (6–12). Patients are typically older than 65 years and lack evidence of hyperestrinism (13–19). Although women with serous carcinoma are less frequently obese and exposed to unopposed estrogen, there is emerging data suggesting that the development of some "type II carcinomas" may not be entirely estrogen independent (20). There is an association with carcinoma of the breast and tamoxifen therapy (15,21–25), pelvic radiation (usually for cervical or rectal carcinoma) (26–31), and rarely, a *BRCA1* germline mutation (32–35). The risk of developing endometrial carcinoma due to a germline *BRCA1* mutation is at most only slightly higher than in patients lacking this mutation.

Serous carcinomas were historically considered type II carcinomas based on Bokhman's epidemiologic and clinical studies of Soviet women in the 1970s and 1980s (13). Several lines of evidence suggest that the dualistic model for endometrial cancer may obscure important differences between different types of endometrial carcinoma and currently may not be applicable. Although obesity (body mass index [BMI] over 30 kg/m^2) is typically cited as a robust risk factor for type I carcinoma, recent observations indicate that obesity is also related to an increased risk of type II carcinomas (16–18). Smoking has been consistently associated with a decreased risk of endometrial cancer possibly due to an antiestrogenic effect (36), but several studies have reported similar risk associations between smoking and risk for both types I and II carcinomas (16,17,19).

Brinton et al. (15) compared risk factors between type I and type II carcinomas (mixed epithelial, clear cell, serous, and carcinosarcoma) in an analysis of 210 tumors by the Gynecologic Oncology Group (GOG) trial. Women with type II carcinomas were older and more often non-Caucasian, multiparous, smokers, or status-post tubal ligation, compared to women with type I carcinomas, and were less often obese and more likely to have a history of breast cancer or tamoxifen exposure. Women with type II carcinomas and a history of breast cancer or tamoxifen use preferentially had serous carcinoma and carcinosarcoma, rather than clear cell carcinoma. These findings underscore the diversity of type II carcinomas and call into question continued use of this simplistic and outmoded dualistic model of endometrial carcinogenesis for diagnostic and investigative purposes.

CLINICAL FEATURES

Approximately two thirds of patients with serous carcinoma are over 65 (median, 70) years of age. Patients often have increased CA125 serum levels and, rarely, paraneoplastic hypercalcemia (37). Most patients present with vaginal bleeding, and less commonly, are asymptomatic. Serous carcinoma may be found in a cervicovaginal cytology or curettage performed for a thickened endometrial stripe in the setting of tamoxifen therapy. The initial manifestation in some patients is extrauterine disease, including ovarian or omental masses, ascites, pleural effusion, or lymphadenopathy.

Compared to other types of endometrial carcinoma, serous carcinoma presents more

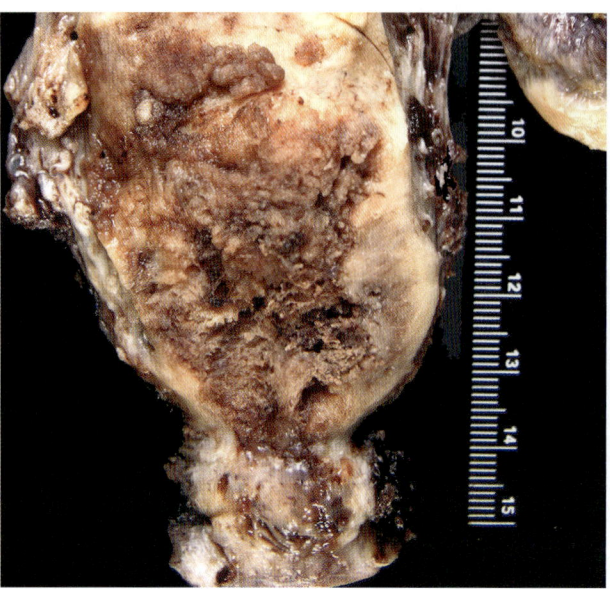
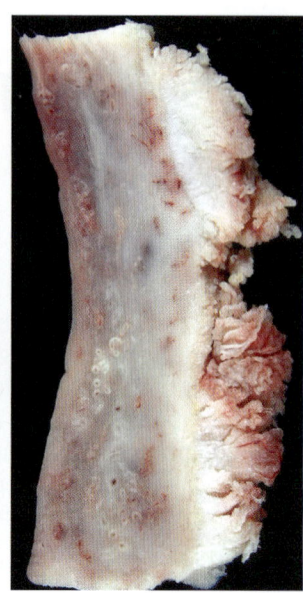

Figure 6-1

UTERINE SEROUS CARCINOMA

The endometrium is replaced by a large, variegated tumor. The cut surface shows multiple papillary excrescences but only minimal myometrial invasion.

commonly with advanced-stage disease, although International Federation of Gynecology and Obstetrics (FIGO) stage IA tumors occur. Approximately 10 percent of patients have carcinoma confined to the endometrium; an additional 30 to 50 percent have myometrial invasive carcinoma confined to the uterus; and the remaining 40 to 60 percent have extrauterine disease. In contrast to endometrioid and clear cell carcinomas, 20 to 40 percent of patients have metastasis to the peritoneum at presentation. When lymph node dissection is performed at the time of hysterectomy, 20 percent have nodal metastases (32,38–42). Even though serous carcinomas are assigned a FIGO stage like other endometrial carcinomas (42), there have been studies that highlight the shortcomings of FIGO 2009 staging for non-endometrioid carcinomas in general and serous carcinomas specifically (42,43).

GROSS FINDINGS

Uteri harboring serous carcinoma tend to be smaller than those with endometrioid carcinomas. The extent of tumor varies from a diffuse coating of the endometrium (fig. 6-1) to involvement limited to an endometrial polyp. Sometimes papillary architecture may be noted on cut section (fig. 6-1). Many serous carcinomas demonstrate myometrial invasion and extension or secondary involvement of the uterine serosa and adnexa.

MICROSCOPIC FINDINGS

Almost all serous carcinomas feature papillary architecture at least focally. The papillae are typically irregular in shape and size, but some are small (micropapillae) (fig. 6-2). They are lined by pseudostratified epithelium associated with prominent cell budding and dyshesion, resulting in ragged or serrated luminal contours (fig. 6-3). Cells are cuboidal to low columnar and severely atypical with high nuclear to cytoplasmic (N:C) ratios, hyperchromatic nuclei, prominent nucleoli, and high mitotic indexes, including abnormal forms. Multinucleation and monstrous cells with smudged chromatin are also common (fig. 6-4).

Endometrial serous carcinomas are by definition high grade in contrast to both low- and high-grade serous carcinomas in the adnexa, and thus, the binary grading scheme in use for ovarian and tubal serous carcinomas is not applicable to those of the endometrium (44). Occasionally, cells with a lower N:C ratio and eosinophilic (squamoid) (fig. 6-5, left) or clear cytoplasm are seen (fig. 6-5, right) (45).

Serous carcinoma may also have glandular or solid architecture. Tumors with glandular architecture (pseudoendometrioid) tend to have "thick" outlines due to the degree of nuclear pseudostratification. They may display incipient clefting, micropapillae within the glands, evidence

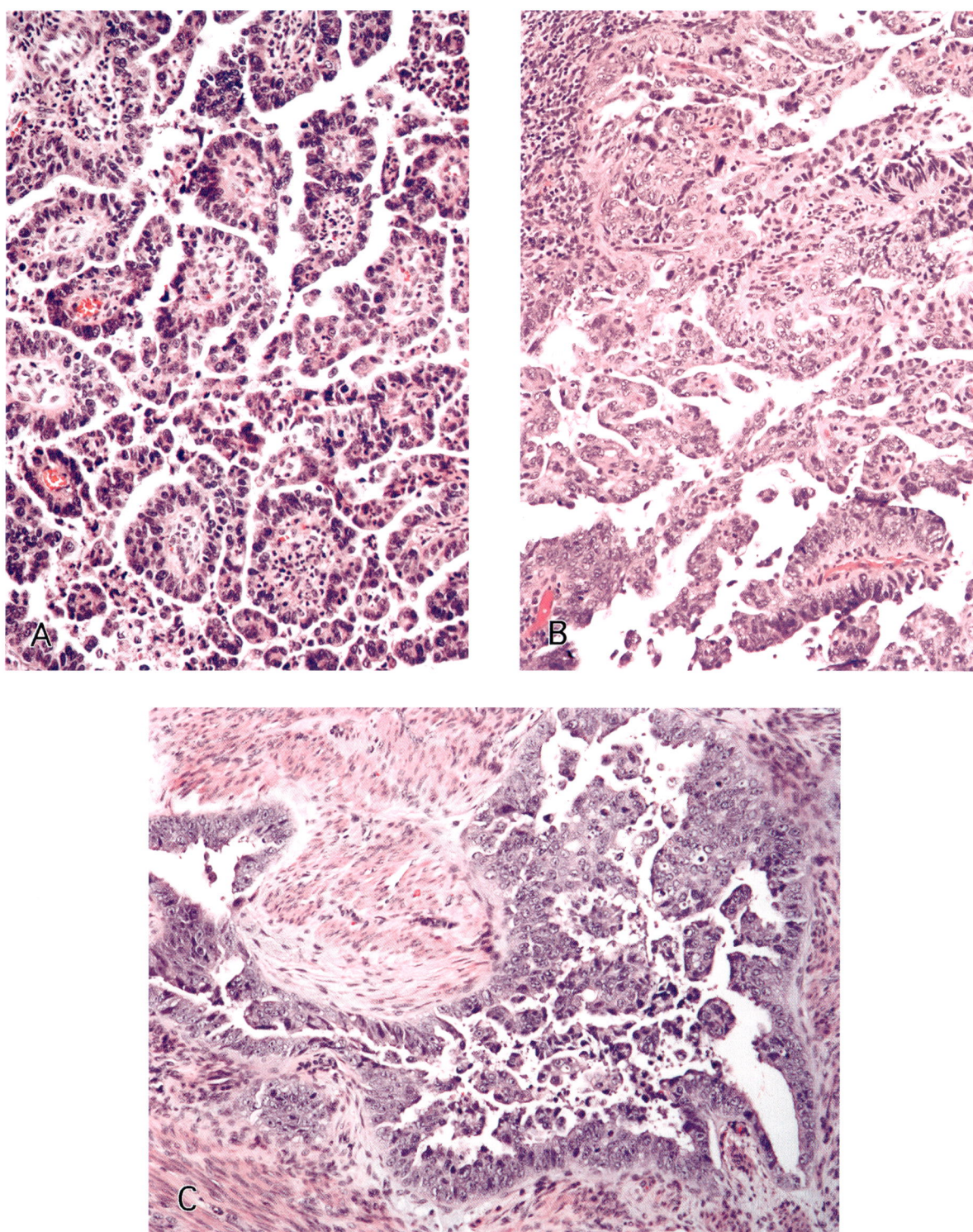

Figure 6-2

PAPILLARY SEROUS CARCINOMA

Papillary architecture is the most classic and common morphology in serous carcinoma. The papillae vary in size (A and B), and may have prominent micropapillary architecture (C).

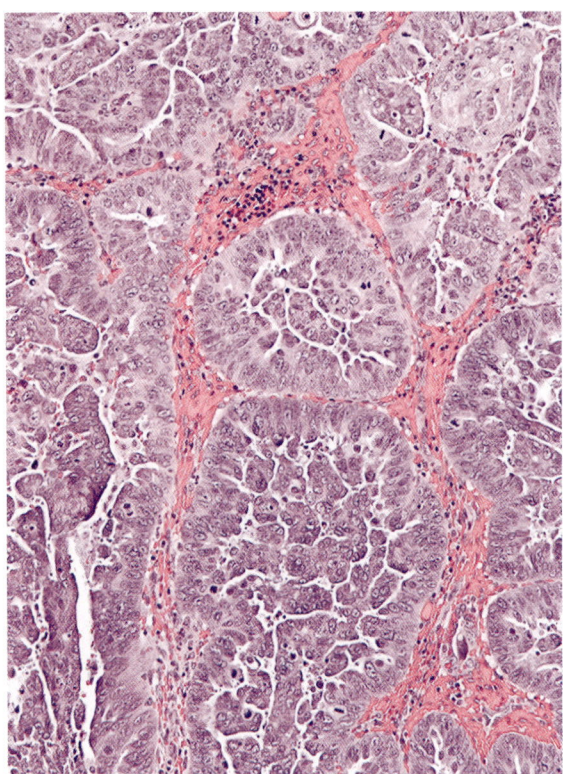 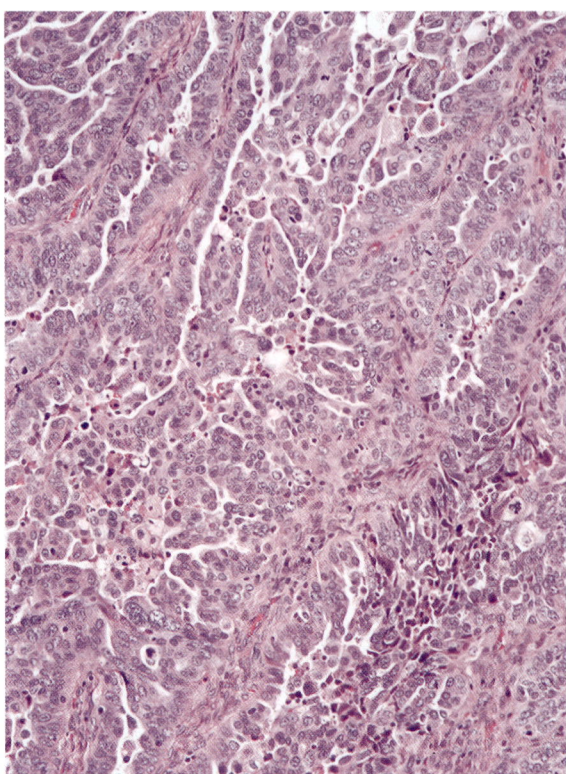

Figure 6-3

SEROUS CARCINOMA

Prominent budding of tumor cells is due to cell dyshesion (left). Clefting is also a characteristic finding (right).

of dyshesion, and altered cellular polarity similar to their papillary counterparts (fig. 6-6) (46–48). A solid component that may contain, at least focally, cleft-like spaces, is often present in association with a papillary component, but in isolation the solid architecture may be difficult to interpret accurately (fig. 6-7).

Psammoma bodies are seen in less than one third of serous carcinomas, far less commonly than in their ovarian counterparts. When invasive, serous carcinomas may display a "gaping gland" appearance within the myometrium (fig. 6-8). Lymphovascular invasion is common.

Endometrial serous carcinoma may arise in or be associated with an endometrial polyp. Invasion of the stroma of the polyp is generally easy to identify, however, colonization of preexisting atrophic endometrial glands within a polyp (fig. 6-9), within atrophic endometrial glands outside the polyp or on the endometrial surface, can be challenging without scrutiny at high magnification (49–54). Thus, *intraepithelial serous carcinoma* is recognized by the presence of cuboidal to columnar cells with high N:C ratios and high-grade cytologic atypia that replaces preexisting endometrial surface or subadjacent endometrial glands with an abrupt transition to non-neoplastic epithelium (fig. 6-10). The appearance is similar to that seen in the precursor to adnexal high-grade serous carcinoma, serous tubal intraepithelial carcinoma. Secondary formation of micropapillae may be seen. Recognition of intraepithelial serous carcinoma is important, since metastases to the peritoneum are found in 20 to 40 percent of cases (52,55), even when obvious stromal or myometrial invasion is not present (56). Transtubal spread is hypothesized to be the mechanism responsible for peritoneal metastases without myometrial invasion (57).

The term *minimal serous carcinoma* has been proposed for intraepithelial serous carcinomas and endometrial stromal-invasive serous carcinomas

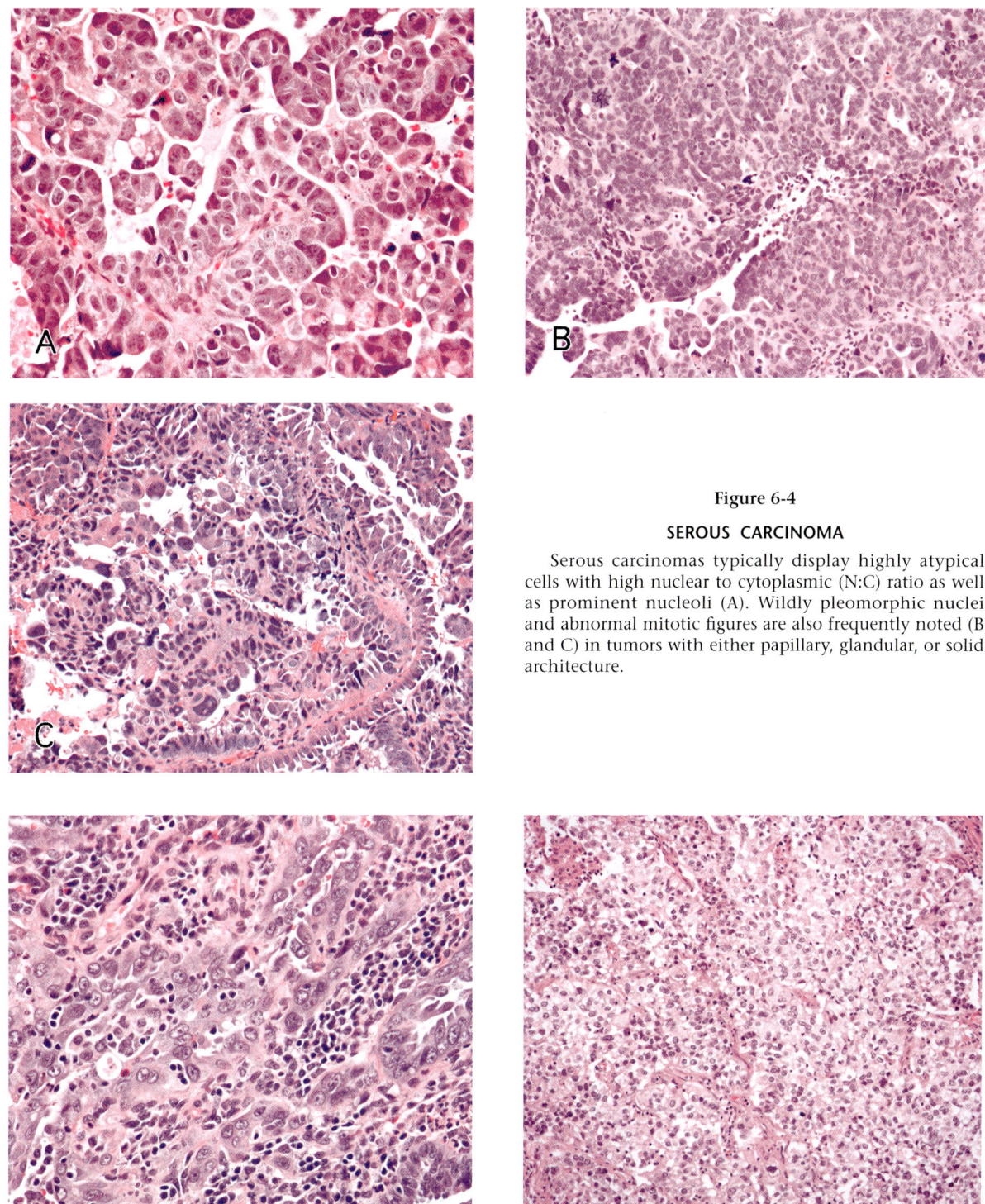

Figure 6-4

SEROUS CARCINOMA

Serous carcinomas typically display highly atypical cells with high nuclear to cytoplasmic (N:C) ratio as well as prominent nucleoli (A). Wildly pleomorphic nuclei and abnormal mitotic figures are also frequently noted (B and C) in tumors with either papillary, glandular, or solid architecture.

Figure 6-5

SEROUS CARCINOMA WITH EOSINOPHILIC OR CLEAR CYTOPLASM

Some serous carcinomas may have a squamoid morphology due to abundant eosinophilic cytoplasm (left). Slit-like architecture, incipient micropapillae, and pleomorphic nuclei, typical of serous carcinoma, are evident. Rarely, cells in serous carcinoma have clear cytoplasm (right).

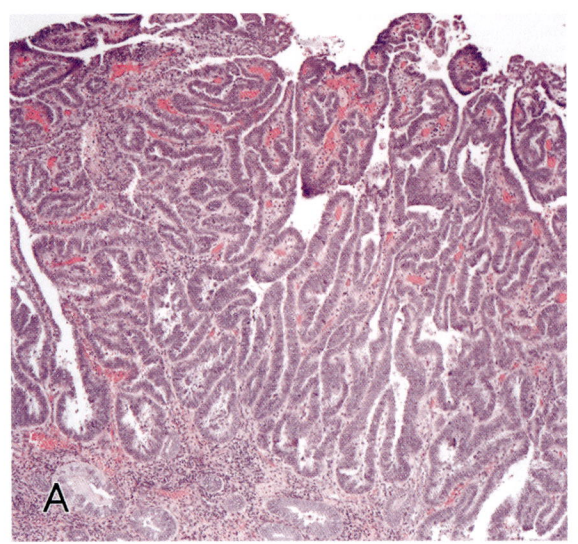
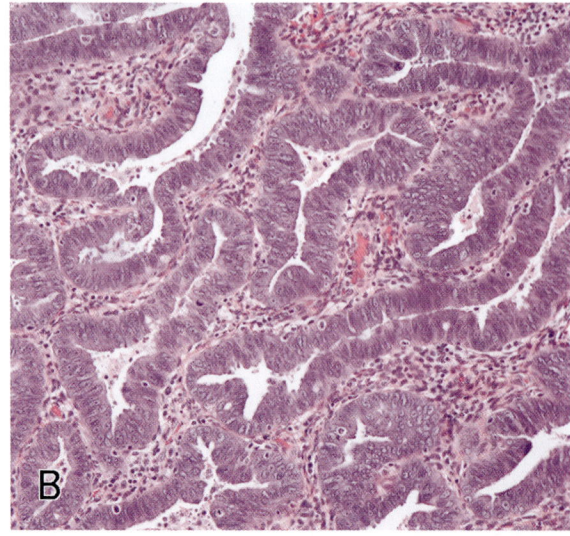

Figure 6-6
SEROUS CARCINOMA: GLANDULAR ARCHITECTURE

Although not easily recognized as serous carcinoma on low power, serous differentiation is suggested by multiple areas in which detached buds of neoplastic cells are noted in lumens (A). Glands show incipient clefting as well as loss of nuclear polarity (B). Abnormal glands may be difficult to appreciate at low power, however, irregular luminal contours, cuboidal cells with high N:C ratio, and enlarged pleomorphic nuclei with prominent nucleoli are seen (C). At low power the architecture of some glandular serous carcinomas mimics low-grade endometrioid carcinoma (D). At high power, "thick" glands (in contrast to adjacent atrophic glands), striking pseudostratification, and cytologic atypia are seen. Overt features of serous carcinoma are difficult to appreciate in tumors with a papillary and glandular architecture. Clues to the correct diagnosis are cells with high N:C ratio, obvious nucleoli, and subtle undulations in luminal contours (E).

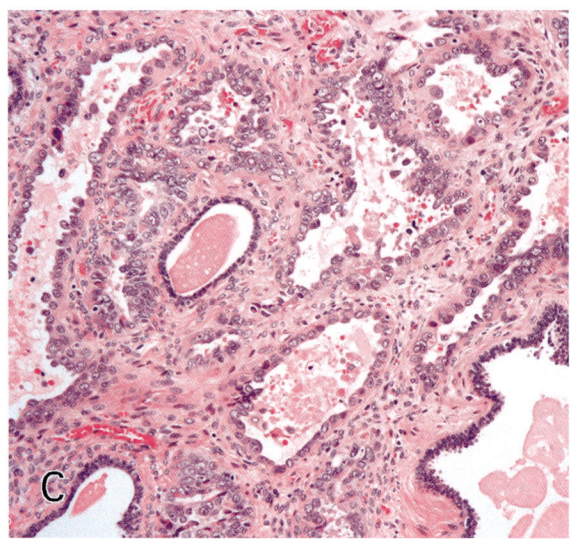
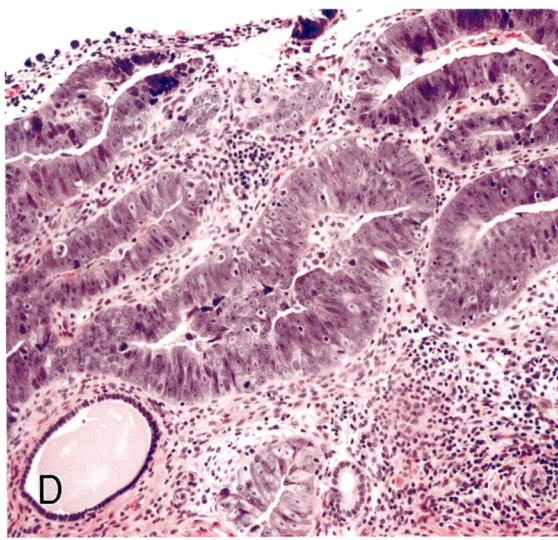
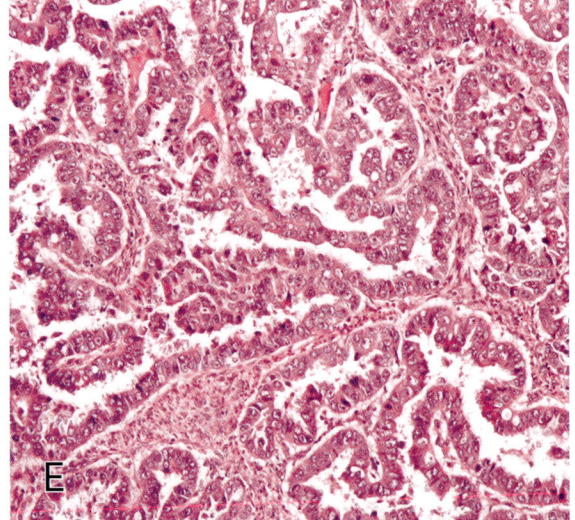

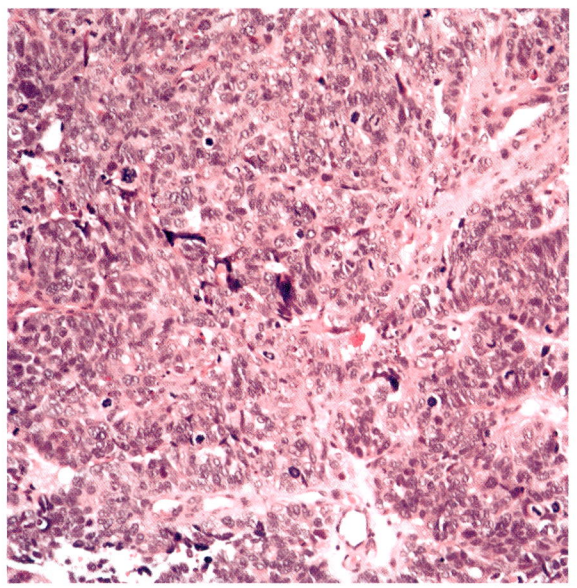

Figure 6-7

SEROUS CARCINOMA: SOLID GROWTH

This pattern is associated with highly pleomorphic cells.

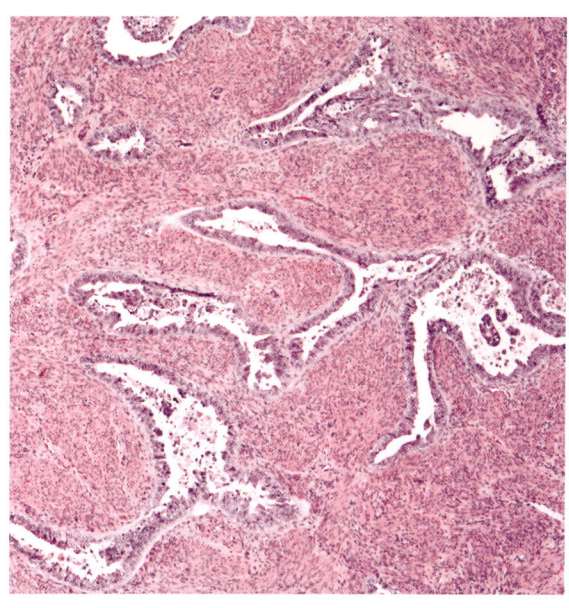

Figure 6-8

SEROUS CARCINOMA: GAPING GLAND INVASION

This is a characteristic, but not pathognomonic, pattern of myometrial invasion.

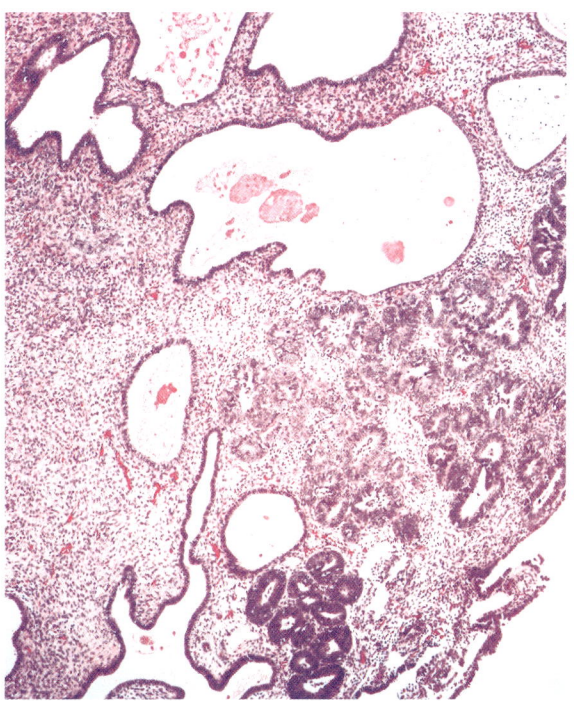

Figure 6-9

SEROUS CARCINOMA IN AN ENDOMETRIAL POLYP

At low-power examination (left), the lesion may simulate the appearance of atypical hyperplasia. The focal presence of a dark blue glandular proliferation in an atrophic polyp should suggest the possibility of serous carcinoma. At high power, the characteristic features of serous carcinoma are seen (right).

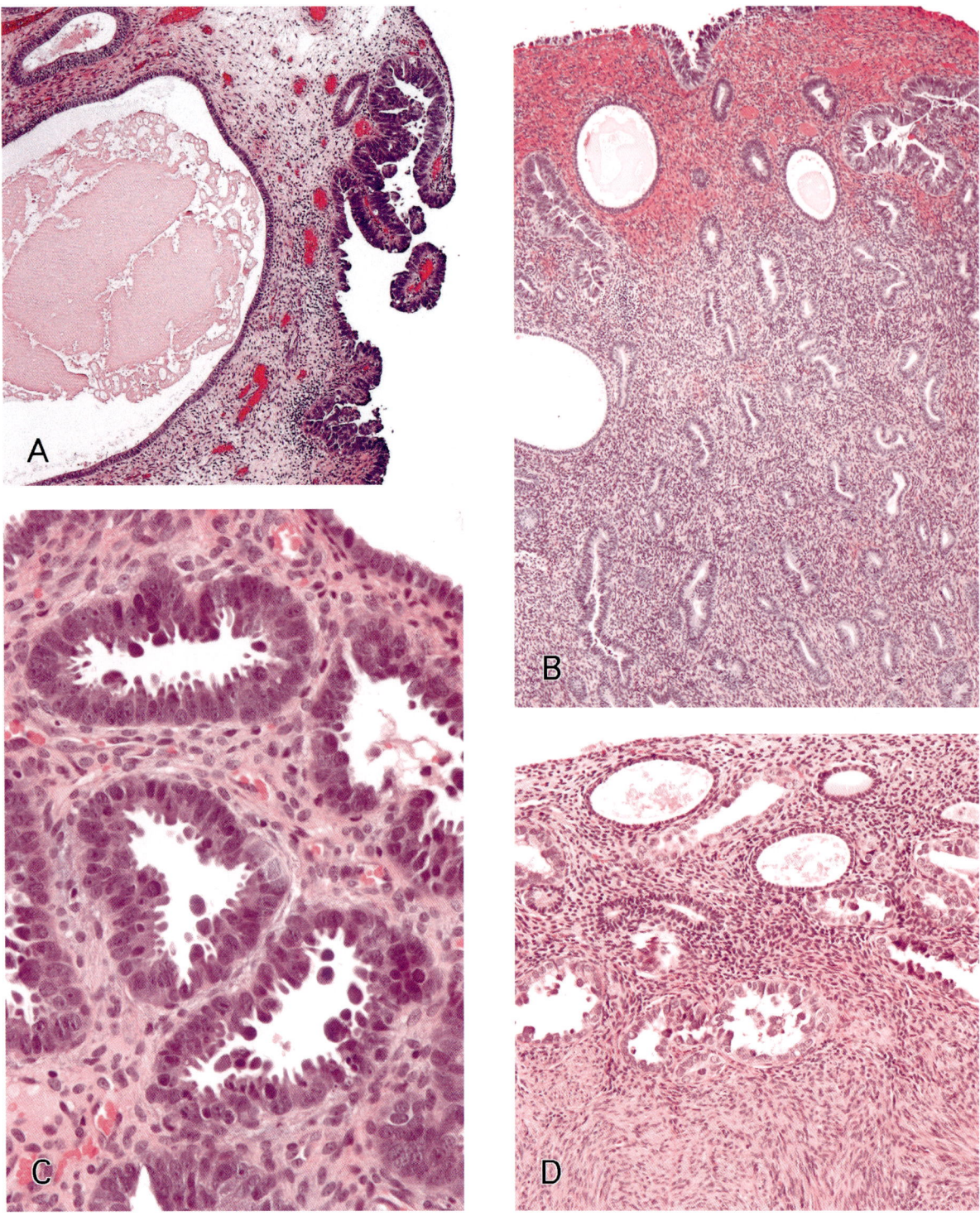

Figure 6-10

INTRAEPITHELIAL SEROUS CARCINOMA

Serous carcinoma colonizes atrophic surface epithelium (A) or atrophic glands (B–D).

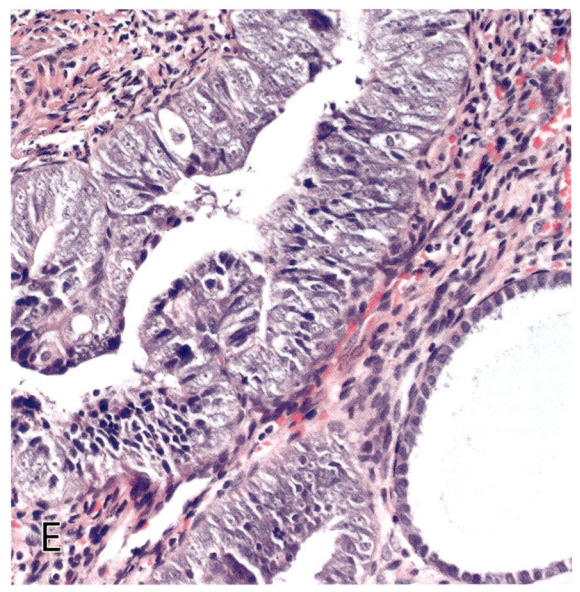

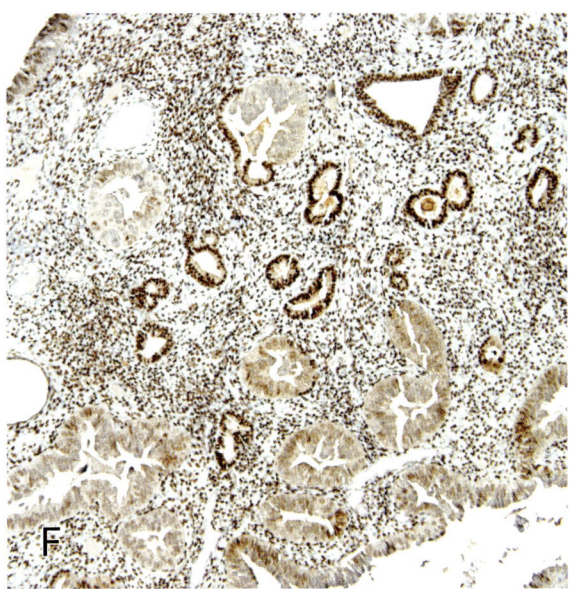

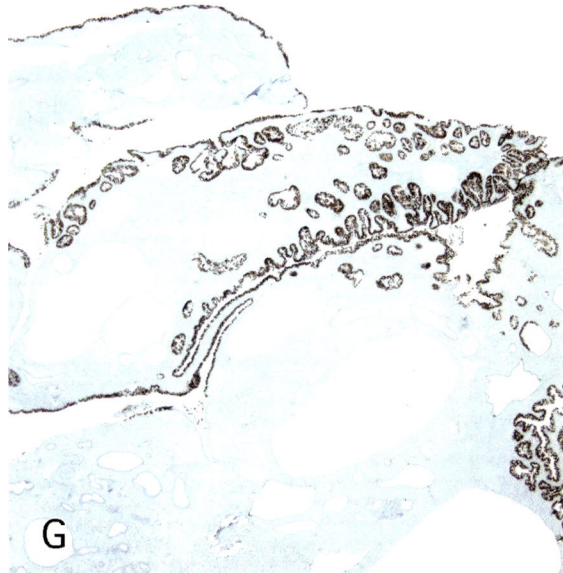

Figure 6-10, continued
Intraepithelial serous carcinoma is difficult to visualize at low power, but the correct diagnosis is suggested by the thickened "blue" epithelium with an irregular contour as well as dyshesion of some cells, irregular luminal contours, hyperchromatism, and high-grade cytologic features (E). Intraepithelial serous carcinoma typically shows minimal to absent expression of estrogen receptor (F) and striking p53 positivity in surface and in small glands (G).

measuring 1 cm or less (52). When there is no myometrial invasion and comprehensive staging surgery is negative for extrauterine tumor, clinical outcomes are excellent in most instances.

Rarely, serous carcinomas are associated with giant cell carcinoma (58) or trophoblastic differentiation (59,60). They may be part of a mixed carcinoma including neuroendocrine carcinoma (61).

SEROUS CARCINOMA PRECURSORS

Although *intraepithelial serous carcinoma*, also referred to as *endometrial intraepithelial carcinoma* or *serous endometrial intraepithelial carcinoma*, has been postulated as a serous carcinoma precursor, it is probably more accurate to state that it is a precursor to invasive or metastatic serous carcinoma. Also, intraepithelial serous carcinoma may behave as an overt malignancy. In some cases, intraepithelial serous carcinoma represents intraepithelial spread of an established endometrial or adnexal serous carcinoma (62,63). Thus, the use of this term could be misleading.

Several investigators have described putative precursors to intraepithelial serous carcinoma (64–69), but this is a controversial area. The abnormalities detected with immunohistochemistry are similar to those described in the fallopian tube as potential serous tubal intraepithelial carcinoma precursors (i.e., p53 signature lesion and others). These lesions can sometimes be found adjacent to obvious examples of serous carcinoma, particularly in endometrial polyps when immunohistochemistry is performed in an attempt to establish a diagnosis of intraepithelial serous carcinoma. If the lesion lacks marked cytologic atypia or mitoses, it is best diagnosed as "nonspecific atypia" after ensuring that the entire lesion has been sampled and examined.

IMMUNOHISTOCHEMICAL AND MOLECULAR GENETIC FINDINGS

Most serous carcinomas co-express PAX8, pancytokeratins, cytokeratin 7 (CK7), and vimentin as well as cell surface glycoproteins such as BerEP4, B72.3, MOC31, CA125, and epithelial membrane antigen (EMA). Approximately 50 percent of serous carcinomas have detectable expression of estrogen receptor (ER) and progesterone receptor (PR), but with lesser extent and intensity than low-grade endometrioid carcinomas and high-grade ovarian serous carcinomas (70–75). Most serous carcinomas are WT1 negative or show weak and patchy positivity, although about 20 percent display diffuse expression (73,76–79).

Serous carcinomas are typically characterized by aberrant p53 expression (50,75,80–84). Approximately 80 percent show overexpression, defined as more than 50, 60 or 75 percent of tumor cell nuclei with uniform and strong intensity (fig. 6-11A,B), while approximately 15 percent display a null pattern of expression with no p53 staining. Rare serous carcinomas do not show an aberrant p53 staining pattern (85). A positive control (with wild-pattern staining) (usually non-neoplastic endometrium, stroma, endothelial cells, or inflammatory cells) should be evaluated concurrently before scoring a tumor as having a null p53 staining pattern.

Approximately 90 percent of tumors overexpress p16, defined by an every-cell staining pattern (fig. 6-11C) (86–88). Patchy staining with p16, even when intense, is not considered sufficient for p16 overexpression.

Loss of expression of PTEN (73,82,89–91), ARID1A, and the DNA mismatch repair (MMR) proteins is exceptional (73). HER2 amplification is found in about 25 percent of serous and clear cell carcinomas (73), which can sometimes be targeted with agents similar to trastuzumab. IMP3, also known as IGF-2 mRNA binding protein 3 (IGF2BP3), is expressed in these tumors, but does not distinguish between serous carcinoma and other high-grade endometrial carcinomas (73,92).

The most commonly dysregulated somatic genes in this subtype of endometrial carcinoma are, in decreasing order of prevalence, *TP53* (missense, nonsense, frameshift mutations), *PPP2R1A*, *PIK3CA*, *FBXW7*, and *HER2* amplification (5). All serous carcinomas map to the copy number-high cluster described in the TCGA study of endometrial carcinoma (5), which translates into a high number of gross chromosomal abnormalities, such as amplifications and deletions, even though the number of deleterious mutations per cell is low. The most common amplification involves *CCNE1*, which encodes cyclin E (5).

DIFFERENTIAL DIAGNOSIS

Endometrioid Carcinoma. Endometrioid carcinoma may contain scattered clusters of highly atypical cells. However, an endometrial carcinoma that shows a diffuse growth of cells with highly atypical nuclei lacking nuclear polarity, well-defined luminal borders, or squamous or mucinous differentiation cannot be diagnosed as endometrioid regardless of the presence of architectural features usually ascribed to these tumors (combinations of glandular, nested, and cribriform growths). Low-grade endometrioid carcinomas may display metaplastic changes that can be mistaken for serous carcinoma. However, the nuclear features are low grade and these metaplastic changes are seen in juxtaposition with areas of conventional endometrioid carcinoma. In exceptional cases, p53 and Ki-67 immunohistochemistry can be used to exclude serous carcinoma.

Colonization of atrophic endometrial glands by intraepithelial serous carcinoma may be confused at low-power microscopy with crowded endometrioid-type glands, leading to an erroneous diagnosis of atypical hyperplasia or FIGO grade 1 endometrioid carcinoma. As this represents an early form of serous carcinoma,

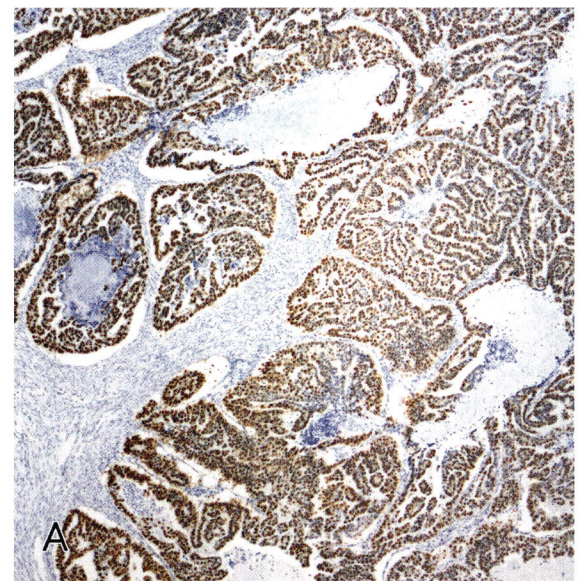
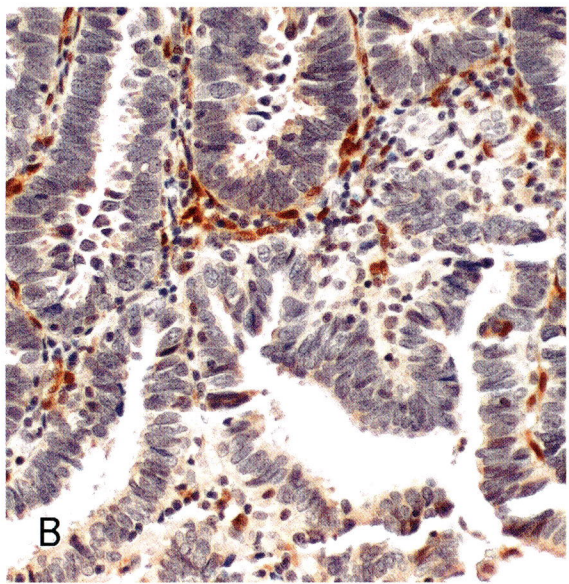
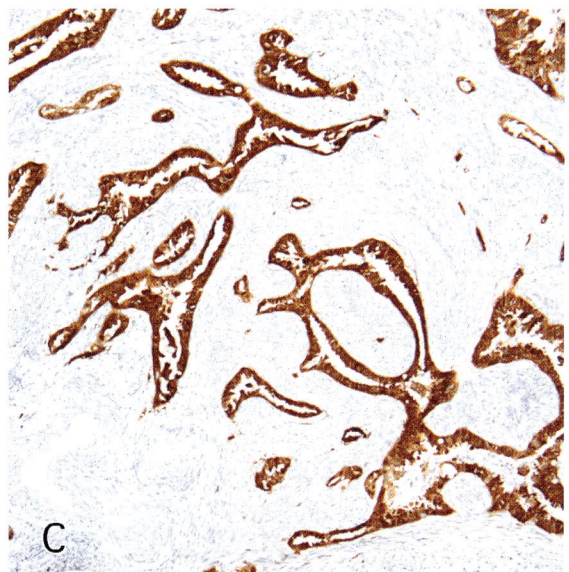

Figure 6-11

SEROUS CARCINOMA: p53 AND p16

p53 overexpression (A) and null phenotype (B) in serous carcinomas. A positive internal control is seen in B. These tumors also typically show diffuse p16 positivity (C).

the full spectrum of architectural and nuclear features may not be apparent. Clues to an accurate diagnosis are the presence of marked pseudostratification, high N:C ratio, and cells with a high proliferation index as well as early clefting and dyshesion. Overexpression or complete absence of p53 (aberrant staining) and a high proliferation index confirm the diagnosis of serous carcinoma (50,51).

Rare examples of endometrioid carcinomas with low-grade serous-like morphology have been reported. They are characterized by delicate papillae that resemble low-grade serous carcinoma of the ovary. However, the cells have at most moderate cytologic atypia and typically merge with conventional areas of endometrioid carcinoma, in contrast to what would be expected in a serous carcinoma of the endometrium. Furthermore, they typically show wild p53 expression and some have *KRAS* mutations (93,94).

Much more difficult is the differentiation of serous carcinoma from a high-grade endometrioid carcinoma since both may display solid growth and severe cytologic atypia. Striking pleomorphism (with monstrous cells), slit-like spaces, coexistent irregular papillae, and absence of clearcut endometrioid glandular formation favor a diagnosis of serous carcinoma. FIGO grade 3 endometrioid carcinomas more characteristically contain nests or thick interanastomosing trabeculae of cells. p53 and p16 should be applied with caution in this differential diagnosis because about 30 percent of high-grade endometrioid carcinomas show diffuse positivity for these markers as typically seen in serous carcinomas (38,78,80,81,86,93,95–99). Even though an aberrant p53 staining pattern does not distinguish high-grade endometrioid from serous carcinoma, a wild-type staining pattern makes a diagnosis of serous carcinoma much less likely. DNA MMR proteins (MLH1, PMS2, MSH2, MSH6 or only PMS2 and MSH6), ARID1A, and PTEN may be more helpful in this differential diagnosis, as loss of expression of these markers supports a diagnosis of endometrioid carcinoma (73).

Clear Cell Carcinoma. As mentioned, serous carcinoma may contain a component of clear cells. This finding should not lead to the misinterpretation of the tumor as a clear cell carcinoma. To make the diagnosis of clear cell carcinoma, the typical architectural patterns should be present, regardless of the finding of clear or hobnail cells. The papillae of clear cell carcinoma are generally round and small, and lined by a monolayer of cuboidal cells, with or without cytoplasmic clearing, in contrast to the larger and irregularly shaped papillae of serous carcinoma, lined by stratified layers of cells with high N:C ratio. The stroma of clear cell carcinoma may be hyalinized or myxoid and contain an obvious plasmacytic infiltrate. In contrast to ovarian clear cell carcinomas, endometrial clear cell carcinomas display a greater range of nuclear atypia and mitotic activity, thus, these features, if present, cannot be used to distinguish clear cell carcinoma from serous carcinoma in the endometrium.

A wild-type pattern of p53 expression favors clear cell carcinoma over serous carcinoma, but 20 to 30 percent of clear cell carcinomas show aberrant p53 expression (75,100–102). In the latter scenario, ER/PR, ARID1A, napsin A, and HNF-1β can be used, although evaluation of the tumor architecture should take precedence. In contrast to serous carcinoma (≈50/positive), clear cell carcinomas are almost always negative for ER/PR (or are very weakly and focally stained), may show loss of ARID1A expression, and frequently stain with napsin A and HNF-1β.

Mixed Carcinomas with a Serous Component. There is emerging evidence that, with only rare exceptions, mixed carcinomas of the endometrium with a serous component are not mixed from a genomic perspective, even when the different components are histologically distinctive (103). A high threshold should be used to diagnose mixed carcinomas. Most of these tumors derive from the same precursor, either an endometrioid carcinoma, which then acquires intratumoral heterogeneity and further gene mutations in the high-grade components, or a serous carcinoma with areas that resemble an endometrioid carcinoma (fig. 6-12). Aberrant p53 expression is usually not found in the former but it is characteristically seen throughout the tumor in the latter.

The clinical significance of a mixed carcinoma with only one component demonstrating aberrant p53 staining is currently uncertain. Some represent *POLE* hotspot mutated endometrioid carcinomas with a highly favorable prognosis, some are microsatellite unstable (MSI-H) endometrioid carcinomas with an intermediate prognosis, and others are low-grade endometrioid carcinomas with tumor progression in the form of serous carcinoma or TP53-mutated high-grade endometrioid carcinoma (94,103). The latter is the only example of a "mixed endometrioid and serous carcinoma" (fig. 6-13). DNA MMR immunohistochemical stains and *POLE* mutational analysis, if available, distinguish between these entities.

A diagnosis of "mixed endometrioid and serous carcinoma" should not be made for a more or less homogeneous-appearing tumor with overlapping features of both endometrioid and serous carcinomas (94,104,105). Some of these tumors are pure serous carcinomas with focal glandular and cribriform architecture and diffuse nuclear atypia but no confirmatory endometrioid features, and show aberrant p53 expression throughout (47). Others are endometrioid carcinomas with intratumoral heterogeneity and patchy nuclear atypia, particularly when no aberrant p53 can be demonstrated (106,107). It is probably a good practice to evaluate for MSI-H or *POLE* hotspot mutations given this latter scenario,

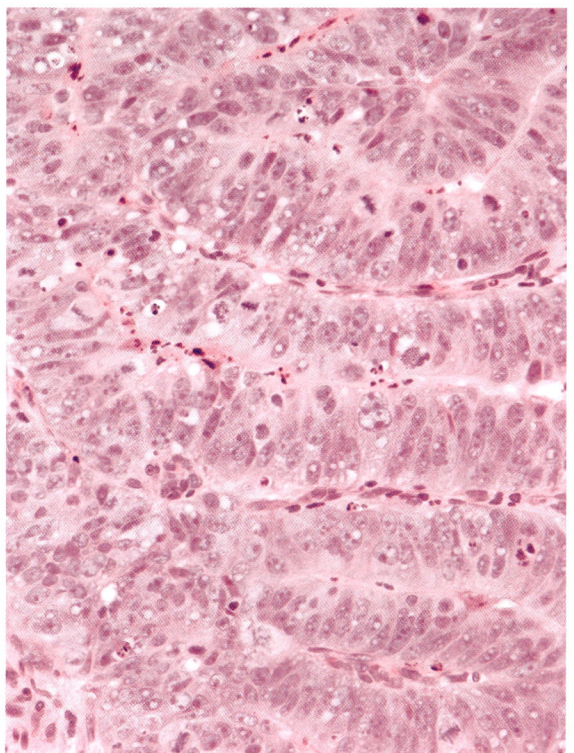 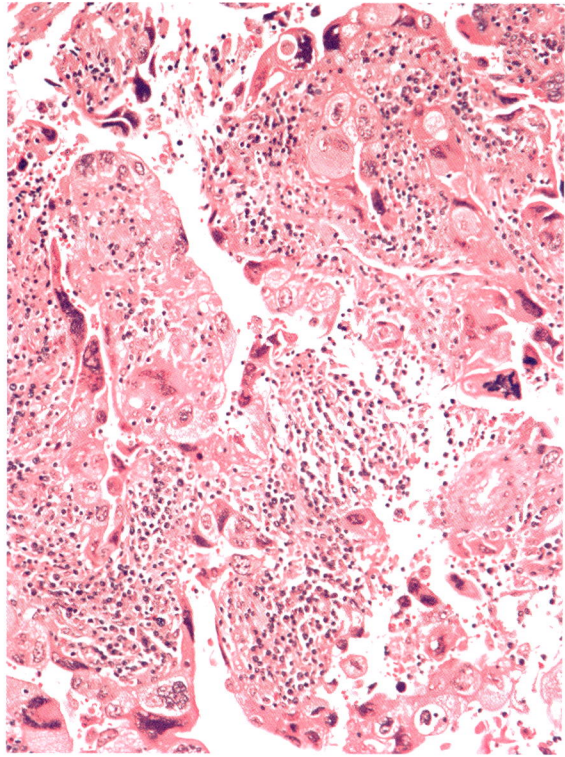

Figure 6-12

SEROUS VERSUS ENDOMETRIOID CARCINOMA

Columnar, eosinophilic cells suggest endometrioid differentiation, but diffusely distributed severe nuclear atypia suggests serous carcinoma (left). Wildly pleomorphic cells suggest serous carcinoma, but a low N:C ratio is not characteristic of most serous carcinomas (right). An obvious lymphocytic infiltrate suggests that this tumor is high microsatellite instability (MSI-H) or *POLE* mutated, features that do not support a diagnosis of serous carcinoma.

since tumors with these abnormalities are known to be either relatively (MSI-H) or highly (*POLE*) prognostically favorable (fig. 6-14).

Carcinosarcoma. According to the most recent World Health Organization (WHO) classification (107a), carcinosarcoma should only be diagnosed when the tumor in question contains histologically high-grade epithelial and mesenchymal components. The high-grade mesenchymal component likely to be encountered given a background of serous carcinoma is a pleomorphic homologous spindle cell proliferation or a heterologous round cell or spindle cell proliferation, frequently with a rhabdomyoblastic component. Even the focal presence of any malignant mesenchymal component would qualify such a tumor as carcinosarcoma. Immunohistochemical stains should not be used to distinguish serous carcinoma and carcinosarcoma, although desmin and myogenin may confirm the presence of skeletal muscle differentiation. An occasional endometrial serous carcinoma evolves to carcinosarcoma in metastatic sites or at recurrence. Anecdotally, metastatic pure rhabdomyosarcoma can also be encountered after a diagnosis of endometrial serous carcinoma.

Drop Metastasis of Serous Carcinoma. The true incidence of drop metastasis from an adnexal (fallopian tube, ovary, or peritoneum) serous carcinoma is unknown since a gold standard diagnostic criterion does not exist. Nevertheless, drop metastasis (fig. 6-15, left) is suggested in the presence of any of the following: high-grade carcinoma with tumor volume in adnexa significantly greater than in endometrium; patient younger than 60 years; presence of serous tubal intraepithelial carcinoma; absence of intraepithelial serous carcinoma; WT1 diffuse

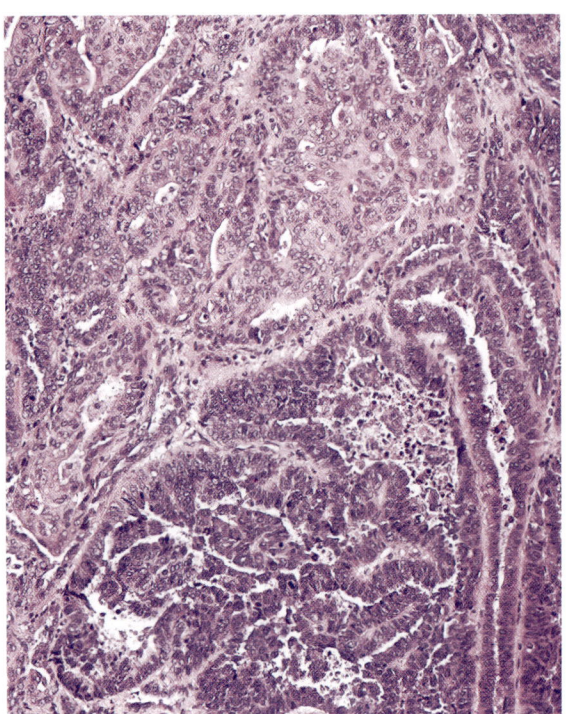 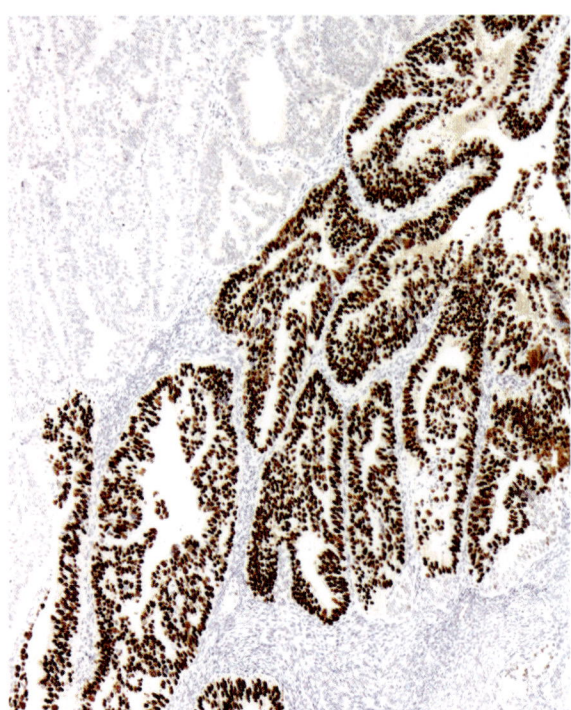

Figure 6-13

MIXED SEROUS AND ENDOMETRIOID CARCINOMA

Serous features are present at the lower right contrasting with endometrioid features at the upper left (left). Aberrant p53 expression helps identify the serous component (right).

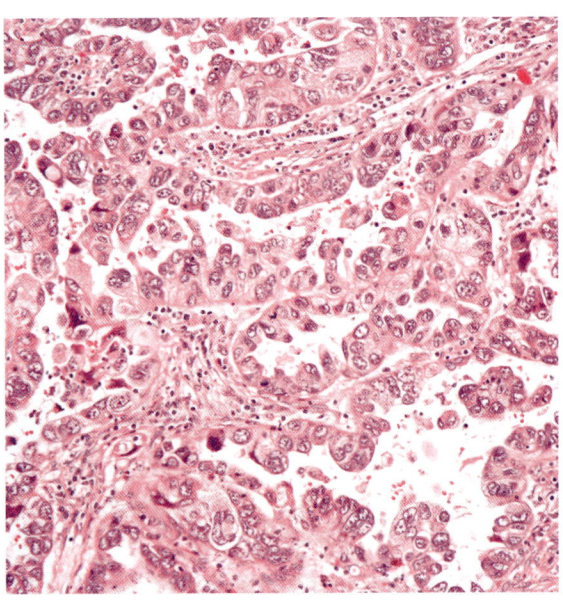

Figure 6-14

POLE-MUTATED CARCINOMA

This heterogeneous endometrial carcinoma contained a component that resembled serous carcinoma (shown here).

positivity (fig. 6-15, right); *BRCA* gene mutation carrier; or small, multifocal tumor deposits in endometrium. Unequivocal WT1 positivity in adnexa and endometrium supports an adnexal origin, but the significance of preferential expression of the marker in only one site or weak, patchy expression is of uncertain significance. The finding of a bona fide low-grade serous carcinoma in the endometrium essentially excludes endometrium as the primary site.

Pleomorphic Undifferentiated Carcinoma. Although purely pleomorphic carcinomas of endometrium undoubtedly exist, anecdotal experience suggests that many, if not most, are merely anaplastic components of high-grade endometrial carcinomas, such as serous or clear cell carcinoma. In the absence of data, there does not seem to be a clear mandate for rigid separation of serous carcinoma with anaplastic features and pleomorphic undifferentiated carcinoma.

Endocervical Adenocarcinoma. Dissociated fragments of high-grade, mucin-poor endocervical carcinoma found in an endometrial or

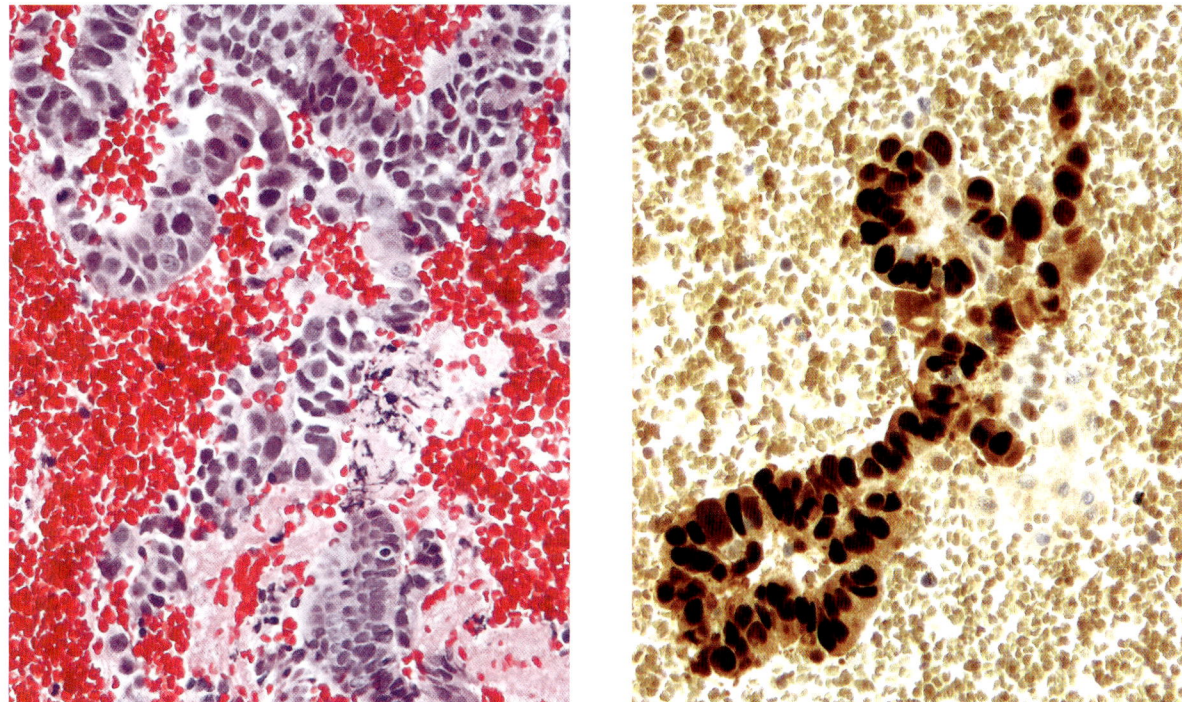

Figure 6-15

ADNEXAL SEROUS CARCINOMA: ENDOMETRIAL DROP METASTASIS

Small, scattered serous carcinoma strips are present adjacent to a non-neoplastic endometrial gland (left). The strips are p53 positive (right). Endometrial serous intraepithelial carcinoma may show similar features.

endocervical curettage might cause concern for serous carcinoma. In a premenopausal or perimenopausal woman, the differential diagnosis includes a drop metastasis of serous carcinoma from the adnexa (discussed above). In a postmenopausal patient with tumor centered in the cervix, the differential diagnosis includes a primary endometrial or adnexal serous carcinoma. Primary serous carcinoma of the endocervix is rare to nonexistent. Strong WT1 expression favors a drop metastasis from the adnexa. p53 and in situ hybridization for high-risk human papillomavirus (HPV) can be applied in this differential diagnosis. Most serous carcinomas and HPV-associated endocervical adenocarcinomas show diffuse p16 overexpression. A tumor with diffuse p16 labeling, aberrant p53 staining, and negative HPV in situ hybridization most likely represents a serous carcinoma, given appropriate morphology.

Reactive Changes. A diagnosis of serous carcinoma may sometimes be considered when atypical cells with hyperchromatic nuclei are found in infarcted endometrial polyps or in surface endometrium subjected to trauma or treatment with radiation. Reactive changes typically represent an incidental and focal finding. Cells show preserved N:C ratios, smudgy chromatin, and only rare or absent mitoses. These changes do not result in aberrant p53 expression and they do not display increased Ki-67 labeling, although a large number of cells with variably intense p53 staining may be present (fig. 6-16) (108,109).

TREATMENT AND PROGNOSIS

Most patients who are determined to have "operable" disease undergo total hysterectomy, bilateral salpingo-oophorectomy, omentectomy, peritoneal biopsies, and either lymphadenectomy or sentinel lymph node biopsies. FIGO stage, patient age, patient performance status, and medical co-morbidities are the most important prognostic factors (110). Interestingly, the impact of race on survival disappears in hospital-based series of serous carcinoma (111).

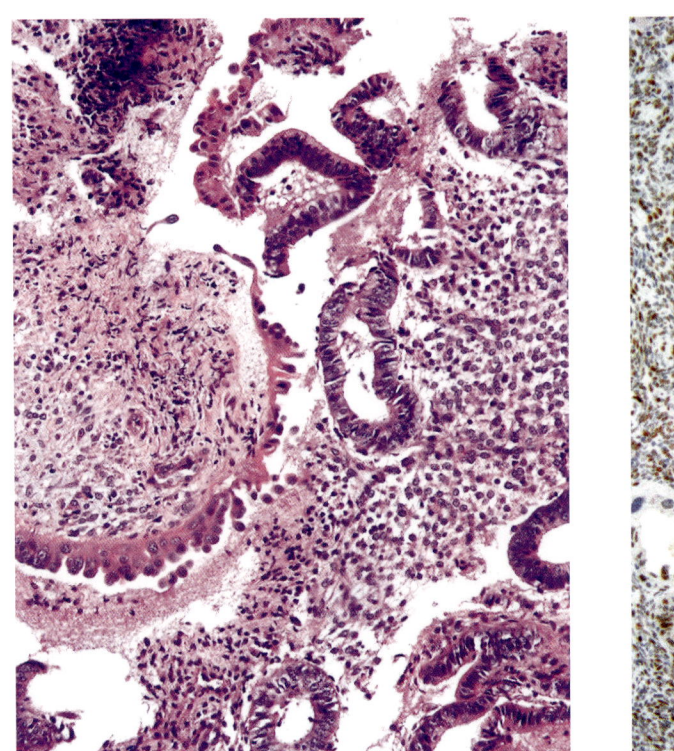 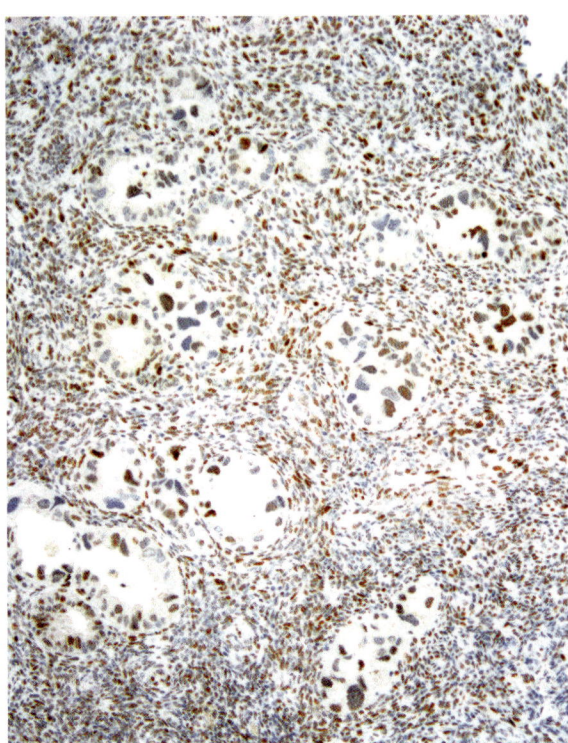

Figure 6-16

MIMICS OF SEROUS CARCINOMA

Hobnail metaplasia (left) may show increased p53 labeling that falls short of "p53 expression," as seen with radiation changes (right). Neither sample would show robust labeling with Ki-67.

Most patients with endometrial serous carcinoma receive adjuvant chemotherapy with carboplatin and taxol. In some centers, pelvic radiation therapy is administered instead of or in combination with chemotherapy. Patients advised not to receive adjuvant chemotherapy include those without residual carcinoma in a well-sampled hysterectomy specimen with good surgical staging and selected patients with residual, but low-volume serous carcinoma confined to the endometrium or endometrial polyp ("minimal serous carcinoma") (112).

The overall 5-year disease-specific survival rate is 40 to 50 percent for patients with serous carcinoma (71,113). Patients who have undergone comprehensive surgical staging with tumor confined to an endometrial polyp have an overall survival rate of about 90 percent, even without chemotherapy (114–120). Other FIGO stage I patients (comprehensively staged and treated with chemotherapy) have a 70 to 80 percent 5-year survival rate, but the presence of extensive lymphovascular invasion may be associated with decreased survival (121). Survival drops to approximately 50 percent with adnexal metastases, 40 percent with pelvic lymph node metastases, and less than 30 percent with omental metastases. Approximately 50 percent of patients will develop recurrences: about 60 percent pelvic, 50 percent abdominal, and 50 percent nodal or visceral. Metastases to lung are not uncommon while brain or liver metastases are less frequent. These values are estimated from studies using large cohorts of patients that have undergone comprehensive staging surgery.

REFERENCES

1. Christopherson WM, Alberhasky RC, Connelly PJ. Carcinoma of the endometrium. II. Papillary adenocarcinoma: a clinical pathological study, 46 cases. Am J Clin Pathol 1982;77:534-40.
2. Hendrickson M, Ross J, Eifel P, Martinez A, Kempson R. Uterine papillary serous carcinoma: a highly malignant form of endometrial adenocarcinoma. Am J Surg Pathol 1982;6:93-108.
3. Lauchlan SC. Tubal (serous) carcinoma of the endometrium. Arch Pathol Lab Med 1981;105:615-8.
4. Walker AN, Mills SE. Serous papillary carcinoma of the endometrium. A clinicopathologic study of 11 cases. Diagn Gynecol Obstet 1982;4:261-7.
5. Cancer Genome Atlas Research Network, Kandoth C, Schultz N, et al. Integrated genomic characterization of endometrial carcinoma. Nature 2013;497:67-73.
6. Randall TC, Armstrong K. Differences in treatment and outcome between African-American and white women with endometrial cancer. J Clin Oncol 2003;21:4200-6.
7. Sherman ME, Devesa SS. Analysis of racial differences in incidence, survival, and mortality for malignant tumors of the uterine corpus. Cancer 2003;98:176-86.
8. Soslow RA, Slomovitz BM, Saqi A, Baergen RN, Caputo TA. Tumor suppressor gene, cell surface adhesion molecule, and multidrug resistance in Mullerian serous carcinomas: clinical divergence without immunophenotypic differences. Gynecol Oncol 2000;79:430-7.
9. Santin AD, Bellone S, Siegel ER, et al. Racial differences in the overexpression of epidermal growth factor type II receptor (HER2/neu): a major prognostic indicator in uterine serous papillary cancer. Am J Obstet Gynecol 2005;192:813-8.
10. Ueda SM, Kapp DS, Cheung MK, et al. Trends in demographic and clinical characteristics in women diagnosed with corpus cancer and their potential impact on the increasing number of deaths. Am J Obstet Gynecol 2008;198:218.e1-6.
11. Wright JD, Fiorelli J, Schiff PB, et al. Racial disparities for uterine corpus tumors: changes in clinical characteristics and treatment over time. Cancer 2009;115:1276-85.
12. Smotkin D, Nevadunsky NS, Harris K, Einstein MH, Yu Y, Goldberg GL. Histopathologic differences account for racial disparity in uterine cancer survival. Gynecol Oncol 2012;127:616-9.
13. Bokhman JV. Two pathogenetic types of endometrial carcinoma. Gynecol Oncol 1983;15:10-7.
14. Felix AS, Weissfeld JL, Stone RA, et al. Factors associated with Type I and Type II endometrial cancer. Cancer Causes Control 2010;21:1851-6.
15. Brinton LA, Felix AS, McMeekin DS, Etiologic heterogeneity in endometrial cancer: evidence from a Gynecologic Oncology Group trial. Gynecol Oncol 2013;129:277-84.
16. Yang HP, Wentzensen N, Trabert B, et al. Endometrial cancer risk factors by 2 main histologic subtypes: the NIH-AARP Diet and Health Study. Am J Epidemiol 2013;177:142-51.
17. Bjorge T, Engeland A, Tretli S, Weiderpass E. Body size in relation to cancer of the uterine corpus in 1 million Norwegian women. Int J Cancer 2007;120:378-83.
18. McCullough ML, Patel AV, Patel R, et al. Body mass and endometrial cancer risk by hormone replacement therapy and cancer subtype. Cancer Epidemiol Biomarkers Preven 2008;17:73-9.
19. Sherman ME, Sturgeon S, Brinton LA, et al. Risk factors and hormone levels in patients with serous and endometrioid uterine carcinomas. Mod Pathol 1997;10:963-8.
20. Setiawan VW, Yang HP, Pike MC, et al. Type I and II endometrial cancers: have they different risk factors? J Clin Oncol 2013;31:2607-18.
21. Magriples U, Naftolin F, Schwartz PE, Carcangiu ML. High-grade endometrial carcinoma in tamoxifen-treated breast cancer patients. J Clin Oncol 1993;11:485-90.
22. Silva EG, Tornos C, Malpica A, Mitchell MF. Uterine neoplasms in patients treated with tamoxifen. J Cell Biochem Suppl 1995;23:179-83.
23. Hoogendoorn WE, Hollema H, van Boven HH, et al. Prognosis of uterine corpus cancer after tamoxifen treatment for breast cancer. Breast Cancer Res Treat 2008;112:99-108.
24. Bland AE, Calingaert B, Secord AA, et al. Relationship between tamoxifen use and high risk endometrial cancer histologic types. Gynecol Oncol 2009;112:150-4.
25. Ferguson SE, Soslow RA, Amsterdam A, Barakat RR. Comparison of uterine malignancies that develop during and following tamoxifen therapy. Gynecol Oncol 2006;101:322-6.
26. Pothuri B, Ramondetta L, Martino M, et al. Development of endometrial cancer after radiation treatment for cervical carcinoma. Obstet Gynecol 2003;101(Pt 1):941-5.

27. Pothuri B, Ramondetta L, Eifel P, et al. Radiation-associated endometrial cancers are prognostically unfavorable tumors: a clinicopathologic comparison with 527 sporadic endometrial cancers. Gynecol Oncol 2006;103:948-51.
28. Fehr PE, Prem KA. Malignancy of the uterine corpus following irradiation therapy for squamous cell carcinoma of the cervix. Am J Obstet Gynecol 1974;119:685-92.
29. Rodriguez J, Hart WR. Endometrial cancers occurring 10 or more years after pelvic irradiation for carcinoma. Int J Gynecol Pathol 1982;1:135-44.
30. Gallion HH, van Nagell JR Jr, Donaldson ES, Powell DE. Endometrial cancer following radiation therapy for cervical cancer. Gynecol Oncol 1987;27:76-83.
31. Parkash V, Carcangiu ML. Uterine papillary serous carcinoma after radiation therapy for carcinoma of the cervix. Cancer 1992;69:496-501.
32. Cirisano FD Jr, Robboy SJ, Dodge RK, et al. Epidemiologic and surgicopathologic findings of papillary serous and clear cell endometrial cancers when compared to endometrioid carcinoma. Gynecol Oncol 1999;74:385-94.
33. Hecht JL, Konstantinopoulos PA, Awtrey CS, Soslow RA. Immunohistochemical loss of BRCA1 protein in uterine serous carcinoma. Int J Gynecol Pathol 2014;33:282-7.
34. Moslehi R, Chu W, Karlan B, et al. BRCA1 and BRCA2 mutation analysis of 208 Ashkenazi Jewish women with ovarian cancer. Am J Hum Genet 2000;66:1259-72.
35. Shu CA, Pike MC, Jotwani AR, et al. Uterine cancer after risk-reducing salpingo-oophorectomy without hysterectomy in women with BRCA mutations. JAMA Oncol 2016;2:1434-40.
36. Zhou B, Yang L, Sun Q, et al. Cigarette smoking and the risk of endometrial cancer: a meta-analysis. Am J Med 2008;121:501-8.e3.
37. Sachmechi I, Kalra J, Molho L, Chawla K. Paraneoplastic hypercalcemia associated with uterine papillary serous carcinoma. Gynecol Oncol 1995;58:378-82.
38. Creasman WT, Kohler MF, Odicino F, Maisonneuve P, Boyle P. Prognosis of papillary serous, clear cell, and grade 3 stage I carcinoma of the endometrium. Gynecol Oncol 2004;95:593-6.
39. Soslow RA, Bissonnette JP, Wilton A, et al. Clinicopathologic analysis of 187 high-grade endometrial carcinomas of different histologic subtypes: similar outcomes belie distinctive biologic differences. Am J Surg Pathol 2007;31:979-87.
40. Hamilton CA, Cheung MK, Osann K, et al. Uterine papillary serous and clear cell carcinomas predict for poorer survival compared to grade 3 endometrioid corpus cancers. Br J Cancer 2006;94:642-6.
41. Cirisano FD Jr, Robboy SJ, Dodge RK, et al. The outcome of stage I-II clinically and surgically staged papillary serous and clear cell endometrial cancers when compared with endometrioid carcinoma. Gynecol Oncol 2000;77:55-65.
42. Seward S, Ali-Fehmi R, Munkarah AR, et al. Outcomes of patients with uterine serous carcinoma using the revised FIGO staging system. Int J Gynecol Cancer 2012;22:452-6.
43. Barlin JN, Soslow RA, Lutz M, et al. Redefining stage I endometrial cancer: incorporating histology, a binary grading system, myometrial invasion, and lymph node assessment. Int J Gynecol Cancer 2013;23:1620-8.
44. Ahmed Q, Hussein Y, Hayek K, et al. Is the two-tier ovarian serous carcinoma grading system potentially useful in stratifying uterine serous carcinoma? A large multi-institutional analysis. Gynecol Oncol 2014;132:372-6.
45. Soslow RA Longacre TA. Uterine pathology: Cambridge illustrated surgical pathology. Cambridge, UK: Cambridge University Press; 2012.
46. Garg K, Soslow RA. Strategies for distinguishing low-grade endometrioid and serous carcinomas of endometrium. Adv Anat Pathol 2012;19:1-10.
47. Garg K, Leitao MM Jr, Wynveen CA, et al. p53 overexpression in morphologically ambiguous endometrial carcinomas correlates with adverse clinical outcomes. Mod Pathol 2010;23:80-92.
48. Lomo L, Nucci MR, Lee KR, et al. Histologic and immunohistochemical decision-making in endometrial adenocarcinoma. Mod Pathol 2008;21:937-42.
49. Ambros RA, Sherman ME, Zahn CM, Bitterman P, Kurman RJ. Endometrial intraepithelial carcinoma: a distinctive lesion specifically associated with tumors displaying serous differentiation. Hum Pathol 1995;26:1260-7.
50. Sherman ME, Bur ME, Kurman RJ. p53 in endometrial cancer and its putative precursors: evidence for diverse pathways of tumorigenesis. Hum Pathol 1995;26:1268-74.
51. Tashiro H, Isacson C, Levine R, Kurman RJ, Cho KR, Hedrick L. p53 gene mutations are common in uterine serous carcinoma and occur early in their pathogenesis. Am J Pathol 1997;150:177-85.
52. Soslow RA, Pirog E, Isacson C. Endometrial intraepithelial carcinoma with associated peritoneal carcinomatosis. Am J Surg Pathol 2000;24:726-32.
53. Zheng W, Schwartz PE. Serous EIC as an early form of uterine papillary serous carcinoma: recent progress in understanding its pathogenesis and current opinions regarding pathologic and clinical management. Gynecol Oncol 2005;96:579-82.

54. Spiegel GW. Endometrial carcinoma in situ in postmenopausal women. Am J Surg Pathol 1995;19:417-32.
55. Euscher ED, Malpica A, Deavers MT, Silva EG. Differential expression of WT-1 in serous carcinomas in the peritoneum with or without associated serous carcinoma in endometrial polyps. Am J Surg Pathol 2005;29:1074-8.
56. Hui P, Kelly M, O'Malley DM, Tavassoli F, Schwartz PE. Minimal uterine serous carcinoma: a clinicopathological study of 40 cases. Mod Pathol 2005;18:75-82.
57. Stewart CJ, Doherty DA, Havlat M, et al. Transtubal spread of endometrial carcinoma: correlation of intra-luminal tumour cells with tumour grade, peritoneal fluid cytology, and extra-uterine metastasis. Pathology 2013;45:382-7.
58. Mulligan AM, Plotkin A, Rouzbahman M, Soslow RA, Gilks CB, Clarke BA. Endometrial giant cell carcinoma: a case series and review of the spectrum of endometrial neoplasms containing giant cells. Am J Surg Pathol 2010;34:1132-8.
59. Horn LC, Hanel C, Bartholdt E, Dietel J. Serous carcinoma of the endometrium with choriocarcinomatous differentiation: a case report and review of the literature indicate the existence of 2 prognostically relevant tumor types. Int J Gynecol Pathol 2006;25:247-51.
60. Horn LC, Hanel C, Bartholdt E, Dietel J. Mixed serous carcinoma of the endometrium with trophoblastic differentiation: analysis of the p53 tumor suppressor gene suggests stem cell origin. Ann Diagn Pathol 2008;12:1-3.
61. Posligua L, Malpica A, Liu J, Brown J, Deavers MT. Combined large cell neuroendocrine carcinoma and papillary serous carcinoma of the endometrium with pagetoid spread. Arch Pathol Lab Med 2008;132:1821-4.
62. Kos Z, Broaddus RR, Djordjevic B. Fallopian tube high-grade serous carcinoma with intramucosal spread and presenting as a malignancy on pap smear. Int J Gynecol Pathol 2014;33:443-8.
63. Euscher E, Malpica A. Use of immunohistochemistry in the diagnosis of miscellaneous and metastatic tumors of the uterine corpus and cervix. Semin Diagn Pathol 2014;31:233-57.
64. Jia L, Liu Y, Yi X, et al. Endometrial glandular dysplasia with frequent p53 gene mutation: a genetic evidence supporting its precancer nature for endometrial serous carcinoma. Clin Cancer Res 2008;14:2263-9.
65. Zheng W, Liang SX, Yu H, Rutherford T, Chambers SK, Schwartz PE. Endometrial glandular dysplasia: a newly defined precursor lesion of uterine papillary serous carcinoma. Part I: morphologic features. Int J Surg Pathol 2004;12:207-23.
66. Liang SX, Chambers SK, Cheng L, Zhang S, Zhou Y, Zheng W. Endometrial glandular dysplasia: a putative precursor lesion of uterine papillary serous carcinoma. Part II: molecular features. Int J Surg Pathol 2004;12:319-31.
67. Zheng W, Liang SX, Yi X, Ulukus EC, Davis JR, Chambers SK. Occurrence of endometrial glandular dysplasia precedes uterine papillary serous carcinoma. Int J Gynecol Pathol 2007;26:38-52.
68. Fadare O, Zheng W. Endometrial glandular dysplasia (EmGD): morphologically and biologically distinctive putative precursor lesions of Type II endometrial cancers. Diagn Pathol 2008;3:6.
69. Zheng W, Xiang L, Fadare O, Kong B. A proposed model for endometrial serous carcinogenesis. Am J Surg Pathol 2011;35:e1-e14.
70. Alkushi A, Clarke BA, Akbari M, et al. Identification of prognostically relevant and reproducible subsets of endometrial adenocarcinoma based on clustering analysis of immunostaining data. Mod Pathol 2007;20:1156-65.
71. Carcangiu ML, Chambers JT. Uterine papillary serous carcinoma: a study on 108 cases with emphasis on the prognostic significance of associated endometrioid carcinoma, absence of invasion, and concomitant ovarian carcinoma. Gynecol Oncol 1992;47:298-305.
72. Chambers JT, Carcangiu ML, Voynick IM, Schwartz PE. Immunohistochemical evaluation of estrogen and progesterone receptor content in 183 patients with endometrial carcinoma. Part II: Correlation between biochemical and immunohistochemical methods and survival. Am J Clin Pathol 1990;94:255-60.
73. Chen W, Husain A, Nelson GS, et al. Immunohistochemical Profiling of Endometrial Serous Carcinoma. Int J Gynecol Pathol 2017;36:128-39.
74. Darvishian F, Hummer AJ, Thaler HT, et al. Serous endometrial cancers that mimic endometrioid adenocarcinomas: a clinicopathologic and immunohistochemical study of a group of problematic cases. Am J Surg Pathol 2004;28:1568-78.
75. Lax SF, Pizer ES, Ronnett BM, Kurman RJ. Comparison of estrogen and progesterone receptor, Ki-67, and p53 immunoreactivity in uterine endometrioid carcinoma and endometrioid carcinoma with squamous, mucinous, secretory, and ciliated cell differentiation. Hum Pathol 1998;29:924-31.
76. Acs G, Pasha T, Zhang PJ. WT1 is differentially expressed in serous, endometrioid, clear cell, and mucinous carcinomas of the peritoneum, fallopian tube, ovary, and endometrium. Int J Gynecol Pathol 2004;23:110-8.
77. Dupont J, Wang X, Marshall DS, et al. Wilms Tumor Gene (WT1) and p53 expression in endometrial carcinomas: a study of 130 cases using a tissue microarray. Gynecol Oncol 2004;94:449-55.

78. Egan JA, Ionescu MC, Eapen E, Jones JG, Marshall DS. Differential expression of WT1 and p53 in serous and endometrioid carcinomas of the endometrium. Int J Gynecol Pathol 2004;23:119-22.
79. Goldstein NS, Uzieblo A. WT1 immunoreactivity in uterine papillary serous carcinomas is different from ovarian serous carcinomas. Am J Clin Pathol 2002;117:541-5.
80. Lax SF, Kendall B, Tashiro H, Slebos RJ, Hedrick L. The frequency of p53, K-ras mutations, and microsatellite instability differs in uterine endometrioid and serous carcinoma: evidence of distinct molecular genetic pathways. Cancer 2000;88:814-24.
81. Soslow RA, Shen PU, Chung MH, Isacson C. Distinctive p53 and mdm2 immunohistochemical expression profiles suggest different pathogenetic pathways in poorly differentiated endometrial carcinoma. Int J Gynecol Pathol 1998;17:129-34.
82. Tashiro H, Blazes MS, Wu R, et al. Mutations in PTEN are frequent in endometrial carcinoma but rare in other common gynecological malignancies. Cancer Res 1997;57:3935-40.
83. Zheng W, Khurana R, Farahmand S, Wang Y, Zhang ZF, Felix JC. p53 immunostaining as a significant adjunct diagnostic method for uterine surface carcinoma: precursor of uterine papillary serous carcinoma. Am J Surg Pathol 1998;22:1463-73.
84. Prat J, Oliva E, Lerma E, Vaquero M, Matias-Guiu X. Uterine papillary serous adenocarcinoma. A 10-case study of p53 and c-erbB-2 expression and DNA content. Cancer 1994;74:1778-83.
85. Fadare O, Roma AA, Parkash V, Zheng W, Walavalkar V. Does a p53 "wild-type" immunophenotype exclude a diagnosis of endometrial serous carcinoma? Adv Anat Pathol 2018;25:61-70.
86. Yemelyanova A, Ji H, Shih IeM, Wang TL, Wu LS, Ronnett BM. Utility of p16 expression for distinction of uterine serous carcinomas from endometrial endometrioid and endocervical adenocarcinomas: immunohistochemical analysis of 201 cases. Am J Surg Pathol 2009;33:1504-14.
87. Reid-Nicholson M, Iyengar P, Hummer AJ, Linkov I, Asher M, Soslow RA. Immunophenotypic diversity of endometrial adenocarcinomas: implications for differential diagnosis. Mod Pathol 2006;19:1091-100.
88. Chiesa-Vottero AG, Malpica A, Deavers MT, Broaddus R, Nuovo GJ, Silva EG. Immunohistochemical overexpression of p16 and p53 in uterine serous carcinoma and ovarian high-grade serous carcinoma. Int J Gynecol Pathol 2007;26:328-33.
89. Sun H, Enomoto T, Fujita M, et al. Mutational analysis of the PTEN gene in endometrial carcinoma and hyperplasia. Am J Clin Pathol 2001;115:32-8.
90. Risinger JI, Hayes K, Maxwell GL, et al. PTEN mutation in endometrial cancers is associated with favorable clinical and pathologic characteristics. Clin Cancer Res 1998;4:3005-10.
91. Garg K, Broaddus RR, Soslow RA, Urbauer DL, Levine DA, Djordjevic B. Pathologic scoring of PTEN immunohistochemistry in endometrial carcinoma is highly reproducible. Int J Gynecol Pathol 2012;31:48-56.
92. Mhawech-Fauceglia P, Yan L, Liu S, Pejovic T. ER+ /PR+ /TFF3+ /IMP3- immunoprofile distinguishes endometrioid from serous and clear cell carcinomas of the endometrium: a study of 401 cases. Histopathology 2013;62:976-85.
93. Soslow RA, Wethington SL, Cesari M, et al. Clinicopathologic analysis of matched primary and recurrent endometrial carcinoma. Am J Surg Pathol 2012;36:1771-81.
94. Espinosa I, D'Angelo E, Palacios J, Prat J. Mixed and ambiguous endometrial carcinomas: a heterogenous group of tumors with different clinicopathologic and molecular genetic features. Am J Surg Pathol 2016;40:972-81.
95. Alkushi A, Abdul-Rahman ZH, Lim P, et al. Description of a novel system for grading of endometrial carcinoma and comparison with existing grading systems. Am J Surg Pathol 2005;29:295-304.
96. Alvarez T, Miller E, Duska L, Oliva E. Molecular profile of grade 3 endometrioid endometrial carcinoma: is it a type I or type II endometrial carcinoma? Am J Surg Pathol 2012;36:753-61.
97. Halperin R, Zehavi S, Habler L, Hadas E, Bukovsky I, Schneider D. Comparative immunohistochemical study of endometrioid and serous papillary carcinoma of endometrium. Eur J Gynaecol Oncol 2001;22:122-6.
98. Riethdorf L, Begemann C, Riethdorf S, Milde-Langosch K, Loning T. Comparison of benign and malignant endometrial lesions for their p53 state, using immunohistochemistry and temperature-gradient gel electrophoresis. Virchows Arch 1996;428:47-51.
99. Zannoni GF, Vellone VG, Arena V, et al. Does high-grade endometrioid carcinoma (grade 3 FIGO) belong to type I or type II endometrial cancer? A clinical-pathological and immunohistochemical study. Virchows Arch 2010;457:27-34.
100. Arai T, Watanabe J, Kawaguchi M, et al. Clear cell adenocarcinoma of the endometrium is a biologically distinct entity from endometrioid adenocarcinoma. Int J Gynecol Cancer 2006;16:391-5.
101. DeLair DF, Burke KA, Selenica P, et al. The genetic landscape of endometrial clear cell carcinomas. J Pathol 2017;243:230-41.

102. Fadare O, Gwin K, Desouki MM, et al. The clinicopathologic significance of p53 and BAF-250a (ARID1A) expression in clear cell carcinoma of the endometrium. Mod Pathol 2013;26:1101-10.
103. Kobel M, Meng B, Hoang LN, et al. Molecular analysis of mixed endometrial carcinomas shows clonality in most cases. Am J Surg Pathol 2016;40:166-80.
104. Soslow RA. Endometrial carcinomas with ambiguous features. Seminars in diagnostic pathology. 2010;27:261-73.
105. Soslow RA. High-grade endometrial carcinomas—strategies for typing. Histopathology 2013;62:89-110.
106. Hussein YR, Broaddus R, Weigelt B, Levine DA, Soslow RA. The genomic heterogeneity of FIGO grade 3 endometrioid carcinoma impacts diagnostic accuracy and reproducibility. Int J Gynecol Pathol 2016;35:16-24.
107. Hussein YR, Weigelt B, Levine DA, et al. Clinicopathological analysis of endometrial carcinomas harboring somatic POLE exonuclease domain mutations. Mod Pathol 2015;28:505-14.
107a. Kurman RJ, Carcangiu ML, Herrington CS, Young RH. WHO classification of tumours of female reproductive organs, 4th ed. Lyon: IARC Press; 2014;6.
108. McCluggage G, McBride H, Maxwell P, Bharucha H. Immunohistochemical detection of p53 and bcl-2 proteins in neoplastic and non-neoplastic endocervical glandular lesions. Int J Gynecol Pathol 1997;16:22-7.
109. McCluggage WG, McBride HA. Papillary syncytial metaplasia associated with endometrial breakdown exhibits an immunophenotype that overlaps with uterine serous carcinoma. Int J Gynecol Pathol 2012;31:206-10.
110. SGO Clinical Practice Endometrial Cancer Working Group, Burke WM, Orr J, et al. Endometrial cancer: a review and current management strategies: part II. Gynecol Oncol 2014;134:393-402.
111. Al-Wahab Z, Ali-Fehmi R, Cote ML, et al. The impact of race on survival in uterine serous carcinoma: a hospital-based study. Gynecol Oncol 2011;121:577-80.
112. Wheeler DT, Bell KA, Kurman RJ, Sherman ME. Minimal uterine serous carcinoma: diagnosis and clinicopathologic correlation. Am J Surg Pathol 2000;24:797-806.
113. Abeler VM, Kjorstad KE. Serous papillary carcinoma of the endometrium: a histopathological study of 22 cases. Gynecol Oncol 1990;39:266-71.
114. van der Putten LJ, Hoskins P, Tinker A, Lim P, Aquino-Parsons C, Kwon JS. Population-based treatment and outcomes of Stage I uterine serous carcinoma. Gynecol Oncol 2014;132:61-4.
115. Desai NB, Kiess AP, Kollmeier MA, et al. Patterns of relapse in stage I-II uterine papillary serous carcinoma treated with adjuvant intravaginal radiation (IVRT) with or without chemotherapy. Gynecol Oncol 2013;131:604-8.
116. Kelly MG, O'Malley D M, Hui P, et al. Improved survival in surgical stage I patients with uterine papillary serous carcinoma (UPSC) treated with adjuvant platinum-based chemotherapy. Gynecol Oncol 2005;98:353-9.
117. Elit L, Kwon J, Bentley J, Trim K, Ackerman I, Carey M. Optimal management for surgically Stage 1 serous cancer of the uterus. Gynecol Oncol 2004;92:240-6.
118. Slomovitz BM, Burke TW, Eifel PJ, et al. Uterine papillary serous carcinoma (UPSC): a single institution review of 129 cases. Gynecol Oncol 2003;91:463-9.
119. Growdon WB, Rauh-Hain JJ, Cordon A, et al. Prognostic determinants in patients with stage I uterine papillary serous carcinoma: a 15-year multi-institutional review. Int J Gynecol Cancer 2012;22:417-24.
120. Huh WK, Powell M, Leath CA 3rd, et al. Uterine papillary serous carcinoma: comparisons of outcomes in surgical Stage I patients with and without adjuvant therapy. Gynecol Oncol 2003;91:470-5.
121. Winer I, Ahmed QF, Mert I, et al. Significance of lymphovascular space invasion in uterine serous carcinoma: what matters more; extent or presence? Int J Gynecol Pathol 2015;34:47-56.

7 CLEAR CELL CARCINOMA

Clear cell carcinoma is a high-grade malignant epithelial neoplasm composed of non- or minimally stratified, cuboidal or flat cells, usually with clear cytoplasm, arranged in papillary, glandular, tubulocystic, and/or solid patterns. The nuclei are malignant but typically uniform in appearance. The combination of architectural, nuclear, and cytoplasmic features is definitional; the presence of clear cytoplasm in isolation, while characteristic, is neither an entirely sensitive nor specific diagnostic feature.

GENERAL FEATURES

Clear cell carcinoma constitutes less than 5 percent of all endometrial carcinomas when a high threshold is applied for its diagnosis (1,2). Little is known about the epidemiologic risk factors due to poor reproducibility in diagnosis. Historically, many clear cell carcinomas were grouped with serous carcinomas because of the assumption that clear cell carcinomas were "type 2 endometrial carcinomas."

CLINICAL FEATURES

Patients with clear cell carcinoma are diagnosed at a median age of 65 to 68 years, although younger patients are also affected. Vaginal bleeding and disease confined to the uterus occur in 40 to 60 percent of patients while about 15 percent have adnexal metastases. The remainder have metastases to regional lymph nodes or omentum (3–8).

Paraneoplastic syndromes, including thromboembolic disease (9–12) and hypercalcemia (11,13,14), are associated manifestations. Progressive cerebellar syndrome (15) and bilateral diffuse uveal melanocytic proliferation (16) have also been reported on occasion. The occurrence of thromboembolic disease may be linked to the expression of tissue factor and heparinase, as well as hepatocyte nuclear factor 1 beta (HNF-1β) (9,17). Clear cell carcinoma can arise in the setting of Lynch syndrome (18–20), accounting for its occasional presentation in patients younger than 60 years, as well as in patients treated with tamoxifen (21).

GROSS FINDINGS

Uteri harboring clear cell carcinomas tend to be smaller than those with endometrioid carcinoma since they are typically seen in postmenopausal patients. The tumors often present as polypoid fleshy masses that extensively involve the endometrium, or they may be found in an endometrial polyp (about 10 percent) (22), but less frequently than serous carcinoma (fig. 7-1). Myometrial invasion is common. Rarely, clear cell carcinoma is centered in the myometrium in association with adenomyosis (23).

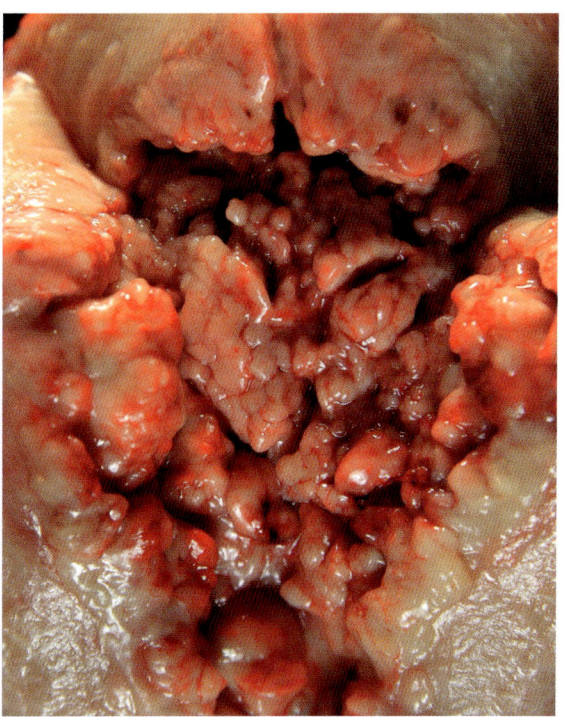

Figure 7-1

CLEAR CELL CARCINOMA

The tumor extensively involves the endometrium, forming multiple polypoid masses.

Figure 7-2

CLEAR CELL CARCINOMA WITH PAPILLARY GROWTH

Multiple round and hyalinized small papillae are lined by a monolayer of cuboidal cells (A). Papillae may have prominent myxoid stroma (B) or be empty "ringlets" (C).

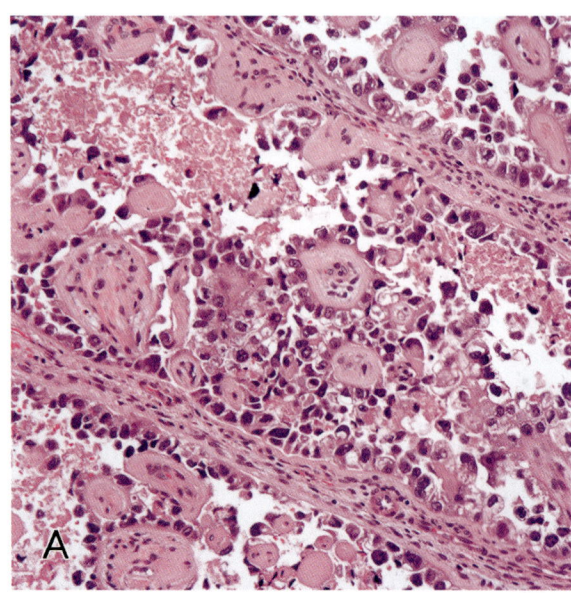
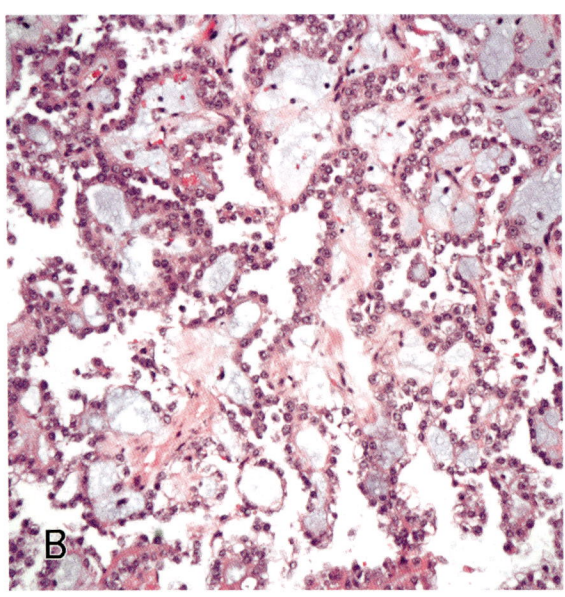
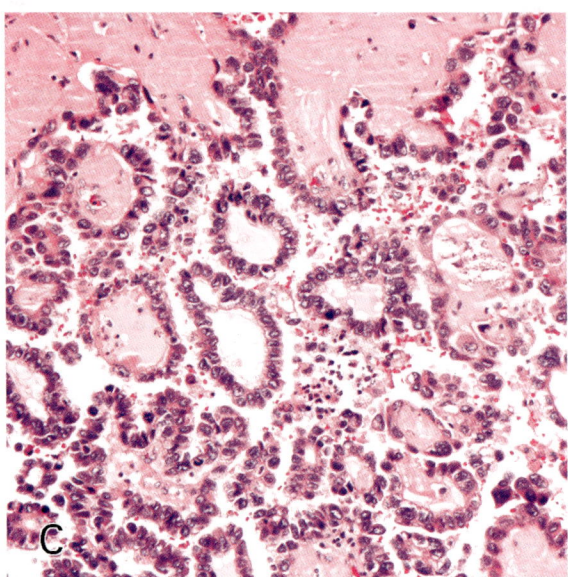

MICROSCOPIC FINDINGS

Previously, a significant number of serous and endometrioid carcinomas were misclassified as clear cell carcinomas due to the finding of cells with clear cytoplasm. Although most clear cell carcinomas have cells with clear cytoplasm, many display only cells with "oxyphilic" cytoplasm (24). The diagnosis of clear cell carcinoma should be based only on the presence of the specific architectural patterns and cytologic features.

A recent study emphasized the following features of clear cell carcinoma that allow for a reproducible diagnosis: 1) glands and papillae lined by cuboidal to flat, noncolumnar cells; 2) nuclear stratification absent or present only focally within glands and papillae; and 3) absence or only focal severe nuclear pleomorphism (22,25). Typically, clear cell carcinomas are not assigned a grade and they are by definition high grade.

Architectural Findings

Clear cell carcinomas display papillary, glandular, tubulocystic, and solid architecture, and commonly more than one pattern is present. Papillae tend to be round and small, and typically lack the extensive branching or cellular

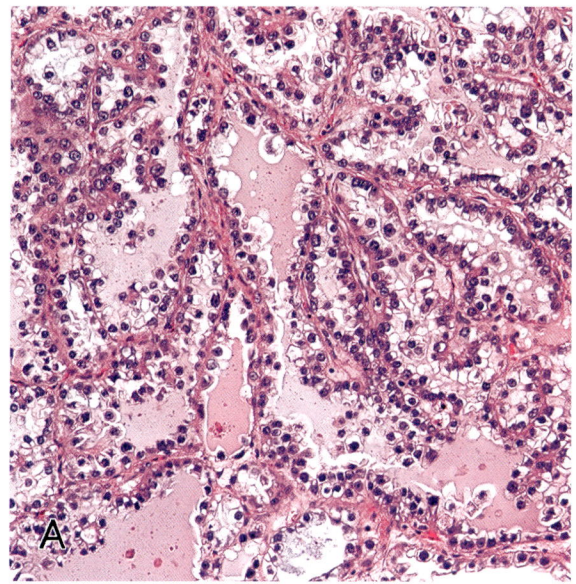
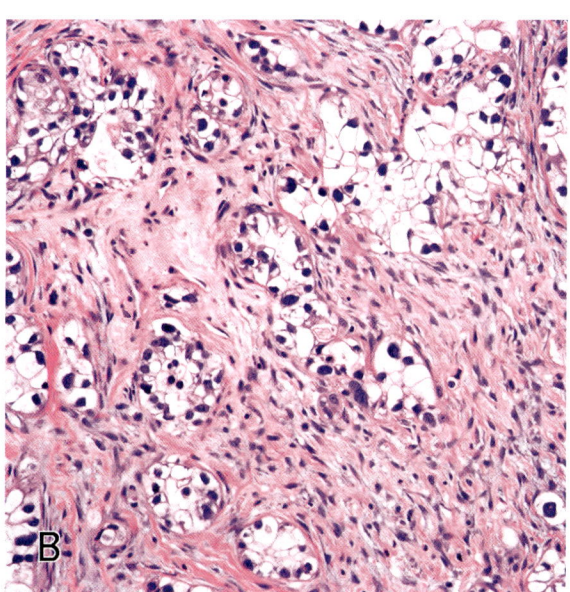
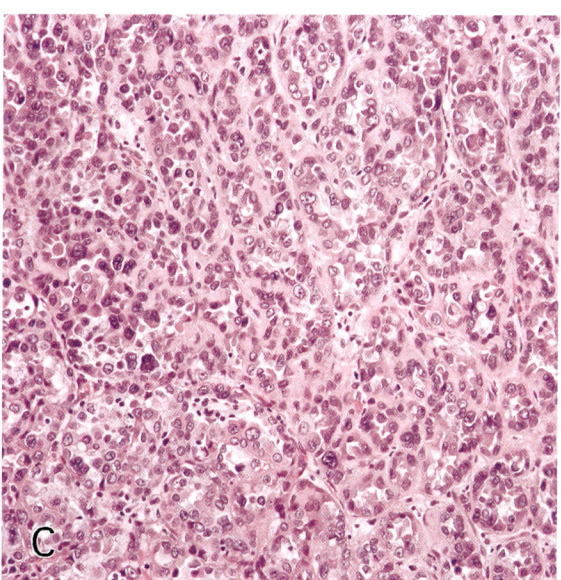

Figure 7-3

CLEAR CELL CARCINOMA WITH GLANDULAR GROWTH

Nondescript glands are closely packed and lined by a monolayer of cuboidal cells with clear cytoplasm and monomorphic nuclei (A). Small irregularly shaped glands have a haphazard distribution in fibroblastic/reactive stroma. They are lined by cuboidal cells with clear cytoplasm that focally fill the lumens (B). Back-to-back glands with collapsed lumens are lined by cuboidal to flattened cells with eosinophilic cytoplasm; rare enlarged nuclei are found (C).

stratification characteristic of serous carcinoma. However, papillae may be larger, irregular in shape, or complex; in these cases, more characteristic round papillae are also present. The cores of the papillae may be hyalinized, but they may be empty (ringlets) or have myxoid stroma (fig. 7-2). A nondescript glandular architecture may be present, but it is usually not extensive (fig. 7-3). The tubulocystic pattern is characterized by variably sized tubules and cysts with luminal eosinophilic or basophilic (mucin) contents (fig. 7-4).

Papillae, glands, tubules, and cysts are lined by a monolayer of cuboidal to flattened cells that lack appreciable budding and detachment. Cellular stratification is present in only about 5 percent of tumors, in contrast to serous carcinomas (22). Clear cell carcinomas with a purely solid growth are uncommon, and if present, it typically coexists with other patterns that usually predominate (figs. 7-5, 7-6). Overall, glands are reportedly present in about 80 percent, papillae in about 70 percent, solid pattern in 50 percent, and tubules and cysts in about 30 percent of clear cell carcinomas of the uterus (22). Combinations of the different patterns are characteristic, as mentioned previously (fig.

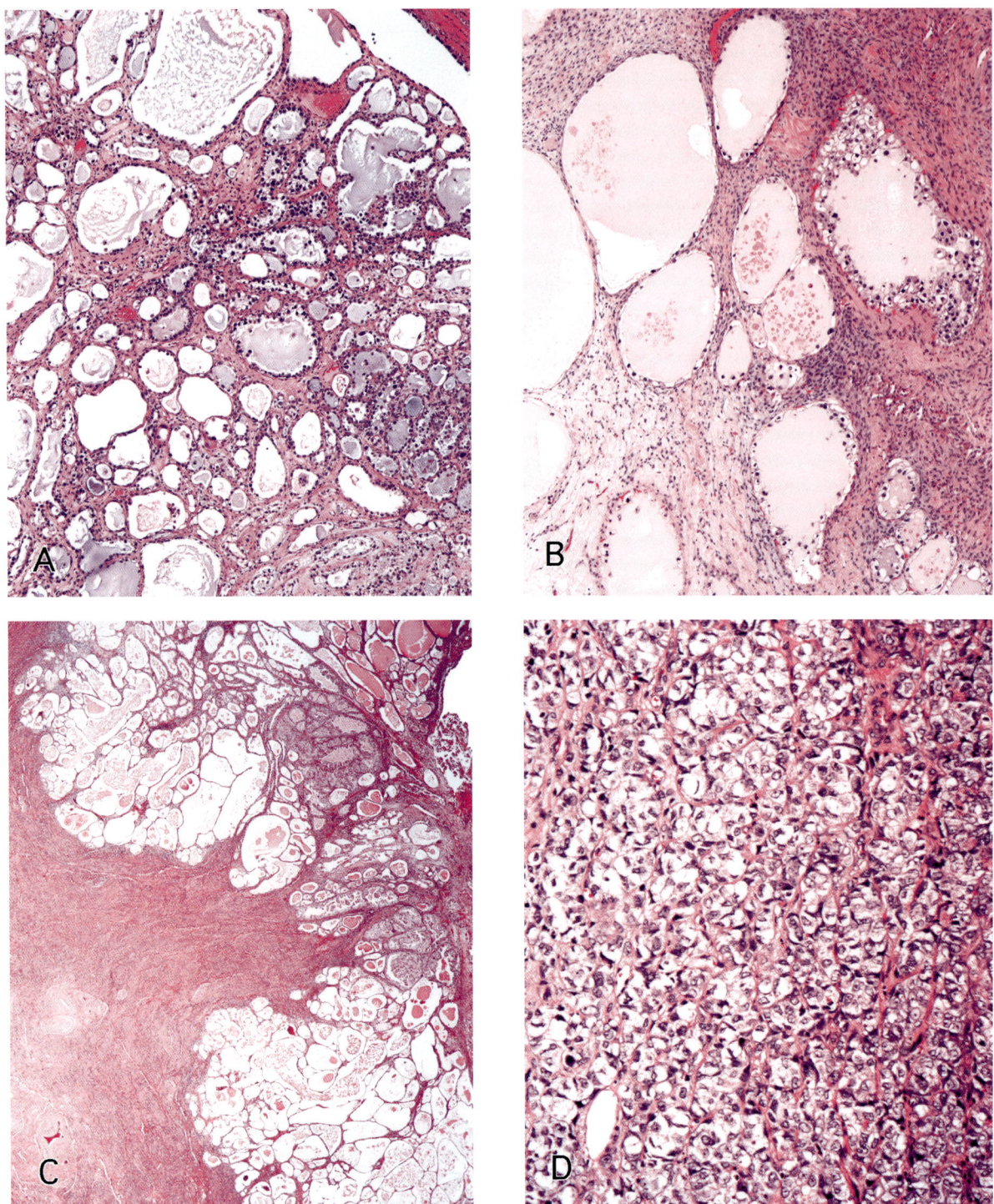

Figure 7-4

CLEAR CELL CARCINOMA WITH TUBULOCYSTIC GROWTH

Tubules and cysts containing predominantly basophilic material are lined by flattened to low cuboidal cells (A). At intermediate magnification, cysts show hobnail and clear cells, with some enlarged, hyperchromatic nuclei (B). Some clear cell carcinomas are predominantly cystic. A confluent growth pattern is seen (C). In some instances, lumens are obliterated by tumor cells (D).

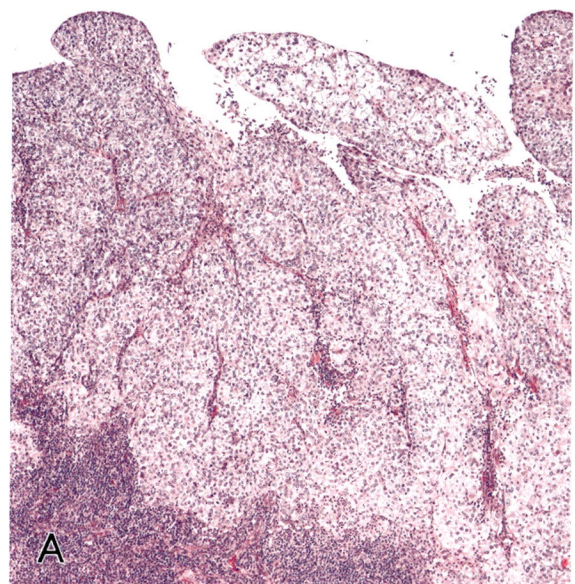
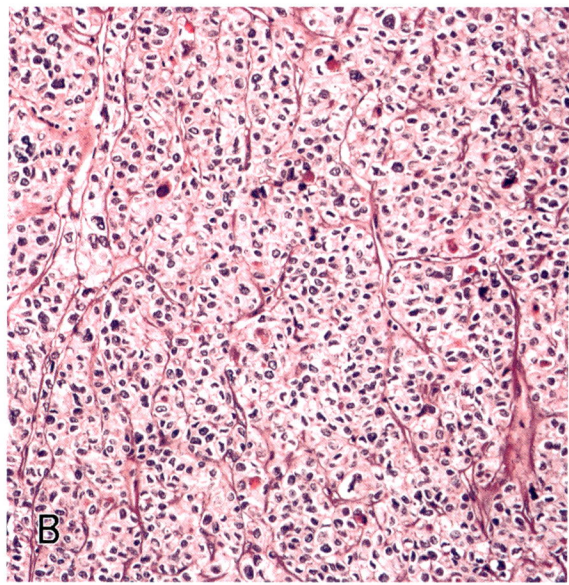
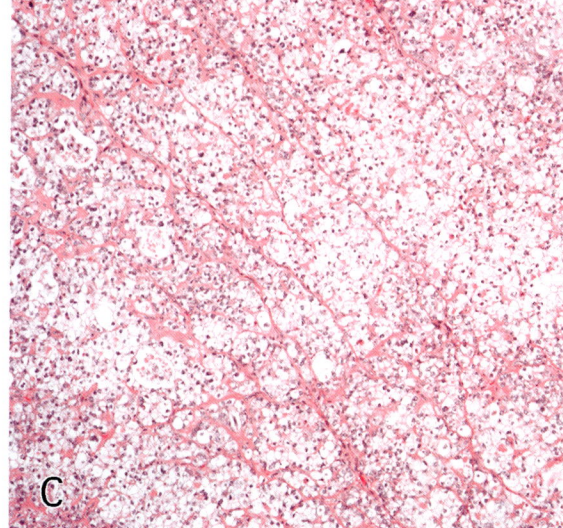

Figure 7-5

CLEAR CELL CARCINOMA WITH SOLID GROWTH

Solid growth is uncommon in clear cell carcinoma and only rarely the predominant component. Shown at low power is a solid clear cell carcinoma with an appearance simulating transitional cell carcinoma. The solid microacini are filled by clear cells (top) and the lymphoplasmacytic infiltrate is tracking along intratumoral septa and at the tumor base (A). Higher-power magnification demonstrates packets of polygonal cells with clear to eosinophilic cytoplasm and variably sized, hyperchromatic and sometimes koilocyte-like nuclei (B). The solid growth may display coalescent large nests and islands of tumor cells (C).

7-6), but 5 to 30 percent of tumors may feature one predominant pattern.

Cytologic Findings

Clear cell carcinomas usually display cuboidal cells (fig. 7-7), but flattened cells are more typically seen with the tubulocystic pattern. It has been reported that clear cells are the sole or predominant cell type in approximately 40 percent of tumors, eosinophilic cells predominate in about 40 percent (although that figure seems higher than what would be estimated based on anecdote), while equal combinations of cells with clear and eosinophilic cytoplasm are seen in the remainder (22). Hobnail cells are easily found in about 60 percent of tumors and the nuclear to cytoplasmic (N:C) ratio may appear increased when compared to nonhobnail cells (22). Hyaline globules and targetoid bodies (mucin droplets within cytoplasmic vacuoles) are common, and psammoma bodies may also be present, most commonly in papillary clear cell carcinomas (fig. 7-8).

Clear cell carcinomas typically feature nuclear uniformity (fig. 7-9). Ninety-five percent of these tumors have an overall nuclear grade of 2 (out of 3) and only less than 5 percent display

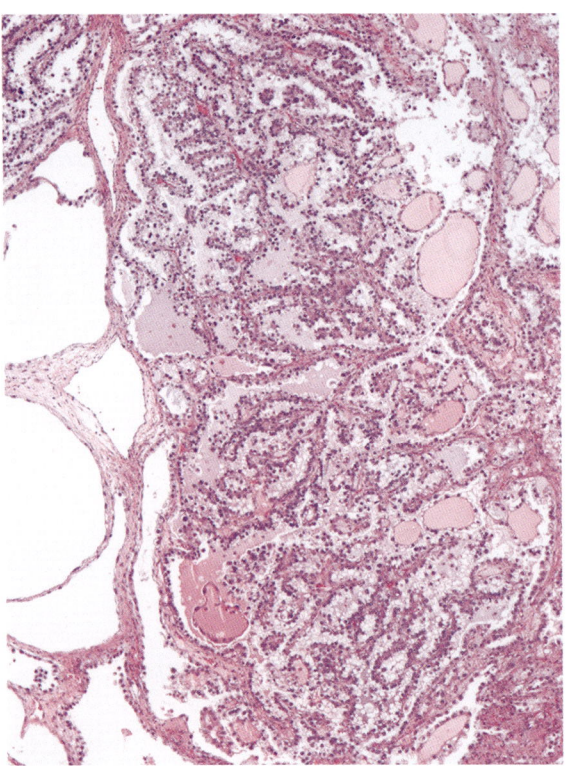 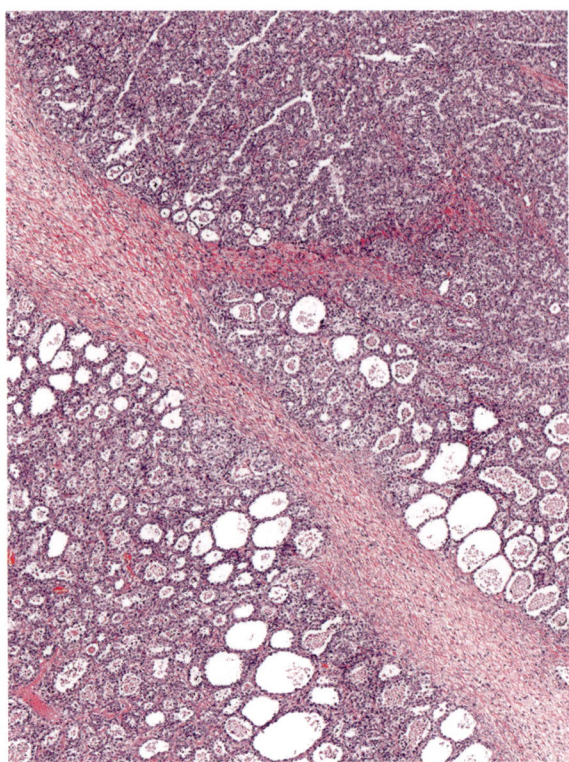

Figure 7-6

CLEAR CELL CARCINOMA

Mixed architectural patterns are frequent, with tubulocystic and papillary being the most common combination (left). An admixture of tubulocystic and solid (top) growth is uncommon (right).

overt diffusely distributed nuclear pleomorphism. More than 50 percent of tumors, however, have enlarged and bizarre nuclei as a minor component (22). Papillary, glandular, and most solid clear cell carcinomas display round nuclei, frequently with a prominent nucleolus, whereas tubulocystic and solid areas and hobnail cells display hyperchromatic nuclei. Some solid tumors have koilocyte-like nuclei, and nuclear pseudoinclusions are found occasionally. The mean and median mitotic indices are 4.5 and 2 per 10 high-power fields, respectively. Nevertheless, approximately 20 percent of tumors have a significantly higher mitotic index, similar to that seen in serous carcinomas (22).

Stromal Features

Although the stroma of clear cell carcinoma can be nondescript, there are several recurrent and characteristic features. These include stromal hyalinization (fig. 7-10) and myxoid deposition, present in about 30 percent and 10 percent of tumors, respectively (22). These features are most striking within the stromal cores of the papillary structures. The stroma is otherwise often fibroblastic or collagenous. Appreciable associated plasma cell inflammation and, much less frequently, neutrophilic infiltrates, are seen (fig. 7-11).

Anaplastic or "Undifferentiated" Clear Cell Carcinoma

Clear cell carcinoma may have an anaplastic appearance in the primary or recurrent setting (personal observation). These tumors contain noncohesive round to polygonal cells with large, bizarre nuclei arranged in sheets, in a background of abundant neutrophils (fig. 7-12). Tumors with these features can only be confidently diagnosed as clear cell carcinoma given a history of clear cell carcinoma or when found as a component of a tumor with characteristic clear cell carcinoma morphology.

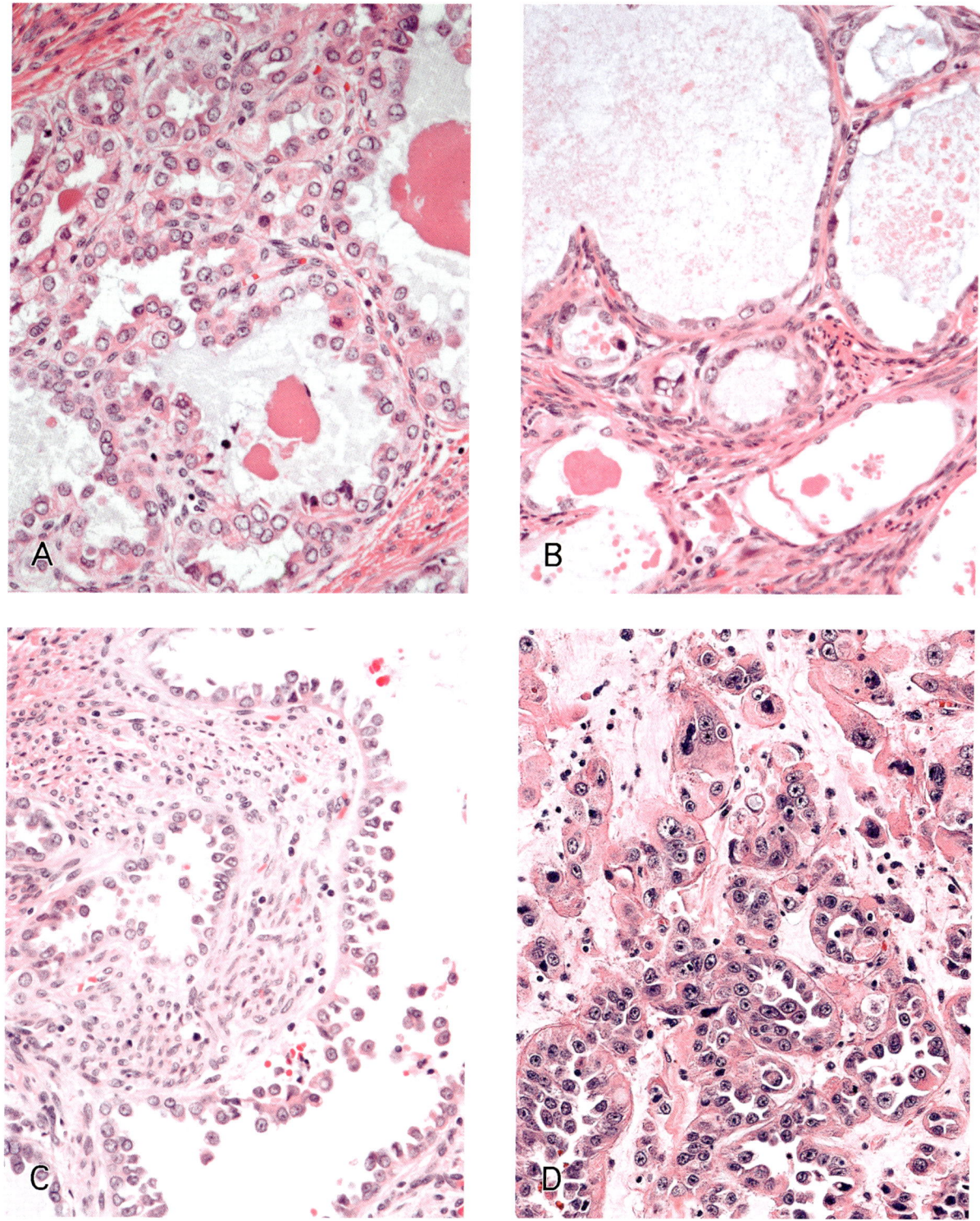

Figure 7-7

CLEAR CELL CARCINOMA

Cells are often cuboidal (A) or flattened (B) and may be hobnail when in cysts or papillae (C). Oxyphilic cells are less common (D).

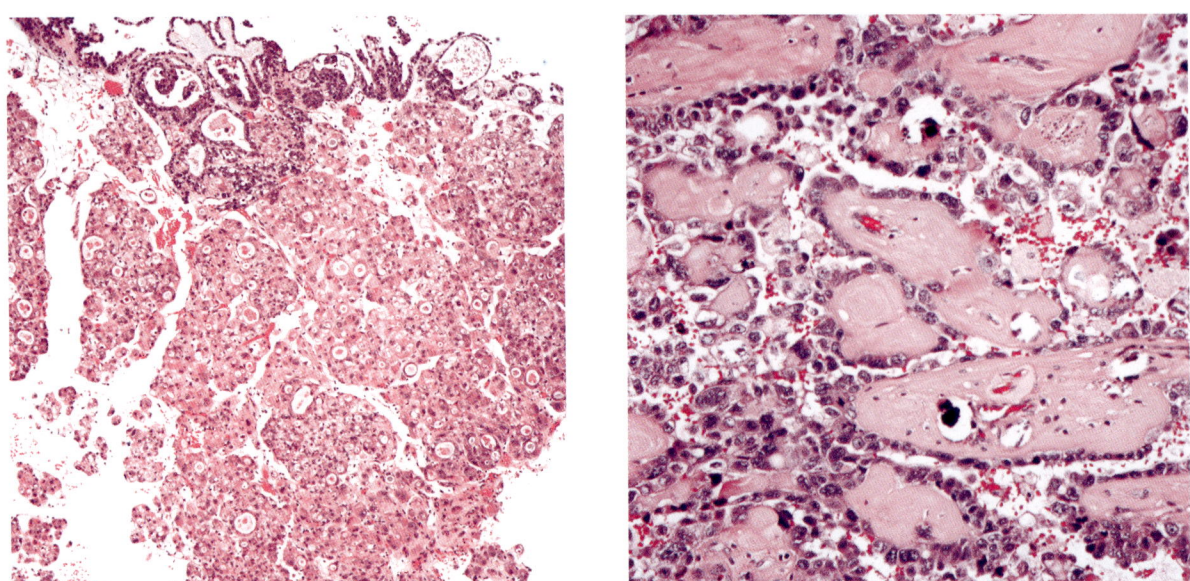

Figure 7-8

CLEAR CELL CARCINOMA

Intracytoplasmic targetoid bodies (left) are characteristic and more common than psammoma bodies (right) in clear cell carcinoma.

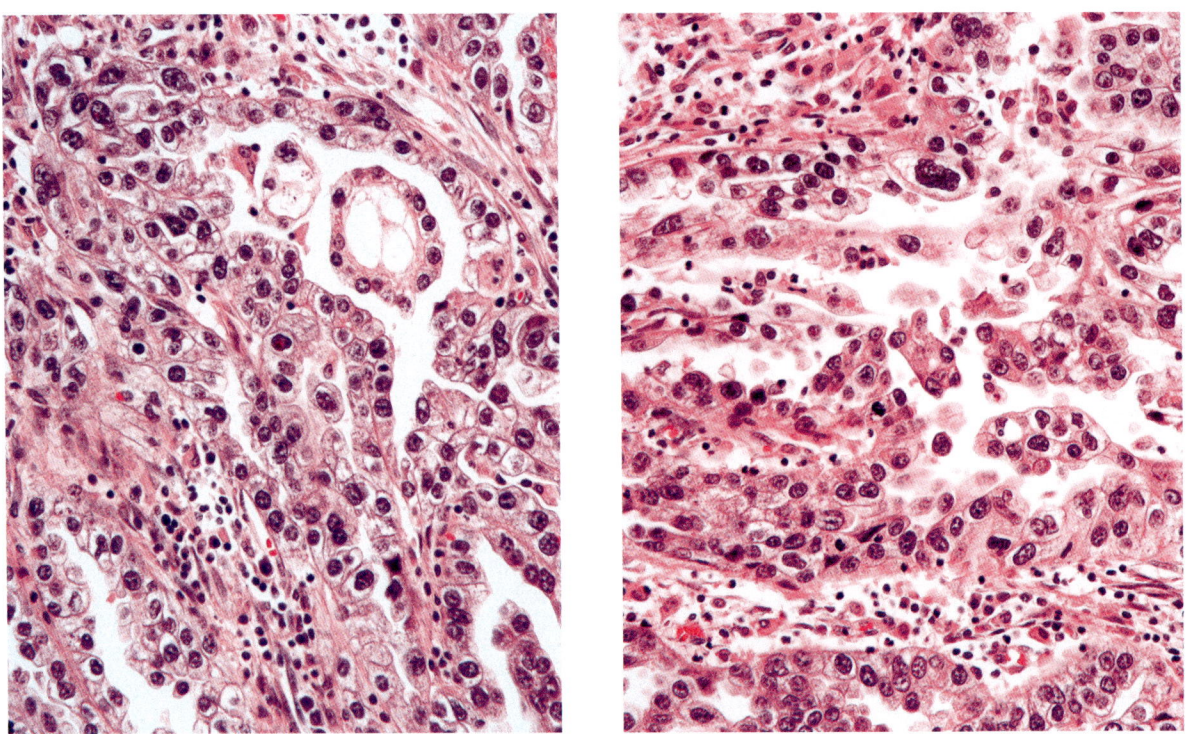

Figure 7-9

CLEAR CELL CARCINOMA

The presence of round nuclei, many containing a single, prominent nucleolus, is a characteristic feature (left). Scattered pleomorphic nuclei are also often noted (right).

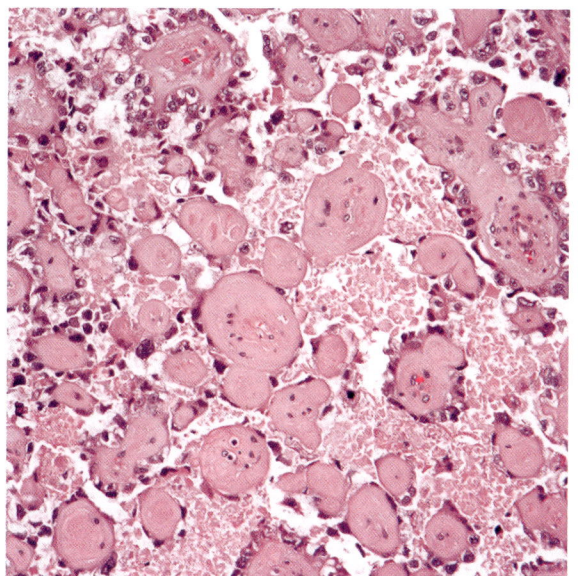 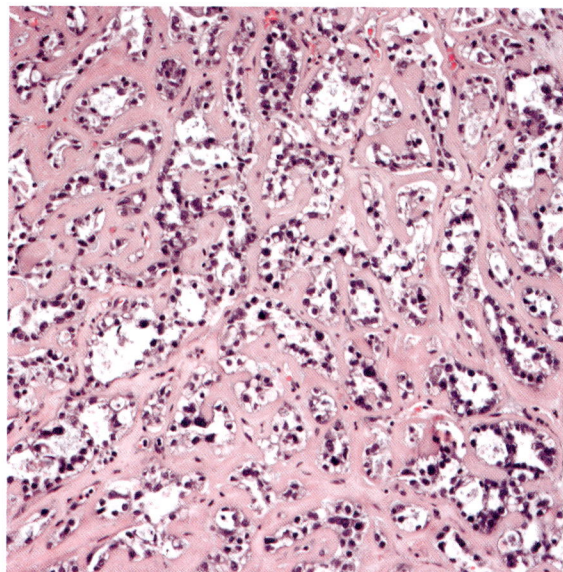

Figure 7-10

CLEAR CELL CARCINOMA

Prominent stromal hyalinization is present within cores of papillae (left) and between the glands (right).

Clear Cell Carcinoma Precursors

Intraepithelial clear cell carcinoma has been described and is reportedly associated with up to 40 percent of clear cell carcinomas (22). Intraepithelial clear cell carcinomas are characterized by an intraepithelial/intraglandular proliferation of cells with a range of nuclear atypia resembling adjacent invasive clear cell carcinoma but maintaining the preexistent architecture of the endometrial glands (26). The significance of this lesion when unaccompanied by invasive clear cell carcinoma is unknown and its diagnostic reproducibility low.

IMMUNOHISTOCHEMICAL FINDINGS

Most clear cell carcinomas coexpress PAX8, pancytokeratins, cytokeratin 7 (CK7), and vimentin. Vimentin is typically expressed in a basolateral pattern, which may be overlooked as "negative" at low-power examination. Most tumors also express cell surface glycoproteins, such as BerEP4, B72.3, MOC31, and CA125, as well as epithelial membrane antigen (EMA) (27). Nearly all clear cell carcinomas are negative for progesterone receptor (PR) and most are negative or only weakly positive for estrogen receptor (ER) (27–30). Loss of ARID1A expression is found in 30 to 50

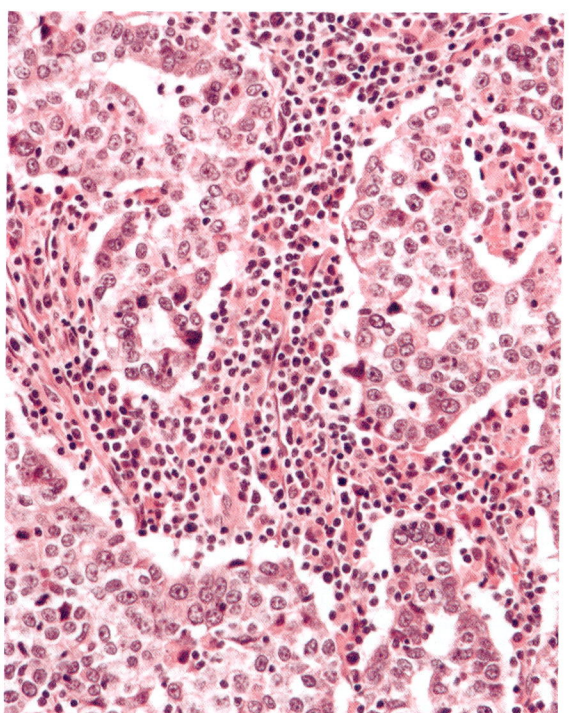

Figure 7-11

CLEAR CELL CARCINOMA

Although nonspecific, the finding of a lymphoplasmacytic infiltrate, often with abundant plasma cells, may be diagnostically helpful.

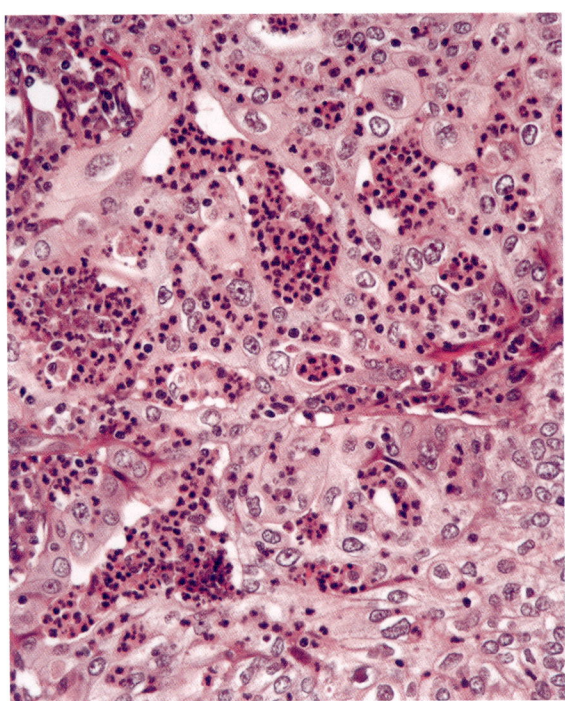 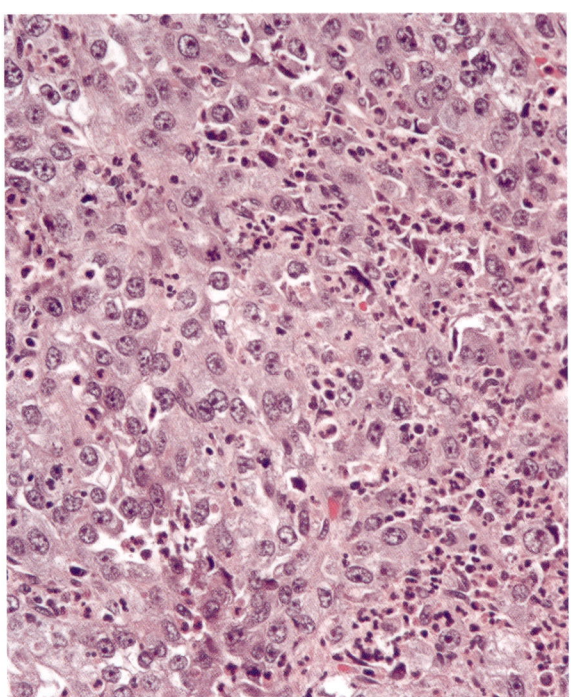

Figure 7-12

CLEAR CELL CARCINOMA WITH ANAPLASTIC APPEARANCE

Sheets of polygonal cells are present in a stroma rich in neutrophils (left and right). Clear cell carcinoma can be diagnosed in the presence of other typical patterns.

percent of clear cell carcinomas (8,31,32), while PTEN and DNA mismatch repair (MMR) protein loss is documented in a significant minority (33).

HNF-1β, napsin A, and α-methylacyl-coenzyme-A racemase (p504s) are expressed in most of tumors (fig. 7-13A,C) and are helpful in the differential diagnosis with other endometrial carcinomas when used in conjunction with ER/PR; napsin A and p504s are more specific than HNF-1β (30,34–39). p53 shows an aberrant expression pattern (most frequently overexpression and less frequently lack of expression) in about 30 percent of tumors (fig. 7-13B) (8,28,40,41). p16 usually shows weak to moderate and patchy expression; however, up to 40 percent of clear cell carcinomas show diffuse and strong expression of this marker (42).

MOLECULAR GENETIC FINDINGS

The most commonly dysregulated somatic genes in clear cell carcinoma are: *TP53* (41,43,44), *PIK3CA*, *PPP2R1A* (41), *FBX7* (41), *ARID1A* (45,46), and DNA MMR *(hMSH2, hMSH6, hMLH1, hPMS2)* (33,36,41,44,47). *ARID1A* is a chromatin remodeling gene, part of the SWI/SNF complex, that acts as a tumor suppressor gene (45,46); it is mutated in subsets of endometrioid, undifferentiated, and clear cell carcinomas of ovary and endometrium, in addition to a small collection of extragonadal tumors. Approximately 20 percent of endometrial clear cell carcinomas are MSI-H and approximately 5 percent have *POLE* (41) or *SMARCA4* mutations (48,49). Exclusive of the microsatellite unstable-high (MSI-H) and *POLE*-mutated cases, the remaining clear cell carcinomas have *TP53* mutations (about 35 percent), or mutations usually associated with endometrioid carcinoma or show a nonspecific genotype (41).

Endometrial clear cell carcinomas are genomically distinctive from ovarian clear cell carcinomas (39) and can be stratified into robust and separable genomic categories, each associated with different clinical outcomes (41), as reported in high-grade endometrioid carcinomas. Previous studies have suggested the existence of at least three clear cell carcinoma subgroups: endometrioid-like, pure or prototypical clear cell, and serous-like (28).

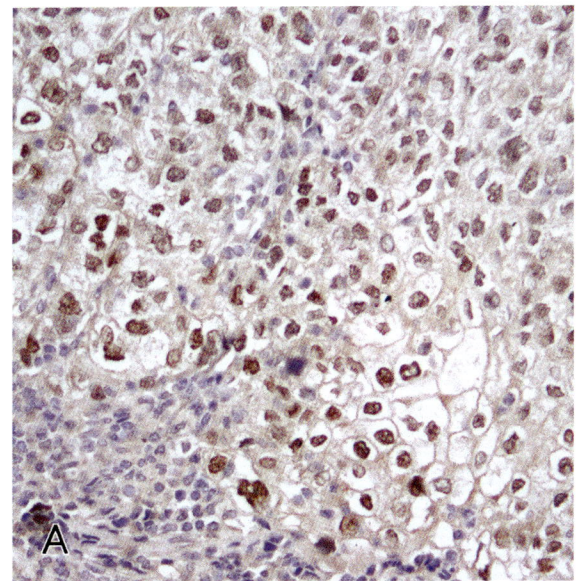
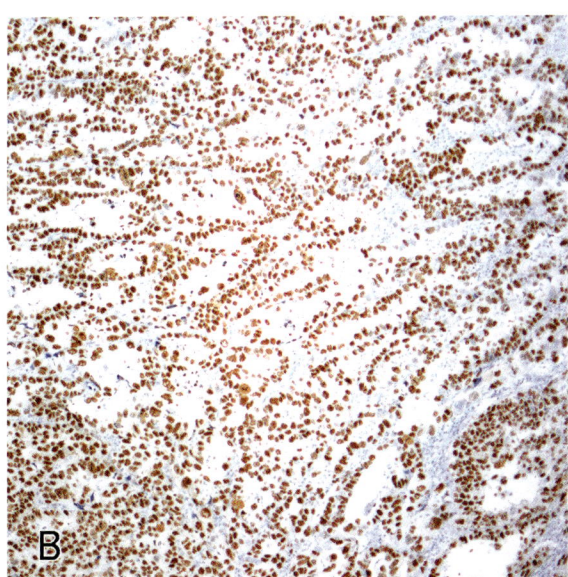
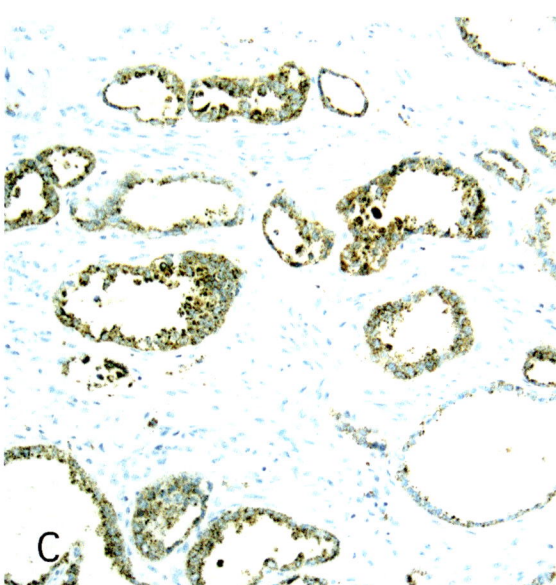
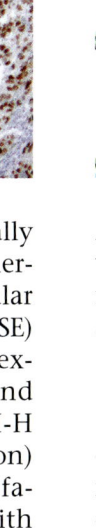

Figure 7-13
CLEAR CELL CARCINOMA: IMMUNOPHENOTYPE

Hepatocyte nuclear factor 1β (HNF-1β), when strongly and diffusely expressed, is a good marker of clear cell carcinoma, but focal and patchy expression can be seen in neoplastic and non-neoplastic endometrium with cytoplasmic clearing; it should, therefore, be used as part of a larger immunohistochemical panel (A). p53 shows an aberrant pattern of staining (in this case, overexpression) in approximately one third of endometrial clear cell carcinomas. This marker conveys prognostic information, but it should not be used alone, since aberrant expression is seen in some high-grade endometrioid carcinomas and almost all serous carcinomas (B). Napsin A shows granular cytoplasmic staining and overall is a better marker than HNF-1β for separating clear cell carcinoma from endometrioid carcinoma, including those with clear cells (C).

Investigators have attempted to genomically classify clear cell carcinomas using next-generation sequencing and the Proactive Molecular Risk Classifier for Endometrial Cancer (PROMISE) algorithm (50). Ultramutated (with *POLE* exonuclease domain hotspot mutations) and hypermutated clear cell carcinomas (MSI-H with aberrant DNA MMR protein expression) segregate together into a prognostically favorable category. Clear cell carcinomas with *TP53* mutations that are not ultramutated or hypermutated constitute the most clinically aggressive group, similar to serous carcinoma. A genomically indeterminate group also exists, with some features suggesting kinship to copy number-low endometrioid carcinoma, but these also are prognostically unfavorable tumors (41).

DIFFERENTIAL DIAGNOSIS

Endometrioid Carcinoma. In contrast to clear cell carcinomas, endometrioid carcinomas, including those with secretory change or cytoplasmic clearing (51), are composed mostly of columnar to polygonal cells (fig. 7-14) and do not demonstrate the characteristic architectural patterns of clear cell carcinoma. Although

Figure 7-14
ENDOMETRIOID ADENOCARCINOMA

The finding of cytoplasmic clearing in the absence of clear cell carcinoma architectural features is not diagnostic of clear cell carcinoma and can be seen in endometrioid carcinomas with glycogenated squamous differentiation (most prominent at right) (A), with nonspecific cytoplasmic clearing (B), or with extensive secretory-like change (C) due to the presence of intracytoplasmic subnuclear or supranuclear vacuoles.

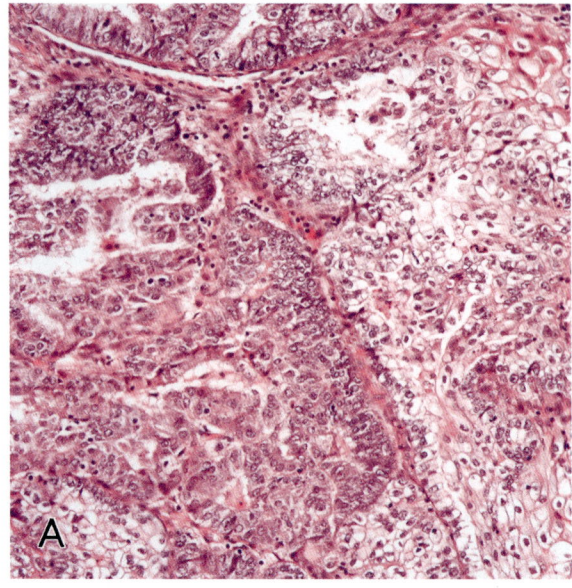

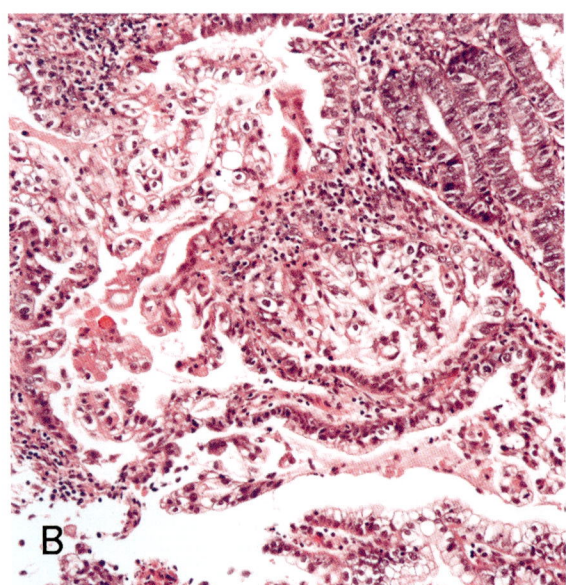

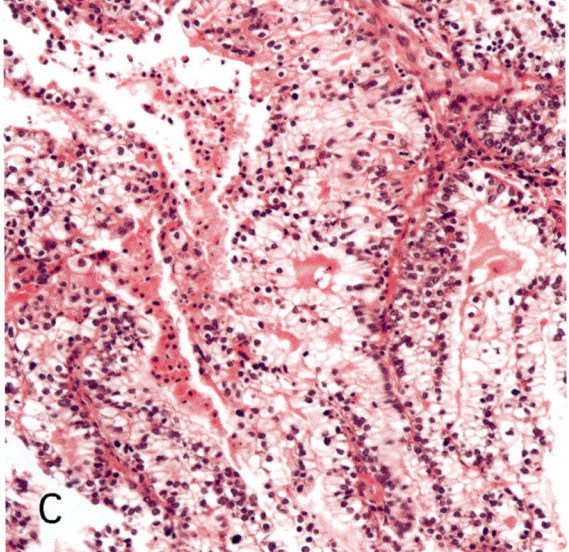

evaluation of endometrioid carcinomas with a preponderance of glands containing cells with cytoplasmic vacuolization may be difficult, endometrioid glands are typically lined by columnar cells in contrast to the cuboidal or flattened cells of clear cell carcinoma. Furthermore, it is unusual for a gland-forming endometrioid carcinoma to have marked although uniform cytologic atypia. A diagnosis of solid clear cell carcinoma should be avoided when clear cells are present in a tumor with background endometrioid characteristics and other typical architectural patterns of clear cell carcinoma are lacking (22).

Immunohistochemistry can be helpful in this differential diagnosis. In contrast to clear cell carcinomas, endometrioid carcinomas tend to be positive for ER/PR, especially if glandular or papillary in architecture. Expression of HNF-1β (more often), as well as napsin A and racemase may be found in endometrioid carcinomas, especially when they have clear cells, thus, it is best to use a panel of immunohistochemical markers (30,34–39). Rare endometrioid carcinomas may recur in the form of clear cell carcinoma (52,53).

Mixed Endometrioid and Clear Cell Carcinoma. Currently, several studies assert that

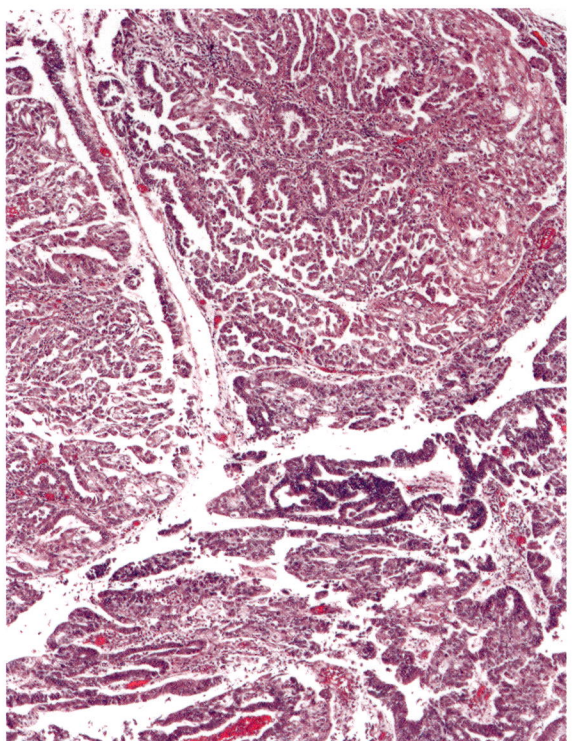 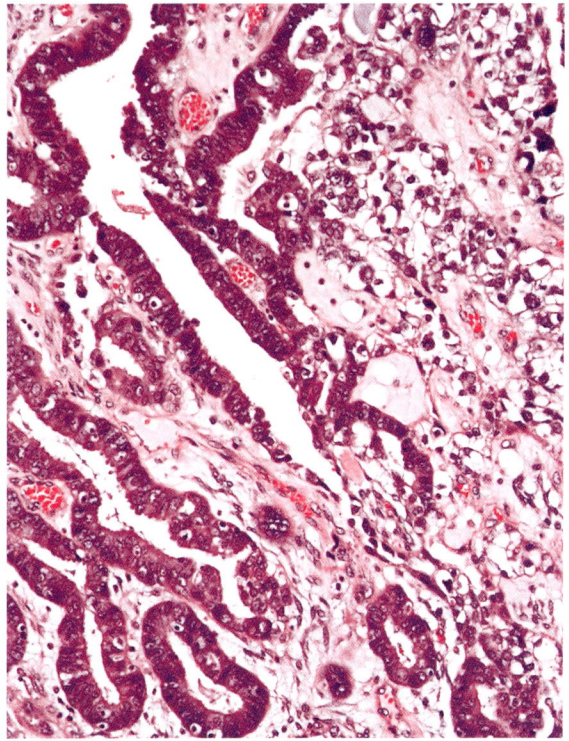

Figure 7-15

MIXED ENDOMETRIOID AND CLEAR CELL CARCINOMA

The clear cell component is recognized by a glandular proliferation of eosinophilic hobnail cells and incipient papillary architecture (top) juxtaposed to the endometrioid carcinoma component (bottom) (left). Seamless fusion of subtly different components is not diagnostic of a mixed carcinoma (right). An abrupt change in cell shape and nuclear features is more characteristic.

most mixed epithelial carcinomas derive from the same precursor, usually an endometrioid carcinoma, which then acquires intratumoral heterogeneity and further gene mutations in the heterogeneous components (54,55). The exception is a mixed endometrioid and clear cell carcinoma that arises in the setting of Lynch syndrome (55), wherein both components may be clonally unrelated. This diagnosis should only be made when the different components are histologically distinctive (figs. 7-15) and should be avoided for a homogeneous-appearing tumor with overlapping features of both endometrioid and clear cell carcinoma.

Serous Carcinoma. Mixed clear cell and serous carcinomas are exceedingly rare and their existence is a matter of debate (fig. 7-16). Clear cell carcinoma can be easily distinguished from serous carcinoma in most cases based on architectural, cytologic, and stromal features (fig. 7-17). The presence of large, branching and irregular papillae, cellular pseudostratification, diffuse nuclear pleomorphism, and a high mitotic index (more than 5 mitoses per 10 high-power fields) favors a diagnosis of serous carcinoma, although a subset of endometrial clear cell carcinomas has proliferative rates as high as those seen in serous carcinomas.

Highly proliferative clear cell carcinomas may also show overlapping cytologic features with serous carcinoma and aberrant p53 expression (25). Napsin A, HNF-1β (30,34–39), WT1, ER/PR, and ARID1A (BAF250a) (8,31,32) are all differentially expressed in serous and clear cell carcinomas, but since there is some degree of overlap, a panel of markers should be used (56). Abnormal PTEN or DNA MMR protein expression, although present in only a minority of clear cell carcinomas (33), is also diagnostically helpful, as serous carcinomas show intact expression. IMP3 can be expressed in both serous and clear cell carcinomas (29),

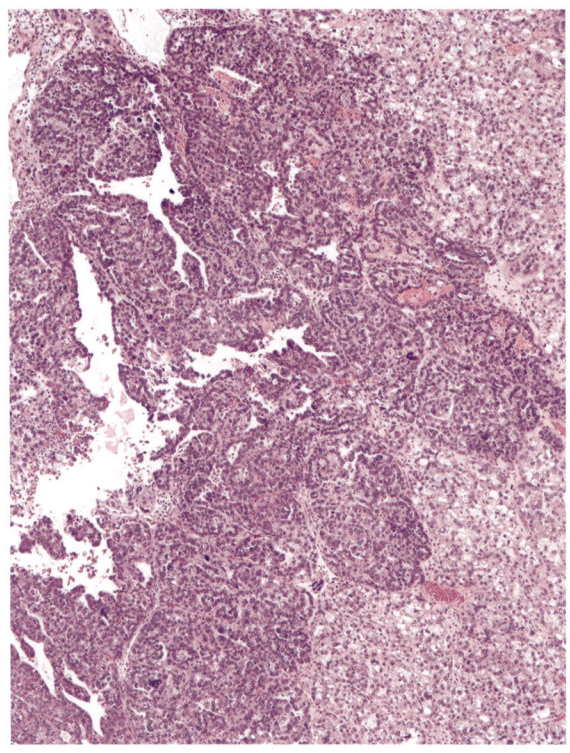

Figure 7-16

MIXED CLEAR CELL AND SEROUS CARCINOMA

Histologically characteristic clear cell carcinoma surrounds an island of serous carcinoma, showing slit-like spaces with tumor cell budding and detachment. Pleomorphic nuclei are present in the serous component.

thus it is not diagnostically helpful in this differential diagnosis.

Arias-Stella and Metaplastic Changes. Gestational endometrium or endometrium from patients treated with progestational agents or tamoxifen may have cells with a clear appearance and hobnail morphology, atypical nuclei, and occasional mitoses (57–59). In contrast to clear cell carcinoma, Arias-Stella reaction is typically an incidental finding that involves glands with preservation of the preexistent architecture, sometimes only with partial involvement. It shows a spectrum of cytologic atypia, with low N:C ratio, degenerative or smudged nuclear appearance, optically clear nuclei (thought to result from biotin accumulation), tiny nucleoli, and nuclear pseudoinclusions; it typically lacks mitotic activity. Although subtle immunohistochemical differences between Arias-Stella change and clear cell carcinoma have been reported, including higher expression of ER and PR in Arias-Stella (60), there is extensive immunohistochemical overlap; therefore, using immunohistochemistry for this differential diagnosis is usually not informative.

Benign hobnail change and eosinophilic metaplasia occasionally suggest clear cell carcinoma. The context in which these changes are found is often diagnostically helpful, as they tend to be seen in association with other metaplastic changes and may be present in an infarcted polyp or in an area of prior curettage, endometrial stromal breakdown, or chronic endometritis (61–66).

Endocervical Adenocarcinoma. Clear cell carcinomas can arise in the endocervix and often display overlapping histologic and immunohistochemical features with their endometrial counterparts. Only clinical imaging and examination of the resection specimen can distinguish gynecologic clear cell carcinomas from different anatomic sites.

Human papillomavirus (HPV)-associated endocervical adenocarcinoma, the most common subtype, usually does not cause problems in the differential diagnosis with clear cell carcinoma. However, endocervical gastric-type carcinoma (67–69), an uncommon tumor, occasionally involves the endometrium, and may be confused with a clear cell carcinoma (70). Both tumors show accentuated cytoplasmic membranes and monolayered architecture, and both may express PAX8, HNF-1β, and carbonic anhydrase IX (71), and are typically ER/PR negative. The architectural features of gastric-type carcinoma are different from clear cell carcinomas as they lack tubulocystic or papillary growth and the cytoplasm is mucin-rich with a pink hue, and stains a magenta color with alcian blue/periodic acid–Schiff (PAS). The presence of gastric-type mucin (alcian blue/PAS and/or HIK1083 immunohistochemistry) and mCEA favors a gastric-type adenocarcinoma (72).

Mesonephric-Like Carcinoma. Occasional clear cell endometrial carcinomas resemble mesonephric adenocarcinomas, which more commonly occur in the cervix but have been rarely reported in the corpus (73). Their morphology, including a tubulocystic and less often a papillary architecture, glands lined by a monolayer of cells, and eosinophilic secretions,

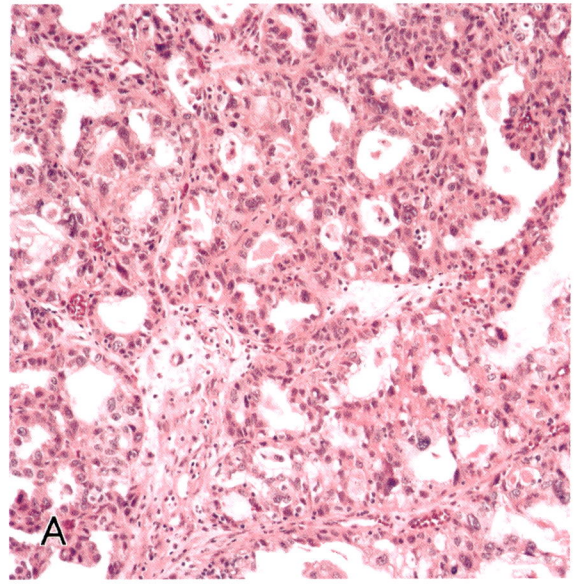

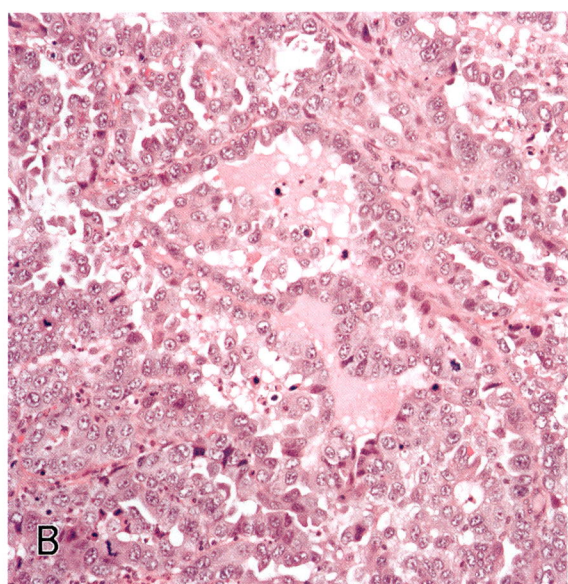

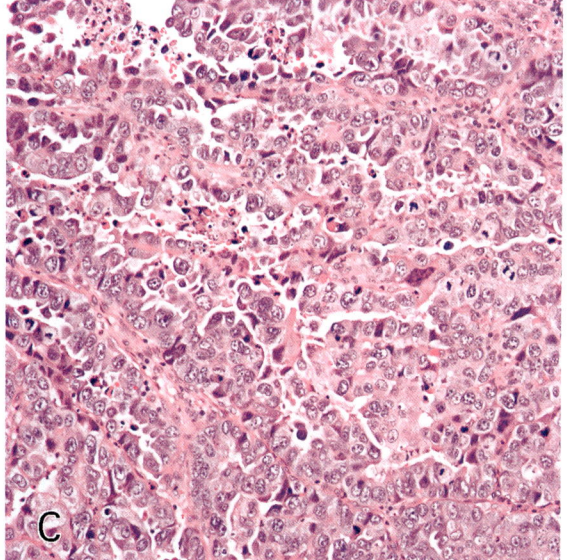

Figure 7-17

HIGH-GRADE ENDOMETRIAL CARCINOMAS WITH SEROUS AND CLEAR CELL FEATURES

The tumor shows glandular spaces lined by a monolayer of cuboidal cells, suggesting clear cell carcinoma with oxyphilic features; however, the degree of nuclear pleomorphism is uncharacteristic of clear cell carcinoma (A).

Tumors with oxyphilic cells show nuclear pleomorphism, cellular stratification, budding, and detachment, along with a high mitotic index, more in keeping with serous carcinoma (B,C).

may overlap with clear cell carcinoma. The immunohistochemical profile may also be similar as both are ER and PR negative and PAX8 positive (74,75), and rarely mesonephric tumors are HNF-1β and napsin A positive (73). Tumors showing mesonephric differentiation may be centered in myometrium; often show other architectural patterns characteristic of mesonephric differentiation, such as glomeruloid and ductal growth, and are GATA3 positive (76,77). The latter marker should be used with caution, as there is no published data on GATA3 expression in clear cell carcinoma.

Perivascular Epithelioid Cell Tumor (PEComa). Most PEComas are composed of epithelioid and spindled cells with clear to eosinophilic cytoplasm and a characteristic sinusoidal vasculature that facilitates their diagnosis. However, if they are mostly composed of clear epithelioid cells, as seen in the TFE3-translocated variant (also referred to as Xp11 PEComa), they may mimic a solid clear cell carcinoma (54,78,79). The morphology and immunophenotype of this tumor are similar to the Xp11 translocation-associated renal carcinomas, with the exception of PAX8 expression, observed in

Xp11 translocation-associated renal carcinomas but lacking in PEComas (54). Clues to this diagnosis include extensive sheets or compact nests of clear cells separated by a delicate sinusoidal vasculature in the absence of glandular or tubulocystic architecture and localization in myometrium rather than endometrium. Occasional tumors display pseudopapillary arrangements, but they do not resemble the typical small, round papillae of clear cell carcinoma. The diagnosis is confirmed with diffuse, strong HMB-45 positivity and lack of staining for epithelial markers. The TFE3 translocation can be suggested with diffuse TFE3 nuclear positivity or a fluorescence in situ hybridization (FISH) assay (54,78,79).

Intermediate-Type Trophoblastic Tumors. Placental-site trophoblastic tumor may show diffuse growth and have clear cells, while epithelioid trophoblastic tumor may display striking cytoplasmic eosinophilia, both potentially resembling the solid pattern of clear cell carcinoma. These tumors are frequently associated with elevated serum beta-human chorionic gonadotropin (hCG) levels. Placental-site trophoblastic tumor recapitulates the placental implantation site, with invasion of myometrium and vascular walls in association with fibrinoid necrosis, while epithelioid trophoblastic tumor is often well circumscribed and shows a nested/diffuse growth of oxyphilic cells, often in a perivascular distribution, with abundant fibrinoid material between the nests. The intermediate trophoblastic tumors show PLAP, CD10, HPL, and inhibin labeling (80–83) and typically express GATA3 (84–86) in contrast to clear cell carcinoma.

Yolk Sac Tumor. This tumor may resemble clear cell carcinoma since both tumors feature cells with clear cytoplasm, but primary pure yolk sac tumor in the endometrium is exceedingly rare. Müllerian carcinomas containing somatic yolk sac tumor (87) have been described, which engender some diagnostic difficulties with clear cell carcinoma. Distinguishing features of yolk sac tumor include reticular, labyrinthine, macrocystic or microcystic architecture in the presence of primitive-appearing nuclei. In contrast to pure clear cell carcinoma, those with yolk sac, are in most instances, negative for CK7 and EMA (88), and show strong SALL4 and glypican-3 expression (89). Occasional clear cell carcinomas, however, show glypican-3 positivity (90) and glandular yolk sac tumors, particularly, can express CK7, EMA, and even PAX8 (91,92). HNF-1β is often positive in both tumors, but napsin-A and racemase are negative in yolk sac tumors (93); therefore, applying a panel of antibodies is preferred given this differential diagnosis. It is best to avoid alpha-fetoprotein (AFP) immunohistochemistry as some clear cell carcinomas are positive for this marker and immunohistochemical results are frequently equivocal due to high background staining.

Other. Tumors that rarely may be considered in the differential diagnosis are epithelioid smooth muscle tumors and alveolar soft part sarcoma (94).

TREATMENT AND PROGNOSIS

Most patients with clear cell carcinoma confined to the uterus undergo total hysterectomy, bilateral salpingo-oophorectomy, omentectomy, peritoneal biopsies, and either lymphadenectomy or sentinel lymph node biopsies. FIGO stage, patient age, patient performance status, and medical co-morbidities are the most robust determinants of prognosis. A recent study showed that, on multivariate analysis, stage and age greater than 65 years were the most important prognostic indicators (22).

Most patients with clear cell carcinoma receive adjuvant chemotherapy with carboplatin and taxol, although most tumors tend to be chemoresistant (95–98). In some centers, pelvic radiation therapy is administered instead of, or in combination with, chemotherapy. Selected patients with FIGO stage I clear cell carcinoma are not considered candidates for chemotherapy.

The 5-year recurrence-free survival rate for patients with clear cell carcinoma is 50 to 60 percent (3–7,99–102), and a recent study reported a 5-year overall survival rate as high as 80 percent (22). When stratified by stage, 5-year overall survival rates were reported as follows: 94 percent for stage I, 87 percent for stage II, 67 percent for stage III, and 43 percent for stage IV tumors. These percentages are in contrast with those reported for serous carcinoma, and similar to those reported for grade 3 endometrioid carcinoma. Approximately 20 percent of patients with clear cell carcinoma experience recurrences. These occur, in order of decreasing incidence in: lung, pelvis (including pelvic soft tissues, pelvic lymph nodes, and vagina), abdomen, liver, distant lymph nodes (including para-aortic and supra-clavicular lymph nodes), kidney, and bone (5,22).

As mentioned previously, clear cell carcinomas have been shown to be associated with different clinical outcomes based on robust and separable genomic categories (41), similar to those reported in grade 3 endometrioid carcinoma. Ultramutated or hypermutated clear cell carcinomas with exonuclease domain POLE hotspot mutations or MSI-H, respectively, cluster together and are associated with a favorable prognosis. Tumors with TP53 mutations and high copy number alterations are highly aggressive, as noted in serous carcinomas and serous-like grade 3 endometrioid carcinomas. These tumors tend to present at an advanced stage and patients have the worst prognosis, with a median progression-free survival period of about 15 months. Patients whose tumors do not map to any of these groups have a median progression-free survival period of about 30 months, significantly shorter than the POLE and MSI-H groups.

REFERENCES

1. Creasman WT, Odicino F, Maisonneuve P, et al., Carcinoma of the corpus uteri. FIGO 26th Annual Report on the Results of Treatment in Gynecological Cancer Int J Gynaecol Obstet 2006;95(Suppl 1):S105-43.
2. National Comprehensive Cancer Network, NCCN Clinical Practice Guidelines in Oncology (NCCN Guidelines®), Version 2.2012. Uterine Neoplasms 2012. http//www.alabmed.com/uploadfile/2014/0126/2014012610903353.pdf
3. Creasman WT, Kohler MF, Odicino F, Maisonneuve P, Boyle P. Prognosis of papillary serous, clear cell, and grade 3 stage I carcinoma of the endometrium. Gynecol Oncol 2004;95:593-6.
4. Cirisano FD Jr, Robboy SJ, Dodge RK, et al. Epidemiologic and surgicopathologic findings of papillary serous and clear cell endometrial cancers when compared to endometrioid carcinoma. Gynecol Oncol 1999;74:385-94.
5. Soslow RA, Bissonnette JP, Wilton A, et al. Clinicopathologic analysis of 187 high-grade endometrial carcinomas of different histologic subtypes: similar outcomes belie distinctive biologic differences. Am J Surg Pathol 2007;31:979-87.
6. Hamilton CA, Cheung MK, Osann K, et al. Uterine papillary serous and clear cell carcinomas predict for poorer survival compared to grade 3 endometrioid corpus cancers. Br J Cancer 2006;94:642-6.
7. Cirisano FD Jr, Robboy SJ, Dodge RK, et al. The outcome of stage I-II clinically and surgically staged papillary serous and clear cell endometrial cancers when compared with endometrioid carcinoma. Gynecol Oncol 2000;77:55-65.
8. Fadare O, Gwin K, Desouki MM, et al. The clinicopathologic significance of p53 and BAF-250a (ARID1A) expression in clear cell carcinoma of the endometrium. Mod Pathol 2013;26:1101-10.
9. Fadare O, Renshaw IL, Liang SX. Expression of tissue factor and heparanase in endometrial clear cell carcinoma: possible role for tissue factor in thromboembolic events. Int J Gynecol Pathol 2011;30:252-61.
10. Rauh-Hain JA, Hariton E, Clemmer J, et al. Incidence and effects on mortality of venous thromboembolism in elderly women with endometrial cancer. Obstet Gynecol 2015;125:1362-70.
11. Lee L, Garrett L, Lee H, Oliva E, Horowitz N, Duska LR. Association of clear cell carcinoma of the endometrium with a high rate of venous thromboembolism. J Reprod Med 2009;54:133-8.
12. Satoh T, Matsumoto K, Uno K, et al. Silent venous thromboembolism before treatment in endometrial cancer and the risk factors. Br J Cancer 2008;99:1034-9.
13. Hiller N, Sonnenblick M, Hershko C. Paraneoplastic hypercalcemia in endometrial carcinoma. Oncology 1989;46:45-8.

14. Savvari P, Peitsidis P, Alevizaki M, Dimopoulos MA, Antsaklis A, Papadimitriou CA. Paraneoplastic humorally mediated hypercalcemia induced by parathyroid hormone-related protein in gynecologic malignancies: a systematic review. Onkologie 2009;32:517-23.
15. Panegyres PK, Graves A. Anti-Yo and anti-glutamic acid decarboxylase antibodies presenting in carcinoma of the uterus with paraneoplastic cerebellar degeneration: a case report. J Med Case Rep 2012;6:155.
16. Mittal R, Cherepanoff S, Thornton S, Kalirai H, Damato B, Coupland SE. Bilateral diffuse uveal melanocytic proliferation: molecular genetic analysis of a case and review of the literature. Ocul Oncol Pathol 2015;2:94-9.
17. Cuff J, Salari K, Clarke N. Integrative bioinformatics links HNF1B with clear cell carcinoma and tumor-associated thrombosis. PLoS One 2013;8: e74562.
18. Bartosch C, Pires-Luís AS, Meireles C, et al. Pathologic findings in prophylactic and non-prophylactic hysterectomy specimens of patients with Lynch syndrome. Am J Surg Pathol 2016;40:1177-91.
19. Broaddus RR, Lynch HT, Chen LM, et al. Pathologic features of endometrial carcinoma associated with HNPCC: a comparison with sporadic endometrial carcinoma. Cancer 2006;106:87-94.
20. Carcangiu ML, Radice P, Casalini P, Bertario L, Merola M, Sala P. Lynch syndrome—related endometrial carcinomas show a high frequency of nonendometrioid types and of high FIGO grade endometrioid types. Int J Surg Pathol 2010;18:21-6.
21. Hoogendoorn WE, Hollema H, van Boven HH, et al. Prognosis of uterine corpus cancer after tamoxifen treatment for breast cancer. Breast Cancer Res Treat 2008;112:99-108.
22. Fadare O, Zheng W, Crispens MA, et al., Morphologic and other clinicopathologic features of endometrial clear cell carcinoma: a comprehensive analysis of 50 rigorously classified cases. Am J Cancer Res 2013;3:70-95.
23. Koshiyama M, Suzuki A, Ozawa M, et al. Adenocarcinomas arising from uterine adenomyosis: a report of four cases. Int J Gynecol Pathol 2002;21:239-45.
24. Young RH, Scully RE. Oxyphilic clear cell carcinoma of the ovary. A report of nine cases. Am J Surg Pathol 1987;11:661-7.
25. Offman SL, Longacre TA. Clear cell carcinoma of the female genital tract (not everything is as clear as it seems). Adv Anat Pathol 2012;19:296-312.
26. Fadare O, Liang SX, Ulukus EC, Chambers SK, Zheng W. Precursors of endometrial clear cell carcinoma. Am J Surg Pathol 2006;30:1519-30.
27. Vang R, Whitaker BP, Farhood AI, Silva EG, Ro JY, Deavers MT. Immunohistochemical analysis of clear cell carcinoma of the gynecologic tract. Int J Gynecol Pathol 2001;20:252-9.
28. Lax SF, Pizer ES, Ronnett BM, Kurman RJ. Clear cell carcinoma of the endometrium is characterized by a distinctive profile of p53, Ki-67, estrogen, and progesterone receptor expression. Hum Pathol 1998;29:551-8.
29. Mhawech-Fauceglia P, Yan L, Liu S, Pejovic T. ER+ /PR+ /TFF3+ /IMP3- immunoprofile distinguishes endometrioid from serous and clear cell carcinomas of the endometrium: a study of 401 cases. Histopathology 2013;62:976-85.
30. Hoang LN, Han G, McConechy M, et al. Immunohistochemical characterization of prototypical endometrial clear cell carcinoma—diagnostic utility of HNF-1beta and oestrogen receptor. Histopathology 2014;64:585-96.
31. Mao TL, Ardighieri L, Ayhan A, et al, Loss of ARID1A expression correlates with stages of tumor progression in uterine endometrioid carcinoma. Am J Surg Pathol 2013;37:1342-8.
32. Wiegand KC, Lee AF, Al-Agha OM, et al. Loss of BAF250a (ARID1A) is frequent in high-grade endometrial carcinomas. J Pathol 2011;224:328-33.
33. Bae HS, Kim H, Young Kwon S, Kim KR, Song JY, Kim I. Should endometrial clear cell carcinoma be classified as type II endometrial carcinoma? Int J Gynecol Pathol 2015;34:74-84.
34. Fadare O, Parkash V, Gwin K, et al. Utility of alpha-methylacyl-coenzyme-A racemase (p504s) immunohistochemistry in distinguishing endometrial clear cell carcinomas from serous and endometrioid carcinomas. Hum Pathol 2013;44:2814-21.
35. Lim D, Ip PP, Cheung AN, Kiyokawa T, Oliva E. Immunohistochemical comparison of ovarian and uterine endometrioid carcinoma, endometrioid carcinoma with clear cell change, and clear cell carcinoma. Am J Surg Pathol 2015;39:1061-9.
36. Han G, Soslow RA, Wethington S, et al. Endometrial carcinomas with clear cells: a study of a heterogeneous group of tumors including interobserver variability, mutation analysis, and immunohistochemistry with HNF-1beta. Int J Gynecol Pathol 2015;34:323-33.
37. Fadare O, Liang SX. Diagnostic utility of hepatocyte nuclear factor 1-beta immunoreactivity in endometrial carcinomas: lack of specificity for endometrial clear cell carcinoma. Appl Immunohistochem Mol Morphol 2012;20:580-7.
38. Fadare O, Desouki MM, Gwin K, et al, Frequent expression of napsin A in clear cell carcinoma of the endometrium: potential diagnostic utility. Am J Surg Pathol 2014;38:189-96.

39. Iwamoto M, Nakatani Y, Fugo K, Kishimoto T, Kiyokawa T. Napsin A is frequently expressed in clear cell carcinoma of the ovary and endometrium. Hum Pathol 2015;46:957-62.
40. Arai T, Watanabe J, Kawaguchi M, et al. Clear cell adenocarcinoma of the endometrium is a biologically distinct entity from endometrioid adenocarcinoma. Int J Gynecol Cancer 2006;16:391-5.
41. DeLair DF, Burke KA, Selenica P, et al. The genetic landscape of endometrial clear cell carcinomas. J Pathol 2017;243:230-41.
42. Reid-Nicholson M, Iyengar P, Hummer AJ, Linkov I, Asher M, Soslow RA. Immunophenotypic diversity of endometrial adenocarcinomas: implications for differential diagnosis. Mod Pathol 2006;19:1091-100.
43. An HJ, Logani S, Isacson C, Ellenson LH. Molecular characterization of uterine clear cell carcinoma. Mod Pathol 2004;17:530-7.
44. Hoang LN, McConechy MK, Meng B, et al. Targeted mutation analysis of endometrial clear cell carcinoma. Histopathology 2015;66:664-74.
45. Wiegand KC, Shah SP, Al-Agha OM, et al. ARID1A mutations in endometriosis-associated ovarian carcinomas. N Engl J Med 2010;363:1532-43.
46. Guan B, Wang TL, Shih IeM. ARID1A, a factor that promotes formation of SWI/SNF-mediated chromatin remodeling, is a tumor suppressor in gynecologic cancers. Cancer Res 2011;71:6718-27.
47. Hoang LN, McConechy MK, Köbel M, et al. Histotype-genotype correlation in 36 high-grade endometrial carcinomas. Am J Surg Pathol 2013;37:1421-32.
48. Conlon N, Silva A, Guerra E, et al. Loss of SMARCA4 expression is both sensitive and specific for the diagnosis of small cell carcinoma of ovary, hypercalcemic type. Am J Surg Pathol 2016;40:395-403.
49. Ramos P, Karnezis AN, Craig DW, et al. Small cell carcinoma of the ovary, hypercalcemic type, displays frequent inactivating germline and somatic mutations in SMARCA4. Nat Genet 2014;46:427-9.
50. Talhouk A, McConechy MK, Leung S, et al. A clinically applicable molecular-based classification for endometrial cancers. Br J Cancer 2015;113:299-310.
51. Silva EG, Young RH. Endometrioid neoplasms with clear cells: a report of 21 cases in which the alteration is not of typical secretory type. Am J Surg Pathol 2007;31:1203-8.
52. Rawish KR, Desouki MM, Crispens MA, Fadare O. Conventional endometrioid adenocarcinomas of the endometrium recurring as clear cell tumors: comparative immunohistochemical analyses. Ann Diagn Pathol 2013;17:270-5.
53. Soslow RA, Wethington SL, Cesari M, et al. Clinicopathologic analysis of matched primary and recurrent endometrial carcinoma. Am J Surg Pathol 2012;36:1771-81.
54. Argani P, Zhong M, Reuter VE, et al. TFE3-fusion variant analysis defines specific clinicopathologic associations among Xp11 translocation cancers. Am J Surg Pathol 2016;40:723-37.
55. Kobel M, Meng B, Hoang LN, et al. Molecular analysis of mixed endometrial carcinomas shows clonality in most cases. Am J Surg Pathol 2016;40:166-80.
56. Chen W, Husain A, Nelson GS, et al. Immunohistochemical profiling of endometrial serous carcinoma. Int J Gynecol Pathol 2017;36:128-39.
57. Arias-Stella J. The Arias-Stella reaction: facts and fancies four decades after. Adv Anat Pathol 2002;9:12-23.
58. Huettner PC, Gersell DJ. Arias-Stella reaction in nonpregnant women: a clinicopathologic study of nine cases. Int J Gynecol Pathol 1994;13:241-7.
59. Nucci MR, Young RH. Arias-Stella reaction of the endocervix: a report of 18 cases with emphasis on its varied histology and differential diagnosis. Am J Surg Pathol 2004;28:608-12.
60. Vang R, Barner R, Wheeler DT, Strauss BL. Immunohistochemical staining for Ki-67 and p53 helps distinguish endometrial Arias-Stella reaction from high-grade carcinoma, including clear cell carcinoma. Int J Gynecol Pathol 2004;23:223-33.
61. Fukuoka K, Hirokawa M, Shimizu M, et al. Oxyphilic cell variant of endometrioid adenocarcinoma. Pathol Int 1998;48:754-6.
62. Hendrickson MR, Kempson RL. Endometrial epithelial metaplasias: proliferations frequently misdiagnosed as adenocarcinoma. Report of 89 cases and proposed classification. Am J Surg Pathol, 1980;4:525-42.
63. Kaku T, Silverberg SG, Tsukamoto N, et al. Association of endometrial epithelial metaplasias with endometrial carcinoma and hyperplasia in Japanese and American women. Int J Gynecol Pathol 1993;12:297-300.
64. Moritani S, Kushima R, Ichihara S, et al. Eosinophilic cell change of the endometrium: a possible relationship to mucinous differentiation. Mod Pathol 2005;18:1243-8.
65. Nicolae A, Preda O, Nogales FF. Endometrial metaplasias and reactive changes: a spectrum of altered differentiation. J Clin Pathol 2011;64:97-106.
66. Pitman MB, Young RH, Clement PB, Dickersin GR, Scully RE. Endometrioid carcinoma of the ovary and endometrium, oxyphilic cell type: a report of nine cases. Int J Gynecol Pathol 1994;13:290-301.

67. Kojima A, Mikami Y, Sudo T, et al. Gastric morphology and immunophenotype predict poor outcome in mucinous adenocarcinoma of the uterine cervix. Am J Surg Pathol 2007;31:664-72.
68. Park KJ, Kiyokawa T, Soslow RA, et al. Unusual endocervical adenocarcinomas: an immunohistochemical analysis with molecular detection of human papillomavirus. Am J Surg Pathol 2011;35:633-46.
69. Karamurzin YS, Kiyokawa T, Parkash V, et al. Gastric-type endocervical adenocarcinoma: an aggressive tumor with unusual metastatic patterns and poor prognosis. Am J Surg Pathol 2015;39:1449-57.
70. Zhang Y, Liang L, Euscher ED, Liu J, Ramalingam P. Gastric-type mucinous adenocarcinoma of the uterine cervix with neoadjuvant therapy mimicking clear cell carcinoma. Int J Clin Exp Pathol 2015;8:11798-803.
71. Carleton C, Hoang L, Sah S, et al. A detailed immunohistochemical analysis of a large series of cervical and vaginal gastric-type adenocarcinomas. Am J Surg Pathol 2016;40:636-44.
72. Stolnicu S, Barsan I, Hoang L, et al. Diagnostic algorithmic proposal based on comprehensive immunohistochemical evaluation of 297 invasive endocervical adenocarcinomas. Am J Surg Pathol 2018;42:989-1000.
73. McFarland M, Quick CM, McCluggage WG. Hormone receptor-negative, thyroid transcription factor 1-positive uterine and ovarian adenocarcinomas: report of a series of mesonephric-like adenocarcinomas. Histopathology 2016;68:1013-20.
74. Goyal A, Yang B. Differential patterns of PAX8, p16, and ER immunostains in mesonephric lesions and adenocarcinomas of the cervix. Int J Gynecol Pathol 2014;33:613-9.
75. Kim SS, Nam JH, Kim GE, Choi YD, Choi C, Park CS. Mesonephric adenocarcinoma of the uterine corpus: a case report and diagnostic pitfall. Int J Surg Pathol 2016;24:153-8.
76. Howitt BE, Emori MM, Drapkin R, et al. GATA3 is a sensitive and specific marker of benign and malignant mesonephric lesions in the lower female genital tract. Am J Surg Pathol 2015;39:1411-9.
77. Roma AA, Goyal A, Yang B. Differential expression patterns of GATA3 in uterine mesonephric and nonmesonephric lesions. Int J Gynecol Pathol 2015;34:480-6.
78. Schoolmeester JK, Dao LN, Sukov WR, et al. TFE3 translocation-associated perivascular epithelioid cell neoplasm (PEComa) of the gynecologic tract: morphology, immunophenotype, differential diagnosis. Am J Surg Pathol 2015;39:394-404.
79. Agaram NP, Sung YS, Zhang L, et al. Dichotomy of genetic abnormalities in PEComas with therapeutic implications. Am J Surg Pathol 2015;39:813-25.
80. Ordi J, Romagosa C, Tavassoli FA, et al. CD10 expression in epithelial tissues and tumors of the gynecologic tract: a useful marker in the diagnosis of mesonephric, trophoblastic, and clear cell tumors. Am J Surg Pathol 2003;27:178-86.
81. Pelkey TJ, Frierson HF Jr, Mills SE, Stoler MH. Detection of the alpha-subunit of inhibin in trophoblastic neoplasia. Hum Pathol 1999;30:26-31.
82. Shih IM, Kurman RJ. Epithelioid trophoblastic tumor: a neoplasm distinct from choriocarcinoma and placental site trophoblastic tumor simulating carcinoma. Am J Surg Pathol 1998;22:1393-403.
83. Shih IM, Kurman RJ. Immunohistochemical localization of inhibin-alpha in the placenta and gestational trophoblastic lesions. Int J Gynecol Pathol 1999;18:144-50.
84. Banet N, Gown AM, Shih IeM, et al. GATA-3 expression in trophoblastic tissues: an immunohistochemical study of 445 cases, including diagnostic utility. Am J Surg Pathol 2015;39:101-8.
85. Miettinen M, McCue PA, Sarlomo-Rikala M, et al. GATA3: a multispecific but potentially useful marker in surgical pathology: a systematic analysis of 2500 epithelial and nonepithelial tumors. Am J Surg Pathol 2014;38:13-22.
86. Mirkovic J, Elias K, Drapkin R, Barletta JA, Quade B, Hirsch MS. GATA3 expression in gestational trophoblastic tissues and tumours. Histopathology 2015;67:636-44.
87. Nogales FF, Bergeron C, Carvia RE, Alvaro T, Fulwood HR. Ovarian endometrioid tumors with yolk sac tumor component, an unusual form of ovarian neoplasm. Analysis of six cases. Am J Surg Pathol 1996;20:1056-66.
88. Ramalingam P, Malpica A, Silva EG, Gershenson DM, Liu JL, Deavers MT. The use of cytokeratin 7 and EMA in differentiating ovarian yolk sac tumors from endometrioid and clear cell carcinomas. Am J Surg Pathol 2004;28:1499-505.
89. Cao D, Guo S, Allan RW, Molberg KH, Peng Y. SALL4 is a novel sensitive and specific marker of ovarian primitive germ cell tumors and is particularly useful in distinguishing yolk sac tumor from clear cell carcinoma. Am J Surg Pathol 2009;33:894-904.
90. Maeda D, Ota S, Takazawa Y, et al. Glypican-3 expression in clear cell adenocarcinoma of the ovary. Mod Pathol 2009;22:824-32.
91. Nogales FF, Preda O, Nicolae A. Yolk sac tumours revisited. A review of their many faces and names. Histopathology 2012;60:1023-33.
92. Sangoi AR, McKenney JK, Brooks JD, Bonventre JV, Higgins JP. Evaluation of putative renal cell carcinoma markers PAX-2, PAX-8, and hKIM-1 in germ cell tumors: a tissue microarray study of 100 cases. Appl Immunohistochem Mol Morphol 2012;20:451-3.

93. Fadare O, Zhao C, Khabele D, et al. Comparative analysis of Napsin A, alpha-methylacyl-coenzyme A racemase (AMACR, P504S), and hepatocyte nuclear factor 1 beta as diagnostic markers of ovarian clear cell carcinoma: an immunohistochemical study of 279 ovarian tumours. Pathology 2015;47:105-11.
94. Schoolmeester JK, Carlson J, Keeney GL, et al. Alveolar soft part sarcoma of the female genital tract: a morphologic, immunohistochemical, and molecular cytogenetic study of 10 cases with emphasis on its distinction from morphologic mimics. Am J Surg Pathol 2017;41:622-32.
95. Abdulfatah E, Sakr S, Thomas S, et al. Clear cell carcinoma of the endometrium: evaluation of prognostic parameters in a multi-institutional cohort of 165 cases. Int J Gynecol Cancer 2017;27:1714-21.
96. Huang CY, Chen CA, Chen YL, et al. Nationwide surveillance in uterine cancer: survival analysis and the importance of birth cohort: 30-year population-based registry in Taiwan. PLoS One 2012;7:e51372.
97. Mahdi H, Lockhart D, Moselmi-Kebria M. Prognostic impact of lymphadenectomy in uterine clear cell carcinoma. J Gynecol Oncol 2015; 26:134-40.
98. Üreyen I, Karalok A, Akdag Cırık D, et al. A comparison of clinico-pathologic characteristics of patients with serous and clear cell carcinoma of the uterus. Turk J Obstet Gynecol 2016;13:137-43.
99. Abeler VM, Vergote IB, Kjørstad KE, Tropé CG. Clear cell carcinoma of the endometrium. Prognosis and metastatic pattern. Cancer 1996;78:1740-7.
100. Carcangiu ML, Chambers JT. Early pathologic stage clear cell carcinoma and uterine papillary serous carcinoma of the endometrium: comparison of clinicopathologic features and survival. Int J Gynecol Pathol 1995;14:30-8.
101. Kurman RJ, Scully RE. Clear cell carcinoma of the endometrium: an analysis of 21 cases. Cancer, 1976;37:872-82.
102. Malpica A, Tornos C, Burke TW, Silva EG. Low-stage clear-cell carcinoma of the endometrium. Am J Surg Pathol 1995;19:769-74.

8 FAMILIAL CANCER SYNDROMES

Many advances have been recently made in the detection of familial cancer syndromes that involve the female genital tract. In this chapter, Lynch and Lynch-like syndromes are discussed because of their prevalence among patients with endometrial carcinoma, the most common carcinoma of the female genital tract and the most common tumor diagnosed in women with Lynch syndrome. DNA polymerase E (POLE), Cowden, and BRCA syndromes are also discussed.

LYNCH SYNDROME

Definition. *Lynch syndrome*, previously referred to as *hereditary nonpolyposis colorectal carcinoma syndrome* (HNPCC), is an autosomal dominant disorder that increases the risk for the development of multiple malignancies (1–3). Among them, endometrial and colon carcinomas are the most frequent, but affected individuals are also at increased risk for ovarian, gastric, urinary, hepatobiliary, and small intestinal carcinomas, as well as gliomas (Table 8-1). Lynch syndrome is currently diagnosed by the presence of one of the following: 1) germline mutation of one of the DNA mismatch repair (MMR) genes (*MLH1, PMS2, MSH2,* and *MSH6*); 2) germline *EPCAM* mutation; or 3) constitutive epimutation.

General Features. Between 2 and 6 percent of endometrial carcinomas are attributable to Lynch syndrome. The lifetime risk for the development of endometrial carcinoma in these patients is 20 to 60 percent (1,2). In women with Lynch syndrome, the risk of developing endometrial and ovarian cancer exceeds that of colorectal cancer; in patients who develop both gynecological and intestinal carcinomas, most develop endometrial or ovarian cancers first (4).

The time to the development of a second cancer varies, with a median of 11 and 5 years for patients first diagnosed with endometrial or ovarian cancer, respectively (5). Surveillance for colorectal carcinoma in known Lynch syndrome patients reduces mortality from this cancer by 65 percent (6–8). Prophylactic hysterectomy and bilateral salpingo-oophorectomy in known carriers are also advantageous. Approximately 25 percent of patients undergoing prophylactic surgery have subclinical endometrial hyperplasia or carcinoma of endometrium and/or ovary (9,10).

Although Lynch syndrome is somewhat heterogeneous, there are some important differences between endometrial cancers associated with Lynch syndrome and those that occur sporadically (11–16). Patients with Lynch syndrome-associated endometrial carcinoma are diagnosed at a younger age than the general population. Up to 10 percent of patients under 40 years of age with endometrial carcinoma have Lynch syndrome (7). Although the incidence of Lynch syndrome increases with age, its prevalence decreases significantly due to the increased incidence of sporadic endometrial carcinoma in the general population. These patients also tend to have lower body mass indices.

Pathophysiology and Genetics. A pathogenic germline mutation of one of the DNA MMR genes is the most commonly encountered

Table 8-1

LIFETIME RISK OF CANCER REPORTED IN FAMILIES WITH AN IDENTIFIED MISMATCH REPAIR GENE MUTATION

Colorectal cancer (men)	28-75%
Colorectal cancer (women)	24-52%
Endometrial cancer	27-71%
Ovarian cancer	4-12%
Gastric cancer	2-13%
Urinary tract cancer	1-12%
Brain tumors	1-4%
Bile duct/gallbladder cancer	2%
Small bowel cancer	4-17%

abnormality in patients with Lynch syndrome. A carrier has one copy of a defective DNA MMR gene in all somatic cells throughout the body. A second "hit" occurs in the target organ, such as the endometrium, leading to loss of a functioning DNA MMR protein, thereby interfering with physiologic DNA MMR. The latter is accomplished by two sets of heterodimers, MLH1 with PMS2 and MSH2 with MSH6. Loss of a functioning DNA MMR protein is usually followed by the accumulation or deletion of multiple short tandem repeats in microsatellites (repetitive and widely dispersed DNA sequences that are normally corrected by an intact DNA MMR system). The length of the microsatellites in the target organ does not match that in tissues unaffected by cancer and this is a marker of defective DNA MMR. Neoplasia develops as errors in replication eventually lead to mutations in driver genes.

DNA MMR gene mutation of *MLH1* or *MSH2* leads to the loss of immunohistochemical expression of the corresponding protein in approximately 90 percent of cases, and their respective partner proteins (i.e., MLH1 with PMS2; and MSH2 with MSH6). Isolated *MSH6* or *PMS2* mutations may occur and lead to loss of MSH6 or PMS2 expression only. Microsatellite instability (MSI) analysis by polymerase chain reaction (PCR) currently uses mononucleotide markers, because the methodology is more sensitive than assays examining mono and dinucleotides. Increased sensitivity is required in order to maximize the ability to recognize MSH6 deficient tumors, many of which appear microsatellite stable or microsatellite instable-low using older techniques (17). An "MSI-high (H)" phenotype is not specific for Lynch syndrome, as it is more commonly seen in sporadic tumors. MSI testing alone is, therefore, not recommended in the initial assay for Lynch syndrome screening.

A pathogenic germline *EPCAM* mutation leads to *MSH2* promoter methylation, with consequent MSH2 inactivation and acquisition of a MSI-H phenotype. Although this scenario is considered part of the spectrum of Lynch syndrome, it has been reported that *EPCAM*-mutant Lynch syndrome families develop carcinomas less commonly than classic Lynch syndrome patients (18,19). Another rare mechanism underpinning the development of Lynch syndrome is the presence of intragenic insertions, deletions, and structural variations in the DNA MMR genes, not always detectable using conventional assays. Next-generation deep DNA sequencing (deep NGS) is more likely to identify these types of abnormalities when compared to Sanger DNA sequencing (20).

Lynch syndrome may also develop by consecutive epimutation, another rare mechanism that yields false-negative results when screening only germline mutation. Constitutive epimutation involves widespread methylation of genes throughout the body, including *MLH1*, with a result thought to be similar to that of sporadic *MLH1* methylation or mutation. Currently, Lynch syndrome is mostly diagnosed by studying tissues unaffected by carcinoma, such as blood, as they contain the germline abnormalities that define the entity without the secondary changes acquired by tumor in the target site.

Lynch syndrome is not only heterogeneous from a molecular perspective, but is also heterogeneous from a clinico-pathologic perspective. This is related to the mechanism underlying the DNA MMR abnormality and the type of mutation present. The latter is associated with the risk of developing endometrial carcinoma and extra-gynecologic cancers, the age at which carcinoma develops, and the presence of MSI (11,13–16,21).

Pathogenic mutations in one of the DNA MMR genes, *MSH6*, are more prevalent in Lynch syndrome-associated endometrial carcinoma than in Lynch syndrome-associated colorectal carcinoma, and this accounts for some of the differences in these two settings. *MSH6* germline mutation carriers present at an older age than other Lynch syndrome patients, and tend to develop endometrial carcinoma more often than colorectal carcinoma. The risk of developing endometrial carcinoma with a germline *MSH6* mutation is also higher than for other mutation types. The average patient with Lynch syndrome-associated endometrial carcinoma is older than the average patient with Lynch syndrome-associated colorectal carcinoma, more likely to have an *MSH6* mutation, less likely to have an MSI-H tumor, and less likely to have a personal or family history of Lynch syndrome-associated carcinomas.

Screening and Diagnosis. Screening is meant to reduce the chance of developing a second lethal malignancy in the index patient

Table 8-2
AMSTERDAM II CRITERIA[a]

Three or more family members with LS/HNPCC[b]-related cancers, one of whom is a first-degree relative of the other two

Two successive affected generations

One or more of the LS/HNPCC-related cancers diagnosed under age 50 years

Familial adenomatous polyposis (FAP) has been excluded

[a]Adapted from table 1 from Vasen HF, Watson P, Mecklin JP, Lynch HT. New clinical criteria for hereditary nonpolyposis colorectal cancer (HNPCC, Lynch syndrome) proposed by the International Collaborative group on HNPCC. Gastroenterology 1999;116:1453-6.
[b]LS/HNPCC = Lynch syndrome/hereditary nonpolyposis colorectal carcinoma syndrome.

Table 8-3
REVISED BETHESDA GUIDELINES[a]

Diagnosed with colorectal cancer before the age of 50 years

Synchronous or metachronous colorectal or other LS/HNPCC[b]-related tumors (which include stomach, bladder, ureter, renal pelvis, biliary tract, brain [glioblastoma], sebaceous gland adenomas, keratoacanthomas, and carcinoma of the small bowel), regardless of age

Colorectal cancer with a high microsatellite instability morphology that was diagnosed before the age of 60 years

Colorectal cancer with one or more first-degree relatives with colorectal cancer or other LS/HNPCC-related tumors. One of the cancers must have been diagnosed before the age of 50 years (this includes adenoma, which must have been diagnosed before the age of 40 years)

Colorectal cancer with two or more relatives with colorectal cancer or other LS/HNPCC-related tumors, regardless of age

[a]Adapted from table 2 from Umar A, Boland CR, Terdiman JP, et al. Revised Bethesda Guidelines for hereditary nonpolyposis colorectal cancer (Lynch syndrome) and microsatellite instability. J Natl Cancer Inst 2004;96:261-8.
[b]LS/HNPCC = Lynch syndrome/hereditary nonpolyposis colorectal carcinoma syndrome.

and provides information to family members who may choose to undergo germline testing themselves. Establishing a diagnosis of Lynch syndrome in a healthy carrier should in men encourage close surveillance colonoscopies and, for women, prophylactic hysterectomy and bilateral salpingo-oophorectomy at the appropriate age. A variety of screening modalities based on patient factors such as age, personal history, and family history have been proposed and tested. The Amsterdam (Table 8-2) and Bethesda (Table 8-3) criteria focus primarily on colorectal carcinoma, and most endometrial cancer patients with Lynch syndrome do not meet either criteria. In one seminal study, 70 percent of patients with Lynch syndrome-associated endometrial adenocarcinoma did not meet the Amsterdam criteria or Bethesda guidelines (13).

The more recently proposed Society of Gynecologic Oncologists (SGO) guidelines for the detection of Lynch syndrome in gynecologic cancer patients (22) focus specifically on gynecologic tumors and state that "All women diagnosed with endometrial carcinoma should undergo systematic clinical screening for Lynch syndrome (review of personal and family history) and/or molecular screening. Molecular screening of endometrial cancer for Lynch syndrome is the preferred strategy, when resources are available." Although it is currently not feasible to perform germline sequencing to detect mutated DNA MMR genes in every endometrial carcinoma patient, universal germline sequencing, which requires patient consent, may become standard in the future.

We currently rely on immunohistochemistry to detect DNA MMR proteins. DNA MMR immunohistochemistry is approximately 90 percent sensitive and specific for a DNA MMR abnormality (15,23–25). DNA MMR immunohistochemistry followed by targeted germline sequencing, has been reported to be the most efficient and cost-effective way to identify endometrial cancer patients with Lynch syndrome (15). If DNA MMR immunohistochemistry shows loss of MSH2 and MSH6 expression, germline sequencing should focus on those genes specifically. Although MSI assays fail to recognize all MSI-H endometrial carcinomas, it is effective when used in conjunction with DNA MMR immunohistochemistry, as the false negative rate drops from 10 percent to approximately 5 percent.

The use of next-generation sequencing has also uncovered novel DNA MMR mutations, some of which have not been confirmed to be pathogenic (commonly referred to as "variant of uncertain [or unknown] significance" [VUS]). Most of these cases would previously have been associated with false-negative assays due to the inability of Sanger sequencing to detect the abnormality. Whether these cases constitute Lynch syndrome is uncertain.

DNA MMR immunohistochemistry is only an indirect method of screening for Lynch syndrome. Confirmatory germline testing is still required for this diagnosis since there are several mechanisms that affect DNA MMR expression aside from germline mutations. The most common mechanism underlying expression loss of DNA MMR proteins is epigenetic silencing of the MLH1 promoter due to methylation, present in 20 to 30 percent of endometrial carcinomas and found in the target organ, but not in normal tissues. Comparatively, less is known about the occasional somatic DNA MMR mutations found only in cancer from the target organ. If a cancer cell harbors one allele with a pathogenic somatic DNA MMR mutation, a second hit needs to occur before damage is done to the DNA MMR system. In many instances, the second hit is another somatic DNA MMR mutation. These abnormalities do not constitute Lynch syndrome.

There is growing consensus that, if resources permit, all endometrial carcinomas should undergo DNA MMR immunohistochemical testing as most selective screening schemes fail to detect all Lynch syndrome-associated endometrial carcinomas (26,27). To limit resource expenditure, an age limit, potentially at 65 years, can be set, beyond which the ratio of Lynch syndrome-associated to sporadic endometrial carcinoma falls dramatically, and a two DNA MMR immunomarker panel (i.e., MSH6 and PMS2) can be used, rather than the more traditional four-marker panel (MLH1, PMS2, MSH2, and MSH6) (24). Recent data, however, have shown that a significant percentage of Lynch syndrome patients develop endometrial carcinoma at an old age, calling into question whether it is reasonable to set an upper age limit for screening. More restrictive screening paradigms can be used (21,27), but as more restrictions are placed on screening and resource expenditure lessens, more Lynch syndrome patients will go unrecognized.

Gross Findings. There is scant reported data on the macroscopic characteristics of Lynch syndrome-associated endometrial carcinomas. Although they mostly arise in the corpus, these carcinomas are over-represented among those centered in the lower uterine segment (10 to 30 percent) (27–29). There are also anecdotal reports of multicentric tumors. Prophylactic hysterectomies that contain carcinoma (about 25 percent) harbor small tumors that tend to be less than 2 cm in size. Synchronous ovarian carcinomas can also be encountered (9,10).

Microscopic Findings. The majority of endometrial carcinomas that arise in the setting of Lynch syndrome are endometrioid carcinomas. Some tumors, however, have a histologically ambiguous appearance and may be difficult to histotype, as occurs in sporadic, MSI-H carcinomas (30–33). This likely accounts for variable prevalence rates of nonendometrioid carcinomas in Lynch syndrome cohorts among different studies. Broaddus et al. (34) reported 40 endometrioid carcinomas among 47 patients with Lynch syndrome-associated endometrial carcinomas, while Carcangiu (35) reported only 12 of 22, with many of the "non-endometrioid carcinomas" occurring at young age. After endometrioid carcinoma (the most common Lynch syndrome-associated endometrial carcinoma, about 80 percent) (fig. 8-1), undifferentiated (fig. 8-2), dedifferentiated (fig. 8-3), and mixed endometrioid/clear cell carcinomas follow in prevalence (36). Carcinosarcomas that occur in the setting of Lynch syndrome have a histologic appearance that differs from prototypical examples since they may contain admixtures of differentiated endometrioid carcinoma, undifferentiated carcinoma, and spindled sarcoma. Pure serous carcinomas demonstrating classic morphology and genotype are either exceedingly rare in Lynch syndrome or, perhaps, nonexistent.

Several studies of MSI-H endometrioid carcinomas, including those associated and unassociated with Lynch syndrome, have consistently demonstrated certain histologic and topographic features that differ from those found in microsatellite stable endometrioid carcinomas (21,37,38). These features include: presence of a prominent Crohns-like peritumoral lymphocytic infiltrate (fig. 8-4); increased tumor-infiltrating lymphocytes (fig. 8-5) (defined as more than 42 per 10 high-power fields and evaluated by identifying hotspots at scanning magnification); tumor heterogeneity (defined as two morphologically distinct tumor populations juxtaposed but not intimately admixed (fig. 8-6), including but not limited to dedifferentiated endometrial carcinoma);

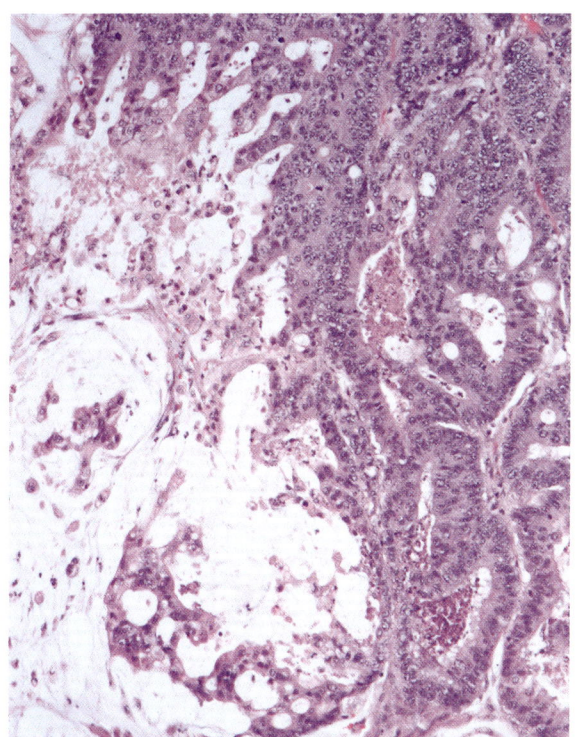
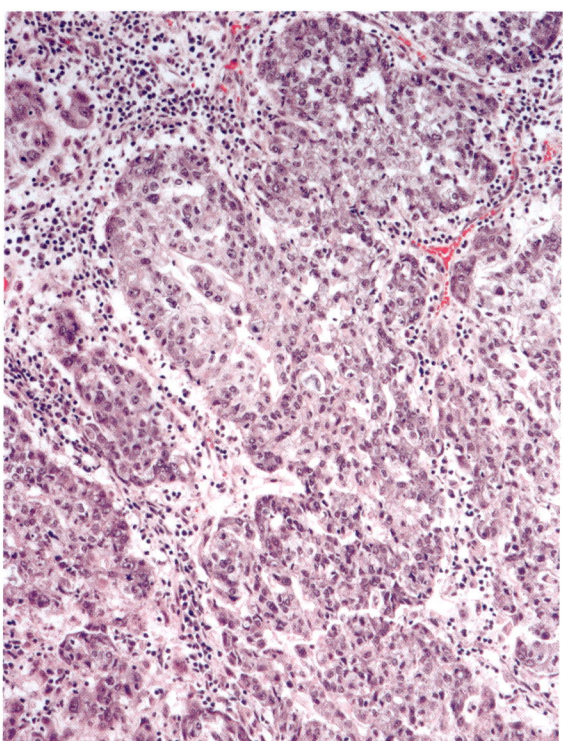

Figure 8-1

LYNCH SYNDROME-ASSOCIATED ENDOMETRIOID ADENOCARCINOMA

Mucinous differentiation (left) and peritumoral lymphocytes (right) are seen.

histologic ambiguity (fig. 8-7); multicentricity; and mucinous differentiation (39). "Histologic ambiguity" describes a tumor with overlapping features of at least two types of carcinoma (32,33,40,41), such as a carcinoma with features of both endometrioid and serous carcinoma.

As mentioned earlier, Lynch syndrome-associated endometrial carcinomas are disproportionately represented in the small group of endometrial cancers that arise or are centered in the lower uterine segment (26,28,29), accounting for 10 to 30 percent of such carcinomas. Synchronous uterine endometrioid carcinoma and ovarian clear cell carcinoma have been seen in association with Lynch syndrome, but there are few reported cases (fig. 8-8) (12,42–44). Rare synchronous endometrioid carcinomas of endometrium and ovary have also been reported (45), although this phenomenon is more commonly found in the sporadic setting. Last, there appears to be an association between Lynch syndrome and endometriosis-associated carcinomas, with or without a synchronous endometrioid carcinoma of endometrium (12,46–48).

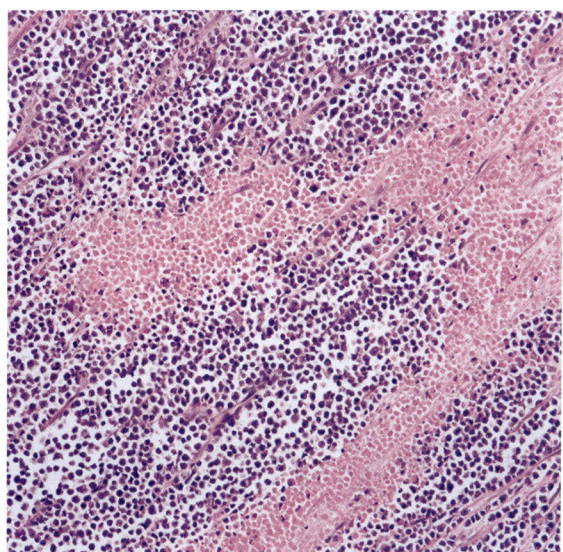

Figure 8-2

LYNCH SYNDROME-ASSOCIATED UNDIFFERENTIATED ENDOMETRIAL CARCINOMA

The tumor resembles a "small blue-cell tumor" with cellular dyshesion and necrosis.

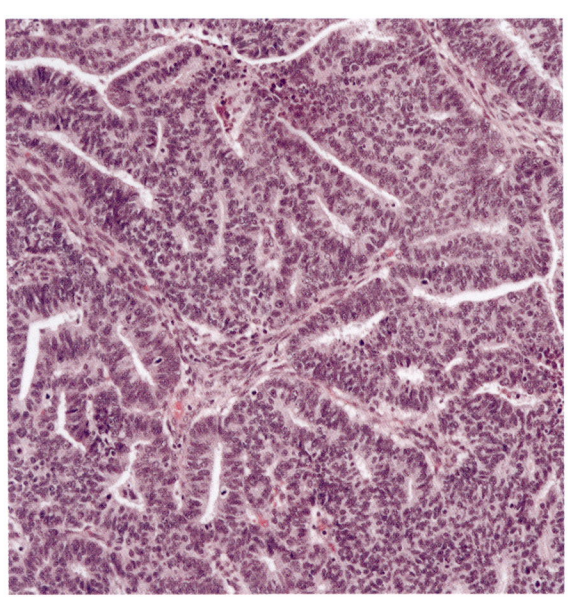 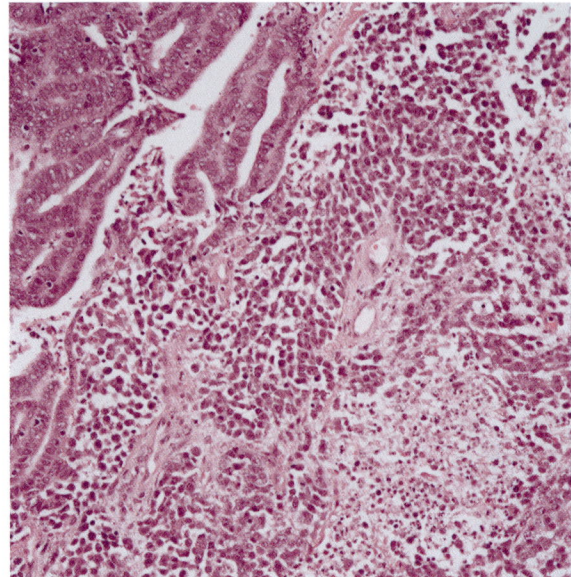

Figure 8-3

LYNCH SYNDROME-ASSOCIATED DEDIFFERENTIATED ENDOMETRIAL CARCINOMA

There are differentiated gland forming (left) and undifferentiated (right) components.

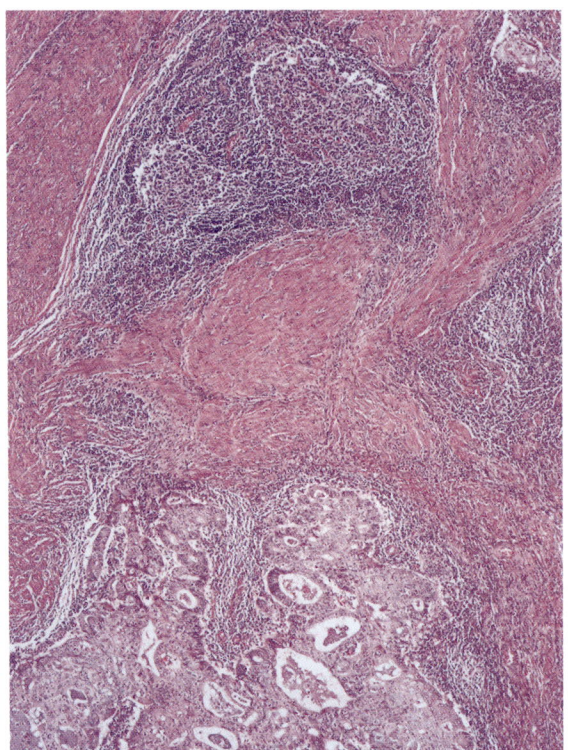 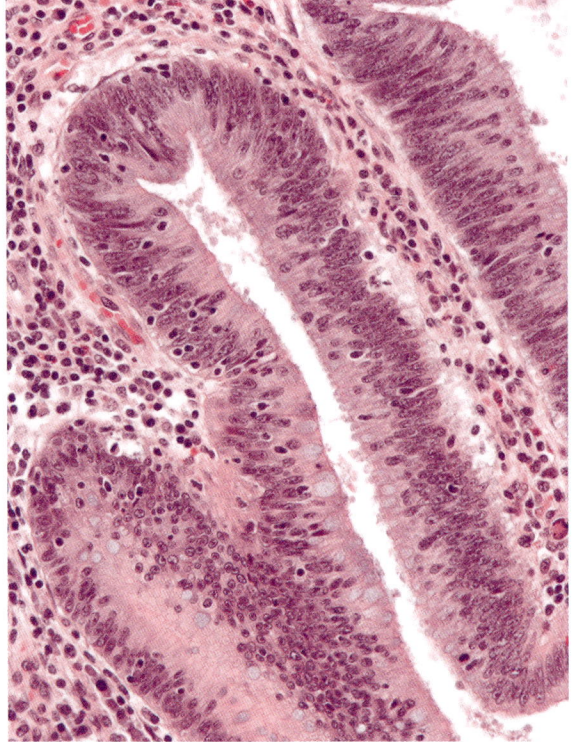

Figure 8-4

MSI-HIGH ENDOMETRIOID CARCINOMA

There is a Crohns-like peritumoral lymphoid infiltrate

Figure 8-5

MSI-HIGH ENDOMETRIOID CARCINOMA

Numerous tumor-infiltrating lymphocytes are seen.

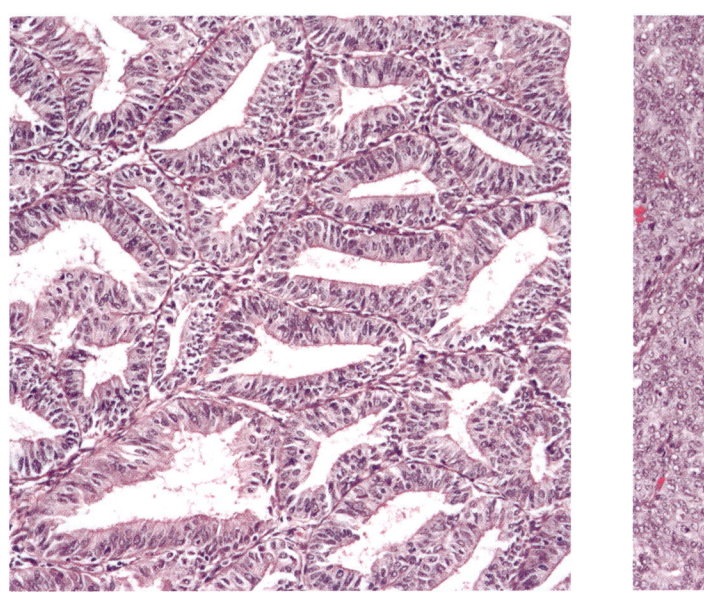
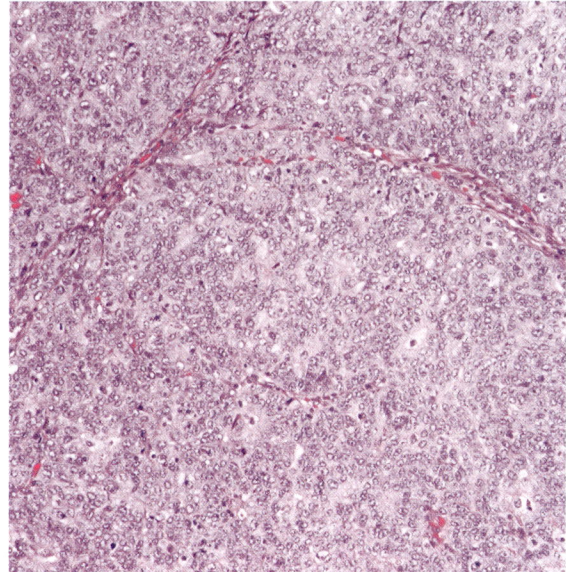

Figure 8-6

MSI-HIGH ENDOMETRIOID CARCINOMA WITH TUMOR HETEROGENEITY
Well-differentiated (left) and poorly differentiated (right) morphologies are present.

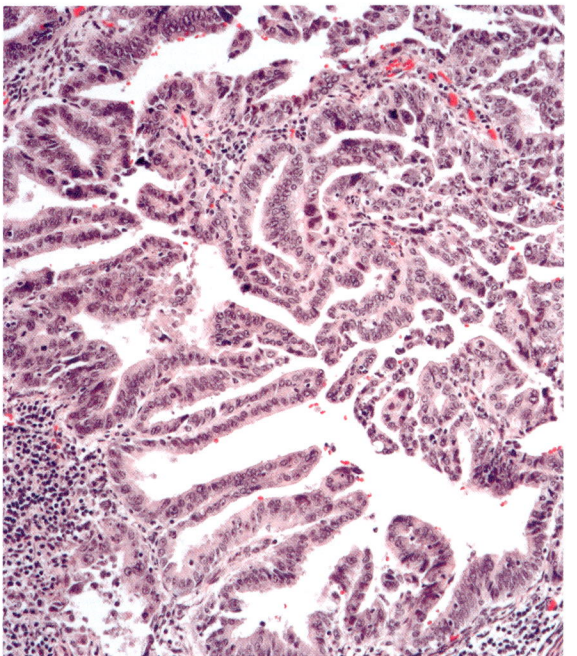
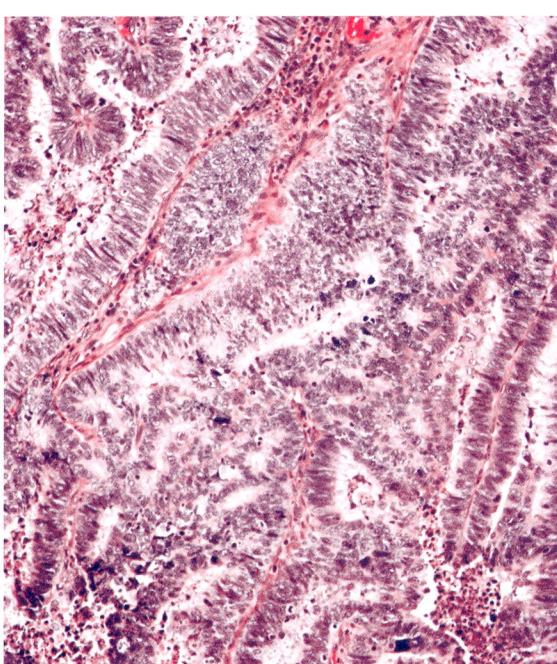

Figure 8-7

MSI-HIGH CARCINOMAS WITH AMBIGUOUS FEATURES

Features suggest endometrioid (at left and bottom) and serous-like differentiation (at upper right). This tumor is best diagnosed as endometrioid adenocarcinoma, although the findings are morphologically ambiguous. Most carcinomas that contain foci diagnostic of low-grade endometrioid carcinoma are endometrioid by genotype (left). An endometrioid carcinoma with striking nuclear stratification, focal loss of polarity, and prominent luminal debris is seen, showing overlapping appearance with serous carcinoma (right).

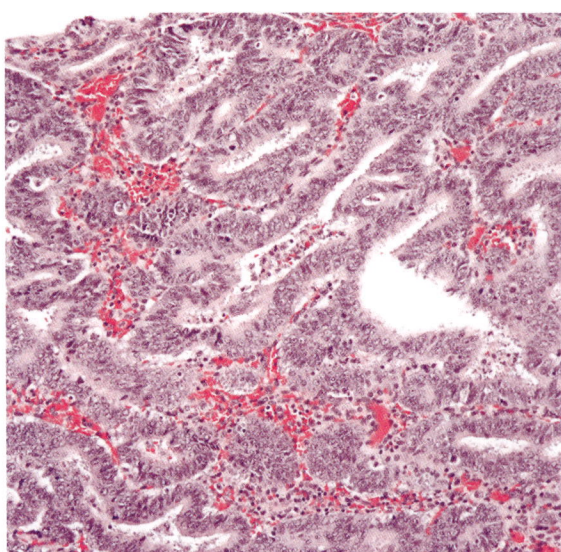 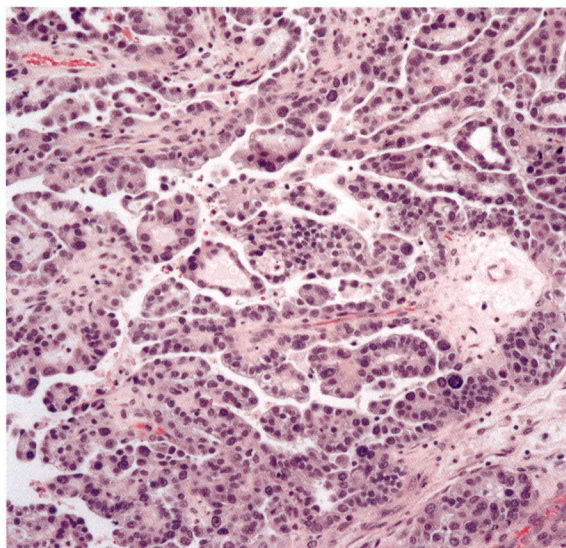

Figure 8-8

MSI-HIGH SYNCHRONOUS ENDOMETRIAL ENDOMETRIOID (left) AND OVARIAN CLEAR CELL (right) CARCINOMAS

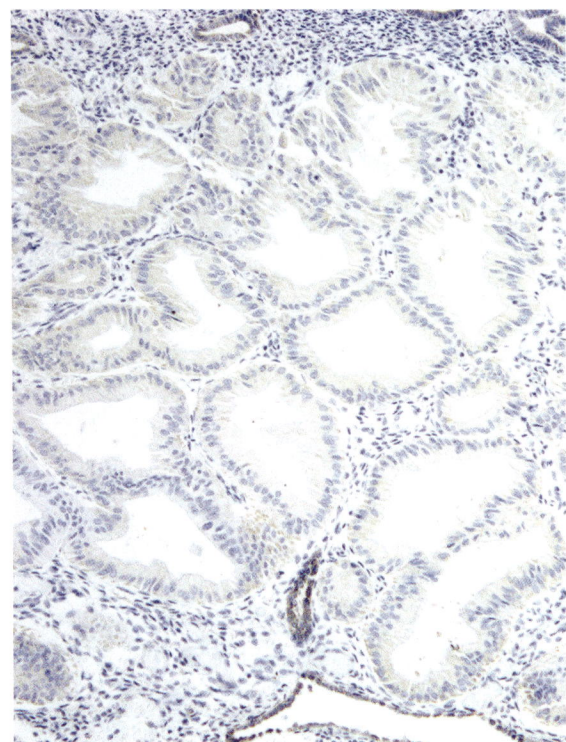

Figure 8-9

LOSS OF EXPRESSION OF MLH1

An atrophic gland provides the positive internal control.

Table 8-4

DNA MISMATCH REPAIR (MMR) IMMUNOHISTOCHEMICAL STAINING PATTERNS AND THEIR SIGNIFICANCE[a]

Diffuse MLH1 and PMS2 loss
  MLH1 promoter methylation>>*MLH1* germline mutation, *MLH1* somatic mutation

Diffuse MSH2 and MSH6 loss
  MSH2 germline mutation, *MSH2* somatic mutation >*EPCAM* deletion

Diffuse MSH6 loss
  MSH6 germline mutation>*MSH6* somatic mutation

Diffuse PMS2 loss
  PMS2 germline mutation or *MLH1* promoter methylation

[a]Adapted from Table 9 from Soslow RA. Practical issues related to uterine pathology: staging, frozen section, artifacts, and Lynch syndrome. Mod Pathol 2016;29(Suppl 1):S59-77.

Immunohistochemical Findings. Loss of DNA MMR expression in tumor cell nuclei is equated to an abnormal DNA MMR immunohistochemical result. To properly score immunostains, an intact internal positive control, usually provided by non-neoplastic stromal cells, endothelium, tumor-infiltrating lymphocytes, and non-neoplastic endometrium, should be present for comparison (fig. 8-9). Table 8-4 compiles the

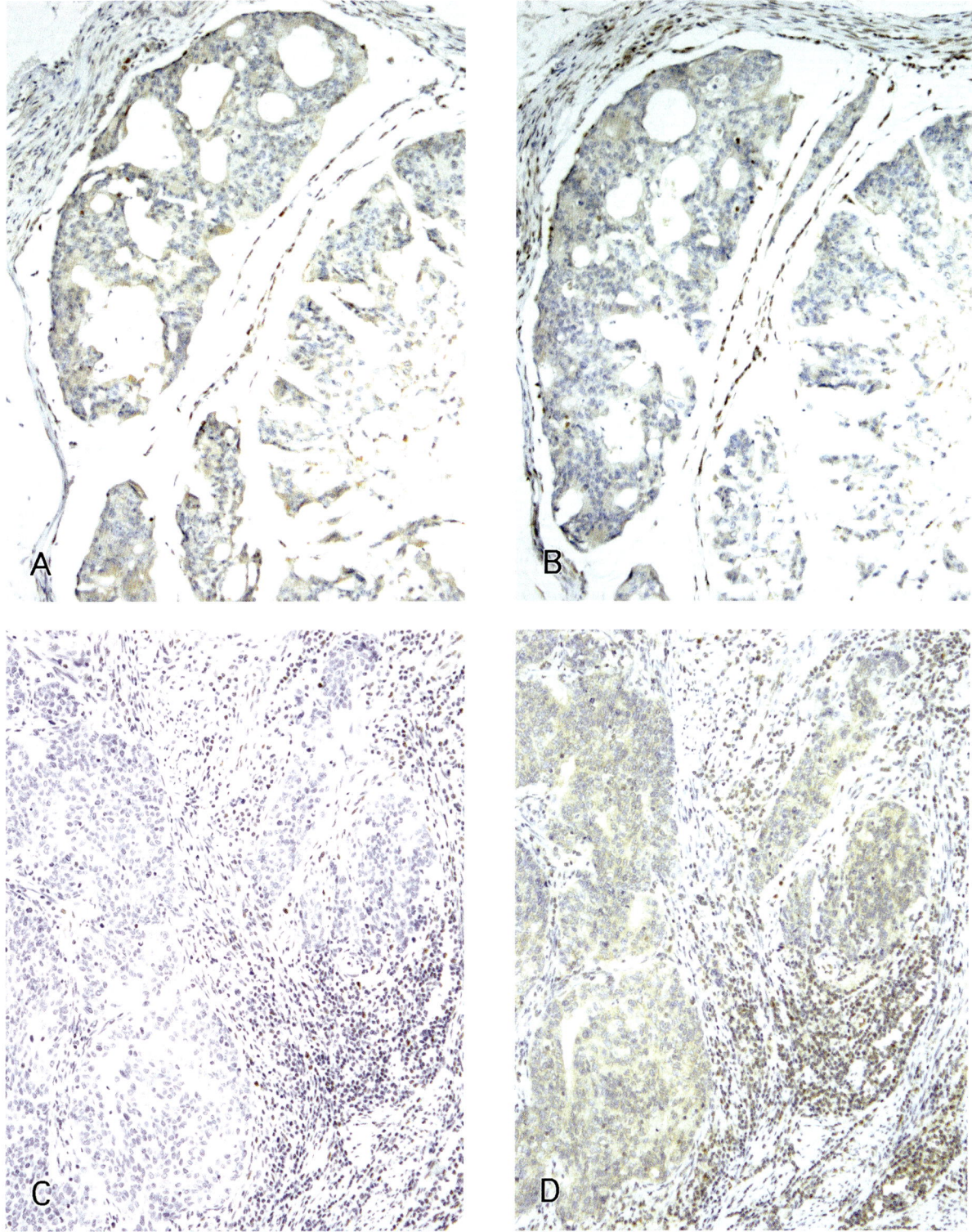

Figure 8-10

CONCORDANT LOSS OF EXPRESSION OF MSH2 AND MSH6 OR MLH1 AND PMS2

Loss of expression of MSH2 (A), MSH6 (B), MLH1 (C), and PMS2 (D) are seen.

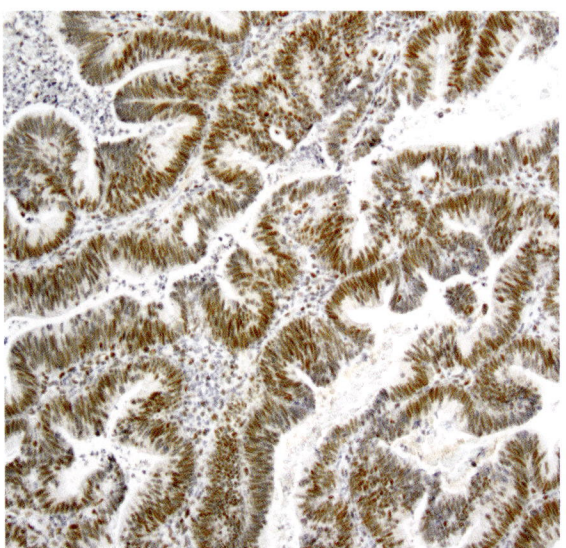 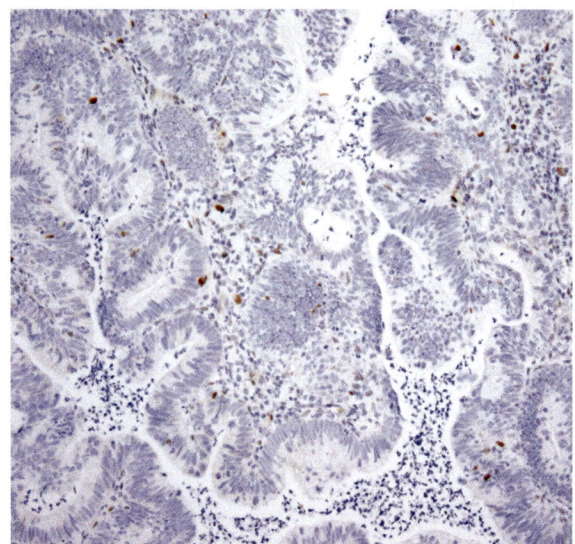

Figure 8-11

DISCORDANT EXPRESSION OF MSH2 AND MSH6

Intact expression of MSH2 (left) and loss of expression of MSH6 (right) are seen in the same tumor.

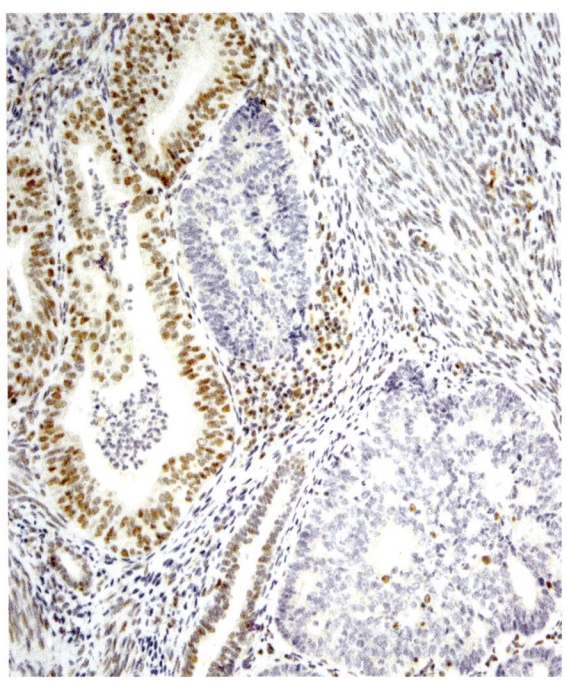

Figure 8-12

GEOGRAPHIC/HETEROGENEOUS LOSS OF MLH1 EXPRESSION

MLH1 staining is lost in morphologically and spatially distinct regions of this carcinoma. This staining pattern is not suggestive of Lynch syndrome. Rather, it can be seen in the presence of subclonal *MLH1* promoter methylation or somatic mutation.

most common abnormal DNA MMR immunohistochemical staining patterns, listed in order of decreasing frequency. The most common involves loss of expression of MLH1/PMS2 or MSH2/MSH6 (fig. 8-10). Less frequently, abnormal PMS2 with intact MLH1 or abnormal MSH6 without MSH2 is found (fig. 8-11). These findings support the use of a two DNA MMR immunomarker panel consisting of PMS2 and MSH6 (21,24,49).

Two other rare abnormal patterns are loss of three or four markers (50) and geographic loss of expression (51,52). The latter, particularly when involving MLH1, is associated with acquisition of promoter methylation in a subclone of the tumor and is unassociated with Lynch syndrome in most instances (fig. 8-12) (51,52). Geographic loss of expression of MSH6 tends to be a pattern associated with *POLE* exonuclease domain hotspot mutations (personal observation), usually a somatic event.

Table 8-5 lists some common pitfalls in the interpretation of DNA MMR immunohistochemistry. The two most common problems are distinguishing weak or equivocal staining from abnormal staining (fig. 8-13), and confusing tumor-infiltrating lymphocytes (fig. 8-14) for tumor cells with intact DNA MMR staining. In the first scenario, the stain should be repeated. Additionally, it is important to

Table 8-5
CHALLENGES IN INTERPRETING DNA MISMATCH REPAIR (MMR) IMMUNOHISTOCHEMISTRY[a]

Challenge	Solution
Weak or equivocal MLH1 staining	Use PMS2 staining pattern to adjudicate
Lacking positive internal control	Look for proliferative cells, particularly lymphocytes; stain another block if necessary
Unexpected staining patterns (cytoplasmic, nucleolar, perinuclear, patchy staining)	Accept only nuclear staining as valid. Any nuclear staining should be scored as "retained/protein present"; be sure not to score positive intratumoral lymphocytes alone as "retained/protein present"

[a]Table 10 from Soslow RA. Practical issues related to uterine pathology: staging, frozen section, artifacts, and Lynch syndrome. Mod Pathol 2016;29(Suppl 1):S59-77.

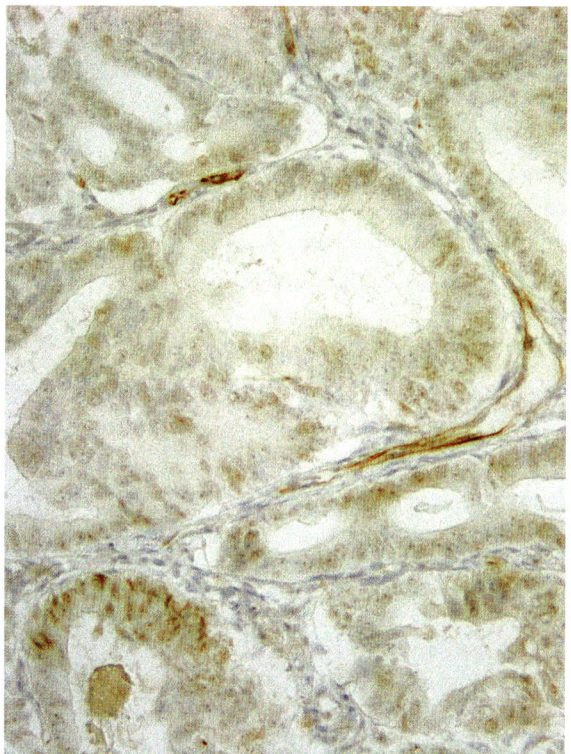 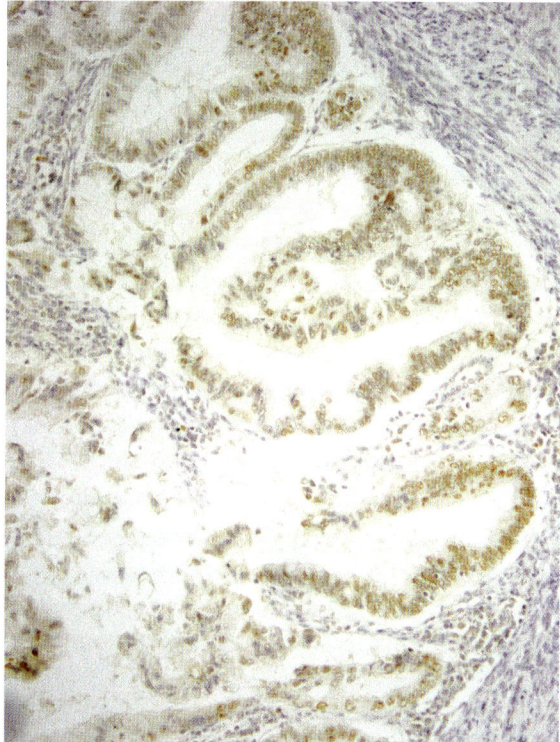

Figure 8-13

WEAK MLH1 EXPRESSION IN TUMOR CELLS

This is confirmed as "retained staining" (left) when PMS2 stain (right) shows unequivocal intact tumor nuclear staining.

evaluate the result for the partner protein (i.e., look at PMS2 if the MLH1 is equivocal), choose another tumor block for staining, or show stains to an experienced colleague. If results remain equivocal, results should be reported as inconclusive rather than "normal" or "abnormal." Distinguishing tumor-infiltrating lymphocytes from tumor cells is generally straightforward once one is aware of this pitfall. Use of leukocyte common antigen immunohistochemistry may be considered.

When DNA MMR immunohistochemistry shows abnormal MLH1 and PMS2 expression, the most commonly encountered abnormal staining pattern, germline genetic testing should not be undertaken without first performing an MLH1 promoter methylation assay (fig. 8-15) (53). As finding MLH1 promoter methylation signifies

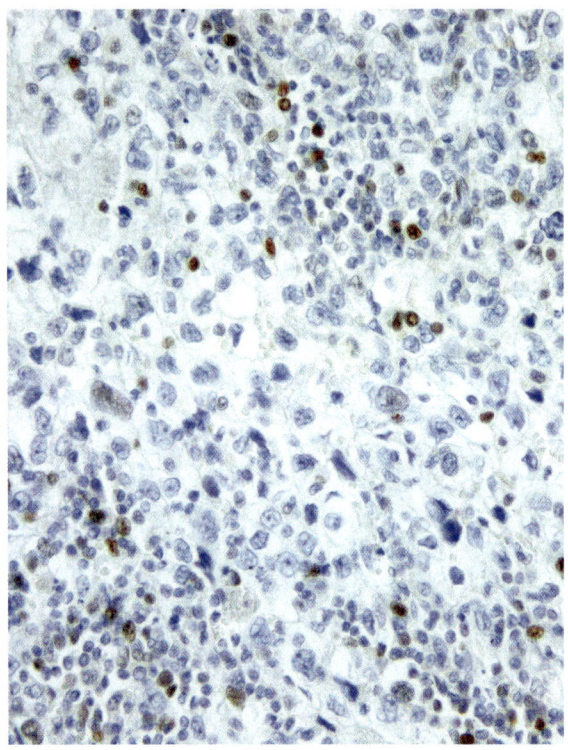

Figure 8-14

MSH6-POSITIVE TUMOR-INFILTRATING LYMPHOCYTES

Lymphocytes are seen in a background of Lynch syndrome-associated endometrioid carcinoma with loss of MSH6 staining.

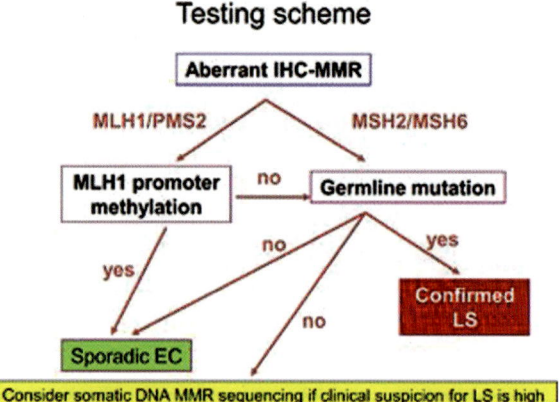

Figure 8-15

Integrated DNA-mismatch repair immunohistochemical staining and genetic testing schema. (Fig. 22 from Soslow RA. Practical issues related to uterine pathology: staging, frozen section, artifacts, and Lynch syndrome. Mod Pathol 2016;29(Suppl 1):S59-77.)

that the patient has the lowest risk for Lynch syndrome, germline genetic testing is generally not performed unless there is a strong family or personal history of Lynch syndrome-related carcinomas. The MLH1 promoter methylation assay replaces BRAF testing, as is performed in colorectal carcinomas, as *BRAF* mutations are almost never found in endometrial carcinomas.

Comprehensive Screening System. The development of a comprehensive screening system for Lynch syndrome warrants a multidisciplinary approach. It is recommended to seek advice and collaboration from medic-legal experts, clinical geneticists, gynecologic surgeons, medical oncologists, and pathologists. Table 8-6 presents a summary of the barriers to identify all endometrial cancer patients with Lynch syndrome and underscores ways in which even a coordinated and motivated team may miss such patients. A uniform approach to Lynch syndrome screening may not be appropriate, but the complexity of any system requires open lines of communication, compliance audits, and further refinements as practitioners learn more about Lynch syndrome. It is uncertain whether this collaborative approach can succeed in low-volume practices and in settings where interdisciplinary teams do not exist or are not highly functional. At a minimum, compliance audits must demonstrate that, regardless of the screening paradigm used, all applicable tumors are tested and all abnormal results are reported to physicians and/or clinical geneticists who can make the best use of the information.

Treatment and Prognosis. Many studies have reported that Lynch syndrome-associated endometrial carcinomas can exhibit adverse prognostic indicators, including nonendometrioid and undifferentiated histology, high FIGO grade, high stage, and lymphovascular invasion (21,34,35,38,54), but the prognostic implications of these findings are uncertain. In fact, some studies have found an association between MMR defects and improved survival, while others have shown no association with survival or worse clinical outcome (55–57). Larger studies with long-term follow-up are required to definitively assess the impact of MMR status on therapy and outcome in endometrial carcinoma patients.

Table 8-6
BARRIERS TO THE IDENTIFICATION OF ENDOMETRIAL CANCER PATIENTS WITH LYNCH SYNDROME

1. Problems with patient selection and testing for Lynch syndrome (LS)
   a. The rationale for detecting LS in endometrial cancer patients is not as well-delineated as it is in colorectal carcinoma patients as it is not yet known whether LS affects the clinical biology of endometrial cancer or whether therapy should be modulated based on LS status. Therefore, screening for LS may appear mostly an academic exercise from a gynecologist's standpoint. It is emphasized that detecting which endometrial cancer patients have LS may save lives because of the benefit of screening colonoscopies that lower death rates from subsequent colorectal carcinomas in the index patient and related carriers, and of prophylactic hysterectomy and bilateral salpingo-oophorectomy in carriers.
   b. Many practitioners still use the term "hereditary nonpolyposis colorectal carcinoma syndrome," which places undue emphasis on colorectal carcinoma. The majority of women with LS develop endometrial and/or ovarian cancer. When they develop both LS-associated endometrial and colorectal carcinomas, many patients present with the gynecologic cancer first.
   c. Many clinicians depend on a simple family history report to roughly screen for LS. Up to 70% of endometrial cancer patients with LS do NOT have a personal or family history of LS. This is in contrast to colorectal carcinoma, where rates are in the 20–30% range.
   d. Current LS screening uses immunohistochemistry for DNA mismatch repair (MMR) proteins on tumor samples. Centers that do the four-marker panel on all endometrial cancers would theoretically have the lowest miss rates for picking up possible LS. This practice:
      i. Uses many resources, not all of which are reimbursed to pathologists.
      ii. Mandates follow-up of an inordinate number of patients who do NOT have LS. Greater than 75% of patients whose tumors have abnormal DNA MMR immunohistochemistry have either a somatic DNA MMR mutation or MLH1 promoter methylation, neither of which constitutes LS. Further testing, given this scenario, requires the MLH1 methylation assay, which is not available at most medical centers, and in some, somatic mutation testing.
   e. As DNA MMR immunohistochemistry is only 90% sensitive, there will be at least a 10% miss rate if the sole screening system is immunohistochemistry. MSI analyses can be performed in addition to immunohistochemistry in order to minimize false negative results.
2. Problems with reporting
   a. The immunohistochemistry report may accompany the main biopsy or hysterectomy report or may be issued as an addendum (issued a few days after the main pathology report). Not finding the report at the right time, and having the wrong physician find the report are all barriers. Examples include the following: the clinician does not compulsively check the electronic medical record every day in order to find the addendum report; the report is generated after the patient's first follow-up visit and the surgeon gets the report, but in many instances, the medical oncologist or clinical geneticist are most appropriate to interpret the report and convey the information to the patient. A quality assurance audit should ensure that every patient with an abnormal report is contacted by a clinical geneticist. A formal clinical genetics consultation is scheduled only after any necessary ancillary tests are performed (i.e., MLH1 promoter methylation testing) and the patient is motivated to attend the consultation.
   b. Related to the terminology used in immunohistochemistry reports, most DNA MMR immunohistochemistry reports avoid the use of the terms "LS" and "germline genetic testing" because then regulators could argue that DNA MMR immunohistochemistry is a germline genetic test that requires patient consent. The report usually talks about "lost" or "retained" expression of DNA MMR proteins, the subtleties of which may be lost on the recipient.
3. Problems with clinical genetics consultation and germline genetic testing
   a. Many endometrial cancer patients are not motivated to attend clinical genetics consultation.
   b. With some uncommon exceptions, germline genetic testing cannot be performed on tumor material presently, thus, normal tissue needs to be procured, usually in the form of a blood sample.
   c. Once MLH1 promoter methylation is excluded, germline genetic testing detects germline mutations in only 40–70% of patients with abnormal DNA MMR immunohistochemistry. Thirty to 40% have somatic mutations, LS with undetectable germline mutations, or germline variants of uncertain significance.

(Appendix 1 from Soslow RA. Practical issues related to uterine pathology: staging, frozen section, artifacts, and Lynch syndrome. Mod Pathol 2016;29(Suppl 1):S59-77.

Currently, patients with Lynch syndrome are treated based on widely accepted norms such as stage and grade. A growing number of clinical trials involve modulation of antitumor immunity using immune checkpoint blockade, and such therapy is now FDA-approved for recurrent, MSI-H endometrial carcinomas. Lynch syndrome-associated carcinomas are thought to be good therapeutic candidates for these trials as they are hypermutated, contain many neo-antigens due to high mutational rates and microsatellite instability, and frequently contain many tumor-infiltrating lymphocytes. It has been recently reported that MMR-deficient endometrial carcinomas may be more sensitive to adjuvant therapy than MMR-proficient tumors (58).

LYNCH-LIKE SYNDROME

Definition. *Lynch-like syndrome* is the development of an MSI-H and/or DNA MMR-deficient carcinoma, lacking MLH1 promoter methylation, without an identifiable pathogenic DNA MMR germline mutation. As we learn more about this provisional category, patients whose tumors have biallelic somatic DNA MMR mutations may be said to have sporadic endometrial carcinomas, rather than "Lynch-like syndrome" (discussed below).

General Features and Epidemiology. Most of the work on this topic has been performed in the setting of colorectal carcinoma, and it is assumed that many of the underlying mechanisms that account for Lynch-like syndrome in endometrial and ovarian carcinomas are probably similar, but other details need confirmation. Lynch-like syndrome patients present at approximately the same age as Lynch syndrome patients (10 to 20 years younger than patients with sporadic carcinomas), have significantly lower rates of developing colorectal carcinoma, and less frequently, have a family or personal history of Lynch syndrome-associated carcinomas (20,59–63).

Lynch-like syndrome carcinomas constitute 30 to 60 percent of all MSI-H carcinomas lacking pathogenic DNA MMR germline mutations and MLH1 promoter methylation (i.e., *EPCAM* mutation). The presence of rare germline abnormalities, discussed above, should be excluded before considering Lynch-like syndrome.

Pathophysiology and Genetics. Literature on colorectal carcinoma and a few recent publications on Lynch-like syndrome-associated endometrial carcinoma have emphasized the importance of bi-allelic pathogenic somatic mutations affecting one of the DNA MMR genes (somatic DNA MMR mutations as both first and second hits in the target organ) as a widespread mechanism for the development of this carcinoma (64–68). It has been postulated that the first hit might occur in a cancer precursor lesion, while the second hit occurs with the development of carcinoma. These patients are thought to lack a heritable cancer syndrome and, thus, it is not necessarily recommended that they undergo close surveillance to detect colorectal carcinoma.

A pathogenic somatic mutation in *polymerase E* or *polymerase D1* (*POLE* or *POLD1*, respectively), with secondary somatic mutations in one or more of the DNA MMR genes (69) has been reported as an uncommon mechanism for the development of a Lynch-like syndrome phenotype. Bi-allelic somatic mutations account for only approximately half of Lynch-like syndrome cases, with the remainder being poorly understood.

A number of epigenetic mechanisms may be responsible for Lynch-like syndrome or a poorly understood Lynch syndrome variant, an example being inhibitory microRNAs that influence transcription of the DNA MMR genes (20). Bi-allelic somatic mutations in the *MUTYH* gene can also be responsible for a Lynch-like syndrome phenotype (70,71). It is currently unknown whether these somatic mutations are a result of an association with a yet obscure germline event.

Lynch syndrome is distinguished from Lynch-like syndrome when well-known and well-understood abnormalities reported in the setting of Lynch syndrome are documented; these are most readily identified using NGS targeting a panel of pertinent genes. Somatic mutations of *POLE* or *POLD1*, or bi-allelic somatic mutation of one or more of the DNA MMR genes may help exclude a diagnosis of Lynch syndrome, however, due to limitations of current sequencing technologies, it is often not possible to determine whether both mutations occur on the same allele. If Lynch syndrome is excluded, these patients do not need the close surveillance of Lynch syndrome patients or other patients in which neither germline nor somatic mutations are found.

There is a spectrum of poorly understood abnormalities that may place the patient and relatives at increased risk for Lynch syndrome-associated carcinomas, such as the presence of a variant of uncertain significance. Affected patients should consult with a clinical geneticist in collaboration with the treating physician to determine whether close clinical surveillance offered to bona fide Lynch-like syndrome patients is warranted.

POLE AND POLD1 GERMLINE MUTATIONS

Endometrial carcinomas with somatic *POLE* mutations involving hotspots in the exonuclease domain are discussed in chapter 5. Germline mutations in *POLE* and *POLD1* have also been reported to predispose to endometrial and colorectal carcinomas (72–75).

POLE mutations are more likely to be somatic compared to *POLD1* mutations. Pathogenic mutations in these genes lead to the "polymerase proofreading-associated polyposis syndrome" of the bowel, a dominantly inherited and highly penetrant syndrome associated with development of colorectal and endometrial carcinomas in young individuals. A recent study focusing on International Federation of Gynecology and Obstetrics (FIGO) grade 3 endometrioid carcinomas in Southeast Asian patients (76) reported two germline *POLE* mutations and two germline *POLD1* mutations in 47 patients tested (i.e., nearly 10 percent of FIGO grade 3 endometrioid carcinomas in this population had a germline mutation affecting one of the polymerase genes). Pathogenic somatic and germline mutations of these genes were associated with 100 percent recurrence-free survival in this study, but several recurrent *POLE*-mutated endometrial carcinomas have been recently described (77). Since there was an apparent association between these mutations and MSI (mostly in *POLE* tumors) and dense peritumoral lymphocytic infiltration, it was suggested that these findings could be used as ancillary features that might prompt evaluation for *POLE* and *POLD1* abnormalities, once Lynch syndrome is excluded.

COWDEN SYNDROME

Cowden syndrome is one of several disorders that are considered part of the PTEN hamartoma tumor syndrome. This autosomal dominant syndrome develops in individuals with pathogenic germline mutations in the phosphatase and tensin homolog gene (*PTEN*), a tumor suppressor located on 10q23.3. Other genes have been implicated, including *SDH-B, SDH-C, SDH-D*, and *KLLN* (78).

Patients with Cowden syndrome are at risk for different types of hamartomas as well as a variety of malignancies, which in decreasing order of incidence are carcinomas of the breast, thyroid gland, endometrium, and kidney. The prevalence of Cowden syndrome is estimated to be approximately 1 in 200,000 to 250,000, but the true incidence is difficult to ascertain due to the subtle and variable presentation in many patients, leading to probable underdiagnosis (79–83).

In addition to endometrial carcinoma, women are also prone to develop uterine leiomyomas and benign ovarian cysts (78,84). Nonmalignant manifestations include multiple hamartomatous tumors, especially in the gastrointestinal tract, mucocutaneous (facial tricholemmomas, papillomatous oral proliferations), benign breast or thyroid gland lesions, and macrocephaly. Significant predictors of germline *PTEN* abnormality in patients with endometrial carcinoma include: carcinoma diagnosed at age 50 years or younger, macrocephaly, and synchronous/metachronous renal cell carcinoma (78).

Cowden syndrome patients have up to a 28 percent lifetime risk of developing endometrial carcinoma (85,86). The prevalence of Cowden syndrome in unselected endometrial carcinoma patients, however, is largely unknown, although it is probably very low as no germline *PTEN* abnormalities were identified in a series of 240 consecutive endometrial carcinoma patients (87). The mean age at diagnosis of endometrial carcinoma (44 years) was reported in only one series of patients with Cowden syndrome (78), but endometrial carcinoma has also been reported in adolescents as young as 14 years who were subsequently diagnosed with Cowden syndrome (84,88,89).

Scant data regarding the histologic subtypes of endometrial carcinoma that occur in patients with Cowden syndrome is available. In a large study of 371 patients with Cowden syndrome, endometrioid carcinoma was the most common (42 percent), followed by serous/clear cell (5 percent) and mucinous (0.3 percent) subtypes. In half of the patients, however, the histologic type was not known (78). There have also been isolated case reports of endometrioid carcinomas occurring in patients with Cowden syndrome (88–91) but large morphologically detailed studies are lacking.

The prognostic significance of a germline *PTEN* mutation is unknown. Cowden syndrome patients, however, have a 7-fold increased risk of a secondary malignancy, compared to the general population (92).

HEREDITARY BREAST AND OVARIAN CANCER SYNDROMES (*BRCA* SYNDROMES)

There are rare reports of endometrial serous carcinoma in Israeli kindreds (93–95) and endometrial serous carcinomas with loss of BRCA1 protein expression (96), suggesting that a rare patient with a *BRCA* germline mutation can develop endometrial serous carcinoma. A recent epidemiologic study reported that patients with *BRCA1* germline mutations are 22 times more likely than controls to develop endometrial serous carcinoma or carcinosarcoma (97), but tamoxifen exposure is also associated with a similar increased risk. The data presented included only four patients with *BRCA1*-associated serous carcinoma (n=3) or carcinosarcoma with a serous epithelial component (n=1). Two serous carcinomas and the one carcinosarcoma were tested with BRCA1 immunohistochemistry and all three tumors showed loss of expression, indicating an abnormality in *BRCA1*, probably with loss of heterozygosity. Another *BRCA1* germline carrier from the same series developed uterine leiomyosarcoma, which was subsequently found to be sporadic and unrelated to the patient's germline *BRCA1* mutation.

Although it is possible that a *BRCA1* germline mutation is etiologically responsible for the development of rare endometrial serous carcinomas and carcinosarcomas, it is also possible that at least some of the reported cases represent drop metastases from occult high-grade serous carcinomas of the fallopian tube or are tamoxifen-induced endometrial serous carcinomas. These recent observations have invoked a discussion regarding whether hysterectomy should be performed at the time of risk-reducing (prophylactic) bilateral salpingo-oophorectomy in known *BRCA1* carriers, but no consensus has been reached. It appears that the overwhelming majority of gynecologists would still not counsel their patients, particularly those of reproductive age, to undergo risk-reducing hysterectomy, based on current evidence.

RARE AND CONTROVERSIAL DRIVERS OF ENDOMETRIAL CARCINOMA

In addition to the germline mutations discussed in this chapter, other germline mutations found in patients with endometrial carcinoma or thought to possibly increase the risk of endometrial carcinoma include *CHEK2*, *MUTYH*, *STK11*, genes involved in Cowden-like syndrome (*SDHB*, *SDHC*, *SDHD*, *AKT1*, *PIK3CA*, *KLLN*, and *SEC23B*), *RINT1*, *NTLH1*, *FAN1*, *APC*, *ATM*, *BRIP1*, *FANCC*, *NBN*, *PALB2*, and *RAD51C* (98). With the exception of genes involved in Cowden-like syndrome, which certainly predispose to the development of endometrial carcinoma, the other genes are likely extremely rare drivers of endometrial carcinoma or not related to endometrial carcinoma at all.

REFERENCES

1. Aarnio M, Sankila R, Pukkala E, et al. Cancer risk in mutation carriers of DNA-mismatch-repair genes. Int J Cancer 1999;81:214-8.
2. Vasen HF, Offerhaus GJ, den Hartog Jager FC, et al. The tumour spectrum in hereditary non-polyposis colorectal cancer: a study of 24 kindreds in the Netherlands. Int J Cancer 1990;46:31-4.
3. Watson P, Lynch HT. The tumor spectrum in HNPCC. Anticancer Res 1994;14:1635-9.
4. Hampel H, de la Chapelle A. The search for unaffected individuals with Lynch syndrome: do the ends justify the means? Cancer Prev Res (Phila) 2011;4:1-5.
5. Lu KH, Dinh M, Kohlmann W, et al. Gynecologic cancer as a "sentinel cancer" for women with hereditary nonpolyposis colorectal cancer syndrome. Obstet Gynecol 2005;105:569-74.
6. Jarvinen HJ, Aarnio M, Mustonen H, et al. Controlled 15-year trial on screening for colorectal cancer in families with hereditary nonpolyposis colorectal cancer. Gastroenterology 2000;118:829-34.
7. Lu KH, Schorge JO, Rodabaugh KJ, et al. Prospective determination of prevalence of lynch syndrome in young women with endometrial cancer. J Clin Oncol 2007;25:5158-64.
8. Pylvanainen K, Lehtinen T, Kellokumpu I, Jarvinen H, Mecklin JP. Causes of death of mutation carriers in Finnish Lynch syndrome families. Fam Cancer 2012;11:467-71.
9. Bartosch C, Pires-Luis AS, Meireles C, et al. Pathologic findings in prophylactic and non-prophylactic hysterectomy specimens of patients with Lynch syndrome. Am J Surg Pathol 2016;40:1177-91.
10. Karamurzin Y, Soslow RA, Garg K. Histologic evaluation of prophylactic hysterectomy and oophorectomy in Lynch syndrome. Am J Surg Pathol 2013;37:579-85.
11. Bonadona V, Bonaiti B, Olschwang S, et al. Cancer risks associated with germline mutations in MLH1, MSH2, and MSH6 genes in Lynch syndrome. JAMA 2011;305:2304-10.
12. Garg K, Shih K, Barakat R, Zhou Q, Iasonos A, Soslow RA. Endometrial carcinomas in women aged 40 years and younger: tumors associated with loss of DNA mismatch repair proteins comprise a distinct clinicopathologic subset. Am J Surg Pathol 2009;33:1869-77.
13. Hampel H, Frankel W, Panescu J, et al. Screening for Lynch syndrome (hereditary nonpolyposis colorectal cancer) among endometrial cancer patients. Cancer Res 2006;66:7810-7.
14. Ramsoekh D, Wagner A, van Leerdam ME, et al. Cancer risk in MLH1, MSH2 and MSH6 mutation carriers; different risk profiles may influence clinical management. Hered Cancer Clin Pract 2009;7:17.
15. Resnick K, Straughn JM Jr, Backes F, Hampel H, Matthews KS, Cohn DE. Lynch syndrome screening strategies among newly diagnosed endometrial cancer patients. Obstet Gynecol 2009;114:530-6.
16. Win AK, Young JP, Lindor NM, et al. Colorectal and other cancer risks for carriers and noncarriers from families with a DNA mismatch repair gene mutation: a prospective cohort study. J Clin Oncol 2012;30:958-64.
17. Zhang L. Immunohistochemistry versus microsatellite instability testing for screening colorectal cancer patients at risk for hereditary nonpolyposis colorectal cancer syndrome. Part II. The utility of microsatellite instability testing. J Mol Diagn 2008;10:301-7.
18. Kang SY, Park CK, Chang DK, et al. Lynch-like syndrome: characterization and comparison with EPCAM deletion carriers. Int J Cancer 2015;136:1568-78.
19. Kuiper RP, Vissers LE, Venkatachalam R, et al. Recurrence and variability of germline EPCAM deletions in Lynch syndrome. Hum Mutat 2011;32:407-14.
20. Buchanan DD, Rosty C, Clendenning M, Spurdle AB, Win AK. Clinical problems of colorectal cancer and endometrial cancer cases with unknown cause of tumor mismatch repair deficiency (suspected Lynch syndrome). Appl Clin Genet 2014;7:183-93.
21. Garg K, Leitao MM Jr, Kauff ND, et al. Selection of endometrial carcinomas for DNA mismatch repair protein immunohistochemistry using patient age and tumor morphology enhances detection of mismatch repair abnormalities. Am J Surg Pathol 2009;33:925-33.
22. SGO Clinical Practice Statement: Screening for Lynch Syndrome in Endometrial Cancer. Society of Gynecologic Oncology 2014. https://www.sgo.org/clinical-practice/guidelines/screening-for-lynch-syndrome-in-endometrial-cancer/
23. Modica I, Soslow RA, Black D, Tornos C, Kauff N, Shia J. Utility of immunohistochemistry in predicting microsatellite instability in endometrial carcinoma. Am J Surg Pathol 2007;31:744-51.
24. Mojtahed A, Schrijver I, Ford JM, Longacre TA, Pai RK. A two-antibody mismatch repair protein immunohistochemistry screening approach for colorectal carcinomas, skin sebaceous tumors, and gynecologic tract carcinomas. Mod Pathol 2011;24:1004-14.
25. Ryan P, Mulligan AM, Aronson M, et al. Comparison of clinical schemas and morphologic features in predicting Lynch syndrome in mutation-positive patients with endometrial cancer encountered in the context of familial gastrointestinal cancer registries. Cancer 2012;118:681-8.

26. Mills AM, Liou S, Ford JM, Berek JS, Pai RK, Longacre TA. Lynch syndrome screening should be considered for all patients with newly diagnosed endometrial cancer. Am J Surg Pathol 2014;38:1501-9.
27. Rabban JT, Calkins SM, Karnezis AN, et al. Association of tumor morphology with mismatch-repair protein status in older endometrial cancer patients: implications for universal versus selective screening strategies for Lynch syndrome. Am J Surg Pathol 2014;38:793-800.
28. Westin SN, Lacour RA, Urbauer DL, et al. Carcinoma of the lower uterine segment: a newly described association with Lynch syndrome. J Clin Oncol 2008;26:5965-71.
29. Mills AM, Liou S, Kong CS, Longacre TA. Are women with endocervical adenocarcinoma at risk for lynch syndrome? Evaluation of 101 cases including unusual subtypes and lower uterine segment tumors. Int J Gynecol Pathol 2012;31:463-9.
30. Hoang LN, Kinloch MA, Leo JM, et al. Interobserver agreement in endometrial carcinoma histotype diagnosis varies depending on The Cancer Genome Atlas (TCGA)-based molecular subgroup. Am J Surg Pathol 2017;41:245-52.
31. Hussein YR, Broaddus R, Weigelt B, Levine DA, Soslow RA. The genomic heterogeneity of FIGO grade 3 endometrioid carcinoma impacts diagnostic accuracy and reproducibility. Int J Gynecol Pathol 2016;35:16-24.
32. Soslow RA. Endometrial carcinomas with ambiguous features. Semin Diagn Pathol 2010;27:261-73.
33. Soslow RA. High-grade endometrial carcinomas—strategies for typing. Histopathology 2013;62:89-110.
34. Broaddus RR, Lynch HT, Chen LM, et al. Pathologic features of endometrial carcinoma associated with HNPCC: a comparison with sporadic endometrial carcinoma. Cancer 2006;106:87-94.
35. Carcangiu ML, Radice P, Casalini P, Bertario L, Merola M, Sala P. Lynch syndrome—related endometrial carcinomas show a high frequency of nonendometrioid types and of high FIGO grade endometrioid types. Int J Surg Pathol 2010;18:21-6.
36. Hussein YR, Garg K, Soslow RA, DeLair D. Endometrial carcinomas with DNA mismatch repair abnormalities: analysis of 75 cases. Mod Pathol 2013;26(Suppl 2):280A.
37. Shia J, Black D, Hummer AJ, Boyd J, Soslow RA. Routinely assessed morphological features correlate with microsatellite instability status in endometrial cancer. Hum Pathol 2008;39:116-25.
38. van den Bos M, van den Hoven M, Jongejan E, et al. More differences between HNPCC-related and sporadic carcinomas from the endometrium as compared to the colon. Am J Surg Pathol 2004;28:706-11.
39. Sloan EA, Moskaluk CA, Mills AM. Mucinous differentiation with tumor infiltrating lymphocytes is a feature of sporadically methylated endometrial carcinomas. Int J Gynecol Pathol 2017;36:205-16.
40. Garg K, Leitao MM Jr, Wynveen CA, et al. p53 overexpression in morphologically ambiguous endometrial carcinomas correlates with adverse clinical outcomes. Mod Pathol 2010;23:80-92.
41. Hussein YR, Weigelt B, Levine DA, et al. Clinicopathological analysis of endometrial carcinomas harboring somatic POLE exonuclease domain mutations. Mod Pathol 2015;28:505-14.
42. Bennett JA, Morales-Oyarvide V, Campbell S, Longacre TA, Oliva E. Mismatch repair protein expression in clear cell carcinoma of the ovary: incidence and morphologic associations in 109 cases. Am J Surg Pathol 2016;40:656-63.
43. Jensen KC, Mariappan MR, Putcha GV, et al. Microsatellite instability and mismatch repair protein defects in ovarian epithelial neoplasms in patients 50 years of age and younger. Am J Surg Pathol 2008;32:1029-37.
44. Seiden MV, Patel D, O'Neill MJ, Oliva E. Case records of the Massachusetts General Hospital. Case 13-2007. A 46-year-old woman with gynecologic and intestinal cancers. New Engl J Med 2007;356:1760-9.
45. Aysal A, Karnezis A, Medhi I, Grenert JP, Zaloudek CJ, Rabban JT. Ovarian endometrioid adenocarcinoma: incidence and clinical significance of the morphologic and immunohistochemical markers of mismatch repair protein defects and tumor microsatellite instability. Am J Surg Pathol 2012;36:163-72.
46. Chui MH, Gilks CB, Cooper K, Clarke BA. Identifying Lynch syndrome in patients with ovarian carcinoma: the significance of tumor subtype. Adv Anat Pathol 2013;20:378-86.
47. Kobayashi Y, Nakamura K, Nomura H, et al. Clinicopathologic analysis with immunohistochemistry for DNA mismatch repair protein expression in synchronous primary endometrial and ovarian cancers. Int J Gynecol Cancer 2015;25:440-6.
48. Aaltonen MH, Staff S, Mecklin JP, Pylvanainen K, Maenpaa JU. Comparison of lifestyle, hormonal and medical factors in women with sporadic and Lynch syndrome-associated endometrial cancer: A retrospective case-case study. Mol Clin Oncol 2017;6:758-64.
49. Hall G, Clarkson A, Shi A, et al. Immunohistochemistry for PMS2 and MSH6 alone can replace a four antibody panel for mismatch repair deficiency screening in colorectal adenocarcinoma. Pathology 2010;42:409-13.
50. Shia J, Zhang L, Shike M, et al. Secondary mutation in a coding mononucleotide tract in MSH6 causes loss of immunoexpression of MSH6 in colorectal carcinomas with MLH1/PMS2 deficiency. Mod Pathol 2013;26:131-8.
51. Pai RK, Plesec TP, Abdul-Karim FW, et al. Abrupt loss of MLH1 and PMS2 expression in endometrial carcinoma: molecular and morphologic analysis of 6 cases. Am J Surg Pathol 2015;39:993-9.

52. Watkins JC, Nucci MR, Ritterhouse LL, Howitt BE, Sholl LM. Unusual mismatch repair immunohistochemical patterns in endometrial carcinoma. Am J Surg Pathol 2016;40:909-16.
53. Soslow RA. Practical issues related to uterine pathology: staging, frozen section, artifacts, and Lynch syndrome. Mod Pathol 2016;29(Suppl 1):S59-77.
54. Honore LH, Hanson J, Andrew SE. Microsatellite instability in endometrioid endometrial carcinoma: correlation with clinically relevant pathologic variables. Int J Gynecol Cancer 2006;16:1386-92.
55. Black D, Soslow RA, Levine DA, et al. Clinicopathologic significance of defective DNA mismatch repair in endometrial carcinoma. J Clin Oncol 2006;24:1745-53.
56. Fiumicino S, Ercoli A, Ferrandina G, et al. Microsatellite instability is an independent indicator of recurrence in sporadic stage I-II endometrial adenocarcinoma. J Clin Oncol 2001;19:1008-14.
57. Zighelboim I, Goodfellow PJ, Gao F, et al. Microsatellite instability and epigenetic inactivation of MLH1 and outcome of patients with endometrial carcinomas of the endometrioid type. J Clin Oncol 2007;25:2042-8.
58. McMeekin DS, Tritchler DL, Cohn DE, et al. Clinicopathologic significance of mismatch repair defects in endometrial cancer: an NRG Oncology/Gynecologic Oncology Group Study. J Clin Oncol 2016;34:3062-8.
59. Carethers JM. Differentiating Lynch-like from Lynch syndrome. Gastroenterology 2014;146:602-4.
60. Hampel H, Bennett RL, Buchanan A, Pearlman R, Wiesner GL, Guideline Development Group, American College of Medical Genetics and Genomics Professional Practice and Guidelines Committee and National Society of Genetic Counselors Practice Guidelines Committee. A practice guideline from the American College of Medical Genetics and Genomics and the National Society of Genetic Counselors: referral indications for cancer predisposition assessment. Genet Med 2015;17:70-87.
61. Mensenkamp AR, Vogelaar IP, van Zelst-Stams WA, et al. Somatic mutations in MLH1 and MSH2 are a frequent cause of mismatch-repair deficiency in Lynch syndrome-like tumors. Gastroenterology 2014;146:643-6.e8.
62. Mills AM, Sloan EA, Thomas M, et al. Clinicopathologic comparison of Lynch syndrome-associated and "Lynch-like" endometrial carcinomas identified on universal screening using mismatch repair protein immunohistochemistry. Am J Surg Pathol 2016;40:155-65.
63. Moline J, Mahdi H, Yang B, et al. Implementation of tumor testing for lynch syndrome in endometrial cancers at a large academic medical center. Gynecol Oncol 2013;130:121-6.
64. Hampel H, Frankel WL, Martin E, et al. Screening for the Lynch syndrome (hereditary nonpolyposis colorectal cancer). N Engl J Med 2005;352:1851-60.
65. Haraldsdottir S, Hampel H, Tomsic J, et al. Colon and endometrial cancers with mismatch repair deficiency can arise from somatic, rather than germline, mutations. Gastroenterology 2014;147:1308-16.e1.
66. Leenen CH, van Lier MG, van Doorn HC, et al. Prospective evaluation of molecular screening for Lynch syndrome in patients with endometrial cancer </= 70 years. Gynecol Oncol 2012;125:414-20.
67. Rodriguez-Soler M, Perez-Carbonell L, Guarinos C, et al. Risk of cancer in cases of suspected lynch syndrome without germline mutation. Gastroenterology 2013;144:926-32.e1; quiz e13-4.
68. Win AK, Buchanan DD, Rosty C, et al. Role of tumour molecular and pathology features to estimate colorectal cancer risk for first-degree relatives. Gut 2015;64:101-10.
69. Billingsley CC, Cohn DE, Mutch DG, Stephens JA, Suarez AA, Goodfellow PJ. Polymerase varepsilon (POLE) mutations in endometrial cancer: clinical outcomes and implications for Lynch syndrome testing. Cancer 2015;121:386-94.
70. Castillejo A, Vargas G, Castillejo MI, et al. Prevalence of germline MUTYH mutations among Lynch-like syndrome patients. Eur J Cancer 2014;50:2241-50.
71. Morak M, Heidenreich B, Keller G, et al. Biallelic MUTYH mutations can mimic Lynch syndrome. Eur J Hum Genet 2014;22:1334-7.
72. Bellido F, Pineda M, Aiza G, et al. POLE and POLD1 mutations in 529 kindred with familial colorectal cancer and/or polyposis: review of reported cases and recommendations for genetic testing and surveillance. Genet Med 2016;18:325-32.
73. Church DN, Briggs SE, Palles C, et al. DNA polymerase epsilon and delta exonuclease domain mutations in endometrial cancer. Hum Mol Genet 2013;22:2820-8.
74. Church JM. Polymerase proofreading-associated polyposis: a new, dominantly inherited syndrome of hereditary colorectal cancer predisposition. Dis Colon Rectum 2014;57:396-7.
75. Palles C, Cazier JB, Howarth KM, et al. Germline mutations affecting the proofreading domains of POLE and POLD1 predispose to colorectal adenomas and carcinomas. Nat Genet 2013;45:136-44.
76. Wong A, Kuick CH, Wong WL, et al. Mutation spectrum of POLE and POLD1 mutations in South East Asian women presenting with grade 3 endometrioid endometrial carcinomas. Gynecol Oncol 2016;141:113-20.

77. Santin AD, Bellone S, Buza N, et al. Regression of chemotherapy-resistant polymerase epsilon (POLE) ultra-mutated and MSH6 hyper-mutated endometrial tumors with Nivolumab. Clin Cancer Res 2016;22:5682-7.
78. Mahdi H, Mester JL, Nizialek EA, Ngeow J, Michener C, Eng C. Germline PTEN, SDHB-D, and KLLN alterations in endometrial cancer patients with Cowden and Cowden-like syndromes: an international, multicenter, prospective study. Cancer 2015;121:688-96.
79. Eng C. Will the real Cowden syndrome please stand up: revised diagnostic criteria. J Med Genet 2000;37:828-30.
80. Haibach H, Burns TW, Carlson HE, Burman KD, Deftos LJ. Multiple hamartoma syndrome (Cowden's disease) associated with renal cell carcinoma and primary neuroendocrine carcinoma of the skin (Merkel cell carcinoma). Am J Clin Pathol 1992;97:705-12.
81. Schrager CA, Schneider D, Gruener AC, Tsou HC, Peacocke M. Clinical and pathological features of breast disease in Cowden's syndrome: an underrecognized syndrome with an increased risk of breast cancer. Hum Pathol 1998;29:47-53.
82. Stadler ZK, Robson ME. Inherited predisposition to endometrial cancer: moving beyond Lynch syndrome. Cancer 2015;121:644-7.
83. Wong A, Ngeow J. Hereditary syndromes manifesting as endometrial carcinoma: how can pathological features aid risk assessment? Biomed Res Int 2015;2015:219012.
84. Tan MH, Mester J, Peterson C, et al. A clinical scoring system for selection of patients for PTEN mutation testing is proposed on the basis of a prospective study of 3042 probands. Am J Hum Genet 2011;88:42-56.
85. Pilarski R, Eng C. Will the real Cowden syndrome please stand up (again)? Expanding mutational and clinical spectra of the PTEN hamartoma tumour syndrome. J Med Genet 2004;41:323-6.
86. Tan MH, Mester JL, Ngeow J, Rybicki LA, Orloff MS, Eng C. Lifetime cancer risks in individuals with germline PTEN mutations. Clin Cancer Res 2012;18:400-7.
87. Black D, Bogomolniy F, Robson ME, Offit K, Barakat RR, Boyd J. Evaluation of germline PTEN mutations in endometrial cancer patients. Gynecol Oncol 2005;96:21-4.
88. Baker WD, Soisson AP, Dodson MK. Endometrial cancer in a 14-year-old girl with Cowden syndrome: a case report. J Obstet Gynaecol Res 2013;39:876-8.
89. Elnaggar AC, Spunt SL, Smith W, Depas M, Santoso JT. Endometrial cancer in a 15-year-old girl: A complication of Cowden Syndrome. Gynecol Oncol Case Rep 2012;3:18-9.
90. Edwards JM, Alsop S, Modesitt SC. Coexisting atypical polypoid adenomyoma and endometrioid endometrial carcinoma in a young woman with Cowden syndrome: case report and implications for screening and prevention. Gynecol Oncol Case Rep 2012;2:29-31.
91. Schmeler KM, Daniels MS, Brandt AC, Lu KH. Endometrial cancer in an adolescent: a possible manifestation of Cowden syndrome. Obstet Gynecol 2009;114(Pt 2):477-9.
92. Ngeow J, Stanuch K, Mester JL, Barnholtz-Sloan JS, Eng C. Second malignant neoplasms in patients with Cowden syndrome with underlying germline PTEN mutations. J Clin Oncol 2014;32:1818-24.
93. Bruchim I, Amichay K, Kidron D, et al. BRCA1/2 germline mutations in Jewish patients with uterine serous carcinoma. Int J Gynecol Cancer 2010;20:1148-53.
94. Hornreich G, Beller U, Lavie O, Renbaum P, Cohen Y, Levy-Lahad E. Is uterine serous papillary carcinoma a BRCA1-related disease? Case report and review of the literature. Gynecol Oncol 1999;75:300-4.
95. Lavie O, Ben-Arie A, Segev Y, et al. BRCA germline mutations in women with uterine serous carcinoma--still a debate. Int J Gynecol Cancer 2010;20:1531-4.
96. Hecht JL, Konstantinopoulos PA, Awtrey CS, Soslow RA. Immunohistochemical loss of BRCA1 protein in uterine serous carcinoma. Int J Gynecol Pathol 2014;33:282-7.
97. Shu CA, Pike MC, Jotwani AR, et al. Uterine cancer after risk-reducing salpingo-oophorectomy without hysterectomy in women with BRCA mutations. JAMA Oncol 2016;2:1434-40.
98. Spurdle AB, Bowman MA, Shamsani J, Kirk J. Endometrial cancer gene panels: clinical diagnostic vs research germline DNA testing. Mod Pathol 2017;30:1048-68.

9 ENDOMETRIAL STROMAL TUMORS

Endometrial stromal neoplasms are the second most frequent mesenchymal tumors of the uterus, following smooth muscle tumors. Within this group, endometrial stromal sarcomas are the most common, accounting for 0.2 to 1.5 percent of all uterine malignancies and approximately 10 percent of all uterine sarcomas (1,2) with an incidence of approximately 2 per million women (3).

Although these tumors are uncommon, the understanding and classification of endometrial stromal tumors have evolved remarkably over the last decades, especially with the discovery of specific molecular alterations that can be correlated with clinical, histologic, and immunohistochemical characteristics. In the latest World Health Organization (WHO) classification, endometrial stromal neoplasms are divided into four categories: 1) endometrial stromal nodule, 2) endometrial stromal sarcoma, 3) high-grade endometrial stromal sarcoma, and 4) undifferentiated uterine sarcoma (4) (Table 9-1). The latter is no longer designated as undifferentiated endometrial stromal sarcoma since some of these tumors have a smooth muscle or other cell of origin. Since the publication of that classification, new categories of high-grade endometrial stromal sarcomas have been identified indicating that this is still a developing classification.

ENDOMETRIAL STROMAL NODULE AND ENDOMETRIAL STROMAL SARCOMA

Definition. Benign (*endometrial stromal nodule*) or low-grade (*endometrial stromal sarcoma*, as designated in the newest WHO classification) (4) mesenchymal tumors of endometrial stromal derivation, cytologically reminiscent of proliferative-phase endometrium, although they may display a wide morphologic spectrum. Endometrial stromal nodule and stromal sarcoma are discussed together because they share morphologic, immunohistochemical, and molecular characteristics, despite differences in their border (noninvasive versus invasive), which dictates prognosis (Table 9-1).

Clinical Features. Endometrial stromal nodules tend to occur in perimenopausal women but they have been reported within a wide age range (20 to 86 years), while endometrial stromal sarcomas tend to be seen in women between 40 and 55 (range, 16 to 83) years, a younger age when compared to other uterine sarcomas (mean, 60 years) (5). Patients present with abnormal uterine bleeding, pelvic/abdominal pain, and sometimes an enlarged uterus or pelvic mass on gynecologic exam. The nodule may be an incidental finding at the time of surgery for other reasons, most commonly for leiomyomas (6–12).

An association with prolonged estrogen or tamoxifen intake as well as pelvic radiation has been reported in patients with endometrial stromal sarcomas (13–16). Occasionally, the first manifestation is metastatic disease, most commonly seen in lungs or ovary (17–19). Rarely, endometrial stromal sarcomas are associated with paraneoplastic syndromes including paraneoplastic consumptive coagulopathy (20).

Gross Findings. *Endometrial Stromal Nodule.* These neoplasms are typically solitary and well circumscribed with pushing borders. They may be centered in the endometrium where they are often polypoid (fig. 9-1) or within the myometrium (although some of the latter reported in the literature may have represented examples of highly cellular leiomyoma). Endometrial stromal nodules vary extensively in size, ranging from less than 1 cm (rare, typically an incidental finding) to 22 cm, with a mean of 4 and 7 cm in the two largest series reported to date. They typically display a solid, fleshy, tan to yellow, homogeneous cut surface (fig. 9-1), often with one or several cysts filled with hemorrhagic fluid; rarely, they are predominantly cystic and filled with necrotic debris. Areas of necrosis and hemorrhage or ulceration may be present (7–9) and should not be considered signs of malignancy.

Table 9-1

ENDOMETRIAL STROMAL NEOPLASMS
(BENIGN OR LOW-GRADE)

Type	Margins	Lymphovascular Invasion
Endometrial stromal nodule	Well-circumscribed or at most <3 protrusions, <3 mm	–
Endometrial stromal tumor with limited infiltration	No overt myometrial permeation	–
Endometrial stromal sarcoma	Overt myometrial invasion	+/–

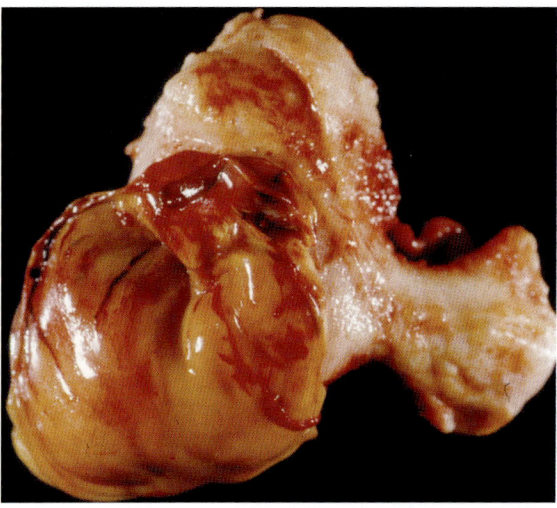

Figure 9-1

ENDOMETRIAL STROMAL NODULE

A large polypoid mass with a homogeneous tan to yellow surface fills the endometrial cavity. It is well circumscribed and separated from the underlying myometrium.

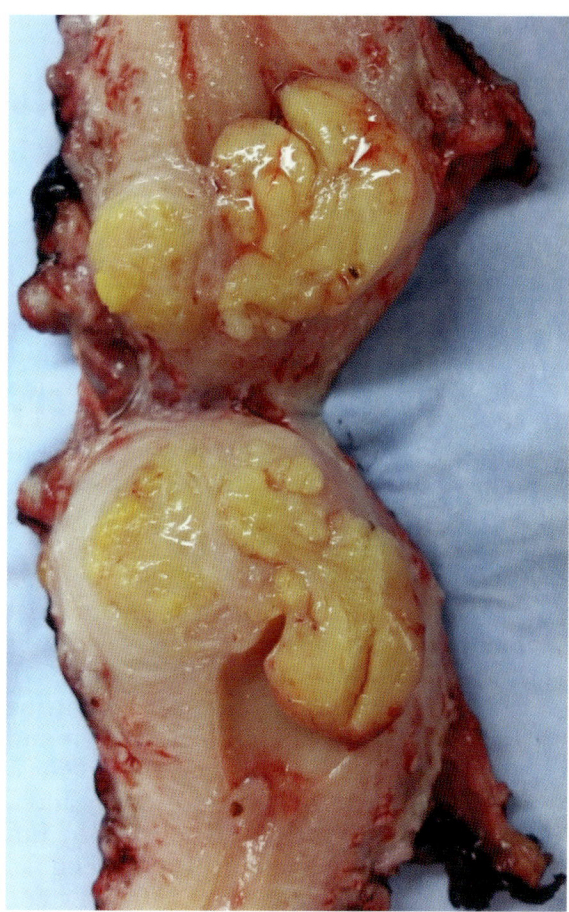

Figure 9-2

ENDOMETRIAL STROMAL SARCOMA

Multiple coalescent, polypoid, yellow nodules displaying an irregular border are present within the endometrium and myometrium.

Endometrial Stromal Sarcoma. These are poorly circumscribed tumors characterized by several variably sized, soft, yellow to tan to whitish coalescent nodules that often have polypoid endometrial and myometrial components (fig. 9-2). Worm-like plugs of tumor may fill and distend myometrial and, not infrequently, parametrial veins (fig. 9-3), the latter easier to identify since they are not compressed by the compacted myometrial muscle. Some tumors have an extrauterine component that is more prominent than the intrauterine tumor due to massive lymphovascular involvement (fig. 9-3), while others are associated with an ill-defined but exuberant thickening of the myometrium that may mimic the trabeculated muscle seen in association with adenomyosis (fig. 9-4). Some endometrial stromal sarcomas are deceivingly well demarcated from the surrounding myometrium, closely mimicking the gross appearance of an endometrial stromal nodule. In any such tumor, extensive sampling of the tumor-myometrial interface is mandatory to appropriately evaluate that margin under the microscope (7). Areas of hemorrhage and necrosis may be seen (9–12); only rarely are endometrial stromal sarcomas predominantly cystic, typically secondary to necrosis.

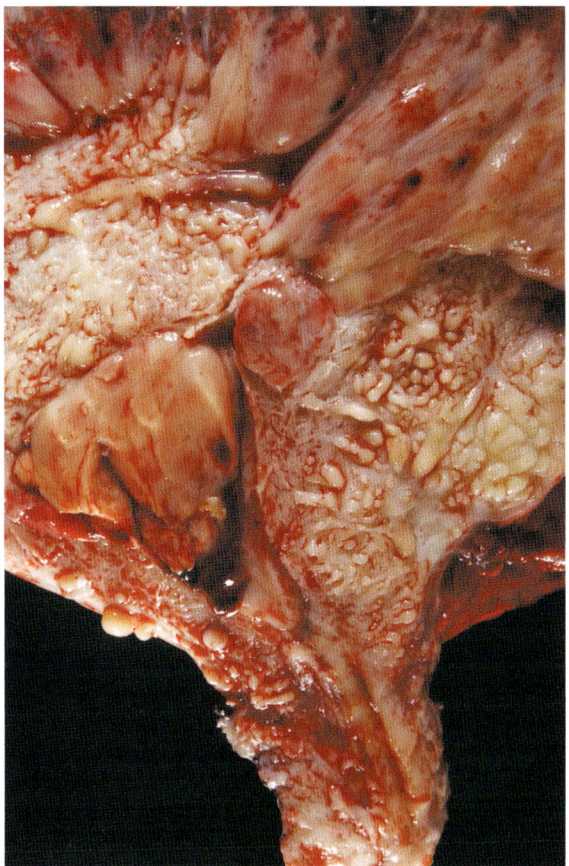

Figure 9-3

ENDOMETRIAL STROMAL SARCOMA

The polypoid intraluminal tumor has dissected between the muscle fibers and has a large serosal component. Striking "worm-like" lymphovascular invasion is present.

Endometrial Stromal Neoplasms with Variant Morphology. These tumors have an appearance that differs from that seen in conventional endometrial stromal neoplasms. Tumors with smooth muscle differentiation may be submucosal and polypoid, centered in the myometrium, or rarely, subserosal. They display a multinodular appearance, alternating soft, tan-yellow and white firm nodules, the latter with the appearance of a leiomyoma. The stromal component often predominates, with small white firm nodules embedded in a soft tan to yellow background (21). Rarely, they have been grossly described as tan, white, whorled, circumscribed nodules as seen in typical leiomyomas (22). Tumors with myxoid or fibroblastic background may be polypoid and predominantly

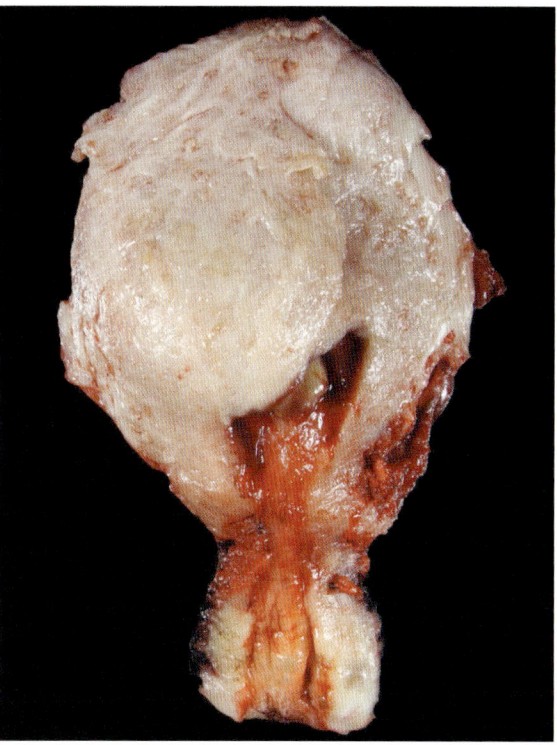

Figure 9-4

ENDOMETRIAL STROMAL SARCOMA

Diffuse permeation of the myometrium associated with poorly demarcated borders imparts a hypertrophic appearance to the myometrium as may be seen in exuberant adenomyosis.

intracavitary or intramyometrial, and when malignant, display multinodular growth within the myometrium as occurs with typical endometrial stromal tumors. Myxoid tumors may have a gelatinous, sticky cut surface while those with a fibroblastic morphology may display a firm and white cut surface that may closely mimic that of a typical leiomyoma (22,23).

Microscopic Findings. *Endometrial stromal nodule* is defined by the WHO as a tumor with well-circumscribed margins (fig. 9-5) and limited irregularities (less than three), seen as finger-like projections or nests of tumor cells immediately adjacent to the main mass measuring less than 3 mm. The presence of lymphovascular invasion excludes the diagnosis of endometrial stromal nodule (4). In contrast, *endometrial stromal sarcoma* is characterized by a "tongue-like" permeative pattern of invasion into the myometrium by irregularly sized and shaped nests of tumor

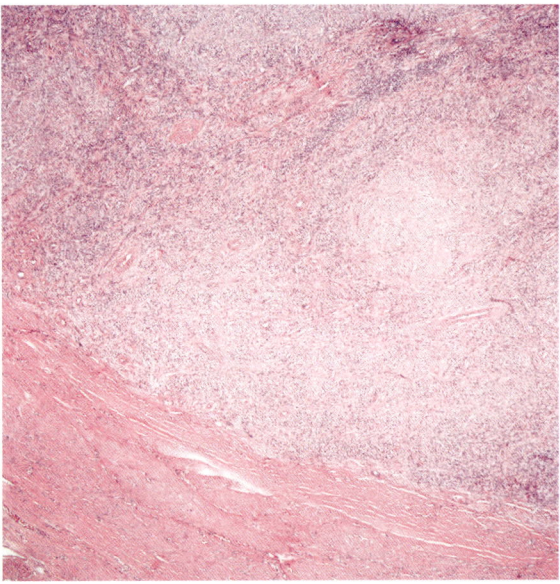

Figure 9-5

ENDOMETRIAL STROMAL NODULE

The tumor shows focal smooth muscle differentiation and has a well-demarcated border with the surrounding myometrium.

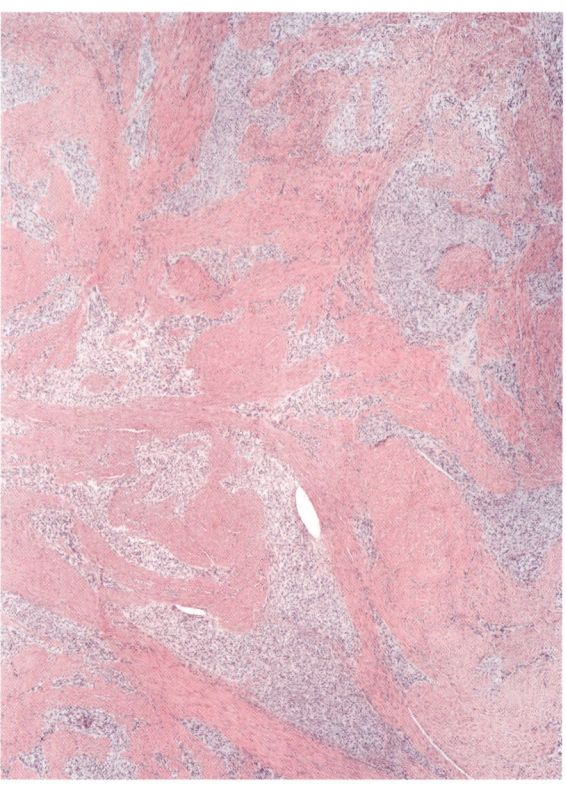

Figure 9-7

ENDOMETRIAL STROMAL SARCOMA

The tumor cells form irregular nests that infiltrate the myometrium without an associated stromal response.

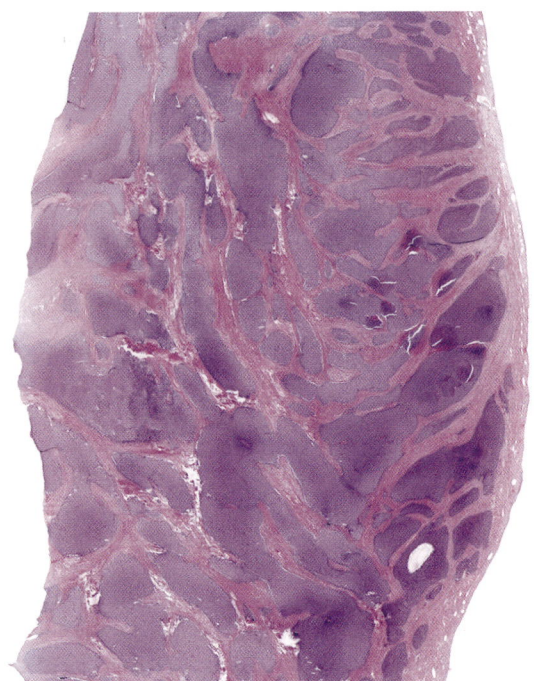

Figure 9-6

ENDOMETRIAL STROMAL SARCOMA

There is striking "tongue-like" permeative infiltration of the myometrium by islands of "blue" tumor cells.

cells, without an associated stromal response, as well as lymphovascular invasion, which is commonly encountered (figs. 9-6–9-9) (4).

Some endometrial stromal sarcomas show limited myometrial infiltration. These tumors can be confused with endometrial stromal nodules on gross examination, but extensive sampling of the tumor-myometrial interface shows more extensive (irregularities up to 9 mm and up to six in number) myometrial infiltration than that allowed in endometrial stromal nodules. Despite the relatively limited extent of myometrial invasion compared to typical endometrial stomal sarcomas, they should still be reported as endometrial stromal sarcomas (7).

On high-power examination, endometrial stromal nodule and endometrial stromal sarcoma have identical morphologic appearances. They are characterized by a diffuse growth of small uniform "blue" cells with scant to moderate amount of amphophilic to eosinophilic

Endometrial Stromal Tumors

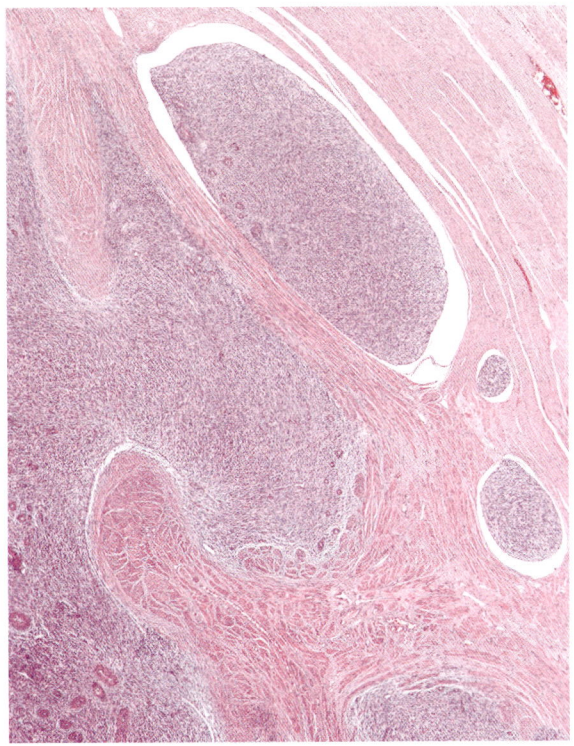

Figure 9-8

ENDOMETRIAL STROMAL SARCOMA

The tumor has an irregular border and it is associated with lymphovascular invasion.

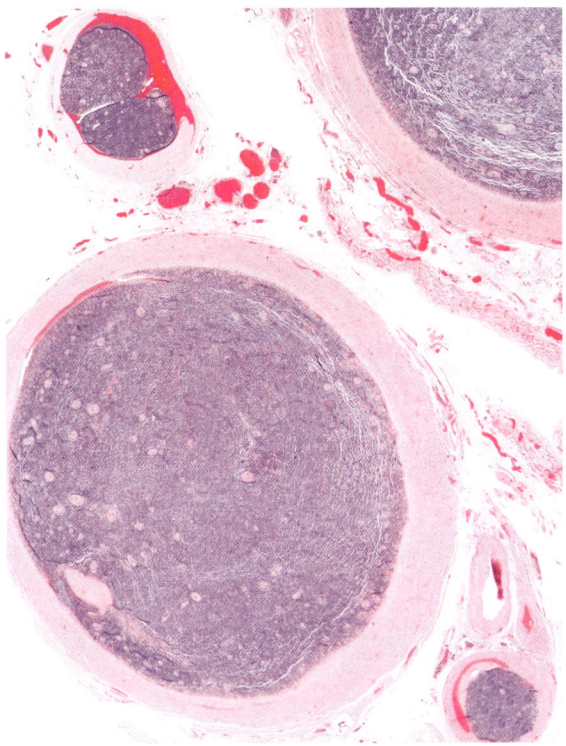

Figure 9-9

ENDOMETRIAL STROMAL SARCOMA

Prominent lymphovascular invasion in the parametrial soft tissues may be easy to identify on gross examination.

cytoplasm, oval to slightly fusiform nuclei, inconspicuous nucleoli, and bland cytologic features. Occasionally, they have abundant amphophilic cytoplasm due to variable degrees of decidualization. This morphology is reminiscent of proliferative phase endometrium (figs. 9-10, 9-11). Mitotic activity is often low (usually less than 5 mitoses per 10 high-power fields) but higher rates have been reported in both endometrial stromal nodules (up to 24 per 10 high-power fields) and endometrial stromal sarcomas (up to 32 per 10 high-power fields). No atypical mitoses are noted.

The mitotic count is no longer used as a stand-alone criterion in the distinction of low- and high-grade endometrial stromal sarcomas. By definition, an infiltrative tumor with a morphologic appearance reminiscent of proliferative phase endometrium should be diagnosed as low-grade endometrial stromal sarcoma regardless of its mitotic count (4). Although endometrial stromal tumors are typically hypercellular,

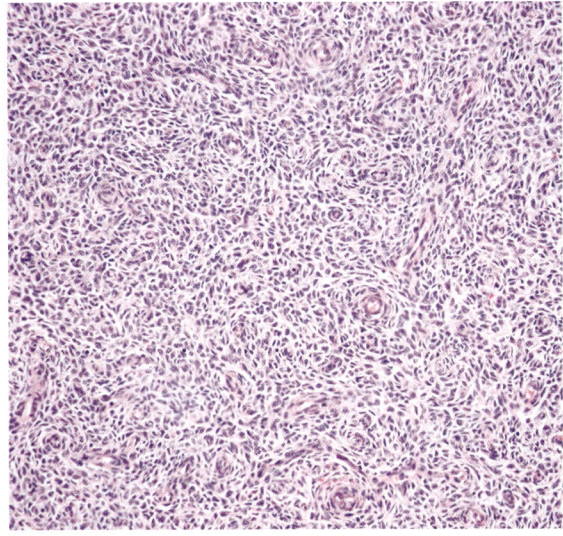

Figure 9-10

ENDOMETRIAL STROMAL NODULE AND SARCOMA

Both tumors are composed of a uniform population of small blue cells that are closely packed and reminiscent of proliferative phase endometrium.

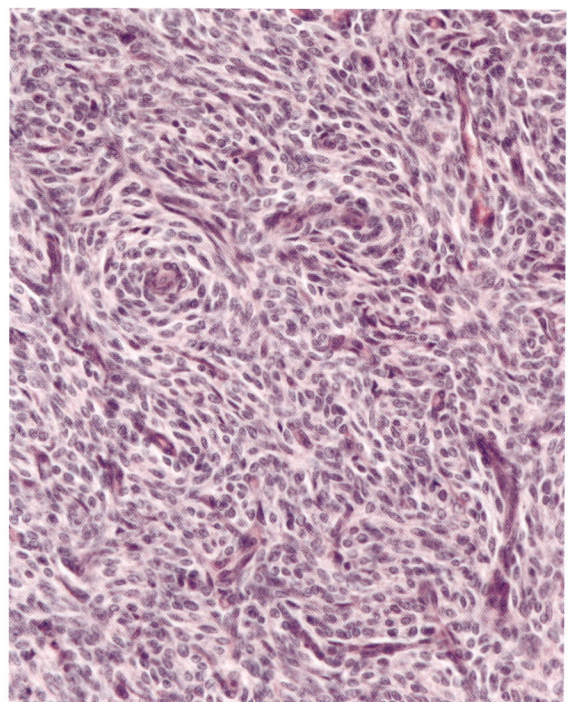

Figure 9-11

ENDOMETRIAL STROMAL NODULE AND SARCOMA

The tumor cells have scant cytoplasm and oval nuclei with inconspicuous nucleoli, and often whorl around small vessels, reminiscent of arterioles as seen in proliferative-type endometrium.

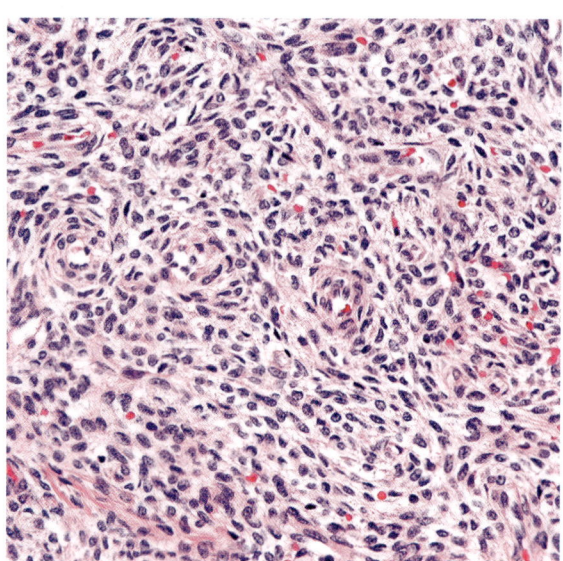

Figure 9-12

ENDOMETRIAL STROMAL NODULE AND SARCOMA

The cellularity in these tumors may not be uniform and intercellular edema may be prominent.

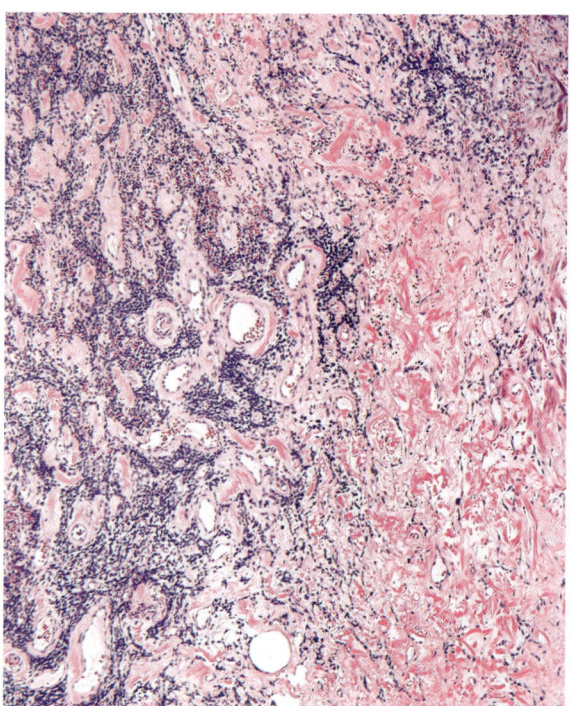

Figure 9-13

ENDOMETRIAL STROMAL NODULE AND SARCOMA

Conspicuous hyalinization, sometimes related to confluence of collagen bands, is seen. Notice hyalinized vessels.

cellularity may vary from area to area due to edema (fig. 9-12) or hyalinization (fig. 9-13).

A rich vascular framework consisting of small vessels reminiscent of spiral arterioles is characteristic but only infrequently conspicuous within a neoplasm (fig. 9-10). Vessels may be hyalinized and more apparent (fig. 9-13). The tumor cells may whorl around these arterioles. Curvilinear, thin (fig. 9-14) or small ectatic vessels or even staghorn vessels are common. Thick and large vessels are rare, and if present, are typically seen at the periphery of the tumor and are likely entrapped (fig. 9-15), although rarely they are seen within the tumor, particularly at the base of intracavitary polypoid tumors.

Irregularly shaped and sized hyaline bands, plaques, or nodules of hyalinized collagen may be seen and are occasionally prominent (fig. 9-16). Cysts, more commonly present in endometrial stromal nodules than sarcomas, are lined by stromal cells, foamy histiocytes, or both, with the latter present in groups, admixed with tumor cells (fig. 9-17) or cholesterol clefts, or rarely, in large

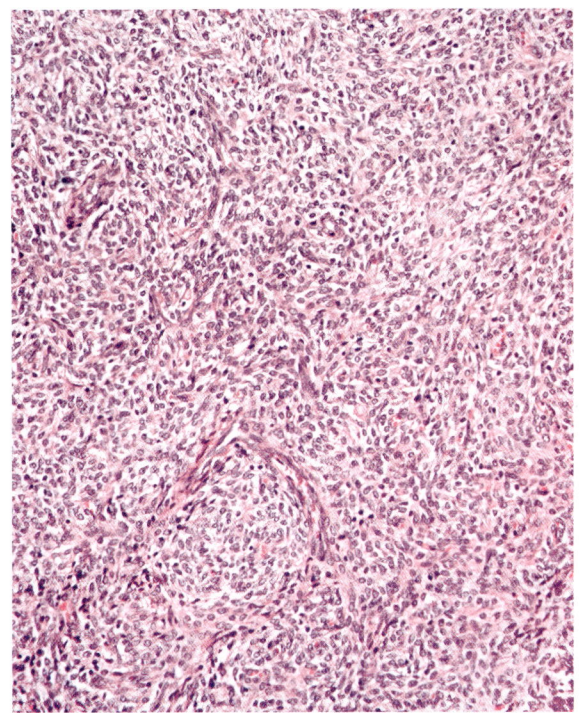

Figure 9-14
ENDOMETRIAL STROMAL NODULE AND SARCOMA
As well as the typical arteriole-like vessels, a thin curvilinear vascular network is common in these tumors.

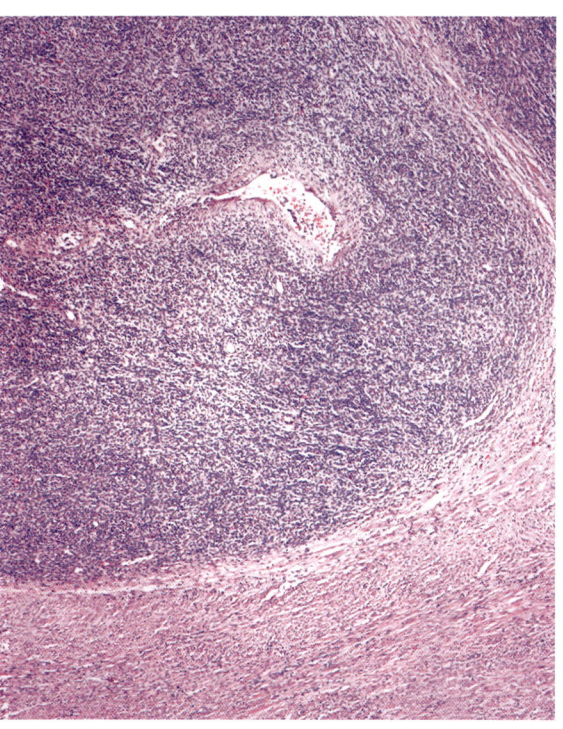

Figure 9-15
ENDOMETRIAL STROMAL NODULE AND SARCOMA
Thick blood vessels are seen more often near the interface with the myometrium but they are uncommon.

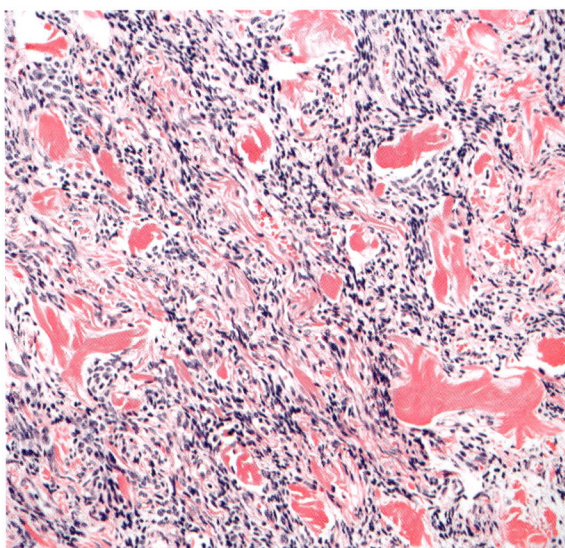

Figure 9-16
ENDOMETRIAL STROMAL NODULE AND SARCOMA
Irregular-sized collagen plaques are characteristic but not pathognomonic of these mesenchymal tumors.

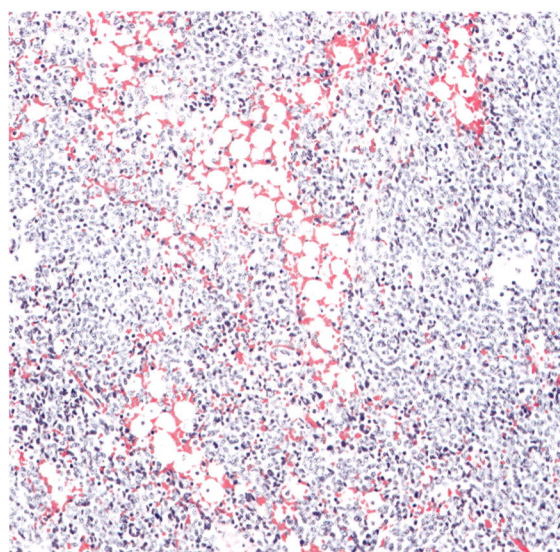

Figure 9-17
ENDOMETRIAL STROMAL NODULE AND SARCOMA
Foamy histiocytes form irregular aggregates and are intimately admixed with the neoplastic endometrial stromal cells.

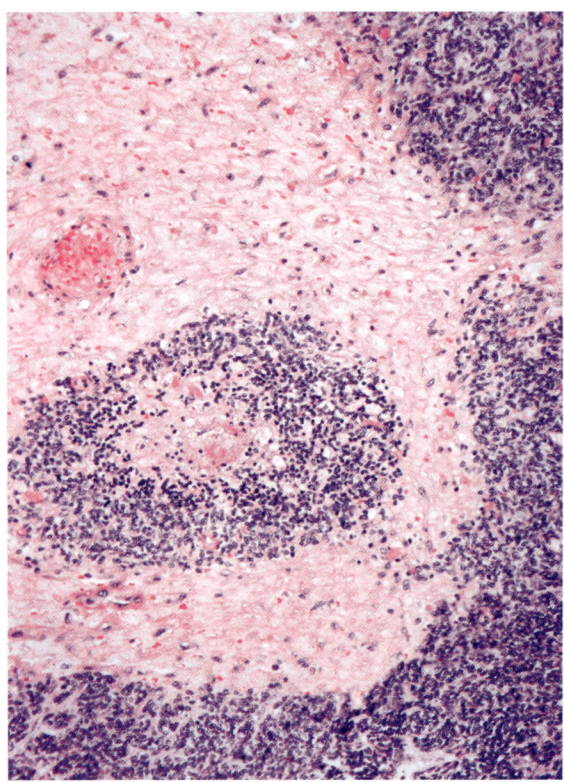 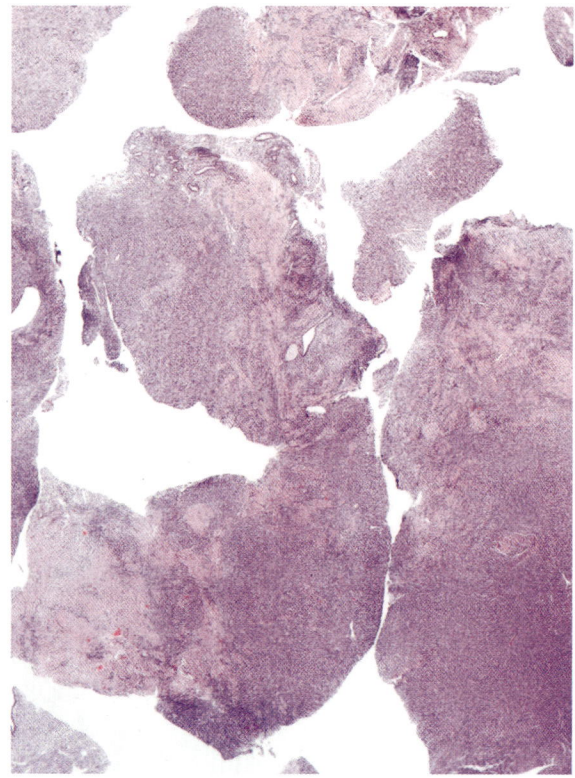

Figure 9-18

ENDOMETRIAL STROMAL TUMOR

There is perivascular necrosis of tumor cells.

Figure 9-19

ENDOMETRIAL STROMAL TUMOR

In a curettage specimen, large fragments composed of only stroma should suggest an endometrial stromal tumor. In these specimens, however, it is almost always impossible to further subclassify the tumor as nodule or sarcoma as margins are not seen.

aggregates. Tumors may contain inflammatory cells, most frequently lymphocytes (8,10,24,25). Necrosis, typically of infarct type and variably associated with recent or old hemorrhage, may be present in both endometrial stromal nodules and sarcomas. However, tumor cell necrosis has also been noted in endometrial stromal sarcomas (fig. 9-18) (2,9). Rarely, areas of calcification or even ossification have been reported.

The morphologic features mentioned above are encountered in both stromal nodule and endometrial stromal sarcoma, thus a specific diagnosis typically cannot be rendered on a curettage specimen, since the margins of the tumor cannot be assessed (fig. 9-19) except in rare occasions when the tumor is really small and enucleated or when it is seen infiltrating the myometrium in a curettage specimen (fig. 9-20) (26,27). The latter scenario may be confounded by the fact that some endometrial stromal tumors show smooth muscle differentiation that may be misinterpreted as myometrium.

Variant morphologic features seen in these two categories of tumors (Table 9-2) include smooth muscle, skeletal muscle, sex cord-like, glandular, and adipocytic (mature appearing) (28) differentiation as well as a fibrous, myxoid, or fibromyxoid background and a pseudopapillary, papillary, rhabdoid, epithelioid, granular (7,29), or clear (30) appearance. Cells with bizarre nuclei (28,29,31,32) and osteoclast-like cells (33) have been reported. More than one feature may be seen within a single tumor and, frequently, smooth muscle and sex cord-like differentiation coexist. These morphologic variants may be seen in the primary or metastatic setting, and a metastatic tumor may have an appearance that differs from the primary uterine tumor (22).

Smooth muscle differentiation has been reported in endometrial stromal tumors. Bird and Willis (34) described the production of

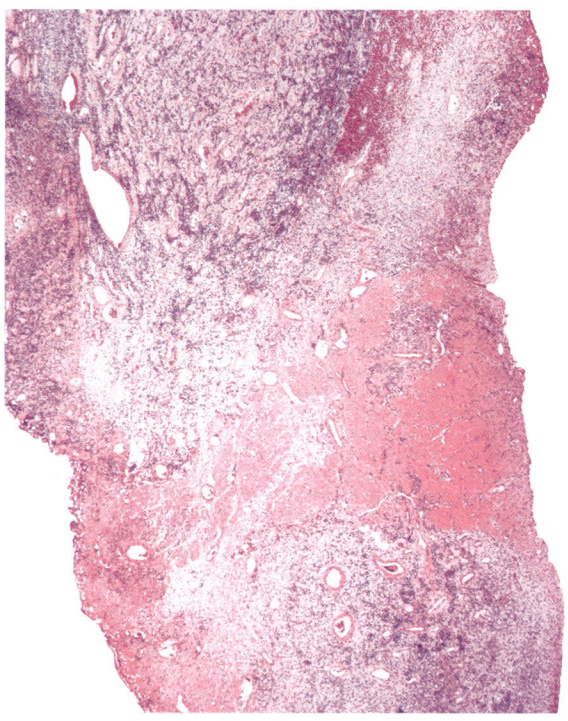

Figure 9-20

ENDOMETRIAL STROMAL SARCOMA

Rarely, invasion of the myometrium establishes a diagnosis of endometrial stromal sarcoma in a curettage specimen.

Table 9-2
TYPES OF DIFFERENTIATION/APPEARANCES IN ENDOMETRIAL STROMAL TUMORS
Smooth muscle
Skeletal muscle
Sex cord-like
Glandular
Fibrous and/or myxoid
Adipocytic
Pseudopapillary or papillary
Rhabdoid
Epithelioid and/or granular
Clear
Cells with bizarre nuclei
Osteoclast-like cells

smooth muscle by normal endometrial stroma and the presence of cells at the endomyometrial junction resembling myofibroblasts during the follicular phase of the menstrual cycle. During the luteal phase, ultrastructural features of these cells include distinct cytoplasmic filaments with dense bodies and plaques, features known to be characteristic of smooth muscle differentiation (35). It has been postulated that multipotent cells within the myometrium are capable of differentiation into endometrial stromal or smooth muscle cells (36). Thus, it is not surprising that smooth muscle differentiation is common within these tumors.

Smooth muscle differentiation is often seen on low-power magnification as an abrupt transition from areas of conventional endometrial stromal neoplasia. The most characteristic morphology is rounded to slightly irregular nodules with prominent central hyalinization from which collagen bands radiate toward the periphery, embedding rounded cells ("starburst pattern"). This appearance transitions to disorganized short fascicles that in turn form longer fascicles of spindle cells (figs. 9-21, 9-22). It should be noted that this morphology is not pathognomonic of this tumor. Variable numbers of large, thick-walled blood vessels are often present in these areas. Less commonly, smooth muscle differentiation is represented by a gradual transition from the endometrial stromal component or is seen as distinct islands with irregular contours within an endometrial stromal background (fig. 9-23). A meningothelial-like morphology has also been reported (37).

The cells within the collagenized nodules typically have scant and clear cytoplasm and round to oval nuclei with inconspicuous nucleoli, while at the periphery of the nodules, where fascicular growth becomes apparent, cells become spindled with eosinophilic cytoplasm, elongated nuclei with small nucleoli, bland cytologic features, and low mitotic activity. The starburst pattern of the smooth muscle component is often seen at the periphery of the tumor in an endometrial stromal nodule (band-like) (fig. 9-24) and when part of an endometrial stromal sarcoma, shows the typical tongue-like pattern of infiltration.

The smooth muscle component may be predominant, may display malignant cytologic features, or may be the sole component at a metastatic site (7,8,21,22,24,38–40). Although focal smooth muscle differentiation has been reported based on morphologic,

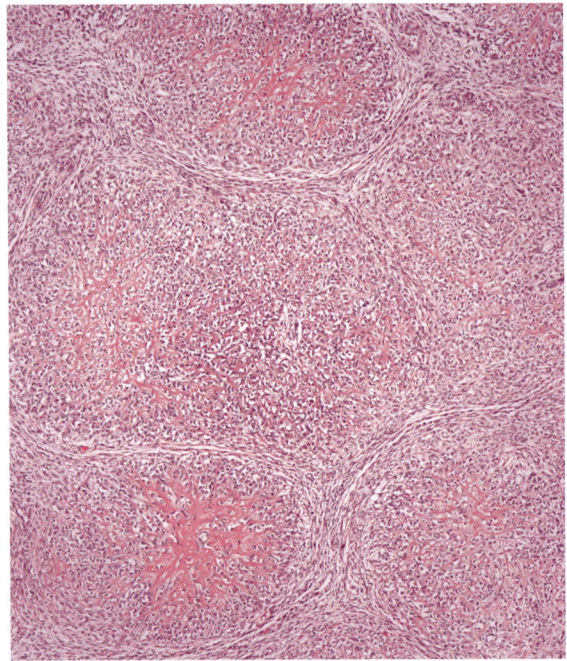

Figure 9-21

ENDOMETRIAL STROMAL SARCOMA WITH SMOOTH MUSCLE DIFFERENTIATION

Smooth muscle differentiation is seen as multiple, poorly defined nodules with a hyalinized center, and a "starburst" appearance.

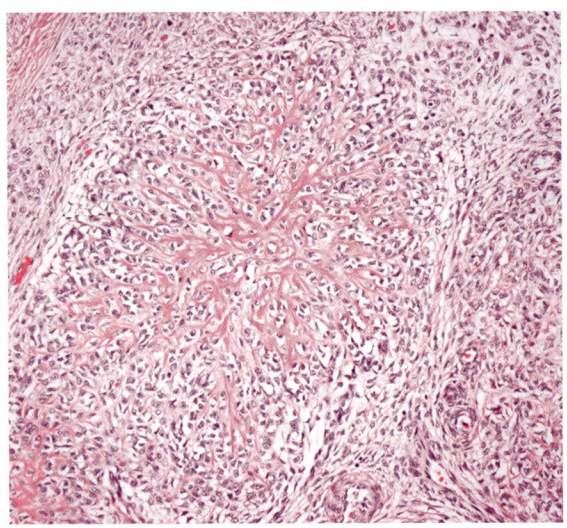

Figure 9-22

ENDOMETRIAL STROMAL SARCOMA WITH SMOOTH MUSCLE DIFFERENTIATION

In the starburst pattern of smooth muscle differentiation, collagen bands radiate toward the periphery, embedding small and round cells, which in turn form small and disorganized fascicles of smooth muscle.

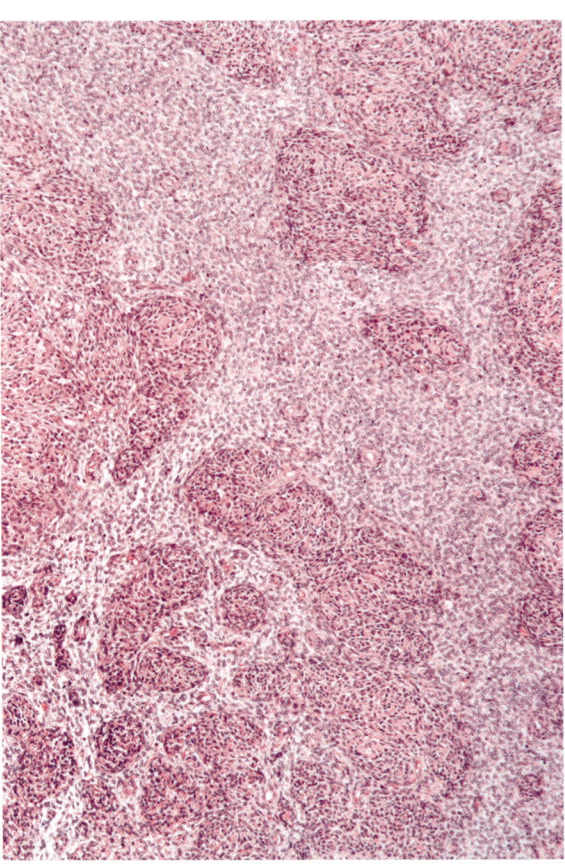

Figure 9-23

ENDOMETRIAL STROMAL SARCOMA WITH SMOOTH MUSCLE DIFFERENTIATION

Less commonly, smooth muscle differentiation is seen as irregularly shaped islands of cells with pink cytoplasm that are embedded in a background of stromal neoplasia.

immunohistochemical, and ultrastructural features (7–10,12,21,22,38,41–44), the current classification requires that more than 30 percent of the tumor should display smooth muscle differentiation on morphologic grounds for a diagnosis of endometrial stromal tumor with smooth muscle differentiation (4).

These tumors should be classified based on their margins and/or the presence of lymphovascular invasion as occurs with typical endometrial stromal tumors. Even when smooth muscle differentiation is focal, the pathology report should mention it as this might be helpful in the diagnosis of a recurrence showing more extensive or only smooth muscle differentiation. The term "stromomyoma" was used in the past to describe this type of differentiation

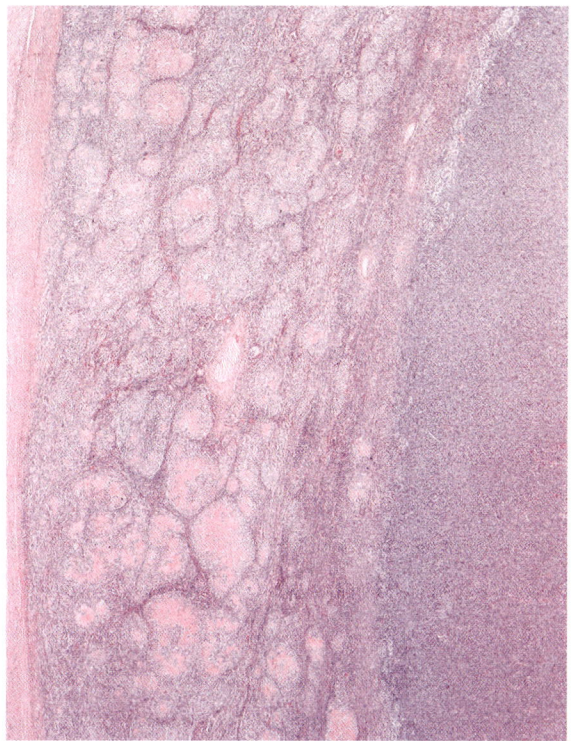

Figure 9-24

ENDOMETRIAL STROMAL NODULE WITH SMOOTH MUSCLE DIFFERENTIATION

Smooth muscle differentiation forms a band at the periphery of the tumor.

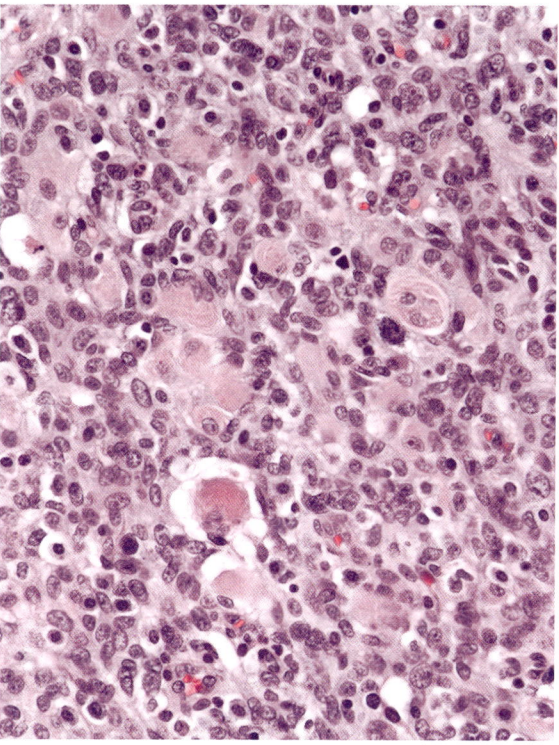

Figure 9-25

ENDOMETRIAL STROMAL TUMOR WITH SKELETAL MUSCLE DIFFERENTIATION

Skeletal muscle differentiation is seen as round cells with abundant eosinophilic cytoplasm due to paranuclear distribution of filaments.

in endometrial stromal tumors, but this term is no longer accepted since it implies that all such tumors are benign, and as mentioned earlier, smooth muscle differentiation can be seen in both endometrial stromal nodules and endometrial stromal sarcomas (45,46).

In contrast to smooth muscle differentiation, skeletal muscle differentiation is rare (fig. 9-25) but it is often seen when the former is present. Cells may be large and round, with abundant bright eosinophilic cytoplasm and filaments in a perinuclear distribution, or they may have strap-shaped morphology and easily identified cross striations (28,44,47).

Sex cord-like differentiation is seen with variable frequency (may be predominant) in a background of endometrial stromal neoplasia. Tumors with this component correspond to Clement and Scully group I tumors (48). Sex cord-like differentiation most often displays anastomosing trabeculae, cords, nests, or islands of cells separated by delicate fibroblastic or hyalinized stroma, recapitulating the morphology of adult granulosa cell tumors (figs. 9-26, 9-27). Rarely, structures reminiscent of Call-Exner bodies are seen. Hollow or solid tubules, including retiform morphology with intraluminal papillae (49), with or without solid growth (morphologies seen in Sertoli-Leydig and Sertoli cell tumors) may also be noted, although not frequently. The neoplastic cells may have scant to abundant cytoplasm depending on the amount of lipid content (reminiscent of luteinized cells), regular nuclei with small nucleoli, without conspicuous nuclear grooves, and variable mitotic activity (10,24,48,50,51). Leydig cells have not been reported. Sex cord-like differentiation may be juxtaposed or intermingled with smooth muscle differentiation.

Rhabdoid morphology, characterized by prominent paranuclear arrays of intermediate filaments, may be noted, especially in areas with an

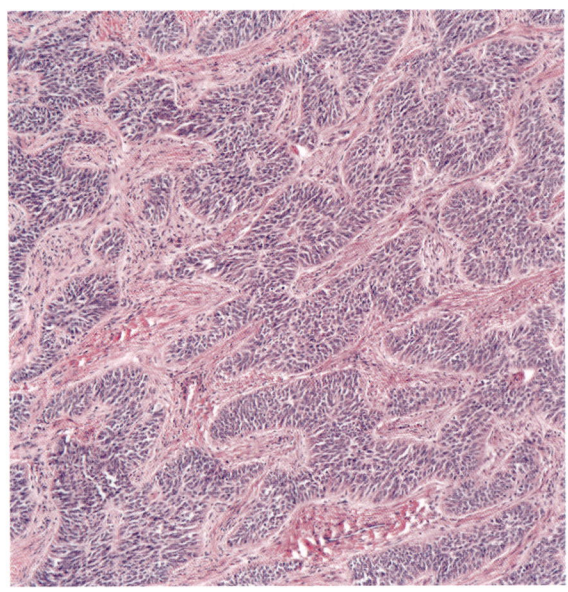

Figure 9-26

ENDOMETRIAL STROMAL NODULE WITH SEX CORD-LIKE DIFFERENTIATION

Interanastomosing trabeculae of cells are reminiscent of a granulosa cell tumor of the ovary.

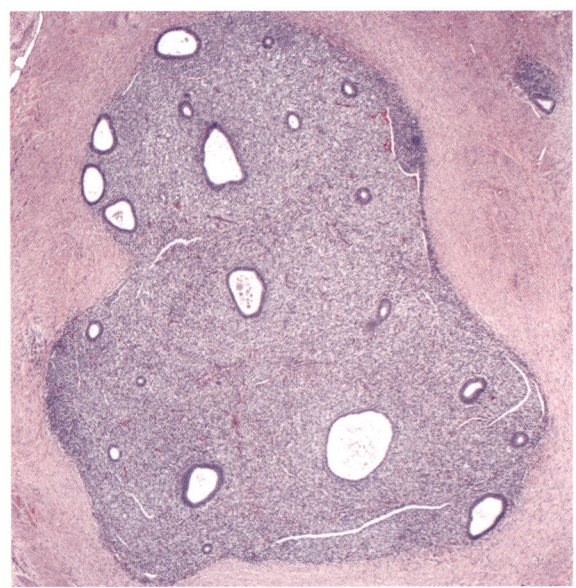

Figure 9-28

ENDOMETRIAL STROMAL SARCOMA WITH GLAND DIFFERENTIATION

The endometrioid-type glands have simple outlines and are lined by one cell layer. The invasive island of endometrial stromal component has an expansile contour.

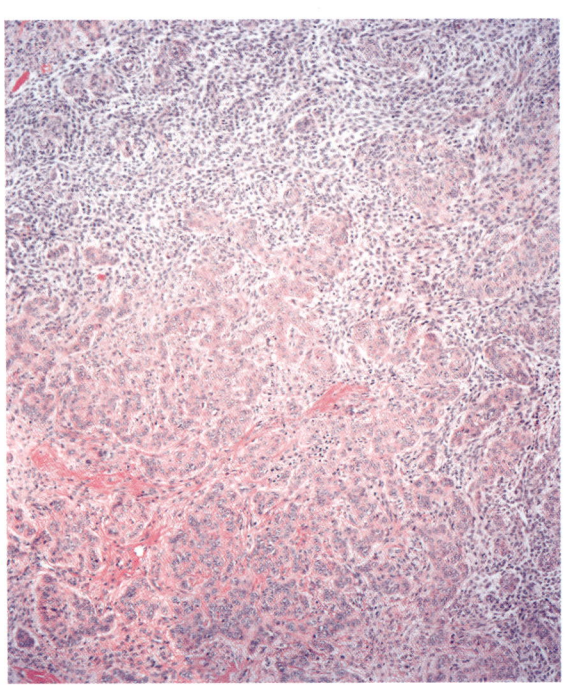

Figure 9-27

ENDOMETRIAL STROMAL SARCOMA WITH SEX CORD-LIKE DIFFERENTIATION

Cords of tumor cells merge with a typical component of endometrial stromal neoplasia.

appearance reminiscent of granulosa cell tumor (52–56). Although rhabdoid morphology often occurs within the sex cord-like elements (52,54), it can also be seen within areas of conventional endometrial stromal neoplasia (57).

Endometrioid glandular differentiation has been described in endometrial stromal nodules and sarcomas. The morphology ranges from benign (fig. 9-28) to atypical to carcinoma, and can vary extensively in amount (8,38,58,59). Papillae and pseudopapillae (not signifying epithelial differentiation) are rarely seen in endometrial stromal tumors but can be the predominant morphology when the myometrium or vascular spaces are involved (figs. 9-29, 9-30). Within papillae and pseudopapillae, typical small uniform cells with bland cytologic features associated with the classic vasculature are noted (60).

A fibrous or myxoid background is uncommon in endometrial stromal tumors and in the past, some of these tumors may have been referred to as myxofibrosarcomas. The most striking feature is the hypocellular appearance of the tumor at low-power magnification, which is in sharp contrast to the hypercellular nature of most

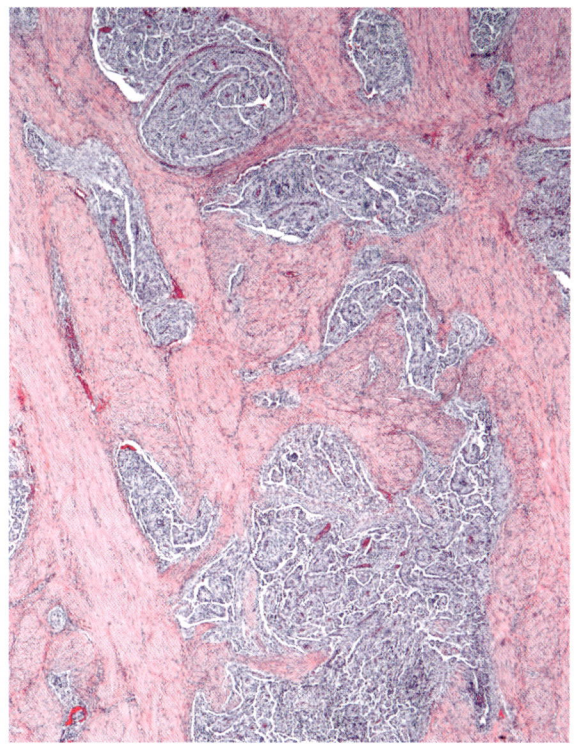

Figure 9-29

ENDOMETRIAL STROMAL SARCOMA WITH PSEUDOPAPILLAE

Pseudopapillae of tumor cells infiltrate the myometrium and are also present within vascular spaces.

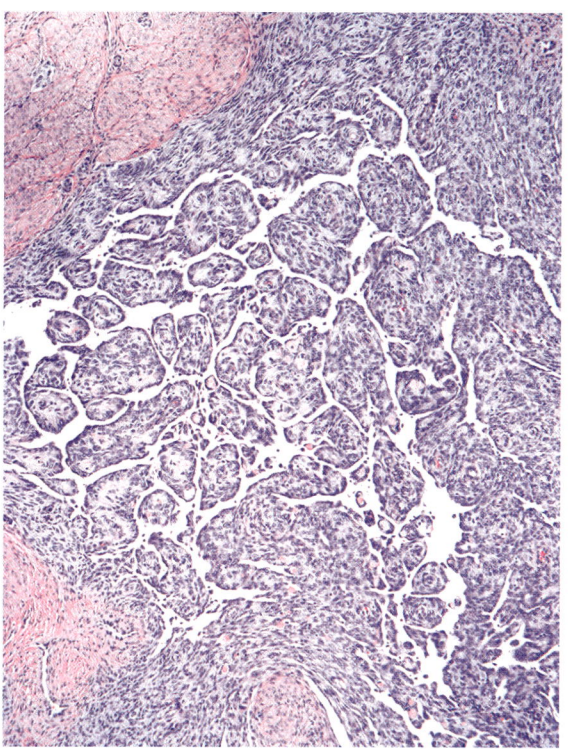

Figure 9-30

ENDOMETRIAL STROMAL SARCOMA WITH PSEUDOPAPILLAE

Uniform small tumor cells associated with the typical vasculature are seen within the pseudopapillae.

endometrial stromal neoplasms (figs. 9-31, 9-32). Although uncommon, they may be pure, lacking a conventional component (8,11,22,23,61–63). Prominent delicate collagen or a myxoid background is characteristic of these tumors. The cells often display a nodular, fascicular (either short and disorganized or long and intersecting) or diffuse (fig. 9-32) architecture in the fibroblastic variant; areas of focal or extensive hyalinization may be seen (fig. 9-33). When myxoid, the tumor cells have a diffuse distribution that may be associated with microcysts (fig. 9-34).

Myxoid and fibrous areas may coexist. In both variants, cells are typically small with oval nuclei, bland cytologic features, and low mitotic activity. Scattered binucleated cells may be noted. The vessels are small and arteriole-like, similar to typical endometrial stromal tumors (fig. 9-35). A tongue-like pattern of infiltration occurs when the tumor is malignant. Tumors may also display glands, sex cord elements, or smooth muscle differentiation (22,23). At metastatic sites, the morphology may be similar to that seen in the uterus, but may be more cellular and reminiscent of a fibrosarcoma. These endometrial stromal tumor variants may be associated with YWHAE-FAM22 high-grade endometrial stromal sarcoma (≈40 to 50 percent) (discussed below) (fig. 9-36) (64).

Epithelioid (fig. 9-37), granular, or clear cytoplasm (fig. 9-38) is seen occasionally in endometrial stromal tumors. The cells tend to be polygonal, with abundant eosinophilic or clear cytoplasm, which may be the predominant morphology of the tumor. The cytoplasm may be granular and periodic acid–Schiff (PAS) and PAS with diastase positive (29,30).

Mononucleated or multinucleated bizarre nuclei, similar to those seen in endometrial polyps with bizarre nuclei (fig. 9-39) (65), have been reported in endometrial stromal tumors with epithelioid morphology and rarely in

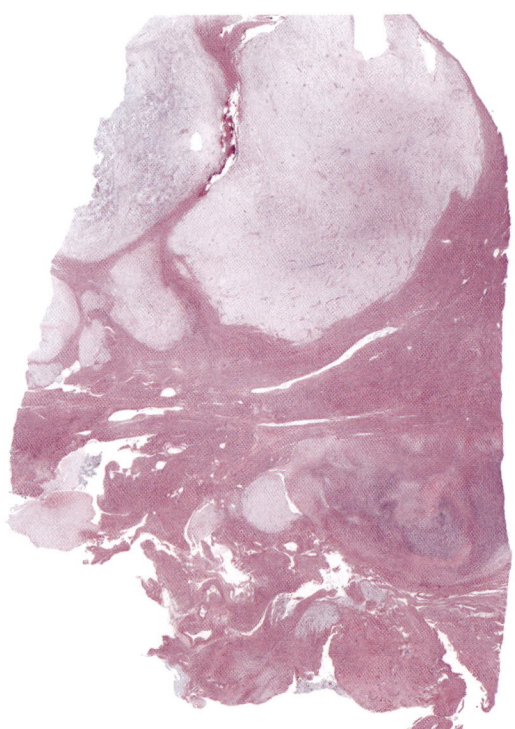
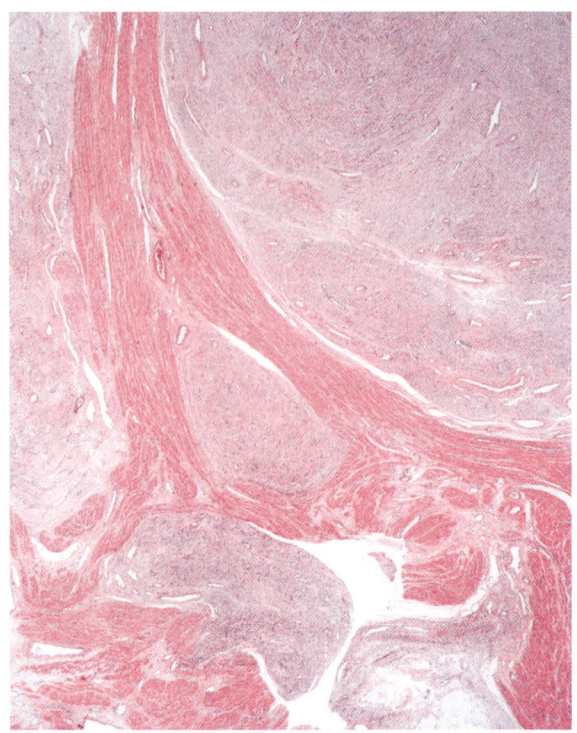

Figure 9-31

ENDOMETRIAL STROMAL SARCOMA WITH MYXOID AND FIBROBLASTIC BACKGROUND

The infiltrating tumor nests appear hypocellular when compared to typical endometrial stromal sarcoma (left and right).

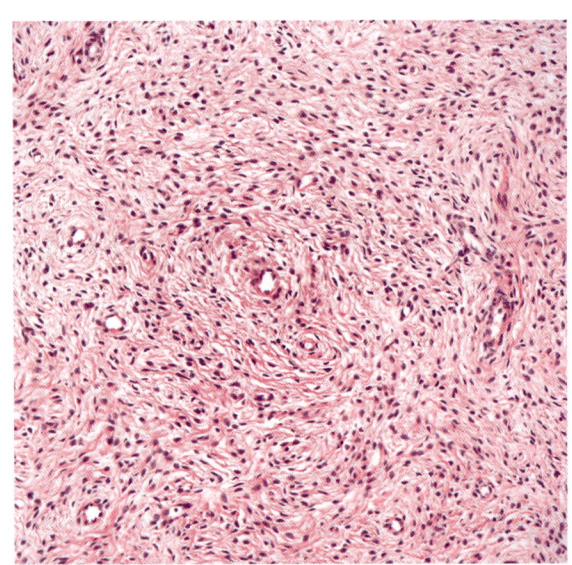
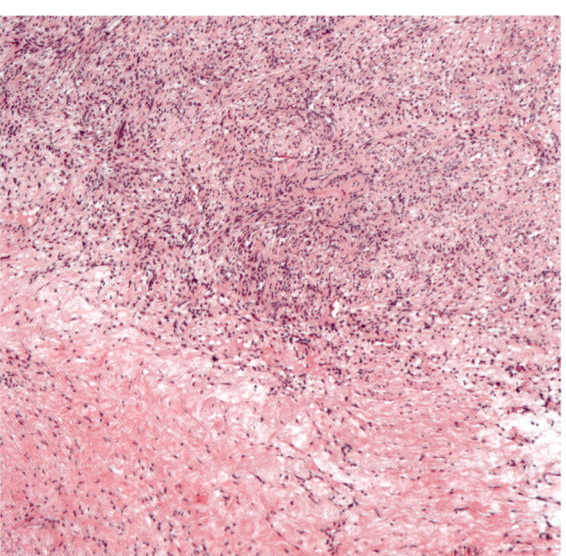

Figure 9-32

ENDOMETRIAL STROMAL SARCOMA WITH FIBROBLASTIC BACKGROUND

The tumor is associated with delicate collagen deposition in between which small uniform cells with oval nuclei and scant cytoplasm display a diffuse growth.

Figure 9-33

ENDOMETRIAL STROMAL SARCOMA WITH FIBROBLASTIC BACKGROUND

The tumor is associated with extensive hyalinization.

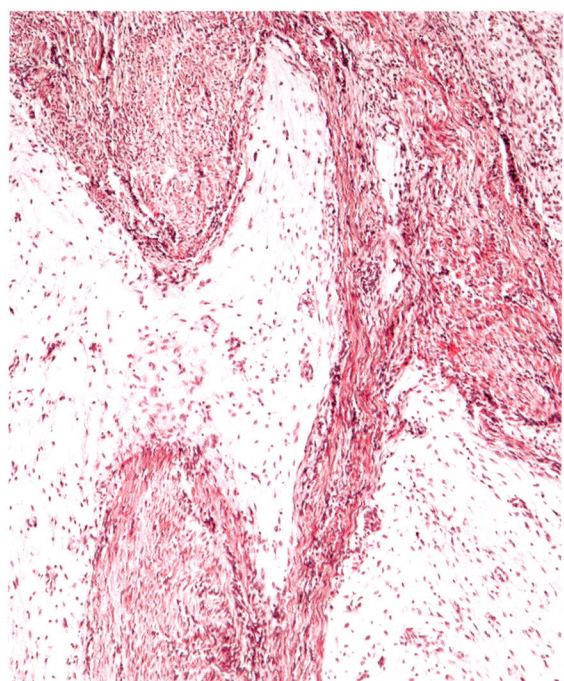

Figure 9-34

ENDOMETRIAL STROMAL SARCOMA WITH MYXOID BACKGROUND

The tumor shows the classic tongue-like pattern of infiltration as well as small arterioles.

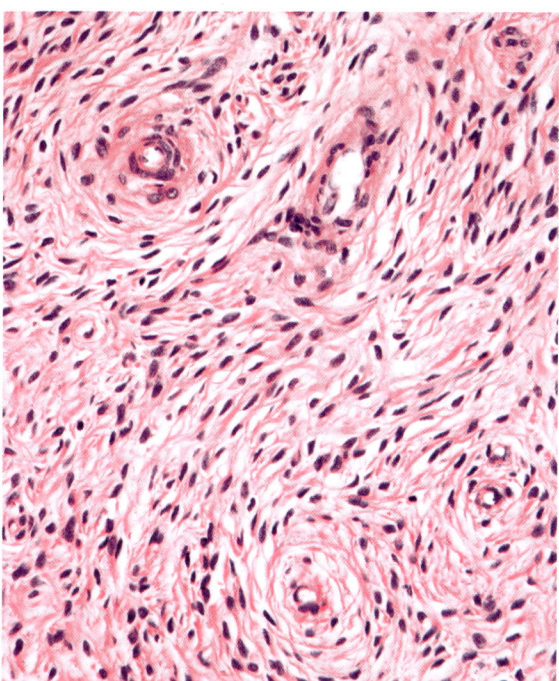

Figure 9-35

ENDOMETRIAL STROMAL SARCOMA WITH FIBROBLASTIC BACKGROUND

The tumor cells whorl around arteriole-like vessels.

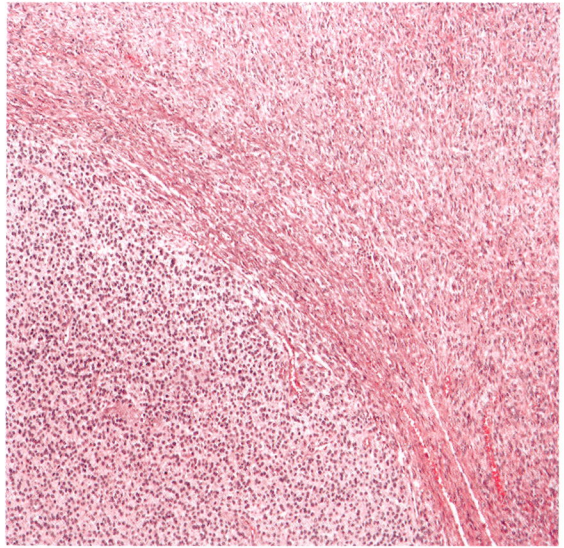

Figure 9-36

ENDOMETRIAL STROMAL SARCOMA TRANSITIONING TO *YWHAE-FAM22* HIGH-GRADE ENDOMETRIAL STROMAL SARCOMA

Two discrete areas are noted: fibroblastic (right) and hypercellular with an epithelioid morphology (left).

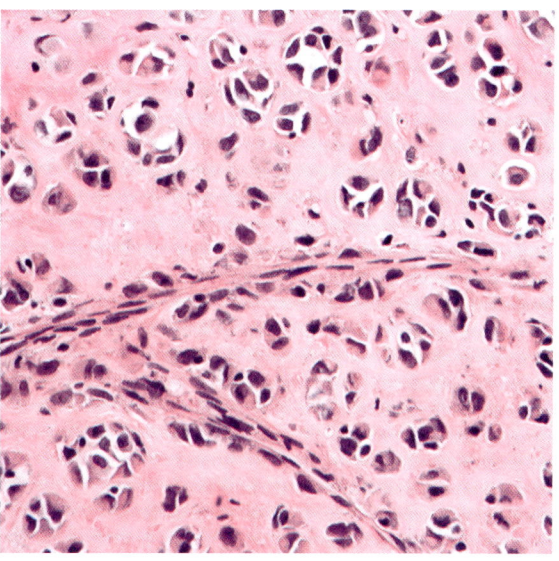

Figure 9-37

ENDOMETRIAL STROMAL SARCOMA WITH EPITHELIOID CELLS

The cells are round, with abundant eosinophilic cytoplasm.

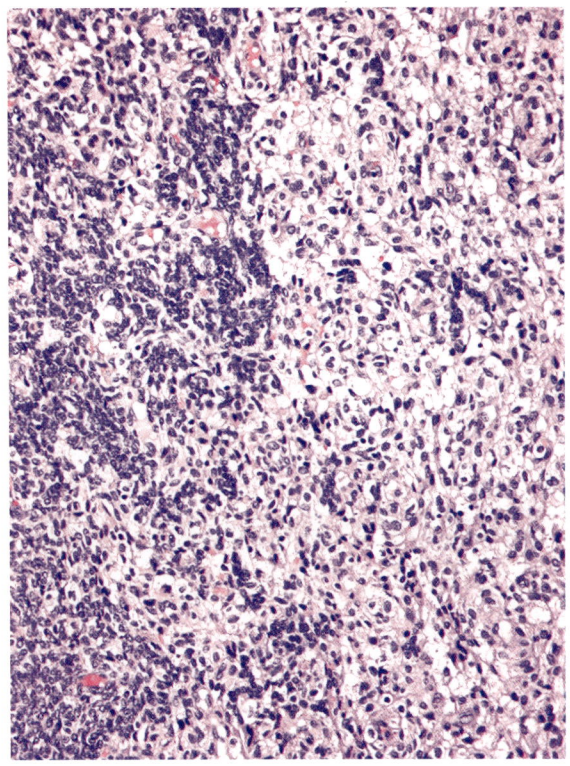

Figure 9-38

ENDOMETRIAL STROMAL SARCOMA WITH CLEAR CELLS

Typical areas of endometrial stromal neoplasia transition to cells with clear cytoplasm.

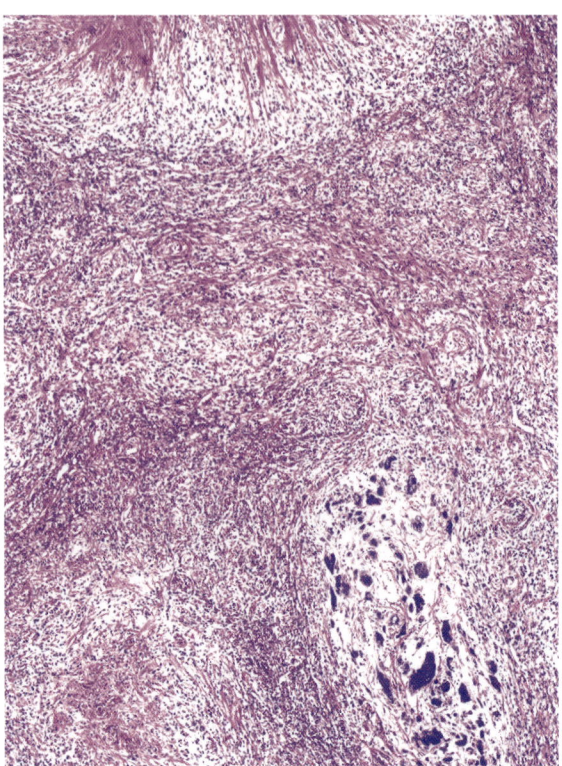

Figure 9-39

ENDOMETRIAL STROMAL SARCOMA WITH BIZARRE NUCLEI

The tumor shows smooth muscle differentiation (starburst pattern, bottom) as well as large and hyperchromatic bizarre nuclei.

tumors with other types of differentiation, including smooth muscle differentiation with a starburst pattern (28,29). Osteoclast-like cells have been described in one endometrial stromal tumor within the areas of smooth muscle differentiation (33). The cells had 2 to 15 bland monomorphic vesicular nuclei with ample cytoplasm and no mitotic activity. These cells were vimentin, alpha-1-antichymotrypsin, and CD68 positive with membranous staining for leukocyte common antigen.

Immunohistochemical Findings. Endometrial stromal nodule and endometrial stromal sarcoma, including variants, are typically positive for CD10 (also known as common acute lymphoblastic leukemia antigen) (fig. 9-40). CD10 functions as a cell surface enzyme that is expressed in a variety of normal tissues and neoplasms including normal endometrial stroma and endometrial stromal neoplasms. Cytoplasmic staining is often strong and diffuse (66), although it may be only focal and weak, and some tumors may be negative (67). This marker was originally thought to be a useful adjunct in the distinction between endometrial stromal and smooth muscle tumors (positive in the former and negative in the latter) with a sensitivity of 75 to 100 percent (66,68–71). It was subsequently reported, however, that CD10 has poor specificity as most tumors with a mesenchymal component, including highly cellular leiomyoma and leiomyosarcoma, may be strongly positive for this marker (up to 60 percent) (69,71–74).

Interferon-inducible transmembrane protein-1 (IFITM1 or CD225) has recently been shown to stain benign and malignant endometrial stroma with moderate to strong and multifocal to diffuse cytoplasmic positivity in the latter (fig. 9-41) (75). Although it was thought that IFITM1 had comparable sensitivity and higher specificity

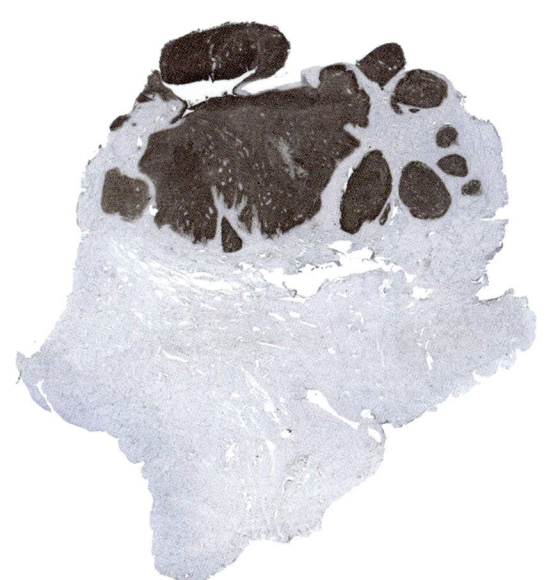 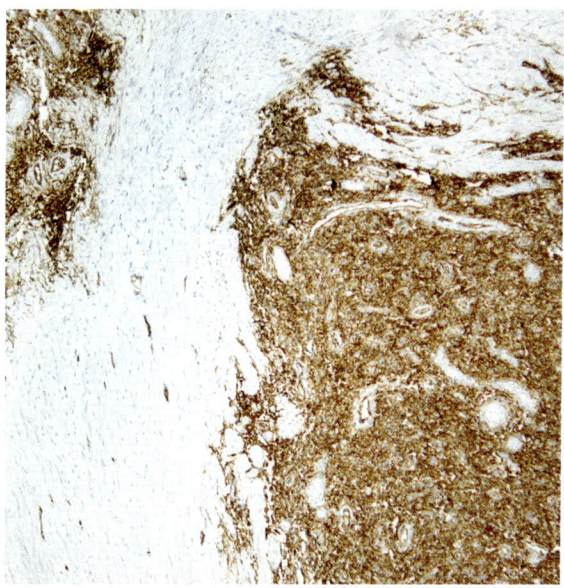

Figure 9-40

ENDOMETRIAL STROMAL SARCOMA

CD10 is strongly positive and highlights the infiltrating islands of tumor cells within the myometrium (left and right).

than CD10 in the diagnosis of these tumors (76), about 20 percent of smooth muscle tumors were also reported to be positive, some with multifocal or strong staining (75). Also, IFITM1 may be positive in other tissues such as ovarian stroma, a potential mimic of endometrial stroma, thus emphasizing the importance of immunohistochemical/morphologic correlation.

Estrogen and progesterone receptors (ER and PR) have heterogeneous expression in endometrial stromal tumors (77). ER is expressed in 40 to 100 percent of all endometrial stromal sarcomas, specifically the isoform α, but not isoform β (fig. 9-42). PR expression ranges from 60 to 100 percent in endometrial stromal sarcomas. It is typically strongly expressed in normal endometrial glands and stroma, but PR isoforms show distinct fluctuations during the menstrual cycle in each compartment, and while PRα and PRβ are equally expressed in the glandular cells, PRα is the major isoform expressed in endometrial stroma and endometrial stromal tumors (77–84). This ratio may change in endometrial stromal tumor variants (82). Marked differences in the PR profile may be noted between primary and recurrent tumors, the latter showing PRβ predominance which may be associated with changes in tumor morphology (22,82).

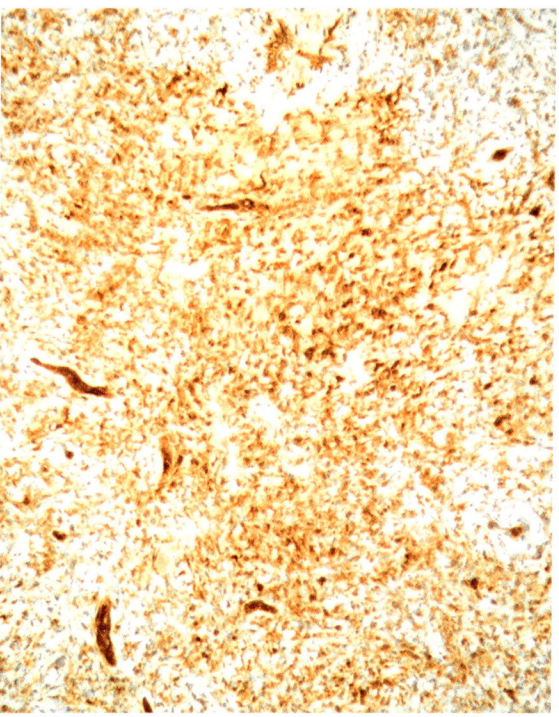

Figure 9-41

ENDOMETRIAL STROMAL NODULE

The tumor cells are diffusely positive for IFITM1, a marker that appears to be more specific than CD10 in the diagnosis of endometrial stromal tumors.

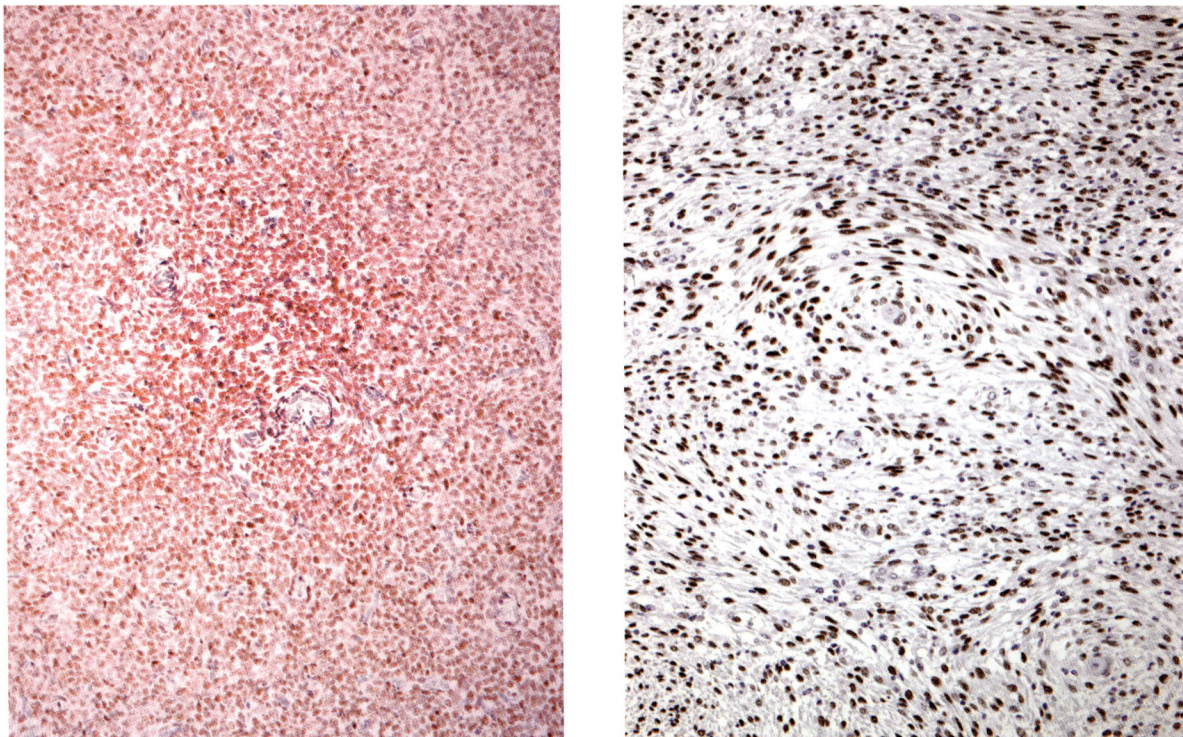

Figure 9-42

ENDOMETRIAL STROMAL SARCOMA

The tumor cells show diffuse and strong positivity for ER in a typical endometrial stromal tumor (left), and in a tumor with fibroblastic morphology (right), but staining varies from tumor to tumor.

Androgen receptor (AR) expression has been less often studied in these tumors, but overall, it is less often expressed when compared to ER and PR (about 50 percent), with a similar heterogenous pattern of staining (85,86). Aromatase is a key enzyme in estrogen biosynthesis, but only less than half of endometrial stromal sarcomas are positive for this marker, often with a heterogeneous pattern of staining (87).

These tumors are also often positive for keratins including AE1/3, CAM5.2 (fig. 9-43, left), MNF116, CK8/18 (41,88,89), and WT1 (90,91). Smooth muscle markers may be positive in conventional areas of endometrial stromal neoplasia, most frequently smooth muscle actin, muscle-specific actin, and calponin (71), uncommonly desmin (fig. 9-44A), and rarely caldesmon, HDCA8, and smooth muscle myosin (68,91–93). Smooth muscle actin, desmin, caldesmon, and HDCA8 are often positive in areas of smooth muscle differentiation (fig. 9-44B) (50,51,71,93–96). Desmin may be positive (sometimes extensive) in endometrial stromal tumors with fibroblastic morphology (fig. 9-44C) (23). Most tumors (nodules and sarcomas) reported in two series show nuclear β-catenin positivity (including some that may be CD10 negative) in contrast to normal endometrial stroma, although this finding has not been confirmed by other investigators. Mutations have been only rarely reported (72,97).

Areas of sex cord differentiation within endometrial stromal tumors may be positive for a variety of sex cord markers including inhibin (more often if abundant/lipidized cytoplasm), calretinin (fig. 9-45), CD99, melan A, and WT1 (42,50,51,60,89,92,98–100). Among these sex cord markers, calretinin appears to be most consistently expressed (50). They also express CD56, but are negative for FOXL2, which is a very specific marker of stromal and sex cord tumors in the ovary (60,100). As occurs with uterine tumors resembling sex cord tumors, areas of sex cord differentiation often are

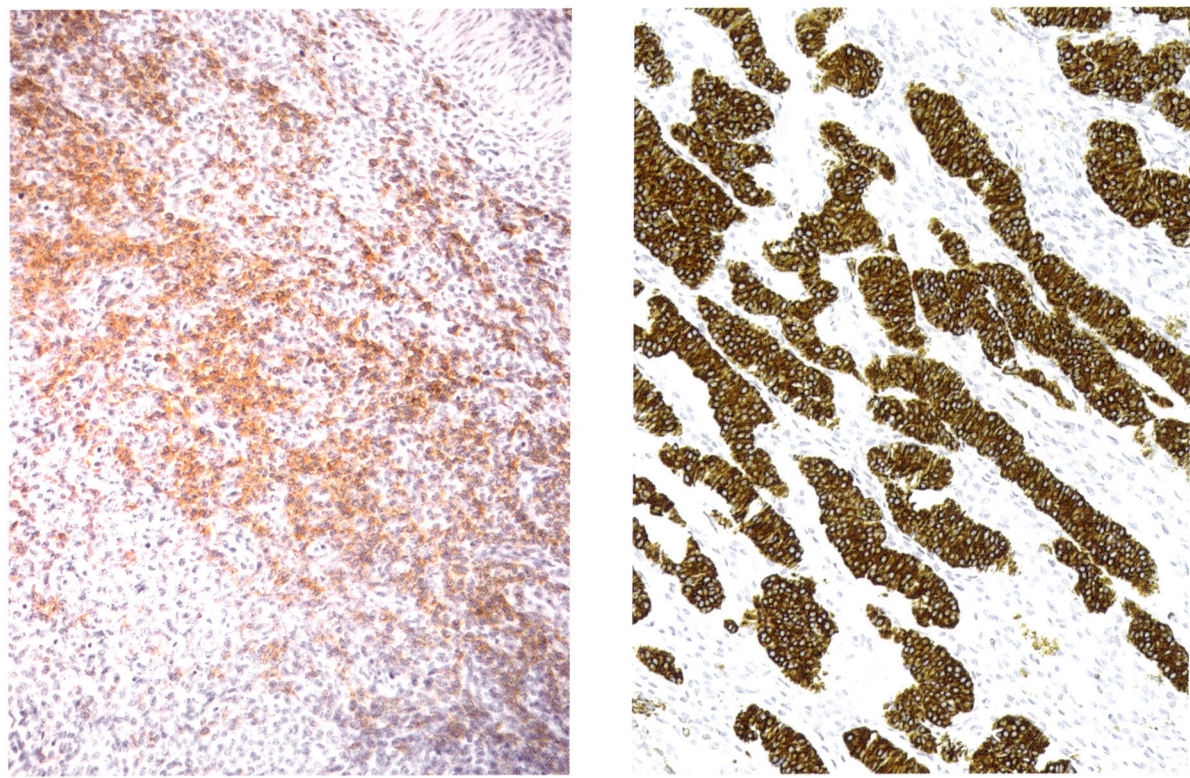

Figure 9-43

ENDOMETRIAL STROMAL SARCOMA

Typical areas of endometrial stromal neoplasia may be positive for keratins, more frequently AE1/3 (left) but areas of sex cord-like differentiation are more often positive (right).

polyphenotypic, with coexpression of sex cord markers, epithelial markers (most commonly keratins [AE1.3/CAM5.2] (fig. 9-43, right) and rarely EMA) (54,92) as well as smooth muscle markers (22,49,53,54,60,89,93,99,101,102). Among the latter, caldesmon, HDCA8, and smooth muscle myosin have not been tested in these areas. ER, PR, and CD10 are often positive in areas of sex cord-like differentiation as occurs in conventional areas of stromal neoplasia and it appears that CD10 positivity in the sex cord areas is higher than that observed in uterine tumors resembling sex cord tumors (50,53,100).

C-KIT positivity may be detected in endometrial stromal sarcomas but it is not associated with *C-KIT* mutations (103,104). Cyclin D1, BCOR, and DOG1 are typically negative, although rare tumors may be positive for cyclin D1 and BCOR (105–107). Endometrial stromal sarcomas are often positive for PDGFR-α but negative for PDGFR-β and unassociated with hotspot mutations (108). Tumors with myxoid background are alcian blue positive and PAS negative (23).

Molecular Genetic Findings. In the last three decades, there have been tremendous advances in the molecular characterization of endometrial stromal tumors. These tumors are genetically heterogeneous and harbor distinct cytogenetic abnormalities that most commonly involve chromosomes 6, 7, and 17. In 1988, Dal Cin et al. (109) reported the first cytogenetic abnormality (ins[10;19]) in an endometrial stromal sarcoma, but 3 years later the well-known t(7,17) (p15;q11) was detected in these tumors (fig. 9-46) (110). Since then, this translocation has been reported in both endometrial stromal nodules (70 percent) and endometrial stromal sarcomas (50 percent), especially those with conventional morphology (111,112). This gene fusion is less commonly identified in endometrial stromal tumors with variant morphology, including those with smooth muscle

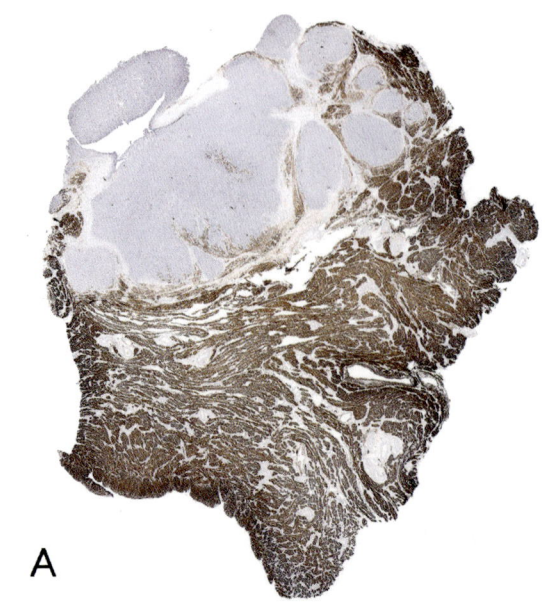

Figure 9-44

ENDOMETRIAL STROMAL SARCOMA

Most typical endometrial stromal tumors are desmin negative but some show some degree of positivity (A). Areas of smooth muscle differentiation are typically positive for desmin (B), while tumors with fibroblastic background are also often positive for desmin (C).

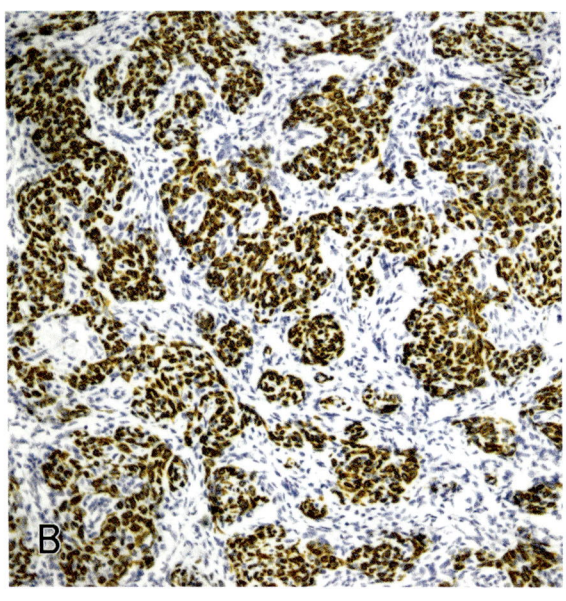
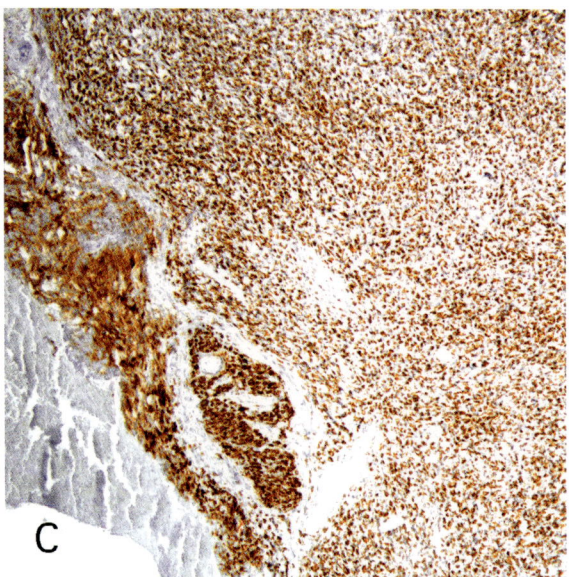

differentiation, sex cord-like differentiation, and with epithelioid, rhabdoid, or fibrous/myxoid morphology (56,105,113–119). Koontz et al. (120) first identified the genes involved in this translocation, encoding two novel proteins with zinc-finger motifs, *JAZF1* on chromosome 7 and *SUZ12* (also known as *JJAZ1*) on chromosome 17. It has been suggested that *JAZF1-SUZ12* fusion is an early event in the development of endometrial stromal tumors, and that endometrial stromal nodule may be the precursor of endometrial stromal sarcoma. The presence of this translocation in occasional undifferentiated sarcomas indicates that some of these tumors represent progression from low-grade tumors, and are, therefore, de-differentiated endometrial stromal sarcomas rather than undifferentiated uterine sarcomas.

Other less common gene fusions reported in tumors with conventional and variant morphology include *JAZF1-PHF1, EPC1-PHF1, MEAF6-PHF1, ZC3H7B-BCOR, MBTD1-CXORF67,* and *BRD8-PHF1*, although disruption of some genes may occur without an associated known partner gene (*JAZF1* or *PHF1*) (112,117,119–133). It has been shown that *JAZF1* is a transcriptional repressor while *SUZ12, PHF1*, and *MBTD1* are members of the polycomb group of proteins also involved in transcriptional repression. It appears that most of the genes involved in these translocations alter transcriptional control in endometrial stromal progenitor cells.

Despite the increasing number of gene fusions reported in these tumors, there seems to be no correlation with specific variant histology except for endometrial stromal tumors with sex cord differentiation (frequently with *PHF1* rearrangements) (fig. 9-46) (56) and fibromyxoid differentiation that may show a *YWHAE-NUTM2A/B* fusion without being associated with high-grade morphology (107,134). When present, these translocations are mutually exclusive, although they are all specific for the diagnosis of endometrial stromal neoplasia among mesenchymal uterine tumors.

The translocations/fusions are detected with traditional cytogenetic techniques, interphase fluorescence in situ hybridization (FISH) and reverse-transcriptase polymerase chain reaction (RT-PCR), but the latter may result in false negative results due to poor tissue preservation using formalin-fixed paraffin-embedded tissue. At present, FISH is the method of choice for the detection of these gene fusions. It has been recently shown that next generation RNA

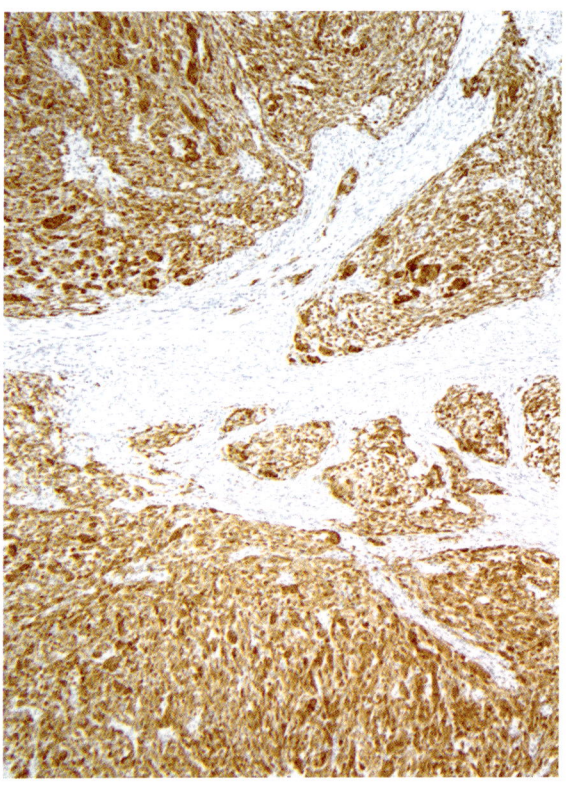

Figure 9-45

ENDOMETRIAL STROMAL SARCOMA WITH SEX CORD DIFFERENTIATION

The sex cord-like areas are often positive for calretinin.

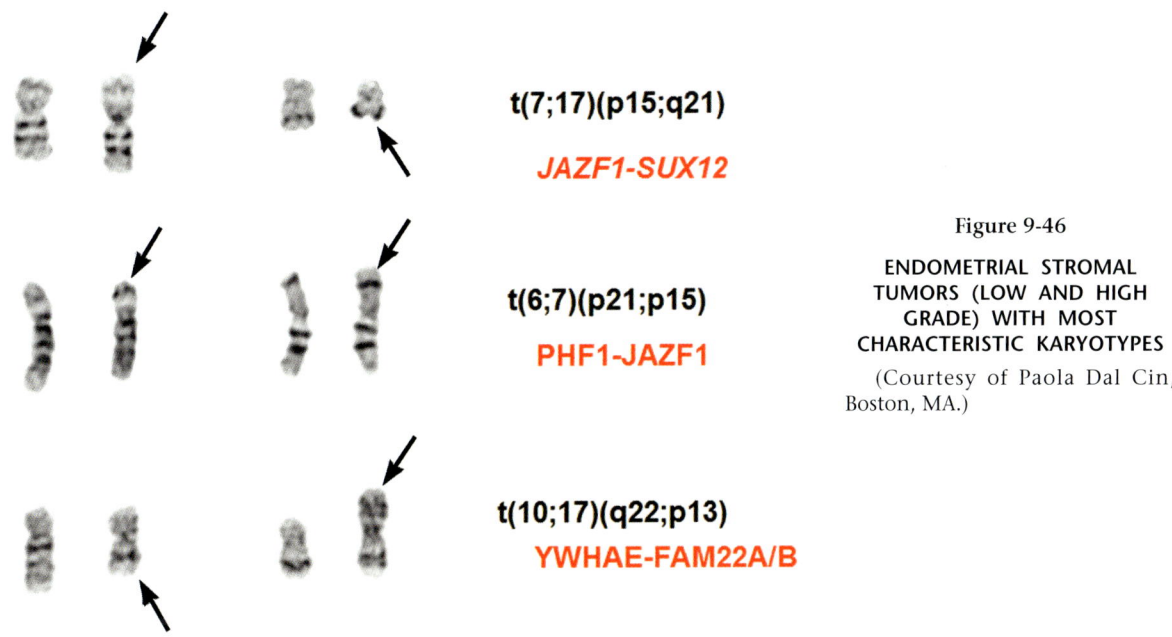

Figure 9-46

ENDOMETRIAL STROMAL TUMORS (LOW AND HIGH GRADE) WITH MOST CHARACTERISTIC KARYOTYPES

(Courtesy of Paola Dal Cin, Boston, MA.)

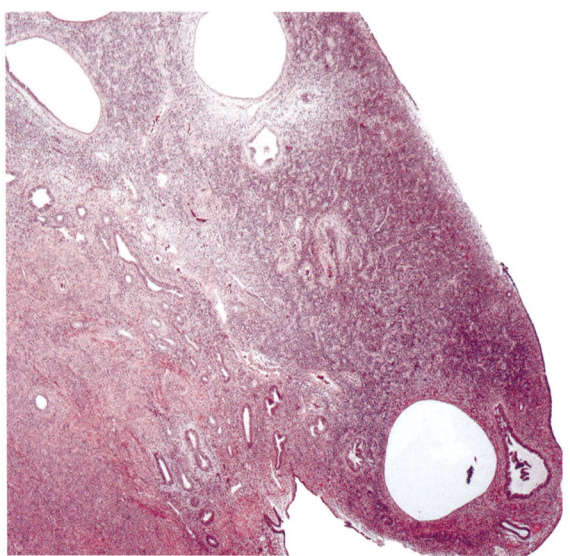 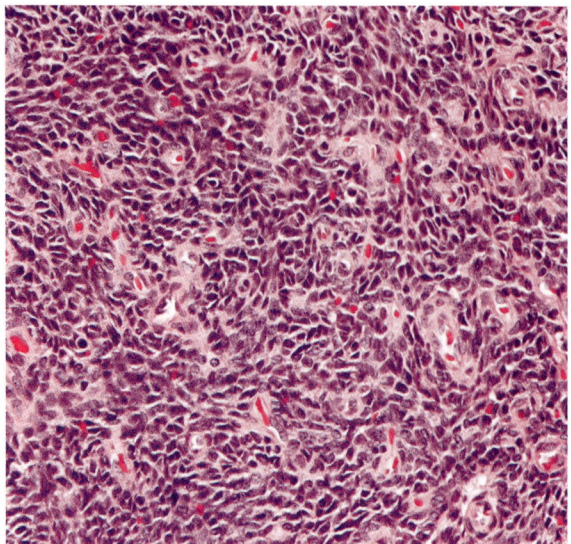

Figure 9-47

CELLULAR ENDOMETRIAL POLYP

In a curettage specimen, these benign lesions may cause concern for an endometrial stromal tumor due to their "blue" appearance and lack of associated endometrial glands in some areas (left). At high-power examination, there is an inactive "compacted" appearance of the stromal cells (right).

sequencing has good sensitivity and specificity for the detection of fusion transcripts in endometrial stromal tumors (135).

PPARG and *IRF4* mutations have been detected in endometrial stromal sarcomas. PPARG encodes peroxisome proliferator-activated receptor gamma, which acts as a tumor suppressor in breast, prostate gland, pituitary gland, and other endocrine organs while in the uterus its activation suppresses estrogen biosynthesis. IRF4 encodes a transcription factor in the interferon regulatory factor family required for endometrial decidualization. It has been hypothesized that *PPARG* and *IRF4* mutations are involved in the development of these tumors (136).

Differential Diagnosis. The differential diagnosis of endometrial stromal tumors is extensive as this group of tumors shows a wide spectrum of morphologic features. Before discussing this differential diagnosis, it is important to emphasize that the distinction between an endometrial stromal nodule and sarcoma can only be accomplished in a hysterectomy specimen, except when the tumor is very small and margins are appreciated in a polypectomy or "myomectomy" specimen. In a curetting, the working diagnosis should be "endometrial stromal tumor" without further classification. As these patients are typically of reproductive age and often want to preserve fertility, a conservative approach may be undertaken in selected instances, which typically includes hormonal treatment with conservative resection and hysteroscopic and radiologic monitoring of the tumor-myometrial interface (137,138).

Among non-neoplastic lesions in the differential diagnosis of endometrial stromal tumors, *cellular endometrial polyps* and *gland-poor or intravascular adenomyosis* are the most common entities, while intravascular endometrial tissue or menses-associated cellular stroma may occasionally suggest an endometrial stromal neoplasm. *Cellular endometrial polyps*, when fragmented and seen in a curettage specimen, may suggest an endometrial stromal tumor (fig. 9-47). In general, the fragments composed of stroma only show stromal cells with an inactive to atrophic "compacted" appearance without mitotic activity; they lack the arteriolar-type vessels characteristic of endometrial stromal tumors but instead display medium to large vessels, at least in some of the fragments, with others showing similar stroma admixed with inactive endometrial glands, providing a clue

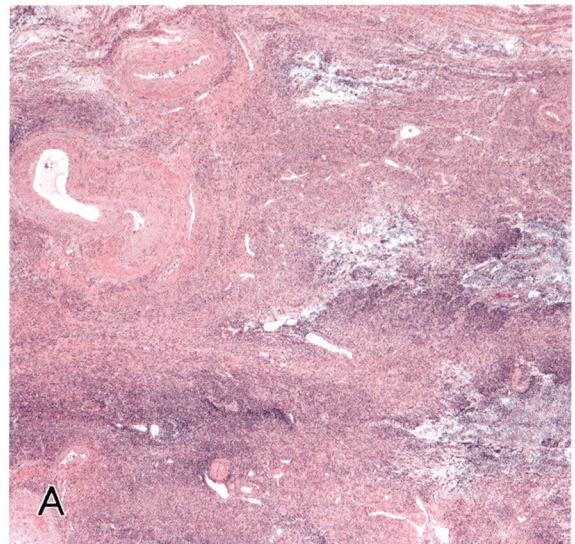

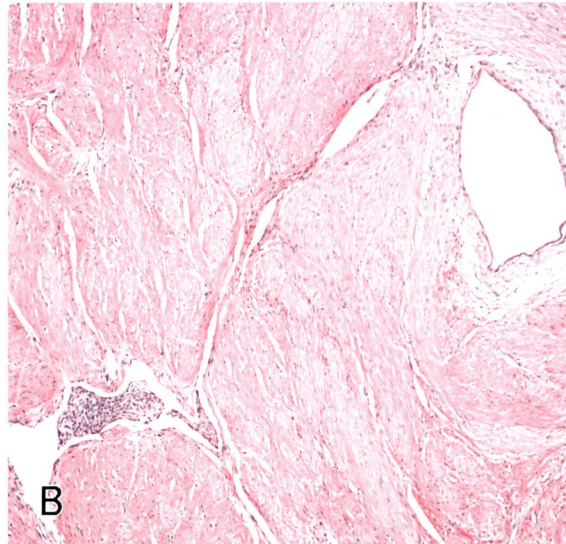
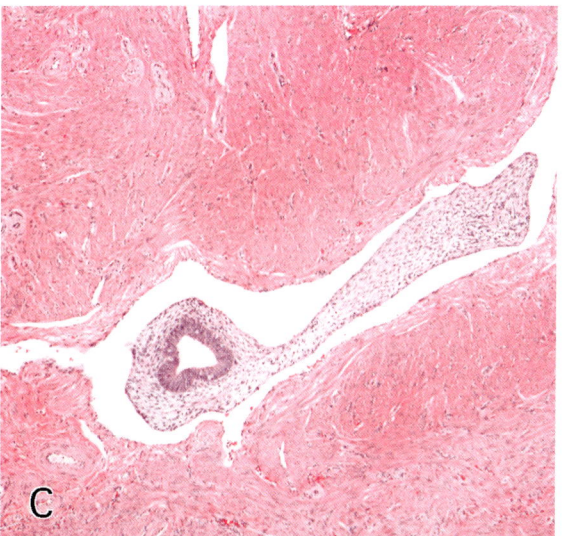

Figure 9-48

GLAND-POOR AND INTRAVASCULAR GLAND-POOR ADENOMYOSIS

Nests of endometrial stromal cells lacking endometrial glands (A), or if intravascular, more often gland poor (B) but sometimes with glands (C), may raise the possibility of an endometrial stromal sarcoma. However, the nests have an inactive to atrophic appearance, are often associated with typical areas of adenomyosis, and typically represent an incidental finding.

to the correct diagnosis (26). One study found that in curettage specimens, most endometrial stromal tumors were represented by fragments containing only or predominantly endometrial stroma measuring more than 5 mm while benign conditions were characterized by smaller fragments (see fig. 9-19). The diagnosis of endometrial stromal tumors becomes easier if one or more of the fragments have variant morphology or there is myometrial infiltration, the latter a rare finding (see fig. 9-20) (139).

The microscopic appearance of *gland-poor or intravascular adenomyosis* may focally overlap with that seen in endometrial stromal sarcoma when evaluating hysterectomy specimens (fig. 9-48). In contrast to the latter, however, no mass is noted on gross examination. Typical areas of adenomyosis, often with an atrophic appearance of the stroma, are present nearby without typical endometrial stromal neoplasia (140).

Endometrial tissue within uterine vessels is seen during the menstrual period (141) and less commonly in uteri with adenomyosis. It may be composed only of endometrial stroma (142). In the first scenario, stromal cells are typically hyperchromatic and associated with apoptotic debris and frequently admixed with inflammatory cells. When associated with adenomyosis the endometrial stroma is more likely to represent gland-poor adenomyosis (fig. 9-48B,C) (142).

Table 9-3

DIFFERENTIAL FEATURES OF ENDOMETRIAL STROMAL SARCOMA AND HIGHLY CELLULAR LEIOMYOMA

Features	Endometrial Stromal Sarcoma	Highly Cellular Leiomyoma
Irregular margins	Common and extensive	Uncommon and focal
Merging with myometrium	–	+
Vasculature	Small, arteriole-like or curvilinear (if large vessels at interface)	Large and thick (may have small vessels, not arteriole-like)
Cleft-like spaces	–	+
Spindle cells with fascicular growth	–	+
CD10	+	+/–
IFITM1	+	– (limited experience)
ER/PR	+	+
WT1	+	+
Keratin	+/–	+/–
Smooth muscle actin	+	+
Desmin	–/+	+
Caldesmon	–	+

The differential diagnosis of typical endometrial stromal tumors, both nodule and sarcoma, includes *highly cellular leiomyoma*, a common and most diagnostically challenging tumor as it shares with the former the findings of dense cellularity and prominent vasculature (Table 9-3). Furthermore, (highly) cellular leiomyomas also have a tan to yellow cut surface, may have a diffuse rather than fascicular growth in the center, may be associated with a prominent component of small vessels, show an irregular margin (fig. 9-49A) with the adjacent myometrium, contain hyaline plaques (fig. 9-49B), and are often positive for CD10 (may be extensive), typical features of endometrial stromal tumors. A correct diagnosis is crucial since this differential frequently arises in the context of a curettage performed in a young woman for vaginal bleeding, and while treatment can be conservative if the diagnosis is that of a highly cellular leiomyoma, the patient will almost always require a hysterectomy if the diagnosis is that of an endometrial stromal tumor.

Features that point toward a highly cellular leiomyoma include fascicular growth of spindle cells which contrasts with the diffuse growth of ovoid cells seen in endometrial stromal tumors, large and thick blood vessels, and cleft-like spaces (fig. 9-49C). Even though the interface with the myometrium in a highly cellular leiomyoma may be irregular, there is merging of the neoplastic cells with the surrounding myometrium. These tumors are also typically extensively positive for desmin, h-caldesmon, and HDAC8 (71,95,143). Oxytocin, although not commonly used, is typically positive in smooth muscle tumors and negative in endometrial stromal tumors (144). Transgelin, a newly developed smooth muscle marker, has been reported to be negative in endometrial stromal tumors and may be useful in this differential diagnosis although more experience is needed before widespread use (145).

When evaluating a "fibroid" uterus, there may be multiple nodules, one or more of which may demonstrate necrosis. It is always important to section thoroughly and evaluate all such areas since they may correspond to an endometrial stromal tumor.

Endometrial stromal tumors with smooth muscle differentiation should be distinguished from smooth muscle tumors when the characteristic starburst pattern is lacking although the overall morphology is different (21). *Adenomyoma* is a mass-forming lesion and rarely may be in the differential diagnosis of an endometrial stromal nodule, but histologic examination reveals not only endometrial stroma but also

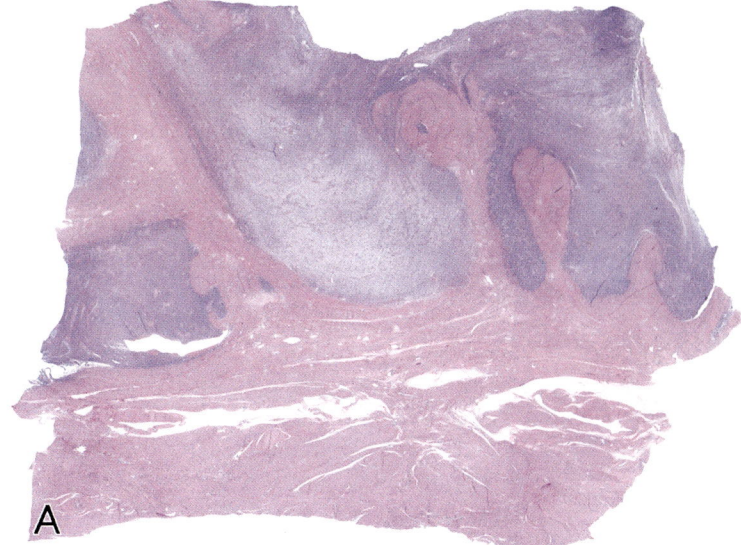

Figure 9-49

HIGHLY CELLULAR LEIOMYOMA

This variant of leiomyoma may show irregular margins (A), and the collagen plaques (B) seen in endometrial stromal tumors, but it also displays large thick blood vessels and cleft-like spaces (C), characteristic of this tumor.

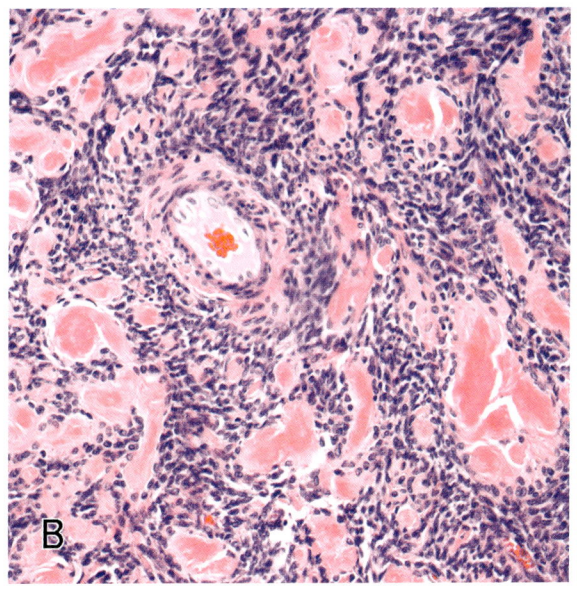

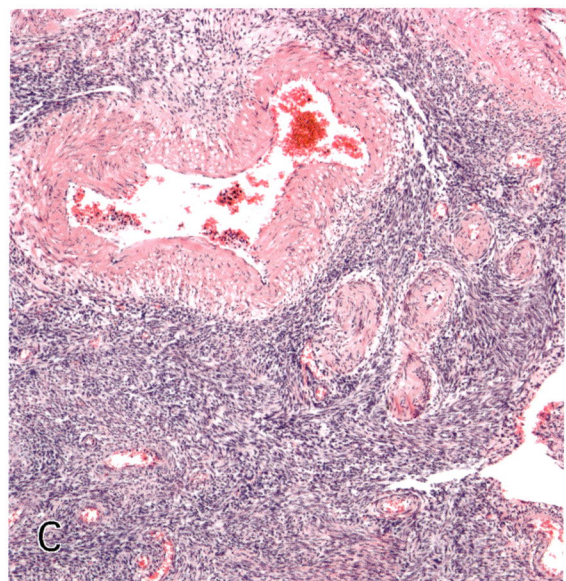

glands and smooth muscle that correlate with a gross appearance closely resembling a smooth muscle tumor (146). Caution should be exercised when applying immunohistochemistry if the differential diagnosis includes an endometrial stromal tumor with smooth muscle differentiation since in this scenario positivity for muscle markers is often noted, mostly in the smooth muscle component. To classify such a tumor as an endometrial stromal tumor, the immunophenotype of areas resembling typical stromal cells should be evaluated, rather than areas of smooth muscle differentiation. As no single marker is entirely sensitive or specific, a panel of immunostains including CD10 and two smooth muscle markers (desmin and h-caldesmon) is most useful in distinguishing between endometrial stromal tumors and smooth muscle neoplasms. A final observation regarding endometrial stromal tumors with smooth muscle differentiation relates to the occasional discrepancy between the macroscopic and microscopic appearance: in an apparently circumscribed tumor, the smooth muscle differentiation may be misconstrued as myometrial invasion. In such cases, it is crucial to evaluate the interface

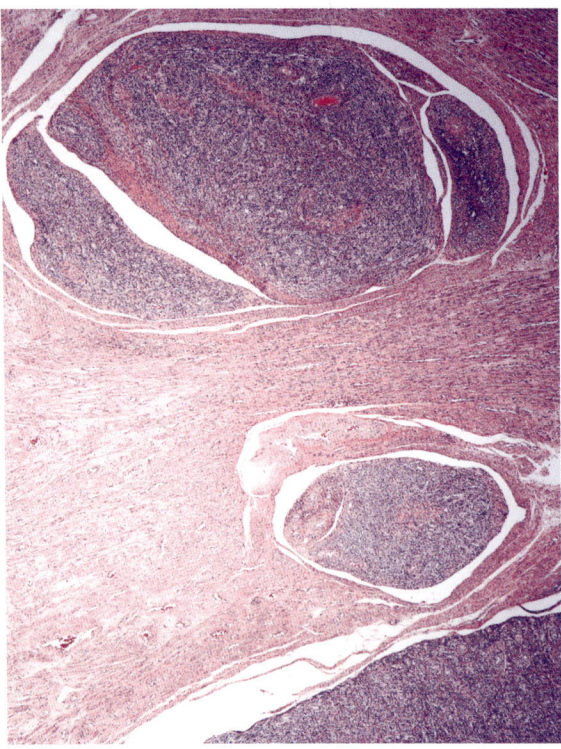

Figure 9-50

CELLULAR INTRAVENOUS LEIOMYOMATOSIS

This tumor may closely mimic an endometrial stromal sarcoma, but large thick blood vessels and cleft-like spaces are typical of this proliferation.

of the tumor with the myometrium on gross as well as on low-power scrutiny (21).

Rarely, *cellular intravenous leiomyomatosis* is confused with endometrial stromal sarcoma since both share dense cellularity, hyaline plaques, and intravascular growth (fig. 9-50). Although cardiac involvement is more commonly seen in intravenous leiomyomatosis, it has been described in endometrial stromal sarcoma (147). In contrast to the latter, intravenous leiomyomatosis shows a fascicular growth of spindle cells, large thick-walled blood vessels, cleft-like spaces (similar to highly cellular and typical leiomyomas), and often a subendothelial proliferation of spindle cells "colonizing" the walls of the veins (148,149). Highly cellular leiomyomas are occasionally associated with small seedling cellular leiomyomas and at low-power examination may vaguely mimic the appearance of an endometrial stromal sarcoma. The features already discussed can be applied in this differential diagnosis (150).

Extensive sex cord-like differentiation in an endometrial stromal tumor may suggest a uterine tumor resembling a sex cord-stromal tumor (48), especially in a curettage specimen. A diagnosis of *uterine tumor resembling a sex cord-stromal tumor* cannot usually be established without a hysterectomy since the possible presence of an endometrial stromal component is difficult or impossible to exclude in this setting (26,27,151,152). Uterine tumors resembling sex cord ovarian tumors may be grossly polypoid and intracavitary or intramural. They have a tan to yellow cut surface, with or without cystic change, areas with solid growth, and rhabdoid cells, features that overlap with those seen in endometrial stromal tumors (153). In a hysterectomy specimen, extensive sampling should fail to reveal an endometrial stromal component. Although the immunophenotype of these two tumor types largely overlaps, it has been reported that uterine tumors resembling sex cord tumors are more frequently positive for markers of sex cord differentiation including calretinin (most common), CD99, melan A, and inhibin when compared to endometrial stromal tumors with sex cord-like differentiation (50). Uterine tumors resembling ovarian sex cord tumors may express FOXL2 in contrast to endometrial stromal tumors with sex cord-like differentiation, which in one study were all negative (100,154). Uterine tumors resembling ovarian sex cord tumors also lack the most common molecular alteration, t(7,17) or *PHF1* gene rearrangements, identified in endometrial stromal tumors including those with sex cord differentiation (155,156). Müllerian adenosarcomas with sex cord-like elements also enter in the differential diagnosis, but typical adenosarcomatous architecture is usually present to establish this diagnosis.

Sex cord-like areas lacking expression of sex cord-stromal-associated markers can be found in *epithelioid smooth muscle tumors* and *endometrioid adenocarcinomas with sertoliform morphology*. This may represent a diagnostic challenge when present in curettage specimens. The immunohistochemical profile of the aforementioned tumors partially overlaps and, thus, is of limited diagnostic utility (157,158). The presence of a spindle component with strong desmin and caldesmon positivity, with or without epithelial membrane antigen (EMA) or wide-spectrum keratin positivity, but negative for sex cord markers, supports a diagnosis of a smooth muscle tumor, over an endometrial stromal tumor with sex cord-like elements (50,71,150,159–161). Endometrial carcinomas are typically positive for epithelial markers, including EMA, but only rarely may be positive for inhibin (157).

YWHAE-FAM22 high-grade endometrial stromal sarcoma may enter the differential diagnosis of tumors with sex cord-like or epithelioid features, since the tumor cells are round and grow in nests. They lack, however, corded, trabecular, or tubular architecture, they display high nuclear to cytoplasmic (N/C) ratios, and there is uniform cytologic atypia with brisk mitotic activity. This contrasts with the low-grade morphology in areas of sex cord-like differentiation in low-grade endometrial stromal neoplasms. The tumor cells of *YWHAE-FAM22* high-grade endometrial stromal sarcoma are cyclin D1 diffusely positive but negative for CD10, ER, PR, and sex cord markers (162). C-KIT is usually expressed in these tumors (163) in contrast to uterine tumors resembling ovarian sex cord tumors (153) in which only occasional positivity has been reported, and endometrial stromal tumors, which are negative, including the few cases with sex cord differentiation that have been tested (71).

Endometrial stromal tumors with glandular differentiation should be distinguished from both benign and malignant processes. *Florid adenomyosis* may enter this differential diagnosis especially if it has an intravascular component. In a study of 434 uteri with adenomyosis, intravascular adenomyosis (fig. 9-48C) was seen in about 12 percent, most frequently represented by stroma only, but one third had both endometrial stroma and glands within vascular spaces (164). More than three vessels were involved in about 35 percent of cases. Similar to gland-poor adenomyosis, and in contrast to endometrial stromal sarcoma, there is no discrete mass. There is, at most, thickening or irregularity of the myometrium on gross examination, areas of typical adenomyosis, nodular smooth muscle hypertrophy surrounding adenomyotic islands (especially striking at low power), and stromal cells with an atrophic appearance, in contrast to the expansile and tongue-like growth seen in endometrial stromal sarcoma (140). *Intravascular adenomyomatosis* is thought to represent a variant of intravenous leiomyomatosis and is typically noted in association with leiomyomas and adenomyosis (165). Among malignant tumors, *low-grade müllerian adenosarcoma* (if glands are benign) or rarely, *carcinosarcoma* (if glands are malignant), may enter in the differential diagnosis. The typical condensation of low-grade malignant stroma, phyllodes architecture, intraluminal projections of stroma, and a variety of müllerian epithelia characteristic of adenosarcoma are lacking in endometrial stromal tumors. Furthermore, adenosarcoma rarely invades the myometrium. If invasive, the stromal component tends to be higher grade when compared to that of endometrial stromal sarcoma. Occasionally, endometrial stromal sarcoma arises in the background of a müllerian adenosarcoma (166). In carcinosarcoma, there is destructive invasion of the myometrium, mostly by the malignant glands, the epithelial and stromal elements show high-grade cytologic features, and frequently, the epithelial component of the tumor is predominant while other features typical of endometrial stromal sarcoma are lacking (59).

Fibrous and myxoid endometrial stromal tumors are often misclassified as *hydropic leiomyomas* or *benign or malignant myxoid smooth muscle tumors*. The latter should display the typical fascicular growth of cells with elongated blunted nuclei at least focally, as well as large thick-walled blood vessels as the predominant vascular component (167,168). Although smooth muscle tumors are usually positive for desmin and caldesmon, the expression pattern is frequently focal/weak or absent, especially for caldesmon, limiting the utility of immunohistochemistry in this differential diagnosis (169). Furthermore, as noted earlier, some fibroblastic endometrial stromal tumors may be desmin positive (22,23). p53 positivity favors a malignant smooth muscle tumor since endometrial stromal sarcomas (low-grade) are typically negative (170,171). Smooth muscle actin is frequently used in the differential diagnosis of smooth muscle and endometrial stromal tumors, but this marker is commonly positive in the latter and thus, not helpful in this distinction.

Other entities in the differential diagnosis are rare, including *nerve sheath tumors, solitary fibrous tumor, myxoid change in* the myometrium, *myxoma, inflammatory myofibroblastic tumor,* and *embryonal rhabdomyosarcoma*. Among nerve sheath tumors, *neurofibromas* typically occur in the setting of neurofibromatosis and are characterized by cells with wavy nuclei present in a fibromyxoid background; cells are typically S-100 protein positive and lack areas of conventional endometrial stromal neoplasia (172,173). *Malignant nerve sheath tumor,* although only reported in the cervix, may have a vague resemblance to endometrial stromal sarcomas including prominent small vessels and either a myxoid or fibroblastic morphology. They are often positive for SOX10 and S-100 protein, and CD34 if fibroblastic (174,175). *Solitary fibrous tumor* has recently been reported to occur in the uterus and may suggest the fibrous variant of endometrial stromal tumors, however, the latter show at least focally the typical vasculature and are STAT6 negative (176,177).

Multifocal myxoid change within the myometrium has been recently reported, in some instances associated with lupus erythematosus or type I neurofibromatosis, although in some cases, with unknown etiology. In patients with lupus erythematosus, the myxoid change is typically acellular and the uterus is homogeneously enlarged and hypertrophic (myxomatosis) (178). In neurofibromatosis, there is multifocal distribution of CD10-positive cells in well-demarcated myxoid nodules within superficial and deep myometrium. The nodules are paucicellular, containing uniform cells with a fibroblastic morphology. The process may also involve the cervix. In contrast to endometrial stromal tumors, no areas of conventional endometrial stromal neoplasia are identified and the cells are CD34 positive (179,180).

Myxomas are rare in the uterus and when encountered they are part of the constellation of Carney syndrome. On microscopic examination, myxoma is difficult to separate from myxoid endometrial stromal tumor. However, myxomas lack the typical vasculature and areas of conventional endometrial stromal neoplasia (181). Although *inflammatory myofibroblastic tumor* is more often confused with a myxoid smooth muscle tumor, it shares with myxoid endometrial stromal tumors the myxoid background, finger-like projections at the infiltrating border, and CD10 positivity. Endometrial stromal tumors lack the striking lymphoplasmacytic inflammatory infiltrate as well as the fasciitis-like appearance seen in inflammatory myofibroblastic tumors and are ALK-1 negative (182,183). *Embryonal rhabdomyosarcomas* may have a prominent myxoid background and small cells. In contrast to endometrial stromal tumors, however, they often have a cambium layer, alternating hypocellular and hypercellular areas, and cells that are highly malignant with hyperchromatic nuclei, brisk mitotic activity, and apoptotic debris (184).

Clear, epithelioid, and granular cytoplasm as well as rhabdoid morphology, bizarre nuclei and adipose metaplasia have been described more often in smooth muscle tumors including leiomyomas and intravenous leiomyomatosis. In these instances, the overall morphologic features of the tumors makes the distinction from endometrial stromal tumor straightforward (148,183,185–189).

Treatment and Prognosis. Endometrial stromal nodules are always benign and typically treated by hysterectomy, except in young patients who can undergo polypectomy or myomectomy with negative margins. Patients with endometrial stromal sarcomas are treated by total hysterectomy and bilateral salpingo-oophorectomy since the risk of recurrence is higher if only hysterectomy is performed (190–192). Omentectomy and lymph node dissection do not seem to influence survival in patients with low-stage endometrial stromal sarcomas (despite rates of lymph node metastases that approach 16 percent) (193,194), although some studies have reported different results (190,195–197). Lymph node metastases are frequently associated with gross extrauterine disease, extensive myoinvasion, and lymphovascular invasion (198). Patients with endometrial stromal sarcomas with limited infiltration likely have a better prognosis than those with typical endometrial stromal sarcomas. They should nevertheless, be diagnosed as having endometrial stromal sarcoma with a note indicating that follow-up information is too limited to draw any consistent conclusions (7).

Radiation therapy, although not the standard of care, is considered by some to control local recurrences but does not appear to improve overall survival in patients with endometrial stromal sarcoma, which is excellent (see below) (199–201). Hormonal therapy is an option in metastatic/recurrent disease, for young patients that want to preserve fertility, or for prevention of recurrences. Options include gonadotropin-releasing hormone (GnRH) analogues, aromatase inhibitors, or progestins (the most widely used) (87,202,203).

As endometrial stromal tumors often occur in the setting of hyperestrogenism, different mechanisms have been linked to the development and progression of these tumors based on estrogen levels. Aromatase inhibitors reduce estrogen levels by inhibition of its synthesis at peripheral sites, resulting in reduced receptor-mediated growth stimulation (87). It has been hypothesized that genetic polymorphisms in the aromatase gene *CYP19* may be associated with increased sensitivity of ER-positive cells to estrone and estradiol and these alterations may be involved in the oncogenesis of endometrial stromal sarcomas (202). Evaluation of ER and PR status is recommended by some at the time of initial diagnosis and recurrences, as loss in the latter may be indicative of more aggressive behavior (203).

Most patients with endometrial stromal sarcoma present with stage I tumors (about 70 percent) while about 20 percent have metastatic disease (9,194,204). These tumors are typically slow growing and associated with an indolent course, with an overall 5-year disease-specific survival rate of over 90 percent for all stages. Patients should be followed for long periods of time as they often develop late recurrences and metastases, resulting in a decline of the survival rate at 10 years to 75 percent (2). Even though stage is the best predictor of outcome in tumors confined to the uterus (9), one third to half of patients with stage I tumors still develop recurrences at 5 years while patients with stage III and IV tumors develop recurrences within 9 months. In the largest series to date, the median time between surgery and recurrence was 5.4 years for stage I tumors and 9 months for stage III and IV tumors (9). It is possible that some of the high-stage tumors with early recurrences reported in this study would now be classified as high-grade endometrial stromal sarcomas, given the authors' descriptions of enlarged nuclear size and increased mitotic rate in such tumors.

Extrauterine disease may involve one or more of the following sites: pelvis, lymph nodes, abdomen, lung, or bone (9,205,206). Although distant metastases are uncommon, lung is the most often affected site (7 to 28 percent) (19). The morphologic appearance of the tumor may change in recurrences, such that it mimics the appearance of primary tumors found in the metastatic site. For example, in the lung, metastatic endometrial stromal sarcoma may have a cystic appearance, leading to confusion with cystic hamartoma or lymphangiomyomatosis (93,207), and in the ovary they may mimic a stromal or sex cord tumor (17). Rarely, the tumor undergoes transformation to a high grade or even heterologous sarcoma, making it difficult to distinguish between a new tumor and transformation of the original tumor.

The significance of prognostic parameters other than stage is debatable, especially in patients with stage I tumors. Among clinical factors, some studies have reported that patients over 50 years (192,208,209), black patients (194,201), multiparity (210), and postmenopausal status (192,211,212) are associated with a worse outcome, but other studies have contradicted these findings (210,213,214). Among pathologic factors, mitotic activity and tumor cell necrosis have been disputed as prognostically relevant. In a study of 85 endometrial stromal sarcomas in a cohort of 419 uterine sarcomas, mitotic activity was found to be an independent prognostic factor in stage I tumors, with tumor cell necrosis and mitotic count of greater than 10 per 10 high-power fields being associated with worst outcome (215). Another study postulated that high proliferation index, measured by mitotic index, Ki-67, or PHH3 may be predictive of recurrences (216). However, in the largest study of these tumors, mitotic activity had no predictive value in stage I tumors by multivariate analysis but it was associated with poorer survival in patients who had extrauterine disease at the time of diagnosis (9). Tumor cell necrosis, one of the well-known defining criteria of leiomyosarcomas, has been associated with poor prognosis in endometrial stromal sarcomas (2). Patients with tumors lacking necrosis had a 96 percent 5-year crude survival rate in contrast to 69.2 percent for those with tumors with necrosis. In another study, patients with tumors with inconspicuous or absent necrosis had 5- and 10-year survival rates of about 90 and 80 percent, dropping to 45 percent in those with extensive necrosis

(217). However, the largest series to date did not find that association (9). It is difficult to objectively interpret data related to mitoses and necrosis in these tumors as it is likely that these studies included tumors that currently would be classified as high-grade endometrial stromal sarcomas. Furthermore, necrosis is a common finding even in endometrial stromal nodules and may have the appearance of tumor cell necrosis. Other parameters, including size, lymphovascular invasion, hormonal status, and ploidy have also shown conflicting results (218).

Although the FDA stipulated that morcellation should not be used for most patients with fibroids due to the potential risk of peritoneal spread of an occult malignant tumor during surgery, including endometrial stromal sarcomas (219), it seems that the consequences of peritoneal dissemination may not be as high as those reported with leiomyosarcoma. Nevertheless, affected patients may need prolonged clinical follow-up since experience with this situation is limited (220).

HIGH-GRADE ENDOMETRIAL STROMAL SARCOMAS

Definition. *High-grade endometrial stromal sarcomas* are tumors that have morphologic features that differ from the "proliferative-type" morphology seen in typical endometrial stromal tumors, although some are associated with a low-grade component. Two well-defined categories of high-grade endometrial stromal sarcoma exist, one described after the most recent WHO classification publication; both have unique morphologic (typically high-grade), immunohistochemical, and molecular features when compared to endometrial stromal tumors (4). A third category should be recognized in which high-grade sarcoma arises in a background of an endometrial stromal sarcoma (Table 9-4).

YWHAE-FAM22 (YWHAE-NUTM2) High-Grade Endometrial Stromal Sarcoma

Clinical Features. Patients with *YWHAE-FAM22 (YWHAE-NUTM2) endometrial stromal sarcomas* range widely in age (25 to 70 years), often presenting with abnormal vaginal bleeding or an enlarged uterus/pelvic or abdominal mass on physical exam. At the time of diagnosis, extrauterine extension is seen in more than half of patients.

Gross Findings. On gross examination, these tumors are often large and bulky (median, 8 cm). The cut surface is white and fleshy, with frequent areas of necrosis and hemorrhage (fig. 9-51) (64).

Microscopic Findings. These tumors are characterized by extensive permeative growth within the myometrium and myometrial veins, as seen in typical endometrial stromal sarcomas. On high-power examination, the tumors are cellular and display round cells with scant to moderately abundant eosinophilic cytoplasm, round to angulated nuclei (at least four times the size of lymphocyte nuclei), finely granular to slightly vesicular chromatin lacking visible nucleoli, and brisk mitotic activity (typically more than 10 mitoses per 10 high-power fields, but often 20 to 30). The cells are typically arranged in a vaguely nested or diffuse growth associated with a delicate capillary sinusoidal vasculature (fig. 9-52A,B). A focal pseudopapillary, cord-like, or rosette-like morphology has been reported (fig. 9-52C) (64,221). Patchy to extensive geographic tumor cell necrosis is common.

Approximately 50 percent of these tumors display a second component characterized in most instances by a low-grade spindle morphology, with or without an associated myxoid background, as typically seen in fibrous/myxoid variants of endometrial stromal sarcomas. This component is hypocellular and displays oval to spindle cells with bland cytologic features embedded in a delicate collagenous or myxoid background along, with the arteriolar vasculature that characterizes typical endometrial stromal tumors (fig. 9-53) (22,23). Rarely, these tumors evolve from a conventional low-grade endometrial stromal sarcoma at a metastatic site. In one case, the original tumor was stage I at time of diagnosis. The patient experienced multiple and early abdominopelvic recurrences and lung metastases that displayed a fibroblastic morphology associated with scattered large atypical cells and tested positive for the *YWHAE-FAM22* rearrangement. Five years after the initial diagnosis, the patient developed scalp metastases with the typical morphology of a *YWHAE-FAM22* high-grade endometrial stromal sarcoma and died of disease (222).

Immunohistochemical and Molecular Genetic Findings. The high-grade component

Table 9-4
HIGH-GRADE ENDOMETRIAL STROMAL SARCOMA TYPES

Type	Morphology	LG Component	ER/PR	CD10	Cyclin D1	BCOR	Other
YWHAE-FAM22 fusion	epithelioid	+/−	−	−	+	+	C-KIT
		fibromyxoid> conventional	+	+	−	−	−
ZC3H7B-BCOR fusion	spindle and myxoid	−	+/−	+/−	+	+	actin>desmin
NOS, rare JAZF1	variable	+	−/+	+/−	− (rare exceptions)	−	p53

of these tumors is typically strongly and diffusely positive for cyclin D1 (over 70 percent of cells) (fig. 9-54A), in contrast to low-grade tumors. They are negative for CD10, ER, and PR (fig. 9-54B) although minimal staining may be seen (162). They may express IFITM1 (75). They also express C-KIT (fig. 9-54C) (without associated mutations) but are negative for DOG1 (106,163). They are positive for BCOR, an antibody that has been found to be a more sensitive marker than cyclin D1 in the detection of these tumors (fig. 9-54D) (106). The low-grade component is characterized by CD10, ER, and PR positivity while it is negative or shows weak and focal cyclin D1 positivity with only some exceptions (162). They may show focal and weak staining with IFITM1 (75,76).

Tumors display t(10;17)(q22;p13) associated with *YWHAE-FAM22* (also known as *YWHAE-NUTM2*), identical to a fusion reported in clear cell sarcoma of the kidney (223,224). Rearrangements can be detected by FISH or RT-PCR analysis. FISH is more sensitive, with a cutoff of at least 20 to 30 percent positive cells. Less positivity may still be indicative of this translocation (124,225). The translocation has also been occasionally detected in endometrial stromal tumors with typical low-grade or variant morphologic features. One such tumor was reported to show striking and extensive cyclin D1 positivity, a low mitotic rate and Ki-67 index, with strong and diffuse positivity for ER and PR (107). Also, tumors without a *YWHAE-FAM22* fusion may rarely display strong positivity for cyclin D1 (226).

Differential Diagnosis. Although the morphologic appearance of this tumor is very

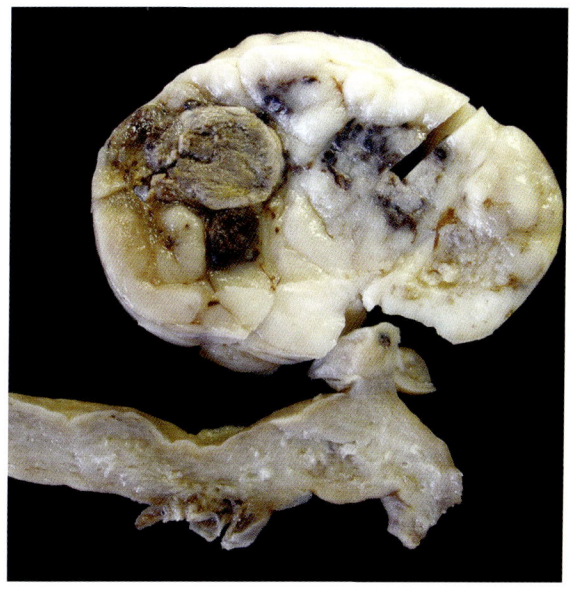

Figure 9-51

YWHAE-FAM22 HIGH-GRADE ENDOMETRIAL STROMAL SARCOMA

The tumor has a fleshy cut surface with extensive areas of necrosis and hemorrhage. It does not resemble the gross appearance of a typical endometrial stromal sarcoma.

characteristic, diagnostic considerations in the uterine corpus, especially in biopsy specimens, include undifferentiated/dedifferentiated carcinoma, epithelioid leiomyosarcoma, primitive neuroectodermal tumor, undifferentiated uterine sarcoma, gastrointestinal tumor (if biopsy of extrauterine mass), or metastases. *Undifferentiated/dedifferentiated carcinomas* are composed of monomorphous, noncohesive, medium-sized round cells that may focally be associated with a myxoid background, frequently show strong

Figure 9-52
YWHAE-FAM22 HIGH-GRADE ENDOMETRIAL STROMAL SARCOMA

The tumor is composed of sheets and closely packed tumor cells separated by a prominent thin sinusoidal vasculature (A). The cells are polygonal with scant cytoplasm and round nuclei with associated brisk mitotic activity (B). Rosette-like formations are seen (C).

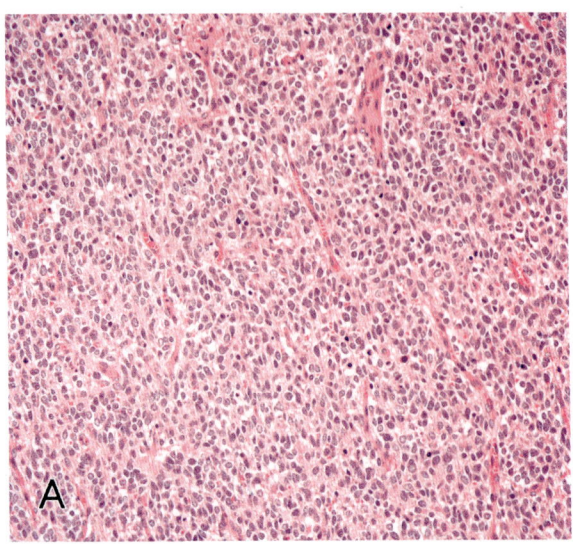

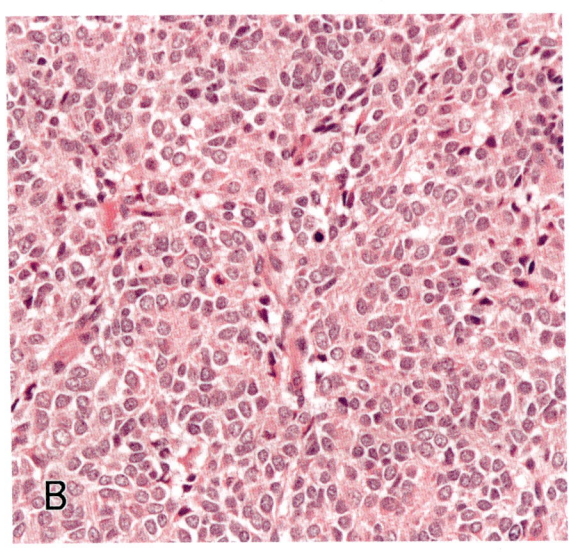

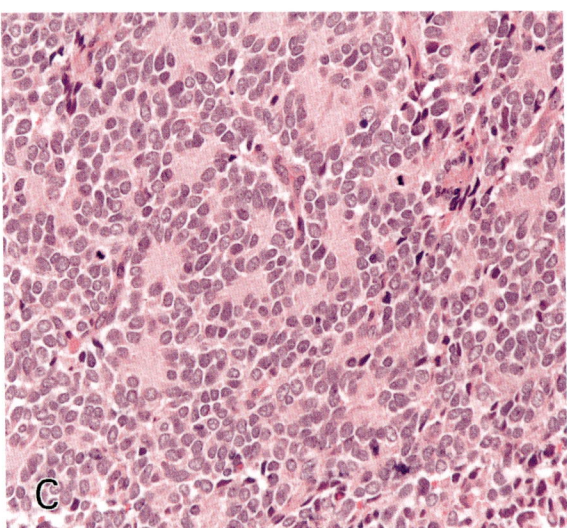

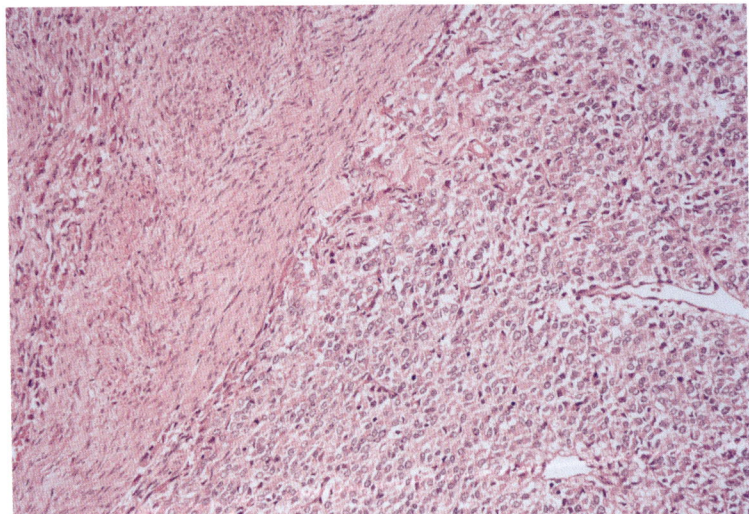

Figure 9-53
YWHAE-FAM22 HIGH-GRADE ENDOMETRIAL STROMAL SARCOMA

The high-grade component is juxtaposed to a low-grade fibroblastic component.

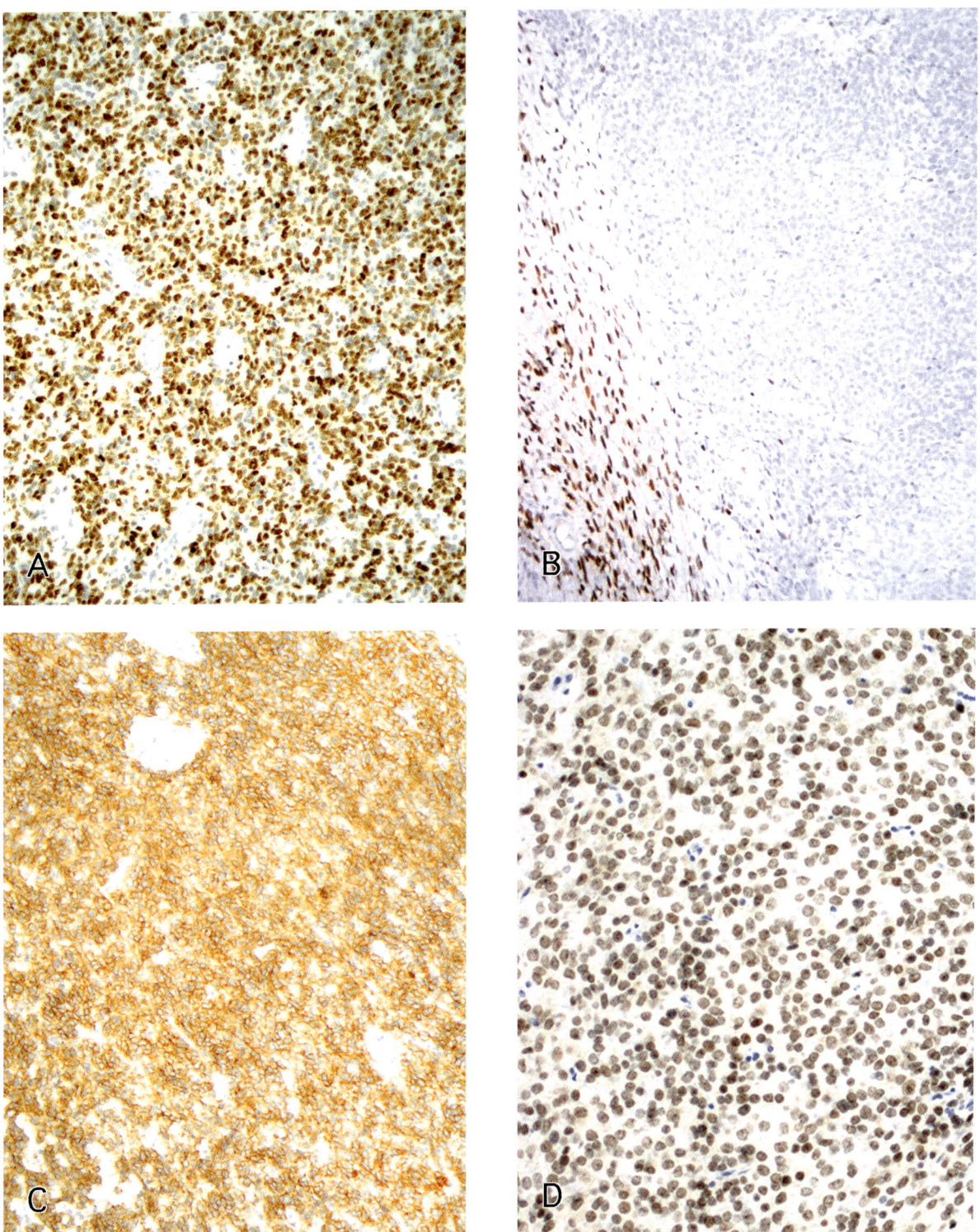

Figure 9-54

***YWHAE-FAM22* HIGH-GRADE ENDOMETRIAL STROMAL SARCOMA**

The high-grade component is diffusely and strongly positive for cyclinD1 (A), lacks positivity for PR (B), ER, and CD10, and is often positive for C-KIT (C) and BCOR (D).

and diffuse cyclin D1 positivity, while being typically negative for PAX8 and EMA. These features overlap with *YWHAE- FAM22* high-grade endometrial stromal sarcoma (227) when no associated low-grade carcinoma is present in a biopsy or curettage. Undifferentiated carcinomas have a strikingly diffuse growth pattern, lack a sinusoidal vasculature, are positive for keratin cocktail and keratin 8/18, and display concurrent loss of MLH1 and PMS2 or loss of E-cadherin and CD44 in about 50 percent (228).

Epithelioid leiomyosarcoma may display round cells and may be occasionally cyclin D1 and BCOR positive (106,162). However, the cells tend to be larger and commonly display an overtly malignant spindle cell component. Positivity for smooth muscle markers including desmin and h-caldesmon and frequent keratin and EMA positivity are seen (160).

Primitive neuroectodermal tumors (PNETs) are exceedingly rare in the uterus but since they are highly cellular and may display rosettes, they enter in the differential diagnosis of *YWHAE-FAM22* high-grade endometrial stromal sarcomas. The latter can, on occasion, express CD99, a common (although nonspecific) marker of PNET tumors. In most PNETs, the cells lack easily identified cytoplasm. Central-type PNETs express glial fibrillary acid protein (GFAP) in about 50 percent of cases, while PNETs of peripheral type are associated with *EWSR1* rearrangement (229,230). Rarer tumors that have morphologic and immunophenotypic features of Ewing sarcoma/peripheral PNET, but lack *EWSR1* rearrangement may enter in the differential diagnosis although they have not yet been reported in the uterus. These *CIC* (capicua transcriptional repressor)-rearranged sarcomas harbor less common alterations affecting *FUS*, *BCOR*, *CCNB3*, *CIC*, or *DUX4* (231).

Undifferentiated sarcomas also enter in the differential diagnosis as they may be extensively positive for cyclin D1. In contrast to *YWHAE- FAM22* high-grade endometrial stromal sarcomas, however, they also show extensive and strong CD10 positivity and they typically display marked pleomorphism as well as destructive myometrial invasion (4,226). Lastly, *epithelioid gastrointestinal stromal tumors* and *YWHAE-FAM22* endometrial stromal sarcomas share C-KIT expression. The latter, however, typically involves the uterus primarily, it lacks *C-KIT* mutations, and DOG1 is usually negative (232,233).

Treatment and Prognosis. Patients typically undergo hysterectomy followed by adjuvant chemotherapy, with or without radiation therapy. Chemotherapy with anthracycline-based drugs was shown to achieve complete radiologic response in a small series recently reported (234). These tumors are detected at higher stage (stage II or III) than typical endometrial stromal sarcomas.

The prognosis is intermediate between that of endometrial stromal sarcomas and undifferentiated uterine sarcomas (64,225). Patients frequently develop recurrences, typically early in the disease course. Peritoneal recurrences and pulmonary metastases are common. The high-grade morphology of *YWHAE-FAM22* endometrial stromal sarcoma may not be present in the primary tumor but may become apparent in concurrent metastases or recurrences (222). Although immunohistochemical or molecular tools may allow detection of low-grade tumors with the *YWHAE-FAM22* fusion, it is currently unknown which tumors evolve to a high-grade *YWHAE-FAM22* endometrial stromal sarcoma.

ZC3H7B-BCOR High-Grade Endometrial Stromal Sarcoma

Although only tumors harboring the t(10, 17)(q22;p13) were recognized in the latest WHO classification as high-grade endometrial stromal sarcomas, a new category, *high-grade ZC3H7B-BCOR endometrial stromal sarcoma*, has been recently described. It is notable for its close resemblance to myxoid leiomyosarcoma (235–237).

Clinical Features. In the only series of 17 tumors reported to date, patients had a wide age range (28 to 71 years), with most developing in the fifth decade (235). A small subgroup characterized by *BCOR* internal tandem duplications (*BCOR-ITD*) occurs in younger patients (18 to 32 years) (219,237). Patients present with nonspecific symptoms, including vaginal bleeding and a pelvic mass. Frequently, they have extrauterine disease, including lymph node metastases or pelvic disease, at the time of diagnosis (235,236).

Gross Findings. On gross examination, all high-grade *ZC3H7B-BCOR* endometrial stromal sarcomas (typical and with *BCOR* internal tandem duplication) are large (mean, 10 cm),

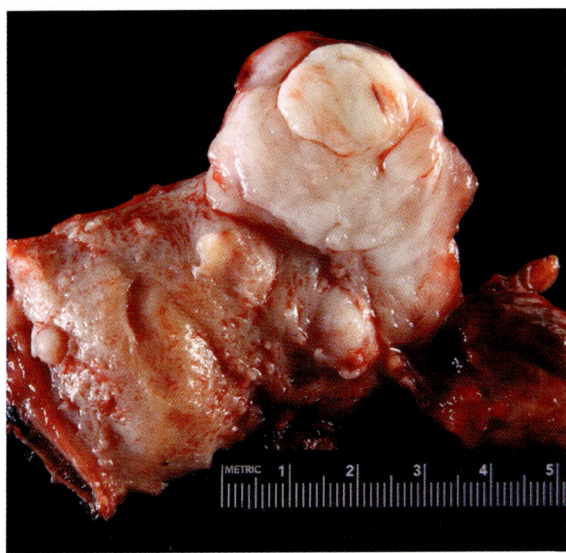

Figure 9-55

ZC3H7B-BCOR HIGH-GRADE ENDOMETRIAL STROMAL SARCOMA

On gross examination, these tumors may be intramyometrial and typically show irregular margins with a soft and fleshy cut surface.

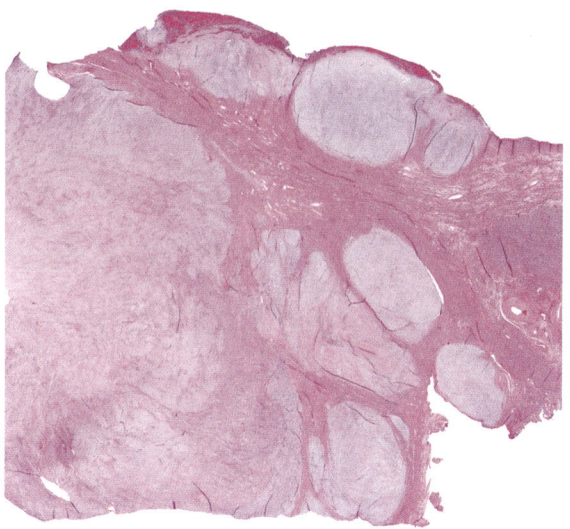

Figure 9-56

ZC3H7B-BCOR HIGH-GRADE ENDOMETRIAL STROMAL SARCOMA

At low power, these tumors may show permeative growth within the myometrium and may be strikingly myxoid.

polypoid, and centered in the endometrium but they can be predominantly intramyometrial and display an irregular border (fig. 9-55). They have a solid, soft, fleshy to rubbery, tan to yellow to pink cut surface and they may be gelatinous.

Microscopic Findings. On low-power microscopic examination, they may show a tongue-like or broad front, destructive (least common) pattern of invasion (fig. 9-56), but usually both are noted. The tumors are typically uniformly cellular, with cells growing in haphazard fascicles. The cells are spindled, with scant to abundant gray to eosinophilic cytoplasm and spindled to ovoid, or less commonly, round nuclei with inconspicuous nucleoli and evenly distributed chromatin without overt pleomorphism (fig. 9-57). *BCOR-ITD* tumors may show closely packed spindle cells that grow either in fascicles or sheets. Often a second component of round epithelioid cells is admixed with the spindle cells (fig. 9-58). The mitotic rate is typically brisk, often more than 15 mitoses per 10 high-power fields. Vascularity varies from case to case, but most often is characterized by small arterioles without striking perivascular whorling of tumor cells. Large and hemangiopericytoma-like vessels are also seen. In *BCOR-ITD* tumors, the vasculature is prominent and consists of numerous small vessels with prominent walls without curvilinear morphology.

The background stroma is either myxoid, including variably sized pools of basophilic material, or collagenous, with frequent collagen plaques (fig. 9-59). Areas of necrosis and lymphovascular invasion are common (235,236). In contrast to *YWHAE-FAM22* high-grade endometrial stromal sarcomas, these tumors are not associated with a conventional or variant component of low-grade endometrial stromal sarcoma.

Immunohistochemical and Molecular Genetic Findings. The immunohistochemical profile of typical *ZC3H7B-BCOR* tumors and those with *BCOR-ITD* closely overlap except for CD10 expression, which is typically positive, often with a diffuse and strong pattern of staining, in typical *ZC3H7B-BCOR* tumors (fig. 9-60A) but negative or only focally positive in the rare *BCOR-ITD* tumors reported (235–237). Cyclin D1 is strongly and diffusely positive in most tumors while BCOR is also typically positive, although paradoxically not to the extent seen in *YWHAE-FAM22* high-grade endometrial stromal sarcomas (fig. 9-60B). Positivity ranges in intensity and extent. There is frequently concordant expression of cyclin D1

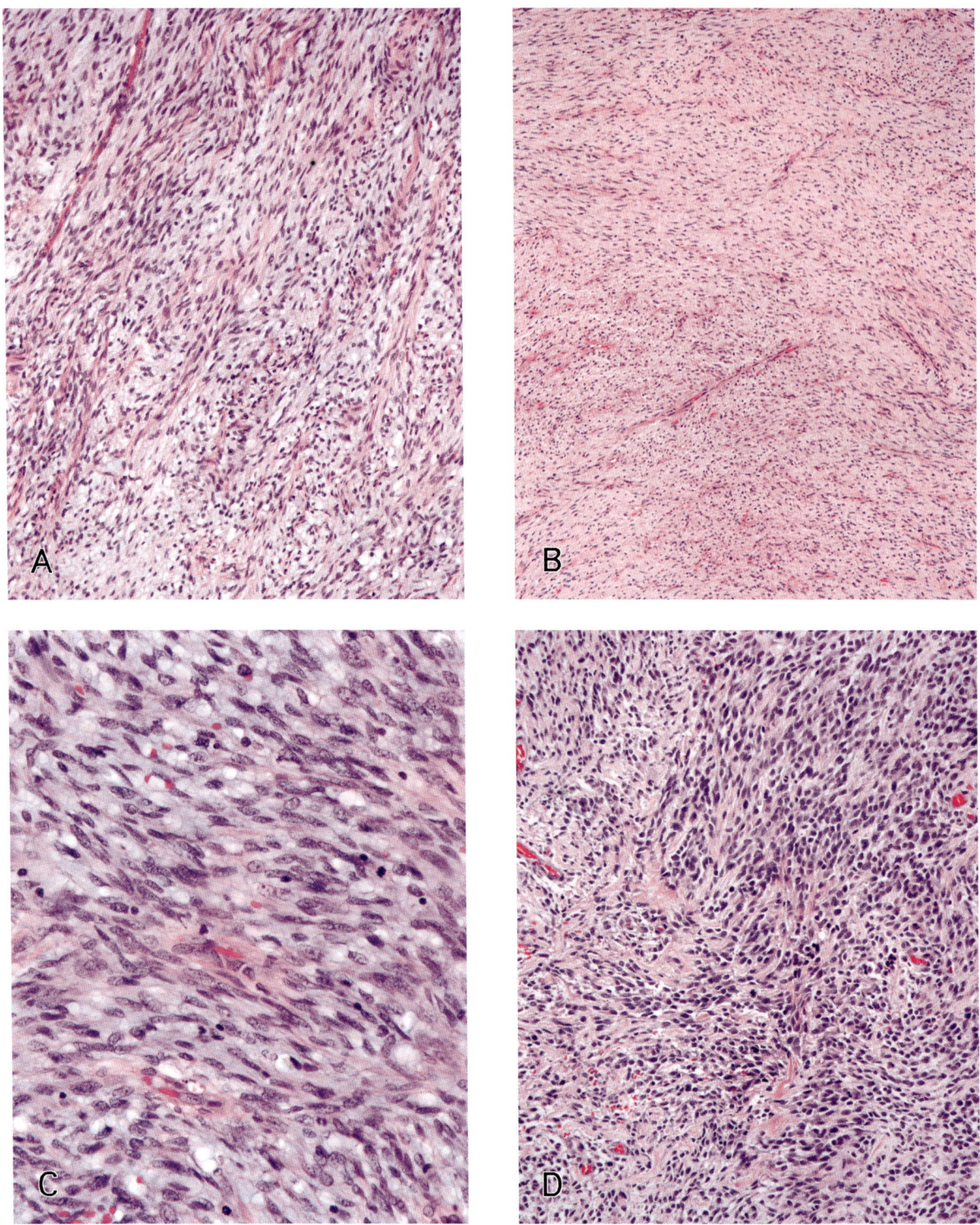

Figure 9-57

ZC3H7B-BCOR HIGH-GRADE ENDOMETRIAL STROMAL SARCOMA

The morphology of the tumor is uniform, consisting of spindle cells growing in fascicles set in a myxoid (A) or collagenous background (B), with abundant cytoplasm, elongated nuclei, and brisk mitotic activity (C). The cells may be round (D).

Endometrial Stromal Tumors

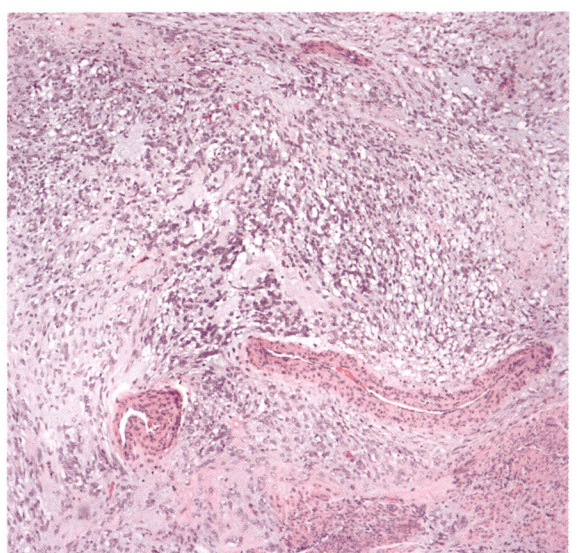
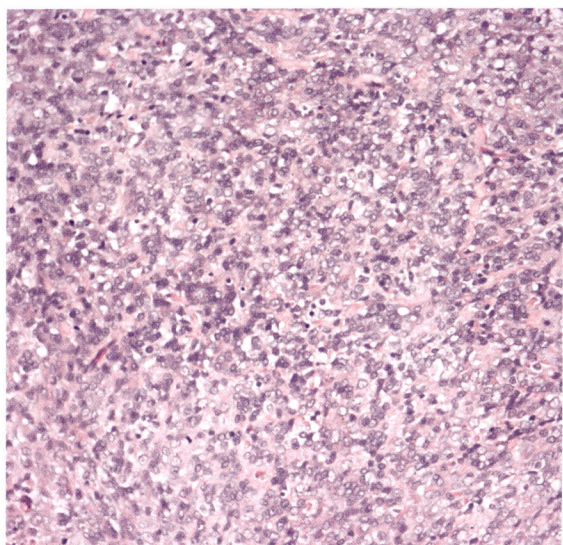

Figure 9-58

BCOR-ITD HIGH-GRADE ENDOMETRIAL STROMAL SARCOMA

The neoplastic cells have a spindled or rounded morphology and are present in a myxoid background.

and BCOR, with rare exceptions (106,235,236). ER and PR are variably positive (fig. 9-60C). Among smooth muscle markers, actin is most frequently positive, but typically focal in distribution, while desmin and caldesmon are almost always negative (fig. 9-60D).

These tumors are characterized by *ZC3H7B-BCOR* rearrangements that result from t(X;22)(p11q13), which can be detected by FISH or PCR. Some tumors show internal tandem duplications (ITDs) involving exon 15 of *BCOR* (235–237). Of note, this abnormality has also been reported in clear cell sarcoma of the kidney (237a).

Differential Diagnosis. Myxoid leiomyosarcoma is the most common entity in the differential diagnosis, and in the past most *ZC3H7B-BCOR* high-grade endometrial stromal sarcomas were likely diagnosed as myxoid leiomyosarcomas. *Leiomyosarcomas*, including the myxoid subtype, may be CD10 positive (71). In the largest series of myxoid leiomyosarcomas reported to date, some tumors were only positive for CD10 while another group showed positivity for CD10 and smooth muscle actin or desmin, potentially representing *ZC3H7B-BCOR* high-grade endometrial stromal sarcomas (169). Although *ZC3H7B-BCOR* tumors may show positivity for smooth muscle markers, they lack caldesmon expression and desmin positivity

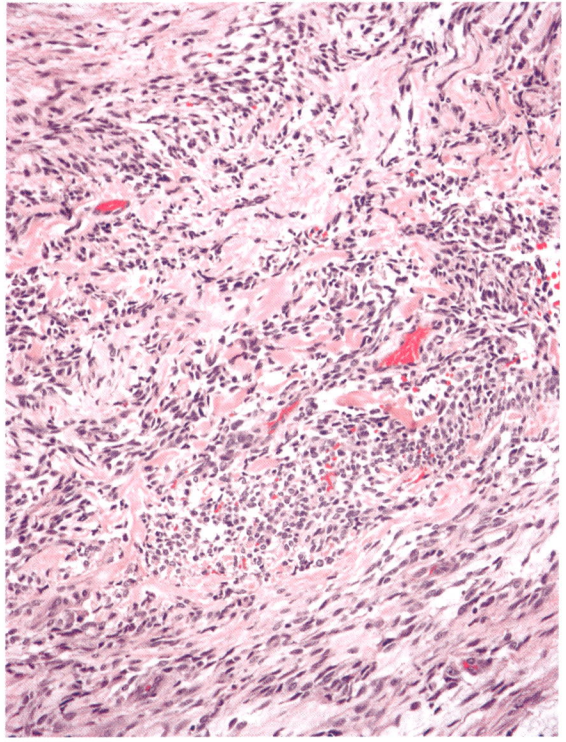

Figure 9-59

ZC3H7B-BCOR HIGH-GRADE ENDOMETRIAL STROMAL SARCOMA

Collagen plaques as seen in low-grade endometrial stromal tumors are present.

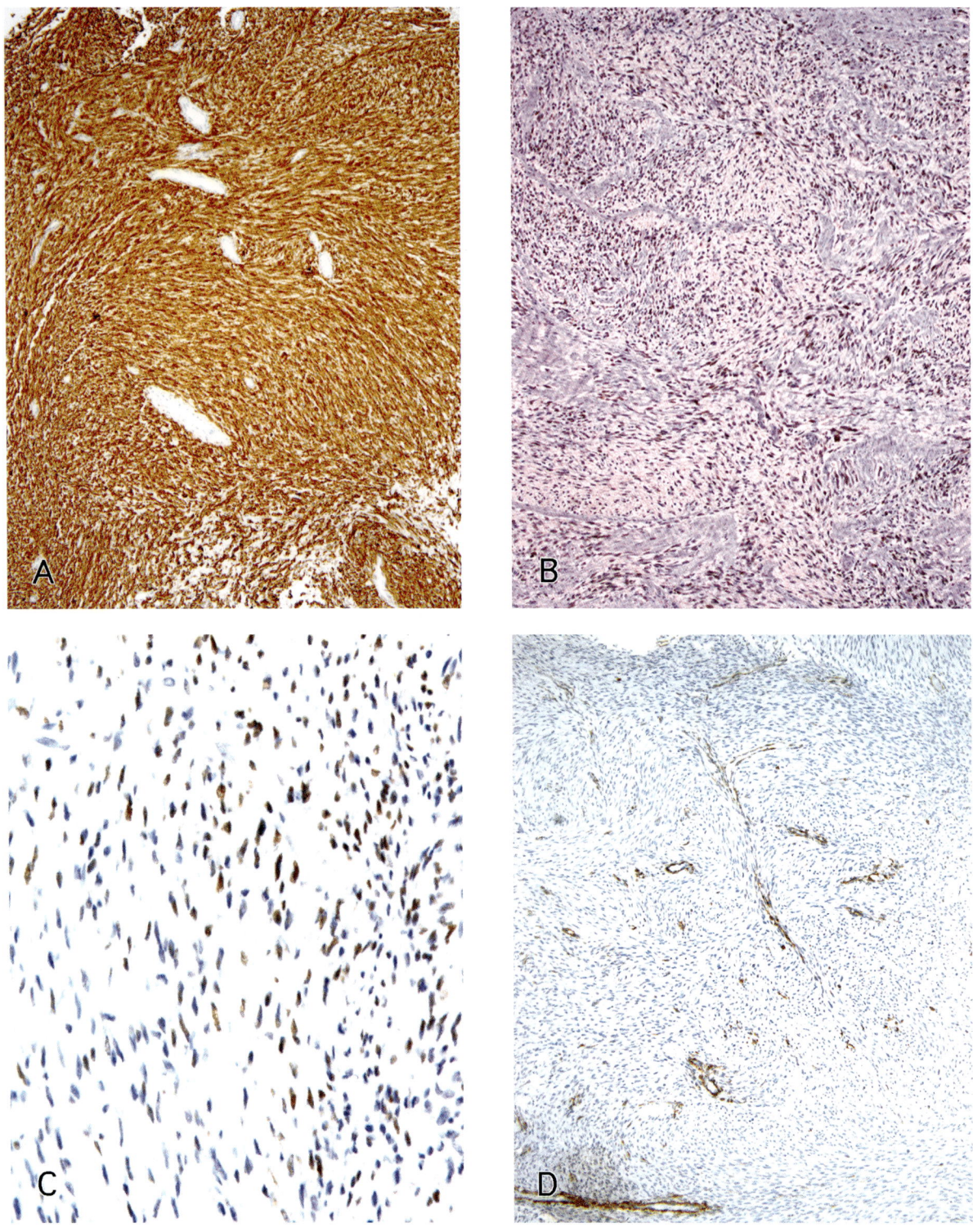

Figure 9-60

ZC3H7B-BCOR **HIGH-GRADE ENDOMETRIAL STROMAL SARCOMA**

These tumors are positive for CD10 (A), BCOR (B), and cyclin D1, and may be ER positive (C) but are typically negative for caldesmon (D).

is typically not diffuse. Furthermore, *ZC3H7B-BCOR* stromal sarcomas lack well-formed fascicles and cells with cigar-shaped nuclei, and are cyclin D1 and BCOR positive. In one study, only 1 of 19 leiomyosarcomas was positive for BCOR (106), while in another, only 1 of 80 such tumors expressed cyclin D1 diffusely (162). Recently, it has been shown that myxoid leiomyosarcomas may have a *PLAG1* gene rearrangement, also helpful in this differential diagnosis (238).

Typical endometrial stromal sarcoma shares with *ZC3H7B-BCOR* high-grade endometrial stromal sarcoma, a tongue-like pattern of myometrial invasion, uniform cytologic features, collagen bands, and in some instances, CD10, ER, and PR positivity. Endometrial stromal sarcomas with a fibroblastic or myxoid morphology are even more problematic, since they may be positive for some smooth muscle markers including desmin (23). However, *BCOR-ITD* and typical *ZC3H7B-BCOR* high-grade endometrial stromal sarcomas lack the typical features reminiscent of proliferative phase endometrium, such as the characteristic vasculature and whorling of the neoplastic cells around the vessels, while they display cytologic atypia and brisk mitotic activity. Typical and variant endometrial stromal sarcomas show CD10, ER, and PR positivity while BCOR and cyclin D1 are typically negative, with rare exceptions (only focal and weak positivity) (106).

Although, *YWHAE-FAM22* endometrial stromal sarcoma is also high grade and shares with *ZC3H7B-BCOR* and *BCOR-ITD* positivity for cyclin D1 and BCOR, its morphology and associated gene rearrangements are distinctive. Small epithelioid cells without an associated spindle component or myxoid background are seen in the high-grade component, although they may be associated with a low-grade myxoid endometrial stromal component. They lack positivity for smooth muscle markers and typically are negative for CD10, ER, and PR, while *ZC3H7B-BCOR* and *BCOR-ITD* tumors show variable positivity for all these markers.

Rarely, *inflammatory myofibroblastic tumor* or *adenosarcoma with sarcomatous overgrowth* are in the differential diagnosis as they may also display a myxoid background. The former, however, is associated with inflammatory infiltrates as well as compacted fascicular architecture, ALK positivity, and associated rearrangements (182,183), while the latter shows characteristic areas of low-grade müllerian adenosarcoma and thus far, no cyclin D1 staining or *BCOR* genetic alterations have been reported (162,239).

Undifferentiated uterine sarcoma may be considered in the differential diagnosis and in fact two out of three *BCOR-ITD* high-grade endometrial stromal sarcomas in one series were originally diagnosed as undifferentiated uterine sarcomas (237). The latter is more pleomorphic and demonstrates destructive invasion without associated collagen plaques.

Treatment and Prognosis. Hysterectomy, bilateral salpingo-oophorectomy, and adjuvant chemotherapy or radiation therapy is the treatment of choice for these patients. Although experience with these tumors is limited, patients with *ZC3H7B-BCOR* high-grade endometrial stromal sarcomas appear to have a prognosis that is similar to those with *YWHAE-FAM22* high-grade sarcomas. Both are associated with high stage at presentation, frequent recurrences, and metastases even when tumors are stage I (235,237).

High-Grade Endometrial Stromal Sarcoma in a Background of Low-Grade Endometrial Stromal Sarcoma

Occasionally, a high-grade sarcoma is seen juxtaposed to a typical endometrial stromal sarcoma. In such scenario, a diagnosis of high-grade endometrial stromal sarcoma can be rendered (60,171,226,240–243) although some investigators use the term dedifferentiated endometrial stromal sarcoma for such cases. The term high-grade endometrial stromal sarcoma, not otherwise specified (NOS) (226), has been used by some for tumors without a low-grade component but the current WHO classifies these tumors as undifferentiated uterine sarcomas (4). Thus, issues in terminology make difficult to unify criteria in the diagnosis of this group of tumors.

Patients often present with nonspecific symptoms and signs, most commonly vaginal bleeding or a uterine mass, and have extrauterine disease at the time of diagnosis. The tumors show a permeative or destructive pattern of invasion into the myometrium. Cells often show a diffuse growth. They may be variably pleomorphic or uniform with epithelioid or spindle morphology,

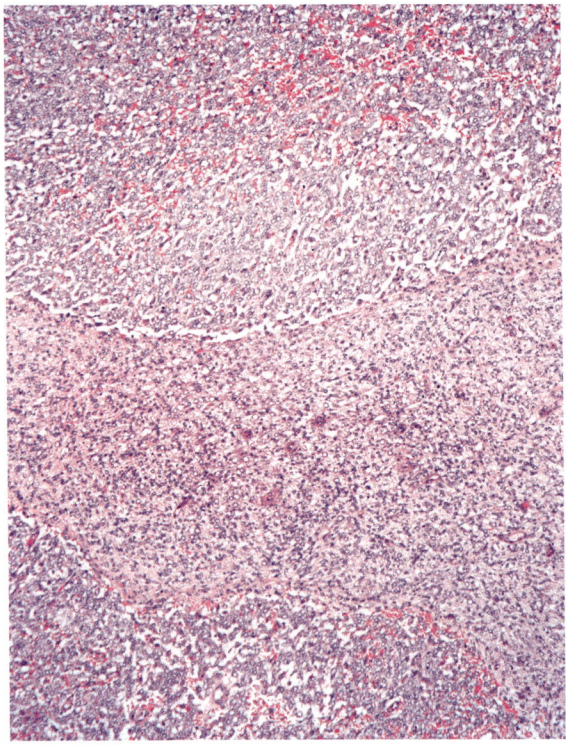

Figure 9-61

HIGH-GRADE ENDOMETRIAL STROMAL SARCOMA ARISING FROM A LOW-GRADE ENDOMETRIAL STROMAL SARCOMA

The high-grade component seen in isolation would be impossible to classify as of endometrial stromal derivation.

variable amounts of cytoplasm, hyperchromatic and irregular nuclei with prominent nucleoli, and high mitotic index including atypical forms (fig. 9-61). Rarely, heterologous differentiation (rhabdomyosarcoma) is seen (171,226). Extensive areas of necrosis are common. Areas of conventional endometrial stromal sarcoma may be present (see fig. 9-65).

CD10, ER, and PR are variably negative in the high-grade component when pleomorphic but typically positive in the low-grade component (226,243). Cyclin D1 may positive or p53 overexpression noted in pleomorphic examples (72,105,171,226,241). High-grade endometrial stromal sarcoma may express AE1/3 and CAM 5.2 (88). Rare fusion of *JAZF1* and *JJAZ1* genes has been identified in these tumors (120,171), suggesting transformation from an occult low-grade component.

UNDIFFERENTIATED UTERINE SARCOMA

Definition. *Undifferentiated uterine sarcomas* are a rare and heterogenous group of malignant mesenchymal tumors defined in the most recent WHO classification as neoplasms arising in the endometrium or myometrium with high-grade cytologic features lacking any resemblance to proliferative-phase endometrial stroma and with no specific differentiation. The diagnosis is one of exclusion since undifferentiated/dedifferentiated carcinoma, adenosarcoma with sarcomatous overgrowth, malignant mixed müllerian tumor with minimal epithelial component, or dedifferentiated leiomyosarcoma need to be ruled out (4).

After the exclusion of the term high-grade endometrial stromal sarcoma from the 2003 WHO classification, Kurihara et al. (171) undertook an analysis of undifferentiated endometrial sarcomas and divided these tumors into uniform and pleomorphic types based on their morphologic, immunohistochemical, and molecular findings. Within the group with uniform cytologic atypia, some tumors expressed ER and PR and had *β-catenin* mutations lacking *p53* mutations and some displayed a component of low-grade endometrial stromal sarcoma; others were ER and PR negative and cyclin D1 diffusely positive. This represented an initial approach toward redefining two of the three categories of high-grade endometrial stromal sarcoma discussed above: high-grade sarcomas with *YWHAE-FAM22* rearrangements and those that can be labeled as high-grade that have an associated low-grade component. Tumors in the pleomorphic category were typically ER, PR, and β-catenin negative and some expressed p53. This latter group, although small, is likely composed of undifferentiated sarcomas (171). Acquisition of new molecular and genetic data may help to reclassify some of the tumors in this group into other tumor types and may influence application of specific molecular targeted therapies.

Clinical Features. Undifferentiated uterine sarcomas typically occur in postmenopausal women who present with vaginal bleeding and signs and symptoms related to a rapidly growing mass or metastatic disease (171,244,245).

Gross Findings. On gross examination, they are typically large fleshy masses that may involve the endometrium, including polypoid growth, and/or the myometrium. They are often associated with extensive areas of hemorrhage and necrosis.

Microscopic Findings. Undifferentiated sarcomas are characterized by a destructive pattern of invasion. As a high-grade sarcoma, the spindled or epithelioid tumor cells grow in sheets or fascicles and have marked cytologic atypia, including multinucleation and brisk mitotic activity with atypical mitoses (fig. 9-62). Focal rhabdoid morphology may be seen (171). Necrosis and lymphovascular invasion are common (24,246).

Immunohistochemical and Molecular Genetic Findings. These tumors may show variable positivity for CD10 as well as IFITM1, but they are typically ER and PR negative (75,171, 246,247). Cyclin D1 may be variably expressed but even if extensively positive (uncommon), the tumors are also CD10 positive (162). They may be p16 and p53 positive (247). Other immunohistochemical markers including keratin, smooth muscle actin, and desmin may be positive, albeit focally (171,246).

Gene expression studies have identified large numbers of differentially expressed genes as well as different chromosomal aberrations when compared to typical endometrial stromal sarcomas. Undifferentiated uterine sarcomas have a higher number of chromosomal alterations and complex karyotypes. These tumors frequently have *p53* alterations. Data suggest that progression from typical endometrial stromal sarcoma to undifferentiated sarcoma is unlikely (248–251). Although *JAZF1-SUZ12* rearrangements occasionally had been detected in undifferentiated uterine sarcomas (120), a recent study failed to identify this rearrangement (83). Those examples may have represented high-grade endometrial stromal sarcomas that were associated with a low-grade component that was not identified with sections taken. Another study identified five copy number alterations encompassing cancer-related genes (*EZR, CDH1, RB1, TP53,* and *PRKAR1A*) with close correlation with gene expression changes in undifferentiated uterine sarcomas, suggesting that they may have some impact in the development of these tumors (136).

Differential Diagnosis. As this is a diagnosis of exclusion, extensive sampling is strongly recommended to identify the morphologic

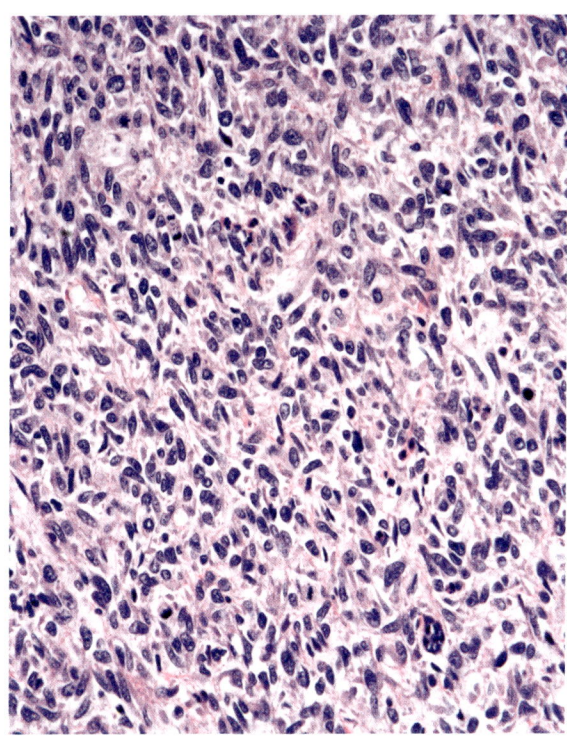

Figure 9-62

UNDIFFERENTIATED UTERINE SARCOMA

The tumor is composed of pleomorphic cells.

features that help to establish the diagnosis of other entities in the differential diagnosis. These tumors include *undifferentiated/dedifferentiated carcinoma, adenosarcoma with sarcomatous overgrowth, malignant mixed müllerian tumor with a minimal epithelial component,* and *dedifferentiated leiomyosarcoma*. CD10 positivity as supporting evidence for a diagnosis of undifferentiated uterine sarcoma should be interpreted with caution as this marker is positive in most tumors (epithelial, mesenchymal, and mixed) that occur in the uterus and are included in this differential diagnosis. Dedifferentiated leiomyosarcoma displays a pleomorphic appearance that may closely overlap with that seen in undifferentiated uterine sarcoma since it lacks smooth muscle differentiation. In contrast to the latter, however, there are areas showing discrete transition to differentiated smooth muscle neoplasia (252).

Recently, a small number of undifferentiated uterine sarcomas have been reported with a rhabdoid morphology and positivity for SMARCA-4. The tumors typically occur in reproductive-aged patients, and display a prominent infiltrative border, lymphovascular invasion, and extrauterine spread. There may be focal positivity for keratins, EMA, CD10, and actin, but most characteristically, truncating mutations in *SMARCA4* are present. Although undifferentiated uterine sarcomas may focally show rhabdoid morphology (171) they differ significantly morphologically, immunohistochemically, and molecularly from *SMARCA4*-deficient undifferentiated uterine sarcoma (malignant rhabdoid tumor of the uterus) (253).

Treatment and Prognosis. Patient outcome is poor, including those with stage I tumors, despite aggressive treatment, since a large number of patients have disease outside the uterus at the time of diagnosis (24,171). Five-year survival rates of 70, 43, and 23 percent, respectively, have been reported for patients with localized, regional, or distant disease (219). A recent study stratified the prognosis of patients with undifferentiated uterine sarcomas based on mitotic index, hormone receptor expression, and *YWHAE-FAM22* translocation status. Tumors with more than 25 mitoses per 10 high-power fields and lacking ER, PR, and *YWHAE-FAM22* translocation were associated with the poorest prognosis (247).

UTERINE TUMORS RESEMBLING OVARIAN SEX CORD TUMORS

Definition. Uterine tumors that may resemble ovarian sex cord tumors, without a recognizable component of endometrial stromal neoplasia (4). Although rare examples of uterine tumors with an appearance resembling granulosa cell tumors of the ovary had been reported in the literature (254,255), these tumors were first described as a group by Clement and Scully in 1976 (48). In that study, the authors described two groups, those with and those without accompanying endometrial stromal neoplasia. The designation *uterine tumor resembling ovarian sex cord tumor* (UTROSCT) subsequently became restricted to the pure category of tumors. Although traditionally thought to be related to stromal neoplasms, their origin remains unknown.

Clinical Features. Patients range in age from 16 to 70 (mean, about 50) years. They commonly present with vaginal bleeding or pelvic pain, but tumors may be discovered incidentally on routine exam or at time of hysterectomy for

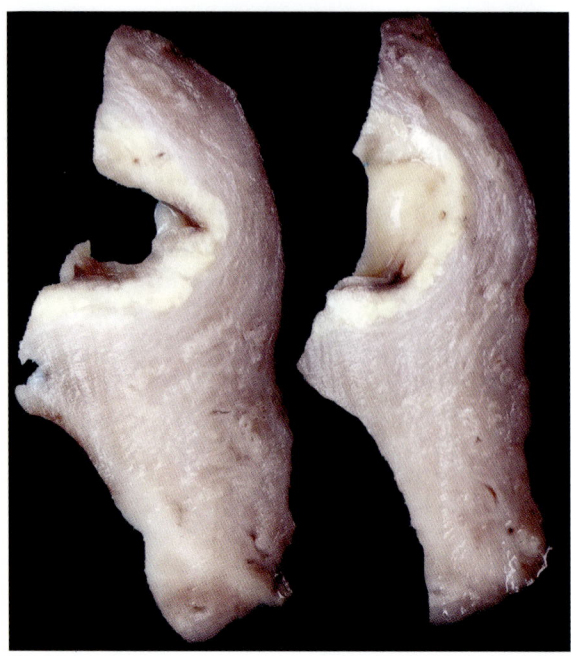

Figure 9-63

UTERINE TUMOR RESEMBLING AN OVARIAN SEX CORD TUMOR

The tumor is well circumscribed. It has a yellow rim but it is predominantly cystic.

fibroids (256). By ultrasound, UTROSCTs are hypoechoic and cannot be distinguished from an endometrial polyp if intracavitary or a leiomyoma if intramyometrial (257).

Gross Findings. The tumors range widely in size, with a median of 5 to 6 cm. Most tumors arise in the uterine fundus but have been rarely reported in the cervix (258). They are either polypoid/submucosal or intramyometrial, and rarely, subserosal. They are typically well circumscribed, but occasionally display infiltrative borders on gross examination. They have a fleshy, yellow to tan to white, firm cut surface, but some tumors may be solid and cystic (fig. 9-63) (48,50,153). Necrosis and hemorrhage are uncommon.

Microscopic Findings. On low-power examination, most UTROSCTs are well circumscribed although nonencapsulated (fig. 9-64). Some tumors overtly infiltrate between smooth muscle, however, in others, the smooth muscle is intrinsic to the tumor, imparting a pseudoinfiltrative appearance (fig. 9-65) (259).

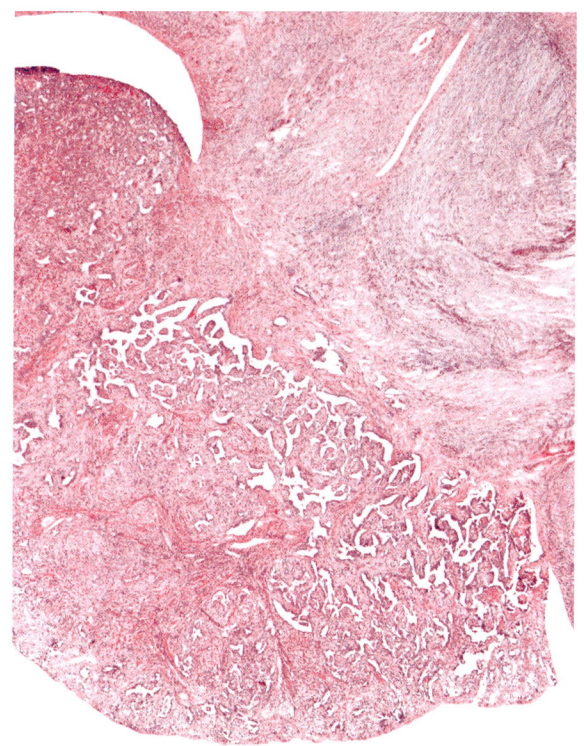

Figure 9-64

UTERINE TUMOR RESEMBLING AN OVARIAN SEX CORD TUMOR

The tumor has a polypoid configuration, is not encapsulated, and is centered in the endometrium.

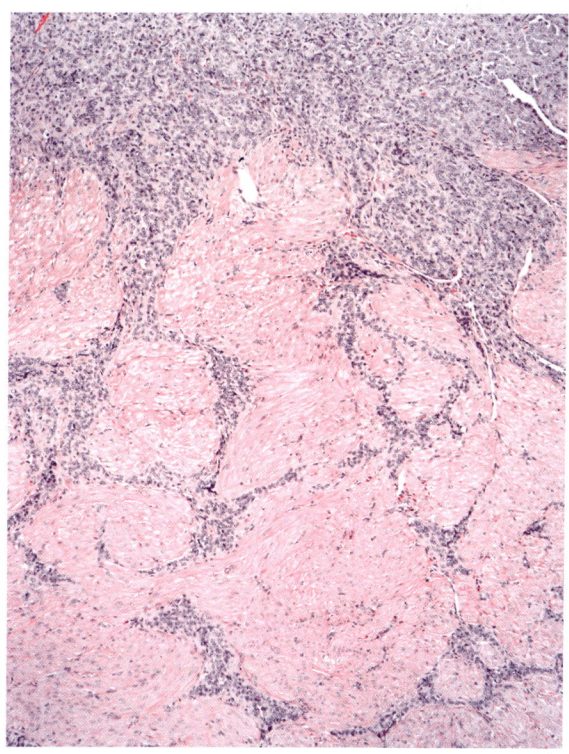

Figure 9-65

UTERINE TUMOR RESEMBLING AN OVARIAN SEX CORD TUMOR

Intermingling of tumor cells with adjacent myometrium confers a pseudoinfiltrative appearance.

There is an array of architectural growth patterns that closely mimic the morphologic appearance of sex cord-stromal tumors of the ovary/testis. They may have interanastomosing cords or trabeculae, small nests, insulae with peripheral palisading, or diffuse growth as seen in adult granulosa cell tumors (fig. 9-66). Call-Exner bodies are rarely seen. They also show hollow or solid tubules, some with a retiform morphology (which may be striking), including intraluminal papillae as seen in Sertoli and Sertoli-Leydig cell tumors (fig. 9-67) (260).

The cells tend to be "epithelioid" in morphology, with scant cytoplasm and round to oval nuclei with some nuclear irregularities, but only rare nuclear grooves and a low mitotic index (fig. 9-68). Some cells have abundant, often vacuolated cytoplasm, more often within tubules, while in some, tumor cells are spindled (fig. 9-68). Cells with rhabdoid morphology have also been reported (fig. 9-69) (261). Foamy histiocytes may be seen, but they are typically only a focal finding. Cells similar to Leydig cells have been occasionally reported (50,262). Tumors with the sole morphology of retiform Sertoli-Leydig cell tumor have also been reported (262). Most importantly, areas of conventional endometrial stromal neoplasia should not be present. The intervening stroma ranges from scant in most tumors to abundant and it may be variably cellular. Hyalinization is sometimes striking, but necrosis and lymphovascular invasion are rare.

Immunohistochemical Findings. UTROSCTs are polyphenotypic since they often coexpress sex cord, epithelial, and smooth muscle markers. They are frequently positive for at least two markers of sex cord-like differentiation, most commonly and extensively calretinin, CD99, SF1, WT1, and FOXL2, and less frequently melan A and inhibin (fig. 9-70) (50,98,100, 153,261,263–265). Melan A is thought to be indicative of steroid-producing cells and may

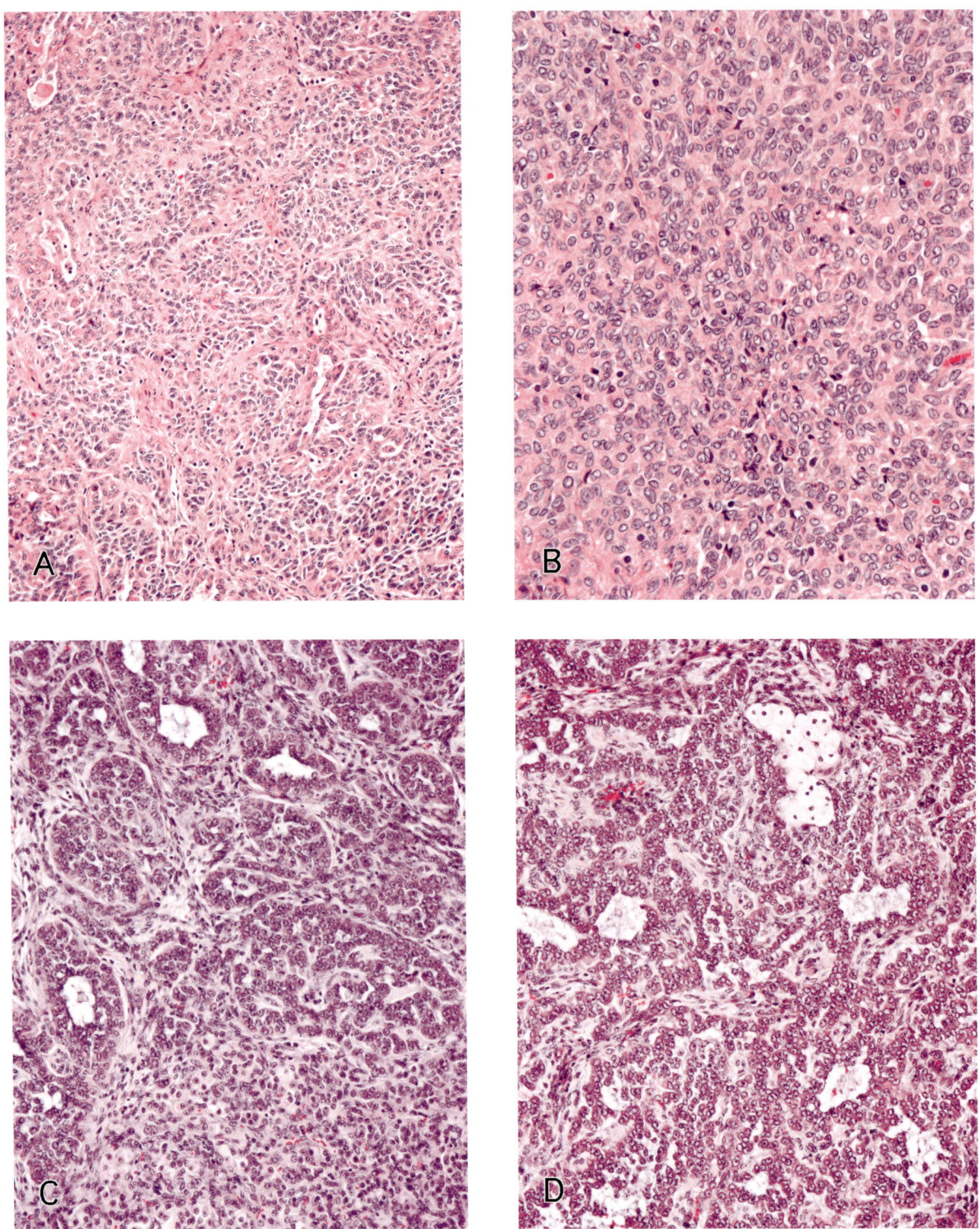

Figure 9-66

UTERINE TUMOR RESEMBLING AN OVARIAN SEX CORD TUMOR

The tumor has a range of morphologies that closely resemble those seen in adult granulosa cell tumors, including the finding of pseudoglands and lipidized cells.

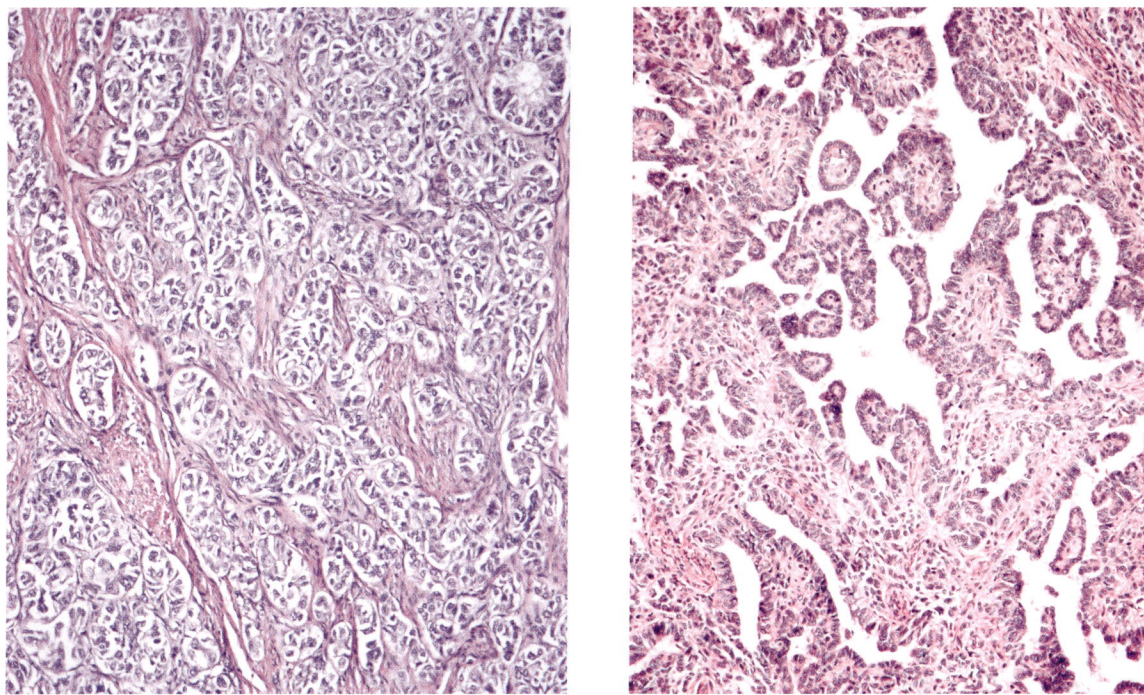

Figure 9-67

UTERINE TUMOR RESEMBLING AN OVARIAN SEX CORD TUMOR

The tumor appearance ranges from hollow to solid Sertoli tubules (left) to a retiform architecture (right).

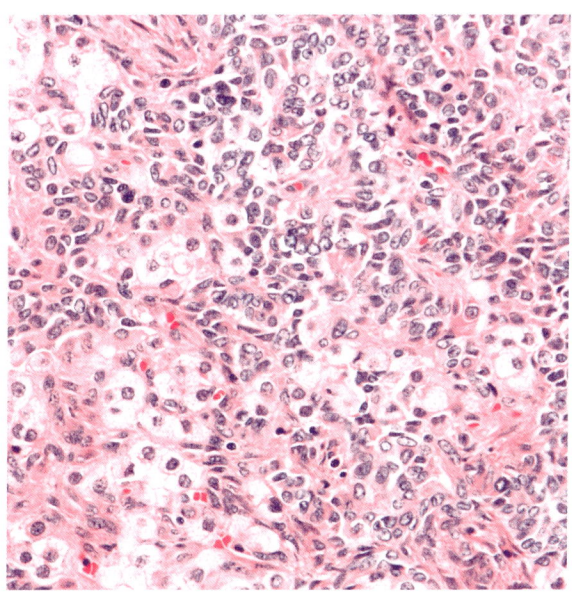

Figure 9-68

UTERINE TUMOR RESEMBLING AN OVARIAN SEX CORD TUMOR

Cells have scant to abundant eosinophilic to vacuolated cytoplasm. The nuclei are angulated or rounded with variable nucleoli.

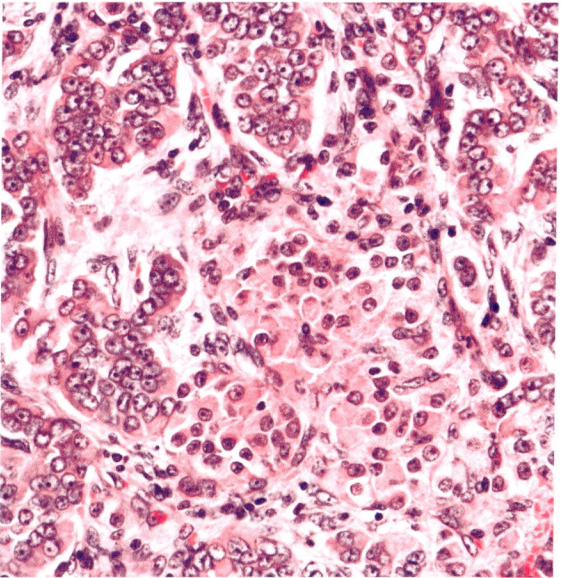

Figure 9-69

UTERINE TUMOR RESEMBLING AN OVARIAN SEX CORD TUMOR

This tumor has a rhabdoid morphology.

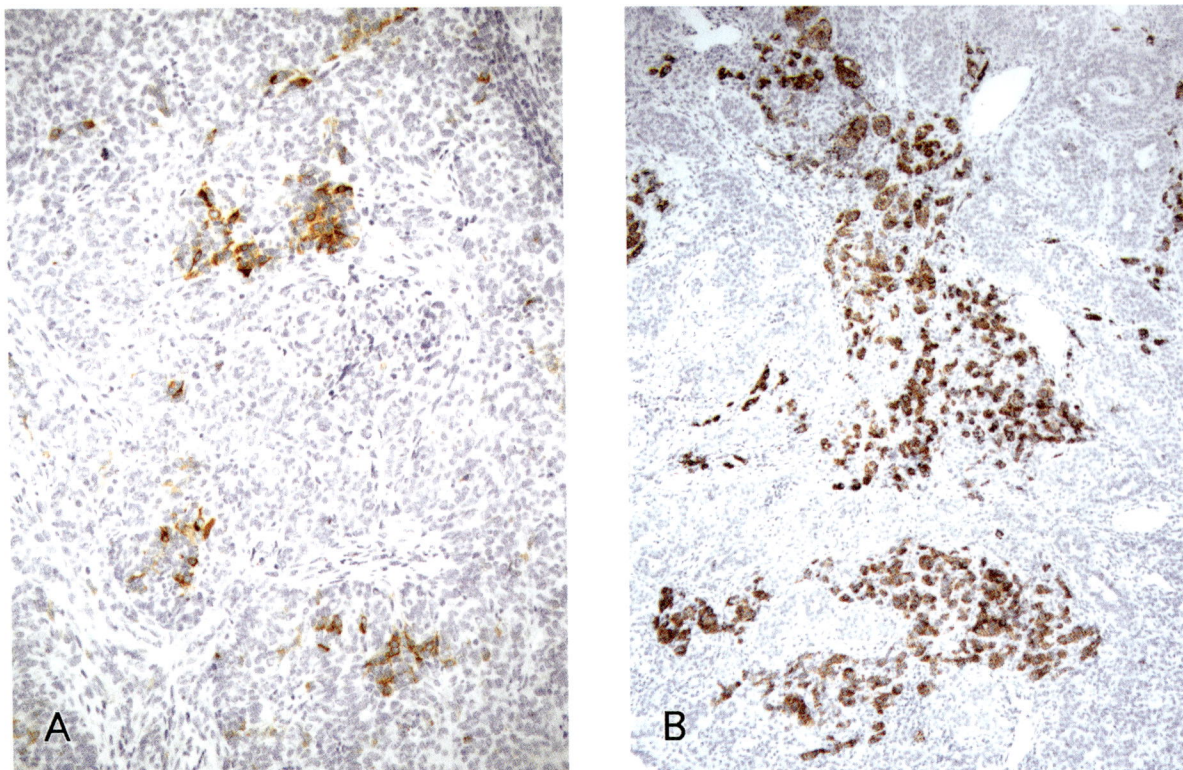

Figure 9-70

UTERINE TUMOR RESEMBLING AN OVARIAN SEX CORD TUMOR

The tumor cells are often positive for sex cord markers, although inhibin tends to be the least positive (A); they are also positive for melan A (B).

be indirect evidence of a specialized gonadal stromal derivation. It tends to be expressed in cells that display abundant lipid (98). CD56 and CD10 are also often positive but they are not helpful in differentiating these tumors from others in the differential diagnosis (100,153).

Among smooth muscle markers, UTROSCTs express smooth muscle actin, desmin, and HDAC8, and less commonly, h-caldesmon and smooth muscle myosin heavy chain (71,98,153, 261,262). They are positive for AE1/3, CAM 5.2, CK7, CK18, and KL1, and less commonly, EMA (153,258,260–262). Most tumors express ER and PR (100,153). Some tumors are focally positive for CD117, and they are negative for S-100 protein and HMB-45 (102,153,261,264).

Ultrastructural Findings. Although an origin from a multipotential mesenchymal cell was originally hypothesized (266), smooth muscle (267), endometrial stromal (25), and sex cord stromal origins (268) have also been postulated. In the largest study to date (13 cases) (269), cytoplasmic lipid droplets were a common finding, while epithelial differentiation was rare and features of smooth muscle differentiation were lacking (no dense bodies, subplasmalemmal densities, or pinocytotic vesicles). The finding of abundant paranuclear filaments did not correlate with positivity for myoid markers. These data suggest that UTROSCTs may be the result of divergent differentiation from endometrial stromal tumors or represent a distinct group of uterine tumors with sex cord differentiation that are perhaps more closely related to ovarian sex cord tumors. The finding of Charcott-Bottcher crystals in the cells of one reported case also suggests that these tumors have true sex cord differentiation (268).

Molecular Genetic Findings. Even though UTROSCTs are frequently FOXL2 positive they lack *FOXL2* and *DICER* mutations (263), two mutations that are defining events of adult

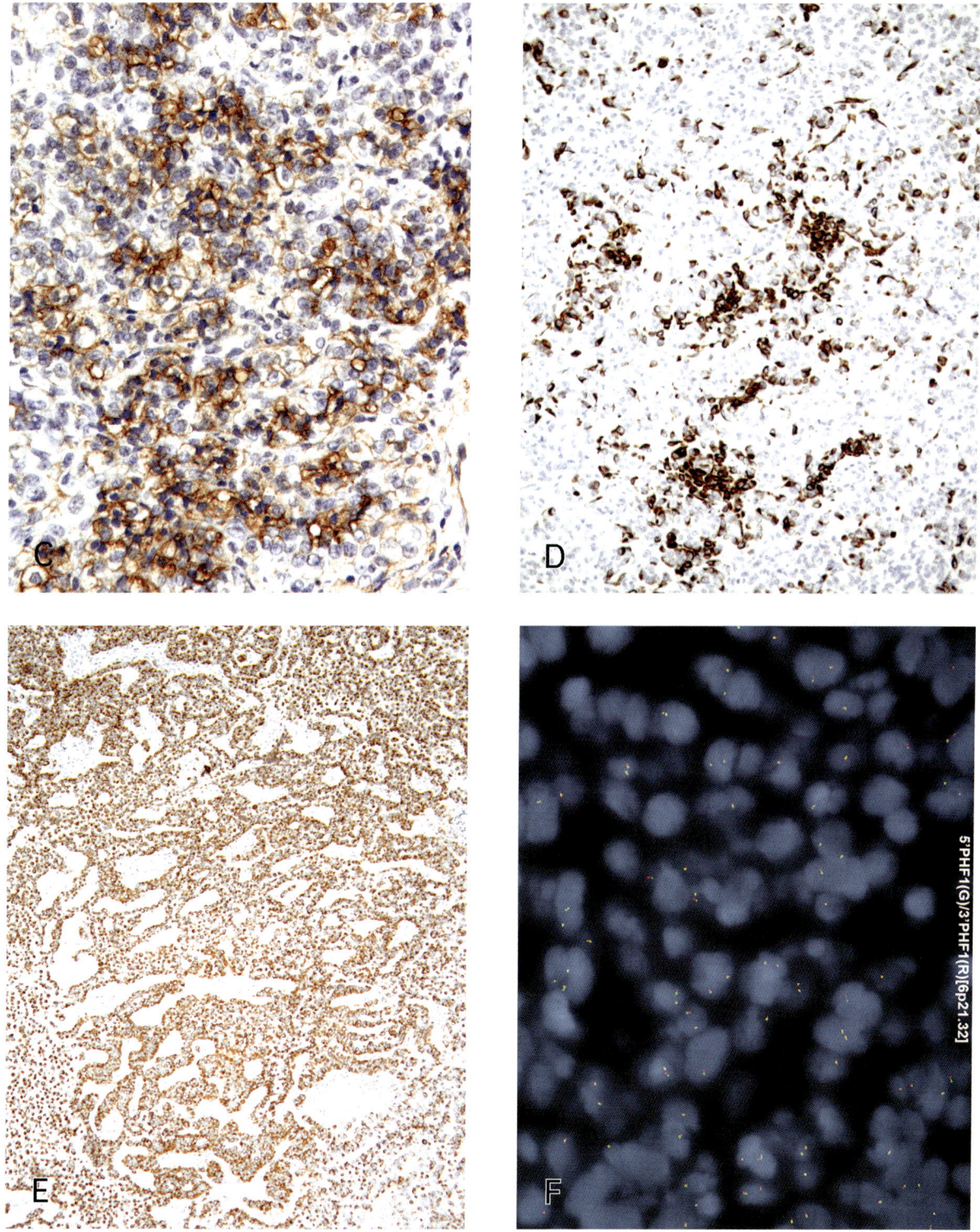

Figure 9-70, continued

Tumor cells are often positive for CD99 (C). They also stain for smooth muscle markers including desmin (D) and epithelial markers, more often AE1/3 (E). They do not show the typical *PHF* rearrangement as seen in endometrial stromal tumors with sex cord differentiation (F).

granulosa cell tumors (270) and intermediate to poorly differentiated Sertoli-Leydig cell tumors, Sertoli cell tumors, and gynandroblastomas (271,272). Although these tumors have been postulated to be related to endometrial stromal tumors, they lack the most frequent t(7,17), which has been reported in almost 60 percent of the later (155). Endometrial stromal tumors with sex cord-like differentiation have been reported to carry rearrangements on the *PHF1* gene, however, this alteration has not been reported in UTROSCTs (fig. 9-70F) (156). Very recently a recurrent NCOA2/3 gene fusion has been reported in these tumors (273). One UTROSCT has been reported to carry a balanced t(X;6)(p22.3;q23.1) and t(4;18)(q21.1;q21.3) (273a). That case, however, did not show positivity for sex cord stromal markers other than WT1.

Differential Diagnosis. These tumors should be distinguished from other mesenchymal and, less often, epithelial or mixed tumors of the uterus. In the distinction from *endometrial stromal tumors with sex cord-like differentiation*, sampling is crucial, thus the distinction from UTROSCT may not be possible in curetting specimens if areas of conventional endometrial stromal neoplasia are not seen (26). The morphology of the sex cord elements overlaps as does the immunoprofile, including positivity for keratin, calretinin, smooth muscle, desmin, and rarely, smooth muscle myosin heavy chain (50,91). Melan A has not been reported in endometrial stromal tumors with sex cord-like differentiation, although the utility of this marker is still limited. Some studies have noted that positivity for sex cord markers in these tumors is less frequent when compared to UTROSCT. SF1 and FOXL2 appear to be negative in areas of sex cord differentiation in endometrial stromal tumors in contrast to UTROSCT, but rare FOXL2 positivity has been recently reported in benign endometrial stroma; thus these results should be interpreted with caution (274). The finding of conventional areas of endometrial stromal neoplasia are most helpful, as well as the presence of NCOA2/3 gene fusion (273).

UTROSCT should also be separated from *epithelioid smooth muscle tumor* as the latter may show a nested, corded, or trabecular architecture. It is typically positive for smooth muscle markers and can be positive for epithelial markers and WT1 (71,91), only rarely for calretinin (275,276), but it is negative for melan A, inhibin, SF1, and FOXL2, in contrast to UTROSCTs. HMB45 expression is nonspecific.

Endometrioid carcinoma may have sex cord-like morphology, either sertoliform (158) or with sex cord-like formations (277), mimicking the appearance of UTROSCT. Some of these tumors are positive for calretinin, less often for WT1 (278), and rarely for inhibin (157,279) and both express epithelial markers (50,71,98,153,261). Squamous and mucinous differentiation, along with EMA and PAX8 expression, help establish the diagnosis of endometrioid carcinoma.

Low-grade müllerian adenosarcoma may have sex cord-like differentiation and rarely this component overgrows and results in rhabdoid-type cells, which can complicate distinction from a UTROSCT, especially in a curettage specimen (280–282). The immunohistochemical profile in areas showing sex cord-like differentiation overlaps and is, therefore, not helpful. In cases consisting of only sex cord elements, a hysterectomy is needed to identify areas of conventional adenosarcoma, which is the component determining classification and prognosis.

Treatment and Prognosis. Although experience with UTROSCTs is limited, patients undergo hysterectomy (usually for diagnostic purposes), yet some patients may be treated conservatively with resection if fertility preservation is desired (283,284). Most UTROSCTs are associated with a benign outcome (48,285,286), but since they can recur or metastasize, they are considered to have uncertain malignant behavior (256,287–290). Features that are associated with poor outcome include increased mitotic activity, lymphovascular invasion, and infiltrative borders, but studies are limited and there is no consensus about parameters that are prognostically important.

REFERENCES

1. Kempson RL, Hendrickson MR. Pure mesenchymal neoplasms of the uterine corpus: selected problems. Semin Diagn Pathol 1988;5:172-98.
2. Abeler VM, Royne O, Thoresen S, Danielsen HE, Nesland JM, Kristensen GB. Uterine sarcomas in Norway. A histopathological and prognostic survey of a total population from 1970 to 2000 including 419 patients. Histopathology 2009;54:355-64.
3. Barakat RR. Contemporary issues in the management of endometrial cancer. CA Cancer J Clin 1998;48:299-314.
4. Oliva E, Carcangiu ML, Carinelli S, et al. Mesenchymal tumours. In: Kurman RJ, Carcangiu ML, Herrington CS, Young RH, eds. WHO classification of tumours of female reproductive organs. Lyons: IARC Press; 2014:135-145.
5. Xue WC, Cheung AN. Endometrial stromal sarcoma of uterus. Best Pract Res Clin Obstet Gynaecol 2011;25:719-32.
6. De Fusco PA, Gaffey TA, Malkasian GD Jr, Long HJ, Cha SS. Endometrial stromal sarcoma: review of Mayo Clinic experience, 1945-1980. Gynecol Oncol 1989;35:8-14.
7. Dionigi A, Oliva E, Clement PB, Young RH. Endometrial stromal nodules and endometrial stromal tumors with limited infiltration: a clinicopathologic study of 50 cases. Am J Surg Pathol 2002;26:567-81.
8. Tavassoli FA, Norris HJ. Mesenchymal tumours of the uterus. VII. A clinicopathological study of 60 endometrial stromal nodules. Histopathology 1981;5:1-10.
9. Chang KL, Crabtree GS, Lim-Tan SK, Kempson RL, Hendrickson MR. Primary uterine endometrial stromal neoplasms. A clinicopathologic study of 117 cases. Am J Surg Pathol 1990;14:415-38.
10. Hart WR, Yoonessi M. Endometrial stromatosis of the uterus. Obstet Gynecol 1977;49:393-403.
11. Norris HJ, Taylor HB. Mesenchymal tumors of the uterus. I. A clinical and pathological study of 53 endometrial stromal tumors. Cancer 1966;19:755-66.
12. Fekete PS, Vellios F. The clinical and histologic spectrum of endometrial stromal neoplasms: a report of 41 cases. Int J Gynecol Pathol 1984;3:198-212.
13. Beer TW, Buchanan R, Buckley CH. Uterine stromal sarcoma following tamoxifen treatment. J Clin Pathol 1995;48:596.
14. Eddy GL, Mazur MT. Endolymphatic stromal myosis associated with tamoxifen use. Gynecol Oncol 1997;64:262-4.
15. Press MF, Scully RE. Endometrial "sarcomas" complicating ovarian thecoma, polycystic ovarian disease and estrogen therapy. Gynecol Oncol 1985;21:135-54.
16. Meredith RF, Eisert DR, Kaka Z, Hodgson SE, Johnston GA Jr, Boutselis JG. An excess of uterine sarcomas after pelvic irradiation. Cancer 1986;58:2003-7.
17. Young RH, Scully RE. Sarcomas metastatic to the ovary: a report of 21 cases. Int J Gynecol Pathol 1990;9:231-52.
18. Young RH, Prat J, Scully RE. Endometrioid stromal sarcomas of the ovary. A clinicopathologic analysis of 23 cases. Cancer 1984;53:1143-55.
19. Aubry MC, Myers JL, Colby TV, Leslie KO, Tazelaar HD. Endometrial stromal sarcoma metastatic to the lung: a detailed analysis of 16 patients. Am J Surg Pathol 2002;26:440-9.
20. Takeda A, Imoto S, Mori M, Nakano T, Nakamura H. Paraneoplastic consumptive coagulopathy related to intramyometrial low-grade endometrial stromal sarcoma coexistent with adenomyosis diagnosed 7 years after laparoscopic-assisted myomectomy. Arch Gynecol Obstet 2010;282:665-70.
21. Oliva E, Clement PB, Young RH, Scully RE. Mixed endometrial stromal and smooth muscle tumors of the uterus: a clinicopathologic study of 15 cases. Am J Surg Pathol 1998;22:997-1005.
22. Yilmaz A, Rush DS, Soslow RA. Endometrial stromal sarcomas with unusual histologic features: a report of 24 primary and metastatic tumors emphasizing fibroblastic and smooth muscle differentiation. Am J Surg Pathol 2002;26:1142-50.
23. Oliva E, Young RH, Clement PB, Scully RE. Myxoid and fibrous endometrial stromal tumors of the uterus: a report of 10 cases. Int J Gynecol Pathol 1999;18:310-9.
24. Evans HL. Endometrial stromal sarcoma and poorly differentiated endometrial sarcoma. Cancer 1982;50:2170-82.
25. Fekete PS, Vellios F, Patterson BD. Uterine tumor resembling an ovarian sex-cord tumor: report of a case of an endometrial stromal tumor with foam cells and ultrastructural evidence of epithelial differentiation. Int J Gynecol Pathol 1985;4:378-87.
26. Oliva E, Clement PB, Young RH. Endometrial stromal tumors: an update on a group of tumors with a protean phenotype. Adv Anat Pathol 2000;7:257-81.
27. Nucci MR. Practical issues related to uterine pathology: endometrial stromal tumors. Mod Pathol 2016;29(Suppl 1):S92-103.
28. Baker PM, Moch H, Oliva E. Unusual morphologic features of endometrial stromal tumors: a report of 2 cases. Am J Surg Pathol 2005;29:1394-8.

29. Oliva E, Clement PB, Young RH. Epithelioid endometrial and endometrioid stromal tumors: a report of four cases emphasizing their distinction from epithelioid smooth muscle tumors and other oxyphilic uterine and extrauterine tumors. Int J Gynecol Pathol 2002;21:48-55.
30. Lifschitz-Mercer B, Czernobilsky B, Dgani R, Dallenbach-Hellweg G, Moll R, Franke WW. Immunocytochemical study of an endometrial diffuse clear cell stromal sarcoma and other endometrial stromal sarcomas. Cancer 1987;59:1494-9.
31. Kibar Y, Aydin A, Deniz H, Balat O, Cebesoy B, Al-Nafussi A. A rare case of low-grade endometrial stromal sarcoma with myxoid differentiation and atypical bizarre cells. Eur J Gynaecol Oncol 2008;29:397-8.
32. Shah R, McCluggage WG. Symplastic atypia in neoplastic and non-neoplastic endometrial stroma: report of 3 cases with a review of atypical symplastic cells within the female genital tract. Int J Gynecol Pathol 2009;28:334-7.
33. Fadare O, McCalip B, Mariappan MR, Hileeto D, Parkash V. An endometrial stromal tumor with osteoclast-like giant cells. Ann Diagn Pathol 2005;9:160-5.
34. Bird CC, Willis RA. The production of smooth muscle by the endometrial stroma of the adult human uterus. J Pathol Bacteriol 1965;90:75-81.
35. Fujii S, Konishi I, Mori T. Smooth muscle differentiation at endometrio-myometrial junction. An ultrastructural study. Virchows Arch A Pathol Anat Histopathol 1989;414:105-12.
36. Scully RE. Smooth-muscle differentiation in genital tract disorders. Arch Pathol Lab Med 1981;105:505-7.
37. Zamecnik M, Sultani K. Meningothelial-like nodules: additional pattern of myoid differentiation in endometrial stromal tumors. Pathol Int 2007;57:632-3.
38. McCluggage WG, Cromie AJ, Bryson C, Traub AI. Uterine endometrial stromal sarcoma with smooth muscle and glandular differentiation. J Clin Pathol 2001;54:481-3.
39. Kim YH, Cho H, Kyeom-Kim H, Kim I. Uterine endometrial stromal sarcoma with rhabdoid and smooth muscle differentiation. J Korean Med Sci 1996;11:88-93.
40. Schammel DP, Silver SA, Tavassoli FA. Combined endometrial stromal/smooth muscle neoplasms of the uterus. A clinicopathologic study of 38 cases [abstract]. Mod Pathol 1999;12:124A.
41. Binder SW, Nieberg RK, Cheng L, al-Jitawi S. Histologic and immunohistochemical analysis of nine endometrial stromal tumors: an unexpected high frequency of keratin protein positivity. Int J Gynecol Pathol 1991;10:191-7.
42. Devaney K, Tavassoli FA. Immunohistochemistry as a diagnostic aid in the interpretation of unusual mesenchymal tumors of the uterus. Mod Pathol 1991;4:225-31.
43. Kim YH, Cho H, Kyeom-Kim H, Kim I. Uterine endometrial stromal sarcoma with rhabdoid and smooth muscle differentiation. J Korean Med Sci 1996;11:88-93.
44. Lloreta J, Prat J. Endometrial stromal nodule with smooth and skeletal muscle components simulating stromal sarcoma. Int J Gynecol Pathol 1992;11:293-8.
45. Khalifa MA, Hansen CH, Moore JL Jr, Rusnock EJ, Lage JM. Endometrial stromal sarcoma with focal smooth muscle differentiation: recurrence after 17 years: a follow-up report with discussion of the nomenclature. Int J Gynecol Pathol 1996;15:171-6.
46. Tang CK, Toker C, Ances IG. Stromomyoma of the uterus. Cancer 1979;43:308-16.
47. Lloreta J, Prat J. Ultrastructure of an endometrial stromal nodule with skeletal muscle. Ultrastruct Pathol 1993;17:405-10.
48. Clement PB, Scully RE. Uterine tumors resembling ovarian sex-cord tumors. A clinicopathologic analysis of fourteen cases. Am J Clin Pathol 1976;66:512-25.
49. Zamecnik M, Michal M. Endometrial stromal nodule with retiform sex-cord-like differentiation. Pathol Res Pract 1998;194:449-53.
50. Irving JA, Carinelli S, Prat J. Uterine tumors resembling ovarian sex cord tumors are polyphenotypic neoplasms with true sex cord differentiation. Mod Pathol 2006;19:17-24.
51. Lillemoe TJ, Perrone T, Norris HJ, Dehner LP. Myogenous phenotype of epithelial-like areas in endometrial stromal sarcomas. Arch Pathol Lab Med 1991;115:215-9.
52. Rosty C, Genestie C, Blondon J, Le Charpentier Y. [Endometrial stromal tumor associated with rhabdoid phenotype and and zones of "sex cord-like" differentiation.] Ann Pathol 1998;18:133-6. [French]
53. Fukunaga M, Miyazawa Y, Ushigome S. Endometrial low-grade stromal sarcoma with ovarian sex cord-like differentiation: report of two cases with an immunohistochemical and flow cytometric study. Pathol Int 1997;47:412-5.
54. McCluggage WG, Date A, Bharucha H, Toner PG. Endometrial stromal sarcoma with sex cord-like areas and focal rhabdoid differentiation. Histopathology 1996;29:369-74.
55. Fitko R, Brainer J, Schink JC, August CZ. Endometrial stromal sarcoma with rhabdoid differentiation. Int J Gynecol Pathol 1990;9:379-82.

56. D'Angelo E, Ali RH, Espinosa I, et al. Endometrial stromal sarcomas with sex cord differentiation are associated with PHF1 rearrangement. Am J Surg Pathol 2013;37:514-21.
57. Tanimoto A, Sasaguri T, Arima N, Hashimoto H, Hamada T, Sasaguri Y. Endometrial stromal sarcoma of the uterus with rhabdoid features. Pathol Int 1996;46:231-7.
58. McCluggage WG, Ganesan R, Herrington CS. Endometrial stromal sarcomas with extensive endometrioid glandular differentiation: report of a series with emphasis on the potential for misdiagnosis and discussion of the differential diagnosis. Histopathology 2009;54:365-73.
59. Clement PB, Scully RE. Endometrial stromal sarcomas of the uterus with extensive endometrioid glandular differentiation: a report of three cases that caused problems in differential diagnosis. Int J Gynecol Pathol 1992;11:163-73.
60. McCluggage WG, Young RH. Endometrial stromal sarcomas with true papillae and pseudopapillae. Int J Gynecol Pathol 2008;27:555-61.
61. Kim HS, Yoon G, Jung YY, Lee YY, Song SY. Fibromyxoid variant of endometrial stromal sarcoma with atypical bizarre nuclei. Int J Clin Exp Pathol 2015;8:3316-21.
62. Park JY, Sung CO, Jang SJ, Song SY, Han JH, Kim KR. Pulmonary metastatic nodules of uterine low-grade endometrial stromal sarcoma: histopathological and immunohistochemical analysis of 10 cases. Histopathology 2013;63:833-40.
63. Kasashima S, Kobayashi M, Yamada M, Oda Y. Myxoid endometrial stromal sarcoma of the uterus. Pathol Int 2003;53:637-41.
64. Lee CH, Mariño-Enriquez A, Ou W, et al. The clinicopathologic features of YWHAE-FAM22 endometrial stromal sarcomas: a histologically high-grade and clinically aggressive tumor. Am J Surg Pathol 2012;36:641-53.
65. Tai LH, Tavassoli FA. Endometrial polyps with atypical (bizarre) stromal cells. Am J Surg Pathol 2002;26:505-9.
66. Chu P, Arber DA. Paraffin-section detection of CD10 in 505 nonhematopoietic neoplasms. Frequent expression in renal cell carcinoma and endometrial stromal sarcoma. Am J Clin Pathol 2000;113:374-82.
67. McCluggage WG, Sumathi VP, Maxwell P. CD10 is a sensitive and diagnostically useful immunohistochemical marker of normal endometrial stroma and of endometrial stromal neoplasms. Histopathology 2001;39:273-8.
68. Chu PG, Arber DA, Weiss LM, Chang KL. Utility of CD10 in distinguishing between endometrial stromal sarcoma and uterine smooth muscle tumors: an immunohistochemical comparison of 34 cases. Mod Pathol 2001;14:465-71.
69. Abeler VM, Nenodovic M. Diagnostic immunohistochemistry in uterine sarcomas: a study of 397 cases. Int J Gynecol Pathol 2011;30:236-43.
70. Toki T, Shimizu M, Takagi Y, Ashida T, Konishi I. CD10 is a marker for normal and neoplastic endometrial stromal cells. Int J Gynecol Pathol 2002;21:41-7.
71. Oliva E, Young RH, Amin MB, Clement PB. An immunohistochemical analysis of endometrial stromal and smooth muscle tumors of the uterus: a study of 54 cases emphasizing the importance of using a panel because of overlap in immunoreactivity for individual antibodies. Am J Surg Pathol 2002;26:403-12.
72. Jung CK, Jung JH, Lee A, et al. Diagnostic use of nuclear beta-catenin expression for the assessment of endometrial stromal tumors. Mod Pathol 2008;21:756-63.
73. Mikami Y, Hata S, Kiyokawa T, Manabe T. Expression of CD10 in malignant mullerian mixed tumors and adenosarcomas: an immunohistochemical study. Mod Pathol 2002;15:923-30.
74. D'Angelo E, Prat J. Uterine sarcomas: a review. Gynecol Oncol 2010;116:131-9.
75. Parra-Herran CE, Yuan L, Nucci MR, Quade BJ. Targeted development of specific biomarkers of endometrial stromal cell differentiation using bioinformatics: the IFITM1 model. Mod Pathol 2014;27:569-79.
76. Busca A, Gulavita P, Parra-Herran C, Islam S. IFITM1 outperforms CD10 in differentiating low-grade endometrial stromal sarcomas from smooth muscle neoplasms of the uterus. Int J Gynecol Pathol 2018;37:372-8.
77. Reich O, Regauer S, Urdl W, Lahousen M, Winter R. Expression of oestrogen and progesterone receptors in low-grade endometrial stromal sarcomas. Br J Cancer 2000;82:1030-4.
78. Navarro D, Cabrera JJ, Leon L, et al. Endometrial stromal sarcoma expression of estrogen receptors, progesterone receptors and estrogen-induced srp27 (24K) suggests hormone responsiveness. J Steroid Biochem Mol Biol 1992;41:589-96.
79. Yoon A, Park JY, Lee YY, et al. Prognostic factors and outcomes in endometrial stromal sarcoma with the 2009 FIGO staging system: a multicenter review of 114 cases. Gynecol Oncol 2014;132:70-5.
80. Chu MC, Mor G, Lim C, Zheng W, Parkash V, Schwartz PE. Low-grade endometrial stromal sarcoma: hormonal aspects. Gynecol Oncol 2003;90:170-6.
81. Sabini G, Chumas JC, Mann WJ. Steroid hormone receptors in endometrial stromal sarcomas. A biochemical and immunohistochemical study. Am J Clin Pathol 1992;97:381-6.

82. Balleine RL, Earls PJ, Webster LR, et al. Expression of progesterone receptor A and B isoforms in low-grade endometrial stromal sarcoma. Int J Gynecol Pathol 2004;23:138-144.
83. Jakate K, Azimi F, Ali RH, et al. Endometrial sarcomas: an immunohistochemical and JAZF1 re-arrangement study in low-grade and undifferentiated tumors. Mod Pathol 2013;26:95-105.
84. Wu TI, Chou HH, Yeh CJ, et al. Clinicopathologic parameters and immunohistochemical study of endometrial stromal sarcomas. Int J Gynecol Pathol 2013;32:482-92.
85. Roy M, Kumar S, Bhatla N, et al. Androgen receptor expression in endometrial stromal sarcoma: correlation with clinicopathologic features. Int J Gynecol Pathol 2017;36:420-7.
86. Moinfar F, Regitnig P, Tabrizi AD, Denk H, Tavassoli FA. Expression of androgen receptors in benign and malignant endometrial stromal neoplasms. Virchows Arch 2004;444:410-4.
87. Reich O, Regauer S. Aromatase expression in low-grade endometrial stromal sarcomas: an immunohistochemical study. Mod Pathol 2004; 17:104-8.
88. Rahimi S, Akaev I, Marani C, Chopra M, Yeoh CC. Immunohistochemical expression of different subtypes of cytokeratins by endometrial stromal sarcoma. Appl Immunohistochem Mol Morphol 2018. [Epub ahead of print]
89. Farhood AI, Abrams J. Immunohistochemistry of endometrial stromal sarcoma. Hum Pathol 1991;22:224-30.
90. Sumathi VP, Al-Hussaini M, Connolly LE, Fullerton L, McCluggage WG. Endometrial stromal neoplasms are immunoreactive with WT-1 antibody. Int J Gynecol Pathol 2004;23:241-7.
91. Agoff SN, Grieco VS, Garcia R, Gown AM. Immunohistochemical distinction of endometrial stromal sarcoma and cellular leiomyoma. Appl Immunohistochem Mol Morphol 2001;9:164-9.
92. Franquemont DW, Frierson HF Jr, Mills SE. An immunohistochemical study of normal endometrial stroma and endometrial stromal neoplasms. Evidence for smooth muscle differentiation. Am J Surg Pathol 1991;15:861-70.
93. Abrams J, Talcott J, Corson JM. Pulmonary metastases in patients with low-grade endometrial stromal sarcoma. Clinicopathologic findings with immunohistochemical characterization. Am J Surg Pathol 1989;13:133-40.
94. Nucci MR, O'Connell JT, Huettner PC, Cviko A, Sun D, Quade BJ. H-caldesmon expression effectively distinguishes endometrial stromal tumors from uterine smooth muscle tumors. Am J Surg Pathol 2001;25:455-63.
95. de Leval L, Waltregny D, Boniver J, Young RH, Castronovo V, Oliva E. Use of histone deacetylase 8 (HDAC8), a new marker of smooth muscle differentiation, in the classification of mesenchymal tumors of the uterus. Am J Surg Pathol 2006;30:319-27.
96. Rush DS, Tan J, Baergen RN, Soslow RA. H-caldesmon, a novel smooth muscle-specific antibody, distinguishes between cellular leiomyoma and endometrial stromal sarcoma. Am J Surg Pathol 2001;25:253-8.
97. Ng TL, Gown AM, Barry TS, et al. Nuclear beta-catenin in mesenchymal tumors. Mod Pathol 2005;18:68-74.
98. Krishnamurthy S, Jungbluth AA, Busam KJ, Rosai J. Uterine tumors resembling ovarian sex-cord tumors have an immunophenotype consistent with true sex-cord differentiation. Am J Surg Pathol 1998;22:1078-82.
99. Baker RJ, Hildebrandt RH, Rouse RV, Hendrickson MR, Longacre TA. Inhibin and CD99 (MIC2) expression in uterine stromal neoplasms with sex-cord-like elements. Hum Pathol 1999;30:671-9.
100. Stewart CJ, Crook M, Tan A. SF1 immunohistochemistry is useful in differentiating uterine tumours resembling sex cord-stromal tumours from potential histological mimics. Pathology 2016;48:434-40.
101. Ohta Y, Suzuki T, Kojima M, Shiokawa A, Mitsuya T. Low-grade endometrial stromal sarcoma with an extensive epithelial-like element. Pathol Int 2003;53:246-51.
102. Horn LC, Stegner HE. [Uterine stromal tumor with ovarian sex cord differentiation.] Pathologe 1995;16:421-5. [German]
103. Klein WM, Kurman RJ. Lack of expression of c-kit protein (CD117) in mesenchymal tumors of the uterus and ovary. Int J Gynecol Pathol 2003;22:181-4.
104. Rushing RS, Shajahan S, Chendil D, et al. Uterine sarcomas express KIT protein but lack mutation(s) in exon 11 or 17 of c-KIT. Gynecol Oncol 2003;91:9-14.
105. Kurihara S, Oda Y, Ohishi Y, et al. Coincident expression of beta-catenin and cyclin D1 in endometrial stromal tumors and related high-grade sarcomas. Mod Pathol 2010;23:225-34.
106. Chiang S, Lee CH, Stewart CJR, et al. BCOR is a robust diagnostic immunohistochemical marker of genetically diverse high-grade endometrial stromal sarcoma, including tumors exhibiting variant morphology. Mod Pathol 2017;30:1251-61.
107. Attygalle AD, Vroobel K, Wren D, et al. An unusual case of YWHAE-NUTM2A/B endometrial stromal sarcoma with confinement to the endometrium and lack of high-grade morphology. Int J Gynecol Pathol 2017;36:165-71.

108. Liegl B, Gully C, Reich O, Nogales FF, Beham A, Regauer S. Expression of platelet-derived growth factor receptor in low-grade endometrial stromal sarcomas in the absence of activating mutations. Histopathology 2007;50:448-52.
109. Dal Cin P, Talcott J, Abrams J, Li FP, Sandberg AA. Ins(10;19) in an endometrial stromal sarcoma. Cancer Genet Cytogenet 1988;36:1-5.
110. Sreekantaiah C, Li FP, Weidner N, Sandberg AA. An endometrial stromal sarcoma with clonal cytogenetic abnormalities. Cancer Genet Cytogenet 1991;55:163-6.
111. Chiang S, Oliva E. Cytogenetic and molecular aberrations in endometrial stromal tumors. Hum Pathol 2011;42:609-17.
112. Hrzenjak A. JAZF1/SUZ12 gene fusion in endometrial stromal sarcomas. Orphanet J Rare Dis 2016;11:15.
113. Oliva E, de Leval L, Soslow RA, Herens C. High frequency of JAZF1-JJAZ1 gene fusion in endometrial stromal tumors with smooth muscle differentiation by interphase FISH detection. Am J Surg Pathol 2007;31:1277-84.
114. Hrzenjak A, Moinfar F, Tavassoli FA, et al. JAZF1/JJAZ1 gene fusion in endometrial stromal sarcomas: molecular analysis by reverse transcriptase-polymerase chain reaction optimized for paraffin-embedded tissue. J Mol Diagn 2005;7:388-95.
115. Huang HY, Ladanyi M, Soslow RA. Molecular detection of JAZF1-JJAZ1 gene fusion in endometrial stromal neoplasms with classic and variant histology: evidence for genetic heterogeneity. Am J Surg Pathol 2004;28:224-32.
116. Ali RH, Al-Safi R, Al-Waheeb S, et al. Molecular characterization of a population-based series of endometrial stromal sarcomas in Kuwait. Hum Pathol 2014;45:2453-62.
117. Chiang S, Ali R, Melnyk N, et al. Frequency of known gene rearrangements in endometrial stromal tumors. Am J Surg Pathol 2011;35:1364-72.
118. Stewart CJ, Leung YC, Murch A, Peverall J. Evaluation of fluorescence in-situ hybridization in monomorphic endometrial stromal neoplasms and their histological mimics: a review of 49 cases. Histopathology 2014;65:473-82.
119. Nucci MR, Harburger D, Koontz J, Dal Cin P, Sklar J. Molecular analysis of the JAZF1-JJAZ1 gene fusion by RT-PCR and fluorescence in situ hybridization in endometrial stromal neoplasms. Am J Surg Pathol 2007;31:65-70.
120. Koontz JI, Soreng AL, Nucci M, et al. Frequent fusion of the JAZF1 and JJAZ1 genes in endometrial stromal tumors. Proc Natl Acad Sci U S A 2001;98:6348-53.
121. Micci F, Gorunova L, Gatius S, et al. MEAF6/PHF1 is a recurrent gene fusion in endometrial stromal sarcoma. Cancer Lett 2014;347:75-8.
122. Dewaele B, Przybyl J, Quattrone A, et al. Identification of a novel, recurrent MBTD1-CXorf67 fusion in low-grade endometrial stromal sarcoma. Int J Cancer 2014;134:1112-22.
123. Panagopoulos I, Thorsen J, Gorunova L, et al. Fusion of the ZC3H7B and BCOR genes in endometrial stromal sarcomas carrying an X;22-translocation. Genes Chromosomes Cancer 2013;52:610-8.
124. Croce S, Hostein I, Ribeiro A, et al. YWHAE rearrangement identified by FISH and RT-PCR in endometrial stromal sarcomas: genetic and pathological correlations. Mod Pathol 2013;26:1390-1400.
125. Panagopoulos I, Micci F, Thorsen J, et al. Novel fusion of MYST/Esa1-associated factor 6 and PHF1 in endometrial stromal sarcoma. PLoS One 2012;7:e39354.
126. Lee CH, Ou WB, Mariño-Enriquez A, et al. 14-3-3 fusion oncogenes in high-grade endometrial stromal sarcoma. Proc Natl Acad Sci U S A 2012;109:929-34.
127. Micci F, Panagopoulos I, Bjerkehagen B, Heim S. Consistent rearrangement of chromosomal band 6p21 with generation of fusion genes JAZF1/PHF1 and EPC1/PHF1 in endometrial stromal sarcoma. Cancer Res 2006;66:107-12.
128. Dal Cin P, Aly MS, De Wever I, Moerman P, Van Den Berghe H. Endometrial stromal sarcoma t(7;17)(p15-21;q12-21) is a nonrandom chromosome change. Cancer Genet Cytogenet 1992;63:43-6.
129. Hennig Y, Caselitz J, Bartnitzke S, Bullerdiek J. A third case of a low-grade endometrial stromal sarcoma with a t(7;17)(p14 approximately 21;q11.2 approximately 21). Cancer Genet Cytogenet 1997;98:84-6.
130. Micci F, Walter CU, Teixeira MR, et al. Cytogenetic and molecular genetic analyses of endometrial stromal sarcoma: nonrandom involvement of chromosome arms 6p and 7p and confirmation of JAZF1/JJAZ1 gene fusion in t(7;17). Cancer Genet Cytogenet 2003;144:119-24.
131. Pauwels P, Dal Cin P, Van de Moosdijk CN, Vrints L, Sciot R, Van den Berghe H. Cytogenetics revealing the diagnosis in a metastatic endometrial stromal sarcoma. Histopathology 1996;29:84-7.
132. Satoh Y, Ishikawa Y, Miyoshi T, Mukai H, Okumura S, Nakagawa K. Pulmonary metastases from a low-grade endometrial stromal sarcoma confirmed by chromosome aberration and fluorescence in-situ hybridization approaches: a case of recurrence 13 years after hysterectomy. Virchows Arch 2003;442:173-8.

133. Micci F, Brunetti M, Dal Cin P, et al. Fusion of the genes BRD8 and PHF1 in endometrial stromal sarcoma. Genes Chromosomes Cancer 2017;56:841-5.
134. Regauer S, Emberger W, Reich O, Pfragner R. Cytogenetic analyses of two new cases of endometrial stromal sarcoma--non-random reciprocal translocation t(10;17)(q22;p13) correlates with fibrous ESS. Histopathology 2008;52:780-3.
135. Li X, Anand M, Haimes JD, et al. The application of next-generation sequencing-based molecular diagnostics in endometrial stromal sarcoma. Histopathology 2016;69:551-9.
136. Choi YJ, Jung SH, Kim MS, et al. Genomic landscape of endometrial stromal sarcoma of uterus. Oncotarget 2015;6:33319-28.
137. Schilder JM, Hurd WW, Roth LM, Sutton GP. Hormonal treatment of an endometrial stromal nodule followed by local excision. Obstet Gynecol 1999;93(Pt 2):805-7.
138. Dong R, Mao H, Zhang P. Conservative management of endometrial stromal sarcoma at stage III: A case report. Oncol Lett 2014;8:1234-6.
139. Stemme S, Ghaderi M, Carlson JW. Diagnosis of endometrial stromal tumors: a clinicopathologic study of 25 biopsy specimens with identification of problematic areas. Am J Clin Pathol 2014;141:133-9.
140. Goldblum JR, Clement PB, Hart WR. Adenomyosis with sparse glands. A potential mimic of low-grade endometrial stromal sarcoma. Am J Clin Pathol 1995;103:218-23.
141. Sampson JA. Metastatic or embolic endometriosis, due to the menstrual dissemination of endometrial tissue into the venous circulation. Am J Pathol 1927;3:93-110.
142. Sahin AA, Silva EG, Landon G, Ordoñez NG, Gershenson DM. Endometrial tissue in myometrial vessels not associated with menstruation. Int J Gynecol Pathol 1989;8:139-46.
143. Oliva E, Young RH, Clement PB, Bhan AK, Scully RE. Cellular benign mesenchymal tumors of the uterus. A comparative morphologic and immunohistochemical analysis of 33 highly cellular leiomyomas and six endometrial stromal nodules, two frequently confused tumors. Am J Surg Pathol 1995;19:757-68.
144. Loddenkemper C, Mechsner S, Foss HD, et al. Use of oxytocin receptor expression in distinguishing between uterine smooth muscle tumors and endometrial stromal sarcoma. Am J Surg Pathol 2003;27:1458-62.
145. Tawfik O, Rao D, Nothnick WB, Graham A, Mau B, Fan F. Transgelin, a novel marker of smooth muscle differentiation, effectively distinguishes endometrial stromal tumors from uterine smooth muscle tumors. Int J Gynecol Obstet Reprod Med Res 2014;1:26-31.
146. Gilks CB, Clement PB, Hart WR, Young RH. Uterine adenomyomas excluding atypical polypoid adenomyomas and adenomyomas of endocervical type: a clinicopathologic study of 30 cases of an underemphasized lesion that may cause diagnostic problems with brief consideration of adenomyomas of other female genital tract sites. Int J Gynecol Pathol 2000;19:195-205.
147. Tabata T, Takeshima N, Hirai Y, Hasumi K. Low-grade endometrial stromal sarcoma with cardiovascular involvement—a report of three cases. Gynecol Oncol 1999;75:495-8.
148. Clement PB, Young RH, Scully RE. Intravenous leiomyomatosis of the uterus. A clinicopathological analysis of 16 cases with unusual histologic features. Am J Surg Pathol 1988;12:932-45.
149. Oliva E. Cellular mesenchymal tumors of the uterus: a review emphasizing recent observations. Int J Gynecol Pathol 2014;33:374-84.
150. Oliva E. Practical issues in uterine pathology from banal to bewildering: the remarkable spectrum of smooth muscle neoplasia. Mod Pathol 2016;29(Suppl 1):S104-20.
151. Baker P, Oliva E. Endometrial stromal tumours of the uterus: a practical approach using conventional morphology and ancillary techniques. J Clin Pathol 2007;60:235-43.
152. Hoang L, Chiang S, Lee CH. Endometrial stromal sarcomas and related neoplasms: new developments and diagnostic considerations. Pathology 2018;50:162-77.
153. de Leval L, Lim GS, Waltregny D, Oliva E. Diverse phenotypic profile of uterine tumors resembling ovarian sex cord tumors: an immunohistochemical study of 12 cases. Am J Surg Pathol 2010;34:1749-61.
154. Chiang S, Staats PN, Senz J, et al. FOXL2 mutation is absent in uterine tumors resembling ovarian sex cord tumors. Am J Surg Pathol 2015;39:618-23.
155. Staats PN, Garcia JJ, Dias-Santagata DC, et al. Uterine tumors resembling ovarian sex cord tumors (UTROSCT) lack the JAZF1-JJAZ1 translocation frequently seen in endometrial stromal tumors. Am J Surg Pathol 2009;33:1206-12.
156. Nucci MR, Schoolmeester JK, Sukov WR, Oliva E. Uterine tumors resembling ovarian sex cord tumor (UTROSCT) lack rearrangement of PHF1 by FISH. Mod Pathol. 2014;27:298A.
157. Liang SX, Patel K, Pearl M, Liu J, Zheng W, Tornos C. Sertoliform endometrioid carcinoma of the endometrium with dual immunophenotypes for epithelial membrane antigen and inhibin alpha: case report and literature review. Int J Gynecol Pathol 2007;26:291-7.

158. Eichhorn JH, Young RH, Clement PB. Sertoliform endometrial adenocarcinoma: a study of four cases. Int J Gynecol Pathol 1996;15:119-26.
159. Rizeq MN, van de Rijn M, Hendrickson MR, Rouse RV. A comparative immunohistochemical study of uterine smooth muscle neoplasms with emphasis on the epithelioid variant. Hum Pathol 1994;25:671-7.
160. Iwata J, Fletcher CD. Immunohistochemical detection of cytokeratin and epithelial membrane antigen in leiomyosarcoma: a systematic study of 100 cases. Pathol Int 2000;50:7-14.
161. Portugal R, Oliva E. Calretinin: diagnostic utility in the female genital tract. Adv Anat Pathol 2009;16:118-24.
162. Lee CH, Ali RH, Rouzbahman M, et al. Cyclin D1 as a diagnostic immunomarker for endometrial stromal sarcoma with YWHAE-FAM22 rearrangement. Am J Surg Pathol 2012;36:1562-70.
163. Lee CH, Hoang LN, Yip S, et al. Frequent expression of KIT in endometrial stromal sarcoma with YWHAE genetic rearrangement. Mod Pathol 2014;27:751-7.
164. Meenakshi M, McCluggage WG. Vascular involvement in adenomyosis: report of a large series of a common phenomenon with observations on the pathogenesis of adenomyosis. Int J Gynecol Pathol 2010;29:117-21.
165. Hirschowitz L, Mayall FG, Ganesan R, McCluggage WG. Intravascular adenomyomatosis: expanding the morphologic spectrum of intravascular leiomyomatosis. Am J Surg Pathol 2013;37:1395-400.
166. Wu RI, Schorge JO, Dal Cin P, Young RH, Oliva E. Mullerian adenosarcoma of the uterus with low-grade sarcomatous overgrowth characterized by prominent hydropic change resulting in mimicry of a smooth muscle tumor. Int J Gynecol Pathol 2014;33:573-80.
167. Burch DM, Tavassoli FA. Myxoid leiomyosarcoma of the uterus. Histopathology 2011;59:1144-55.
168. King ME, Dickersin GR, Scully RE. Myxoid leiomyosarcoma of the uterus. A report of six cases. Am J Surg Pathol 1982;6:589-98.
169. Parra-Herran C, Schoolmeester JK, Yuan L, et al. Myxoid leiomyosarcoma of the uterus: a clinicopathologic analysis of 30 cases and review of the literature with reappraisal of its distinction from other uterine myxoid mesenchymal neoplasms. Am J Surg Pathol 2016;40:285-301.
170. Schaefer IM, Hornick JL, Sholl LM, Quade BJ, Nucci MR, Parra-Herran C. Abnormal p53 and p16 staining patterns distinguish uterine leiomyosarcoma from inflammatory myofibroblastic tumour. Histopathology 2017;70:1138-46.
171. Kurihara S, Oda Y, Ohishi Y, et al. Endometrial stromal sarcomas and related high-grade sarcomas: immunohistochemical and molecular genetic study of 31 cases. Am J Surg Pathol 2008;32:1228-38.
172. Gersell DJ, Fulling KH. Localized neurofibromatosis of the female genitourinary tract. Am J Surg Pathol 1989;13:873-8.
173. Gomez-Laencina AM, Martinez Diaz F, Izquierdo Sanjuanes B, Vicente Sanchez EM, Fernandez Salmeron R, Meseguer Peña F. Localized neurofibromatosis of the female genital system: a case report and review of the literature. J Obstet Gynaecol Res 2012;38:953-6.
174. Mills AM, Karamchandani JR, Vogel H, Longacre TA. Endocervical fibroblastic malignant peripheral nerve sheath tumor (neurofibrosarcoma): report of a novel entity possibly related to endocervical CD34 fibrocytes. Am J Surg Pathol 2011;35:404-12.
175. Keel SB, Clement PB, Prat J, Young RH. Malignant schwannoma of the uterine cervix: a study of three cases. Int J Gynecol Pathol 1998;17:223-30.
176. Yang EJ, Howitt BE, Fletcher CDM, Nucci MR. Solitary fibrous tumour of the female genital tract: a clinicopathological analysis of 25 cases. Histopathology 2018;72:749-59.
177. Strickland KC, Nucci MR, Esselen KM, et al. Solitary fibrous tumor of the uterus presenting with lung metastases: a case report. Int J Gynecol Pathol 2016;35:25-9.
178. Veras E, Junkins-Hopkins JM, Marinis S, Vang R. Myometrial myxoidosis: a report of 2 cases of a distinctive type of secondary myometrial hypertrophy in patients with lupus erythematosus. Int J Gynecol Pathol 2009;28:164-71.
179. McCluggage WG, Young RH. Myxoid change of the myometrium and cervical stroma: description of a hitherto unreported non-neoplastic phenomenon with discussion of myxoid uterine lesions. Int J Gynecol Pathol 2010;29:351-7.
180. Pugh A, McCluggage WG, Hirschowitz L. Multifocal uterine myxoid change: a newly recognized association with neurofibromatosis type 1. Int J Gynecol Pathol 2012;31:580-3.
181. Barlow JF, Abu-Gazeleh S, Tam GE, et al. Myxoid tumor of the uterus and right atrial myxomas. S D J Med 1983;36:9-13.
182. Parra-Herran C, Quick CM, Howitt BE, Dal Cin P, Quade BJ, Nucci MR. Inflammatory myofibroblastic tumor of the uterus: clinical and pathologic review of 10 cases including a subset with aggressive clinical course. Am J Surg Pathol 2015;39:157-68.

183. Bennett JA, Nardi V, Rouzbahman M, Morales-Oyarvide V, Nielsen GP, Oliva E. Inflammatory myofibroblastic tumor of the uterus: a clinicopathological, immunohistochemical, and molecular analysis of 13 cases highlighting their broad morphologic spectrum. Mod Pathol 2017;30:1489-1503.

184. Li RF, Gupta M, McCluggage WG, Ronnett BM. Embryonal rhabdomyosarcoma (botryoid type) of the uterine corpus and cervix in adult women: report of a case series and review of the literature. Am J Surg Pathol 2013;37:344-55.

185. Kurman RJ, Norris HJ. Mesenchymal tumors of the uterus. VI. Epithelioid smooth muscle tumors including leiomyoblastoma and clear-cell leiomyoma: a clinical and pathologic analysis of 26 cases. Cancer 1976;37:1853-65.

186. Parker RL, Young RH, Clement PB. Skeletal muscle-like and rhabdoid cells in uterine leiomyomas. Int J Gynecol Pathol 2005;24:319-25.

187. Han HS, Park IA, Kim SH, Lee HP. The clear cell variant of epithelioid intravenous leiomyomatosis of the uterus: report of a case. Pathol Int 1998;48:892-6.

188. Mentzel T, Wadden C, Fletcher CD. Granular cell change in smooth muscle tumours of skin and soft tissue. Histopathology 1994;24:223-31.

189. McDonald AG, Dal Cin P, Ganguly A, et al. Liposarcoma arising in uterine lipoleiomyoma: a report of 3 cases and review of the literature. Am J Surg Pathol 2011;35:221-7.

190. Feng W, Hua K, Malpica A, Zhou X, Baak JP. Stages I to II WHO 2003-defined low-grade endometrial stromal sarcoma: how much primary therapy is needed and how little is enough? Int J Gynecol Cancer 2013;23:488-93.

191. Li N, Wu LY, Zhang HT, An JS, Li XG, Ma SK. Treatment options in stage I endometrial stromal sarcoma: a retrospective analysis of 53 cases. Gynecol Oncol 2008;108:306-11.

192. Nordal RR, Kristensen GB, Kaern J, Stenwig AE, Pettersen EO, Trope CG. The prognostic significance of surgery, tumor size, malignancy grade, menopausal status, and DNA ploidy in endometrial stromal sarcoma. Gynecol Oncol 1996;62:254-9.

193. Shah JP, Bryant CS, Kumar S, Ali-Fehmi R, Malone JM Jr, Morris RT. Lymphadenectomy and ovarian preservation in low-grade endometrial stromal sarcoma. Obstet Gynecol 2008;112:1102-8.

194. Chan JK, Kawar NM, Shin JY, et al. Endometrial stromal sarcoma: a population-based analysis. Br J Cancer 2008;99:1210-15.

195. Thomas MB, Keeney GL, Podratz KC, Dowdy SC. Endometrial stromal sarcoma: treatment and patterns of recurrence. Int J Gynecol Cancer 2009;19:253-6.

196. Amant F, De Knijf A, Van Calster B, et al. Clinical study investigating the role of lymphadenectomy, surgical castration and adjuvant hormonal treatment in endometrial stromal sarcoma. Br J Cancer 2007;97:1194-99.

197. Signorelli M, Fruscio R, Dell'Anna T, et al. Lymphadenectomy in uterine low-grade endometrial stromal sarcoma: an analysis of 19 cases and a literature review. Int J Gynecol Cancer 2010;20:1363-6.

198. Dos Santos LA, Garg K, Diaz JP, et al. Incidence of lymph node and adnexal metastasis in endometrial stromal sarcoma. Gynecol Oncol 2011;121:319-22.

199. Gadducci A, Sartori E, Landoni F, et al. Endometrial stromal sarcoma: analysis of treatment failures and survival. Gynecol Oncol 1996;63:247-53.

200. Barney B, Tward JD, Skidmore T, Gaffney DK. Does radiotherapy or lymphadenectomy improve survival in endometrial stromal sarcoma? Int J Gynecol Cancer 2009;19:1232-8.

201. Leath CA 3rd, Huh WK, Hyde J Jr, et al. A multi-institutional review of outcomes of endometrial stromal sarcoma. Gynecol Oncol 2007;105:630-4.

202. Reich O, Regauer S. Hormonal therapy of endometrial stromal sarcoma. Curr Opin Oncol 2007;19:347-52.

203. Gadducci A, Cosio S, Romanini A, Genazzani AR. The management of patients with uterine sarcoma: a debated clinical challenge. Crit Rev Oncol Hematol 2008;65:129-42.

204. Felix AS, Cook LS, Gaudet MM, et al. The etiology of uterine sarcomas: a pooled analysis of the epidemiology of endometrial cancer consortium. Br J Cancer 2013;108:727-34.

205. Mansi JL, Ramachandra S, Wiltshaw E, Fisher C. Endometrial stromal sarcomas. Gynecol Oncol 1990;36:113-8.

206. Fukunaga M, Endo Y. Pelvic bone involvement in low-grade endometrial stromal sarcoma with ovarian sex cord-like differentiation. Histopathology 1996;29:391-3.

207. Itoh T, Mochizuki M, Kumazaki S, Ishihara T, Fukayama M. Cystic pulmonary metastases of endometrial stromal sarcoma of the uterus, mimicking lymphangiomyomatosis: a case report with immunohistochemistry of HMB45. Pathol Int 1997;47:725-9.

208. Bodner K, Bodner-Adler B, Obermair A, et al. Prognostic parameters in endometrial stromal sarcoma: a clinicopathologic study in 31 patients. Gynecol Oncol 2001;81:160-5.

209. Akahira J, Tokunaga H, Toyoshima M, et al. Prognoses and prognostic factors of carcinosarcoma, endometrial stromal sarcoma and uterine leiomyosarcoma: a comparison with uterine endometrial adenocarcinoma. Oncology 2006;71:333-40.
210. Albrektsen G, Heuch I, Wik E, Salvesen HB. Prognostic impact of parity in 493 uterine sarcoma patients. Int J Gynecol Cancer 2009;19:1062-7.
211. Chauveinc L, Deniaud E, Plancher C, et al. Uterine sarcomas: the Curie Institut experience. Prognosis factors and adjuvant treatments. Gynecol Oncol 1999;72:232-7.
212. Park JY, Kim DY, Suh DS, et al. Prognostic factors and treatment outcomes of patients with uterine sarcoma: analysis of 127 patients at a single institution, 1989-2007. J Cancer Res Clin Oncol 2008;134:1277-87.
213. Koivisto-Korander R, Butzow R, Koivisto AM, Leminen A. Clinical outcome and prognostic factors in 100 cases of uterine sarcoma: experience in Helsinki University Central Hospital 1990-2001. Gynecol Oncol 2008;111:74-81.
214. Brooks SE, Zhan M, Cote T, Baquet CR. Surveillance, epidemiology, and end results analysis of 2677 cases of uterine sarcoma 1989-1999. Gynecol Oncol 2004;93:204-8.
215. Feng W, Malpica A, Skaland I, et al. Can proliferation biomarkers reliably predict recurrence in world health organization 2003 defined endometrial stromal sarcoma, low grade? PLoS One 2013;8:e75899.
216. Feng W, Malpica A, Yinhua Y, et al. Diagnostic and prognostic morphometric features in who2003 invasive endometrial stromal tumours. Histopathology 2013;62:688-94.
217. Feng W, Malpica A, Robboy SJ, et al. Prognostic value of the diagnostic criteria distinguishing endometrial stromal sarcoma, low grade from undifferentiated endometrial sarcoma, 2 entities within the invasive endometrial stromal neoplasia family. Int J Gynecol Pathol 2013;32:299-306.
218. Chew I, Oliva E. Endometrial stromal sarcomas: a review of potential prognostic factors. Adv Anat Pathol 2010;17:113-21.
219. American Cancer Society, Inc. Survival rates of uterine sarcoma by stage. Last revised: November 13, 2017. https://www.cancer.org/cancer/uterine-sarcoma/detection-diagnosis-staging/survival-rates.html).
220. Von Bargen EC, Grimes CL, Mishra K, et al. Prevalence of occult pre-malignant or malignant pathology at the time of uterine morcellation for benign disease. Int J Gynaecol Obstet 2017;137:123-8.
221. Amant F, Tousseyn T, Coenegrachts L, Decloedt J, Moerman P, Debiec-Rychter M. Case report of a poorly differentiated uterine tumour with t(10;17) translocation and neuroectodermal phenotype. Anticancer Res 2011;31:2367-71.
222. Aisagbonhi O, Harrison B, Zhao L, Osgood R, Chebib I, Oliva E. YWHAE rearrangement in a purely conventional low-grade endometrial stromal sarcoma that transformed over time to high-grade sarcoma: importance of molecular testing. Int J Gynecol Pathol 2018;37:441-7.
223. Punnett HH, Halligan GE, Zaeri N, Karmazin N. Translocation 10;17 in clear cell sarcoma of the kidney. A first report. Cancer Genet Cytogenet 1989;41:123-8.
224. Rakheja D, Weinberg AG, Tomlinson GE, Partridge K, Schneider NR. Translocation (10;17)(q22;p13): a recurring translocation in clear cell sarcoma of kidney. Cancer Genet Cytogenet 2004;154:175-9.
225. Kruse AJ, Croce S, Kruitwagen RF, et al. Aggressive behavior and poor prognosis of endometrial stromal sarcomas with YWHAE-FAM22 rearrangement indicate the clinical importance to recognize this subset. Int J Gynecol Cancer 2014;24:1616-22.
226. Sciallis AP, Bedroske PP, Schoolmeester JK, et al. High-grade endometrial stromal sarcomas: a clinicopathologic study of a group of tumors with heterogenous morphologic and genetic features. Am J Surg Pathol 2014;38:1161-72.
227. Shah VI, McCluggage WG. Cyclin D1 does not distinguish YWHAE-NUTM2 high-grade endometrial stromal sarcoma from undifferentiated endometrial carcinoma. Am J Surg Pathol 2015;39:722-4.
228. Ramalingam P, Masand RP, Euscher ED, Malpica A. Undifferentiated carcinoma of the endometrium: an expanded immunohistochemical analysis including PAX-8 and basal-like carcinoma surrogate markers. Int J Gynecol Pathol 2016;35:410-8.
229. Chiang S, Snuderl M, Kojiro-Sanada S, et al. Primitive neuroectodermal tumors of the female genital tract: a morphologic, immunohistochemical, and molecular study of 19 cases. Am J Surg Pathol 2017;41:761-72.
230. Euscher ED, Deavers MT, Lopez-Terrada D, Lazar AJ, Silva EG, Malpica A. Uterine tumors with neuroectodermal differentiation: a series of 17 cases and review of the literature. Am J Surg Pathol 2008;32:219-28.
231. Hung YP, Fletcher CD, Hornick JL. Evaluation of NKX2-2 expression in round cell sarcomas and other tumors with EWSR1 rearrangement: imperfect specificity for Ewing sarcoma. Mod Pathol 2016;29:370-80.

232. Miettinen M, Lasota J. Histopathology of gastrointestinal stromal tumor. J Surg Oncol 2011;104:865-73.
233. Novelli M, Rossi S, Rodriguez-Justo M, et al. DOG1 and CD117 are the antibodies of choice in the diagnosis of gastrointestinal stromal tumours. Histopathology 2010;57:259-70.
234. Hemming ML, Wagner AJ, Nucci MR, et al. YWHAE-rearranged high-grade endometrial stromal sarcoma: two-center case series and response to chemotherapy. Gynecol Oncol 2017;145:531-5.
235. Lewis N, Soslow RA, Delair DF, et al. ZC3H7B-BCOR high-grade endometrial stromal sarcomas: a report of 17 cases of a newly defined entity. Mod Pathol 2018;31:674-84.
236. Hoang LN, Aneja A, Conlon N, et al. Novel high-grade endometrial stromal sarcoma: a morphologic mimicker of myxoid leiomyosarcoma. Am J Surg Pathol 2017;41:12-24.
237. Mariño-Enriquez A, Lauria A, Przybyl J, et al. BCOR internal tandem duplication in high-grade uterine sarcomas. Am J Surg Pathol 2018;42:335-41.
237a. Ueno-Yokohata H, Okita H, Nakasato K, et al. Consistent in-frame internal tandem duplications of BCOR characterize clear cell sarcoma of the kidney. Nat Genet 2015;47:861-3.
238. Arias-Stella JA, 3rd, Benayed R, Oliva E, et al. Novel PLAG1 Gene rearrangement distinguishes a subset of uterine myxoid leiomyosarcoma from other uterine myxoid mesenchymal tumors. Am J Surg Pathol [In press]
239. Howitt BE, Sholl LM, Dal Cin P, et al. Targeted genomic analysis of mullerian adenosarcoma. J Pathol 2015;235:37-49.
240. Amant F, Woestenborghs H, Vandenbroucke V, et al. Transition of endometrial stromal sarcoma into high-grade sarcoma. Gynecol Oncol 2006;103:1137-40.
241. Ohta Y, Suzuki T, Omatsu M, et al. Transition from low-grade endometrial stromal sarcoma to high-grade endometrial stromal sarcoma. Int J Gynecol Pathol 2010;29:374-7.
242. Cheung AN, Ng WF, Chung LP, Khoo US. Mixed low grade and high grade endometrial stromal sarcoma of uterus: differences on immunohistochemistry and chromosome in situ hybridisation. J Clin Pathol 1996;49:604-7.
243. Malpica A, Deavers MT, Silva EG. High grade sarcoma in endometrial stromal sarcoma: dedifferentiated endometrial stromal sarcoma. [Abstract]. Mod Pathol 2006;19:188A.
244. Tanner EJ, Garg K, Leitao MM Jr, Soslow RA, Hensley ML. High grade undifferentiated uterine sarcoma: surgery, treatment, and survival outcomes. Gynecol Oncol 2012;127:27-31.
245. Prat J, Mbatani. Uterine sarcomas. Int J Gynaecol Obstet 2015;131(Suppl 2):S105-10.
246. Bartosch C, Exposito MI, Lopes JM. Low-grade endometrial stromal sarcoma and undifferentiated endometrial sarcoma: a comparative analysis emphasizing the importance of distinguishing between these two groups. Int J Surg Pathol 2010;18:286-91.
247. Gremel G, Liew M, Hamzei F, et al. A prognosis based classification of undifferentiated uterine sarcomas: identification of mitotic index, hormone receptors and YWHAE-FAM22 translocation status as predictors of survival. Int J Cancer 2015;136:1608-18.
248. Gil-Benso R, Lopez-Gines C, Navarro S, Carda C, Llombart-Bosch A. Endometrial stromal sarcomas: immunohistochemical, electron microscopical and cytogenetic findings in two cases. Virchows Arch 1999;434:307-14.
249. Micci F, Gorunova L, Agostini A, et al. Cytogenetic and molecular profile of endometrial stromal sarcoma. Genes Chromosomes Cancer 2016;55:834-46.
250. Flicker K, Smolle E, Haybaeck J, Moinfar F. Genomic characterization of endometrial stromal sarcomas with array comparative genomic hybridization. Exp Mol Pathol 2015;98:367-74.
251. Halbwedl I, Ullmann R, Kremser ML, et al. Chromosomal alterations in low-grade endometrial stromal sarcoma and undifferentiated endometrial sarcoma as detected by comparative genomic hybridization. Gynecol Oncol 2005;97:582-7.
252. Chen E, O'Connell F, Fletcher CD. Dedifferentiated leiomyosarcoma: clinicopathological analysis of 18 cases. Histopathology 2011;59:1135-43.
253. Kolin DL, Dong F, Baltay M, et al. SMARCA4-deficient undifferentiated uterine sarcoma (malignant rhabdoid tumor of the uterus): a clinicopathologic entity distinct from undifferentiated carcinoma. Mod Pathol 2018.
254. Langley FA, Smith JP, Woodcock AS. Debatable uterine tumours. Acta Obstet Gynecol Scand 1953;32:143-69.
255. Morehead RP, Bowman MC. Heterologous mesodermal tumors of the uterus: report of a neoplasm resembling a granulosa cell tumor. Am J Pathol 1945;21:53-61.
256. Liu CY, Shen Y, Zhao JG, Qu PP. Clinical experience of uterine tumors resembling ovarian sex cord tumors: a clinicopathological analysis of 6 cases. Int J Clin Exp Pathol 2015;8:4158-64.
257. Franco A, Aquino NM, Malik SL, Navarro C. Sonographic presentation of uterine sex cord-stromal tumor. J Clin Ultrasound 1999;27:199-201.

258. Kabbani W, Deavers MT, Malpica A, et al. Uterine tumor resembling ovarian sex-cord tumor: report of a case mimicking cervical adenocarcinoma. Int J Gynecol Pathol 2003;22:297-302.
259. Rollins S, Clement PB, Young RH. Uterine tumors resembling ovarian sex cord tumors frequently have incorporated mature smooth muscle imparting a pseudoinfiltrative appearance. Mod Pathol. 2007;20:212A.
260. Nogales FF, Stolnicu S, Harilal KR, Mooney E, Garcia-Galvis OF. Retiform uterine tumours resembling ovarian sex cord tumours. A comparative immunohistochemical study with retiform structures of the female genital tract. Histopathology 2009;54:471-7.
261. Hurrell DP, McCluggage WG. Uterine tumour resembling ovarian sex cord tumour is an immunohistochemically polyphenotypic neoplasm which exhibits coexpression of epithelial, myoid and sex cord markers. J Clin Pathol 2007;60:1148-54.
262. Czernobilsky B, Mamet Y, David MB, Atlas I, Gitstein G, Lifschitz-Mercer B. Uterine retiform Sertoli-Leydig cell tumor: report of a case providing additional evidence that uterine tumors resembling ovarian sex cord tumors have a histologic and immunohistochemical phenotype of genuine sex cord tumors. Int J Gynecol Pathol 2005;24:335-40.
263. Croce S, de Kock L, Boshari T, et al. Uterine tumor resembling ovarian sex cord tumor (UTROSCT) commonly exhibits positivity with sex cord markers FOXL2 and SF-1 but lacks FOXL2 and DICER1 mutations. Int J Gynecol Pathol 2016;35:301-8.
264. Sutak J, Lazic D, Cullimore JE. Uterine tumour resembling an ovarian sex cord tumour. J Clin Pathol 2005;58:888-90.
265. Hauptmann S, Nadjari B, Kraus J, Turnwald W, Dietel M. Uterine tumor resembling ovarian sex-cord tumor--a case report and review of the literature. Virchows Arch 2001;439:97-101.
266. Mazur MT, Kraus FT. Histogenesis of morphologic variations in tumors of the uterine wall. Am J Surg Pathol 1980;4:59-74.
267. McCluggage WG, Shah V, Walsh MY, Toner PG. Uterine tumour resembling ovarian sex cord tumour: evidence for smooth muscle differentiation. Histopathology 1993;23:83-5.
268. Kantelip B, Cloup N, Dechelotte P. Uterine tumor resembling ovarian sex cord tumors: report of a case with ultrastructural study. Hum Pathol 1986;17:91-4.
269. Gupta M, de Leval L, Selig M, Oliva E, Nielsen GP. Uterine tumors resembling ovarian sex cord tumors: an ultrastructural analysis of 13 cases. Ultrastruct Pathol 2010;34:16-24.
270. Shah SP, Kobel M, Senz J, et al. Mutation of FOXL2 in granulosa-cell tumors of the ovary. N Engl J Med 2009;360:2719-29.
271. Wang Y, Karnezis AN, Magrill J, et al. DICER1 hotspot mutations in ovarian gynandroblastoma. Histopathology 2018.
272. Conlon N, Schultheis AM, Piscuoglio S, et al. A survey of DICER1 hotspot mutations in ovarian and testicular sex cord-stromal tumors. Mod Pathol 2015;28:1603-12.
273. Dickson BC, Childs TJ, Colgan TJ, et al. Uterine tumor resembling ovarian sex cord tumor: a distinct entity characterized by recurrent NCOA2/3 gene fusions. Am J Surg Pathol 2019;43:178-86.
273a. Wang J, Blakey GL, Zhang L, Bane B, Torbenson M, Li S. Uterine tumor resembling ovarian sex cord tumor: report of a case with t(X;6)(p22.3;q23.1) and t(4;18)(q21.1;q21.3). Diagn Mol Pathol 2003;12:174-80.
274. Croce S, Chibon F. MED12 and uterine smooth muscle oncogenesis: state of the art and perspectives. Eur J Cancer 2015;51:1603-10.
275. Shah VI, Freites ON, Maxwell P, McCluggage WG. Inhibin is more specific than calretinin as an immunohistochemical marker for differentiating sarcomatoid granulosa cell tumour of the ovary from other spindle cell neoplasms. J Clin Pathol 2003;56:221-4.
276. Pusiol T, Parolari AM, Piscioli F. Uterine leiomyoma with tubules. Int Semin Surg Oncol 2008;5:15.
277. Murray SK, Clement PB, Young RH. Endometrioid carcinomas of the uterine corpus with sex cord-like formations, hyalinization, and other unusual morphologic features: a report of 31 cases of a neoplasm that may be confused with carcinosarcoma and other uterine neoplasms. Am J Surg Pathol 2005;29:157-66.
278. Lugli A, Forster Y, Haas P, et al. Calretinin expression in human normal and neoplastic tissues: a tissue microarray analysis on 5233 tissue samples. Hum Pathol 2003;34:994-1000.
279. McCluggage WG, Maxwell P. Adenocarcinomas of various sites may exhibit immunoreactivity with anti-inhibin antibodies. Histopathology 1999;35:216-20.
280. Stolnicu S, Balachandran K, Aleykutty MA, et al. Uterine adenosarcomas overgrown by sex-cord-like tumour: report of two cases. J Clin Pathol 2009;62:942-4.
281. Mohammadizadeh F, Rajabi P, Behnamfar F, Hani M, Bagheri M. Extensive overgrowth of sex cord-like differentiation in uterine mullerian adenosarcoma: a rare and challenging entity. Int J Gynecol Pathol 2016;35:153-61.

282. Stolnicu S, Molnar C, Barsan I, Boros M, Nogales FF, Soslow RA. The impact on survival of an extensive sex cord-like component in mullerian adenosarcomas: a study comprising 6 cases. Int J Gynecol Pathol 2016;35:147-52.
283. Hillard JB, Malpica A, Ramirez PT. Conservative management of a uterine tumor resembling an ovarian sex cord-stromal tumor. Gynecol Oncol 2004;92:347-52.
284. Berretta R, Patrelli TS, Fadda GM, Merisio C, Gramellini D, Nardelli GB. Uterine tumors resembling ovarian sex cord tumors: a case report of conservative management in young women. Int J Gynecol Cancer 2009;19:808-10.
285. Pang LC. Endometrial stromal sarcoma with sex cord-like differentiation associated with tamoxifen therapy. South Med J 1998;91:592-4.
286. Miliaras D, Bontis J. Uterine tumor resembling sex-cord ovarian tumors: one more case of the pure type suggests a neoplasm with benign behavior. Eur J Gynaecol Oncol 1997;18:133-5.
287. Blake EA, Sheridan TB, Wang KL, et al. Clinical characteristics and outcomes of uterine tumors resembling ovarian sex-cord tumors (UTROSCT): a systematic review of literature. Eur J Obstet Gynecol Reprod Biol 2014;181:163-70.
288. Biermann K, Heukamp LC, Buttner R, Zhou H. Uterine tumor resembling an ovarian sex cord tumor associated with metastasis. Int J Gynecol Pathol 2008;27:58-60.
289. Gomes JR, Carvalho FM, Abrao M, Maluf FC. Uterine tumors resembling ovarian sex-cord tumor: a case-report and a review of literature. Gynecol Oncol Rep 2016;15:22-4.
290. Umeda S, Tateno M, Miyagi E, et al. Uterine tumors resembling ovarian sex cord tumors (UTROSCT) with metastasis: clinicopathological study of two cases. Int J Clin Exp Pathol 2014;7:1051-9.

10 SMOOTH MUSCLE AND OTHER MESENCHYMAL TUMORS

LEIOMYOMA AND VARIANTS

Definition. *Leiomyoma* is a benign mesenchymal tumor composed of smooth muscle cells with a spectrum of gross and microscopic features and a variety of growth patterns (Table 10-1) (1).

Epidemiology and General Features. Smooth muscle tumors, specifically leiomyomas, are the most common mesenchymal tumors of the uterus, and overall, the most common solid tumor of the female genital tract (2). Leiomyomas are noted in 70 to 80 percent of hysterectomies performed for noncancer-related conditions (3) although they are only apparent in about 25 percent of women (4). They represent the most common indication for gynecologic surgery in the United States. They are responsible for approximately 200,000 hysterectomies (5), 33 percent to over 40 percent of the about 600,000 hysterectomies done each year, surpassing the number of hysterectomies performed for all types of gynecologic cancers combined (6,7).

The lifetime risk for women developing leiomyomas is as high as 75 percent. Leiomyomas are present in 20 to 30 percent of women over 30 years of age and in more than 40 percent of women older than 40 years. Approximately 42 per 10,000 women between 15 and 54 years of age are hospitalized every year for leiomyoma-related treatments (6), indicating the important repercussions of this disease.

The frequency of uterine leiomyomas varies among ethnic groups: Caucasian women have a much lower incidence than African-American women, who typically tend to have leiomyomas at a younger age that are more often multiple and typically larger, and therefore, have more severe symptoms, signifying the presence of an underlying genetic predisposition or other potential influences. A subset of leiomyomas is associated with the *hereditary leiomyomatosis and renal cell carcinoma* (HLRCC) *syndrome* (Reed *syndrome*), a rare autosomal dominant syndrome with high penetrance caused by germline mutations of the fumarate hydratase gene (*FH*, 1q43). The mutations lead to the development of multiple cutaneous and uterine leiomyomas as well as an increased risk of developing renal papillary cell carcinoma, type II, in 20 to 25 percent of patients; the latter is responsible for the high mortality rate. Uterine leiomyomas in this setting occur in about 80 percent and cutaneous leiomyomas in about 70 percent of female carriers (8). As occurs with African-American women, these patients present at an earlier age and often have multiple leiomyomas associated with more severe symptoms, often leading to earlier surgical intervention compared to those with conventional leiomyomas (9).

Alport, Proteus, and Cowden syndromes may be associated with leiomyomas, although they

Table 10-1

LEIOMYOMA VARIANTS

1. With bizarre nuclei
2. Fumarate hydratase deficient
3. Cellular
4. Mitotically active
5. With hydropic change including perinodular
6. Dissecting including cotyledonoid
7. Apoplectic
8. Other drug-related changes
9. Epithelioid
10. Myxoid
11. With heterologous elements
12. With unusual growth:
    Diffuse leiomyomatosis
    Parasitic leiomyoma
    Diffuse peritoneal leiomyomatosis
    Intravenous leiomyomatosis
    Benign metastasizing leiomyoma

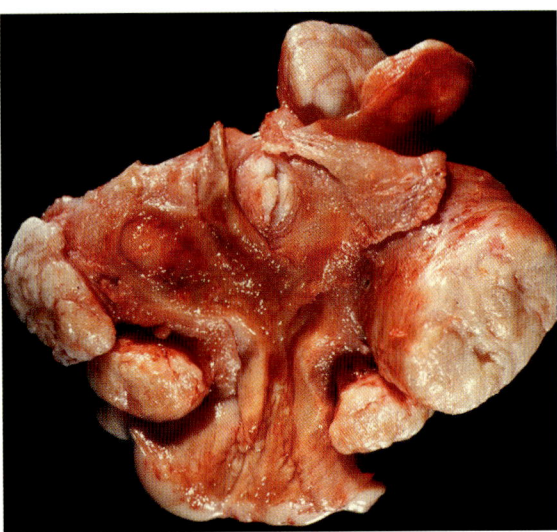

Figure 10-1

TYPICAL LEIOMYOMAS

Variably sized tumors are seen in submucosal, intramyometrial, and subserosal locations, distorting the uterus. They have a homogeneous, bulging, white to slightly pink and whorled cut surface.

are rare. In Alpert syndrome, a small number of women develop numerous uterine leiomyomas (*diffuse leiomyomatosis*) (10). Proteus syndrome is characterized by excessive and asymmetric growth of numerous tissues and organs, and uterine leiomyomas also develop (11), while in patients with Cowden syndrome, the development of leiomyomas is a minor criterion for the diagnosis (12). Familial factors, hormones, and obesity also increase the frequency of leiomyomas (13,14).

Clinical Features. Leiomyomas are seen at any age but are most common during the reproductive years. FH-related tumors present in patients in their twenties (15). Although most patients are asymptomatic, when symptoms/signs occur, they often correlate with location, size, and presence of associated degenerative changes.

Manifestations are divided into three main categories: abnormal uterine bleeding, pelvic pressure/pain, and those related to fertility (16). Abnormal uterine bleeding is by far the most common presenting sign, typically as menorrhagia, hypermenorrhea, or prolonged excessive menstruation; those in a submucosal location more commonly cause symptoms. Secondarily, patients may develop severe iron-deficiency anemia.

Pelvic/abdominal pain often occurs when the uterus increases in size; symptoms relate to the location of the leiomyoma. Leiomyomas in which torsion occurs, those that protrude through the cervical canal, and those associated with secondary acute hemorrhage (*apoplectic leiomyomas*) also cause pain. If the myoma is large, the patient may present with a pelvic mass and secondary gastrointestinal or urinary symptoms due to compression.

Patients may have a history of infertility, increased rates of spontaneous abortions, and pregnancy related complications, especially when there is a submucosal myoma or a markedly distorted uterus (including diffuse leiomyomatosis) with secondary involvement of the endometrium. Leiomyomas that rapidly enlarge may cause clinical concern for malignancy, although the most likely diagnosis is still leiomyoma.

Patients with *FH* germline mutations develop symptoms at an early age (median, 28 years) as tumors are often large, and they undergo hysterectomy before 30 years of age (17–20). About 30 percent of patients with HLRCC also have secondary infertility or recurrent miscarriages (20).

Rarely, patients, including pregnant and postpartum women, with leiomyomas present with acute abdomen or hemoperitoneum due to rupture of their leiomyomas (21). Benign metastasizing leiomyomas may be an incidental finding in patients undergoing X-ray evaluation for another issue, or they appear as solitary or multiple pulmonary nodules that may enhance homogeneously if solid but may be cystic (22).

Leiomyomas are markedly affected by estrogen and progesterone cyclical hormonal changes. Thus, they are rarely reported in adolescents. Patients become symptomatic at 30 to 40 years of age and often symptoms are ameliorated with menopause. Some leiomyoma variants, including diffuse peritoneal leiomyomatosis, are seen more frequently in pregnant or postpartum women, or those taking oral contraceptives, including progestogens, gonadotropin-releasing hormone agonist (GnRHa), and tranexamic acid (23,24). The use of morcellation as a surgical technique has increased the number of cases of iatrogenic parasitic myomas and diffuse peritoneal leiomyomatosis, which impart an appearance similar to that seen in pregnant women (25–30).

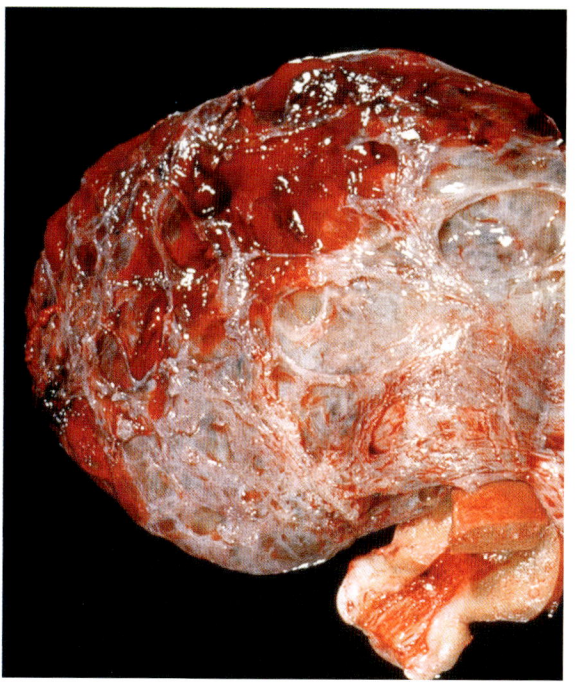 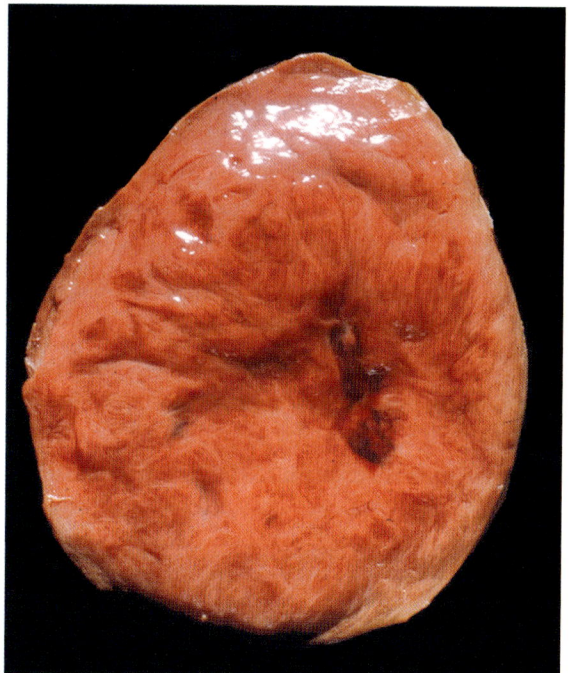

Figure 10-2

LEIOMYOMA WITH SECONDARY CHANGES

Edematous and focally hemorrhagic cut surface with cyst formation may cause concern for malignancy (left). Diffuse dusky color with a minimal rim of viable smooth muscle (red degeneration) as seen in pregnancy or postpartum (right).

Patients with intravenous leiomyomatosis may occasionally present with cardiac manifestations due to tumor extension into the inferior vena cava and right heart, and undergo complete clinical regression after presentation during pregnancy (31). Other less frequent signs and symptoms include secondary erythrocytosis, infection, and ascites (pseudomeig syndrome) (32,33).

Gross Findings. Leiomyomas occur more commonly in the uterine fundus and rarely in the lower uterine segment or cervix. They are typically intramural, less frequently submucosal or subserosal, and often multiple, distorting the uterus (fig. 10-1). If subserosal, the leiomyoma may be pedunculated and twist, with secondary detachment from the uterus, in some instances, becoming attached to adjacent pelvic structures (*parasitic leiomyoma*).

Leiomyomas are characteristically sharply circumscribed and can easily be shelled out from the neighboring myometrium. A bulging white to slightly pink, firm and whorled cut surface is typical, but ulceration (mainly if submucosal), edema, hemorrhage, cyst formation (fig. 10-2, left), and less frequently, calcification or ossification occur. Red degeneration is characteristic of pregnancy or postpartum (fig. 10-2, right).

Leiomyomas show a wide spectrum of gross appearances, especially within leiomyoma variants. Some are related to their constituents and others related to their growth patterns. When handling typical leiomyomas, therefore, it is not necessary to sample each one rigorously, but any tumor with an unusual appearance should be carefully studied and sampled generously as some of these features are also seen in malignant tumors. For example, mitotically active leiomyomas frequently display soft, fleshy or cystic areas with foci of hemorrhage, and they are frequently submucosal (24,34,35). Apoplectic or hemorrhagic leiomyomas show one or more areas of stellate and discrete hemorrhage that may be accompanied by cystic change or necrosis if hemorrhage is extensive or confluent (fig. 10-3). Its color may be different from typical leiomyoma and it may involve more than one leiomyoma (21,36,37). Leiomyomas with

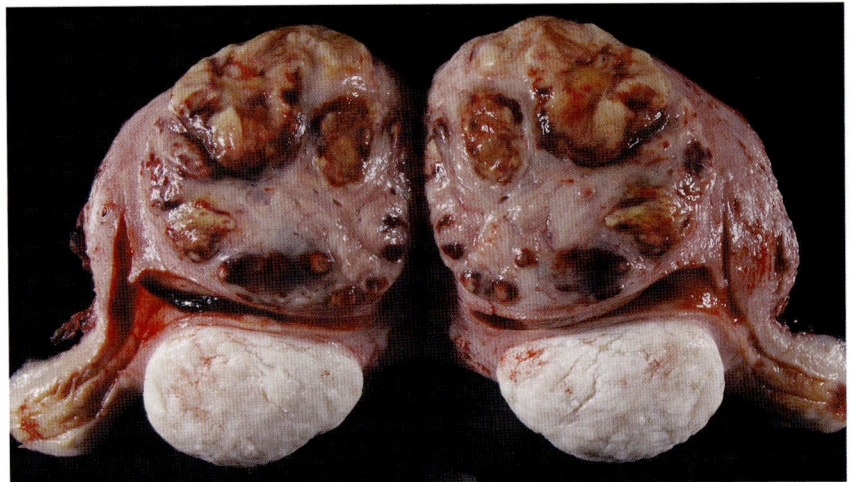

Figure 10-3
APOPLECTIC LEIOMYOMA

Multiple, discrete, rounded nodules have a tan to hemorrhagic cut surface. This appearance contrasts with the homogeneous, white and firm cut surface of an adjacent typical leiomyoma.

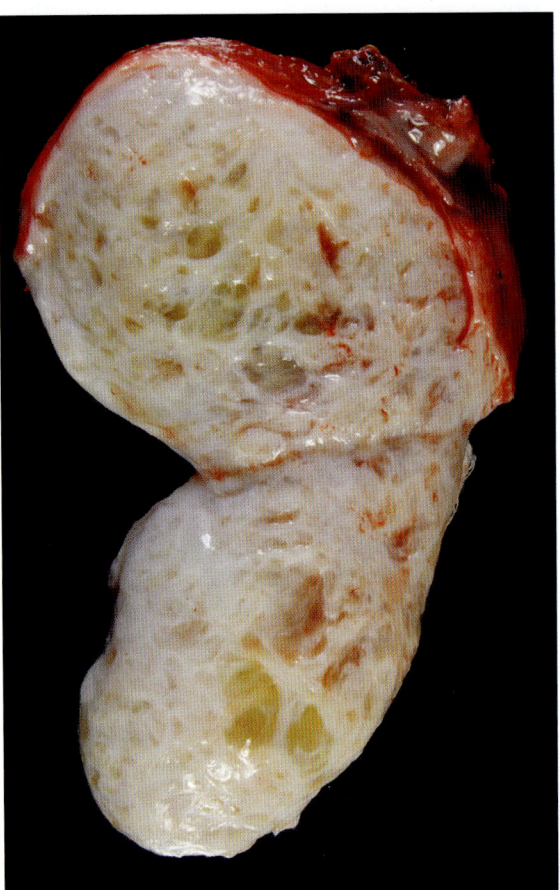
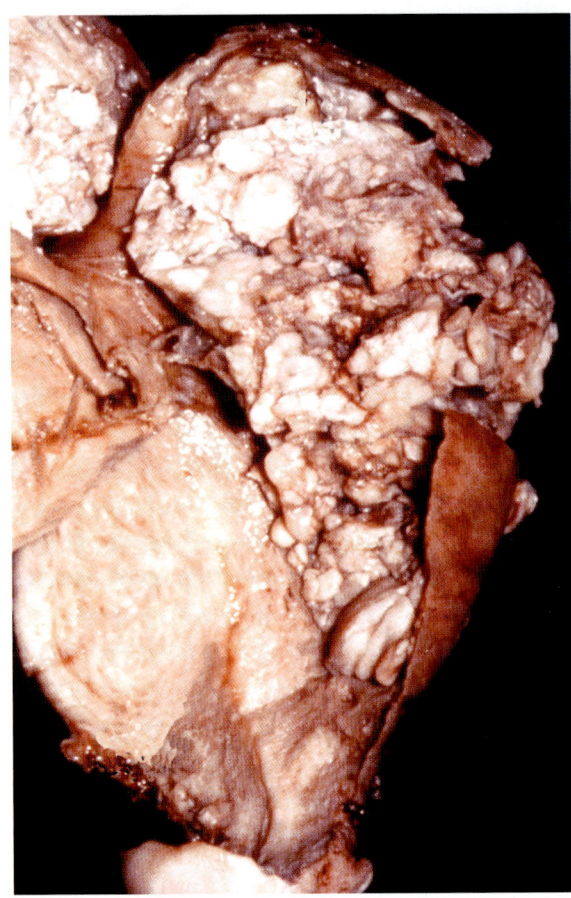

Figure 10-4
HYDROPIC LEIOMYOMA

The tumor has a soft and uniformly pale rather than firm, whorled, white cut surface secondary to abundant edema fluid, which lead to the formation of irregular cystic spaces (left). Multiple small white nodules are separated by empty spaces due to exudation of edema (perinodular). This appearance can be grossly misinterpreted as intravenous leiomyomatosis. The typical cut surface is seen at the bottom half of the tumor (right).

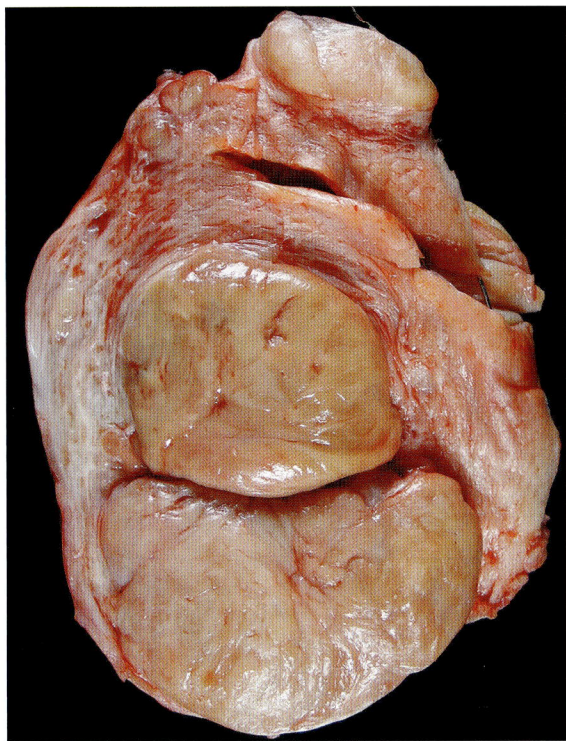

Figure 10-5

HIGHLY CELLULAR LEIOMYOMA

Well-circumscribed nodule with a homogeneous tan and soft cut surface.

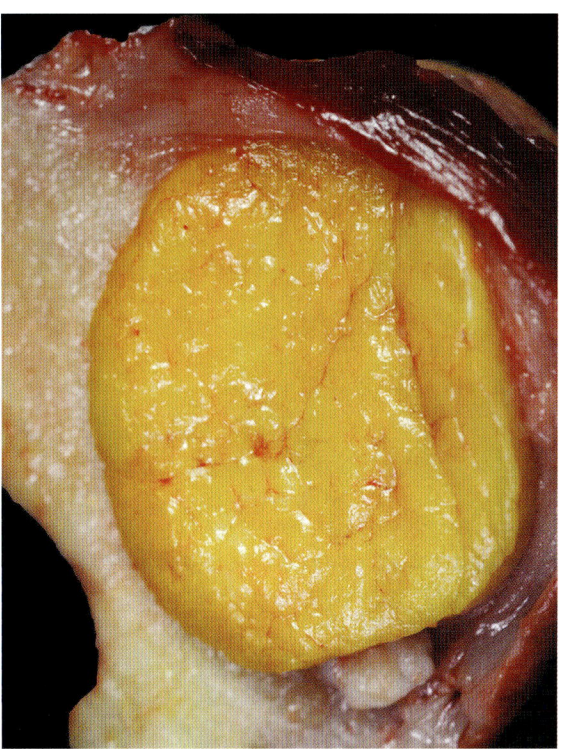

Figure 10-6

LIPOLEIOMYOMA

The tumor has abundant fat and a gross appearance similar to that of a lipoma.

hydropic change may exudate watery fluid on cut section and have cystic spaces (fig. 10-4, left). Some tumors in this group may show a striking nodular appearance, with white to tan nodules separated by edematous tissue (*perinodular hydropic leiomyoma*) (fig. 10-4, right) (38). Leiomyomas with bizarre nuclei frequently have a white and firm cut surface and can be yellow (39,40). Highly cellular leiomyomas are often tan to yellow and soft (fig. 10-5), epithelioid leiomyomas may have a soft cut surface (41), and lipoleiomyoma may display grossly visible yellow soft areas that correspond to the adipose component randomly present between white and firm areas (fig. 10-6). FH-related leiomyomas, which have the typical appearance of leiomyomas, tend to be multiple and large. Myxoid leiomyoma often has a homogeneous, soft, gray, jelly-like cut surface.

Benign smooth muscle proliferations that are associated with unusual growth include *dissecting leiomyoma* (including those with intramyometrial or extrauterine extension [*cotyledonoid leiomyoma, Sternberg tumor*]), *diffuse leiomyomatosis, diffuse leiomyomatosis peritonealis, intravenous leiomyomatosis,* and *benign metastasizing leiomyoma.* Cotyledonoid dissecting leiomyomas project from the uterine serosa and have a striking bosselated and congested appearance that has been described as placental-like (fig. 10-7). They tend to be large (average, 15.4 cm) and nodules are attached to each other by thin membranes (42). *Dissecting noncotyledonoid leiomyomas* are typically intramyometrial, with an irregular lobulated appearance, without an exophytic component (43). *Diffuse leiomyomatosis* displays a diffuse regular thickening of the myometrium due to multiple, often smaller than 1 cm, poorly circumscribed nodules which often blend with each other (fig. 10-8). *Diffuse peritoneal leiomyomatosis* is characterized by studding of the omentum and other peritoneal surfaces by well-demarcated, small (typically less than 2 cm, rarely larger, but always less than 10 cm), white firm nodules (fig. 10-9).

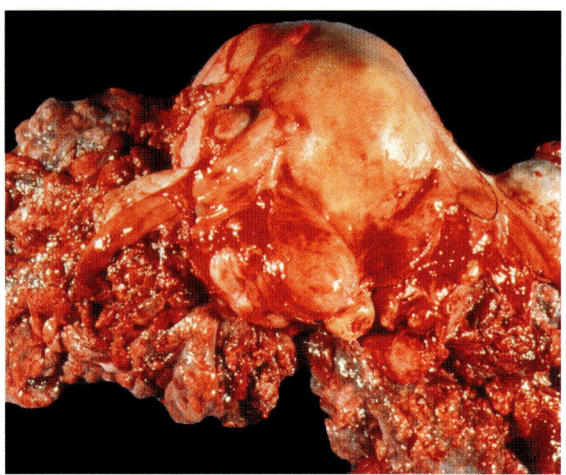

Figure 10-7

DISSECTING COTYLEDONOID LEIOMYOMA

There is a prominent exophytic component with a multinodular growth and hemorrhagic appearance that is reminiscent of placental tissue.

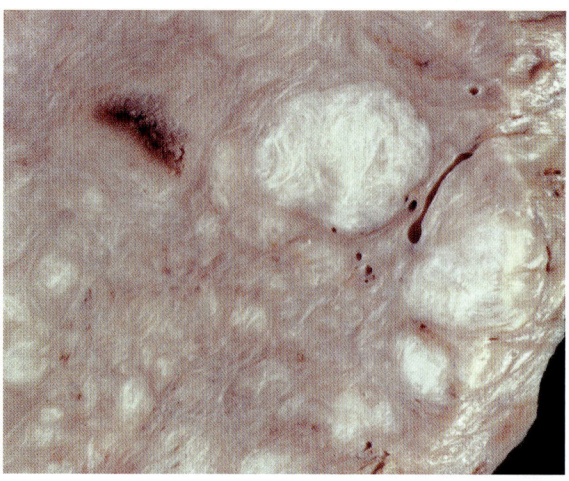

Figure 10-8

DIFFUSE LEIOMYOMATOSIS

Multiple, coalescent, small white whorled nodules are present within the myometrium.

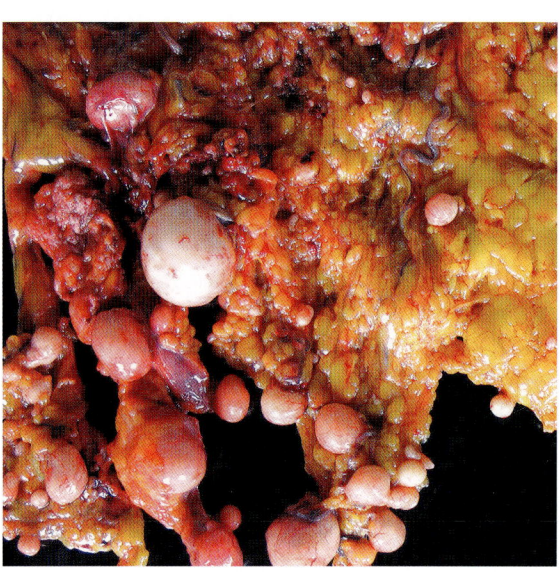

Figure 10-9

DIFFUSE PERITONEAL LEIOMYOMATOSIS

Multiple, well-circumscribed, variably sized (most less than 2 cm) nodules are present within the omentum. The nodules may be microscopic in size, cellular, and have a tendency to coalesce.

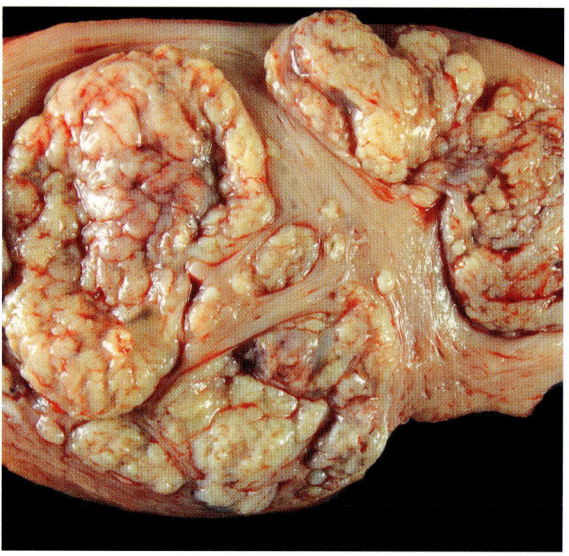

Figure 10-10

INTRAVENOUS LEIOMYOMATOSIS

Multiple rounded nodules with an irregular distribution are noted in the myometrium. Only those more peripheral suggest intravascular growth as they appear to bulge, and on close examination may be seen within veins.

Intravenous leiomyomatosis is seen as multiple, rounded nodules in the myometrium, with or without involvement of parametrial tissues, that at first glance may be grossly diagnosed as leiomyoma (fig. 10-10). In 80 percent of cases, tumor extends beyond the uterus and may be seen in extrauterine veins. The nodules range up to 18 cm, are white to tan to yellow, and are rubbery to spongy. However, especially if tumor is present outside the uterus, coiled worm-like plugs of white tissue may be seen, sometimes distending vascular spaces. Intravenous leiomyomatosis may coexist with leiomyomas but typically is present outside them (44). *Benign metastasizing leiomyoma* is characterized by the finding of one or more extrauterine small (rarely up to 10 cm), white, firm nodules most frequently in the lungs (fig. 10-11) (and less commonly in retroperitoneal and mediastinal lymph nodes, soft tissues, and bone) in women who have had typical uterine leiomyomas, leiomyomas with vascular invasion, or intravenous leiomyomatosis.

Microscopic Findings. Classic leiomyomas are microscopically often well circumscribed. Cells with abundant eosinophilic cytoplasm and elongated "cigar"-shaped nuclei form interweaving fascicles that are separated by varying amounts of collagen (fig. 10-12). If cells are cut transversely, the nuclei appear round, sometimes with an associated paranuclear vacuole. The nuclei display no cytologic atypia and low

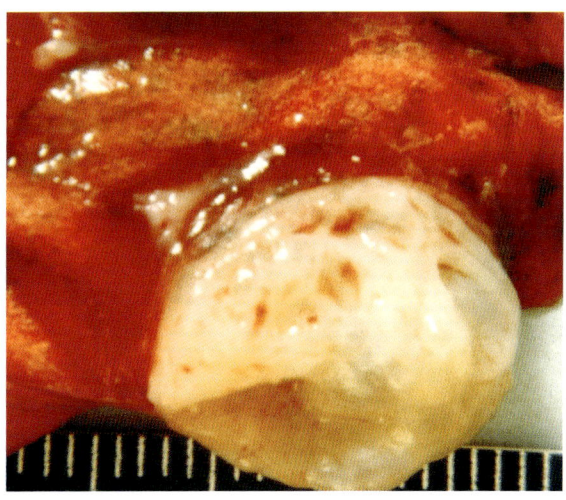

Figure 10-11

BENIGN METASTASIZING LEIOMYOMA

A well-circumscribed nodule bulges from the surrounding lung parenchyma. It has a homogeneous cut surface with associated small cysts.

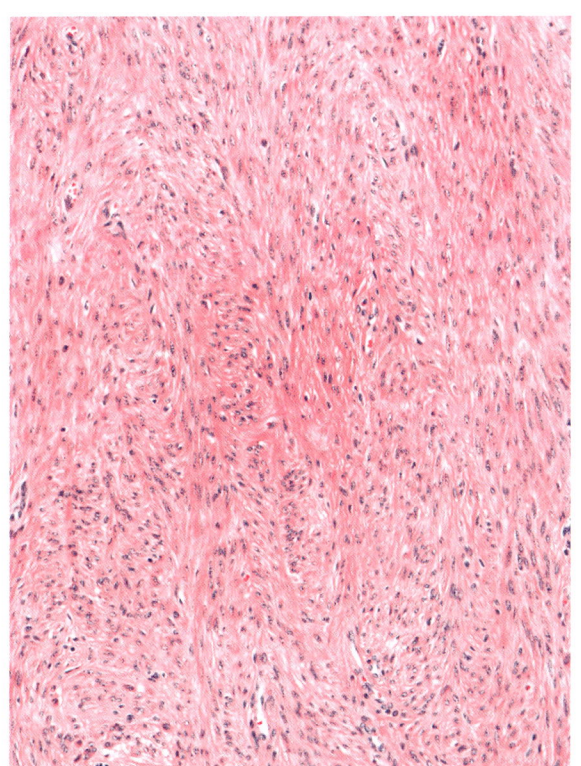 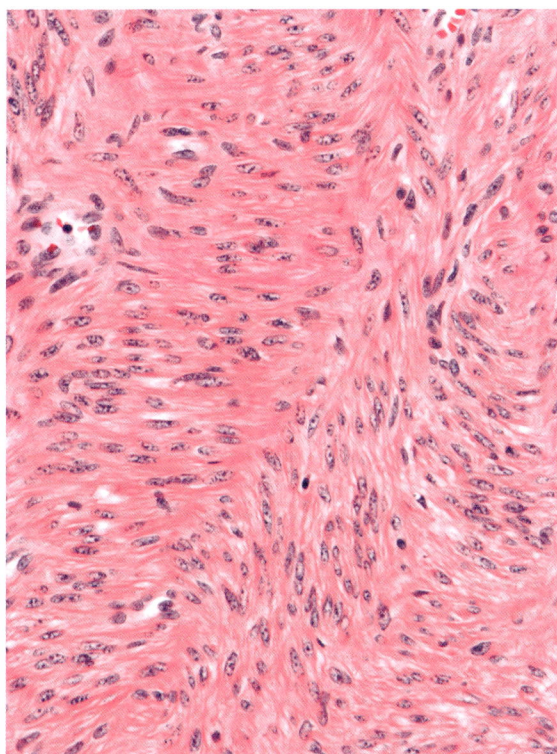

Figure 10-12

TYPICAL LEIOMYOMA

There is a fascicular growth of spindle cells with abundant eosinophilic cytoplasm (left). The nuclei have a cigar-shaped appearance, with homogeneous, delicate chromatin and tiny nucleoli (right).

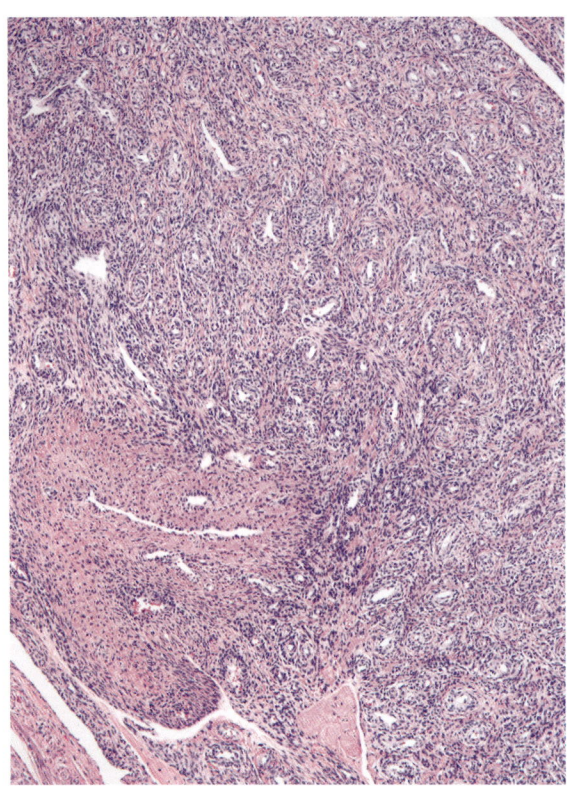 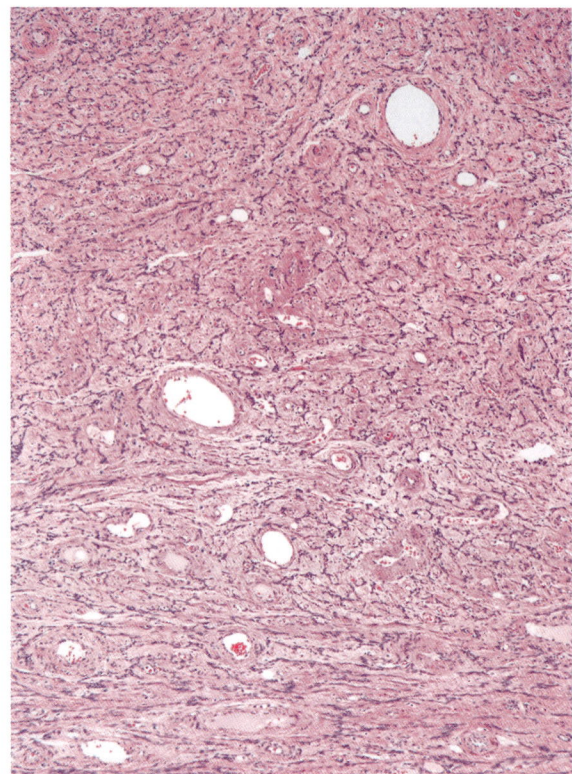

Figure 10-13

TYPICAL LEIOMYOMA

Small vessels mimic those seen in endometrial stromal tumors (left). Thin cords of neoplastic smooth muscle cells are present between a prominent component of vessels, some of which are ectatic (right).

mitotic activity is noted. Several specific variant patterns of leiomyomas have received unique designations such as apoplectic or mitotically active among others, and these are considered under separate headings (below).

Other variant appearances are seen in leiomyomas and occasionally cause confusion. Leiomyomas may contain abundant vasculature, and when displaying thick muscular walls, have been termed *angioleiomyomas* (45) although most do not use that term. The vessels may also be small (fig. 10-13, left). The smooth muscle fibers may not form typical fascicles, but thin cords between the vessels that may impart an unusual appearance (fig. 10-13, right). Palisading of the nuclei, as seen more commonly in benign nerve sheath tumors (neurilemoma-like), may occur (fig. 10-14, left) (46). Skeletal-like or rhabdoid cells with abundant eosinophilic cytoplasm are seen on occasion in leiomyomas without bizarre nuclei (47). Collagen bands may be present (fig. 10-14, right) and rarely, amianthoid-like fibers as seen in myofibroblastoma (48). Typical leiomyomas may contain foci of extramedullary hematopoiesis (49,50) and striking collections of lymphocytes (fig. 10-15) (51,52), mast cells (53,54), eosinophils (55), or histiocytes (56), the latter especially seen in patients taking gonadotropin-releasing hormone agonists (GnRHa). Some leiomyomas become infected, and large amounts of acute inflammatory cells may form abscesses (*pyomyoma*) (57,58). The term *seedling leiomyoma* is applied to tiny leiomyomas that are present at the periphery of a larger leiomyoma (59,60).

Leiomyomas may undergo ulceration and subsequent necrosis secondary to trauma (especially submucosal leiomyomas) and infarct-type necrosis. The latter is characterized by the finding of necrotic tissue with a "mummified" and

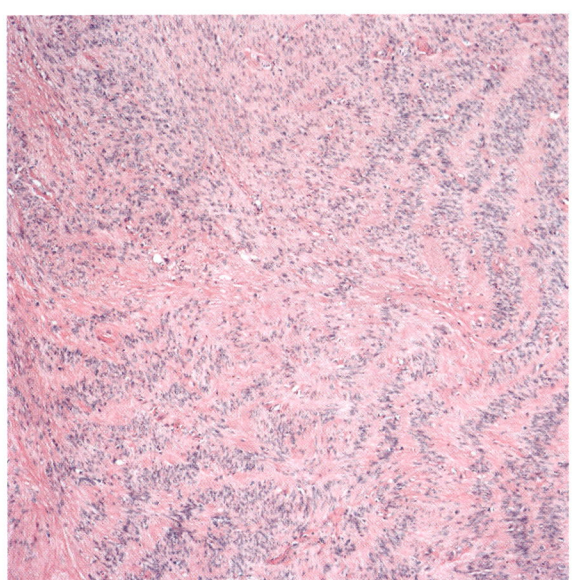
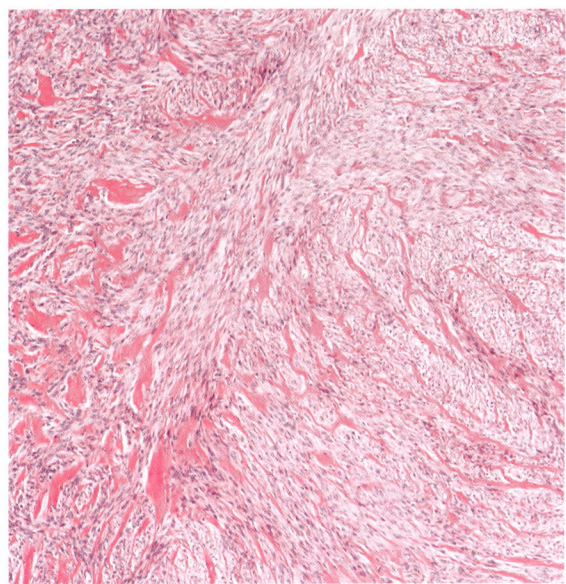

Figure 10-14

TYPICAL LEIOMYOMA

Striking palisading of nuclei (left). Irregular collagen bands are seen between fascicles of smooth muscle cells (right).

homogeneous appearance where tumor cells as well as vessels appear dead. There is an area of transition between the nonviable and viable tumor that is composed of granulation tissue or hyalinized tissue depending on the age of the infarct and may be associated with areas of recent hemorrhage (fig. 10-16A). There is no perivascular growth of tumor cells (with rare exceptions) or a dirty necrotic background, in contrast to tumor cell necrosis. Infarct-type necrosis is seen in both leiomyomas and leiomyosarcomas (61–63).

Leiomyoma with Bizarre Nuclei ("Symplastic" Leiomyoma). In the past, symplastic and atypical leiomyoma were synonymous of leiomyoma with bizarre nuclei, however, in the most recent 2014 World Health Organization (WHO) classification, the term "atypical leiomyoma" has been eliminated (1). On low-power examination, these tumors are typically well circumscribed and are associated with moderate to high cellularity (fig. 10-17). The cardinal and defining feature of these tumors is the presence of cells with atypical "worrisome" nuclei, frequently multinucleated but sometimes mononucleated, with focal, multifocal, or diffuse, albeit most frequently "spotty" distribution, and with low or intermediate density of the

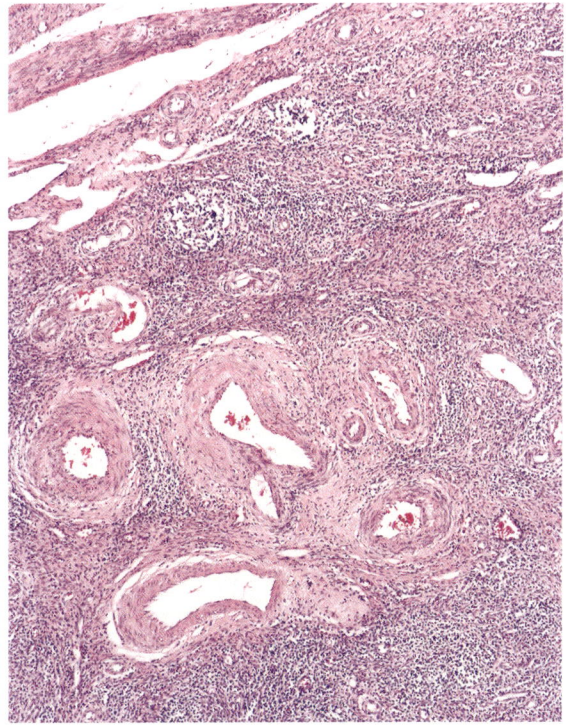

Figure 10-15

TYPICAL LEIOMYOMA

Lymphoid aggregates are present throughout the tumor.

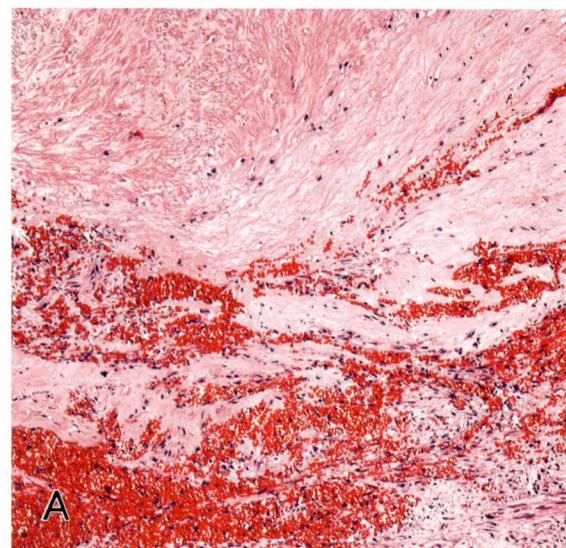

Figure 10-16

INFARCT-TYPE NECROSIS IN LEIOMYOMA

There is a central area of mummified smooth muscle neoplasia where ghost cells from tumor and vessels are seen. A rim of recent hemorrhage associated with some collagen separates that area from viable tumor (A). Areas close to infarct-type necrosis show increased Ki-67 expression (B) and increased p16 expression (C).

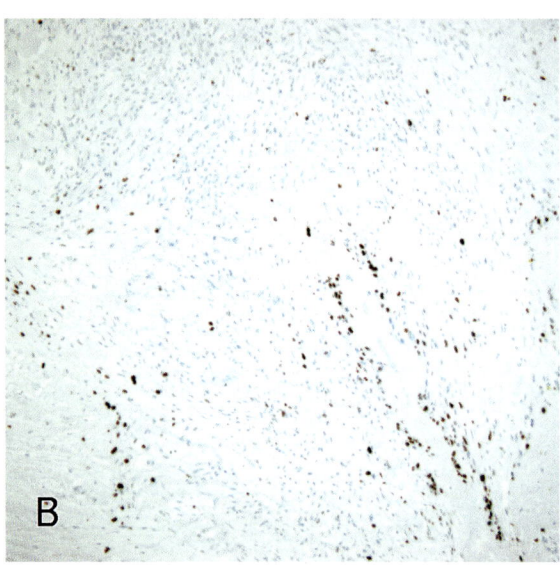
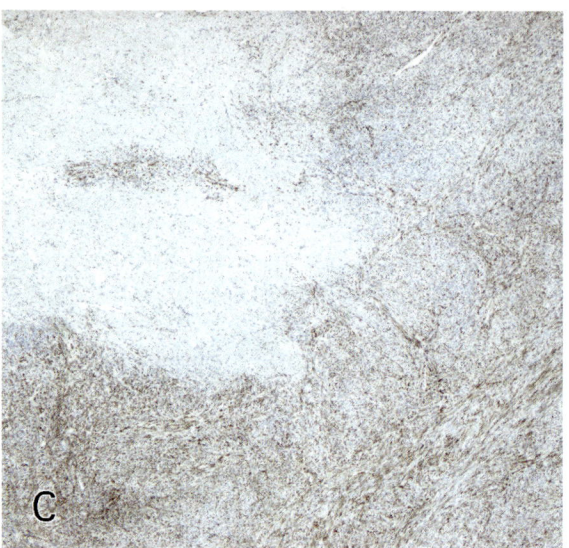

bizarre nuclei in most tumors (fig. 10-18A,B) (39,40,61,64,65). In the past tumors with such cells were considered malignant, but Evans first highlighted that this morphologic feature is not associated with poor outcome in smooth muscle tumors (66). The nuclei may show clear or eosinophilic nuclear pseudoinclusions, which may be striking, or may be pyknotic, with dense smudged chromatin (fig. 10-18A,B). They frequently show prominent nucleoli, coarse chromatin, and mitotic activity as high as 7 to 8 per 10 high-power fields (average 1 to 2 mitoses). Karyorrhectic nuclei are often noted and may be striking (fig. 10-18C). The latter may simulate abnormal mitotic figures, however, caution should be exercised before making that interpretation in a smooth muscle tumor with very low mitotic activity. In karyorrhectic cells, the chromatin is typically coarse while the cell cytoplasm is dense and often shows retraction artifact (fig. 10-18C) (39,40). The cytoplasm of most cells is abundant and eosinophilic, and some contain eosinophilic globules, imparting a rhabdoid appearance (representing whorls of intermediate filaments) without cross striations (47). The associated nonbizarre background cells are spindled, with cigar-shaped nuclei and uniform bland cytologic features (fig. 10-19, left).

Smooth Muscle and Other Mesenchymal Tumors

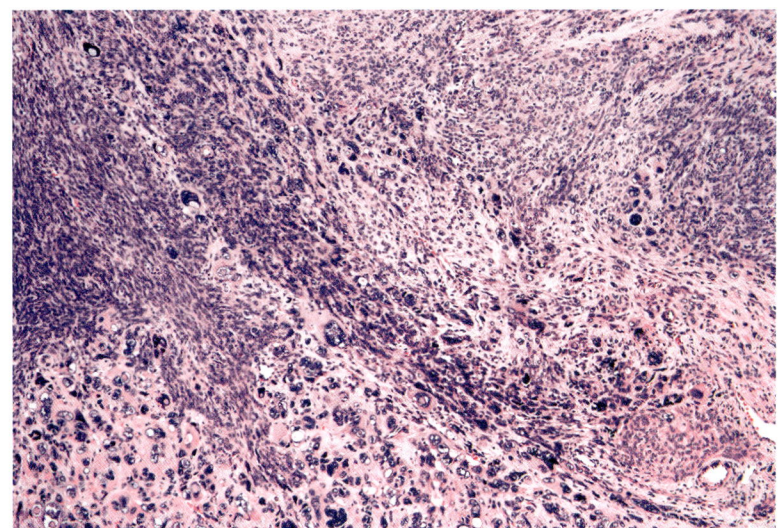

Figure 10-17

LEIOMYOMA WITH BIZARRE NUCLEI

There is increased cellularity with multifocal distribution of cells with bizarre nuclei in a background of typical leiomyoma.

Figure 10-18

LEIOMYOMA WITH BIZARRE NUCLEI

Atypical multinucleated and mononucleated cells display prominent nuclear pseudoinclusions, prominent nucleoli, smudged chromatin, and dense eosinophilic cytoplasm (A–C). A karyorrhectic cell has coarse chromatin as well as dense and retractile eosinophilic cytoplasm (C).

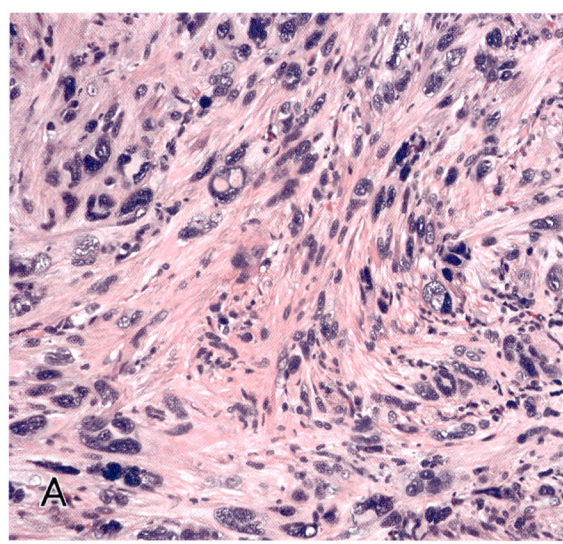
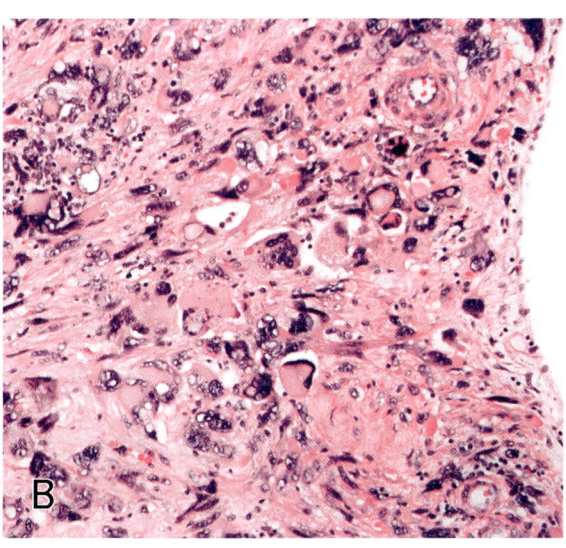
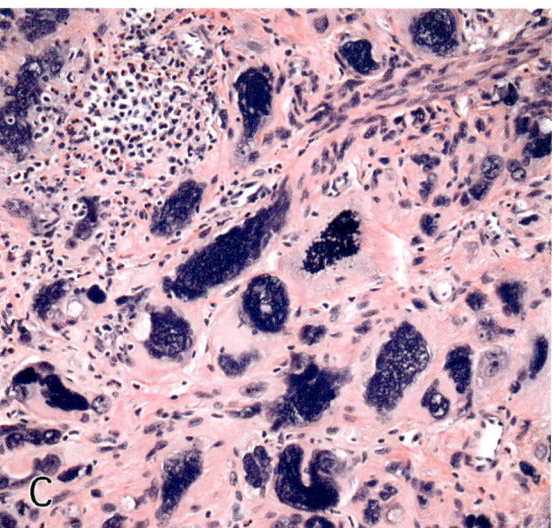

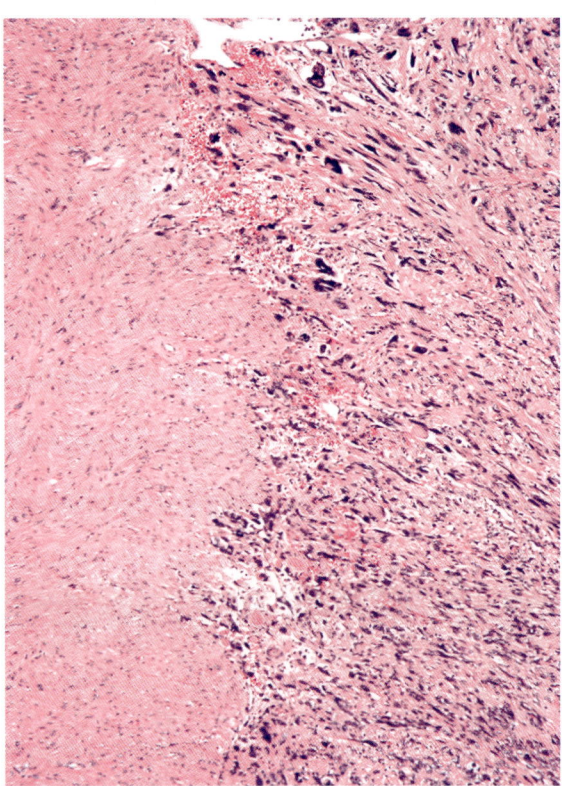 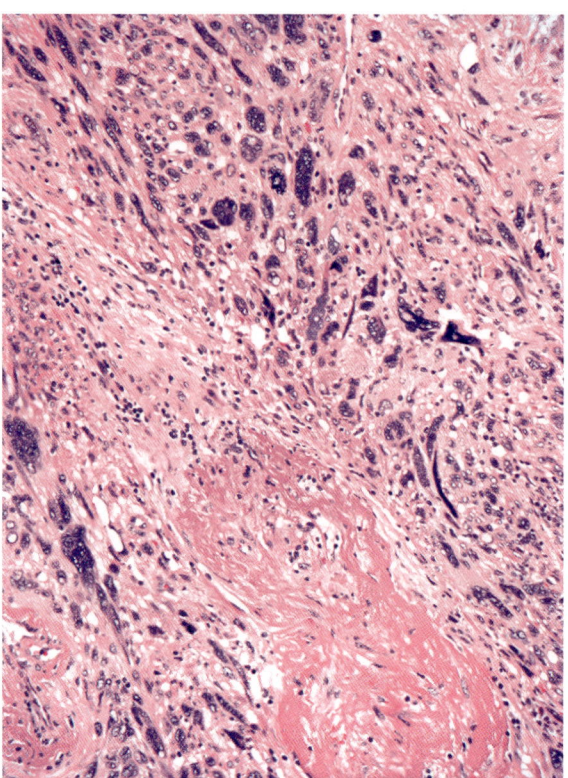

Figure 10-19

LEIOMYOMA WITH BIZARRE NUCLEI

The nonbizarre smooth muscle cells have banal cytologic features and the two components appear juxtaposed, although more frequently they are closely admixed (left). Fibrinoid change is seen within a large blood vessel associated with sparkling of lymphocytes (right).

Most tumors contain large and thick blood vessels, frequently associated with fibrinoid necrosis, perivascular lymphocytic infiltrates, or luminal obliteration (fig. 10-19, right). As seen in other leiomyomas, areas of hyalinization or hydropic change may occur. The striking degenerative nuclear atypia likely correlates with the presence of abundant heterochromatin, which is known to be associated with inactivated DNA (67).

Fumarate Hydratase (FH)-Deficient Leiomyoma. This leiomyoma variant was in the past classified as leiomyoma with bizarre nuclei since it shares the presence of cells with bizarre nuclei. Recently, however, leiomyomas with these cells have been divided in two types. Leiomyomas associated with deficient FH (type I) have a higher density and diffuse distribution of cells with bizarre nuclei; multinucleation is more common than bizarre atypia when compared to those unassociated with FH deficiency (type II; typical leiomyomas with bizarre nuclei) (68).

FH-deficient tumors are typically well circumscribed. At low-power magnification, they often have a prominent vascular component of staghorn (hemangiopericytoma-like) vessels (fig. 10-20, left) as well as a delicate fibrillary background corresponding to cells cytoplasm (fig. 10-20, right). The finding of orangiophilic (inclusion-like) nucleoli surrounded by a perinucleolar halo is one of the morphologic hallmarks of these tumors (fig. 10-21), also seen in renal tumors but not in cutaneous leiomyomas within the HLRCC syndrome (Reed syndrome) (69–73). The nuclei tend to be round with vesicular chromatin imparting a vague epithelioid appearance. Mitoses range from 3 to 4 per 10 high-power fields (71). Eosinophilic cytoplasmic globules that impart a rhabdoid appearance (fig. 10-22, left) and alveolar-type edema (fig. 10-

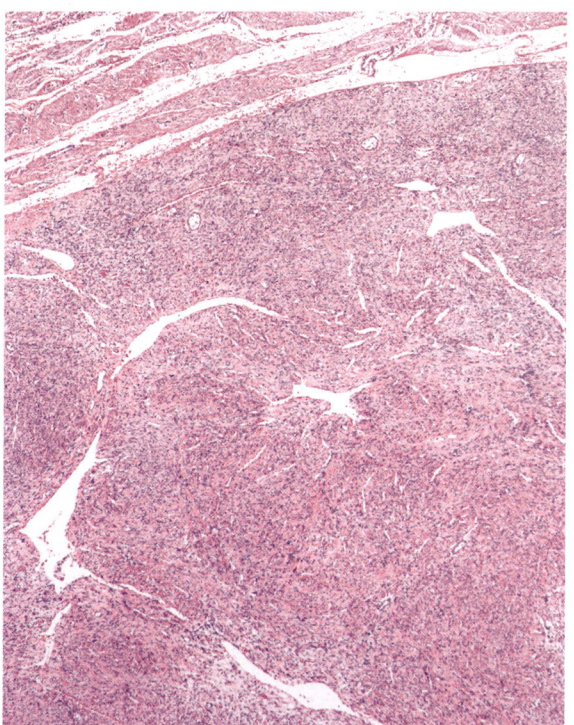
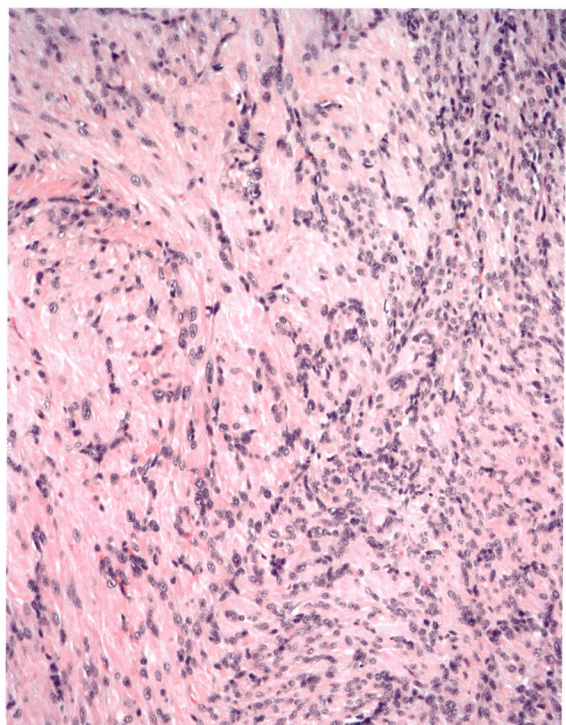

Figure 10-20

FUMARATE HYDRATASE-DEFICIENT LEIOMYOMA

The tumor is hypercellular and shows a striking staghorn vasculature (left). The cytoplasm is abundant and eosinophilic, with a fibrillary appearance (right).

22, right) are characteristic features. The latter is typically a focal or multifocal microscopic finding and consists of striking edema seen between thin muscle fibers; the appearance vaguely resembles pulmonary alveoli (72). All these features may be only focally present within the tumor (74,75) and do not correlate accurately with the presence of somatic or germline mutations, although in one study, staghorn vessels correlated with abnormal FH expression by multivariate analysis (72).

Cellular Leiomyoma. The degree of cellularity within a cellular leiomyoma ranges from more cellular than the surrounding myometrium to comparable to that seen in endometrial stromal tumors (highly cellular), although the term highly cellular has been excluded from latest WHO classification (1). When highly cellular, tumors typically have a diffuse growth of cells in the center (fig. 10-23A) that merges with a fascicular growth at the periphery. Cells range from oval (in the center) to spindle-shaped (at

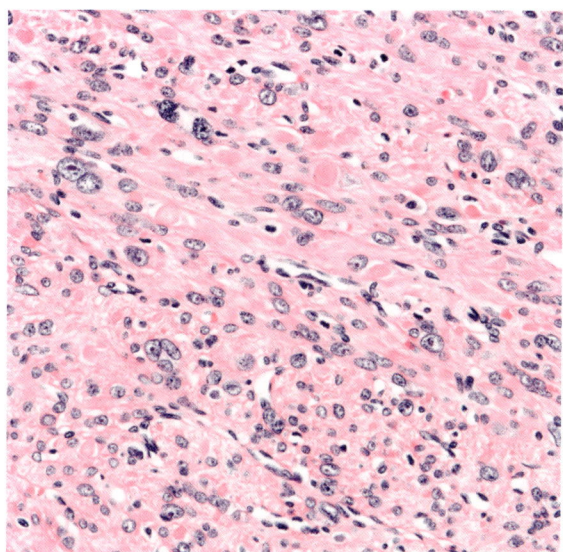

Figure 10-21

FUMARATE HYDRATASE-DEFICIENT LEIOMYOMA

Cells display large nuclei with delicate chromatin and prominent orangeophilic nucleoli associated with a perinucleolar halo.

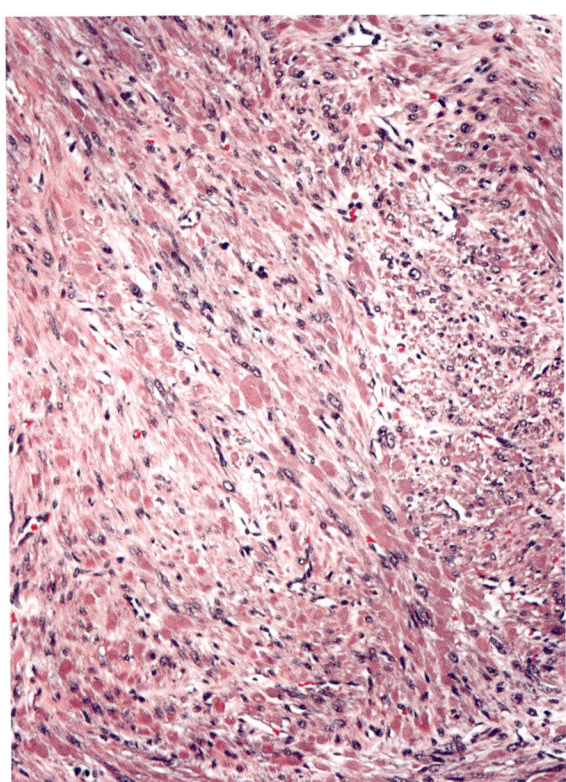 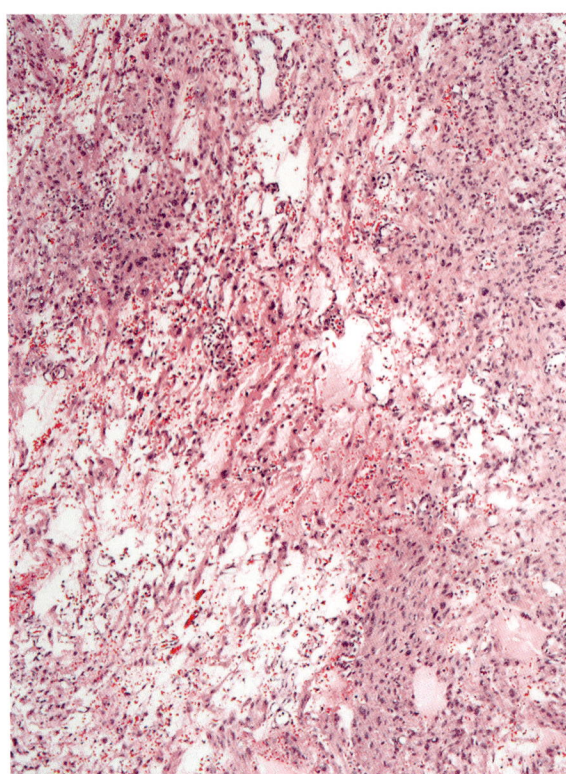

Figure 10-22

FUMARATE HYDRATASE-DEFICIENT LEIOMYOMA

Many eosinophilic intracytoplasmic globules impart a rhabdoid appearance (left). Focal edema has an appearance reminiscent of pulmonary alveoli (alveolar edema) (right).

the periphery), and have scant cytoplasm. Cytologic atypia and mitotic activity are minimal to absent, but tumors rarely may be mitotically active, display bizarre nuclei, or comprise a variable area of a conventional leiomyoma.

Large and thick blood vessels are typically a striking feature (fig. 10-23B) while small vessels may also be seen, sometimes mimicking the appearance of arterioles. Cleft-like spaces are a characteristic and often conspicuous feature (fig. 10-23B) of these tumors, either the result of compressed vessels if lined by endothelial cells or retraction artifact secondary to edema if endothelial cells are lacking. Areas of hyalinization or hemorrhage can be seen.

Although the margin of the tumor is often well circumscribed, irregular extension to the myometrium may be seen (fig. 10-23C); at closer magnification, neoplastic cells at the periphery of the tumor merge imperceptibly with the surrounding myometrium, a clue to determine its smooth muscle nature (41). Sometimes, multiple cellular leiomyomas are seen, with one being predominant and the other small and peripheral (seedling leiomyomas), an appearance that may cause concern for an endometrial stromal sarcoma (fig. 10-24).

Mitotically Active Leiomyoma. This leiomyoma variant is variably cellular (and may be markedly cellular), with a low-power appearance typically identical to that seen in a conventional leiomyoma. At high power, however, it is typically characterized by an increased number of mitoses (5 to 15 per 10 high-power fields) (fig. 10-25) (24,34,35,76) without atypical mitoses (34,35). In one study, most of these leiomyomas had 10 mitoses per 10 high-power fields (35).

The most important criterion in the diagnosis of a mitotically active leiomyoma is the absence of cytologic atypia (fig. 10-25). Rarely, more than one leiomyoma is mitotically active in the same patient (35). As originally pointed out by

Smooth Muscle and Other Mesenchymal Tumors

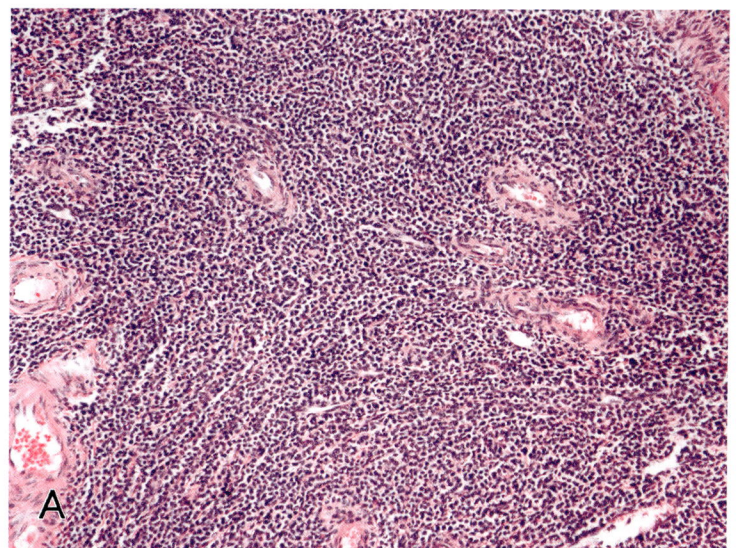

Figure 10-23
HIGHLY CELLULAR LEIOMYOMA
This is a highly cellular "blue" tumor. The cellularity is comparable to that seen in conventional endometrial stromal tumors (A). Thick and large blood vessels and cleft-like spaces are characteristic of these tumors (B). An irregular border with the surrounding myometrium may cause concern for infiltration, but tumor cells merge with the surrounding myometrium (C).

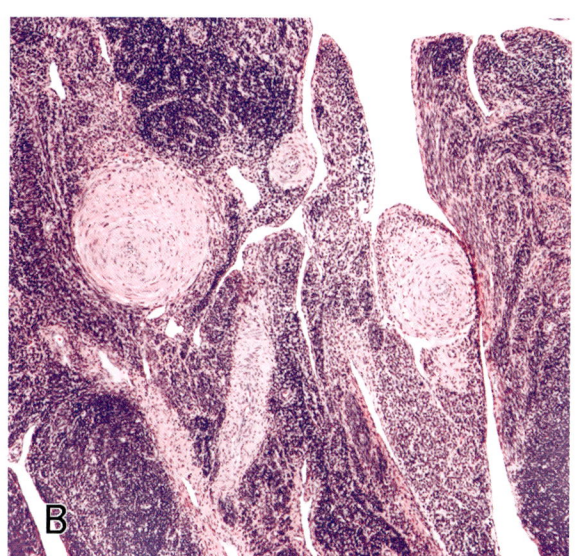
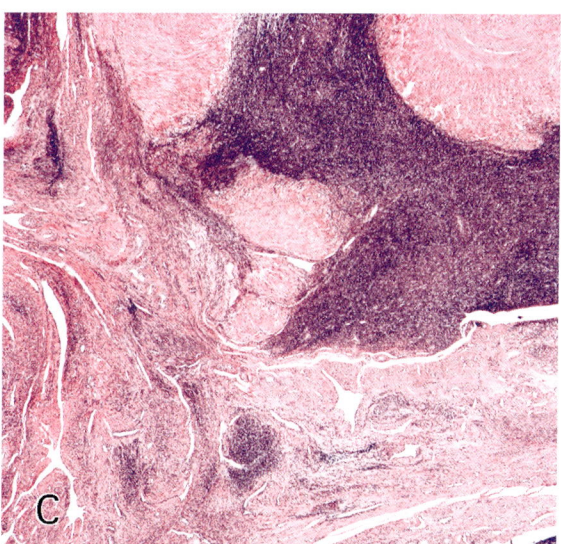

Figure 10-24
HIGHLY CELLULAR LEIOMYOMA WITH SEEDLING CELLULAR LEIOMYOMAS
The small cellular leiomyomas may be interpreted at low power as endometrial stromal sarcoma. (Fig. 3 from Oliva E. Cellular mesenchymal tumors of the uterus: a review emphasizing recent observations. Int J Gynecol Pathol 2014;33:374-84.)

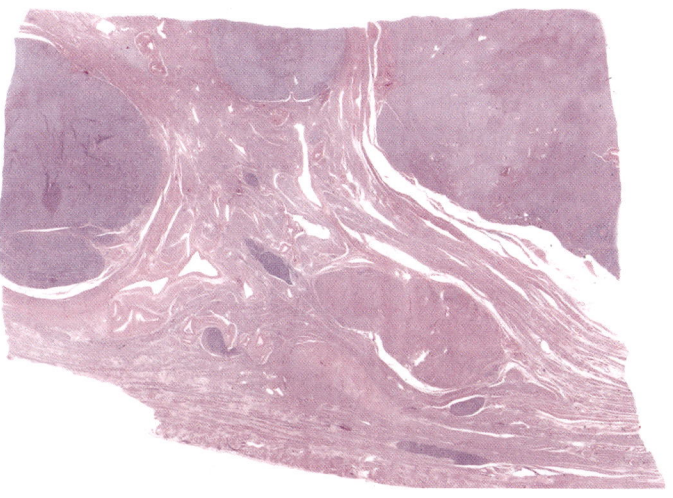

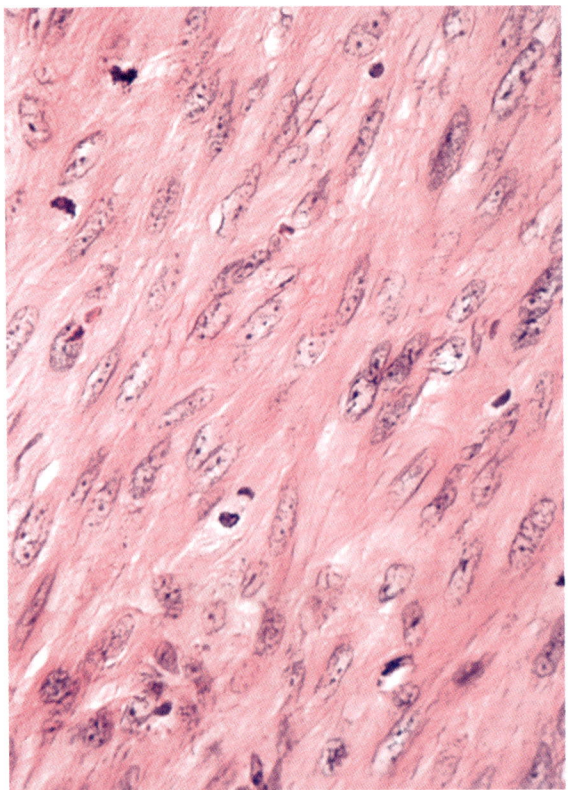

Figure 10-25

MITOTICALLY ACTIVE LEIOMYOMA

Spindle cells are associated with brisk mitotic activity. There is no cytologic atypia.

Silverberg (77) and later on, by Hart and Billman (78), mitotic activity is not a reliable indicator of prognosis when isolated from other factors in evaluating typical (spindle) smooth muscle tumors. These tumors are well circumscribed and although there may be infarct-type necrosis, they lack, by definition, tumor cell necrosis. Extensive sampling should exclude foci of cytologic atypia or tumor cell necrosis that would establish a diagnosis of leiomyosarcoma.

Rarely, a banal-appearing smooth muscle tumor has a mitotic count over 15 mitoses per 10 high-power fields. As experience with these tumors is limited, the designation of smooth muscle tumor with increased mitotic index or smooth muscle tumor of uncertain malignant behavior may be appropriate (61). Increased mitotic activity in these tumors may be related to the mitogenic effect of progesterone in the myometrium during the menstrual cycle since secretory-type endometrium is seen at time of resection of the leiomyoma in 50 to 60 percent of cases (34).

Leiomyoma with Hydropic (Including Diffuse and Perinodular) Change. Hydropic change is reported in about half of leiomyomas (79). It is defined by the finding of edematous fluid (alcian blue negative or at most faintly positive) within poorly demarcated areas of connective tissue that alternate with areas of compact smooth muscle neoplasia (38,80–82). The edematous areas show a dropout of smooth muscle cells, are typically hypocellular, and display scattered fibroblasts associated with collagen bands and blood vessels of variable thickness. The smooth muscle component within these areas may be absent or present as thin and elongated cords or plexiform arrangements of spindle cells, representing a very minor component. Sometimes, cords of neoplastic smooth muscle cells may be seen around thick blood vessels (fig. 10-26A).

Often, areas of edema are juxtaposed to areas of hyalinization but the latter can also be seen away from these areas. Hyalinization imparts a corded morphology to the smooth muscle cells that may be misconstrued as epithelioid (fig. 10-26B). When hydropic change has a perinodular distribution, it divides part or all (diffuse) of the leiomyoma into multiple, small, round, compact smooth muscle nodules. If this hypocellular edematous tissue is minimal or absent around the nodules of smooth muscle, it may create the false impression that individual nodules are free floating within spaces, although the latter are not lined by endothelial cells (fig. 10-27).

Areas not involved by edema or hyalinization have the appearance of a spindle or, rarely, an epithelioid smooth muscle tumor, which may be cellular, with banal cytologic features and rare to absent mitotic figures. Striking vascularity is noted (fig. 10-26C). Even though these tumors are mainly well circumscribed, hydropic change may focally extend to the surrounding myometrium. Microscopic foci of intravenous leiomyomatosis are also seen (38).

"Dissecting" Leiomyoma Including Cotyledonoid Leiomyoma ("Sternberg Tumor"). These tumors are characterized by disorganized swirled fascicles of smooth muscle that dissect the myometrium. Myometrial dissection may be a feature of standard leiomyomas or highly cellular leiomyomas (43). A specific subgroup

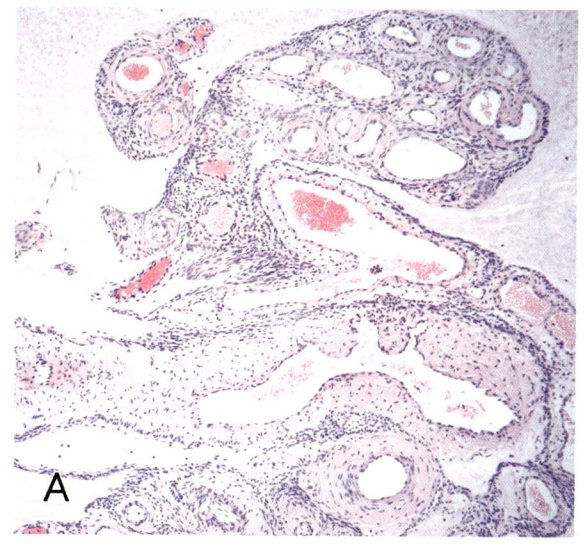
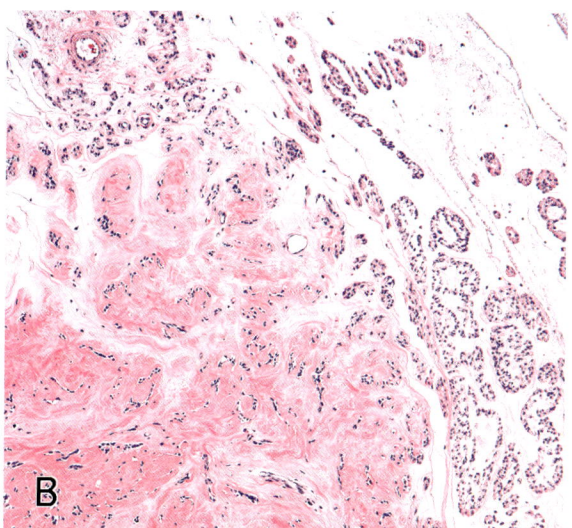
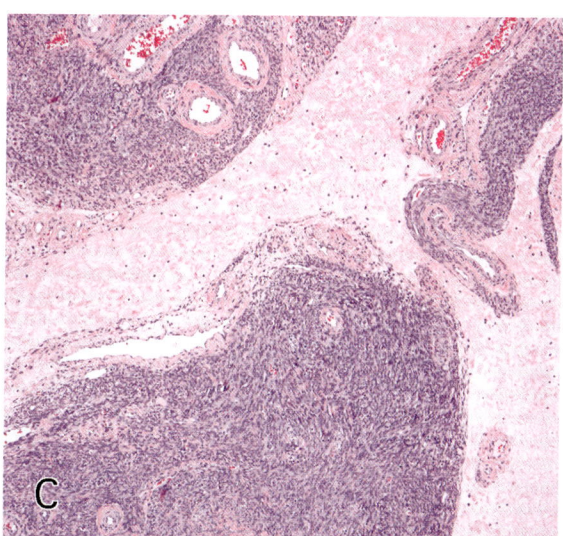

Figure 10-26
HYDROPIC LEIOMYOMA

An irregular island of smooth muscle neoplasia is juxtaposed to prominent edema with dropout of cells. The blood vessels are large and thick (A). Hyalinization alternates with edema, imparting a corded appearance to the smooth muscle cells, which may be confused with an epithelioid appearance (right) (B). Nodules of highly cellular smooth muscle are sharply demarcated from edematous areas. The vasculature is prominent in both components (C).

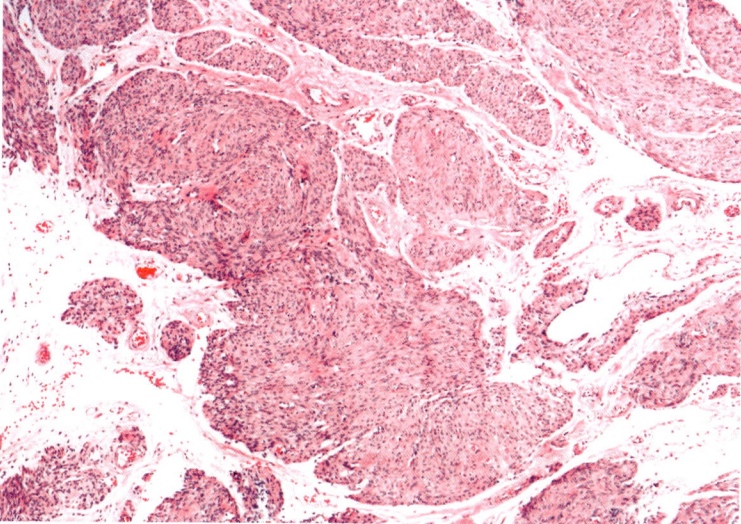

Figure 10-27
PERINODULAR HYDROPIC CHANGE

Multiple nodules of mature smooth muscle are associated with retraction artifact, simulating intravascular growth. The spaces, however, lack an endothelial lining.

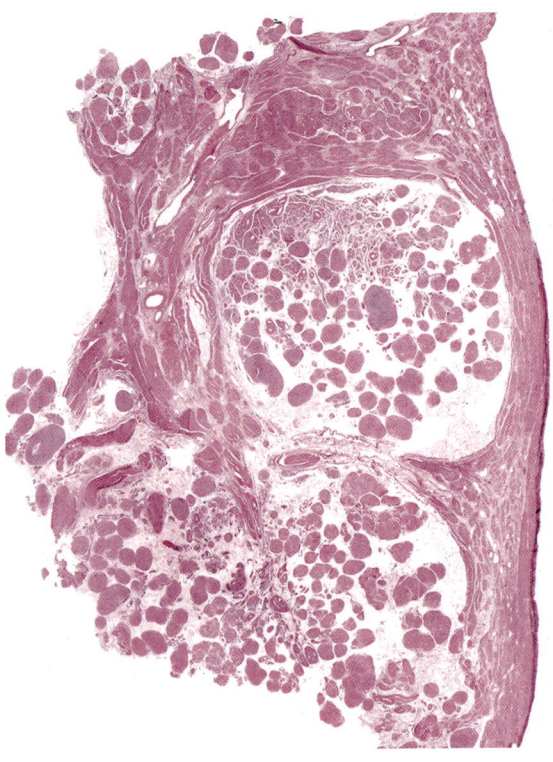

Figure 10-28

DISSECTING COTYLEDONOID LEIOMYOMA

Disorganized swirled fascicles dissect the myometrium (top). The nodular architecture is as seen in hydropic perinodular change (center and bottom).

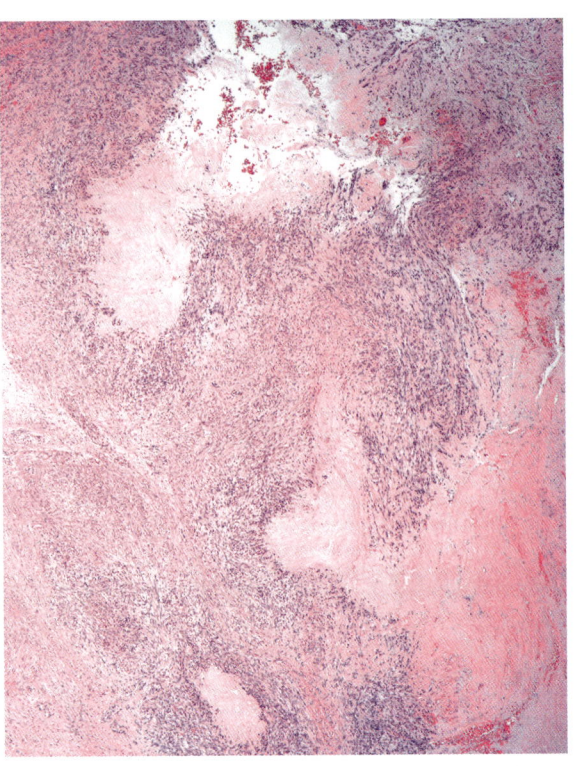

Figure 10-29

APOPLECTIC LEIOMYOMA

Irregularly shaped confluent nodules with a hypercellular rim associated with recent hemorrhage and reorganization impart a worrisome low-power appearance.

associated with a predominant serosal or subserosal component of the leiomyoma, and often associated with hydropic change and placental-like gross features, has been designated dissecting cotyledonoid leiomyoma (42). In the past, these tumors were termed "grape-like" leiomyomas (83). These tumors have a variably hyalinized to hydropic matrix which separates the smooth muscle nodules and is associated with prominent vascularity. The latter typically consists of large muscular vessels (fig. 10-28). The most superficial extrauterine component of the tumor is covered by loose connective tissue associated with dilated and congestive vessels. Rarely, these tumors lack the dissecting myometrial component (cotyledonoid leiomyoma) (84).

Dissecting leiomyomas show intramyometrial dissection by tight swirled fascicles with a micronodular configuration that is typically a focal finding (43). Some tumors are associated with intravenous growth (intravenous leiomyomatosis). Even though the cells are typically spindled, there are reports of epithelioid dissecting leiomyomas and rare adipocytic leiomyomas (42,85–93).

Hemorrhagic Cellular "Apoplectic" Leiomyoma. The term "apoplectic" was first introduced by Myles and Hart in 1985 (36) to highlight the two main features of these tumors: the acute clinical symptomatology and the pathologic features dominated by recent hemorrhage. This leiomyoma variant is characterized by discrete but irregularly shaped foci of hemorrhage in different phases of organization, surrounded by areas of hypercellularity, which at low power may impart a vague nodular architecture, especially if multiple foci are present (fig. 10-29) (21,23,36,37,94–96). The nodules typically have stellate or ovoid contours. Hemorrhage is often but not necessarily recent (fig. 10-30A), and when hemorrhage or secondary necrosis

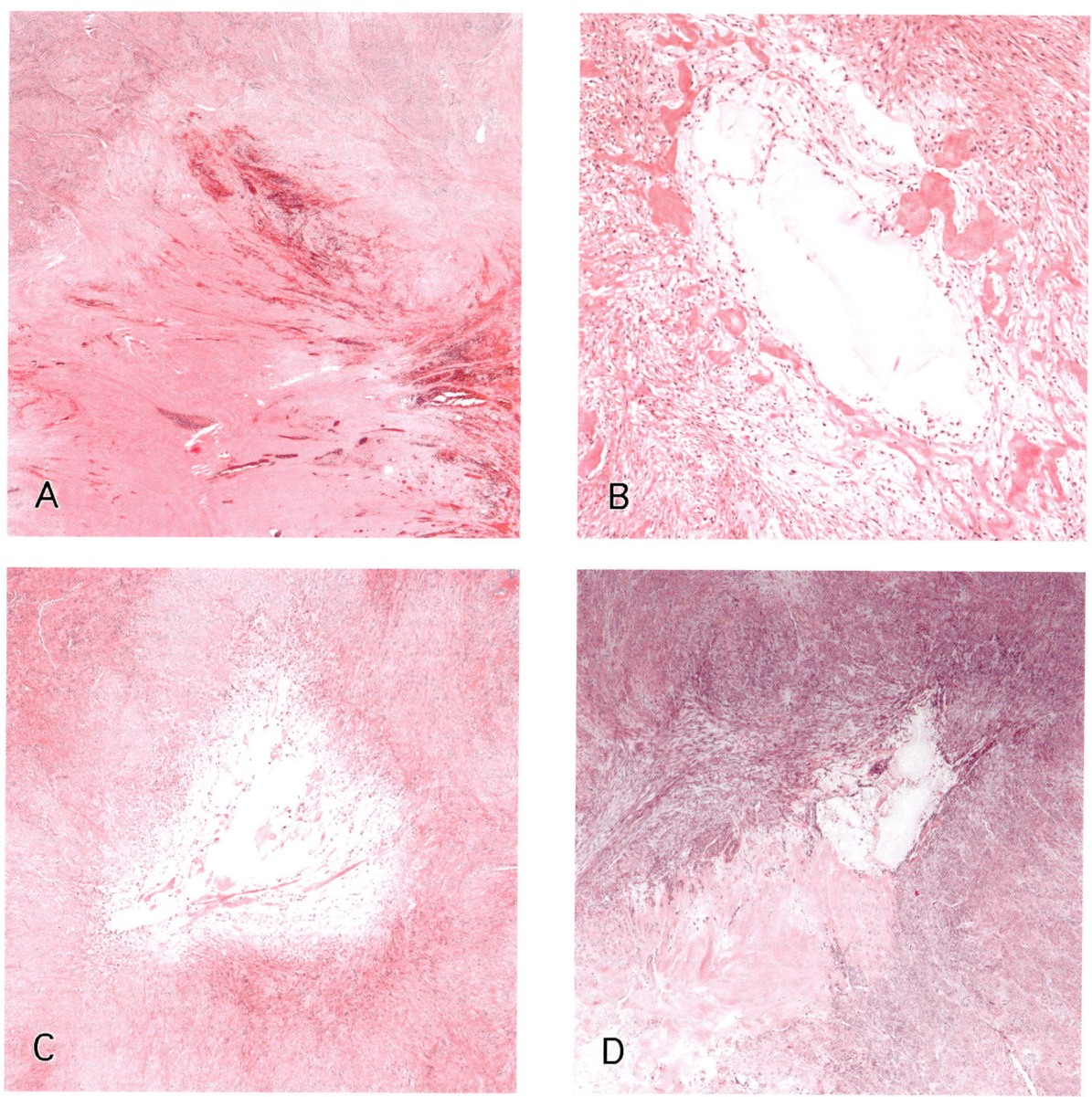

Figure 10-30

APOPLECTIC LEIOMYOMA

The infarcted areas are mummified, associated with linear hemorrhage, and have angulated borders (A). There is dropout of cells and mucoid material in the center of an infarcted focus (B). The nidus of apoplectic change shows dropout of tumor cells and adjacent hypercellular smooth muscle neoplasia. The associated myxoid background may cause concern for a myxoid neoplasm (C). Foci of hyalinization, a reflection of early organization of the infarcted tissue, are seen (D).

is reabsorbed and reorganized, these areas may show a dropout of tissue (cyst formation) (fig. 10-30B). The dropout area may be filled with "myxoid" material (fig. 10-30C) or associated with hyalinization (fig. 10-30D), entrapping preexisting smooth muscle cells. Less common-

ly, hemosiderin-laden macrophages, fibrin, and foamy histiocytes are seen (37).

Around hemorrhagic foci, the smooth muscle tumor is hypercellular and the cells may appear slightly enlarged, with "plump" nuclei displaying nucleoli. The cells may have an epithelioid

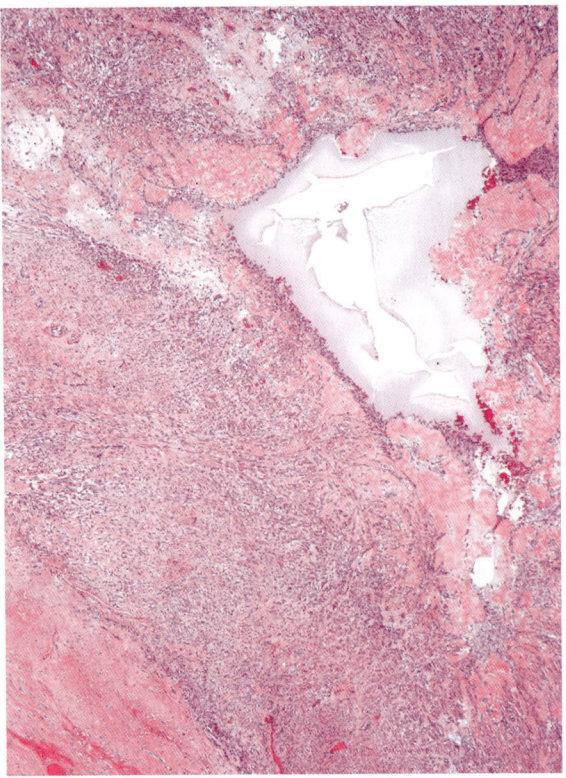

Figure 10-31

APOPLECTIC LEIOMYOMA

When advanced, areas around the infarcted focus may be hypercellular. The cells may be plump and mitoses may be seen.

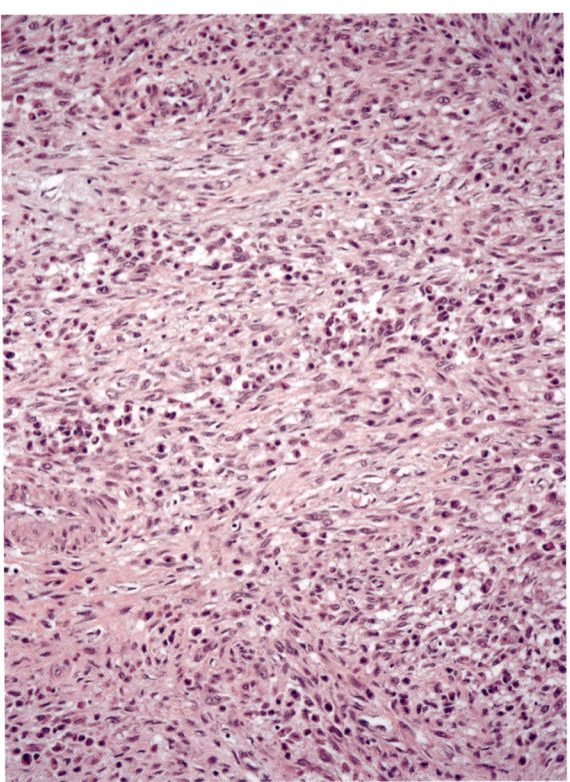

Figure 10-32

APOPLECTIC LEIOMYOMA

Numerous apoptotic cells are seen as noncohesive, shrunken, small rounded cells with dense eosinophilic cytoplasm and irregular pyknotic nuclei. This appearance may be mistaken for epithelioid morphology and may cause concern for malignancy.

appearance but often alternate with spindle cells (fig. 10-31). Some cells show dense eosinophilic cytoplasm and dark chromatin, or irregularly shaped nuclei secondary to apoptoses (fig. 10-32). Mitotic activity is increased when compared to areas distant from hemorrhage (as high as 14 mitoses per 10 high-power fields in the largest study) but atypical mitoses are not noted. The background stroma may be strikingly myxoid within the hypercellular areas while edema is also common and more often displays a hydropic appearance. Intracellular edema may impart a signet ring cell morphology to the smooth muscle cells (21,36,37). In early apoplectic change, while the vague nodular appearance is patent, only scattered red blood cells associated with pyknotic cells are seen, making the diagnosis more difficult. Distant areas display the typical morphology of leiomyomas, with minimal mitotic activity, overall imparting a low-power appearance that is termed "zonation" phenomenon (63).

Drug-Related Changes in Leiomyomas. GnRHa causes pituitary desensitization by the downregulation of GnRH receptors and reduction of estrogen production (artificial menopause) secondary to reduction of luteinizing and follicle-stimulating hormones. This results in variable shrinkage of leiomyomas, mostly within the first month of treatment. Changes that have been associated with GnRHa include tumor size reduction, increased cellularity, nuclear crowding, and ischemic necrosis. Some studies also have found vascular changes (including vasculitis, intimal and medial fibrosis, and wall thickening), edema, hyalinization, increased mitotic activity and apoptotic index, and increased lymphocytic infiltrates. Results, however, are not consistent among studies, and some show no differences between patients treated with GnRHa and controls (97–108). It has been hypothesized that those leiomyomas with more collagen respond less to treatment (98). No cytologic atypia is seen. In contrast, leiomyomas removed several weeks after withdrawal of GnRHa treatment increase rapidly in size and mitotic activity due to estrogenic effect (109,110). In patients treated with GnRHa for "leiomyoma" that turned out to be leiomyosarcoma, the main morphologic features of the tumor were not affected by the treatment including cytologic atypia, brisk mitotic activity, and tumor cell necrosis, making their recognition easy (111).

Leiomyomas may be treated by uterine artery embolization with polyvinyl alcohol (PVA) particles or microspheres, trisacryl gelatin microspheres (TGM), or a combination (112). A recent study with review of the literature has shown that TGM is more efficient than PVA in the treatment of leiomyomas (113). Aggregates of PVA or TGM are seen within necrotic leiomyomas and throughout the myometrium, and may be seen outside the uterus. Both are associated with infarct-type necrosis of the leiomyoma, which varies from case to case, but can also cause infarction of the remainder of the uterus. Foreign body-type giant cells and mononuclear macrophages may be seen (114–120).

It is well known that progestogens and oral contraceptives commonly cause necrosis in leiomyomas. Tranexamic acid, an antifibrinolytic agent used in the treatment of abnormal bleeding including when secondary to fibroids, also results in infarct-type necrosis within leiomyomas. When given less than 2 weeks before surgery, infarct-type necrosis may be difficult to distinguish from tumor cell necrosis. Variable degrees of vascular thrombosis, with thrombi in different stages of recanalization, and rarely fibrinoid change accompanied with abundant subintimal foamy macrophages, can also be seen (121,122).

Epithelioid Leiomyoma. The WHO defines this leiomyoma as displaying rounded to polygonal cells with an epithelial-like morphology (1). At least 50 percent of the tumor should have an epithelioid morphology to belong to this category of smooth muscle neoplasms. These tumors have been referred in the literature to as leiomyoblastoma (if solid growth), and clear

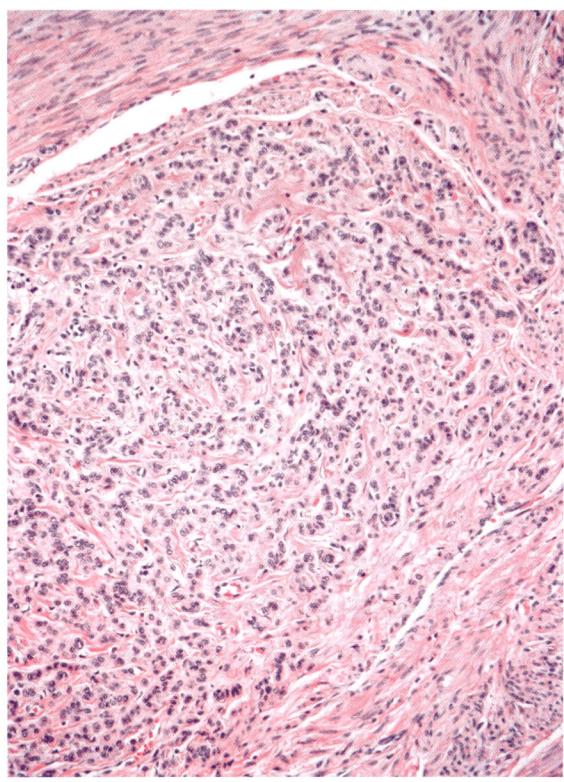

Figure 10-33

EPITHELIOID TUMORLET

The tumor is small (less than 1 cm) and well demarcated, and has an epithelioid morphology. Cells form cords, some interanastomosing, between loose collagen.

cell and plexiform (if cord-like or trabecular growth) leiomyomas based on their architectural and cytologic characteristics (123–127). Currently, they are all termed epithelioid leiomyomas except when less than 1 cm showing a plexiform architecture (fig. 10-33), in which case they are designated as *plexiform tumorlets*. These may be multiple and although they are more frequently found in the myometrium, they may occur in the endometrium. They are not well demarcated and are associated with loose collagen (128–131).

Epithelioid leiomyomas grow in sheets, nests, cords, and trabeculae, or more frequently, a combination of these (fig. 10-34). Rarely, pseudoglandular spaces containing eosinophilic secretions are seen. Variable degrees of stromal hyalinization may also be present. A second spindled component is often seen. Cells have abundant eosinophilic, granular, and less

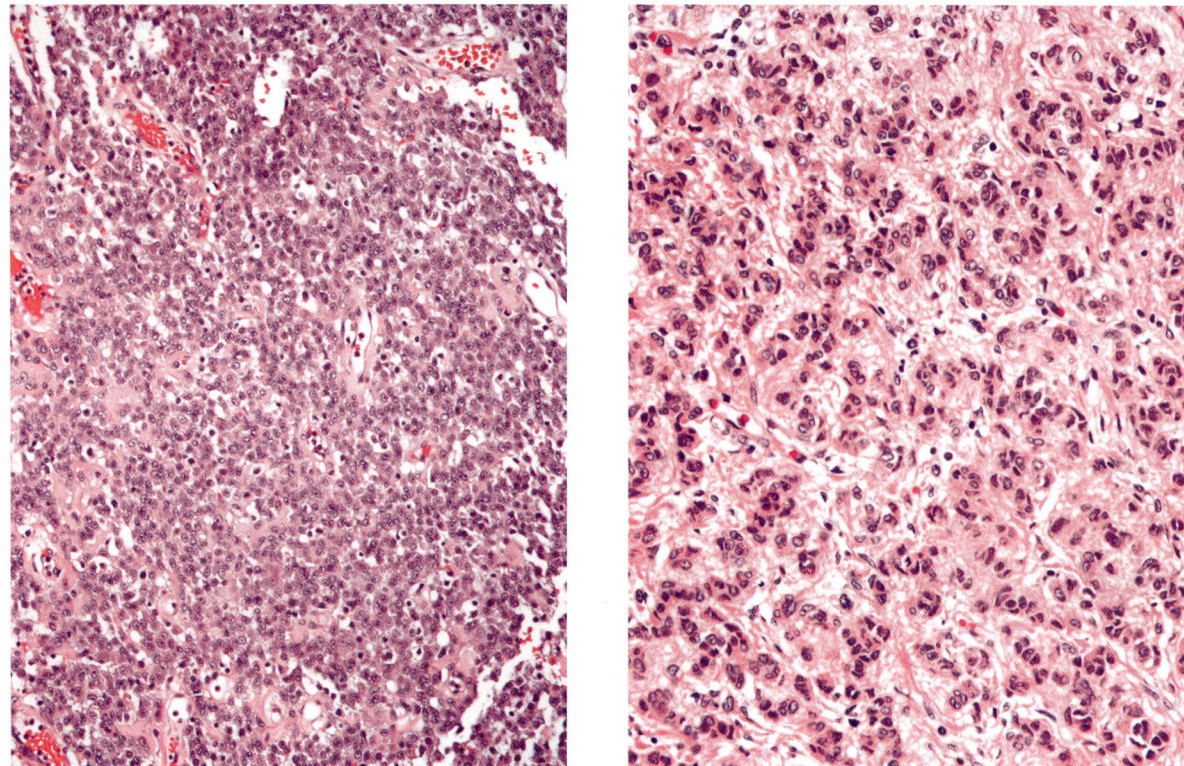

Figure 10-34

EPITHELIOID LEIOMYOMA

The tumor cells have diffuse (left), corded, and nested (right) growth patterns. They show eosinophilic cytoplasm and uniform banal nuclear features.

commonly, clear or vacuolated cytoplasm (due to glycogen or lipid content). They display, at most, mild cytologic atypia and low mitotic activity (less than 3 mitoses per 10 high-power fields). Infarct-type but not tumor cell necrosis may be seen. These tumors should be extensively sampled in order to exclude areas with increased mitotic activity or cytologic activity, which would exclude the diagnosis of benign epithelioid smooth muscle tumor.

Myxoid Leiomyoma. This is defined by abundant myxoid matrix (rich in acid mucins and positive for alcian blue or colloidal iron) within a leiomyoma that is fairly well demarcated and smaller than 6 cm (132–136). Tumors tend to be hypocellular and cells are oval to elongated or stellate, with bland cytologic features and absent to rare mitoses. These tumors are rarely purely myxoid. They often have a component of typical leiomyoma which is helpful in establishing the diagnosis of benign smooth muscle tumor (fig. 10-35). One example with bizarre nuclei has been reported (133). This is an exceedingly rare subtype of leiomyoma and before making this diagnosis, the possibility of leiomyoma with focal myxoid change or leiomyosarcoma should be excluded (see differential diagnosis section).

Leiomyoma with Heterologous Elements. Adipose tissue is the most common heterologous component in benign smooth muscle tumors. Such tumors are classified as *lipoleiomyoma*. They have an incidence of 0.35 to 2.1 percent of patients undergoing treatment for uterine leiomyomas (137,138). The percentage of the lipomatous component varies but is usually minor, with the presence of mature adipocytes either in isolation or in groups between fascicles of banal-appearing spindle smooth muscle cells. Rarely, there is plexiform architecture or bizarre nuclei (fig. 10-36) (138–145). The leiomyoma may contain brown fat (*leiomyohybernoma*), with cells containing multiple small vacuoles and centrally located

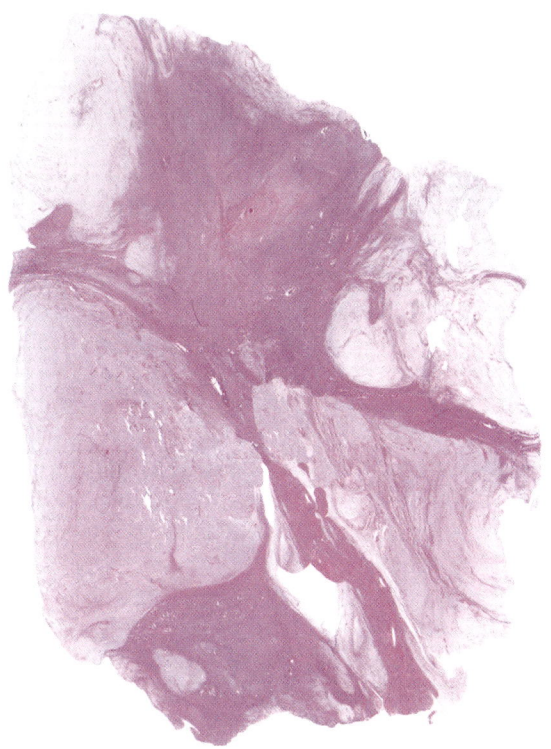

Figure 10-35

MYXOID LEIOMYOMA

The tumor is largely hypocellular, with a prominent myxoid matrix. Nonmyxoid areas have the appearance of a typical leiomyoma, suggesting a benign diagnosis. This tumor was small and well circumscribed (margins not seen).

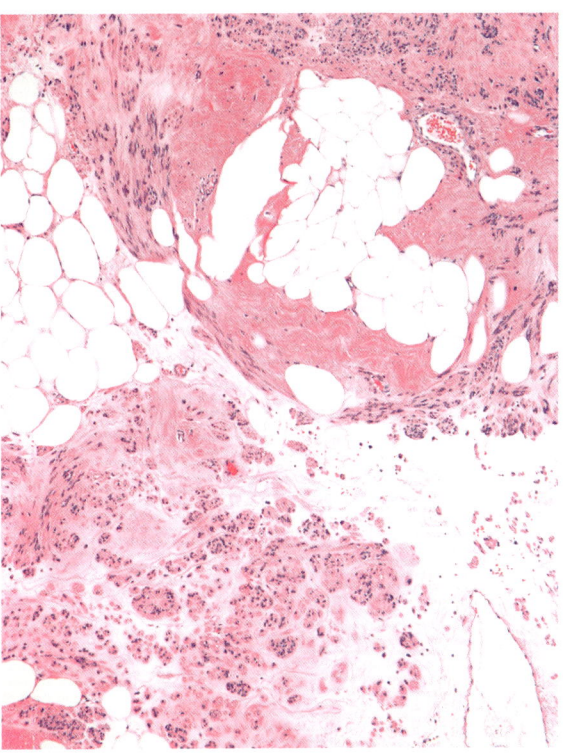

Figure 10-36

LIPOLEIOMYOMA

The benign smooth muscle cells are associated with hydropic change and mature adipocytes.

bland nuclei that may be admixed with mature adipocytes in a myxoid background (146). The adipose component may undergo malignant transformation to liposarcoma (147).

Different theories have been proposed to explain the presence of adipose tissue in the uterine corpus including metaplasia (most accepted), misplacement of embryonic adipocytes, differentiation from progenitor connective tissue cells, secondary infiltration by periuterine adipose soft tissue, and iatrogenic displacement (148). Some tumors have an associated vascular component and are termed as *angiolipoleiomyoma* (140). Rarely, leiomyomas show skeletal muscle (149,150), osseous (151), or cartilaginous (152,153) differentiation.

Diffuse Leiomyomatosis. This is an unusual growth characterized by extensive to massive replacement of the myometrium by numerous closely packed, small nodules of benign smooth muscle that typically lack circumscription and frequently merge imperceptibly with each other and with the surrounding myometrium to resemble nodular hyperplasia (154). The nodules are composed of spindle cells that are cytologically bland with minimal to absent mitotic activity (fig. 10-37). Cellularity may vary but often they are cellular and the spindled cells have at least focally a perivascular arrangement that may also be seen in the adjacent myometrium. There may be increased vascularity seen as small capillaries in the center of the nodules. Diffuse leiomyomatosis is not associated with hydropic, myxoid, or hemorrhagic degenerative changes other than hyalinization (155–158). Rarely, there is extrauterine extension (159). It can be seen as part of Alport syndrome (160).

Parasitic Leiomyoma. This leiomyoma has an original subserosal location and after torsion loses its attachment to the uterus and becomes vascularized by adjacent tissues. The microscopic appearance is that of a typical or variant leiomyoma (22,161).

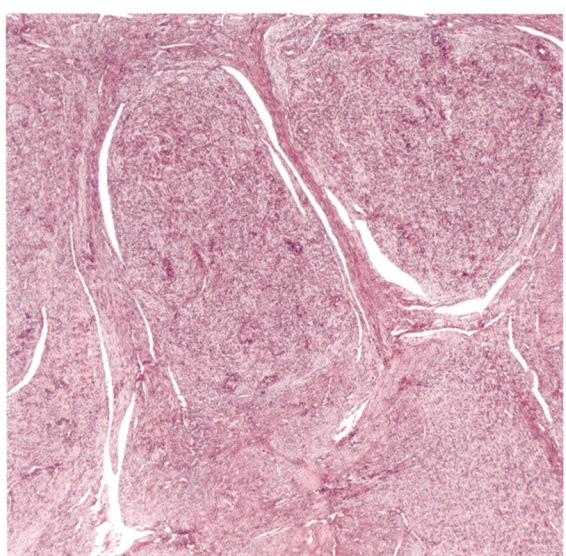

Figure 10-37

DIFFUSE LEIOMYOMATOSIS

Small nodules of benign smooth muscle merge with each other.

Diffuse Peritoneal Leiomyomatosis. Variably sized nodules composed of benign appearing smooth muscle cells with minimal mitotic activity are present in superficial subperitoneal tissues of the pelvis and abdomen, with an appearance identical to typical uterine leiomyomas (fig. 10-38). A component of decidual cells may be noted. Malignant transformation of one of the nodules may occur but is rare (162). This process is considered to originate from metaplastic transformation of submesothelial mesenchymal cells into smooth muscle cells under the hormonal influence of pregnancy or contraceptives (163–167).

Leiomyoma with Vascular Invasion. The microscopic appearance is of a typical leiomyoma or leiomyoma variant associated with microscopic intravascular growth within its confines (168,169). Some authors have hypothesized that a leiomyoma with vascular invasion represents the initial stage of intravenous leiomyomatosis, with the intravenous

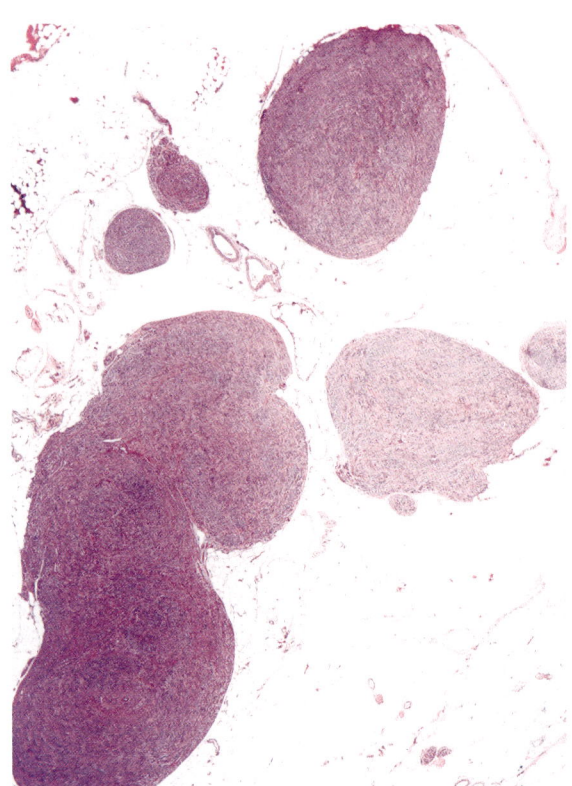
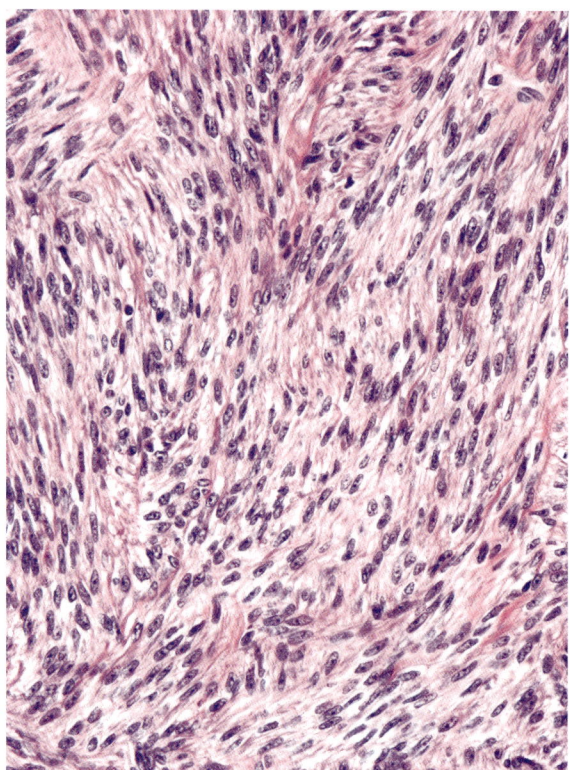

Figure 10-38

DIFFUSE PERITONEAL LEIOMYOMATOSIS

Sharply demarcated nodules (left) composed of spindle cells form fascicles with banal cytologic features (right).

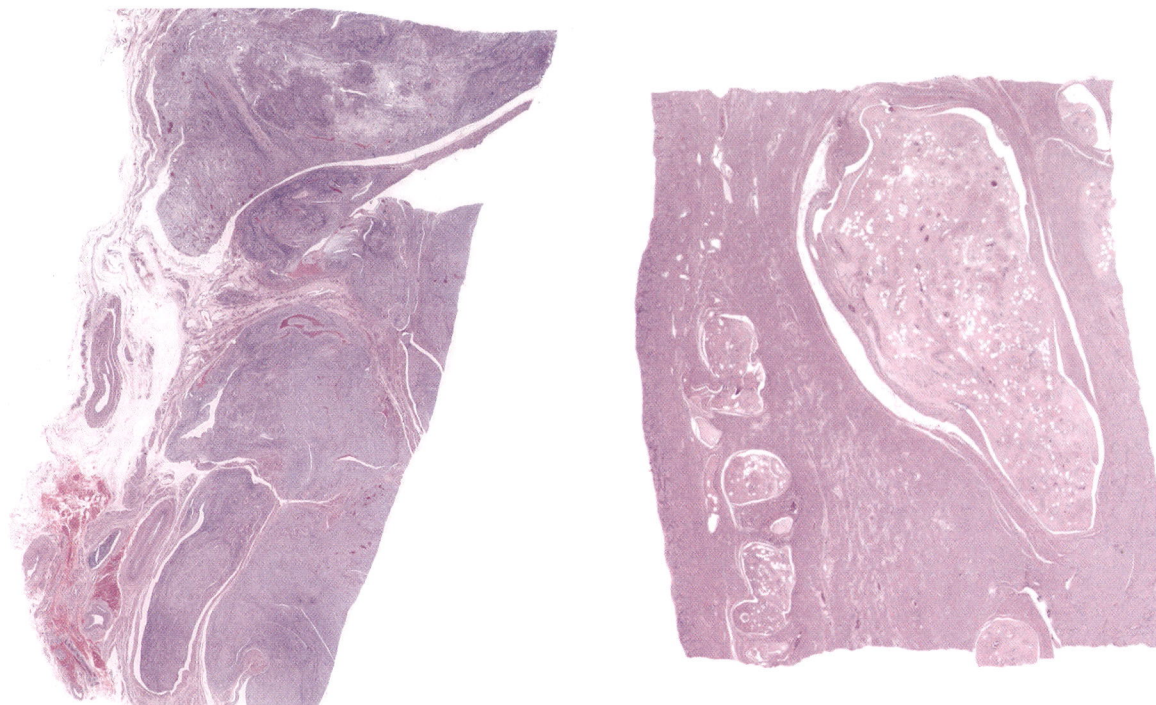

Figure 10-39

INTRAVENOUS LEIOMYOMATOSIS

The intravascular tumor is hypercellular, as seen in the highly cellular leiomyoma, and associated with the characteristic clefting (left). The irregular intramyometrial nodules are difficult to identify within the vascular spaces, but a serpiginous growth is noted in the myometrium. This appearance should suggest intravenous leiomyomatosis. Close examination shows subtle, rounded, intravascular growth (bottom of left figure). The intravascular growth is associated with adipose tissue (intravascular lipoleiomyomatosis) and is extensively hyalinized (right).

component originating in the wall of vessels within the leiomyoma in the uterus, or outside the uterus (170). Leiomyoma with vascular invasion is also associated with benign-appearing smooth muscle nodules within the lungs.

Intravenous Leiomyomatosis. This unusual smooth muscle proliferation is defined by the presence of benign smooth muscle cells resembling either typical or variant leiomyoma (fig. 10-39) within vascular spaces (either free floating or partially attached) outside the confines, or in the absence of a leiomyoma. The estimated amount of intravascular tumor ranges from 5 to 100 percent (171). The involved vascular spaces are typically veins, or less commonly, lymphatic spaces but not arteries.

The intravascular proliferations are composed of spindle cells arranged in intersecting fascicles, an appearance similar to that of typical leiomyoma, at least focally. Thick-walled vessels and cleft-like spaces, the latter imparting a lobulated contour (fig. 10-39, left), are common, but small vessels can also impart an "angiomatoid pattern" (169,172–177). Other common histologic features include extensive hyalinization (fig. 10-39, right), collagen plaques (fig. 10-40A), and hydropic change (as seen in hydropic leiomyoma) (fig. 10-40B). The tumor may be hypercellular (fig. 10-40C), and the cells may be epithelioid (with clear or eosinophilic cytoplasm) or have bizarre nuclei. Sometimes, myxoid (fig. 10-40D), adipocytic (fig. 10-39, right), and glandular (with or without a stromal component) changes, abundant inflammatory cells, or associated histiocytes are seen (169,172–174,178–180). Mitoses are usually rare (fewer than 2 per 10 high-power fields), but have been reported as high as 4 mitoses per 10 high-power fields (169).

In some examples, a subendothelial proliferation of benign smooth muscle merges with

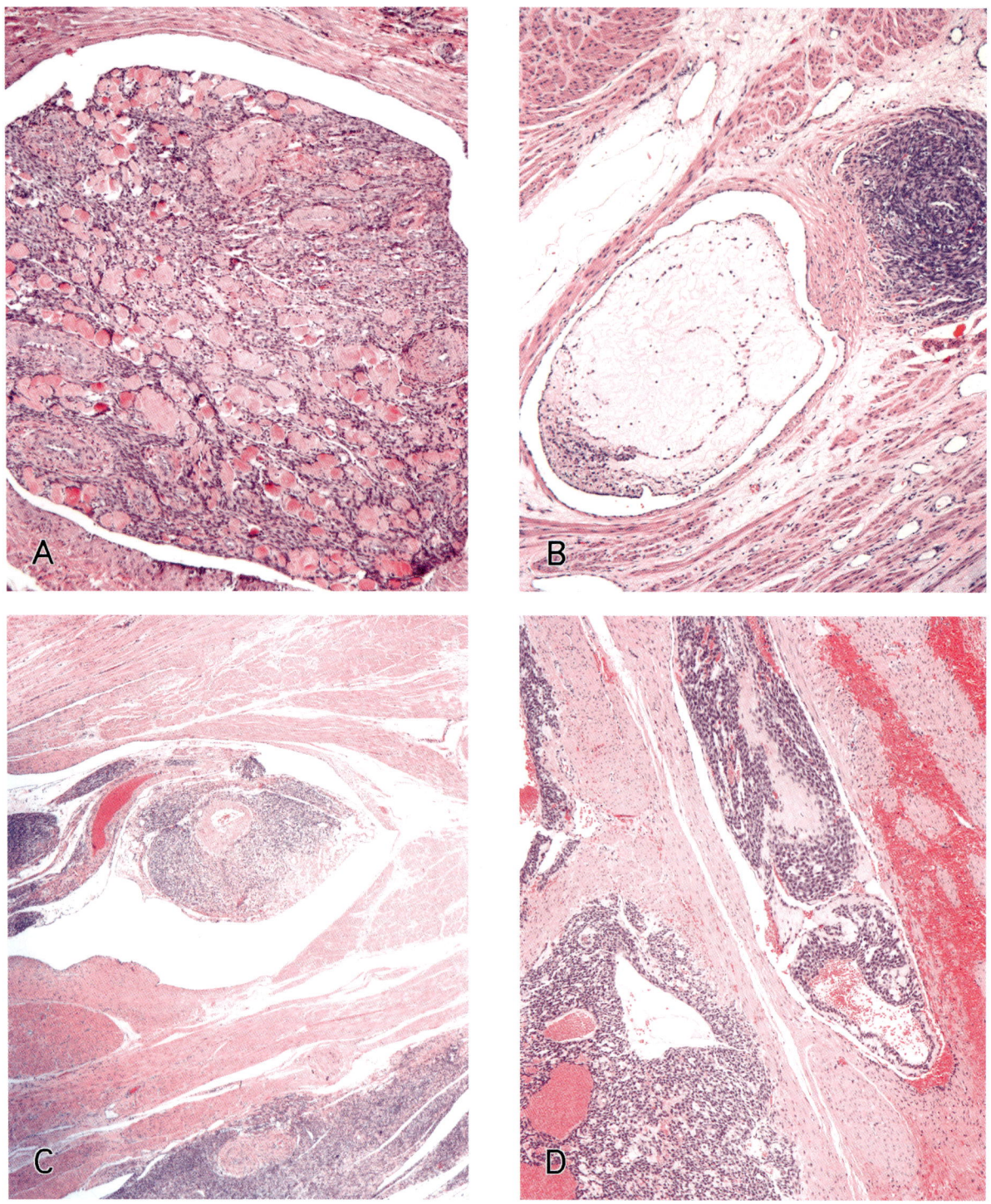

Figure 10-40

INTRAVENOUS LEIOMYOMATOSIS

There are large thick blood vessels as often seen in benign smooth muscle proliferations. Striking collagen plaques may be seen but are more often associated with endometrial stromal sarcoma (A). Hydropic change (B) as well as increased cellularity (C) are seen, similar to the appearance of leiomyoma variants. Focal clefted contours and cystic degeneration are seen, the latter associated with mucoid material (D).

Smooth Muscle and Other Mesenchymal Tumors

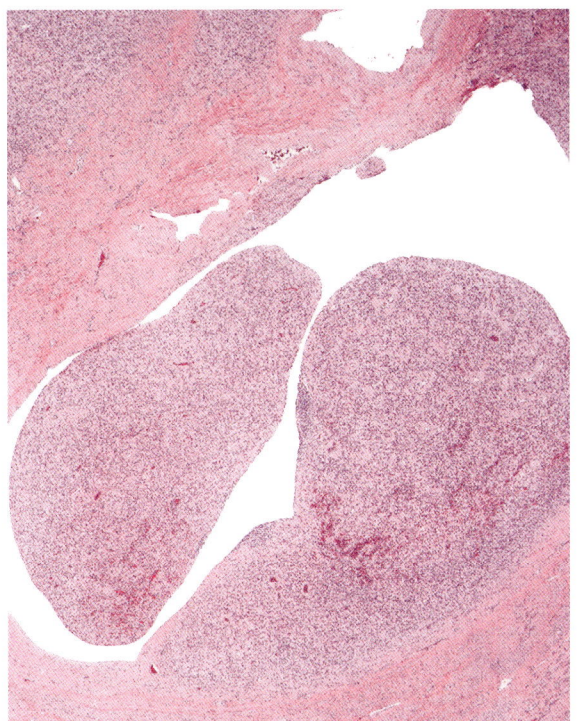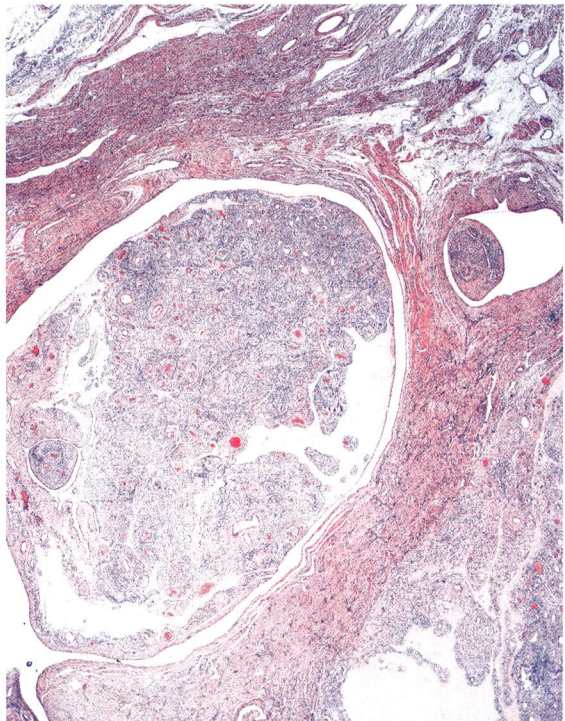

Figure 10-41

INTRAVENOUS LEIOMYOMATOSIS

The intravascular growth is associated with subendothelial growth of smooth muscle (left) and present outside the confines of a cellular leiomyoma (right).

the intravascular tumor if this is attached to the vessel wall. It has been postulated that this is the origin of intravenous leiomyomatosis (fig. 10-41, left) (168,169,181). In some cases, the diagnosis of intravenous leiomyomatosis is first reached on microscopic examination since it may be grossly subtle and confounded by the presence of multiple leiomyomas (fig. 10-41, right). In other cases, suspicion should be raised when finding serpiginous growth within the myometrium even though tumor is not clearly seen within vacular spaces. If in doubt, it is important to reexamine the uterus, focusing on areas that may be suspicious for intravascular growth.

Benign Metastasizing Leiomyoma. Several hypotheses have been proposed to explain the origin of these tumors including that they represent: secondary deposits from intravenous leiomyomatosis or uterine leiomyoma with vascular invasion (favored), underdiagnosed low-grade leiomyosarcoma, iatrogenic leiomyoma secondary to surgery (in more recent years), independent growths (multifocal disease), or primary lung lesions (182). Metastases occur more frequently to the lungs (fig. 10-42, left), but may also involve abdominopelvic and/or mediastinal lymph nodes, soft tissues, bone, skin, and heart (183–188).

Benign metastasizing leiomyomas are composed of fascicles of cytologically bland smooth muscle cells with minimal to absent mitotic activity (fig. 10-42, right). Hydropic change has been reported. They tend to have a peribronchiolar pattern of growth and may entrap alveolar spaces at the periphery (182,183,189–193). They may be pure or admixed with mature adipocytes (194). The diagnosis of benign metastasizing leiomyoma should only be rendered when the uterine tumor has been thoroughly sampled to exclude the possibility of leiomyosarcoma.

Immunohistochemical Findings. A number of smooth muscle markers, including alpha-smooth muscle actin, desmin, smooth muscle myosin, calponin, HDCA8, and h-caldesmon (fig. 10-43, left) are typically positive in leiomyomas

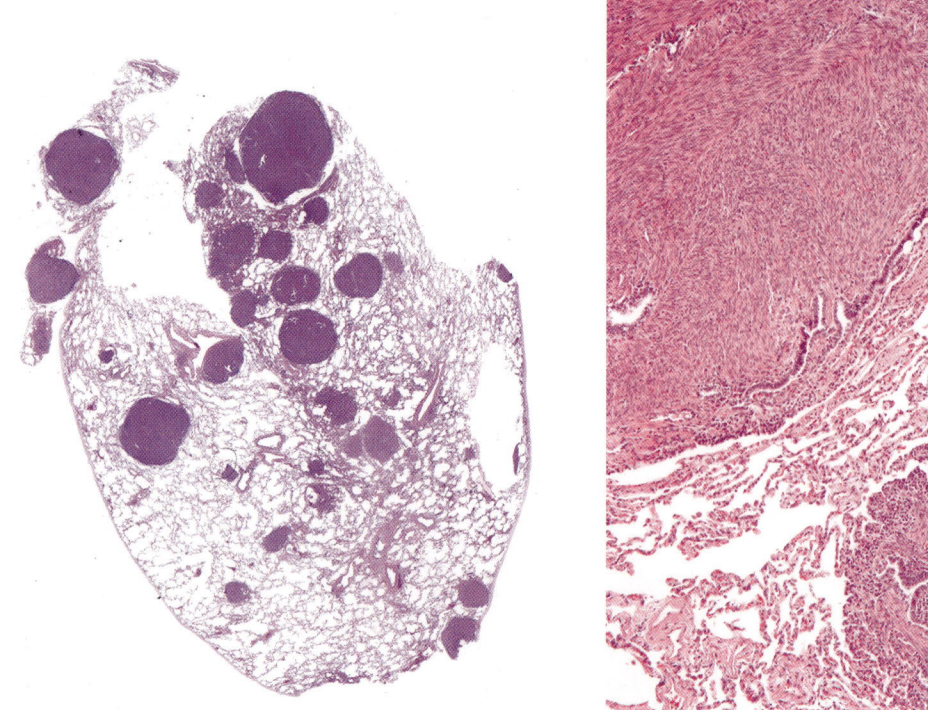

Figure 10-42

BENIGN METASTASIZING LEIOMYOMA

Well-demarcated, variably sized nodules are present within the lung parenchyma (left). The nodules are composed of fascicles of spindle smooth muscle cells with banal cytologic features (right).

(195–203), although positivity may be more limited in myxoid tumors. Smoothelin has been studied in uterine leiomyomas, with most tumors showing nuclear and cytoplasmic positivity (204). Transgelin is new marker expressed in smooth muscle tumors but experience with this antibody is limited (205,206).

Leiomyomas frequently express wide spectrum keratins and epithelial membrane antigen (EMA) (especially if epithelioid morphology) while CD10 shows variable positivity, more often and more extensive in highly cellular leiomyomas (fig. 10-43, right) (165,196–199,202,207–209). WT1 can also be positive, with cytoplasmic staining more common than nuclear staining (198). Estrogen and progesterone receptors (ER and PR) are expressed in almost all uterine leiomyomas, androgen receptor (AR) is positive in about 30 percent (206,210–214), and oxytocin receptor is typically positive (195). Oncofetal proteins IMP3 and stathmin 1 have been studied in rare series comparing expression in leiomyomas and leiomyosarcomas. The former is absent in leiomyomas in contrast to leiomyosarcomas in one published study (215) while stathmin 1 shows typically weaker as well as less frequent positivity in leiomyomas when compared to leiomyosarcomas, limiting its use (216). CD34 may be positive in smooth muscle tumors, more frequently if spindled (202).

MIB-1 expression is typically low in leiomyomas (217) except in mitotically active leiomyomas and those with bizarre nuclei, which may show overlapping rates with those observed in leiomyosarcomas (218). Areas close to infarct-type necrosis also show increased Ki-67 positivity (see fig. 10-16B). Among other proliferative markers that have been used for leiomyomas, phosphohistone-H3 (PHH3) is the most common (219,220). Although expression of p16 has been typically associated with leiomyosarcomas, leiomyomas are also positive, although less commonly (217, 221,222) except in areas next to infarct-type necrosis (see fig. 10-16C)

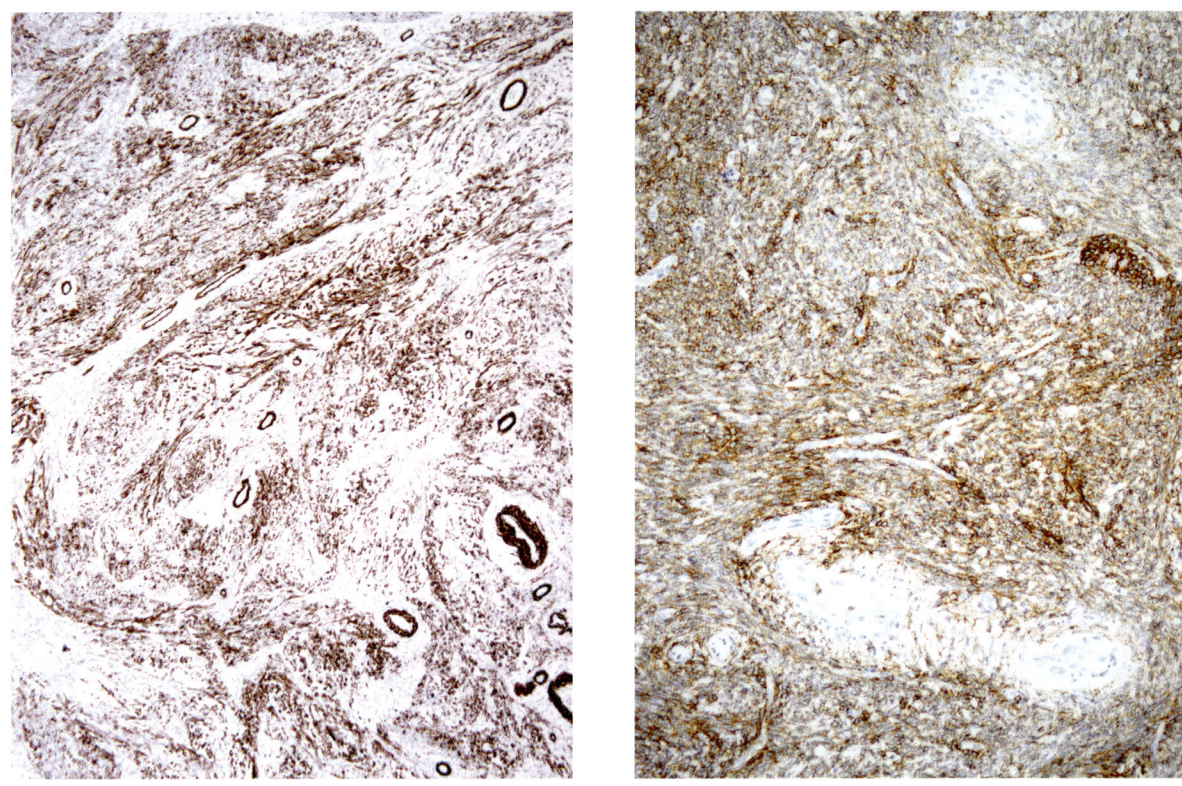

Figure 10-43

HIGHLY CELLULAR LEIOMYOMA

The tumor cells show extensive and strong positivity for caldesmon (left) and CD10 (right).

(223) or in leiomyomas with bizarre nuclei where staining can be strong and diffuse (fig. 10-44, left) (39,68,72,218,224,225). p53 staining is typically minimal (wild-type) except in leiomyomas with bizarre nuclei which may show diffuse and strong positivity (fig. 10-44, right) (39,72,218,225,226), especially with type II tumors (68). HMGA2 has been reported to be overexpressed in 10 to 15 percent of tumors, more frequently in leiomyomas that are cellular or have bizarre nuclei (68,227).

Loss of expression of FH is seen in leiomyomas with bizarre nuclei (type I, fumarate hydratase-deficient leiomyoma) (fig. 10-45) (68,72,74,228–231) and rarely in conventional leiomyomas (74,75,229). Altered FH leads to intracellular accumulation in affected cells, with secondary formation of S-(2-succino)-cysteine (S2C). Tumors that show markedly decreased or absence of cytoplasmic FH expression typically show cytoplasmic S2C expression. Loss of FH expression, however, does not perfectly correlate with *FH* mutational status. It has been reported that 2SC staining (not commercially available) is more sensitive than loss of FH staining to detect *FH* gene aberrations since some tumors have impaired but detectable FH due to missense mutations (229,230,232). *FH* somatic mutations are more frequent than germline mutations but both scenarios share similar morphologic features (74,75). Studies of patients with leiomyomas based on *FH* germline status are necessary to identify morphologic features that are predictive of this syndrome (15). Thus, abnormal FH/2SC staining is not necessarily indicative of HLRCC. When determining which patients should undergo genetic counseling, patient age at presentation (young) as well as other clinical features (finding of cutaneous leiomyomas) are most relevant in the context of abnormal FH/2SC staining (72).

Molecular Genetic Findings. Forty to 50 percent of leiomyomas have detectable cytogenetic rearrangements, typically reported as simple karyotypic abnormalities, in contrast to leiomyosarcomas which commonly have complex

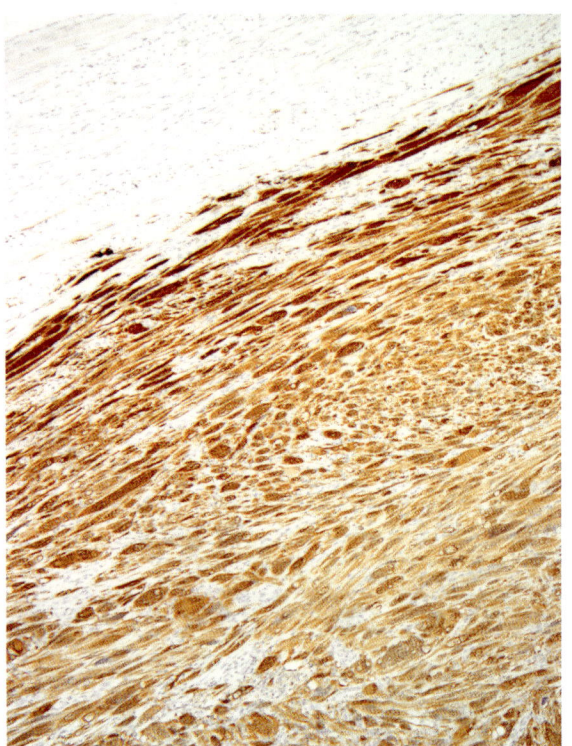 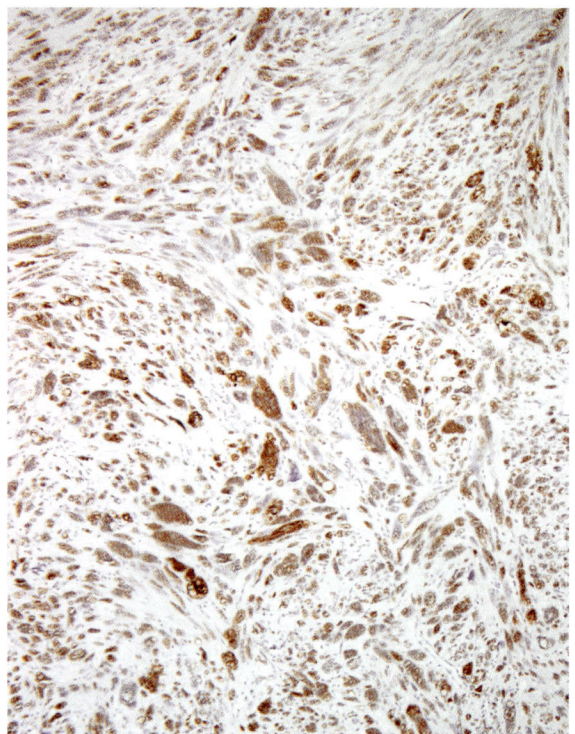

Figure 10-44

LEIOMYOMA WITH BIZARRE NUCLEI

There is strong and diffuse positivity for p16 (left) and p53 (right), mimicking the immunoprofile of leiomyosarcoma.

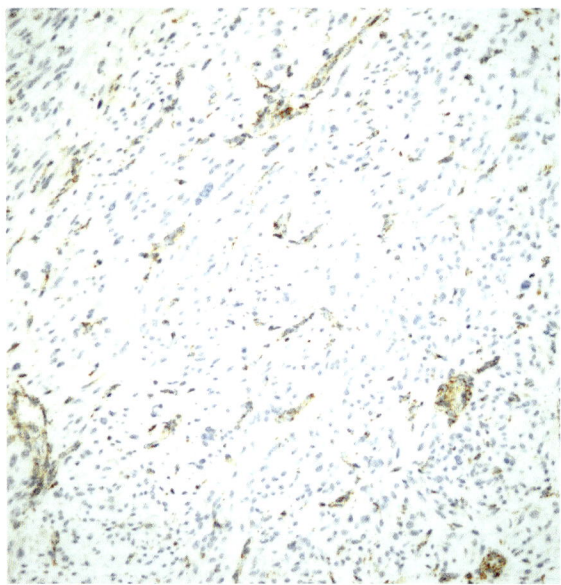

Figure 10-45

FUMARATE HYDRATASE-DEFICIENT LEIOMYOMA

Fumarate hydratase staining is absent in the neoplastic cells with a positive control in blood vessels.

karyotypic abnormalities. The most common recurrent chromosome aberrations are t(12;14)(q15;q24)(*HMGA2;RAD51B*), 7q deletions (*CUX1*), and 6p21 rearrangements (*HMGA1*) occurring in 20, 17, and 5 percent of karyotypically abnormal leiomyomas, respectively (233–235). Other less frequent aberrations involve 1p36, 1q43 (*FH*), 3q, 10q22, 17q24 and 22q (236).

Next-generation sequencing has allowed further insight into the genetics of these tumors including the finding of transcription mediator *MED12* mutations (mostly affecting exon 2) in 70 percent of leiomyomas (237) as well as the presence of "complex chromosomal rearrangements," some of which resemble chromothripsis which were not apparent by conventional methods (234). The latter phenomenon occurs predominantly in leiomyomas lacking *MED12* mutations with intact *TP53*, despite the reported association of chromothripsis with poor prognosis and *TP53* mutations in malignant tumors (238). 12q15 (*HMGA2*) rearrangements and *MED12* mutations are mutually exclusive, with distinct gene expression profiles, and together they are found in 80 to 90 percent of all leiomyomas (239). FH-deficient leiomyomas (sporadic or associated with dominantly inherited HLRCC) also display a unique gene expression profile different from these two molecular subtypes (234). Distinct recurrent alterations with distinct molecular profiles in leiomyomas will likely help further delineate the classification of these tumors.

Cytogenetic studies on disseminated peritoneal leiomyomatosis are limited for both sporadic and iatrogenic forms, but they show aberrations similar to those seen in leiomyomas including alterations in 7q, 12q15, 1q43, and 3q (240–243). In one study, several nodules displayed a non-random X-chromosome inactivation pattern consistent with monoclonal neoplastic growth (244).

Intravenous leiomyomatosis is reported to have a characteristic derivative chromosome (der(14)t(12;14)(q15;q24)) by karyotype that involves the same locus as leiomyomas with 12q15 (*HMGA2*) rearrangements (245,246). A molecular cytogenetic analysis showed recurrent 12q15 rearrangements (58 percent) by fluorescence in situ hybridization (FISH), which was also associated with elevated HMGA2 expression as well as loss of chromosome 22 in two out of three cases analyzed by karyotype (242). A copy number analysis showed recurrent 22q12q13 deletions (66 percent) and 10q22 duplications (33 percent) (247). In addition, hierarchical cluster analysis of the gene expression profiles revealed segregation of these smooth muscle proliferations with leiomyosarcoma rather than with myometrium or leiomyomas (242). These findings suggest that intravenous leiomyomatosis shares some molecular cytogenetic characteristics with uterine leiomyoma (recurrent 12q15 rearrangement, less complicated karyotype in comparison to leiomyosarcomas), and expression profiles similar to those seen in leiomyosarcoma, further supporting their intermediate behavior.

Benign metastasizing leiomyoma shows alterations of 1p36, 6p21, 7q, 3q, and 22q by karyotyping and copy number analyses, which are some of the less frequent aberrations detected in leiomyomas. When available, matched leiomyoma samples from these patients also showed the same rearrangements (182,248–250). On the other hand, sequencing studies showed unique mutations in benign metastasizing leiomyomas that were not detected in their matched leiomyomas; one case showed a *PTEN* mutation and another a *BMP8B* mutation (251,252). These studies suggest that benign metastasizing leiomyomas may have a common origin with leiomyomas detected in the same individual, but acquire additional mutations as they metastasize.

MED12 mutations are common in uterine leiomyomas including mitotically active leiomyomas (between 50 and 90 percent). They usually affect exon 2, being either missense or in-frame-insertion deletions (14,227,237,239, 253–263). A smaller number of leiomyomas (about 10 percent), including cellular leiomyomas, display *HGM2* aberrations (253,264). It appears that *MED12* and *HGMA2* abnormalities are mutually exclusive, as stated earlier. Tumors with either abnormality are associated with distinct gene expression profiles, suggesting that there is a different pathogenesis (234,265).

Leiomyomas with bizarre nuclei often display somatic mutations in *FH, TP53, MED12, FOXA1*, and *KMT2A*. Interestingly, tumors with altered FH/2SC expression have been reported more often to show somatic rather than germline mutations and homozygous deletions affecting the *FH* gene (72,231,266), while tumors with preserved pattern of FH/2SC expression more frequently harbor *TP53* or *RB1* mutations. In contrast to typical leiomyomas, leiomyomas with bizarre nuclei are only rarely associated with *MED12* hotspot mutations (68,72).

FH-deficient leiomyomas do not have *HMGA2* aberrations. A novel point mutation in the *FH* gene has been recently reported in siblings with early onset uterine leiomyomas with the typical morphologic and immunohistochemical findings (267).

Other rare alterations include *COL4A5-COL4A6* (Alport syndrome) and *KAT6B* (Ohdo syndrome) (268), which do not appear to occur with *MED12*, *HMGA2*, or *FH*. Finally, there is one group of leiomyomas with 1p36 deletions that appear to cluster with leiomyosarcomas and may explain the progression/transformation in some benign smooth muscle tumors (269).

Differential Diagnosis. Typical leiomyomas are rarely difficult to diagnose. The one tumor that may enter the differential diagnosis is adenomatoid tumor, which on gross examination

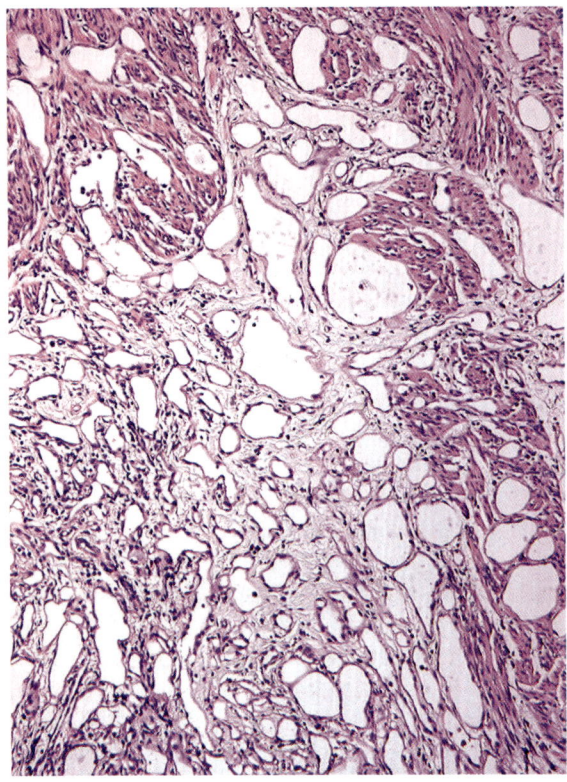

Figure 10-46

ADENOMATOID TUMOR

Variably sized spaces lined by flat to cuboidal mesothelial cells, some with a signet ring morphology, are associated with a mild sprinkling of lymphocytes. The background is edematous and spaces are surrounded by smooth muscle.

vaguely resembles a leiomyoma although its margins are much less defined and it does not bulge from the surrounding myometrium as do typical leiomyomas. At low-power microscopic examination, the tumor is often associated with prominent smooth muscle hyperplasia, and if mostly composed of cystically dilated spaces, the latter may be misconstrued as vessels, and the tumor diagnosed as leiomyoma. At high-power examination, even though the spaces are lined by flattened epithelium that may mimic endothelial cells, they are often associated smaller tubules or nests of cells with abundant cytoplasm, oval to round nuclei, small nucleoli (epithelial appearance), and cells displaying a signet ring cell morphology (fig. 10-46). If subserosal, they may show a focally papillary architecture. The intervening stroma is edematous and often contains lymphocytes, which may form small aggregates at the tumor periphery (270,271). In contrast to leiomyomas, they are positive for calretinin, D2-40, and CK5/6 (272) and are associated with *TRAF7* mutations (273).

In contrast to typical leiomyomas, leiomyoma variants frequently display unusual gross or microscopic features that suggest leiomyosarcoma or, less commonly, other uterine neoplasms. Gross worrisome features include large size, irregular margins, unusual consistency or color, extensive areas of hemorrhage or necrosis, striking edema, or unusual growth patterns as seen for example in cotyledonoid dissecting leiomyoma and intravenous leiomyomatosis. Evaluation of the tumor-myometrium interface, extensive sampling of the tumor from different areas, and a clinical history are crucial in these cases.

Leiomyoma with bizarre nuclei is likely the leiomyoma variant that most often is misdiagnosed as leiomyosarcoma due to the associated striking cytologic atypia, which may be extensive, and the finding of "atypical" mitoses. However, leiomyosarcomas only rarely display degenerative cytologic atypia while brisk mitotic activity and other features of malignancy are seen. Leiomyomas with bizarre nuclei may show significant Ki-67 expression and extensive or diffuse p16 and p53 positivity, and they have a much lower frequency of *MED12* mutations, a profile that closely overlaps with leiomyosarcoma (217,218,221,225,226,254,259,274–276). Thus, these markers should be used with caution in this differential diagnosis. The gross appearance of leiomyomas with bizarre nuclei is often closer to that observed in typical leiomyomas.

Mitotically active leiomyoma should be distinguished from leiomyosarcoma, however, the former lacks any degree of cytologic atypia or tumor cell necrosis. Mitotic activity, an important morphologic criterion in separating benign from malignant smooth muscle tumors in the past, has been shown that in isolation is not necessarily indicative of malignancy. Nevertheless, mitotic activity may be difficult to ascertain on regular histologic sections, thus, markers of proliferation including Ki-67 and PHH3 are used in this distinction (219). Mitotically active leiomyomas that have more than 10 mitoses per 10 high-power fields may cause concern for leiomyosarcoma. In such cases, it is more helpful to evaluate other key histologic features as much as to sample extensively the tumor as some leiomyosarcomas are associated with benign-appearing areas and others are only deceptively malignant (277). When in doubt, the term "smooth muscle tumor of uncertain malignant potential" with an explanatory note may be acceptable so that the patient can be followed appropriately.

Apoplectic leiomyomas can also cause concern for leiomyosarcoma, especially when multiple ill-defined areas of hemorrhage/necrosis are present. Worrisome features include multifocal hypercellularity, epithelioid-like morphology of cells with visible nucleoli and mitoses, pyknotic nuclei, and associated myxoid change near the hemorrhagic/necrotic areas. Ki-67 and p16 expression are often increased in these areas, further suggesting malignancy (223). The gross appearance can also be a confounding feature. However, in contrast to leiomyosarcoma, away from these areas, the tumors have the appearance of a typical leiomyoma, and hemorrhage/necrosis in different phases of reabsorption/reorganization are characteristic of this leiomyoma variant but not seen in leiomyosarcomas. It is important to be aware of the wide morphologic spectrum of these tumors and to inquire about a history of contraceptive intake (37).

Another leiomyoma variant, hydropic leiomyoma, is often clinically suspected to be a leiomyosarcoma, specifically myxoid, due to its rapid growth and gross appearance. The one pathologic feature of concern is the common misinterpretation of edema as myxoid background either on gross or microscopic examination. Some tumors are multinodular, a feature that may be misconstrued as invasion. In contrast to the "sticky" thick myxoid matrix, hydropic leiomyoma has a watery background that is easy to squeeze, the tumor is typically well circumscribed, and there are edematous areas with dropout of smooth muscle cells that alternate with nodules or nests of smooth muscle, typically associated with large and thick blood vessels in contrast to the more commonly evenly distributed myxoid background between the tumor cells in myxoid tumors (278). Alcian blue is negative or only faintly positive. When a hydropic leiomyoma has a striking nodular architecture (diffuse perinodular change) it may be erroneously misinterpreted grossly and microscopically as intravenous leiomyomatosis. However, in contrast to the latter, the nodules of smooth muscle are in spaces that lack endothelial cells, being CD31 negative (38).

Highly cellular leiomyoma is likely the only leiomyoma variant that is typically confused with non-smooth muscle tumors, specifically endometrial stromal tumors. There are striking gross and microscopic similarities as well as some immunohistochemical overlap including yellow to tan color, some margin irregularity, dense cellularity, scant cell cytoplasm, prominent vascularity, and positivity for CD10, muscle actin, WT1, ER, and PR. A final confounding feature in these tumors is the finding of cellular seedling (tiny) leiomyomas at their periphery, increasing the concern at low power for an endometrial stromal sarcoma. In general, smooth muscle tumors have large, thick, muscular-walled blood vessels. Although small vessels may be seen, they lack the characteristic arteriole-like morphology seen in endometrial stromal tumors. Other helpful features lacking in stromal tumors include cleft-like spaces and focal merging of the highly cellular areas with typical fascicular smooth muscle neoplasia and neighboring myometrium. Strong and multifocal or diffuse immunoreactivity for smooth muscle markers, including desmin and h-caldesmon, confirms the smooth muscle nature of the tumor (197,199). It is important not to use one marker but a panel of antibodies in this differential diagnosis.

Epithelioid morphology in smooth muscle tumors elicits a wide differential diagnosis, including leiomyomas with a pseudoepithelioid appearance and other tumor types with true epithelioid morphology. Epithelial-like morphology may be a secondary result from a variety of scenarios including infarct-type necrosis (in apoplectic leiomyomas), hydropic change or hyalinization (with corded morphology) or rhabdoid cells, or due to progesterone effect in tumors occurring in pregnant women. After determining that the tumor has true epithelioid morphology, leiomyosarcoma is likely the main entity in the differential diagnosis. The finding of moderate to severe cytologic atypia, more than 4 mitoses per 10 high-power fields, or tumor cell necrosis, is diagnostic of epithelioid leiomyosarcoma. Although experience with epithelioid tumors is limited and criteria for malignancy in this category of smooth muscle tumors are not as well established as in spindle cell tumors, the mitotic count to establish a diagnosis of malignancy is much lower than in spindle leiomyosarcoma (10 mitoses per 10 high-power fields in the latter) (124–126). Other tumors in the differential diagnosis include PEComa, trophoblastic tumors (placental-site trophoblastic tumor and epithelioid trophoblastic tumor), and, although uncommon, uterine tumor resembling an ovarian sex-cord tumor should also be excluded (discussed in leiomyosarcoma section).

Since myxoid leiomyomas are exceedingly rare, a variety of other entities should be considered before making such a diagnosis (279). The most common scenario is the misinterpretation of a leiomyoma with hydropic change as a myxoid smooth muscle tumor (discussed above). After ascertaining the myxoid nature of the background matrix, focal myxoid change in conventional leiomyomas should be ruled out (seen in up to 13 percent of leiomyomas in different series, often secondary to pregnancy or hormonal treatment). This finding within a smooth muscle tumor does not qualify for a diagnosis of myxoid leiomyoma (21,96). To establish a diagnosis of myxoid smooth muscle tumor, extensive areas should have a myxoid background (more than 30 percent but in some series more than 50 percent) (279). When evaluating a tumor with a myxoid matrix, the two main entities to consider are myxoid leiomyosarcoma and inflammatory myofibroblastic tumor as both, although rare, are more common than myxoid leiomyoma. Myxoid leiomyosarcoma may be fairly well circumscribed and is often hypocellular as occurs with its benign counterpart. Large size, infiltrative borders, cytologic atypia, or more than 2 mitoses per 10 high-power fields are features that establish a diagnosis of leiomyosarcoma. However, as tumors with bland cytology and less than 2 mitoses per 10 high-power fields have recurred, caution should be exercised before making a diagnosis of myxoid leiomyoma; extensive sampling should be performed to identify other features, as for example, infiltrative borders, that can help in establishing a diagnosis of malignancy (136,280). Of course, no single feature but a constellation of features establishes a diagnosis of malignancy. The other entity, inflammatory myofibroblastic tumor, may have an extensive myxoid background, spindle and epithelioid cells, and positivity for smooth muscle markers. However, these tumors typically have a variably prominent inflammatory component of lymphocytes and plasma cells and are often ALK-1 positive (266,281,281a). Rarely, an endometrial stromal nodule may be extensively myxoid; however, it is composed of small oval cells with scant cytoplasm that focally whorl around arterioles, and often areas of conventional endometrial stromal neoplasia are seen at least focally. Immunohistochemical and molecular studies may also help in this differential diagnosis (282,283).

Among benign smooth muscle proliferations with unusual growth patterns, diffuse uterine leiomyomatosis should be separated from the rare uterine lymphangioleiomyomatosis, usually in patients with tuberous sclerosis. The latter is characterized by numerous microscopic ill-defined nodules of smooth muscle surrounding lymphatics and protruding into their lumens, often associated with bright and dense hyaline bands (284,285). The cells typically have clear to granular and eosinophilic cytoplasm and are HMB-45 and melan A positive (285,286).

Diffuse peritoneal leiomyomatosis should be distinguished from primary or metastatic leiomyosarcoma and gastrointestinal stromal tumor. The finding of any degree of cytologic atypia as well as infiltrative growth should exclude a benign diagnosis. Even though gastrointestinal stromal tumors may be positive for actin and desmin, they are typically positive for C-KIT and DOG1 (287). Rarely, diffuse peritoneal leiomyomatosis is mistaken for peritoneal carcinomatosis at the time of cesarian section but mostly on gross examination (288).

Intravenous leiomyomatosis should be distinguished from leiomyoma with vascular invasion and endometrial stromal sarcoma. It shares with the former the finding of smooth muscle tumor within vascular spaces; however, by definition, intravascular growth should occur outside the confines of the leiomyoma. The distinction from an endometrial stromal sarcoma may be challenging, especially if intravenous leiomyomatosis is cellular. Both display intravascular growth and prominent vascularity. Low-grade endometrial stromal sarcoma usually lacks lobulated contours, thick-walled vessels, and hydropic change in its intravascular component, and usually there is an accompanying "tongue-like" pattern of infiltration by the tumor. Other entities in the differential diagnosis of intravenous leiomyomatosis include diffuse perinodular hydropic leiomyoma, cotyledonoid leiomyoma, and diffuse leiomyomatosis if associated with retraction artifact. In the latter, CD31 is negative since there are no endothelial cells, in contrast to intravenous leiomyomatosis (fig. 10-47).

Before making a diagnosis of benign metastasizing leiomyoma, metastatic leiomyosarcoma, primary pulmonary smooth muscle tumors or hamartomas with a prominent smooth muscle component, and lymphangioleiomyomatosis should be excluded. For leiomyosarcoma, it is important to compare the lesion to the prior hysterectomy specimen if available since they may have a deceptive appearance. Pulmonary hamartomas show other histologic components and rarely are multiple. Primary smooth muscle tumors are the rarest benign tumors of the lung and tend to be unifocal (289). Lymphangiomyomatosis is a diffuse process seen exclusively in females that can exhibit a rapidly progressive and fatal course. In contrast to benign metastasizing leiomyoma that has a peribronchiolar distribution, lymphangioleiomyomatosis is centered around vessels. It typically does not form gross nodules and cells are HMB-45 and melan A positive (285).

Rare extrauterine malignancies, typically carcinomas, metastasize to a leiomyoma, imparting an unusual morphology that may potentially be misconstrued as a biphasic tumor within the uterus (290). A prior clinical history and the malignant nature of the epithelial component as well as the presence of tumor outside the leiomyoma are helpful in establishing the correct diagnosis.

Treatment and Prognosis. Leiomyomas are benign tumors that are treated medically or surgically, depending on patient age, symptoms, associated risk factors, number, size, and location of the tumors (International Federation of Gynecology and Obstetrics [FIGO] leiomyoma classification system). Medical treatment is an alternative to surgery or may be implemented preoperatively to improve surgical results but typically represents a short-term option. Phar-

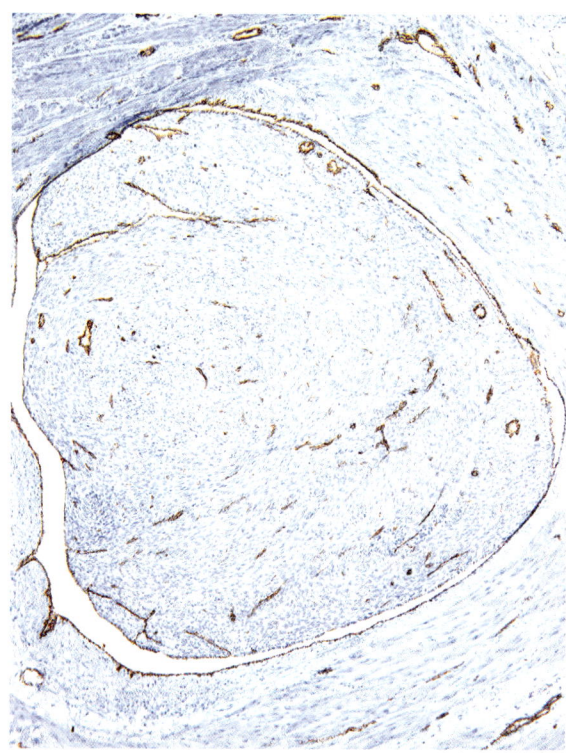

Figure 10-47

INTRAVENOUS LEIOMYOMATOSIS

The intravascular nodules are surrounded by endothelial cells as highlighted by CD31.

macologic therapies include oral contraceptives/progesterone, GnRH agonists and antagonists, aromatase inhibitors, selective estrogen or progesterone receptor modulators, and antifibrinolytic agents. These drugs reduce the symptoms associated with fibroids and some of them also induce a temporary reduction in tumor size (291). Other nonsurgical options are ablation and uterine artery embolization (292).

Surgical options include myomectomy, hysterectomy, or morcellation. Although the latter is associated with reduced hospital time and overall fewer complications (293–295), an increase of parasitic leiomyomas and diffuse peritoneal leiomyomatosis correlates with the use of this surgical modality (26–30). Furthermore, as tumors cannot be sampled by preoperative curettage since they are often intramyometrial, the possibility of leiomyosarcoma cannot be excluded; if a leiomyosarcoma is treated with this modality, the tumor becomes disseminated, impacting severely on patient survival (296–298).

Myomectomy is the gold standard of treatment for patients who want to preserve fertility, while hysterectomy is the standard of treatment for those that have completed childbearing. Reported complications associated with myomectomy are similar to those associated with hysterectomy and include intraoperative conversion to hysterectomy in 3 to 4 percent of myomectomies. The latter is associated with a higher morbidity than hysterectomy, including adhesions and increased risk of uterine rupture, which may affect future pregnancies (299). Studies have shown that the 5-year recurrence rate for fibroids treated with local excision may be as high as 60 percent. The risk is lower in patients with a single fibroid, smaller total uterine size, and those who subsequently had a successful pregnancy (300,301). Leiomyoma variants associated with a benign outcome include tumors mitotically active or those with bizarre nuclei with long follow-up (mean, 15 years) (39,40,61,65).

Among the unusual growth patterns seen in benign smooth muscle proliferations, diffuse leiomyomatosis has been successfully treated by extreme myomectomy since these patients are typically in their reproductive ages (155). Diffuse peritoneal leiomyomatosis may regress spontaneously after pregnancy but if symptomatic, the patient may undergo conservative resection of the masses. If clinically mistaken for peritoneal carcinomatosis at the time of cesarian section, the patient may undergo unnecessary radical surgery (288). Lesions may also regress with hormonal therapy (164,302).

Intravenous leiomyomatosis is probably the only lesion that requires hysterectomy and excision of any extrauterine tumor, if technically feasible, with bilateral adnexectomy since the lesion is estrogen dependent. In most cases, the intravascular growth is likely inconsequential, especially when not extensive, but extrauterine extension is common and cardiac extension has been reported in up to 10 percent, especially in the older literature (169,303). In one study of 16 patients with a mean follow-up of 7.5 years, most had a favorable outcome. Some patients, however, develop pelvic or cardiac recurrences or lung metastases up to 15 years after hysterectomy since the tumor may continue to grow within vessels (173). Currently, it is believed that the risk of recurrence of intravenous leiomyomatosis is low (less than 5 percent) (154). Postoperative imaging studies may be helpful in monitoring tumor regrowth and GnRHa may control nonresectable tumor.

Benign metastasizing leiomyoma is histologically benign (slow growing and hormone sensitive), and most patients have a benign clinical outcome. Treatment options include surgical removal or hormone treatment and some also consider bilateral salpingo-oophorectomy (304,305). After surgical resection, patients frequently require hormonal treatment since lesions may continue to grow (306).

LEIOMYOSARCOMA

Definition. *Leiomyosarcoma* is a malignant smooth muscle tumor, most often displaying spindle cell morphology, but occasionally with epithelioid or myxoid features (1).

Epidemiology and General Features. Leiomyosarcomas are common soft tissue sarcomas, comprising approximately 25 percent of all sarcomas and are most common in the retroperitoneum and uterus (307,308). Leiomyosarcoma is the most common uterine sarcoma in the female genital tract and represents 40 to 50 percent of all uterine sarcomas but only 1 percent of all uterine malignancies (309). Incidence rates are 6.4 per million based on data from nine cancer registries (Surveillance, Epidemiology, and End Results [SEER] data, 1973-1981) (310).

Leiomyosarcoma is the malignant counterpart of uterine leiomyoma, however, the incidence of malignant transformation of leiomyomas is very low, ranging between 0.13 and 0.80, while the incidence ratio of leiomyomas to leiomyosarcomas has been estimated to be 800 to 1. In one study, 1 percent of women between 40 and 60 years (8 of 817) with presumed uterine leiomyomas and symptoms requiring hysterectomy had leiomyosarcoma (311). There seems to be an increased incidence of leiomyosarcoma among African-American women, although not as pronounced as reported for leiomyomas (312). There is an increased incidence in women on tamoxifen therapy for breast cancer (313) and in patients with hereditary retinoblastoma and Li-Fraumeni syndrome (314,315). Although leiomyosarcomas may be part of the HLRCC syndrome, some may represent FH-deficient leiomyomas that have been misdiagnosed as leiomyosarcoma due to their atypical features (316).

Clinical Features. Patients with leiomyosarcoma are often diagnosed at 50 to 60 years of age, one decade later than those with leiomyomas, although they can occur at an earlier age. In some series, up to 40 percent of patients were premenopausal (317) and only 15 percent were younger than 40 years (318,319).

Signs and symptoms have variable duration and include, in order of frequency, abnormal vaginal bleeding (56 percent), palpable pelvic mass on routine gynecologic exam (54 percent), and pelvic/abdominal pain (22 percent). Less frequently, patients present with hemoperitoneum secondary to tumor rupture, or symptoms resulting from extrauterine extension including bowel or urinary obstruction (about 35 percent of patients) or metastases (most often to lung in about 10 percent). Patients may present with nonspecific symptoms including weight loss, weakness, and fever or rarely, they are asymptomatic (317,320).

Rapid uterine growth is always clinically worrisome, but it most often corresponds to leiomyomas in reproductive age women. However, a leiomyosarcoma should be suspected in postmenopausal women with a rapidly growing mass or those with "fibroids" that continue to grow on treatment with GnRHa. Leiomyosarcomas have no known risk factors but some patients may have a prior history of radiation therapy or tamoxifen treatment (321,322).

On physical examination, the uterus is typically enlarged. Preoperative uterine size ranged from 8 to 20 weeks' gestational size in one study (311). Serum cancer antigen 125 or lactate dehydrogenase may be elevated but these markers are not specific (323). Patients occasionally present with hematologic manifestations including thrombotic thrombocytopenic purpura (324), systemic eosinophilia (325) with secondary amyloidosis (326), hyperphosphatemia (327), or hypercalcemia related to secretion of parathyroid hormone-related protein (328). Paraneoplastic syndromes associated with uterine leiomyosarcoma are extremely rare, with only few cases reported in the literature, including ANNA-1-associated encephalitis (329), myasthenia gravis and Lambert-Eaton myasthenic syndrome (330), Lesser-Trélat sign (multiple seborrheic keratosis) (331), and Guillain-Barré syndrome (136); serum beta-hCG may be elevated (136,329–332).

Currently, available radiologic techniques cannot reliably distinguish leiomyomas, other than typical ones, from leiomyosarcomas, as extensive overlap exists. When an endometrial biopsy/curettage is performed it often yields no diagnostic information except if the tumor is submucosal, making preoperative diagnosis of leiomyosarcoma unreliable, and thus, this possibility cannot be excluded when performing a morcellation procedure (297,333).

Gross Findings. Most leiomyosarcomas are centered in the myometrium or endomyometrium, but about 5 percent are subserosal or centered in the cervix (334). In the cervix, although rare, leiomyosarcomas are the most common type of sarcoma (335). They can be seen in the anterior or posterior wall or within the uterine fundus or isthmus. They are typically the largest or the only uterine mass in 80 to 95 percent of cases (336,337). They can be pedunculated with a broad base if submucosal.

Leiomyosarcomas have a mean diameter of 6 to 10 cm (317,319,337–339). They have typically poorly circumscribed borders but may be well circumscribed with a soft and fleshy cut surface that may be multilobulated and frequently is associated with areas of necrosis and hemorrhage (fig. 10-48) (317,334). Some tumors, however, have a firm consistency, with a white cut surface as typically seen in leiomyomas (77). If myxoid, the cut surface may be gelatinous, imparting a "sticky" or "mucoid" texture (fig. 10-49) (136,280,340,341). Cystic degeneration may be noted (136). If arising in a background of leiomyoma, the leiomyosarcoma component may display a distinctive gross appearance (342,343). Although rare, intravascular growth may be seen grossly if prominent (*intravenous leiomyosarcomatosis*) (344).

When evaluating any smooth muscle tumor, gross and microscopic features should be considered equally important. An irregular/infiltrative margin with the surrounding myometrium, an unusual growth pattern, or unusual cut surface should prompt extensive tumor sampling to identify microscopic features, which may not be uniform or may be subtle, that help in the diagnosis of leiomyosarcoma, especially in uncommon subtypes.

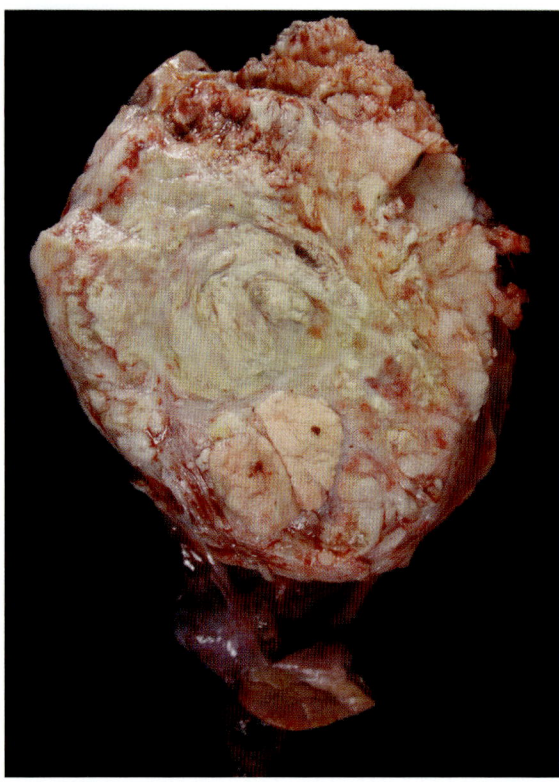

Figure 10-48

SPINDLED LEIOMYOSARCOMA

A large tumor has replaced the entire uterus. It has a gray fleshy appearance and is associated with extensive areas of necrosis.

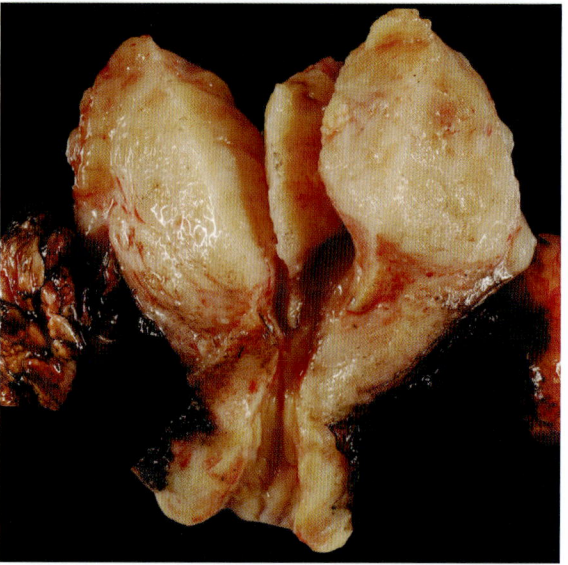

Figure 10-49

MYXOID LEIOMYOSARCOMA

The tumor has a well-circumscribed border and a gelatinous cut surface. (Courtesy of Drs F. Alameda and B. Lloveras, Barcelona, Spain.)

Microscopic Findings. Leiomyosarcomas are mainly divided into three categories: spindled, epithelioid, and myxoid. Although spindle cell leiomyosarcoma is the most common, combinations of patterns occur, more often containing a spindle cell component (1).

Spindle cell (conventional) leiomyosarcomas often display at least focally irregular, variable destructive invasion of the adjacent myometrium but may be well circumscribed. They are composed of long, compact, and often hypercellular intersecting fascicles of spindle cells with eosinophilic fibrillary or, less commonly, clear cytoplasm (fig. 10-50A,B). Paranuclear vacuoles can be seen. Sometimes cells are small, with minimal cytoplasm (fig. 10-50C). Blunt-shaped nuclei are enlarged, often with multifocal or diffuse, moderate to marked atypia, hyperchromatic or pleomorphic nuclei, and one or more prominent nucleoli. However, hypocellular areas or areas reminiscent of a leiomyoma can be seen (fig. 10-51A) (277,345), and leiomyosarcomas with low-grade cytologic atypia exist although are rare (fig. 10-51B) (346). Brisk mitotic activity, often over 10 mitoses per 10 high-power fields, with or without atypical mitoses, is common, but as mentioned for cytologic atypia, tumors with lower mitotic counts also exist. Mono- or multinucleated neoplastic cells with degenerative-type atypia may be focally seen. Rarely, a leiomyosarcoma arises within a leiomyoma, with the two components being sharply demarcated (fig. 10-51C).

Tumor cell necrosis is present in less than half of leiomyosarcomas and this finding should prompt extensive sampling to identify other features of malignancy. Tumor cell necrosis is characterized by an abrupt transition from viable to nonviable tumor without an intervening zone of granulation tissue or hyalinized tissue. There is typically perivascular growth of viable tumor cells while some preserved atypical cells as well as apoptotic cells are still seen within the necrotic foci (fig. 10-52) (61). Even though tumor cell necrosis is important in establishing the diagnosis of leiomyosarcoma, when present, other diagnostic features of malignancy

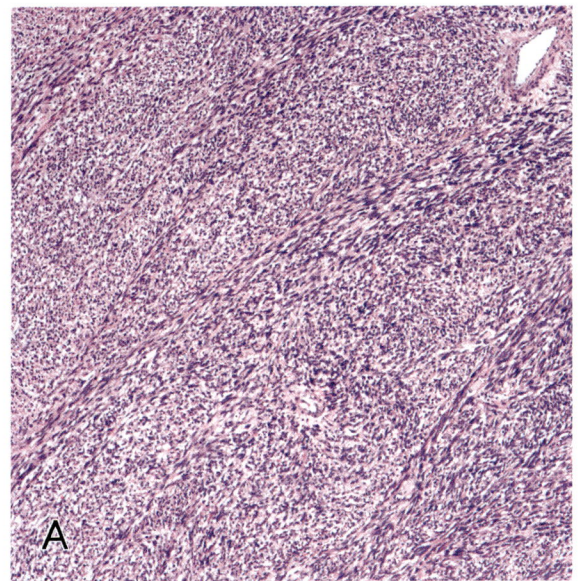

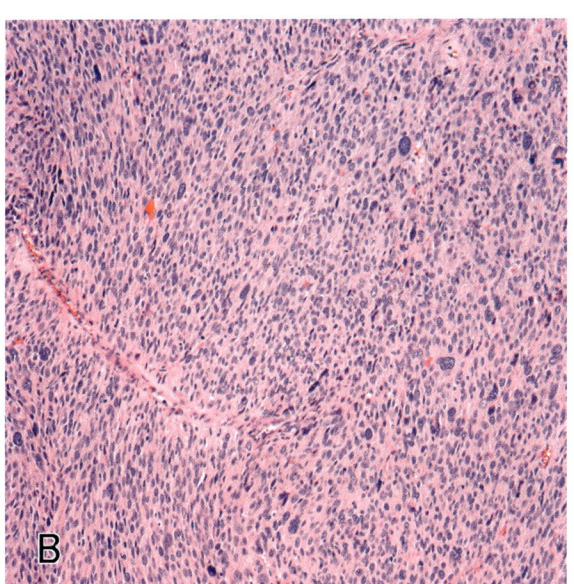
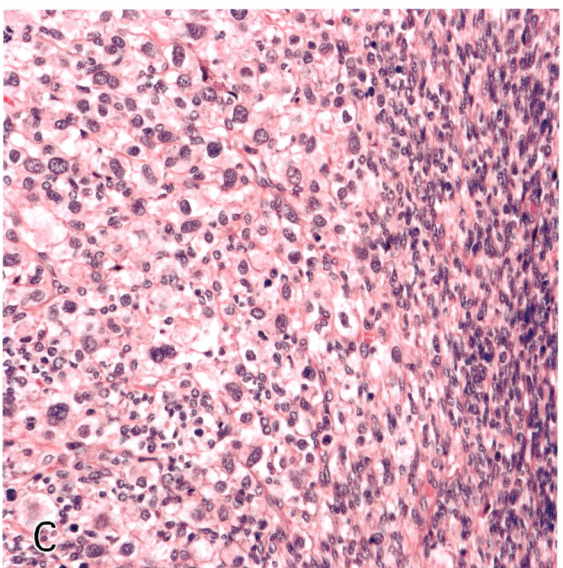

Figure 10-50

SPINDLED LEIOMYOSARCOMA

Compact growth of long hypercellular fascicles is seen (A). The fascicular architecture and cytologic atypia involving all neoplastic cells are appreciated at low-power magnification (B). A component of small spindle cells (uncommon) is juxtaposed with an epithelioid component (C).

(mitotic activity and cytologic atypia) are typically identified in the tumor. Infarct-type necrosis is also frequently seen in leiomyosarcomas and it may be difficult to distinguish from tumor necrosis (63). Infarct-type necrosis is characterized by the presence of granulation or hyalinized tissue between viable and nonviable areas of tumor, frequently associated with recent hemorrhage or hemosiderin deposition. Nonviable areas have a mummified appearance, with easily identified devitalized tumor cells and vessels, and "ghost" tumor cells. In a series of 27 patients with uterine leiomyosarcoma, tumor cell necrosis was observed in 12 (44 percent), with most tumors also exhibiting infarct-type necrosis (346). Interobserver agreement in the interpretation of tumor cell necrosis is at most fair among experienced gynecologic pathologists, highlighting the intrinsic difficulty in obtaining a correct diagnosis, and introducing ambiguous terminology for final tumor classification (347). Evaluation of the extracellular matrix is useful in some cases to distinguish tumor cell from infarct-type necrosis. In one study, the pattern of reticulin staining differed significantly between nonviable areas in leiomyosarcoma

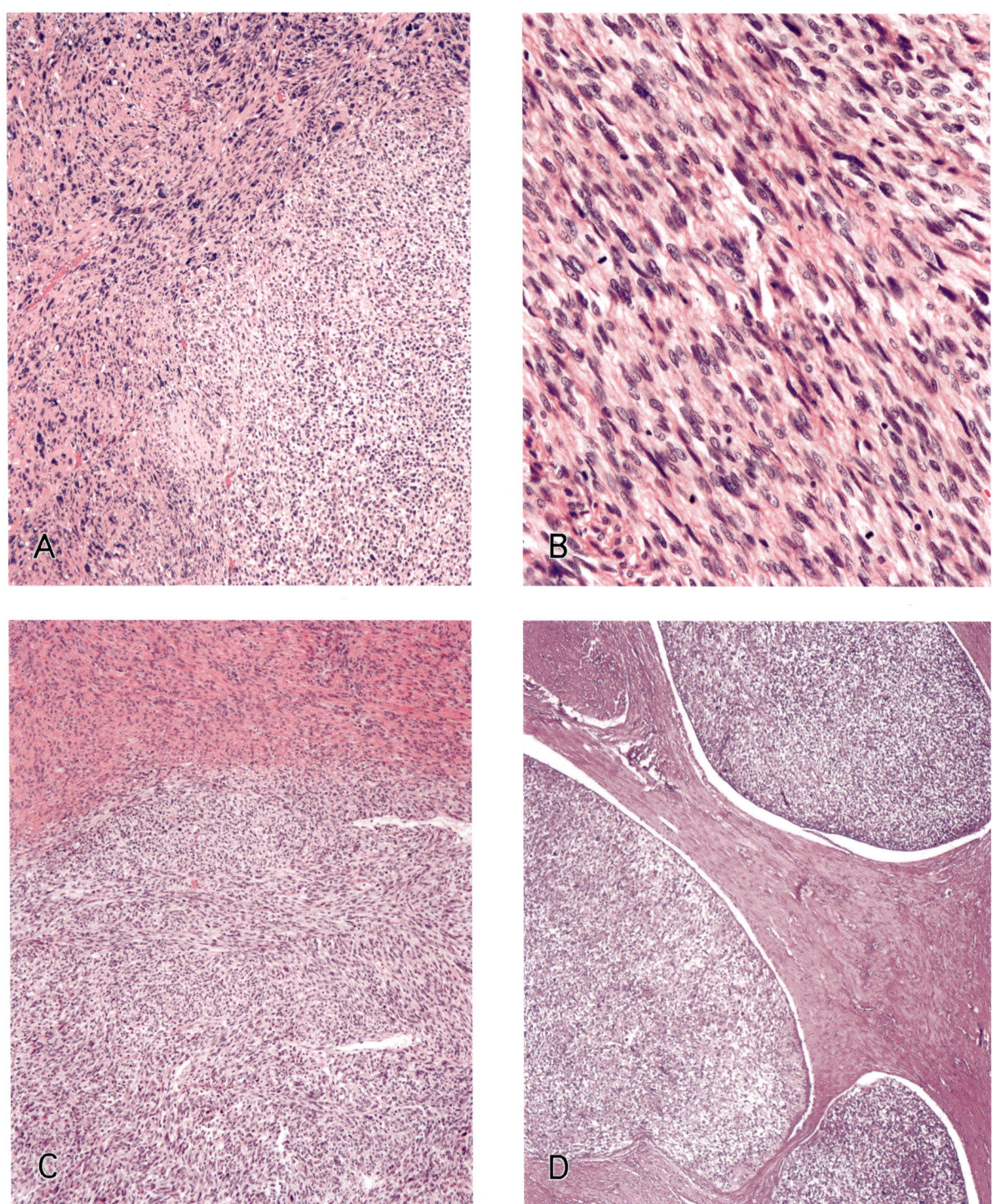

Figure 10-51

SPINDLED LEIOMYOSARCOMA

Areas closely simulating a leiomyoma with bizarre nuclei are juxtaposed to the overtly malignant areas. Cytoplasmic vacuolization is present (A). Brisk mitotic activity is noted in an area without significant cytologic atypia (B). Spindle cell leiomyosarcoma arising in a leiomyoma. Hypercellular fascicular growth of atypical spindle cells and conventional leiomyoma are juxtaposed (C). Prominent intravascular growth is noted (D).

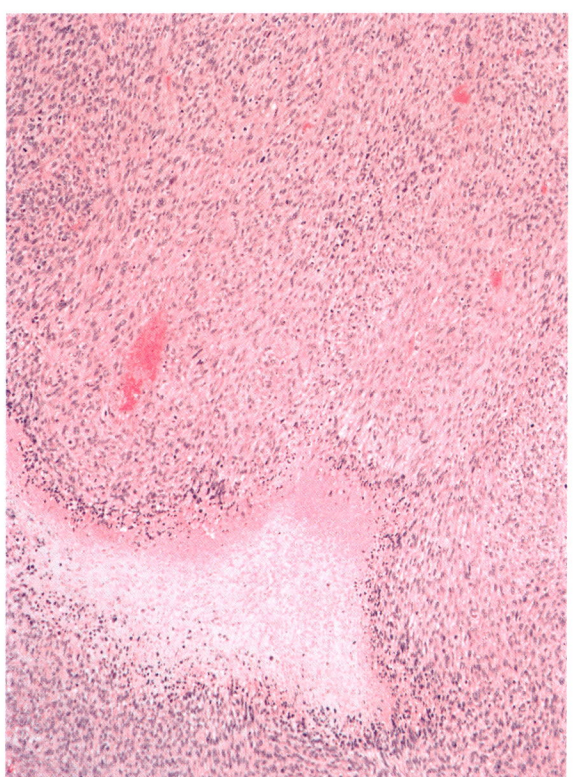 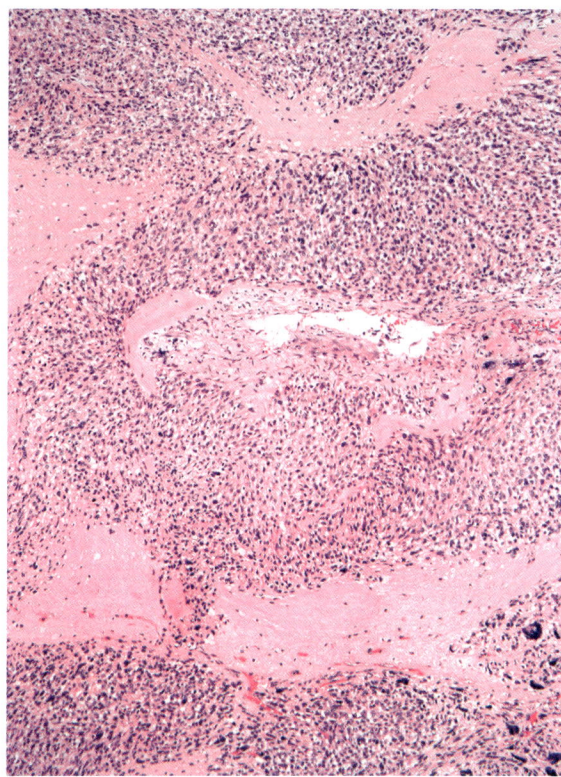

Figure 10-52

SPINDLED LEIOMYOSARCOMA

The tumor is hypercellular and associated with early tumor cell necrosis, which only focally develops around a vessel (left). Tumor cell necrosis has a well-developed perivascular distribution. There is diffuse cytologic atypia as well as scattered malignant multinucleated giant cells (bottom of right figure).

and leiomyoma, with preserved honey-comb pattern in leiomyosarcoma but lost in areas of infarct-type necrosis within leiomyomas (91 versus 39 percent). It was also noted that mitotic activity in leiomyosarcomas increases away from the areas of necrosis (348).

Originally, diagnostic criteria for leiomyosarcoma were based on mitotic activity and cytologic atypia (64,77,349,350), however, tumor cell necrosis was added to the algorithm (61,351). Currently, the diagnosis of spindle leiomyosarcoma is established when a combination of two of the following three features is present: diffuse moderate to severe atypia, more than 10 mitoses per 10 high-power fields and tumor cell necrosis (61,352,353). These features, however, only detect high-grade leiomyosarcomas. Even though low-grade leiomyosarcomas exist, there are currently no well-established criteria for their diagnosis, and likely most are diagnosed as smooth muscle tumors of low or uncertain malignant potential. Tumors originally classified as low-grade leiomyosarcoma consist of two groups of tumors in one study. One group was histologically indistinguishable from conventional leiomyosarcomas, apart from a lower prevalence of tumor cell necrosis (with similar patient outcome). The second was an heterogeneous group including atypical smooth muscle tumors as well as endometrial stromal sarcomas with smooth muscle differentiation among others (354).

Vascular invasion is detected in approximately 20 percent of leiomyosarcomas (355) but some tumors show prominent intravascular growth (fig. 10-51D), simulating intravenous leiomyomatosis (*intravenous leiomyosarcomatosis*) (344). Rarely, a spindle cell leiomyosarcoma with fully developed malignant features is associated with a leiomyoma (fig. 10-51C) (342,343).

Figure 10-53
EPITHELIOID LEIOMYOSARCOMA

A diffuse and compact nested architecture is noted. Scattered cells have severe cytologic atypia (A). Nodular architecture is juxtaposed to infarct-type necrosis (B). Corded growth with squeezed cells is secondary to associated hyalinization (C).

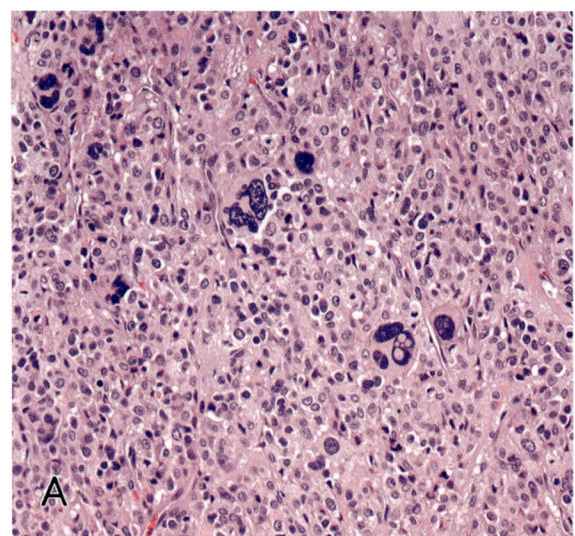

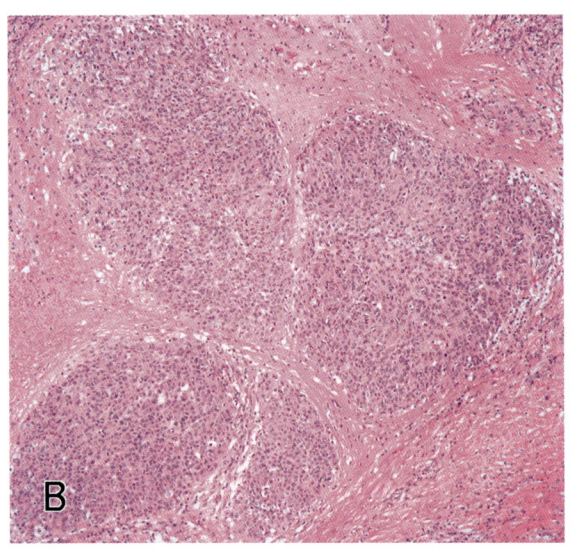

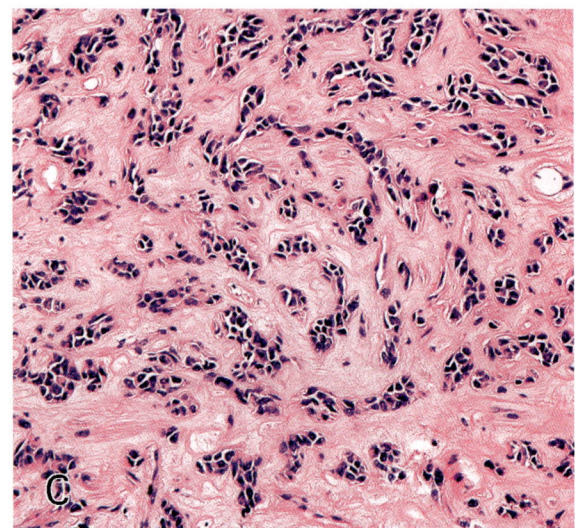

Epithelioid Leiomyosarcoma. This variant is uncommon. To establish this diagnosis, more than 50 percent of the cells of the leiomyosarcoma should have an "epithelial-like" appearance as defined in its benign counterpart (1). As seen with spindle cell leiomyosarcomas, there may be an infiltrative border but many are well circumscribed.

The cells are arranged in diffuse, nodular, nested, or corded growth patterns (fig. 10-53), but more than one pattern is often noted in the same tumor. Pseudoglandular spaces filled with light eosinophilic material may be seen (fig. 10-54) (123,124,126,356–362). Hyalinization is common and may be extensive, especially when tumors have a plexiform or corded growth. Cells are polygonal, with abundant eosinophilic (fig. 10-55), granular, amphophilic, or clear cytoplasm (363), but are occasionally small (360). The nuclei are often round and centrally located, but may be eccentric, occasionally mimicking signet ring cells or even lipoblasts, especially if the cytoplasm is vacuolated. Cells with rhabdoid morphology can be seen (124,362,364). The vasculature tends to be delicate. A component of spindle cells and, less commonly, myxoid leiomyosarcoma can be seen (346). Tumor cell or infarct-type necrosis may be noted. Even though criteria predictive of malignancy are less well established when compared to conventional leiomyosarcomas, the finding of 4 or more mitoses per 10 high-power fields (much lower threshold than in spindled subtype), with

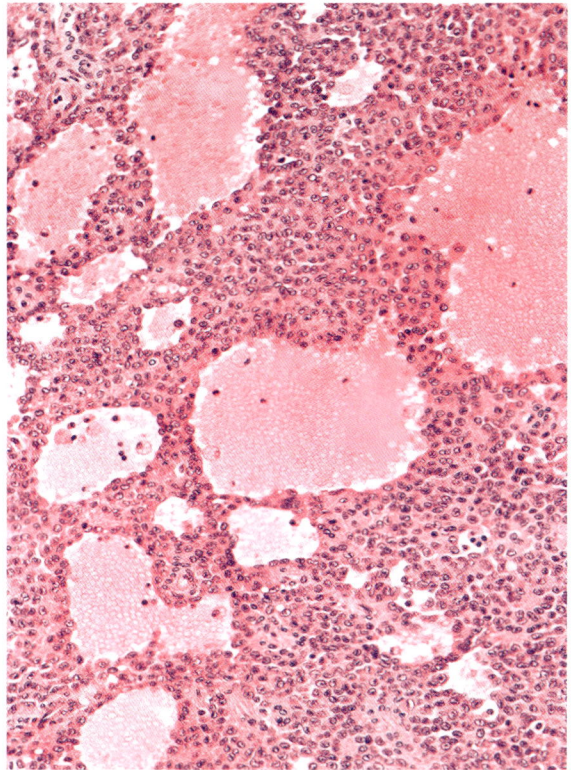

Figure 10-54

EPITHELIOID LEIOMYOSARCOMA

Follicle-like spaces filled with eosinophilic material are seen within the diffuse growth of tumor cells.

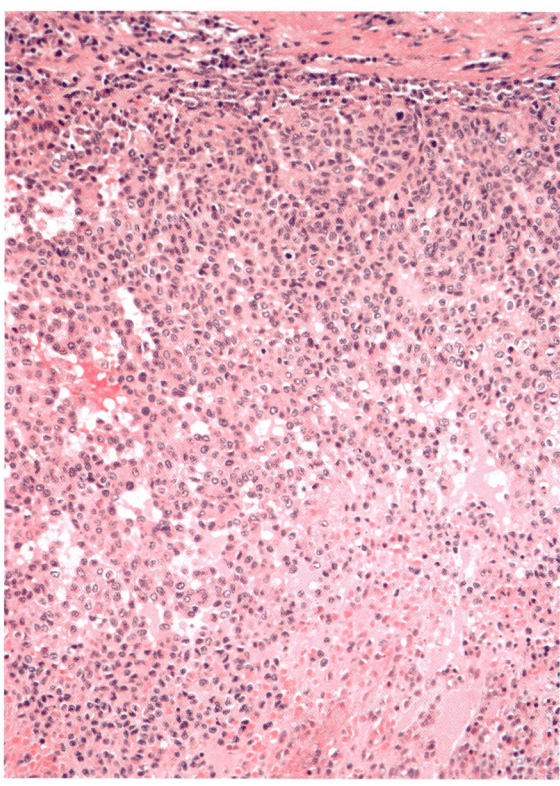

Figure 10-55

EPITHELIOID LEIOMYOSARCOMA

The cells have abundant eosinophilic cytoplasm and slightly irregular-shaped nuclei. Cytologic atypia is not striking but there is brisk mitotic activity and associated necrosis establishing the diagnosis of leiomyosarcoma.

diffuse moderate to severe cytologic atypia or tumor cell necrosis warrants a diagnosis of epithelioid leiomyosarcoma (124,365).

Myxoid Leiomyosarcoma. These tumors typically invade the surrounding myometrium in a destructive, bulbous (fig. 10-56), or tongue-like pattern, although invasion may be limited or deceptive and rarely, tumors are well circumscribed as occurs with other subtypes of leiomyosarcoma. In contrast to the latter, they are often hypocellular due to an abundant extracellular myxoid matrix rich in hyaluronic acid. The threshold of myxoid matrix required for the diagnosis of myxoid smooth muscle tumor ranges from over 30 to over 50 percent in different studies (136,280,340,341,356,365). The tumor cells are seen throughout the myxoid stroma in a diffuse or vaguely nodular pattern (most common), may form thin or loose fascicles, or less commonly, well-defined intersecting fascicles or clusters (fig. 10-57A,B).

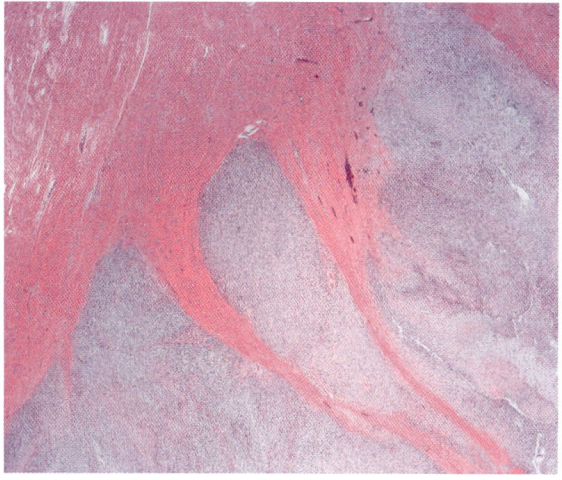

Figure 10-56

MYXOID LEIOMYOSARCOMA

The tumor shows a bulbous infiltrative border into the myometrium and has a prominent myxoid matrix.

Figure 10-57

MYXOID LEIOMYOSARCOMA

Myxoid hypocellular areas with scattered spindle cells are next to conventional areas of leiomyosarcoma, facilitating the diagnosis (A). The cells form thin cords separated by abundant myxoid matrix forming pools of mucin (B). Most cells are spindled and some stellate with mitoses but without prominent cytologic atypia (C).

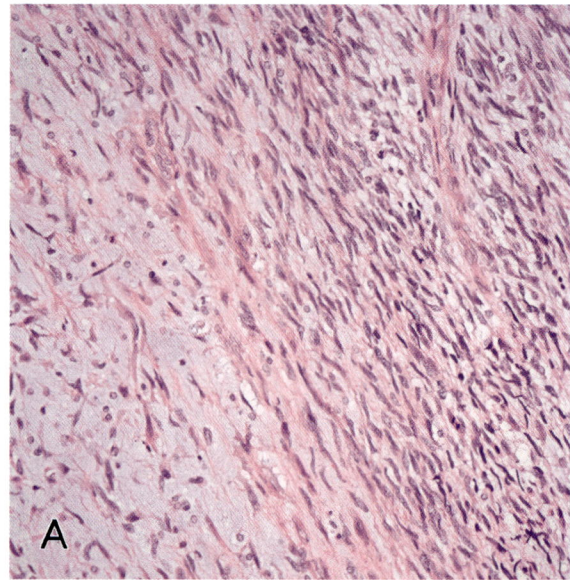

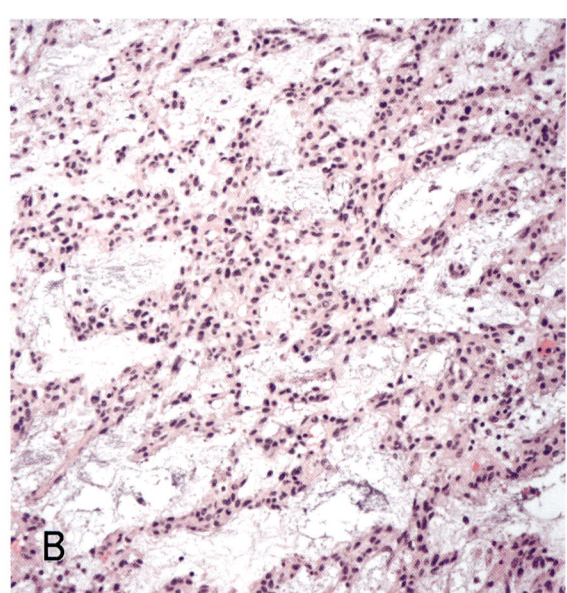

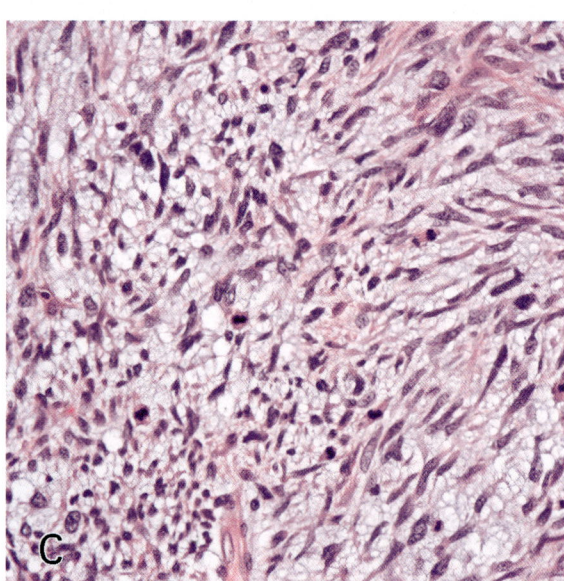

Cellularity varies among neoplasms and within a neoplasm: some tumors are hypercellular and some have large pools of myxoid matrix with minimal cellularity. Variably sized cystic spaces are common, with condensation of cells around cysts imparting a pseudoepithelial appearance. Cells have stellate, spindle, or epithelioid morphology and may be small with oval to spindle-shaped often hyperchromatic nuclei with variably present nucleoli and a variable degree of cytologic atypia. Multinucleated cells may be seen (366). Mitotic activity ranges from inconspicuous to brisk (fig. 10-57C). The vessels are often thin and delicate or ectatic (136,280,340–342,349,365,367–369).

The myxoid material is either weakly eosinophilic or basophilic, since it is strongly positive with alcian blue at pH of 2.5 or colloidal iron and only minimally positive or negative with periodic acid–Schiff (PAS) and mucicarmine (340). Hyalinization may occur and the associated inflammatory infiltrate is typically minimal. A component of spindle or epithelioid leiomyosarcoma may be seen.

As occurs with other types of leiomyosarcoma, tumor cell or infarct-type necrosis may be seen but is not common (tumor cell necrosis is less common). Originally it was reported that tumors with over 2 mitoses per 10 high-power fields should be diagnosed as myxoid leiomyosarcomas in the absence of marked cytologic atypia or tumor cell necrosis (365). However, some myxoid leiomyosarcomas with less than 2 mitoses are also associated with aggressive behavior. Caution should be exercised when evaluating a myxoid smooth muscle tumor, and extensive sampling is crucial, including sections of the tumor myometrium interface, to evaluate margins and detect any area with cytologic atypia or increased mitotic activity (136,280,340,341).

Dedifferentiated (Pleomorphic) Leiomyosarcoma. This tumor has intersecting fascicles of spindle cells with cigar-shaped nuclei and brightly eosinophilic cytoplasm associated with a discrete undifferentiated component lacking morphologic or immunohistochemical myogenic differentiation (370). This leiomyosarcoma variant, although rare, has been reported in the uterus. The dedifferentiated areas often have a morphologic appearance reminiscent of so-called malignant fibrous histiocytoma, with pleomorphic spindle cells admixed with large bizarre atypical cells. Rarely, it displays an epithelioid or rhabdomyoblastic-like morphology and may contain heterologous elements including cartilage or osteoid (370–372).

Other. Rare leiomyosarcomas have a component of osteoclastic-type giant cells that may be more conspicuous in areas of hemorrhage or may resemble a malignant giant cell tumor. Xanthomatous cells with abundant cytoplasm, including lipid vacuoles, and multiple or multilobulated nuclei sometimes disposed in a wreath-like arrangement have also been described (373–377). Leiomyosarcomas occasionally show rhabdomyoblastic or lipoblastic differentiation (378–381).

Immunohistochemical Findings. Mitotic activity is one of the main criteria in the diagnosis of malignancy in smooth muscle tumors of the uterus. However, mitotic counts are frequently difficult to reproduce among pathologists due to technical issues and the common finding of apoptotic cells with karyorrhectic nuclei often misinterpreted as true mitoses (61,382,383). Thus, different proliferating markers have been used to more accurately assess mitotic rate in smooth muscle tumors. Leiomyosarcomas frequently display high Ki-67 indices (217,225,274,384–386). However, Ki-67 typically overestimates mitotic rate and substantial overlap exists between leiomyosarcoma and leiomyoma with bizarre nuclei, the most problematic leiomyoma variant in the differential diagnosis. In one study, positivity in leiomyosarcomas ranged from 6 to 50 percent (mean, 25 percent) and from 0 to 25 percent (mean, 2 percent) in leiomyomas with bizarre nuclei (218). PHH3 is consistently positive in dividing cells but negative in interphase cells (219,220,387,388). It also helps to identify the most mitotically active areas within the tumor (389). One study showed that mitotic counts obtained with PHH3 were almost always higher than by regular counts (220). One potential pitfall is that PHH3 positivity can be detected in nuclei that are not yet dividing since histone H3 phosphorylation starts before real division (220). Thus, correlation with the morphologic findings is always important.

Leiomyosarcomas, when displaying their most characteristic appearance, are easy to diagnose with no need for immunohistochemistry. These tumors are characterized by positivity for a variety of smooth muscle markers, including actins, desmin, h-caldesmon, HDCA8, calponin, and smooth muscle myosin; however, myxoid and poorly differentiated subtypes may show less positivity for these markers (195–197,199, 207,390,391). Transgelin, a new marker for smooth muscle tumors, is positive in leiomyosarcomas although experience is limited (206,392), while smoothelin is much less frequently positive (about 5 percent) when compared to leiomyomas (204).

Leiomyosarcomas are often positive for CAM5.2-AE1/AE3 and EMA, especially when spindled or epithelioid (fig. 10-58, left) (197,203, 209,393) and may express CD10, often focally but occasionally in a diffuse pattern (197,391, 394,395). Expression of ER, PR, and AR varies depending on the degree of differentiation and leiomyosarcoma subtype, ranging from 30 to 40 percent, frequencies typically much lower than those reported in leiomyomas (fig. 10-58, right) (213,214,384,386,396–403). Uterine

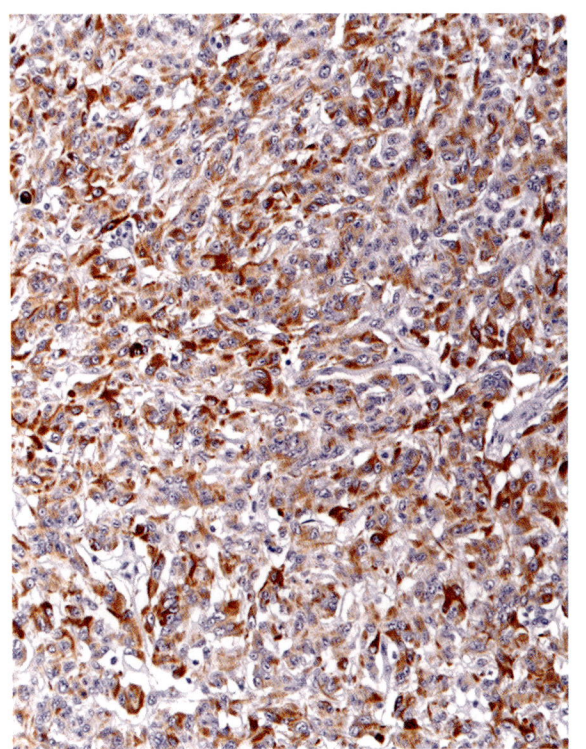 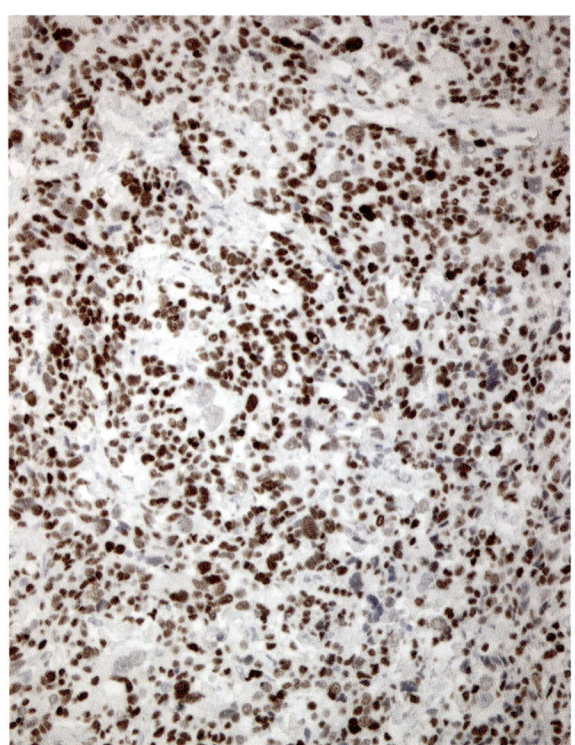

Figure 10-58

LEIOMYOSARCOMA

Keratin is extensively positive in an epithelioid leiomyosarcoma (left). The tumor cells show strong nuclear ER positivity (right).

leiomyosarcomas have higher expression of ER-β than ER-α (the latter more commonly evaluated) in contrast to myometrium and leiomyomas (212). Oxytocin is expressed much less commonly in leiomyosarcomas compared to leiomyomas (195).

HMB-45 can be focally positive in leiomyosarcomas but melan-A is negative (391,404,405). Cathepsin K has not been studied extensively in smooth muscle tumors, but in one series, all uterine leiomyomas tested were negative while another study showed that cathepsin K may be extensively expressed in some leiomyosarcomas (406,407). CD117 (C-KIT) positivity has been reported in some studies (408–410), but not in others (411). *C-KIT* mutations have not been detected (410), and tumors are typically DOG1 negative (287). Leiomyosarcomas are often strongly and diffusely p16 and p53 positive (217, 221,225,275,369,384,386,387,399,412–417). They are also frequently IMP3 and HMGA2 positive (215,227,369), but ALK-1 and S-100 protein negative (413).

Molecular Genetic Findings. Numerical or structural cytogenetic abnormalities have been detected in more than 60 percent of uterine leiomyosarcomas. As it occurs with extrauterine leiomyosarcomas, they are associated with complex numerical and structural chromosomal aberrations including losses on 10q, 11q, 13q, 22q, 6q, and 2p, and gains on Xp, 1q, 5p, 8q, and 17p (264,418–427). One recent study has shown that 5p or 17p gain and chromosome 13 loss are associated with poor prognosis (428).

Mutational status in leiomyosarcomas has been extensively evaluated. Mutations in *TP53* have been implicated in leiomyosarcoma pathogenesis over a decade ago (429). *TP53* mutations are common in uterine leiomyosarcomas compared to extrauterine tumors; *RB1*, *MDM2*, *CDKN2A*, *FABP3*, and *TAGLN* are other affected genes reported in these tumors (227,277,425,430,431). Exome sequencing has revealed that the most frequently mutated genes in leiomyosarcoma are *TP53* (32 percent), alpha thalassemia/mental retardation syndrome X-linked (*ATRX*) (26 percent), and *MED12* (21 percent) (432). *ATRX* inactivating mutations are typically nonsense or frameshift, accompanied by reduction of ATRX immunoexpression and associated with alternative lengthening of telomeres, one of the mechanisms of telomere maintenance in approximately 60 percent of leiomyosarcomas. This phenotype appears to be correlated with aggressive histologic features including tumor cell necrosis and poor clinical outcome (430,433). *MED12* mutations were first described in uterine leiomyomas, but they can also be seen with a much lower frequency in leiomyosarcomas. This finding had led to the hypothesis that some leiomyosarcomas arise from leiomyomas (253–255,258,260,262,434). *MED12* mutations are also found in metastatic tumors (260,261) and some investigators have shown that *MED12* mutations are noted in uterine but not in extrauterine smooth muscle tumors (254). *MED12* mutations can coexist with *TP53* or *ATRX* mutations (432). *HMGA2* mutations have been also reported in uterine leiomyosarcomas, but as occurs with leiomyomas, they are mutually exclusive with *MED12* mutations (227). Although there is limited literature on alterations specific to uncommon histologic subtypes, it has been recently reported that myxoid leiomyosarcomas harbor translocations involving *PLAG1* (435).

Gene expression studies have highlighted potential prognostic characteristics of uterine leiomyosarcomas. Molecular classification of leiomyosarcomas from different sites based on RNA sequencing identified three clinical relevant subtypes. Uterine tumors commonly belong to subtype I, which expresses genes associated with muscle function including *CASQ2*, *ACTG2*, *MYLK*, *SLMAP*, and *CFL2* and appears to be associated with a better outcome when compared to other subtypes (436,437).

Different gene expression profiles as well as microRNA signatures are seen when comparing leiomyomas and leiomyosarcoma (438–440). Specifically, uterine leiomyosarcomas show overexpression of genes related to cell cycle (including *DC7*, *CDC20*, *GTSE1*, *CCNA2*, *CCNB1*, and *CCNB2*), hypomethylation through extensive genomic regions, and common hypermethylation at the polycomb group target genes and protocadherin genes, similar to other malignant solid tumors (438,439). The microRNA signatures of leiomyosarcomas are more closely related to mesenchymal stem cells than leiomyomas (440). MicroRNA and gene expression analyses have also shown differences between primary and metastatic leiomyosarcomas (440–442).

Differential Diagnosis. Uterine leiomyosarcomas have a wide differential diagnosis that includes benign and malignant tumors as well as rare non-neoplastic processes. Spindle cell leiomyosarcoma causes the most problems in the differential diagnosis with leiomyoma variants. The gross features of some leiomyoma variants may be worrisome for malignancy, but the diagnosis becomes straightforward under the microscope. On microscopic examination, issues most often arise with leiomyomas with bizarre (symplastic) nuclei and those with increased mitotic activity or with apoplectic change.

Spindle leiomyosarcoma and leiomyomas with bizarre nuclei share the findings of extensive atypical cells, and in most cases, hypercellularity. Furthermore, karyorrhectic nuclei in leiomyomas with bizarre nuclei may mimic atypical mitoses, increasing concern for malignancy. Expression of Ki-67, p16, and p53 may also overlap. The gross appearance of the tumor, banal cytology of background cells, degenerative morphology of the atypical cells (bizarre), low mitotic activity, and absence of tumor cell necrosis should help in their distinction from leiomyosarcoma. Mitotically active leiomyomas share with leiomyosarcoma the finding of brisk mitotic activity; however, they lack any degree of cytologic atypia and the mitotic activity is usually less than 10 mitoses per 10 high-power fields. Apoplectic change in a leiomyoma is seen in reproductive age pregnant or postpartum women or those taking oral contraceptives. Although infarct-type necrosis may not be fully developed and cause concern for tumor cell necrosis, while nearby areas are hypercellular, mitotically active, show some degree of cytologic atypia as well as increased Ki-67 and p16 expression, there is a well-defined zonation phenomenon with areas away from necrosis having the typical appearance of a leiomyoma, helping to separate this leiomyoma variant from spindle leiomyosarcoma (63). Thus, the sampling of any smooth muscle tumor with unusual microscopic findings is crucial.

Spindle cell leiomyosarcoma should be distinguished from spindle cell (if better differentiated) or pleomorphic (if poorly/dedifferentiated) rhabdomyosarcoma. Spindle cell rhabdomyosarcoma is characterized by spindled cells with elongated nuclei, a microscopic appearance that closely overlaps with that observed in spindle cell leiomyosarcoma. Occasional cells with cytoplasmic cross striations and the finding of a component of conventional embryonal rhabdomyosarcoma are helpful in the diagnosis. Pleomorphic rhabdomyosarcoma shows an admixture of round to polygonal to spindled pleomorphic cells typically admixed with aggregates of large rhabdomyoblasts. Both subtypes are positive for skeletal muscle markers.

Undifferentiated uterine sarcoma, a high-grade sarcoma with no specific differentiation, may mimic a poorly differentiated spindled or dedifferentiated leiomyosarcoma (1). Sampling is most important in this scenario since immunostains may not be helpful. Other entities in the differential diagnosis are solitary fibrous tumor, gastrointestinal stromal tumor, or metastases.

Epithelioid leiomyosarcoma may show overlapping morphologic features with epithelial, mesenchymal, and trophoblastic tumors. Among them, PEComa is responsible for most problems in the differential diagnosis since the tumor cells have abundant clear or eosinophilic cytoplasm with oval to round nuclei, they are disposed in sheets or small nests or cords, they may have an associated spindle cell component, and they may express smooth muscle markers (443–446). Furthermore, rare leiomyosarcomas express HMB-45 (405). In contrast to smooth muscle tumors, however, PEComas are characteristically positive for HMB-45, melan A, cathepsin K, and TFE-3 (if they have clear cytoplasm) and may be associated with tuberous sclerosis and lymphangioleiomyomatosis (446).

Epithelioid leiomyosarcoma should also be distinguished from poorly differentiated carcinoma. Most carcinomas exhibit, at least focally, glandular or squamous differentiation. As epithelioid smooth muscle tumors are frequently positive for keratin and EMA, and ER, PR, p16, and p53 may be positive in both, a panel of antibodies is recommended in this differential diagnosis including PAX8 and muscle markers.

Uterine tumors resembling ovarian sex-cord tumors, although uncommon, may have an appearance similar to that seen in epithelioid smooth muscle tumors, especially in biopsy or curettage specimens. They also show extensive immunohistochemical overlap, with shared expression of epithelial (keratin) and smooth muscle markers (actin and desmin > caldesmon). However, epithelial differentiation is typically more pronounced in uterine tumors resembling ovarian sex cord tumors, with tubular or even retiform architecture and common expression of at least some sex cord markers, more frequently calretinin and CD99, and less frequently inhibin and melan A (197,447).

Placental trophoblastic tumors, placental site and epithelioid trophoblastic tumor, may enter the differential diagnosis when sample is limited and a diffuse growth of cells with abundant eosinophilic or clear cytoplasm is seen. Finding neoplastic cells infiltrating vessels walls associated with fibrinoid necrosis and dissecting preexisting smooth muscle bundles, as seen in normal implantation site, favors a diagnosis of a placental-site trophoblastic tumor. In contrast, a well-circumscribed margin with nested growth around vessels and extensive areas of geographic necrosis support a diagnosis of epithelioid trophoblastic tumor. As trophoblastic and smooth muscle tumors may express epithelial markers, immunoreactivity for CK18, inhibin, placental lactogen (in both trophoblastic tumors), and p63 (in epithelioid trophoblastic tumor) are helpful in establishing a diagnosis of trophoblastic tumor. A history of a recent pregnancy and elevated serum hCG level are also helpful (448).

Metastatic and, less commonly, primary malignant melanomas as well as alveolar soft part sarcomas are excluded among others by their immunoreactivity for S-100 protein, SOX10, HMB-45, and TFE-3 and lack of reactivity for smooth muscle markers (449). Other tumors with epithelioid morphology include epithelioid endometrial stromal sarcoma, gastrointestinal stromal tumor, and rhabdoid tumor.

Myxoid leiomyosarcoma should be distinguished from several entities including leiomyoma with hydropic change, myxoid leiomyoma, inflammatory myofibroblastic tumor, and endometrial stromal sarcoma (63). Leiomyoma with hydropic change is in the differential diagnosis due to its rapid growth clinically concerning for malignancy, and its edematous content, often confused with myxoid matrix. On gross examination, fluid can be easily "squeezed" from the tumor, which does not have the "sticky" texture of myxoid tumors. In areas not affected by edema, the tumor consists of compacted growth of smooth muscle cells and has the appearance of a conventional leiomyoma. When in doubt, alcian blue and colloidal iron are helpful as hydropic leiomyomas are negative for these markers.

Myxoid leiomyoma is much less frequent than myxoid leiomyosarcoma. To establish this diagnosis, the tumor should be small (<6 cm), well circumscribed, and extensively sampled to ensure that no cytologic atypia and minimal to absent mitotic activity are seen (136,280). Intravenous leiomyomatosis may show myxoid change, and due to its intravascular growth may raise the possibility of myxoid leiomyosarcoma, but as discussed for myxoid leiomyoma, no cytologic atypia and minimal to absent mitoses are seen.

Inflammatory myofibroblastic tumor is often misdiagnosed as myxoid leiomyosarcoma as both may be gelatinous on gross examination, and both are myxoid with a fascicular architecture microscopically. The former may also show cytologic atypia, necrosis, and infiltrative borders as seen in leiomyosarcoma. Many inflammatory myofibroblastic tumors likely have been diagnosed as myxoid leiomyosarcomas in the past. Although leiomyosarcomas rarely stain for ALK and show *ALK* amplifications (450), inflammatory myofibroblastic tumors often have an associated lymphoplasmacytic infiltrate, may have ganglion-like cells, and are ALK-1 positive with *ALK-1* rearrangements, in contrast to myxoid leiomyosarcoma (266,281,281a). Some investigators have applied an algorithm including p53, p16, and ALK to separate these two categories of tumors (413).

Endometrial stromal sarcomas, either low or high grade, may also be myxoid. Low-grade tumors often are associated with a conventional component of endometrial stromal neoplasia, cells display a diffuse growth and are small with oval nuclei, in contrast to the spindle cells that may form loose fascicles in myxoid leiomyosarcoma. Leiomyosarcomas can be CD10 positive and myxoid/fibrous endometrial stromal tumors may be desmin positive (197,282). A new subset of high-grade endometrial stromal sarcomas closely mimic the appearance of myxoid leiomyosarcomas. They may have fascicular growth, although frequently disorganized, variable myxoid background, and variable positivity for actins and desmin. In contrast to myxoid leiomyosarcomas, they may show collagen bands, are associated with diffuse cyclin D1 and BCOR nuclear expression, and display *ZC3H7B-BCOR* fusion (451).

Other rare tumors that may be myxoid and enter in the differential diagnosis include nerve sheath tumors and myxomas. Rarely myxoid change occurs in the myometrium and suggests a myxoid smooth muscle tumor in small samples. However, there is no mass lesion, and cells are positive for CD34 and CD10 and negative for desmin. A clinical association with neurofibromatosis and lupus erythematosus may be seen (452–454).

Dedifferentiated leiomyosarcoma should be distinguished from undifferentiated uterine sarcoma, a diagnosis of exclusion. Sampling is important to identify better developed areas of leiomyosarcoma. Tumors containing giant cells should be distinguished from rare pure malignant giant cell tumors of the uterus, as the latter can show a spindle and epithelioid component and they may be positive for actin and desmin. However, they typically have a prominent nodular growth, are often associated with hemorrhage, are negative for caldesmon, and diffusely positive for CD68 and CD163 (455).

Treatment and Prognosis. Hysterectomy is the mainstay of treatment in patients with leiomyosarcoma, with possible debulking of associated extrauterine tumors. Although ovarian and lymph node metastases have been detected in approximately 4 percent and 8 to 11 percent of patients, respectively, the role of oophorectomy and lymph node evaluation is controversial, with no survival advantage (319,339,456,457). Radiation and chemotherapy have not yet been demonstrated to impact survival in these patients, although radiation may help to control local recurrences. Chemotherapy (most often gemcitabine/docetaxel and doxorubicin) plays an important role in advanced or recurrent disease (458–461). Rarely, aromatase inhibitors have been employed to stabilize disease progression (462). Specific therapeutic targets are under investigation including PI3K/AKT/mTOR inhibitors and others (463,464).

Patients with leiomyosarcomas have an overall poor prognosis. Stage is the most important prognostic factor, although patient age, tumor size and grade, cytologic atypia, mitotic rate, and tumor cell necrosis have also been postulated to influence survival (77,219,274,318,339,351,362, 417,465–467). The 5-survival rates range from 12 to 40 percent for patients with all stages to 50 to 70 percent for those with tumors confined to the uterus (317,319,337–339,346,417,465,468–470). In the largest study to date (339), with a cohort of 208 patients and a mean follow-up of almost 8 years, 20 and 60 percent survival rates were reported for patients with advanced disease and disease confined to the uterus, respectively. In that study, stage was the most important prognostic factor, while patient age over 51 years, tumor size over 5 cm, and menopausal status also were associated with reduced overall survival, at least by univariate analysis.

Leiomyosarcomas used to be staged by the modified 1988 FIGO criteria for endometrial cancer. However, leiomyosarcomas tend to spread hematogenously and are often associated with distant metastases, in contrast to endometrial carcinoma. In the past years, a new FIGO staging system has been adopted incorporating tumor size and local/regional tumor extension as in soft tissue sarcomas (American Joint Committee on Cancer [AJCC] staging system) and disregarding cervical or serosal involvement (471,472). In one retrospective large study of leiomyosarcomas with data obtained from the SEER database between 1988 and 2005, tumor size over 5 cm seemed to play an important prognostic role, supporting the addition of this parameter in the new FIGO staging system. Some studies have found a cut-off of 5 cm as prognostically significant in leiomyosarcomas (362), although other studies have shown no advantage in better stratifying patients with this new staging system, with neither system being ideal for staging uterine leiomyosarcomas (469,470,473). It appears that no single parameter can predict outcome in patients with leiomyosarcoma, and thus, some investigators have proposed nomograms that include clinical and pathologic parameters with the aim to improve prediction of outcome (474).

Since most leiomyosarcomas are confined to the uterus at the time of diagnosis, studies also have looked at potential prognostic factors in this group of patients. Some investigators have postulated that a staging system using only grade and size can identify low-, intermediate-, and high-risk patients (456). However, low-grade leiomyosarcomas are exceedingly rare and the new FIGO staging system does not take grade into account, as most leiomyosarcomas are high-grade based on current criteria (61). Furthermore, although low-grade tumors exist, most represent leiomyoma variants or other uterine mesenchymal tumors (354). In another study of 27 stage I leiomyosarcomas based on the old FIGO staging system, no definitive differences in clinicopathologic parameters were observed between patients with favorable and adverse outcomes, although spindle cell morphology was associated with longer overall survival and diffuse high-grade cytologic atypia was related to poorer prognosis (346). Yet, in another study, among tumors confined to the uterus, size over 10 cm and mitotic rate over 10 mitoses per 10 high-power fields allowed for patient stratification into three risk groups: low-risk included patients with tumors 10 cm or smaller and 10 mitoses or less per 10 high-power fields; the medium-risk group was composed of tumors either larger than 10 cm or with more than 10 mitoses per 10 high-power fields; and in the high-risk group, tumors were larger than 10 cm with more than 10 mitoses per 10 high-power fields. Patients in the latter two groups had a 1.9- and 5.3-fold increased risk of death, respectively (351). Overall, clinicopathologic parameters do not reliably predict survival in patients with uterine leiomyosarcoma, including those with stage I tumors.

Most of the literature regarding prognosis in uterine leiomyosarcomas is based on studies of spindle cell leiomyosarcomas. Experience with epithelioid and myxoid leiomyosarcomas is more limited. Although they have also been shown to be aggressive tumors, the interval time to recurrence seems to be much longer than their spindle cell counterpart. The threshold for establishing a diagnosis of malignancy in these tumors is much lower than for spindle cell leiomyosarcomas (123,124,126,136,280,340,346,351,362).

Most patients with confined disease and almost all with extrauterine disease have recurrences within 2 years after initial diagnosis, although exceptions exist. Patients with recurrent disease have a poor prognosis (318,475).

Leiomyosarcomas follow a hematogenous pattern of spread and distant metastases are more common than local recurrences, with lung being the most common site (318,319,373,476,477). In the Gynecology Oncology Group (GOG) study, lung recurrences occurred in 40 percent, with pelvic recurrences in only 13 percent of the patients (319). Other common sites of distant metastases include liver and bone, and much less frequently, soft tissue and skin. In one study, lung metastases were frequently associated with metastases at other sites (373).

Nonclinicopathologic prognostic parameters evaluated in leiomyosarcomas have included ER, PR, p53, p21, p27, p16, BCL-2, metalloproteases, and ploidy, with contradictory results (274,338,396,403,417,478–483). Although ER and PR do not influence overall survival when corrected for stage, PR expression was associated with longer survival in one recent study (403) and some patients may respond to hormonal treatment (396,398,417). The presence of large numbers of macrophages secondary to an increase of colony-stimulating factor-1 may be associated with poor prognosis in nongynecologic and gynecologic leiomyosarcomas (484,485). Also, tumors associated with the ALT (alternative lengthening of telomerases) phenotype have an associated poor outcome (433).

The use of manual or power morcellation techniques has been shown to increase peritoneal dissemination of unexpected malignancies, including leiomyosarcoma. A meta-analysis of 133 studies showed a prevalence of leiomyosarcoma of approximately 1 in 2000 (0.05 percent) surgeries (486). Patients with morcellated leiomyosarcomas should undergo additional peritoneal examination to evaluate for secondary peritoneal dissemination which impacts patient survival (296,297,333,487,488).

SMOOTH MUSCLE TUMORS OF UNCERTAIN MALIGNANT POTENTIAL (ATYPICAL LEIOMYOMA)

Definition. These smooth muscle tumors have features that preclude an unequivocal diagnosis of leiomyosarcoma but do not fulfill the criteria for leiomyoma or its variants, and raise concern that the neoplasm may behave in a malignant fashion. In the latest WHO classification, the term *atypical leiomyoma* is used as a synonym for *smooth muscle tumor of uncertain malignant potential* (1). Atypical leiomyoma has been used loosely for leiomyoma variants, most commonly leiomyoma with bizarre nuclei or mitotically active leiomyoma, when the observer has limited experience with these types of tumors. The term smooth muscle tumor of uncertain malignant potential should be used sparingly and every effort should be made to properly classify a smooth muscle tumor into a specific category when possible.

These tumors are uncommon (489), with only a limited number of series reported. The clinical presentation and gross features are similar to those reported for typical leiomyomas (217,224,386,412,490–497).

The term smooth muscle tumor of uncertain malignant potential was first introduced by Kempson (498) for tumors that were clinically malignant but could not be classified as such using pathologic criteria. In a detailed study of 213 smooth muscle tumors by Bell and colleagues (61), smooth muscle tumors with problematic features were divided into five categories based on cytologic atypia, mitotic count (cut-off 10 mitoses per 10 high-power fields), and tumor cell necrosis. The term "atypical leiomyoma with limited experience" was applied to tumors with focal to multifocal cytologic atypia and up to 10 mitoses per 10 high-power fields. The term "atypical leiomyoma with low risk of recurrence" was used for tumors with similar characteristics but with diffuse cytologic atypia, while "mitotically active leiomyoma with limited experience" was used for tumors with no cytologic atypia and no tumor cell necrosis but with 20 or more mitoses per 10 high-power fields. The term "smooth muscle tumor of low malignant potential" was used for neoplasms that showed tumor cell necrosis with no or minimal cytologic atypia and less than 10 mitoses per 10 high-power fields. One of the four patients in that category had an adverse outcome. That tumor had less than 5 mitoses per 10 high-power fields while three other patients with tumors showing tumor cell necrosis and less than 10 mitoses were alive with no evidence of disease at 29, 46, and 165 months (61). It is important to note that there are often problems in the interpretation of necrosis even among experienced gynecologic pathologists and early infarct-type necrosis is commonly confused with tumor cell necrosis (347) even when special stains (reticulin and trichome) are used (348). Thus, a diagnosis of smooth muscle tumor of uncertain malignant potential based on "tumor cell necrosis" may not be reliable. When evaluating a smooth muscle tumor with unusual features, thorough sampling is mandatory as diagnostic features may only be present focally within the tumor. Rare patients within the other groups in that study (61) had an adverse outcome but most of the tumors in these categories are considered benign by the most recent WHO classification.

Ip et al. (224) in their series also classified their 16 tumors based on the Bell criteria. In this series, the only two patients with recurrences had tumors with diffuse cellularity, multifocal atypia, and up to 5 mitoses per 10 high-power fields. Other pathologists establish the diagnosis of smooth muscle tumor of uncertain malignant potential if the tumor has an infiltrative border, if atypical mitoses are noted, and for myxoid and epithelioid tumors with features between what has been defined for benign and malignant tumors (491). In the latest WHO classification, the term is applied for a variety of scenarios including: tumors with mitotic counts higher than expected for leiomyomas but lower than typical leiomyosarcoma; uncertainty on type of necrosis; and epithelioid or myxoid tumors with inconclusive features of malignancy (1).

In a recent study of 22 smooth muscle tumors of uncertain malignant potential, predictors of adverse outcome, seen in 8 of 22 patients, included infiltrative border (in 5), vascular invasion (in 3), atypical mitoses (in 2), and epithelioid differentiation (in 1), although association with outcome was not strong for any parameter (491). In that study, the finding of cytologic atypia, although not discriminatory, appeared to be common among patients with adverse outcome while tumor cell necrosis did not have such an association. Nonetheless, this category of smooth muscle tumors is still very heterogeneous as no single known morphologic criterion appears to be clearly associated with the development of recurrent or metastatic disease (154,499,500).

Immunohistologic markers, including p16, p53, Mib-1, p21, BCL-2, ER, and PR have been used to more accurately classify these tumors without much success, although some studies have shown that tumors that recurred displayed diffuse p53 and p16 positivity (217,219,224, 275,384,386,399,412,501,502). One study evaluating 18 smooth muscle tumors of uncertain malignant potential found 3 out of 6 with loss of ATRX or death domain associated protein (DAXX) expression, which conferred an adverse outcome (489). The authors hypothesized that loss of ATRX or DAXX expression can be used as an adjunct to predict adverse outcome in at least a subset of these tumors. A recent study evaluating smooth muscle lesions from 76 patients concluded that "genomic index" (defined as A2/C, where A is the total number of segmental gains/losses and C is the number of involved chromosomes) can be used as a predictor of recurrence (428). In this study, 14 tumors were molecularly categorized into two groups, one with simple (genomic index of less than 10, n=2) and another with complex genomic profiles (genomic index of 10 or greater, n=12), similar to leiomyomas and leiomyosarcomas, respectively. A genomic index greater than 35 and 5p gain, 17p gain, and chromosome 13 loss were identified as poor prognostic factors.

The differential diagnosis of smooth muscle tumors of uncertain malignant potential includes primarily leiomyoma variants and leiomyosarcoma. Every attempt should be made to establish a diagnosis of benign or malignant smooth muscle tumor, integrating gross and microscopic features of the tumor with generous sampling in unusual cases. In one study, some tumors originally diagnosed as smooth muscle tumors of uncertain malignant potential were reclassified as inflammatory myofibroblastic tumor after rereview and ALK studies, some of them having a myxoid content (503).

Reported adverse outcomes occur in 5 to 26 percent of patients depending on the morphologic criteria applied. In contrast to leiomyosarcoma, that interval to recurrence (s) is longer (average 47 months), with a median survival of 5.5 years (504).

OTHER MESENCHYMAL TUMORS

PEComa

Definition. *PEComa* is a mesenchymal tumor that typically contains epithelioid cells with clear to eosinophilic granular cytoplasm and

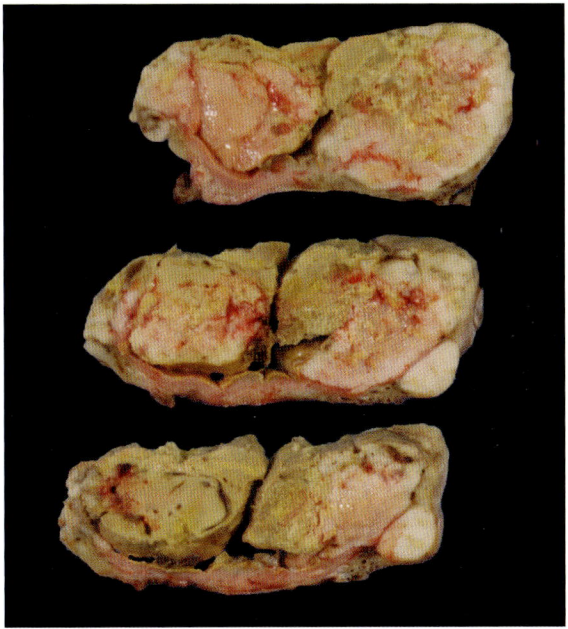
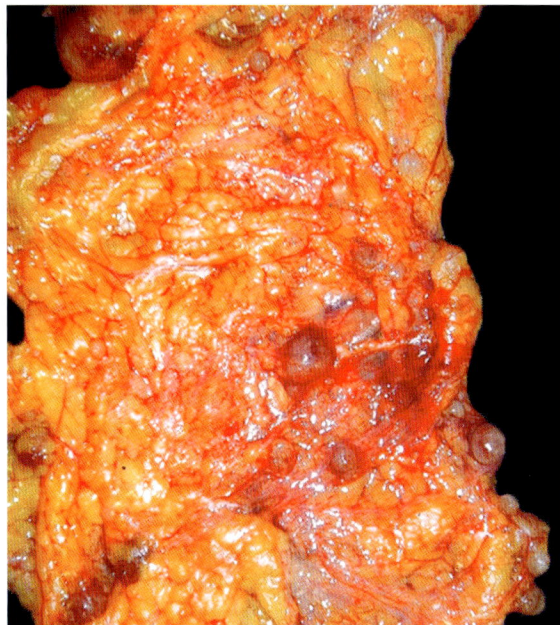

Figure 10-59

PECOMA

The tumor is large and polypoid, and deeply infiltrates the myometrium. It shows prominent necrosis (left). Multiple, variably sized and well-demarcated nodules of PEComa are seen in omentum (right). (Courtesy of Dr. I. Alvarado, Mexico City, Mexico.)

demonstrates melanocytic and smooth muscle differentiation. It is thought to be derived from the so-called perivascular epithelioid cell (PEC) (1).

Epidemiology and General Features. The term PEComa was introduced by Bonetti et al. (505). This family of tumors includes renal and extrarenal angiomyolipomas (506,507), pulmonary and extrapulmonary clear cell "sugar tumor" (508–510), pulmonary and extrapulmonary lymphangioleiomyomatosis (511–514), clear cell myelomelanocytic tumor of ligamentum teres (515), and abdominopelvic sarcoma of PEC (516). These tumors have been reported in multiple other locations, including gastrointestinal tract (517), bone (518), skin (519), adrenal gland, genitourinary tract including urinary bladder (520), prostate gland, urethra, testis (521), breast (522), and soft tissues (444).

Within the female genital tract, PEComas occur more commonly in the uterine corpus (443–446,523–525) but have also been reported in the ovary (445,526–529), uterine cervix (530,531), fallopian tube or broad ligament (532,533), vagina (445), and vulva (508). In patients with tuberous sclerosis, multiple macroscopic and microscopic tumor nodules may involve several gynecologic organs as well as peritoneum (*"PEComatosis"*) (530,534,535).

Clinical Features. Patients are often perimenopausal or postmenopausal, but tumors occur within a wide age range. They most frequently present with vaginal bleeding or pelvic pain and may have a history of tuberous sclerosis complex, an autosomal dominant disease due to losses of *TSC2* (16p13.3) and less commonly *TSC1* (9q34) genes. These losses lead to impaired production of tuberin and hamartin, respectively, which seem to have a role in the regulation of the rapamycin (mTOR) pathway. The association of PEComa and tuberous sclerosis is uncommon in the female genital tract, while the *TFE-3* subgroup of PEComas is characteristically not associated with this syndrome.

Gross Findings. Tumors range from microscopic to over 20 cm. They have a gray-white to tan or yellow, firm or fleshy cut surface (fig. 10-59, left) and are either well- or poorly-circumscribed. Rarely, more than one tumor is noted.

Microscopic Findings. They may be well circumscribed or have a tongue-like permeative (as seen in low-grade endometrial stromal sarcomas) or an overtly infiltrative border (443,445,446).

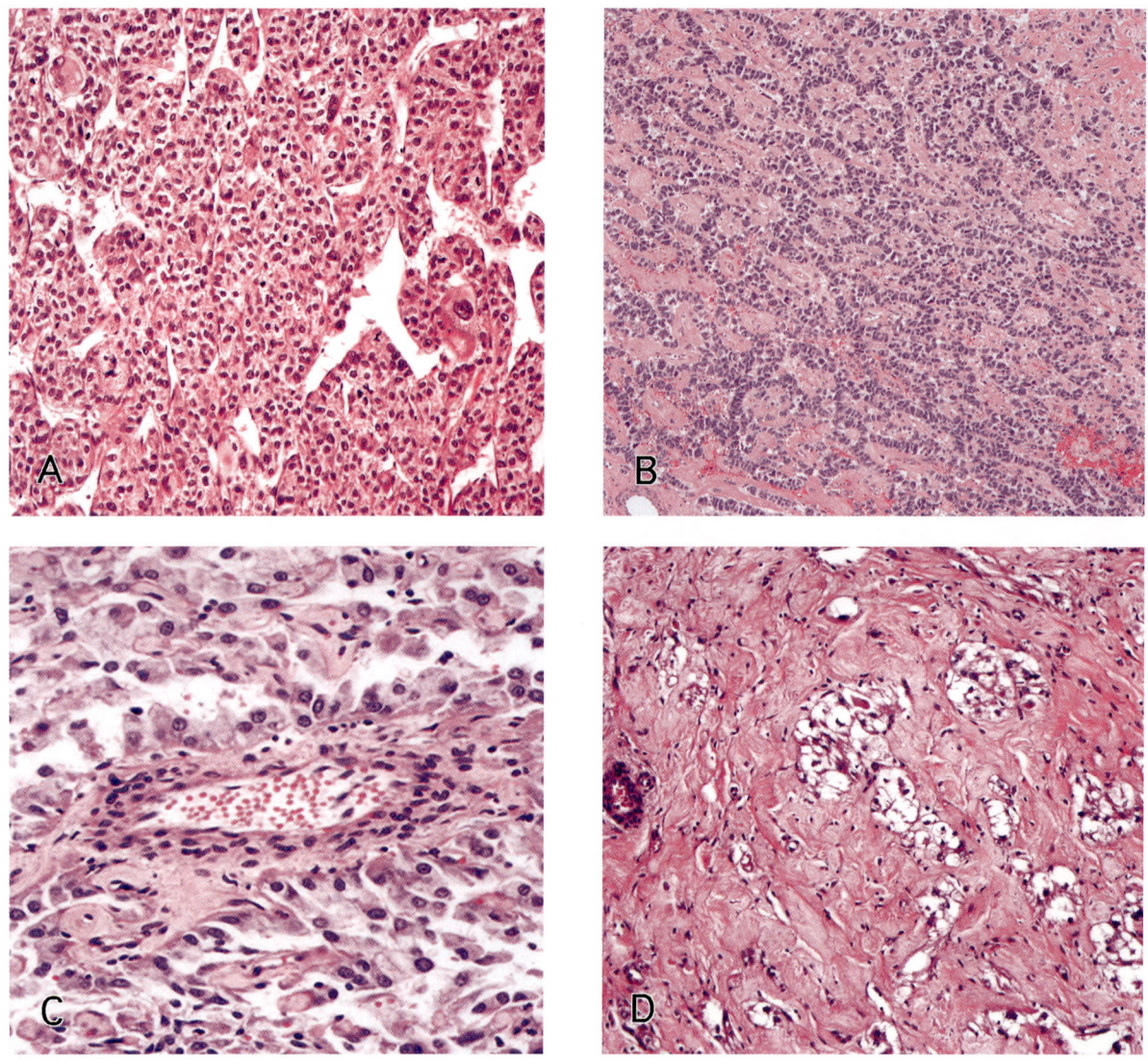

Figure 10-60

PECOMA

The tumor has a striking nested architecture and spotty cytologic atypia. A delicate sinusoidal vasculature is seen surrounding the nests of neoplastic cells (A). Interanastomosing cords are seen (B). The tumor cells have a perivascular radial distribution (C). (Figure 4F from Bennett JA, Braga AC, Pinto A, et al. Uterine PEComas: a morphologic, immunohistochemical, and molecular analysis of 32 tumors. Am J Surg Pathol 2018;42:1370-83.) Extensive hyalinization is present between tumor cells (hyalinized PEComa) (D).

The neoplasms are often hypercellular. The tumor cells grow in nests (more common) or sheets, and less often in cords or fascicles (fig. 10-60A,B). They may display a perivascular radial arrangement, imparting a lymphangioleiomyomatous-like pattern (fig. 10-60C). Most PEComas are predominantly composed of epithelioid cells, but they can show an admixture of epithelioid and spindle cells, or be predominantly spindled (conventional variant). The epithelioid cells commonly have a noncohesive appearance, abundant pale eosinophilic to clear granular cytoplasm (rarely densely eosinophilic), medium-sized round nuclei with small nucleoli, and dispersed chromatin (fig. 10-61A,B). Some neoplasms are purely composed of epithelioid

Smooth Muscle and Other Mesenchymal Tumors

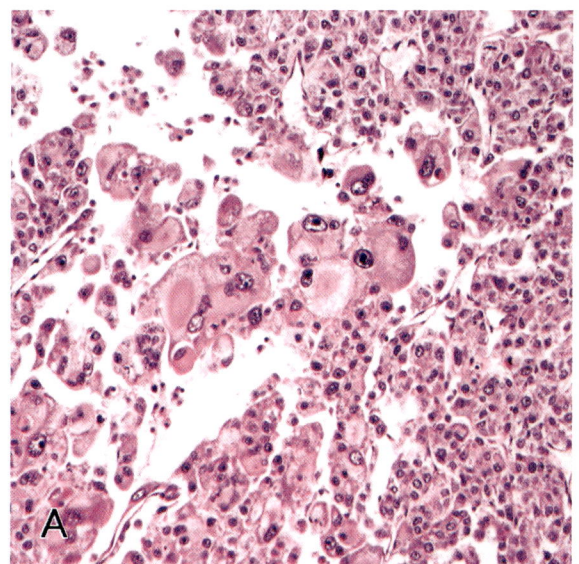

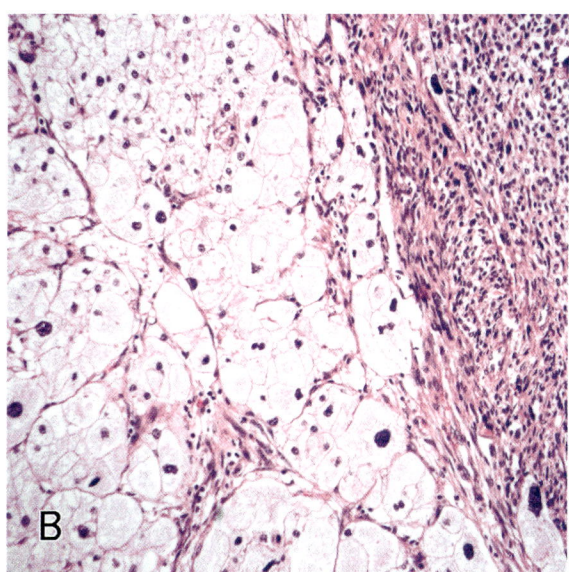

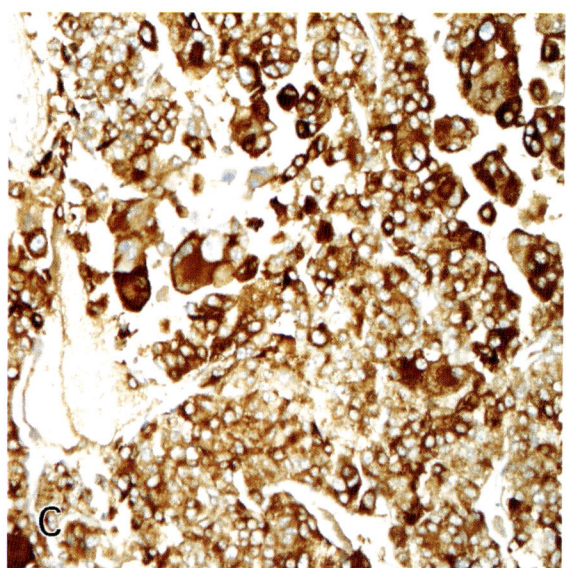

Figure 10-61

PECOMA

Tumor cells have abundant eosinophilic cytoplasm and some show prominent cytologic atypia as well as mitoses (left) (A). Cells with exuberant vacuolated cytoplasm are juxtaposed to a spindle cell component, closely mimicking a smooth muscle tumor (B). (Figure 3F from Bennett JA, Braga AC, Pinto A, et al. Uterine PEComas: a morphologic, immunohistochemical, and molecular analysis of 32 tumors. Am J Surg Pathol 2018;42:1370-83.) Cells are extensively HMB-45 positive although positivity may be only focal (C).

clear cells displaying a striking alveolar architecture (*TFE-3* rearranged variant) (fig. 10-62). Nuclear pseudoinclusions, prominent nucleoli, benign-appearing multinucleated tumor cells, malignant multinucleated giant cells, and spider cells may be seen (444–446,523). Some tumors contain variable intracytoplasmic melanin pigment. Mitotic activity is typically low to absent but a brisk mitotic rate and prominent cytologic atypia may be seen (fig. 10-61A). Necrosis, hemorrhage, and lymphovascular invasion may also be present.

A delicate sinusoidal vasculature (fig. 10-60A), similar to that seen in clear cell renal carcinomas, may be prominent, but hyalinized arterioles and hemangiopericytoma-like vessels may also be seen. The stroma ranges from minimal to extensive (sclerosing variant) (fig. 10-60D). When extensive, scattered nests or cords of epithelioid tumor cells are present in a striking collagenous/hyalinized background (286,446,532,536).

The histologic features associated with adverse outcome include size of 5 cm or greater, tumor necrosis, lymphovascular invasion, significant nuclear atypia, and mitotic activity more than 1 mitosis per 50 high-power fields. Tumors with malignant behavior, defined by recurrence or metastases, have at least three of these features

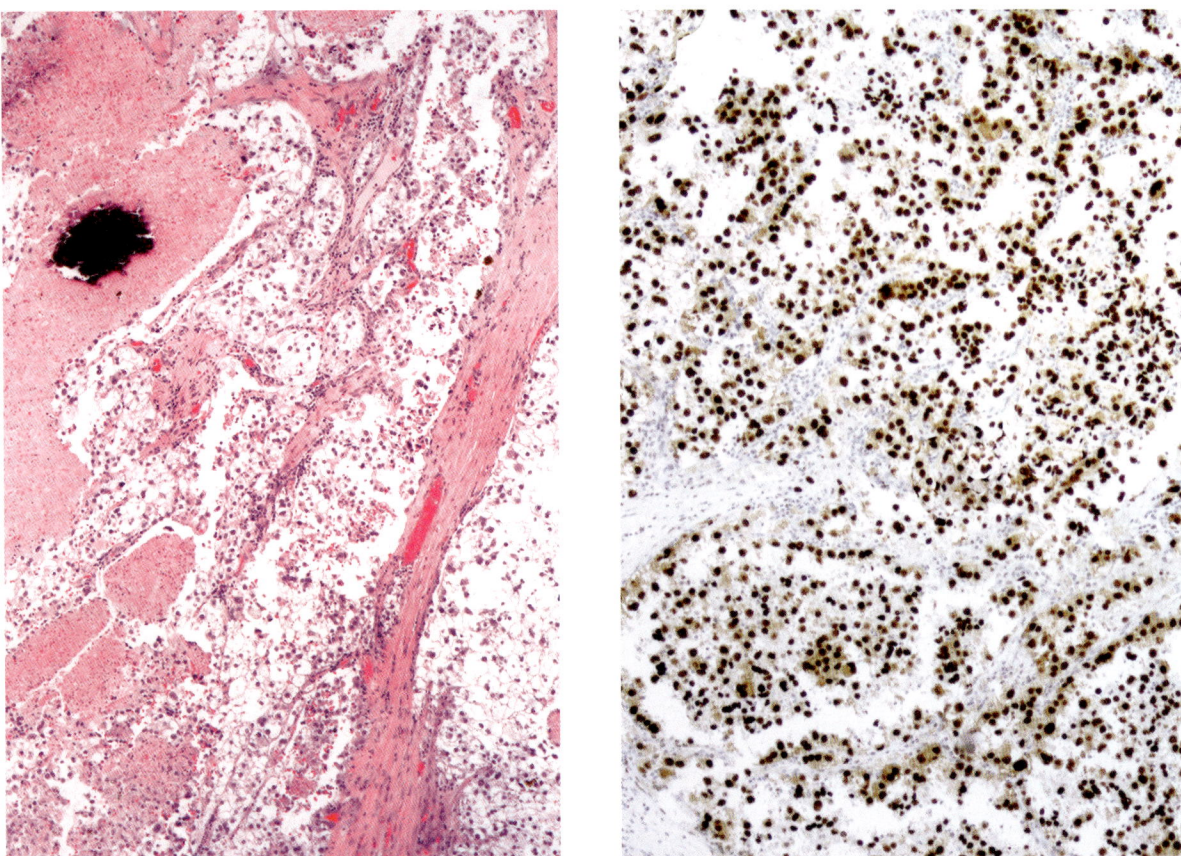

Figure 10-62

TFE-3-REARRANGED PECOMA

The tumor cells have clear cytoplasm (left) and are strongly TFE-3 positive (right). (Courtesy of Dr. R. A. Soslow, New York, NY.)

(444,446,537). These features differ slightly from those used for PEComas in other sites.

PEComas are seen in association with *lymphangiomyomatosis* involving the uterus or the lymph nodes, PEComatosis, or rarely, uterine angiomyolipomas (286). *Lymphangioleiomyomatosis* occurs exclusively in women. It is characterized by an admixture of spindle and epithelioid cells with clear to pale eosinophilic and often vacuolated cytoplasm and bland-appearing nuclei. They are associated with dense hyaline collagen plaques typically arranged around irregularly shaped and often dilated lymphatic channels imparting a slit-like appearance (fig. 10-63). Usually, lymphangiomyomatosis involves the lung and retroperitoneal or pelvic lymph nodes (284,285), although it rarely occurs in the uterus (286,514,538,539). In one study, only patients with pulmonary lymphangiomyomatosis had uterine involvement (284). All patients with uterine lymphangiomyomatosis also had involvement of pelvic lymph nodes or retroperitoneum. When associated with tuberous sclerosis, involvement of the myometrium was diffuse when compared to only outer myometrium in sporadic cases. As with PEComa, lymphangiomyomatosis may or may not occur in association with tuberous sclerosis. Uterine involvement often represents an incidental microscopic finding but it occasionally forms a mass lesion if extensive and secondarily causes bleeding (514). The cells are typically positive for HMB-45 and β-catenin, however, the former typically shows focal staining in contrast to the diffuse and strong cytoplasmic (not nuclear) positivity for β-catenin (285).

Pecomatosis is defined by the presence of multiple tumor nodules involving several

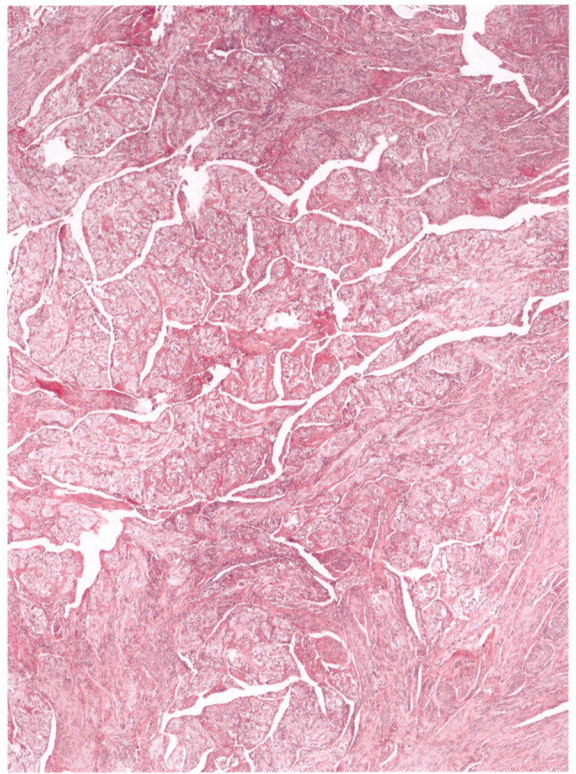

Figure 10-63

LYMPHANGIOMYOMATOSIS

Spindled and epithelioid pale cells form fascicles. They are associated with prominent cleft-like spaces as well as bright collagen bands.

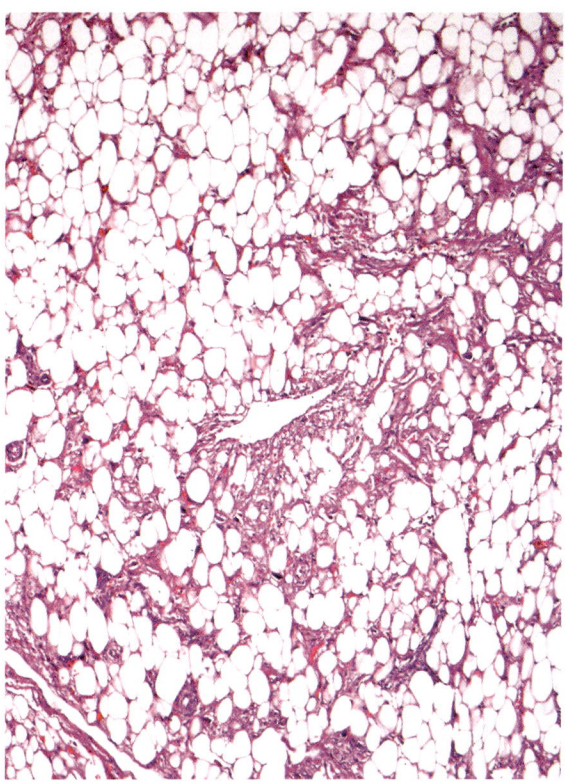

Figure 10-64

ANGIOMYOLIPOMA

A predominant component of mature adipocytes is admixed with scattered vessels (center) and spindle cells with clear cytoplasm.

gynecologic sites. A dominant mass is often found within the uterus; other sites of involvement include ovary, lymph nodes, broad ligament, omentum, and peritoneal surfaces (fig. 10-59, right). The variably sized nodules frequently show an admixture of epithelioid and spindle cells, with the typical immunohistochemical profile. In most reported cases, patients appear to follow a benign course and typically have tuberous sclerosis (530,534,535).

Angiomyolipomas are rare in the uterus (286, 540–542). As in other more common locations, these tumors are composed of mature adipocytes, blood vessels, and benign smooth muscle cells in varying proportions (fig. 10-64). Angiomyolipomas may be negative for HMB-45 (543).

Immunohistochemical Findings. PEComas are characterized by coexpression of melanocytic (HMB-45, melan A, MiTF, cathepsin K) and smooth muscle (desmin> actin> caldesmon) markers. Expression of these two groups of immunohistochemical markers varies depending on the predominant morphology within the tumor. Neoplasms with an epithelioid morphology more often display extensive positivity for melanocytic markers, especially HMB-45 (fig. 10-61C), with only focal positivity for melan A and minimal expression of smooth muscle markers. Sclerosing PEComa shows minimal HMB-45 expression in contrast to its conventional counterpart (536).

Cathepsin K, a transcriptional target of the MiTF family, has recently been shown to be an excellent marker in identifying PEComas, however, it is important to remember that smooth muscle tumors, the most common neoplasms in the differential diagnosis, can also be positive for this marker, limiting its use in this setting (406,544,545).

TFE-3, one of four members of the MiTF family, known to be expressed in melanoma, clear cell sarcoma, alveolar soft part sarcoma, and

Table 10-2

DIFFERENTIAL FEATURES OF EPITHELIOID LEIOMYOSARCOMA AND PECOMA

	Epithelioid LMS	PEComa
Tuberous sclerosis	-	+/-
Pseudoglandular spaces	+/-	-
Prominent hyalinization	-	+/-
Radial perivascular growth	-	+
Sinusoidal vasculature	-	+
Lymphangioleiomyomatosis	-	-/+
Melanin pigment	-	-/+
HMB-45	-/+ (few cells)	+ (few cells to diffuse)
Melan A	-	+
Cathepsin K	-/+	+
TFE-3	-	+
Epithelial markers	+/-	-[a]
ER/PR	+/-	-
P16	+	-

[a]With rare exceptions.

translocation-associated renal cell carcinomas, is also strongly positive in a subset of PEComas composed exclusively of epithelioid clear cells. These tumors characteristically show *TFE-3* rearrangements and lack *TSC2* inactivating mutations (*TFE-3* rearranged variant) (fig. 10-62) (537,546). They also show diffuse positivity for HMB-45, cathepsin K, and TFE-3 while melan A, MiTF, and smooth muscle markers are minimally positive or negative (537,547). Rare tumors with epithelioid and spindle morphology have a mixed immunohistochemical profile (446). CD10 and S-100 protein (one third) positivity may be seen (444) but SOX10 is negative (548).

To establish a diagnosis of PEComa, the tumor should show characteristic morphologic features as well as at least focal strong positivity for two melanocytic markers (HMB-45, melan A, MiTF, cathepsin K) with or without positivity for smooth muscle markers. Rarely, tumors express C-KIT and focal keratin (444). CD1a, a Langerhans cell-associated transmembrane glycoprotein involved in antigen presentation, has been reported by some to be positive in PEComas, while it has been shown by others to represent aberrant positivity (549).

Rare PEComas have a *RAD51B* rearrangement, a finding associated with aggressive behavior (446). Electron microscopic studies have described cytoplasmic melanosomes or premelanosomes in most tumors. PEComas have shown several chromosomal imbalances including losses in chromosomes 19, 16p, 17p, 1p, and 18p and gains on chromosomes X, 12q, 3q, 5q and 2q. The frequent deletion of 16p supports PEComa as a TSC2-linked neoplasm (550).

Differential Diagnosis. PEComas are frequently confused with *benign* or *malignant epithelioid,* and less commonly, *spindle smooth muscle tumors* since their morphologic appearance shows striking overlap (Table 10-2). However, the sinusoidal vasculature seen in PEComas is typically lacking in smooth muscle tumors. Smooth muscle tumors may show some degree of positivity for HMB-45 and a subset may be positive for cathepsin K (406,407), but they are typically negative for melan A (404,551), and show weak to negative TFE-3 expression.

Placental-site trophoblastic tumor may be in the differential diagnosis as both tumors share the finding of epithelioid cells with clear to pale eosinophilic cytoplasm with scattered multinucleated cells, and grow in sheets or cords. In contrast to PEComas, trophoblastic cells typically invade vessels walls, replace endothelial cells, and are associated with fibrinoid necrosis as seen in the normal implantation site. They lack expression of melanocytic markers but typically express keratin, HPL, and inhibin (448).

PEComas may have an infiltrative growth pattern similar to that seen in *low-grade endometrial stromal sarcomas*. The latter, however, rarely are composed of epithelioid or spindle cells, have a characteristic arteriolar vascular network, and lack positivity for melanocytic markers with rare exceptions (552) but show diffuse CD10 expression (553).

Other tumors in the differential diagnosis include clear cell carcinoma, either primary or metastatic, alveolar soft part sarcoma, and secondary involvement by a gastrointestinal tumor. *Clear cell carcinomas* of *endometrium* or *kidney* may be confused with TFE-3 PEComa. Uterine clear cell carcinomas have characteristic architectural patterns including tubulocystic and papillary, show positivity for PAX8, HNF-1B, and napsin-A but are negative for melanocytic markers if primary. Metastatic clear cell renal cell carcinoma may show a similar vasculature to PEComa but it is PAX8 positive as well as CD10, RCC, and CA-IX positive. Often a past history is known. Metastatic Xp11.2 renal cell carcinoma potentially could enter in the differential diagnosis as it has clear cytoplasm and strong TFE-3 and cathepsin K positivity, however, it typically has a prominent papillary architecture and may be positive for cytokeratin, EMA, and vimentin (554). *Alveolar soft part sarcoma* may have a striking alveolar/nested architecture and strongly TFE-3-positive tumor cells, but it is negative for melanocytic markers. These tumors are associated with a specific *ASP-SCR1-TFE3* translocation (449). *Gastrointestinal stromal tumor* may secondarily involve the uterus and may show epithelioid and spindle cells that grow in nests, sheets, and fascicles. However, cells with palely eosinophilic cytoplasm lack the granular quality seen in PEComa. Smooth muscle actin and rarely desmin may be positive in gastrointestinal stromal tumors, albeit usually focally. These tumors are typically positive for C-KIT as well as DOG1 and CD34 but negative for melanocytic markers while PEComas, although rarely C-KIT positive, are CD34 and DOG negative (444,517).

Lymphangiomyomatosis should be distinguished from intravenous leiomyomatosis, diffuse leiomyomatosis, benign metastasizing leiomyoma, and epithelioid leiomyosarcoma. *Intravenous leiomyomatosis* grows characteristically within vascular spaces and not around them, and plugs of tumor filling and distending veins within the myometrium and parametrial spaces are often seen on gross examination (172,173). Furthermore, these lesions are often characterized by HMGA2 expression (242) and lack positivity for melanocytic markers. *Diffuse leiomyomatosis* of the uterus is characterized by symmetric thickening of the uterus due to the presence of numerous confluent leiomyomatous nodules that may be associated with focal proliferation of perivascular smooth muscle cells, both within the nodules and in the surrounding myometrium. However, the cells have a spindle morphology and are not associated with slit-like spaces (157). *Benign metastasizing leiomyoma* can potentially be confused with lymphangiomyomatosis in the setting of pulmonary disease.

In contrast to lymphangioleiomyomatosis, there are multiple, discrete, rounded pulmonary nodules with a spindle morphology that grow around the airway spaces. They are often characterized by a 19q and 22q terminal deletion (182). *Leiomyosarcoma* may have poorly defined borders and epithelioid morphology as seen in lymphangioleiomyomatosis. However, it typically forms a discrete mass and also displays long intersecting fascicles of cells with overt cytologic atypia and brisk mitotic activity without associated perivascular growth. Leiomyosarcomas may show focal HMB-45 (404,405) and cathepsin K positivity but are negative for other PEComa markers.

When involving the uterus and extrauterine sites, especially lymph nodes, lymphangioleiomyomatosis may be confused with *diffuse peritoneal leiomyomatosis*. The latter has the morphology seen in typical smooth muscle tumors and shows the same immunohistochemical profile.

The differential diagnosis of angiomyolipomas includes *lipoleiomyoma, lipoma,* and *angiolipoleiomyoma*. Although these tumors may closely resemble angiomyolipomas, they do not express melanocytic markers. However, it is important to be aware that approximately 20 percent of angiomyolipomas do not stain for HMB-45 (543).

Treatment and Prognosis. Hysterectomy is the treatment of choice for patients with PEComas. As mTOR alterations of tuberous sclerosis complex have been reported in 10 percent of patients, some may benefit from mTOR inhibitors, especially if disease is advanced (446,537).

Of the reported primary uterine tumors, approximately 15 percent have been associated with metastases at the time of diagnosis (555). Initially reported adverse prognostic factors in PEComas included size of 5 cm or greater, infiltration, high-grade nuclear features not symplastic, mitotic rate of 1 or more mitoses per 50 high-power fields, necrosis, and lymphovascular invasion. The presence of two of these features was associated with aggressive behavior (444). A study evaluating uterine tumors found that the presence of four of the following features was indicative of malignancy: size of 5 cm or greater, high-grade nuclear features, mitotic rate of 1 mitosis per 50 high-power fields, necrosis, and lymphovascular invasion (445). The largest

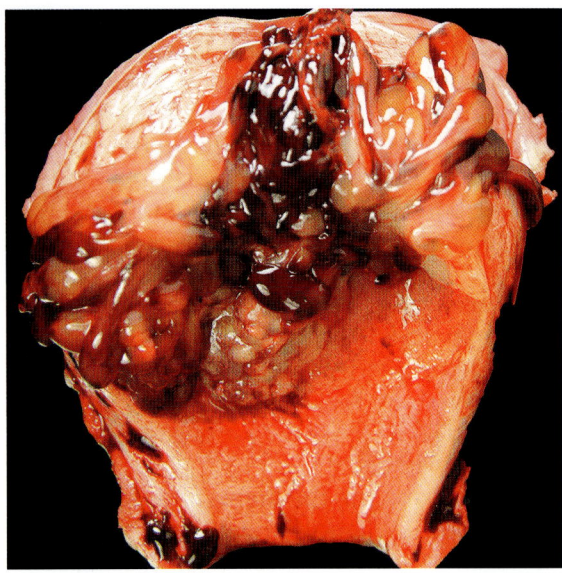

Figure 10-65

EMBRYONAL RHABDOMYOSARCOMA

Multiple polypoid and hemorrhagic ("grape-like") excrescences fill the endometrial cavity.

series reported to date has shown that a modified algorithm using the same criteria but with a threshold of three features establishes the diagnosis of malignancy most accurately in these tumors (446).

Rhabdomyosarcoma

Definition. *Rhabdomyosarcoma* is the most common heterologous sarcoma that shows evidence of skeletal muscle differentiation within the uterus. It is more common in the cervix than the corpus (556–563). There are a variety of morphologies and several subtypes exist: *embryonal*, *spindle*, *pleomorphic*, and *alveolar* (564).

Clinical Features. The age at presentation varies widely, with pleomorphic rhabdomyosarcoma typically seen in postmenopausal women and embryonal rhabdomyosarcoma more commonly in adult patients. Patients present with vaginal bleeding, abdominal distension, and pain or acute abdomen (558–562,565–567). CA125 may be elevated (566).

Gross Findings. The tumors tend to form large polypoid masses (average, 8 to 9 cm) that may show a "grape-like" appearance (*botryoid rhabdomyosarcomas*). The cut surface is white to gray and fleshy, with prominent areas of hemorrhage and necrosis (fig. 10-65). Myometrial invasion may be seen, and is more striking in pleomorphic rhabdomyosarcomas.

Microscopic Findings. Low-power microscopy in embryonal rhabdomyosarcoma shows the characteristic condensation of hypercellular stroma ("cambium layer") under the surface epithelium and around preexisting inactive-appearing endometrial glands (typically few in number) (fig. 10-66A). There are alternating hypocellular and hypercellular areas away from the glands. The hypercellular areas display poorly formed clusters of hyperchromatic primitive cells with a high nuclear to cytoplastic ratio (fig. 10-66B), brisk mitotic activity, and variable rhabdomyoblastic differentiation, with visible cross striations seen in over 50 percent of tumors (fig. 10-66C). The hypocellular areas have a myxoid to edematous to hyalinized background. Fetal-type cartilage is present in up to 50 percent of embryonal rhabdomyosarcomas. Rare tumors are associated with a primitive neuroectodermal tumor (568,569).

Spindle cell rhabdomyosarcoma often has a compact fascicular or storiform growth of spindle cells. Myxoid stroma as well as a component of conventional embryonal rhabdomyosarcoma may be focally seen. Rare rhabdomyoblasts are present (fig. 10-67) (567).

Pleomorphic rhabdomyosarcoma is characterized by a diffuse growth of round to polygonal to spindled pleomorphic cells, typically admixed with aggregates of large rhabdomyoblasts. Smaller cells are also seen (fig. 10-68). Tumor giant cells have been reported. The neoplastic cells have brisk mitotic activity, focal myxoid change, and often, necrosis and hemorrhage (557,560,562,563,567).

Alveolar rhabdomyosarcoma shows a uniform alveolar, nested, or pseudopapillary architecture. Lining cells tend to be noncohesive, with abundant polygonal, eosinophilic cytoplasm. Multinucleated cells may be seen (fig. 10-69) (565,566).

Immunohistochemical and Molecular Genetic Findings. Tumors are typically positive for smooth muscle actin, muscle-specific actin, desmin, MyoD-1, myogenin, myosin, and myoglobin (570). They are often also positive for CD10 (560). Some rhabdomyosarcomas express CD99 and WT1 (571) and aberrant expression of epithelial (wide-spectrum keratin)

Smooth Muscle and Other Mesenchymal Tumors

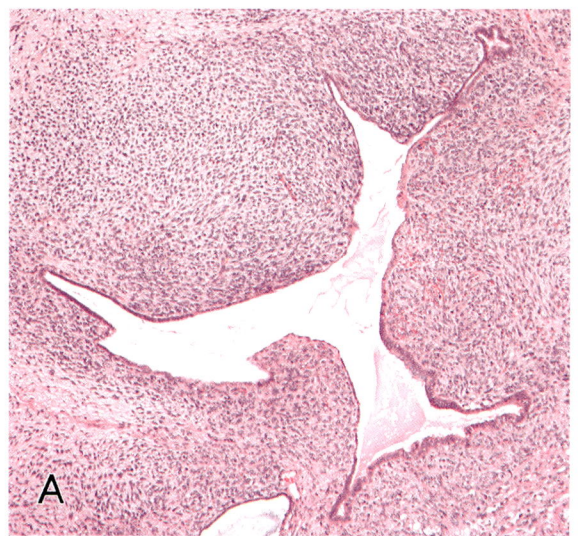

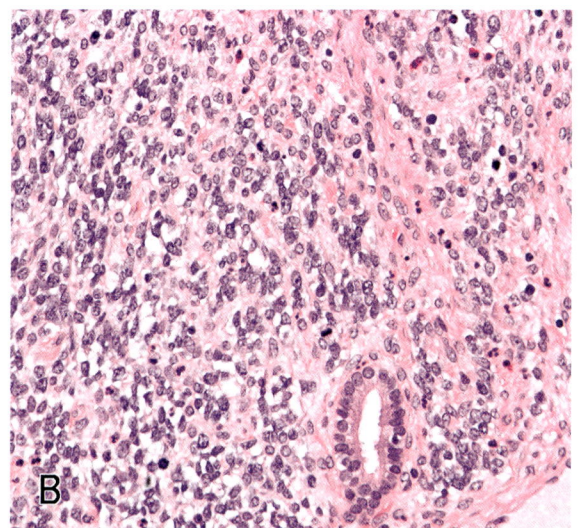

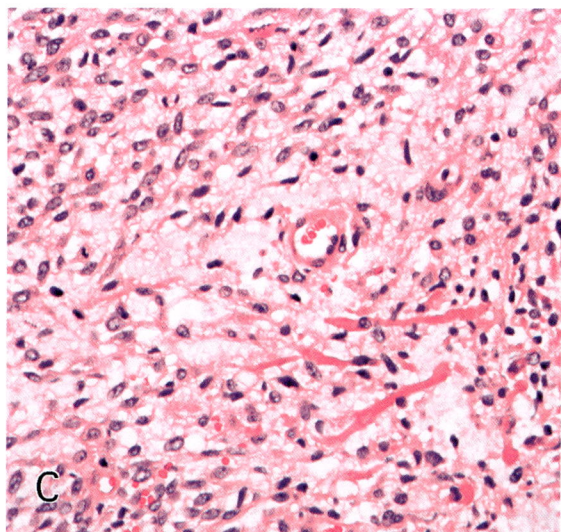

Figure 10-66

EMBRYONAL RHABDOMYOSARCOMA

There is condensation of "blue" cells around preexisting epithelium, imparting a low-power architecture pattern that may overlap with low-grade adenosarcoma (A). However, in contrast to the latter, the tumor cells have a primitive appearance, are small and hyperchromatic, and are associated with brisk mitotic activity. The entrapped glands have a flat and inactive appearance (most typical) (B). The tumor cells are present in a myxoid background; scattered rhabdomyoblasts are seen (C).

and neuroendocrine (synaptophysin and chromogranin) markers has been reported (572).

Alveolar rhabdomyosarcoma is the only subtype associated with chromosomal alterations, typically t(2;13)(q35;q14) or t(1;13)(q36;q14). t(2;13) and t(1;13) are seen in 80 percent of alveolar rhabdomyosarcomas, which are more aggressive. Tumors without these translocations may have a clinical course similar to that reported in embryonal rhabdomyosarcoma (573).

Differential Diagnosis. Entities in the differential diagnosis differ depending on the rhabdomyosarcoma subtype. Embryonal rhabdomyosarcoma is more commonly confused with *low-grade müllerian adenosarcoma* since both have condensation of cells around glands and may be associated with fetal-type cartilage. Rare glands in rhabdomyosarcoma may have a phyllodes-like configuration (fig. 10-66A). However, glands are sparse since they are typically entrapped but not an intrinsic component of the tumor, while in adenosarcoma they are one of the two components of the tumor and are often numerous. Furthermore, the epithelium in adenosarcoma tends to be active and hyperplastic, and may show a variety of metaplastic changes while in rhabdomyosarcoma, the lining epithelium in glands is typically flat and inactive. The stromal cells in adenosarcoma, although atypical and condensating around

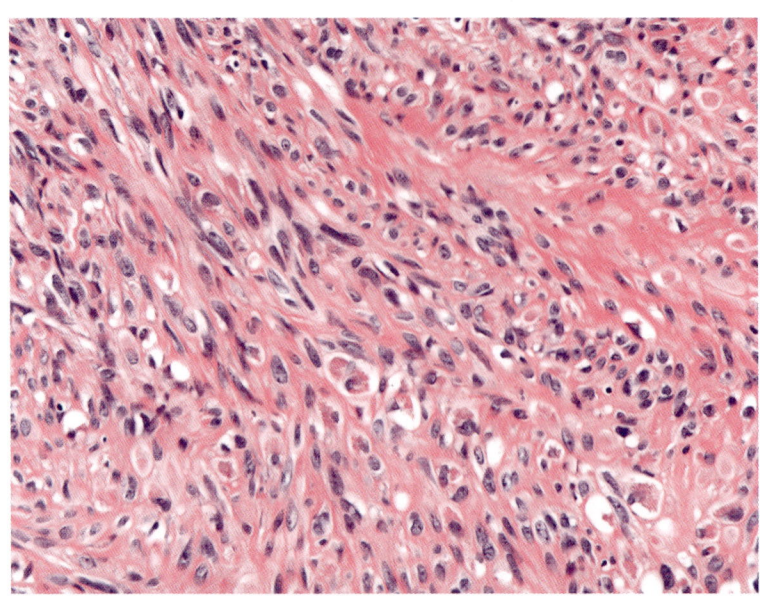

Figure 10-67

SPINDLED RHABDOMYOSARCOMA

Spindle cells with bland morphology are reminiscent of a smooth muscle neoplasm. Rhabdomyoblasts are a focal finding.

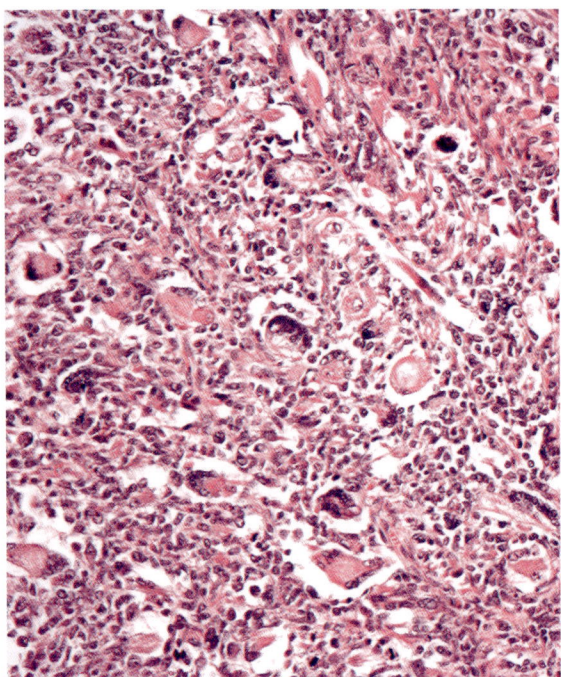

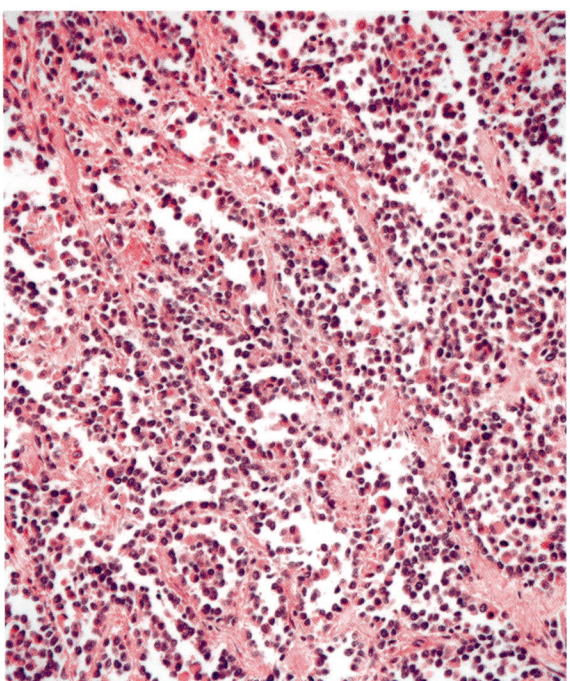

Figure 10-68

PLEOMORPHIC RHABDOMYOSARCOMA

Polygonal to spindled cells are admixed with large and pleomorphic rhabdomyoblasts. No intervening stroma is seen.

Figure 10-69

ALVEOLAR RHABDOMYOSARCOMA

The tumor displays a striking alveolar architecture. The lining cells have a hobnail configuration, and have pink cytoplasm and hyperchromatic nuclei.

glands, lack the primitive appearance, hyperchromatism, apoptotic debris, and brisk mitotic activity seen in rhabdomyosarcoma. The gross appearance of these tumors is also different; even though adenosarcoma has a polypoid growth pattern, it often displays a spongy but not fleshy cut surface if sarcomatous overgrowth is not present (574).

Other tumors that may be considered in the differential diagnosis include *primitive neuroectodermal tumor, lymphoma, small cell* or *undifferentiated carcinoma,* and *malignant melanoma.* In such cases, a wide panel of antibodies should be applied based on the potential diagnostic considerations.

The main entity in the differential diagnosis of spindle rhabdomyosarcoma is *spindle leiomyosarcoma* since both tumors have a spindle morphology and are positive for muscle markers. Focal rhabdomyoblasts, and sometimes, a component of usual embryonal rhabdomyosarcoma as well as positivity for skeletal muscle markers, are seen in spindle cell rhabdomyosarcoma.

Pleomorphic rhabdomyosarcoma should be distinguished from *adenosarcoma* with *sarcomatous overgrowth* and *carcinosarcoma* with prominence of this heterologous component. The former has areas with a typical biphasic growth and show positivity for ER and PR; PR is typically negative in rhabdomyosarcoma (575). Although carcinosarcomas may have a prominent sarcomatous component that contains rhabdomyosarcoma, a biphasic growth of highly malignant epithelium and stroma is typically present. Before establishing a diagnosis of pleomorphic rhabdomyosarcoma, extensive sampling should be performed to exclude these two entities. Other rare tumors in the differential diagnosis include *epithelioid leiomyosarcoma* with *rhabdoid-like features, hybrid leiomyosarcoma-rhabdomyosarcoma, undifferentiated uterine sarcoma,* and *rhabdoid tumor* (370,379,576–579).

Alveolar rhabdomyosarcoma should be primarily distinguished from *alveolar soft part sarcoma.* The latter has cells with abundant granular cytoplasm, large nuclei, and prominent nuclei in contrast to the smaller cells in alveolar rhabdomyosarcoma. Cells in alveolar soft part sarcoma display PAS with diastase (PAS-D) granules and crystals, are TFE-3 positive, and are associated with Der(17)t(X;17)(p11.2;q25) (449).

Treatment and Prognosis. Patients typically undergo total hysterectomy, with or without adjuvant therapy or chemotherapy. The prognosis is related to the histologic subtype. Patients with embryonal rhabdomyosarcoma have a good prognosis since the tumor is typically confined to the uterus and is associated with minimal myometrial and no vascular invasion. Patients with pleomorphic rhabdomyosarcomas have a poor prognosis, which is independent of stage, with at least half dying within a year of the diagnosis. Alveolar rhabdomyosarcoma is also associated with a poor prognosis, similar to that reported for its soft tissue counterpart (556,557).

Inflammatory Myofibroblastic Tumor

Definition and General Features. *Inflammatory myofibroblastic tumor* is a rare tumor, with less than 50 cases reported in the literature (281,281a,580–588) and recognized in the WHO 2014 classification (1). Within the uterus, inflammatory myofibroblastic tumor is more common in the corpus, followed by lower uterine segment and cervix. Although it was considered a reactive or inflammatory lesion, Dehner (589) first proposed the term "inflammatory myofibroblastic tumor" since the immunohistochemical and ultrastructural features of the tumor were indicative of myofibroblastic derivation. More recently, characteristic molecular features, including frequent genetic rearrangements of the *ALK* gene, have been reported (590).

Clinical Features. Tumors occur in patients over a wide age range (6 to 63 years) but are more common in reproductive age women. Patients present with nonspecific manifestations including vaginal bleeding and/or pelvic mass, or constitutional symptoms. Rarely, the tumor is an incidental finding or patients present with metastatic disease (281,281a,581,582).

Gross Findings. Tumors range from 1 to over 20 cm in size and may be well circumscribed (fig. 10-70, left), infiltrative or multinodular. They may massively involve the myometrium, with cervical or parametrial extension (281,581,582). They have either a white and whorled (leiomyoma-like) or yellow, soft, and sometimes gelatinous or fleshy cut surface. Areas of necrosis or hemorrhage can be seen.

Microscopic Findings. The tumors show a spindle cell proliferation that may be hypocellular (fig. 10-70, right), with cells loosely distributed with a fasciitis-like morphology (fig. 10-71A) or hypercellular with compact fascicular growth closely mimicking the appearance of a leiomyoma (fig. 10-71B,C). An associated myxoid background is common but is typically more striking in hypocellular areas (281,281a,581). Less commonly, there is prominent hyalinization between the tumor cells (580,581,591).

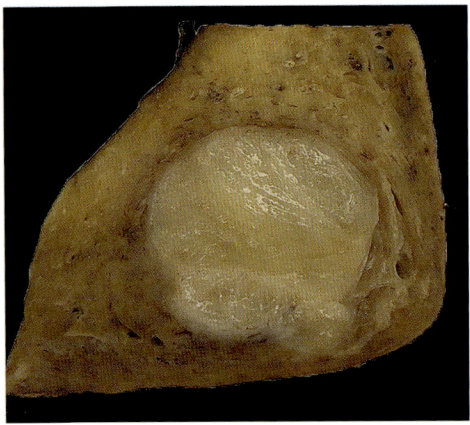 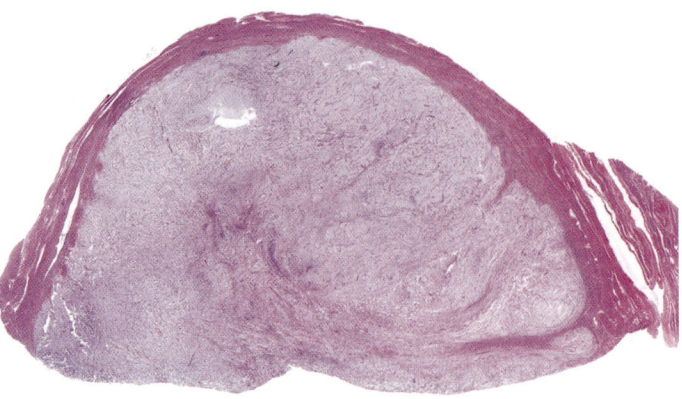

Figure 10-70

INFLAMMATORY MYOFIBROBLASTIC TUMOR

The tumor is well circumscribed and has a striking gelatinous cut surface (left) which correlates with a prominent myxoid background on microscopic examination (right).

Although cells are often spindled with pale eosinophilic and fibrillar cytoplasm, elongated nuclei with vesicular chromatin and small nucleoli, stellate, and epithelioid cells, the latter with round morphology reminiscent of "ganglion cells," may be seen and be extensive. Cytologic atypia is typically mild to moderate but may be striking in malignant tumors, while mitotic activity is often less than 6 mitoses per 10 high-power fields.

A characteristic feature and a clue to the diagnosis is the finding of a lymphoplasmacytic infiltrate, which may be patchy or diffuse and may form discrete aggregates, in which plasma cells are the most striking component (fig. 10-71D). Neutrophils are also common, while eosinophils and mast cells are less frequently seen (281,281a,581,582). The vessels tend to be thin-walled and branching. Necrosis is uncommon.

Features associated with adverse outcome include larger tumor size, cytologic atypia, and tumor cell necrosis (281,281a). Some found that the presence of an infiltrative border and extensive myxoid (versus compact in another study) background were associated with an adverse outcome (281,281a).

Immunohistochemical Findings. The tumors are typically positive for ALK, displaying often strong cytoplasmic staining, although heterogeneous and often not diffuse, but typically in more than 25 percent of cells, a frequency higher than that seen at other sites (fig. 10-72A) (281,281a, 581,588,591). Smooth muscle markers, desmin and smooth muscle actin, are more frequently and strongly positive than h-caldesmon, which is at most focally positive (fig. 10-72B) (583). Interestingly, ALK expression may be stronger in myxoid areas whereas smooth muscle marker expression may be stronger in fascicular areas. A distinct nuclear membrane or perinuclear pattern of ALK positivity is associated with round or epithelioid cell morphology in these tumors outside the uterus and appears to be associated with aggressive behavior (592), but this has not been shown in uterine tumors (281a).

CD10 is typically moderately to strongly positive. Cytokeratin may be positive but EMA is typically negative as well as ER, PR, S-100 protein, and CD117 (580,583,586,588). Ki-67 expression is variable but can be higher in areas with ganglion-like cells (583).

Molecular Genetic Findings. *ALK* rearrangements are seen in approximately 60 percent of tumors, depending on location, but often seen in the uterus (fig. 10-72C). Some tumors may be positive for ALK with negative molecular studies or vice versa (281,281a,581,588,591). This could be explained by the fact that other rearrangements may occur including *ROS-1* or *RET* rearrangements or *EML4-ALK* inversion, at least in soft tissue tumors (593). ROS1 expression correlates with *ROS1* rearrangement in inflammatory myofibroblastic tumors that lack *ALK* rearrangements (594). Rare *RET* rearrangements

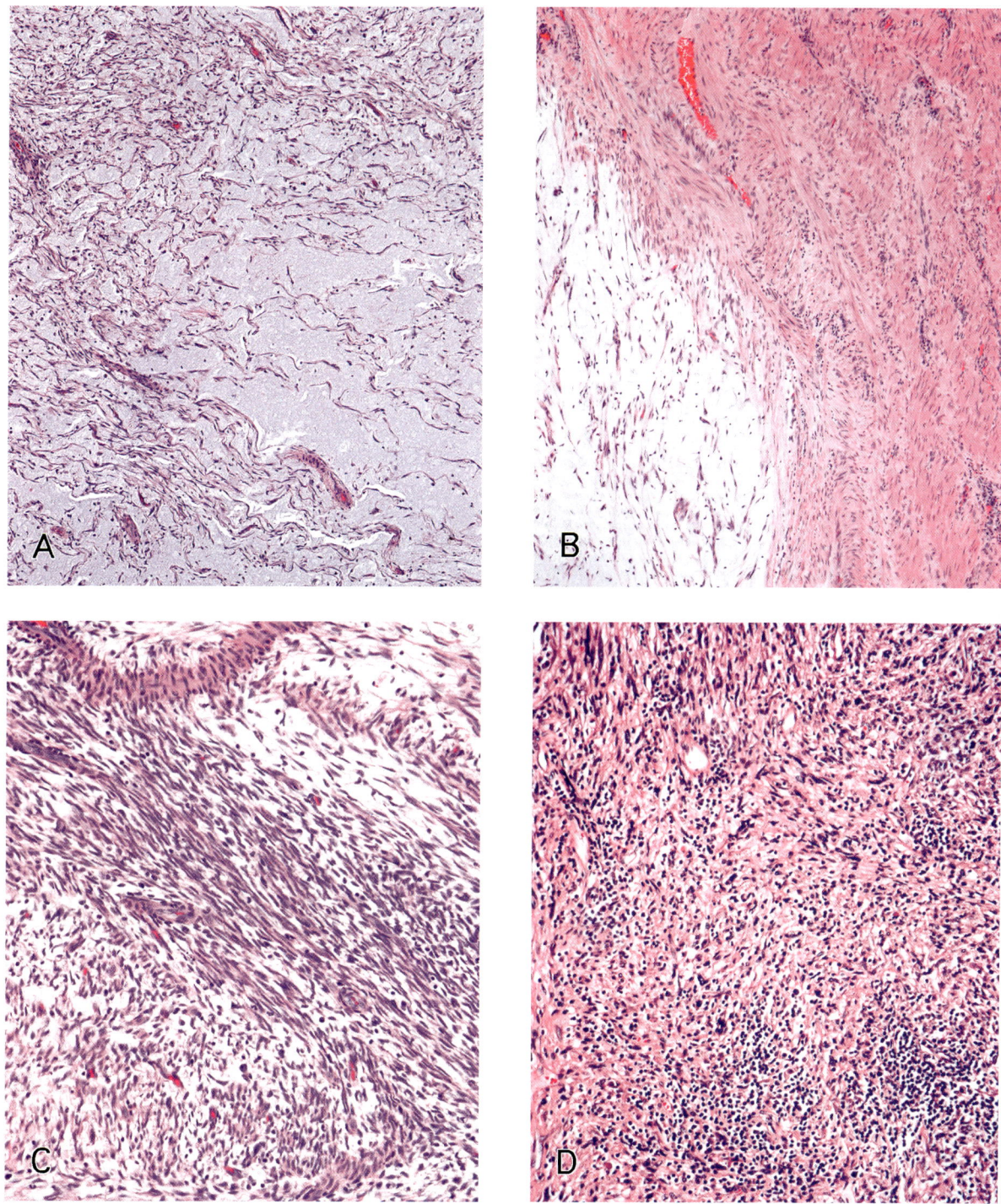

Figure 10-71

INFLAMMATORY MYOFIBROBLASTIC TUMOR

The tumor is hypocellular secondary to prominent myxoid matrix and is frequently misinterpreted as myxoid leiomyosarcoma (A). A myxoid area is juxtaposed to a smooth muscle-like area which may be misconstrued as a myxoid tumor infiltrating the myometrium. There is a sprinkling of lymphocytes in both areas (B). Cells with spindled (right) and some with plump (left) morphology are associated with delicate vasculature (C). The prominent lymphoplasmacytic inflammatory background obscures the neoplastic cells (D).

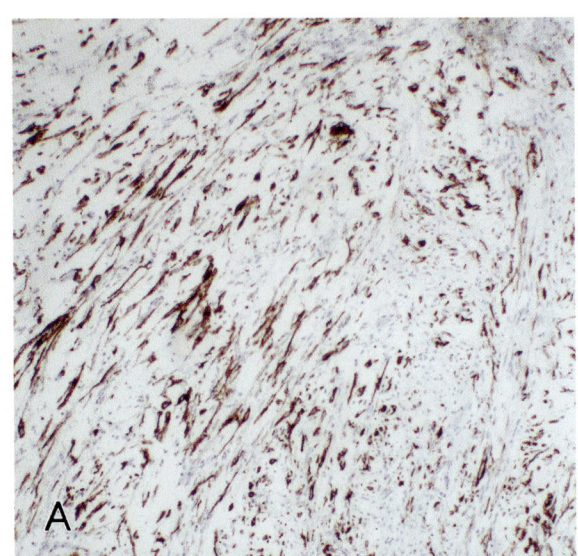

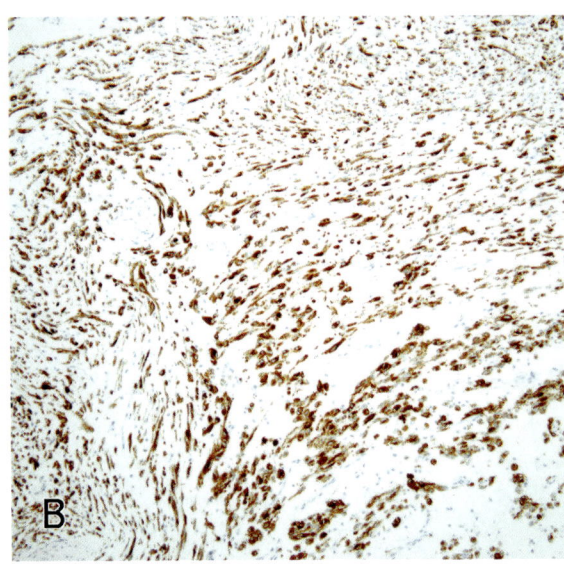

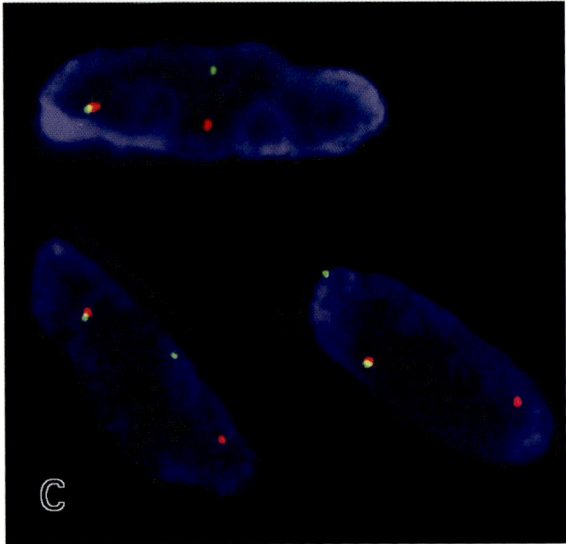

Figure 10-72

INFLAMMATORY MYOFIBROBLASTIC TUMOR

Many tumor cells show strong ALK-1 cytoplasmic positivity (A) but the tumor is also desmin positive (B) and displays *ALK* rearrangement (C).

have been reported in extragenital sites but no *ROS1* or *RET* rearrangements have been reported in uterine locations (593). p53 is often overexpressed in these tumors but its significance is uncertain (595), however, uterine tumors appear to lack mutations and thus, abnormal staining (413).

Ultrastructural Findings. By electron microscopy, cells show scattered nondilated rough endoplasmic reticulum, scattered thin filaments with peripheral dense bodies, pinocytic vesicles, occasional Golgi, and lipid droplets. The cells are surrounded by basal lamina-like material (582).

Differential Diagnosis. Benign and malignant tumors within the smooth muscle category are the most common diagnostic problem (Table 10-3). *Leiomyomas* with a *lymphoid infiltrate* (51) are characterized by an infiltrate of lymphocytes with scattered larger lymphoid cells, sometimes forming germinal centers, and occasionally, numerous plasma cells. Most tumors also show focal to extensive areas of sclerosis. The gross and microscopic features may overlap with inflammatory myofibroblastic tumor. Lack of ganglion-like cells and a myxoid background, positivity for smooth muscle markers, and negative ALK staining support the diagnosis of leiomyoma with lymphoid infiltrate.

Inflammatory myofibroblastic tumor is frequently misdiagnosed as a *myxoid smooth muscle tumor*, in particular, myxoid leiomyosarcoma, since both may show irregular borders, variable myxoid background, cytologic atypia, and mitotic activity. Myxoid leiomyosarcoma has a conventional or epithelioid component (often high grade), which if associated with an inflammatory infiltrate, tends to be minimal. Furthermore, it lacks the characteristic nuclei with vesicular chromatin seen in inflammatory myofibroblastic tumor. Although leiomyosarcomas may stain for ALK and show *ALK* amplifications (450), the finding of *ALK* rearrangements excludes this possibility (136,280). Some show PLAG1 rearrangements (435). A panel of antibodies including p53, p16, and ALK help in this differential diagnosis (413). Distinction is important as leiomyosarcomas are associated with poor prognosis despite aggressive treatment.

Another uterine mesenchymal tumor that may have a prominent myxoid background is *low-grade endometrial stromal sarcoma*. Some are associated with sclerosis, as seen in some inflammatory myofibroblastic tumors. However, endometrial stromal tumors display a tongue-like pattern of invasion, characteristic arteriolar vasculature, small oval cells that sometimes whorl around vessels, and lack the typical lymphoplasmacytic infiltrate seen in inflammatory myofibroblastic tumors (282). *ZC3H7B-BCOR high-grade endometrial stromal sarcomas* may rarely enter in the differential diagnosis. Although myxoid, they lack compact areas as well as inflammatory infiltrate. These sarcomas have collagen plaques and are cyclin D1 and BCOR positive, but ALK negative (451).

Rarely, *nerve sheath tumors*, either benign or malignant, occur in the uterus. Cells grow in fascicles or have a plexiform growth and may be epithelioid with a myxoid background, features that may overlap with an inflammatory myofibroblastic tumor (596,597). However, involvement of the gynecologic tract is exceedingly rare (the vulva is most commonly affected) and most tumors occur in patients with type I neurofibromatosis (598). Other typical morphologic features of nerve sheath tumors as well as positivity for S-100 protein should help in this differential diagnosis.

If myofibroblastic inflammatory tumor extends outside the uterus, a *gastrointestinal stromal tumor* may be a consideration, especially when myxoid. However, these tumors are typically centered in or around the gastrointestinal tract or are retroperitoneal, and associated with characteristic morphologic features including common cytoplasmic vacuolization as well as positivity for C-KIT, DOG-1, and CD34, and are ALK negative (599).

Treatment and Prognosis. Treatment typically consists of hysterectomy if the tumor is confined to the uterus (281,281a). Targeted therapy with tyrosine kinase inhibitors (due to *ALK* mutations) has been used in isolated cases outside the uterus (600). Although inflammatory myofibroblastic tumor is considered to have an intermediate biological behavior, in the female genital tract the two largest studies to date have shown different features to be associated with aggressive behavior. In the first study, larger size, higher proportion of myxoid stroma, and higher mitotic activity were more often seen in aggressive tumors compared to indolent ones, while tumor cell necrosis was only present in tumors associated with adverse outcome (281). In the second, study however, only a size of 8 cm or larger was found to be significantly associated with aggressive behavior by univariate analysis, while mitotic index over 7, presence of lymphovascular invasion, and compact predominance approached statistical significance (281a).

Table 10-3

DIFFERENTIAL FEATURES OF MYXOID SMOOTH MUSCLE TUMOR (SMT) AND INFLAMMATORY MYOFIBROBLASTIC TUMOR (IMT)

	Myxoid SMT	IMT
Fasciitis-like	-	+/-
Ganglion-like cells	-	+/-
Lymphoplasmacytic infiltrate	- (minimal if present)	+ (variable)
Thin branching vessels	-	+/-
Smooth muscle markers	+/-	+/-
ER/PR	+/-	-
P16	+	-
P53	+	-
ALK-1	-[a]	+
ALK-1 rearrangement	-	+
PLAG1 rearrangements	+/-	-

[a]With rare exceptions.

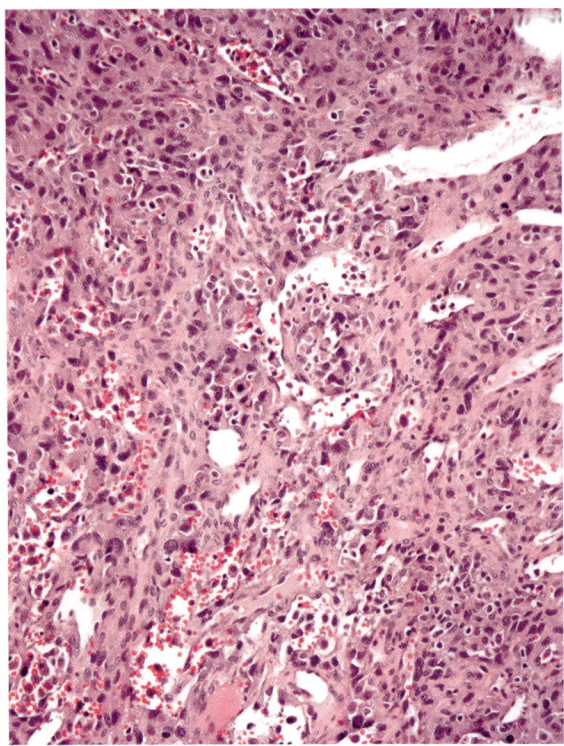

Figure 10-73

ANGIOSARCOMA

The tumor cells form irregular-shaped and -sized spaces that contain red blood cells. The cytoplasm is abundant. Marked cytologic atypia and mitotic activity are seen.

Vascular Tumors

Pure vascular tumors are rare. A prominent vascular component is sometimes part of a leiomyoma. The most common vascular uterine tumor is an *arteriovenous malformation*. *Angiomas* are rare, may be responsible for severe uterine bleeding, and have an appearance similar to that seen at other sites (601–603). *Angiosarcoma*, its malignant counterpart, is an aggressive tumor that can occur anywhere within the female genital tract, more commonly in the ovary followed by the uterus, and rarely in the vagina and vulva (604).

Patients with angiosarcoma are commonly postmenopausal and present with vaginal bleeding secondary to a rapidly growing mass. Patients may have a history of prior radiation (605,606). On gross examination, tumors are frequently hemorrhagic and necrotic. On microscopic examination, tumor cells grow in sheets, fascicles, or nests. They may be spindled or epithelioid, form poorly developed vascular spaces (sometimes slit-like), and contain intracytoplasmic lumens. Angiosarcomas are typically associated with marked cytologic atypia and brisk mitotic activity (fig. 10-73) (607–609). They may originate de novo or arise in a background of a leiomyoma or adenosarcoma (610,611). Tumor cells are positive for CD31, factor VIII, and CD34.

The most common neoplasms in the differential diagnosis of angiosarcoma are leiomyosarcoma and poorly differentiated carcinoma. Although treatment is not standardized, patients typically undergo total abdominal hysterectomy and bilateral salpingo-oophorectomy (as if tumor spreads outside the uterus, it frequently involves the ovaries), with adjuvant chemotherapy and possible radiation therapy. Despite aggressive treatment, the prognosis is dismal (607).

Alveolar Soft Part Sarcoma

Less than 20 cases of *alveolar soft part sarcoma*, a tumor that typically affects soft tissues of the extremities in young adults, have been reported involving the uterine corpus (380,612–618). In the largest series of 9 tumors, 3 were located in the corpus and 3 in the lower uterine segment-cervix (612), although tumors appear to be more commonly seen in the uterine cervix than the corpus (618).

Patients range in age from 14 to 50 (mean, 38) years and they typically present with abnormal uterine bleeding. In some instances, the tumor is an incidental finding when the patient is undergoing hysterectomy for uterine leiomyomas. The tumors range in size from microscopic to 7 cm. They are well circumscribed and have a tan to yellow or yellow-white cut surface. Foci of hemorrhage can be seen.

On microscopic examination, alveolar soft part sarcomas often have a pushing but well-circumscribed or slightly irregular margin. They consistently have prominent alveolar growth that may be admixed with a variable solid component associated with scant stroma. Delicate fibrous septa may become thicker or hyalinized. The tumor cells are polygonal, with abundant vacuolated, granular eosinophilic cytoplasm and large and vesicular nuclei with prominent nucleoli. Cytologic atypia is not striking and mitotic activity is typically low (fig. 10-74, left).

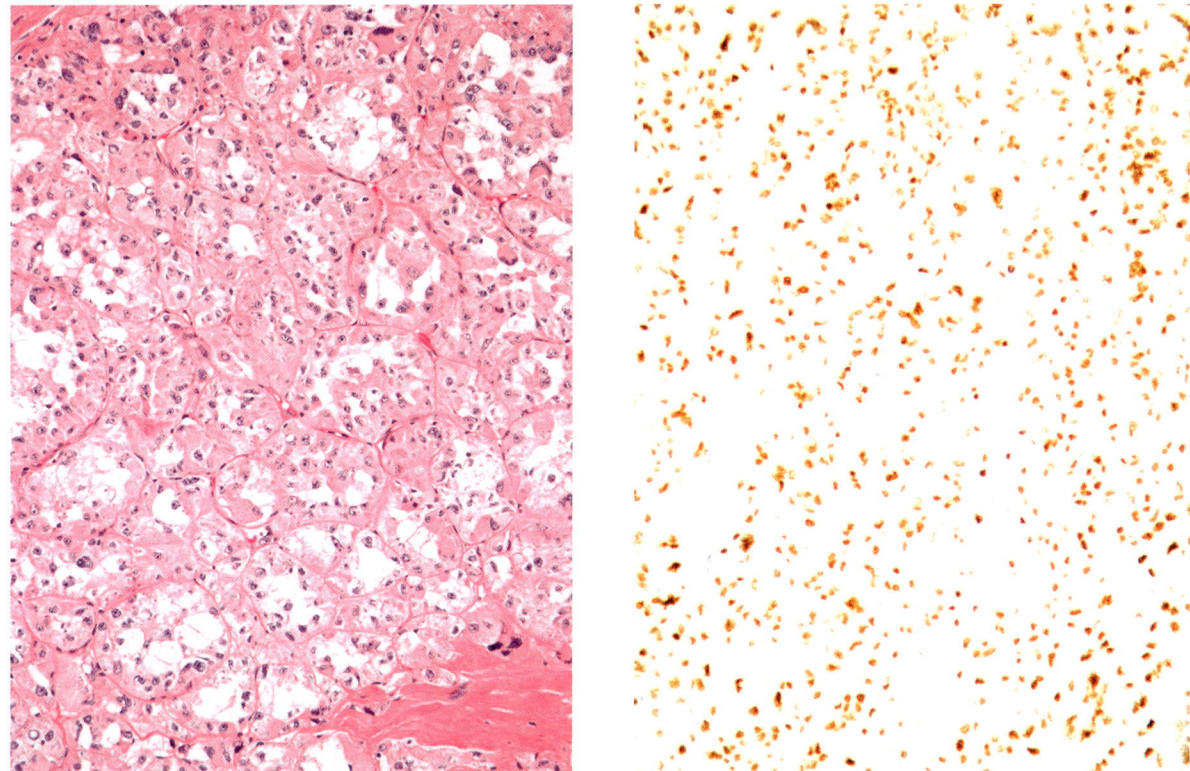

Figure 10-74

ALVEOLAR SOFT PART SARCOMA

The tumor has a striking nested architecture with minimal intervening stroma (left). Cells have abundant pale eosinophilic cytoplasm, large nuclei, and prominent nucleoli with uniform cytologic features. The tumor cells show diffuse and strong TFE-3 nuclear positivity (right).

PAS-positive diastase-resistant intracytoplasmic granules or crystals are present in some cells in most tumors.

Tumor cells are typically strongly and diffusely positive for TFE-3 (fig. 10-74, right). Rare tumors are positive for PR and CD10 (613). They are negative for vimentin, smooth muscle actin, desmin, myoglobin, S-100 protein, HMB-45, melan A, keratins, and EMA as well as for chromogranin and synaptophysin with rare exceptions (380,612,613,615).

By electromicroscopy, cells have rod-like or rhomboid crystals or may only show membrane-bound granules. The tumors are thought to have a myogenic origin, although not with absolute certainty, since it appears that the characteristic crystals are composed of transporter proteins that are especially common in cardiac and skeletal muscle where these tumors have a predilection to occur (619).

The differential diagnosis includes in order of frequency *epithelioid smooth muscle tumor*, *PEComa*, and *metastatic clear cell renal carcinoma*. The former often shows an admixture of epithelioid cells that form nests and spindle cells that grow in fascicles. Cells are positive for muscle markers and may show positivity for keratins and EMA but are negative for TFE-3. Striking morphologic, immunohistochemical, and molecular overlap can occur with PEComas. However, the latter are positive for melanocytic markers and often also positive for smooth muscle markers; most lack the characteristic *ASPSCR1-TFE3* fusion of alveolar soft part sarcomas. Clear cell carcinoma is characterized by nests of tumor cells with variation on nuclear grade and often contain recent hemorrhage. They are positive for PAX8, CA-IX, and RCC markers.

In a multivariate analysis from a review of 251 patients with alveolar soft part sarcoma, older

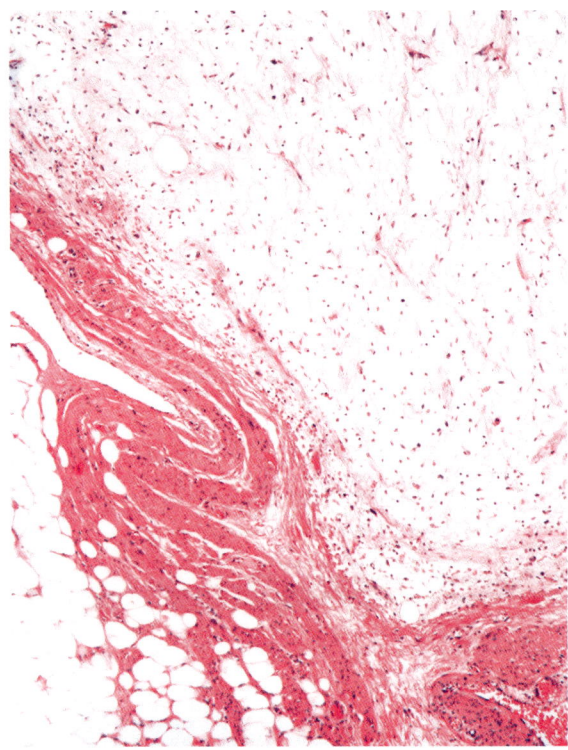

Figure 10-75

MYXOID LIPOSARCOMA

The tumor is associated with a prominent myxoid background and delicate vasculature. A juxtaposed lipoleiomyoma (bottom) is seen.

age, tumor size over 10 cm, distant metastases at diagnosis, and truncal location were identified as independent factors predictive of worse overall survival (620). In the gynecologic tract, tumors appear to be associated with a good prognosis, which has been postulated to be related to the small size of most tumors. Only one patient with a uterine corpus tumor developed lymph node metastases at the time of initial surgery, even though the tumor was less than 3 cm (618). Follow-up is limited in most patients.

Lipoma and Liposarcoma

Lipomas and *liposarcomas* are rare in the uterus in pure form when excluding a lipomatous component, typically benign, admixed with a smooth muscle tumor (lipoleiomyoma). The incidence of lipoma is less than 0.12 percent. Its features are similar to lipomas in soft tissue locations (621–623).

Liposarcoma is the most common soft tissue sarcoma in adults, typically arising in the retroperitoneum or extremities but rare in the female genital tract. The uterus is the most common location (147,380,624–626). Patients often are perimenopausal or postmenopausal and present with uterine bleeding. On gross examination, liposarcomas are centered in the myometrium, and are as large as 20 cm. They are well circumscribed, with pushing borders, and have a nonspecific fleshy appearance or show a sticky-gelatinous cut surface, with or without areas of hemorrhage or necrosis. In contrast to a soft tissue location where well-differentiated liposarcoma is most common, myxoid/round cell types are prevalent within the uterus (147).

Myxoid liposarcoma is typically hypocellular and associated with a prominent myxoid background as well as a conspicuous delicate branching capillary network. Bland spindle cells and rare lipoblasts are seen (fig. 10-75). Pleomorphic cells are typically present if there is a pleomorphic component. S-100 protein is positive and MDM2 may be positive in tumors with a pleomorphic component. Myxoid/round cell liposarcomas are associated with t(12,16).

Liposarcomas may merge with a lipoleiomyoma component, but other associations including lipoleiomyosarcoma, spindled leiomyosarcoma, or leiomyoma have been reported (147,380,627,628). Behavior appears to be more aggressive in patients with pleomorphic or round cell liposarcoma components (147).

Solitary Fibrous Tumor

Solitary fibrous tumor was originally described in the thoracic cavity but has been reported in a variety of extrapleural sites including the uterine corpus, although it is rare in this location (629–632). Patients are often postmenopausal and present with hypoglycemia secondary to the production of high molecular weight insulin-like growth factor II by the tumor cells (629). Some present with signs and symptoms related to the uterine mass (630–632).

Solitary fibrous tumors are typically large (up to 25 cm) and have a firm gray to yellow, uniform cut surface. On microscopic examination, there are alternating hypocellular and hypercellular areas with a patternless growth of tumor cells associated with a "hemangiopericytoma" vasculature and collagen bands (629–632). Rarely, there is a prominent myxoid background (629). The neoplastic cells are spindled, with oval to spindle-shaped nuclei and bland cytologic features. Tumors are typically positive for vimentin, CD34, BCL-2, and STAT6 (secondary to *NAB2/STAT6* fusion) (633). They are negative for epithelial and smooth muscle markers.

The differential diagnosis includes *benign* or *malignant smooth muscle tumors*. Even though the latter tumors may have staghorn-like vessels, overall morphologic features, including spindle cells forming fascicles that are positive for muscle markers, help in this distinction. Rarely, *endometrial stromal sarcoma* may be in the differential diagnosis since cells are oval with scant cytoplasm and may show hypercellular and hypocellular areas. However, vessels are arteriole-like and cells are positive for CD10 but negative for CD34 and STAT6.

Most tumors follow a benign course, but rare tumors metastasize (630). The features recently reported to be associated with malignancy in either intrathoracic or extrathoracic tumors include patient age, tumor size, and mitoses (634). Tumors occurring in patients over 55 years, larger than 15 cm, and with more than 4 mitoses per 10 high-power fields have a high-risk of metastases, but tumors without these features may also have an unfavorable course. Solitary fibrous tumor, therefore, should be considered to have an uncertain malignant potential.

Other Mesenchymal Tumors

Other rare mesenchymal tumors that occur within the uterine corpus (564) are *nerve sheath tumors* (although rare, more common if benign; may be associated with neurofibromatosis) (203,635), *primitive neuroectodermal tumors* (chapter 12), *chondrosarcoma* (636), *osteosarcoma* (637–639), and *malignant rhabdoid tumor/SMARCA-4 deficient (undifferentiated) uterine sarcoma* (576–579).

REFERENCES

1. Oliva E, Carcangiu ML, Carinelli SG, et al. Mesenchymal tumours. In: Kurman RJ, Carcangiu ML, Herrington CS, Young RH, eds. WHO classification of tumours of female reproductive organs, 4th ed. Lyons: IARC 2014;135-47.
2. Baird DD, Dunson DB, Hill MC, Cousins D, Schectman JM. High cumulative incidence of uterine leiomyoma in black and white women: ultrasound evidence. Am J Obstet Gynecol 2003;188:100-7.
3. Cramer SF, Patel A. The frequency of uterine leiomyomas. Am J Clin Pathol 1990;94:435-8.
4. Buttram VC Jr, Reiter RC. Uterine leiomyomata: etiology, symptomatology, and management. Fertil Steril 1981;36:433-45.
5. Farquhar CM, Steiner CA. Hysterectomy rates in the United States 1990-1997. Obstet Gynecol 2002;99:229-34.
6. Wechter ME, Stewart EA, Myers ER, Kho RM, Wu JM. Leiomyoma-related hospitalization and surgery: prevalence and predicted growth based on population trends. Am J Obstet Gynecol 2011;205:492.e1-5.
7. Wu JM, Wechter ME, Geller EJ, Nguyen TV, Visco AG. Hysterectomy rates in the United States, 2003. Obstet Gynecol 2007;110:1091-5.
8. Launonen V, Vierimaa O, Kiuru M, et al. Inherited susceptibility to uterine leiomyomas and renal cell cancer. Proc Natl Acad Sci U S A 2001;98:3387-92.
9. Lehtonen HJ. Hereditary leiomyomatosis and renal cell cancer: update on clinical and molecular characteristics. Fam Cancer 2011;10:397-411.
10. Nozu K, Minamikawa S, Yamada S, et al. Characterization of contiguous gene deletions in COL4A6 and COL4A5 in alport syndrome-diffuse leiomyomatosis. J Hum Genet 2017;62:733-5.
11. Cohen MM Jr. Proteus syndrome: an update. Am J Med Genet C Semin Med Genet 2005;137C:38-52.
12. Pilarski R, Eng C. Will the real Cowden syndrome please stand up (again)? Expanding mutational and clinical spectra of the PTEN hamartoma tumour syndrome. J Med Genet 2004;41:323-6.
13. Flake GP, Andersen J, Dixon D. Etiology and pathogenesis of uterine leiomyomas: a review. Environ Health Perspect 2003;111:1037-54.

14. Commandeur AE, Styer AK, Teixeira JM. Epidemiological and genetic clues for molecular mechanisms involved in uterine leiomyoma development and growth. Hum Reprod Update 2015;21:593-5.
15. Garg K, Karnezis AN, Rabban JT. Uncommon hereditary gynaecological tumour syndromes: pathological features in tumours that may predict risk for a germline mutation. Pathology 2018;50:238-56.
16. Stewart EA. Uterine fibroids. Lancet 2001;357:293-8.
17. Toro JR, Nickerson ML, Wei MH, et al. Mutations in the fumarate hydratase gene cause hereditary leiomyomatosis and renal cell cancer in families in North America. Am J Hum Genet 2003;73:95-106.
18. Stewart L, Glenn GM, Stratton P, et al. Association of germline mutations in the fumarate hydratase gene and uterine fibroids in women with hereditary leiomyomatosis and renal cell cancer. Arch Dermatol 2008;144:1584-92.
19. Wei MH, Toure O, Glenn GM, et al. Novel mutations in FH and expansion of the spectrum of phenotypes expressed in families with hereditary leiomyomatosis and renal cell cancer. J Med Genet 2006;43:18-27.
20. Alam NA, Barclay E, Rowan AJ, et al. Clinical features of multiple cutaneous and uterine leiomyomatosis: an underdiagnosed tumor syndrome. Arch Dermatol 2005;141:199-206.
21. Norris HJ, Hilliard GD, Irey NS. Hemorrhagic cellular leiomyomas ("apoplectic leiomyoma") of the uterus associated with pregnancy and oral contraceptives. Int J Gynecol Pathol 1988;7:212-24.
22. Cohen DT, Oliva E, Hahn PF, Fuller AF Jr, Lee SI. Uterine smooth-muscle tumors with unusual growth patterns: imaging with pathologic correlation. AJR Am J Roentgenol 2007;188:246-55.
23. Ip PP, Lim D, Cheung ANY, Oliva E. Immunoexpression of p16 in uterine leiomyomas with infarct-type necrosis: an analysis of 35 cases. Histopathology 2017;71:743-50.
24. O'Connor DM, Norris HJ. Mitotically active leiomyomas of the uterus. Hum Pathol 1990;21:223-7.
25. Nezhat C, Kho K. Iatrogenic myomas: new class of myomas? J Minim Invasive Gynecol 2010;17:544-50.
26. Nguyen D, Maheshwary R, Tran C, Rudkin S, Treaster L. Diffuse peritoneal leiomyomatosis status post laparoscopic hysterectomy with power morcellation: a case report with review of literature. Gynecol Oncol Rep 2017;19:59-61.
27. Ordulu Z, Dal Cin P, Chong WW, et al. Disseminated peritoneal leiomyomatosis after laparoscopic supracervical hysterectomy with characteristic molecular cytogenetic findings of uterine leiomyoma. Genes Chromosomes Cancer 2010;49:1152-60.
28. Anand N, Handler M, Khan A, Wagreich A, Calhoun S. Disseminated peritoneal leiomyomatosis status post laparoscopic hysterectomy with morcellation. J Radiol Case Rep 2016;10:12-8.
29. Lete I, Gonzalez J, Ugarte L, Barbadillo N, Lapuente O, Alvarez-Sala J. Parasitic leiomyomas: a systematic review. Eur J Obstet Gynecol Reprod Biol 2016;203:250-9.
30. Kho KA, Nezhat C. Parasitic myomas. Obstet Gynecol 2009;114:611-5.
31. Horstmann JP, Pietra GG, Harman JA, Cole NG, Grinspan S. Spontaneous regression of pulmonary leiomyomas during pregnancy. Cancer 1977;39:314-21.
32. Oguma T, Yamasaki N, Nakanishi K, Kinoshita D, Mitsuhashi T, Nakagawa S. Pseudo-Meigs' syndrome associated with hydropic degenerating uterine leiomyoma: a case report. J Obstet Gynaecol Res 2014;40:1137-40.
33. Buka NJ. Eosinophilia associated with uterine leiomyomas. Can Med Assoc J 1965;93:163-5.
34. Prayson RA, Hart WR. Mitotically active leiomyomas of the uterus. Am J Clin Pathol 1992;97:14-20.
35. Perrone T, Dehner LP. Prognostically favorable "mitotically active" smooth-muscle tumors of the uterus. A clinicopathologic study of ten cases. Am J Surg Pathol 1988;12:1-8.
36. Myles JL, Hart WR. Apoplectic leiomyomas of the uterus. A clinicopathologic study of five distinctive hemorrhagic leiomyomas associated with oral contraceptive usage. Am J Surg Pathol 1985;9:798-805.
37. Bennett JA, Lamb C, Young RH. Apoplectic leiomyomas: a morphologic analysis of 100 cases highlighting unusual features. Am J Surg Pathol 2016;40:563-8.
38. Clement PB, Young RH, Scully RE. Diffuse, perinodular, and other patterns of hydropic degeneration within and adjacent to uterine leiomyomas. Problems in differential diagnosis. Am J Surg Pathol 1992;16:26-32.
39. Croce S, Young RH, Oliva E. Uterine leiomyomas with bizarre nuclei: a clinicopathologic study of 59 cases. Am J Surg Pathol 2014;38:1330-9.
40. Downes KA, Hart WR. Bizarre leiomyomas of the uterus: a comprehensive pathologic study of 24 cases with long-term follow-up. Am J Surg Pathol 1997;21:1261-70.
41. Oliva E, Young RH, Clement PB, Bhan AK, Scully RE. Cellular benign mesenchymal tumors of the uterus. A comparative morphologic and immunohistochemical analysis of 33 highly cellular leiomyomas and six endometrial stromal nodules, two frequently confused tumors. Am J Surg Pathol 1995;19:757-68.
42. Roth LM, Reed RJ, Sternberg WH. Cotyledonoid dissecting leiomyoma of the uterus. The Sternberg tumor. Am J Surg Pathol 1996;20:1455-61.

43. Roth LM, Reed RJ. Dissecting leiomyomas of the uterus other than cotyledonoid dissecting leiomyomas: a report of eight cases. Am J Surg Pathol 1999;23:1032-9.
44. Clement PB. Selected miscellaneous ovarian lesions: small cell carcinomas, mesothelial lesions, mesenchymal and mixed neoplasms, and non-neoplastic lesions. Mod Pathol 2005;18(Suppl 2):S113-29.
45. McCluggage WG, Boyde A. Uterine angioleiomyomas: a report of 3 cases of a distinctive benign leiomyoma variant. Int J Surg Pathol 2007;15:262-5.
46. Gisser SD, Young I. Neurilemoma-like uterine myomas: an ultrastructural reaffirmation of their non-Schwannian nature. Am J Obstet Gynecol 1977;129:389-92.
47. Parker RL, Young RH, Clement PB. Skeletal muscle-like and rhabdoid cells in uterine leiomyomas. Int J Gynecol Pathol 2005;24:319-25.
48. Zamecnik M, Kascak P. Uterine leiomyoma with amianthoid-like fibers. Cesk Patol 2011;47:125-7.
49. Schmid C, Beham A, Kratochvil P. Haematopoiesis in a degenerating uterine leiomyoma. Arch Gynecol Obstet 1990;248:81-6.
50. Cui X, Peker D, Greer HO, Conner MG, Novak L. Extramedullary hematopoiesis in uterine leiomyoma associated with numerous intravascular thrombi. Case Rep Pathol 2014;2014:957395.
51. Ferry JA, Harris NL, Scully RE. Uterine leiomyomas with lymphoid infiltration simulating lymphoma. A report of seven cases. Int J Gynecol Pathol 1989;8:263-70.
52. Chuang SS, Lin CN, Li CY, Wu CH. Uterine leiomyoma with massive lymphocytic infiltration simulating malignant lymphoma. A case report with immunohistochemical study showing that the infiltrating lymphocytes are cytotoxic T cells. Pathol Res Pract 2001;197:135-8.
53. Orii A, Mori A, Zhai YL, Toki T, Nikaido T, Fujii S. Mast cells in smooth muscle tumors of the uterus. Int J Gynecol Pathol 1998;17:336-42.
54. Crow J, Wilkins M, Howe S, More L, Helliwell P. Mast cells in the female genital tract. Int J Gynecol Pathol 1991;10:230-7.
55. Vang R, Medeiros LJ, Samoszuk M, Deavers MT. Uterine leiomyomas with eosinophils: a clinicopathologic study of 3 cases. Int J Gynecol Pathol 2001;20:239-43.
56. Adany R, Fodor F, Molnar P, Ablin RJ, Muszbek L. Increased density of histiocytes in uterine leiomyomas. Int J Gynecol Pathol 1990;9:137-44.
57. Manchana T, Sirisabya N, Triratanachat S, Niruthisard S, Tannirandorn Y. Pyomyoma in a perimenopausal woman with intrauterine device. Gynecol Obstet Invest 2007;63:170-2.
58. Das SS, Dogra M, Bala Y. Abscess in fibromyoma following instrumentation. Int J Gynaecol Obstet 1994;45:285-7.
59. Cramer SF, Mann L, Calianese E, Daley J, Williamson K. Association of seedling myomas with myometrial hyperplasia. Hum Pathol 2009;40:218-25.
60. Cramer SF, Horiszny J, Patel A, Sigrist S. The relation of fibrous degeneration to menopausal status in small uterine leiomyomas with evidence for postmenopausal origin of seedling myomas. Mod Pathol 1996;9:774-80.
61. Bell SW, Kempson RL, Hendrickson MR. Problematic uterine smooth muscle neoplasms. A clinicopathologic study of 213 cases. Am J Surg Pathol 1994;18:535-58.
62. Toledo G, Oliva E. Smooth muscle tumors of the uterus: a practical approach. Arch Pathol Lab Med 2008;132:595-605.
63. Oliva E. Practical issues in uterine pathology from banal to bewildering: the remarkable spectrum of smooth muscle neoplasia. Mod Pathol 2016;29(Suppl 1):S104-20.
64. Evans N. Malignant myomata and related tumors of the uterus. Surg Gynecol Obstet 1920;30:225-39.
65. Ly A, Mills AM, McKenney JK, et al. Atypical leiomyomas of the uterus: a clinicopathologic study of 51 cases. Am J Surg Pathol 2013;37:643-9.
66. Kefeli M, Caliskan S, Kurtoglu E, Yildiz L, Kokcu A. Leiomyoma with bizarre nuclei: clinical and pathologic features of 30 patients. Int J Gynecol Pathol 2018;37:379-87.
67. Downes Ka, Tubbs RT, Hart WR. Bizarre uterine leiomyomas: ki-67 activity and DNA ploidy. Mod Pathol 1999;12:116A.
68. Ubago JM, Zhang Q, Kim JJ, Kong B, Wei JJ. Two subtypes of atypical leiomyoma: clinical, histologic, and molecular analysis. Am J Surg Pathol 2016;40:923-33.
69. Sanz-Ortega J, Vocke C, Stratton P, Linehan WM, Merino MJ. Morphologic and molecular characteristics of uterine leiomyomas in hereditary leiomyomatosis and renal cancer (HLRCC) syndrome. Am J Surg Pathol 2013;37:74-80.
70. Garg K, Tickoo SK, Soslow RA, Reuter VE. Morphologic features of uterine leiomyomas associated with hereditary leiomyomatosis and renal cell carcinoma syndrome: a case report. Am J Surg Pathol 2011;35:1235-7.
71. Reyes C, Karamurzin Y, Frizzell N, et al. Uterine smooth muscle tumors with features suggesting fumarate hydratase aberration: detailed morphologic analysis and correlation with S-(2-succino)-cysteine immunohistochemistry. Mod Pathol 2014;27:1020-7.
72. Bennett JA, Weigelt B, Chiang S, et al. Leiomyoma with bizarre nuclei: a morphological, immunohistochemical and molecular analysis of 31 cases. Mod Pathol 2017;30:1476-88.
73. Wei JJ. Atypical leiomyoma with features suggesting of fumarate hydratase mutation. Int J Gynecol Pathol 2016;35:531-6.

74. Harrison WJ, Andrici J, Maclean F, et al. Fumarate hydratase-deficient uterine leiomyomas occur in both the syndromic and sporadic settings. Am J Surg Pathol 2016;40:599-607.
75. Miettinen M, Felisiak-Golabek A, Wasag B, et al. Fumarase-deficient uterine leiomyomas: an immunohistochemical, molecular genetic, and clinicopathologic study of 86 cases. Am J Surg Pathol 2016;40:1661-9.
76. Dgani R, Piura B, Ben-Baruch G, et al. Clinical-pathological study of uterine leiomyomas with high mitotic activity. Acta Obstet Gynecol Scand 1998;77:74-7.
77. Silverberg SG. Leiomyosarcoma of the uterus. A clinicopathologic study. Obstet Gynecol 1971;38:613-28.
78. Hart WR, Billman JK Jr. A reassessment of uterine neoplasms originally diagnosed as leiomyosarcomas. Cancer 1978;41:1902-10.
79. Zaloudek C, Norris HJ. Mesenchymal tumors of the uterus. In: Kurman RJ, ed. Blaustein's pathology of the female genital tract, 4th ed. New York: Springer-Verlag 1994;487-528.
80. Coad JE, Sulaiman RA, Das K, Staley N. Perinodular hydropic degeneration of a uterine leiomyoma: a diagnostic challenge. Hum Pathol 1997;28:249-51.
81. Coard K, Plummer J. Massive multilocular cystic leiomyoma of the uterus: an extreme example of hydropic degeneration. South Med J 2007;100:309-12.
82. Ceyhan K, Simsir C, Dolen I, Calyskan E, Umudum H. Multinodular hydropic leiomyoma of the uterus with perinodular hydropic degeneration and extrauterine extension. Pathol Int 2002;52:540-3.
83. David MP, Homonnai TZ, Deligdish L, Loewenthal M. Grape-like leiomyomas of the uterus. Int Surg 1975;60:238-9.
84. Roth LM, Reed RJ. Cotyledonoid leiomyoma of the uterus: report of a case. Int J Gynecol Pathol 2000;19:272-5.
85. Saeed AS, Hanaa B, Faisal AS, Najla AM. Cotyledonoid dissecting leiomyoma of the uterus: a case report of a benign uterine tumor with sarcomalike gross appearance and review of literature. Int J Gynecol Pathol 2006;25:262-7.
86. Cheuk W, Chan JK, Liu JY. Cotyledonoid leiomyoma: a benign uterine tumor with alarming gross appearance. Arch Pathol Lab Med 2002;126:210-3.
87. Shelekhova KV, Kazakov DV, Michal M. Cotyledonoid dissecting leiomyoma of the uterus with intravascular growth: report of two cases. Virchows Arch 2007;450:119-21.
88. Jordan LB, Al-Nafussi A, Beattie G. Cotyledonoid hydropic intravenous leiomyomatosis: a new variant leiomyoma. Histopathology 2002;40:245-52.
89. Roth LM, Kirker JA, Insull M, Whittaker J. Recurrent cotyledonoid dissecting leiomyoma of the uterus. Int J Gynecol Pathol 2013;32:215-20.
90. Soleymani Majd H, Ismail L, Desai SA, Reginald PW. Epithelioid cotyledonoid dissecting leiomyoma: a case report and review of the literature. Arch Gynecol Obstet 2011;283:771-4.
91. Blake EA, Cheng G, Post MD, Guntupalli S. Cotyledonoid dissecting leiomyoma with adipocytic differentiation: a case report. Gynecol Oncol Rep 2015;11:7-9.
92. Kim NR, Park CY, Cho HY. Cotyledonoid dissecting leiomyoma of the uterus with intravascular luminal growth: a case study. Korean J Pathol 2013;47:477-80.
93. Smith CC, Gold MA, Wile G, Fadare O. Cotyledonoid dissecting leiomyoma of the uterus: a review of clinical, pathological, and radiological features. Int J Surg Pathol 2012;20:330-41.
94. Goldzieher JW, Maqueo M, Ricaud L, Aguilar JA, Canales E. Induction of degenerative changes in uterine myomas by high-dosage progestin therapy. Am J Obstet Gynecol 1966;96:1078-87.
95. Fechner RE. Atypical leiomyomas and synthetic progestin therapy. Am J Clin Pathol 1968;49:697-703.
96. Boyd C, McCluggage WG. Unusual morphological features of uterine leiomyomas treated with progestogens. J Clin Pathol 2011;64:485-9.
97. Crow J, Gardner RL, McSweeney G, Shaw RW. Morphological changes in uterine leiomyomas treated by GnRH agonist goserelin. Int J Gynecol Pathol 1995;14:235-42.
98. Gutmann JN, Thornton KL, Diamond MP, Carcangiu ML. Evaluation of leuprolide acetate treatment on histopathology of uterine myomata. Fertil Steril 1994;61:622-6.
99. Colgan TJ, Pendergast S, LeBlanc M. The histopathology of uterine leiomyomas following treatment with gonadotropin-releasing hormone analogues. Hum Pathol 1993;24:1073-7.
100. Sreenan JJ, Prayson RA, Biscotti CV, Thornton MH, Easley KA, Hart WR. Histopathologic findings in 107 uterine leiomyomas treated with leuprolide acetate compared with 126 controls. Am J Surg Pathol 1996;20:427-32.
101. Deligdisch L, Hirschmann S, Altchek A. Pathologic changes in gonadotropin releasing hormone agonist analogue treated uterine leiomyomata. Fertil Steril 1997;67:837-41.
102. Demopoulos RI, Jones KY, Mittal KR, Vamvakas EC. Histology of leiomyomata in patients treated with leuprolide acetate. Int J Gynecol Pathol 1997;16:131-7.

103. Ueki M, Okamoto Y, Tsurunaga T, Seiki Y, Ueda M, Sugimoto O. Endocrinological and histological changes after treatment of uterine leiomyomas with danazol or buserelin. J Obstet Gynaecol (Tokyo 1995) 1995;21:1-7.
104. Upadhyaya NB, Doody MC, Googe PB. Histopathological changes in leiomyomata treated with leuprolide acetate. Fertil Steril 1990;54:811-4.
105. McCluggage WG, Bharucha H. Cellular leiomyoma mimicking endometrial stromal neoplasm in association with GnRH agonist goserelin. Histopathology 1999;34:184-6.
106. Ohmori T, Wakamoto R, Lu LM, Okada K, Nose M. Immunohistochemical study of a case of uterine leiomyoma showing massive lymphoid infiltration and localized vasculitis after LH-RH derivant treatment. Histopathology 2002;41:276-7.
107. Kalir T, Wu H, Gordon RE, Gil J. Morphometric and electron microscopic analyses of the effect of gonadotropin-releasing hormone agonist treatment on arteriole size in uterine leiomyomas. Arch Pathol Lab Med 2000;124:1295-8.
108. Rutgers JL, Spong CY, Sinow R, Heiner J. Leuprolide acetate treatment and myoma arterial size. Obstet Gynecol 1995;86:386-8.
109. Friedman AJ, Harrison-Atlas D, Barbieri RL, Benacerraf B, Gleason R, Schiff I. A randomized, placebo-controlled, double-blind study evaluating the efficacy of leuprolide acetate depot in the treatment of uterine leiomyomata. Fertil Steril 1989;51:251-6.
110. Friedman AJ, Rein MS, Harrison-Atlas D, Garfield JM, Doubilet PM. A randomized, placebo-controlled, double-blind study evaluating leuprolide acetate depot treatment before myomectomy. Fertil Steril 1989;52:728-33.
111. Meyer WR, Mayer AR, Diamond MP, Carcangiu ML, Schwartz PE, DeCherney AH. Unsuspected leiomyosarcoma: treatment with a gonadotropin-releasing hormone analogue. Obstet Gynecol 1990;75(Pt 2):529-32.
112. Marshburn PB, Matthews ML, Hurst BS. Uterine artery embolization as a treatment option for uterine myomas. Obstet Gynecol Clin North Am 2006;33:125-44.
113. Jiang W, Shen Z, Luo H, Hu X, Zhu X. Comparison of polyvinyl alcohol and tris-acryl gelatin microsphere materials in embolization for symptomatic leiomyomas: a systematic review. Minim Invasive Ther Allied Technol 2016;25:289-300.
114. McCluggage WG, Ellis PK, McClure N, Walker WJ, Jackson PA, Manek S. Pathologic features of uterine leiomyomas following uterine artery embolization. Int J Gynecol Pathol 2000;19:342-7.
115. Lund N, Justesen P, Elle B, Thomsen SG, Floridon C. Fibroids treated by uterine artery embolization. A review. Acta Obstet Gynecol Scand 2000;79:905-10.
116. Colgan TJ, Pron G, Mocarski EJ, Bennett JD, Asch MR, Common A. Pathologic features of uteri and leiomyomas following uterine artery embolization for leiomyomas. Am J Surg Pathol 2003;27:167-77.
117. Dundr P, Mara M, Maskova J, Fucikova Z, Povysil C, Tvrdik D. Pathological findings of uterine leiomyomas and adenomyosis following uterine artery embolization. Pathol Res Pract 2006;202:721-9.
118. Chiesa AG, Hart WR. Uterine artery embolization of leiomyomas with trisacryl gelatin microspheres (TGM): pathologic features and comparison with polyvinyl alcohol emboli. Int J Gynecol Pathol 2004;23:386-92.
119. Spies JB, Ascher SA, Roth AR, Kim J, Levy EB, Gomez-Jorge J. Uterine artery embolization for leiomyomata. Obstet Gynecol 2001;98:29-34.
120. Katsumori T, Bamba M, Kobayashi TK, Moritani S, Urabe M, Nakajima K, et al. Uterine leiomyoma after embolization by means of gelatin sponge particles alone: report of a case with histopathologic features. Ann Diagn Pathol 2002;6:307-11.
121. Ip PP, Lam KW, Cheung CL, et al. Tranexamic acid-associated necrosis and intralesional thrombosis of uterine leiomyomas: a clinicopathologic study of 147 cases emphasizing the importance of drug-induced necrosis and early infarcts in leiomyomas. Am J Surg Pathol 2007;31:1215-24.
122. Kudose S, Krigman HR. Intratumoral vasculopathy in leiomyoma treated with tranexamic acid. Int J Gynecol Pathol 2017;36:364-8.
123. Kurman RJ, Norris HJ. Mesenchymal tumors of the uterus. VI. Epithelioid smooth muscle tumors including leiomyoblastoma and clear-cell leiomyoma: a clinical and pathologic analysis of 26 cases. Cancer 1976;37:1853-65.
124. Prayson RA, Goldblum JR, Hart WR. Epithelioid smooth-muscle tumors of the uterus: a clinicopathologic study of 18 patients. Am J Surg Pathol 1997;21:383-91.
125. Mills AM, Longacre TA. Smooth muscle tumors of the female genital tract. Surg Pathol Clin 2009;2:625-77.
126. Oliva E, Nielsen GP, Clement PB, Young RH, Scully RE. Epitheloid smooth muscle tumors of the uterus. A clinicopathologic analysis of 80 cases. Mod Pathol 1997;10:107A.
127. Watanabe K, Ogura G, Suzuki T. Leiomyoblastoma of the uterus: an immunohistochemical and electron microscopic study of distinctive tumours with immature smooth muscle cell differentiation mimicking fetal uterine myocytes. Histopathology 2003;42:379-86.

128. Kaminski PF, Tavassoli FA. Plexiform tumorlet: a clinical and pathologic study of 15 cases with ultrastructural observations. Int J Gynecol Pathol 1984;3:124-34.
129. Balaton AJ, Vuong PN, Vaury P, Baviera EE. Plexiform tumorlet of the uterus: immunohistological evidence for a smooth muscle origin. Histopathology 1986;10:749-54.
130. Seidman JD, Thomas RM. Multiple plexiform tumorlets of the uterus. Arch Pathol Lab Med 1993;117:1255-6.
131. Nuñez-Alonso C, Battifora HA. Plexiform tumors of the uterus: ultrastructural study. Cancer 1979;44:1707-14.
132. Mazur MT, Kraus FT. Histogenesis of morphologic variations in tumors of the uterine wall. Am J Surg Pathol 1980;4:59-74.
133. Toon C, McGahan S, Henderson P, Russell P. Myxoid symplastic leiomyoma of the uterus. Pathology 2006;38:275-7.
134. Chesnais AL, Watkin E, Beurton D, Devouassoux-Shisheboran M. [Myxoid mesenchymal tumors of uterus: endometrial stromal and smooth muscle tumors, myxoid variant]. Ann Pathol 2011;31:152-8. [French]
135. Kamra HT, Dantkale SS, Birla K, Sakinlawar PW, Narkhede RR. Myxoid leiomyoma of cervix. J Clin Diagn Res 2013;7:2956-7.
136. Goh R, Dal Cin P, Chiang S, Young RH, Oliva E. Myxoid smooth muscle tumors of the uterus: clinicopathologic study of 40 cases. Mod Pathol 2016;29(suppl 2): 285A.
137. Aung T, Goto M, Nomoto M, et al. Uterine lipoleiomyoma: a histopathological review of 17 cases. Pathol Int 2004;54:751-8.
138. Wang X, Kumar D, Seidman JD. Uterine lipoleiomyomas: a clinicopathologic study of 50 cases. Int J Gynecol Pathol 2006;25:239-42.
139. Shintaku M. Lipoleiomyomatous tumors of the uterus: a heterogeneous group? Histopathological study of five cases. Pathol Int 1996;46:498-502.
140. Sieinski W. Lipomatous neometaplasia of the uterus. Report of 11 cases with discussion of histogenesis and pathogenesis. Int J Gynecol Pathol 1989;8:357-63.
141. Terada T. Giant subserosal lipoleiomyomas of the uterine cervix and corpus: a report of 2 cases. Appl Immunohistochem Mol Morphol 2015;23e1-3.
142. Lin M, Hanai J. Atypical lipoleiomyoma of the uterus. Acta Pathol Jpn 1991;41:164-9.
143. Akbulut M, Gundogan M, Yorukoglu A. Clinical and pathological features of lipoleiomyoma of the uterine corpus: a review of 76 cases. Balkan Med J 2014;31:224-9.
144. Morelli L, Pusiol T, Parolari AM, Piscioli I. Plexiform lipoleiomyoma of the uterus: first case report. Arch Gynecol Obstet 2006;274:117-8.
145. Brooks JJ, Wells GB, Yeh IT, LiVolsi VA. Bizarre epithelioid lipoleiomyoma of the uterus. Int J Gynecol Pathol 1992;11:144-9.
146. Chen KT. Uterine leiomyohibernoma. Int J Gynecol Pathol 1999;18:96-7.
147. McDonald AG, Dal Cin P, Ganguly A, et al. Liposarcoma arising in uterine lipoleiomyoma: a report of 3 cases and review of the literature. Am J Surg Pathol 2011;35:221-7.
148. Fadare O, Khabele D. Pleomorphic liposarcoma of the uterine corpus with focal smooth muscle differentiation. Int J Gynecol Pathol 2011;30:282-7.
149. Martin-Reay DG, Christ ML, LaPata RE. Uterine leiomyoma with skeletal muscle differentiation. Report of a case. Am J Clin Pathol 1991;96:344-7.
150. Fornelli A, Pasquinelli G, Eusebi V. Leiomyoma of the uterus showing skeletal muscle differentiation: a case report. Hum Pathol 1999;30:356-9.
151. Chander B, Shekhar S. Osseous metaplasia in leiomyoma: a first in a uterine leiomyoma. J Cancer Res Ther 2015;11:661.
152. Yamadori I, Kobayashi S, Ogino T, Ohmori M, Tanaka H, Jimbo T. Uterine leiomyoma with a focus of fatty and cartilaginous differentiation. Acta Obstet Gynecol Scand 1993;72:307-9.
153. Volpe R, Canzonieri V, Gloghini A, Carbone A. Lipoleiomyoma with metaplastic cartilage (benign mesenchymoma) of the uterine cervix. Pathol Res Pract 1992;188:799-801.
154. Ip PP, Tse KY, Tam KF. Uterine smooth muscle tumors other than the ordinary leiomyomas and leiomyosarcomas: a review of selected variants with emphasis on recent advances and unusual morphology that may cause concern for malignancy. Adv Anat Pathol 2010;17:91-112.
155. Fedele L, Bianchi S, Zanconato G, Carinelli S, Berlanda N. Conservative treatment of diffuse uterine leiomyomatosis. Fertil Steril 2004;82:450-3.
156. Mulvany NJ, Ostor AG, Ross I. Diffuse leiomyomatosis of the uterus. Histopathology 1995;27:175-9.
157. Clement PB, Young RH. Diffuse leiomyomatosis of the uterus: a report of four cases. Int J Gynecol Pathol 1987;6:322-30.
158. Grignon DJ, Carey MR, Kirk ME, Robinson ML. Diffuse uterine leiomyomatosis: a case study with pregnancy complicated by intrapartum hemorrhage. Obstet Gynecol 1987;69(pt 2):477-80.
159. Robles-Frias A, Severin CE, Robles-Frias MJ, Garrido JL. Diffuse uterine leiomyomatosis with ovarian and parametrial involvement. Obstet Gynecol 2001;97(Pt 2):834-5.
160. An YS, Kim DY. 18F-fluorodeoxyglucose PET/CT in a patient with esophageal and genital leiomyomatosis. Korean J Radiol 2009;10:632-4.

161. Kelly HA, Cullen TS. Myomata of the uterus. Philadelphia: W. B. Saunders company, 1909.
162. Akkersdijk GJ, Flu PK, Giard RW, van Lent M, Wallenburg HC. Malignant leiomyomatosis peritonealis disseminata. Am J Obstet Gynecol 1990;163:591-3.
163. Lashgari M, Behmaram B, Ellis M. Leiomyomatosis peritonealis disseminata. A report of two cases. J Reprod Med 1994;39:652-4.
164. Butnor KJ, Burchette JL, Robboy SJ. Progesterone receptor activity in leiomyomatosis peritonealis disseminata. Int J Gynecol Pathol 1999;18:259-64.
165. Bucher M, Pusztaszeri M, Bouzourene H. [Leiomyomatosis peritonealis disseminata: immunohistochemical profile and origin.] Ann Pathol 2006;26:207-10. [French]
166. Hardman WJ 3rd, Majmudar B. Leiomyomatosis peritonealis disseminata: clinicopathologic analysis of five cases. South Med J 1996;89:291-4.
167. Tavassoli FA, Norris HJ. Peritoneal leiomyomatosis (leiomyomatosis peritonealis disseminata): a clinicopathologic study of 20 cases with ultrastructural observations. Int J Gynecol Pathol 1982;1:59-74.
168. Harper RS, Scully RE. Intravenous leiomyomatosis of the uterus. A report of four cases. Obstet Gynecol 1961;18:519-29.
169. Norris HJ, Parmley T. Mesenchymal tumors of the uterus. V. Intravenous leiomyomatosis. A clinical and pathologic study of 14 cases. Cancer 1975;36:2164-78.
170. Canzonieri V, D'Amore ES, Bartoloni G, Piazza M, Blandamura S, Carbone A. Leiomyomatosis with vascular invasion. A unified pathogenesis regarding leiomyoma with vascular microinvasion, benign metastasizing leiomyoma and intravenous leiomyomatosis. Virchows Arch 1994;425:541-5.
171. Clement PB. Intravenous leiomyomatosis of the uterus. Pathol Annu 1988;23(pt 2):153-83.
172. Mulvany NJ, Slavin JL, Ostor AG, Fortune DW. Intravenous leiomyomatosis of the uterus: a clinicopathologic study of 22 cases. Int J Gynecol Pathol 1994;13:1-9.
173. Clement PB, Young RH, Scully RE. Intravenous leiomyomatosis of the uterus. A clinicopathological analysis of 16 cases with unusual histologic features. Am J Surg Pathol 1988;12:932-45.
174. Nogales FF, Navarro N, Martinez de Victoria JM, et al. Uterine intravascular leiomyomatosis: an update and report of seven cases. Int J Gynecol Pathol 1987;6:331-9.
175. Du J, Zhao X, Guo D, Li H, Sun B. Intravenous leiomyomatosis of the uterus: a clinicopathologic study of 18 cases, with emphasis on early diagnosis and appropriate treatment strategies. Hum Pathol 2011;42:1240-6.
176. Tang L, Lu B. Intravenous leiomyomatosis of the uterus: a clinicopathologic analysis of 13 cases with an emphasis on histogenesis. Pathol Res Pract 2018;214:871-5.
177. Andrade LA, Torresan RZ, Sales JF Jr, Vicentini R, De Souza GA. Intravenous leiomyomatosis of the uterus. A report of three cases. Pathol Oncol Res 1998;4:44-7.
178. Hirschowitz L, Mayall FG, Ganesan R, McCluggage WG. Intravascular adenomyomatosis: expanding the morphologic spectrum of intravascular leiomyomatosis. Am J Surg Pathol 2013;37:1395-400.
179. Brescia RJ, Tazelaar HD, Hobbs J, Miller AW. Intravascular lipoleiomyomatosis: a report of two cases. Hum Pathol 1989;20:252-6.
180. Han HS, Park IA, Kim SH, Lee HP. The clear cell variant of epithelioid intravenous leiomyomatosis of the uterus: report of a case. Pathol Int 1998;48:892-6.
181. Evans HL, Chawla SP, Simpson C, Finn KP. Smooth muscle neoplasms of the uterus other than ordinary leiomyoma. A study of 46 cases, with emphasis on diagnostic criteria and prognostic factors. Cancer 1988;62:2239-47.
182. Nucci MR, Drapkin R, Dal Cin P, Fletcher CD, Fletcher JA. Distinctive cytogenetic profile in benign metastasizing leiomyoma: pathogenetic implications. Am J Surg Pathol 2007;31:737-43.
183. Kayser K, Zink S, Schneider T, et al. Benign metastasizing leiomyoma of the uterus: documentation of clinical, immunohistochemical and lectin-histochemical data of ten cases. Virchows Arch 2000;437:284-92.
184. Williams M, Salerno T, Panos AL. Right ventricular and epicardial tumors from benign metastasizing uterine leiomyoma. J Thorac Cardiovasc Surg 2016;151:e21-4.
185. Berti AF, Santillan A, Velasquez LA. Benign metastasizing leiomyoma of the cervical spine 31 years after uterine leiomyoma resection. J Clin Neurosci 2015;22:1491-2.
186. Tori M, Akamatsu H, Mizutani S, et al. Multiple benign metastasizing leiomyomas in the pelvic lymph nodes and biceps muscle: report of a case. Surg Today 2008;38:432-5.
187. Abell MR, Littler ER. Benign metastasizing uterine leiomyoma. Multiple lymph nodal metastases. Cancer 1975;36:2206-13.
188. Barter JF, Szpak C, Creasman WT. Uterine leiomyomas with retroperitoneal lymph node involvement. South Med J 1987;80:1320-2.
189. Esteban JM, Allen WM, Schaerf RH. Benign metastasizing leiomyoma of the uterus: histologic and immunohistochemical characterization of primary and metastatic lesions. Arch Pathol Lab Med 1999;123:960-2.

190. Jautzke G, Müller-Ruchholtz E, Thalmann U. Immunohistological detection of estrogen and progesterone receptors in multiple and well differentiated leiomyomatous lung tumors in women with uterine leiomyomas (so-called benign metastasizing leiomyomas). A report on 5 cases. Pathol Res Pract 1996;192:215-23.

191. Cho KR, Woodruff JD, Epstein JI. Leiomyoma of the uterus with multiple extrauterine smooth muscle tumors: a case report suggesting multifocal origin. Hum Pathol 1989;20:80-3.

192. Prayson RA, Hart WR. Pathologic considerations of uterine smooth muscle tumors. Obstet Gynecol Clin North Am 1995;22:637-57.

193. Gal AA, Brooks JS, Pietra GG. Leiomyomatous neoplasms of the lung: a clinical, histologic, and immunohistochemical study. Mod Pathol 1989;2:209-16.

194. Fukunaga M. Benign "metastasizing" lipoleiomyoma of the uterus. Int J Gynecol Pathol 2003;22:202-4.

195. Loddenkemper C, Mechsner S, Foss HD, et al. Use of oxytocin receptor expression in distinguishing between uterine smooth muscle tumors and endometrial stromal sarcoma. Am J Surg Pathol 2003;27:1458-62.

196. Nucci MR, O'Connell JT, Huettner PC, Cviko A, Sun D, Quade BJ. h-Caldesmon expression effectively distinguishes endometrial stromal tumors from uterine smooth muscle tumors. Am J Surg Pathol 2001;25:455-63.

197. Oliva E, Young RH, Amin MB, Clement PB. An immunohistochemical analysis of endometrial stromal and smooth muscle tumors of the uterus: a study of 54 cases emphasizing the importance of using a panel because of overlap in immunoreactivity for individual antibodies. Am J Surg Pathol 2002;26:403-12.

198. Sumathi VP, Al-Hussaini M, Connolly LE, Fullerton L, McCluggage WG. Endometrial stromal neoplasms are immunoreactive with WT-1 antibody. Int J Gynecol Pathol 2004;23:241-7.

199. de Leval L, Waltregny D, Boniver J, Young RH, Castronovo V, Oliva E. Use of histone deacetylase 8 (HDAC8), a new marker of smooth muscle differentiation, in the classification of mesenchymal tumors of the uterus. Am J Surg Pathol 2006;30:319-27.

200. Agoff SN, Grieco VS, Garcia R, Gown AM. Immunohistochemical distinction of endometrial stromal sarcoma and cellular leiomyoma. Appl Immunohistochem Mol Morphol 2001;9:164-9.

201. Hyde KE, Geisinger KR, Marshall RB, Jones TL. The clear-cell variant of uterine epithelioid leiomyoma. An immunohistologic and ultrastructural study. Arch Pathol Lab Med 1989;113:551-3.

202. Rizeq MN, van de Rijn M, Hendrickson MR, Rouse RV. A comparative immunohistochemical study of uterine smooth muscle neoplasms with emphasis on the epithelioid variant. Hum Pathol 1994;25:671-7.

203. Devaney K, Tavassoli FA. Immunohistochemistry as a diagnostic aid in the interpretation of unusual mesenchymal tumors of the uterus. Mod Pathol 1991;4:225-31.

204. Mayhall KG Jr, Oertling E, Lewin E, et al. The use of smoothelin and other antibodies in the diagnosis of uterine and soft tissue smooth muscle tumors. Appl Immunohistochem Mol Morphol 2017. [Epub ahead of print]

205. Tawfik O, Rao D, Nothnick WB, Graham A, Mau B, Fan F. Transgelin, a novel marker of smooth muscle differentiation, effectively distinguishes endometrial stromal tumors from uterine smooth muscle tumors. Int J Gynecol Obstet Reprod Med Res 2014;1:26-31.

206. Hwang H, Matsuo K, Duncan K, et al. Immunohistochemical panel to differentiate endometrial stromal sarcoma, uterine leiomyosarcoma and leiomyoma: something old and something new. J Clin Pathol 2015;68:710-7.

207. Rush DS, Tan J, Baergen RN, Soslow RA. h-Caldesmon, a novel smooth muscle-specific antibody, distinguishes between cellular leiomyoma and endometrial stromal sarcoma. Am J Surg Pathol 2001;25:253-8.

208. Norton AJ, Thomas JA, Isaacson PG. Cytokeratin-specific monoclonal antibodies are reactive with tumours of smooth muscle derivation. An immunocytochemical and biochemical study using antibodies to intermediate filament cytoskeletal proteins. Histopathology 1987;11:487-99.

209. Iwata J, Fletcher CD. Immunohistochemical detection of cytokeratin and epithelial membrane antigen in leiomyosarcoma: a systematic study of 100 cases. Pathol Int 2000;50:7-14.

210. Zhao Y, Zhang W, Wang S. The expression of estrogen receptor isoforms alpha, beta and insulin-like growth factor-I in uterine leiomyoma. Gynecol Endocrinol 2008;24:549-54.

211. Xie J, Ubango J, Ban Y, Chakravarti D, Kim JJ, Wei JJ. Comparative analysis of AKT and the related biomarkers in uterine leiomyomas with MED12, HMGA2 and FH mutations. Genes Chromosomes Cancer 2018;57:485-94.

212. Rodriguez Y, Baez D, de Oca FM, et al. Comparative analysis of the ERalpha/ERbeta ratio and neurotensin and its high-affinity receptor in myometrium, uterine leiomyoma, atypical leiomyoma, and leiomyosarcoma. Int J Gynecol Pathol 2011;30:354-63.

213. Leitao MM, Soslow RA, Nonaka D, et al. Tissue microarray immunohistochemical expression of estrogen, progesterone, and androgen receptors in uterine leiomyomata and leiomyosarcoma. Cancer 2004;101:1455-62.
214. Zhang Q, Kanis MJ, Ubago J, et al. The selected biomarker analysis in 5 types of uterine smooth muscle tumors. Hum Pathol 2018;76:17-27.
215. Cornejo K, Shi M, Jiang Z. Oncofetal protein IMP3: a useful diagnostic biomarker for leiomyosarcoma. Hum Pathol 2012;43:1567-72.
216. Allen MM, Douds JJ, Liang SX, Desouki MM, Parkash V, Fadare O. An immunohistochemical analysis of stathmin 1 expression in uterine smooth muscle tumors: differential expression in leiomyosarcomas and leiomyomas. Int J Clin Exp Pathol 2015;8:2795-801.
217. O'Neill CJ, McBride HA, Connolly LE, McCluggage WG. Uterine leiomyosarcomas are characterized by high p16, p53 and MIB1 expression in comparison with usual leiomyomas, leiomyoma variants and smooth muscle tumours of uncertain malignant potential. Histopathology 2007;50:851-8.
218. Mills AM, Ly A, Balzer BL, et al. Cell cycle regulatory markers in uterine atypical leiomyoma and leiomyosarcoma: immunohistochemical study of 68 cases with clinical follow-up. Am J Surg Pathol 2013;37:634-42.
219. Chow KL, Tse KY, Cheung CL, et al. The mitosis-specific marker phosphohistone-H3 (PHH3) is an independent prognosticator in uterine smooth muscle tumours: an outcome-based study. Histopathology 2017;70:746-55.
220. Veras E, Malpica A, Deavers MT, Silva EG. Mitosis-specific marker phospho-histone H3 in the assessment of mitotic index in uterine smooth muscle tumors: a pilot study. Int J Gynecol Pathol 2009;28:316-21.
221. Gannon BR, Manduch M, Childs TJ. Differential immunoreactivity of p16 in leiomyosarcomas and leiomyoma variants. Int J Gynecol Pathol 2008;27:68-73.
222. Hakverdi S, Gungoren A, Yaldiz M, Hakverdi AU, Toprak S. Immunohistochemical analysis of p16 expression in uterine smooth muscle tumors. Eur J Gynaecol Oncol 2011;32:513-5.
223. Ip PP, Lim D, Cheung AN, Oliva E. Immunoexpression of p16 in uterine leiomyomas with infarct-type necrosis: an analysis of 35 cases. Histopathology 2017;71:743-50.
224. Ip PP, Cheung AN, Clement PB. Uterine smooth muscle tumors of uncertain malignant potential (STUMP): a clinicopathologic analysis of 16 cases. Am J Surg Pathol 2009;33:992-1005.
225. Chen L, Yang B. Immunohistochemical analysis of p16, p53, and Ki-67 expression in uterine smooth muscle tumors. Int J Gynecol Pathol 2008;27:326-32.
226. Sung CO, Ahn G, Song SY, Choi YL, Bae DS. Atypical leiomyomas of the uterus with long-term follow-up after myomectomy with immunohistochemical analysis for p16INK4A, p53, Ki-67, estrogen receptors, and progesterone receptors. Int J Gynecol Pathol 2009;28:529-34.
227. Bertsch E, Qiang W, Zhang Q, et al. MED12 and HMGA2 mutations: two independent genetic events in uterine leiomyoma and leiomyosarcoma. Mod Pathol 2014;27:1144-53.
228. Carter CS, Skala SL, Chinnaiyan AM, et al. Immunohistochemical characterization of Fumarate Hydratase (FH) and Succinate Dehydrogenase (SDH) in cutaneous leiomyomas for detection of familial cancer syndromes. Am J Surg Pathol 2017;41:801-9.
229. Joseph NM, Solomon DA, Frizzell N, Rabban JT, Zaloudek C, Garg K. Morphology and immunohistochemistry for 2SC and FH aid in detection of fumarate hydratase gene aberrations in uterine leiomyomas from young patients. Am J Surg Pathol 2015;39:1529-39.
230. Buelow B, Cohen J, Nagymanyoki Z, et al. Immunohistochemistry for 2-Succinocysteine (2SC) and Fumarate Hydratase (FH) in cutaneous leiomyomas may aid in identification of patients with HLRCC (Hereditary Leiomyomatosis and Renal Cell Carcinoma Syndrome). Am J Surg Pathol 2016;40:982-8.
231. Zhang Q, Poropatich K, Ubago J, et al. Fumarate hydratase mutations and alterations in leiomyoma with bizarre nuclei. Int J Gynecol Pathol 2017. [Epub ahead of print]
232. Bardella C, El-Bahrawy M, Frizzell N, et al. Aberrant succination of proteins in fumarate hydratase-deficient mice and HLRCC patients is a robust biomarker of mutation status. J Pathol 2011;225:4-11.
233. Ligon AH, Morton CC. Genetics of uterine leiomyomata. Genes Chromosomes Cancer 2000;28:235-45.
234. Mehine M, Kaasinen E, Mäkinen N, et al. Characterization of uterine leiomyomas by whole-genome sequencing. N Engl J Med 2013;369:43-53.
235. Ordulu Z. Fibroids: Genotype and phenotype. Clin Obstet Gynecol 2016;59:25-9.
236. Sandberg AA. Updates on the cytogenetics and molecular genetics of bone and soft tissue tumors: leiomyoma. Cancer Genet Cytogenet 2005;158:1-26.
237. Makinen N, Mehine M, Tolvanen J, et al. MED12, the mediator complex subunit 12 gene, is mutated at high frequency in uterine leiomyomas. Science 2011;334:252-5.

238. Forment JV, Kaidi A, Jackson SP. Chromothripsis and cancer: causes and consequences of chromosome shattering. Nat Rev Cancer 2012;12:663-70.
239. Markowski DN, Bartnitzke S, Loning T, Drieschner N, Helmke BM, Bullerdiek J. MED12 mutations in uterine fibroids--their relationship to cytogenetic subgroups. Int J Cancer 2012;131:1528-36.
240. Mark J, Havel G, Dahlenfors R, Wedell B. Cytogenetics of multiple uterine leiomyomas, parametrial leiomyoma and disseminated peritoneal leiomyomatosis. Anticancer Res 1991;11:33-9.
241. Miyake T, Enomoto T, Ueda Y, et al. A case of disseminated peritoneal leiomyomatosis developing after laparoscope-assisted myomectomy. Gynecol Obstet Invest 2009;67:96-102.
242. Ordulu Z, Nucci MR, Dal Cin P, et al. Intravenous leiomyomatosis: an unusual intermediate between benign and malignant uterine smooth muscle tumors. Mod Pathol 2016;29:500-10.
243. Quade BJ, McLachlin CM, Soto-Wright V, Zuckerman J, Mutter GL, Morton CC. Disseminated peritoneal leiomyomatosis. Clonality analysis by X chromosome inactivation and cytogenetics of a clinically benign smooth muscle proliferation. Am J Pathol 1997;150:2153-66.
244. Baschinsky DY, Isa A, Niemann TH, Prior TW, Lucas JG, Frankel WL. Diffuse leiomyomatosis of the uterus: a case report with clonality analysis. Hum Pathol 2000;31:1429-32.
245. Dal Cin P, Quade BJ, Neskey DM, Kleinman MS, Weremowicz S, Morton CC. Intravenous leiomyomatosis is characterized by a der(14) t(12;14)(q15;q24). Genes Chromosomes Cancer 2003;36:205-6.
246. Quade BJ, Dal Cin P, Neskey DM, Weremowicz S, Morton CC. Intravenous leiomyomatosis: molecular and cytogenetic analysis of a case. Mod Pathol 2002;15:351-6.
247. Buza N, Xu F, Wu W, Carr RJ, Li P, Hui P. Recurrent chromosomal aberrations in intravenous leiomyomatosis of the uterus: high-resolution array comparative genomic hybridization study. Hum Pathol 2014;45:1885-92.
248. Hodge JC, Morton CC. Genetic heterogeneity among uterine leiomyomata: insights into malignant progression. Hum Mol Genet 2007;16:R7-13.
249. Wu RC, Chao AS, Lee LY, et al. Massively parallel sequencing and genome-wide copy number analysis revealed a clonal relationship in benign metastasizing leiomyoma. Oncotarget 2017;8:47547-54.
250. Bowen JM, Cates JM, Kash S, et al. Genomic imbalances in benign metastasizing leiomyoma: characterization by conventional karyotypic, fluorescence in situ hybridization, and whole genome SNP array analysis. Cancer Genet 2012;205:249-54.
251. Jiang J, He M, Hu X, Ni C, Yang L. Deep sequencing reveals the molecular pathology characteristics between primary uterine leiomyoma and pulmonary benign metastasizing leiomyoma. Clin Transl Oncol 2018;20:1080-6.
252. Soritsa D, Teder H, Roosipuu R, et al. Whole exome sequencing of benign pulmonary metastasizing leiomyoma reveals mutation in the BMP8B gene. BMC Med Genet 2018;19:20.
253. Makinen N, Kampjarvi K, Frizzell N, Butzow R, Vahteristo P. Characterization of MED12, HMGA2, and FH alterations reveals molecular variability in uterine smooth muscle tumors. Mol Cancer 2017;16:101.
254. Perot G, Croce S, Ribeiro A, et al. MED12 alterations in both human benign and malignant uterine soft tissue tumors. PLoS One 2012;7:e40015.
255. de Graaff MA, Cleton-Jansen AM, Szuhai K, Bovee JV. Mediator complex subunit 12 exon 2 mutation analysis in different subtypes of smooth muscle tumors confirms genetic heterogeneity. Hum Pathol 2013;44:1597-604.
256. Makinen N, Vahteristo P, Kampjarvi K, Arola J, Butzow R, Aaltonen LA. MED12 exon 2 mutations in histopathological uterine leiomyoma variants. Eur J Hum Genet 2013;21:1300-3.
257. Rieker RJ, Agaimy A, Moskalev EA, et al. Mutation status of the mediator complex subunit 12 (MED12) in uterine leiomyomas and concurrent/metachronous multifocal peritoneal smooth muscle nodules (leiomyomatosis peritonealis disseminata). Pathology 2013;45:388-92.
258. Matsubara A, Sekine S, Yoshida M, et al. Prevalence of MED12 mutations in uterine and extrauterine smooth muscle tumours. Histopathology 2013;62:657-61.
259. McGuire MM, Yatsenko A, Hoffner L, Jones M, Surti U, Rajkovic A. Whole exome sequencing in a random sample of North American women with leiomyomas identifies MED12 mutations in majority of uterine leiomyomas. PLoS One 2012;7:e33251.
260. Ravegnini G, Mariño-Enriquez A, Slater J, et al. MED12 mutations in leiomyosarcoma and extrauterine leiomyoma. Mod Pathol 2013;26:743-9.
261. Schwetye KE, Pfeifer JD, Duncavage EJ. MED12 exon 2 mutations in uterine and extrauterine smooth muscle tumors. Hum Pathol 2014;45:65-70.
262. Liegl-Atzwanger B, Heitzer E, Flicker K, et al. Exploring chromosomal abnormalities and genetic changes in uterine smooth muscle tumors. Mod Pathol 2016;29:1262-77.

263. Heinonen HR, Sarvilinna NS, Sjöberg J, et al. MED12 mutation frequency in unselected sporadic uterine leiomyomas. Fertil Steril 2014;102:1137-42.
264. Sandberg AA. Updates on the cytogenetics and molecular genetics of bone and soft tissue tumors: leiomyosarcoma. Cancer Genet Cytogenet 2005;161:1-19.
265. Hodge JC, Kim TM, Dreyfuss JM, et al. Expression profiling of uterine leiomyomata cytogenetic subgroups reveals distinct signatures in matched myometrium: transcriptional profilingof the t(12;14) and evidence in support of predisposing genetic heterogeneity. Hum Mol Genet 2012;21:2312-29.
266. Vocke CD, Ricketts CJ, Merino MJ, et al. Comprehensive genomic and phenotypic characterization of germline FH deletion in hereditary leiomyomatosis and renal cell carcinoma. Genes Chromosomes Cancer 2017;56:484-92.
267. Gunnala V, Pereira N, Irani M, et al. Novel fumarate hydratase mutation in siblings with early onset uterine leiomyomas and hereditary leiomyomatosis and renal cell cancer syndrome. Int J Gynecol Pathol 2018;37:256-61.
268. Clayton-Smith J, O'Sullivan J, Daly S, et al. Whole-exome-sequencing identifies mutations in histone acetyltransferase gene KAT6B in individuals with the Say-Barber-Biesecker variant of Ohdo syndrome. Am J Hum Genet 2011;89:675-81.
269. Christacos NC, Quade BJ, Dal Cin P, Morton CC. Uterine leiomyomata with deletions of Ip represent a distinct cytogenetic subgroup associated with unusual histologic features. Genes Chromosomes Cancer 2006;45:304-12.
270. Nogales FF, Isaac MA, Hardisson D, et al. Adenomatoid tumors of the uterus: an analysis of 60 cases. Int J Gynecol Pathol 2002;21:34-40.
271. Livingston EG, Guis MS, Pearl ML, Stern JL, Brescia RJ. Diffuse adenomatoid tumor of the uterus with a serosal papillary cystic component. Int J Gynecol Pathol 1992;11:288-92.
272. Sangoi AR, McKenney JK, Schwartz EJ, Rouse RV, Longacre TA. Adenomatoid tumors of the female and male genital tracts: a clinicopathological and immunohistochemical study of 44 cases. Mod Pathol 2009;22:1228-35.
273. Goode B, Joseph NM, Stevers M, et al. Adenomatoid tumors of the male and female genital tract are defined by TRAF7 mutations that drive aberrant NF-kB pathway activation. Mod Pathol 2018;31:660-73.
274. D'Angelo E, Espinosa I, Ali R, et al. Uterine leiomyosarcomas: tumor size, mitotic index, and biomarkers Ki67, and Bcl-2 identify two groups with different prognosis. Gynecol Oncol 2011;121:328-33.
275. Bodner-Adler B, Bodner K, Czerwenka K, Kimberger O, Leodolter S, Mayerhofer K. Expression of p16 protein in patients with uterine smooth muscle tumors: an immunohistochemical analysis. Gynecol Oncol 2005;96:62-6.
276. Croce S, Chibon F. MED12 and uterine smooth muscle oncogenesis: state of the art and perspectives. Eur J Cancer 2015;51:1603-10.
277. Mittal KR, Chen F, Wei JJ, et al. Molecular and immunohistochemical evidence for the origin of uterine leiomyosarcomas from associated leiomyoma and symplastic leiomyoma-like areas. Mod Pathol 2009;22:1303-11.
278. Baker P, Oliva E. Intraoperative consultation during gynecologic pathology (vagina, vulva, uterine cervix, and corpus). In: Marchevsky AM, Abdul-Karim FW, Balzer BL, eds. Intraoperative consultation. Philadelphia: Elsevier Saunders; 2015:292-309.
279. Busca A, Parra-Herran C. Myxoid mesenchymal tumors of the uterus: an update on classification, definitions, and differential diagnosis. Adv Anat Pathol 2017;24:354-61.
280. Parra-Herran C, Schoolmeester JK, Yuan L, et al. Myxoid leiomyosarcoma of the uterus: a clinicopathologic analysis of 30 cases and review of the literature with reappraisal of its distinction from other uterine myxoid mesenchymal neoplasms. Am J Surg Pathol 2016;40:285-301.
281. Parra-Herran C, Quick CM, Howitt BE, Dal Cin P, Quade BJ, Nucci MR. Inflammatory myofibroblastic tumor of the uterus: clinical and pathologic review of 10 cases including a subset with aggressive clinical course. Am J Surg Pathol 2015;39:157-68.
281a. Bennett JA, Nardi V, Rouzbahman M, Morales-Oyarvide V, Nielsen GP, Oliva E. Inflammatory myofibroblastic tumor of the uterus: a clinicopathological, immunohistochemical, and molecular analysis of 13 cases highlighting their broad morphologic spectrum. Mod Pathol 2017;30:1489-503.
282. Oliva E, Young RH, Clement PB, Scully RE. Myxoid and fibrous endometrial stromal tumors of the uterus: a report of 10 cases. Int J Gynecol Pathol 1999;18:310-9.
283. Chiang S, Oliva E. Cytogenetic and molecular aberrations in endometrial stromal tumors. Hum Pathol 2011;42:609-17.
284. Hayashi T, Kumasaka T, Mitani K, et al. Prevalence of uterine and adnexal involvement in pulmonary lymphangioleiomyomatosis: a clinicopathologic study of 10 patients. Am J Surg Pathol 2011;35:1776-85.

285. Schoolmeester JK, Park KJ. Incidental nodal lymphangioleiomyomatosis is not a harbinger of pulmonary lymphangioleiomyomatosis: a study of 19 cases with evaluation of diagnostic immunohistochemistry. Am J Surg Pathol 2015;39:1404-10.
286. Lim GS, Oliva E. The morphologic spectrum of uterine PEC-cell associated tumors in a patient with tuberous sclerosis. Int J Gynecol Pathol 2011;30:121-8.
287. Novelli M, Rossi S, Rodriguez-Justo M, et al. DOG1 and CD117 are the antibodies of choice in the diagnosis of gastrointestinal stromal tumours. Histopathology 2010;57:259-70.
288. Poulsen TD. Leiomyomatosis peritonealis disseminata. Ann Chir Gynaecol 1988;77:41-4.
289. White SH, Ibrahim NB, Forrester-Wood CP, Jeyasingham K. Leiomyomas of the lower respiratory tract. Thorax 1985;40:306-11.
290. Rush SK, Toukatly MN, Kilgore MR, Urban RR. Metastases from lung adenocarcinoma within a leiomyoma: a case report. Gynecol Oncol Rep 2017;20:27-9.
291. Faustino F, Martinho M, Reis J, Aguas F. Update on medical treatment of uterine fibroids. Eur J Obstet Gynecol Reprod Biol 2017;216:61-8.
292. Laughlin-Tommaso SK. Alternatives to hysterectomy: management of uterine fibroids. Obstet Gynecol Clin North Am 2016;43:397-413.
293. Parker WH, Kaunitz AM, Pritts EA, et al. U.S. Food and Drug Administration's guidance regarding morcellation of leiomyomas: well-intentioned, but is it harmful for women? Obstet Gynecol 2016;127:18-22.
294. Siedhoff MT, Wheeler SB, Rutstein SE, et al. Laparoscopic hysterectomy with morcellation vs abdominal hysterectomy for presumed fibroid tumors in premenopausal women: a decision analysis. Am J Obstet Gynecol 2015;212:591.e1-8.
295. Stine JE, Clarke-Pearson DL, Gehrig PA. Uterine morcellation at the time of hysterectomy: techniques, risks, and recommendations. Obstet Gynecol Surv 2014;69:415-25.
296. George S, Barysauskas C, Serrano C, et al. Retrospective cohort study evaluating the impact of intraperitoneal morcellation on outcomes of localized uterine leiomyosarcoma. Cancer 2014;120:3154-8.
297. Oduyebo T, Rauh-Hain AJ, Meserve EE, et al. The value of re-exploration in patients with inadvertently morcellated uterine sarcoma. Gynecol Oncol 2014;132:360-5.
298. Pritts EA, Parker WH, Brown J, Olive DL. Outcome of occult uterine leiomyosarcoma after surgery for presumed uterine fibroids: a systematic review. J Minim Invasive Gynecol 2015;22:26-33.
299. Stewart EA. Clinical practice. Uterine fibroids. N Engl J Med 2015;372:1646-55.
300. Marret H, Fritel X, Ouldamer L, et al. Therapeutic management of uterine fibroid tumors: updated French guidelines. Eur J Obstet Gynecol Reprod Biol 2012;165:156-64.
301. American College of Obstetricians and Gynecologists. ACOG practice bulletin. Alternatives to hysterectomy in the management of leiomyomas. Obstet Gynecol 2008;112(Pt 1):387-400.
302. Hales HA, Peterson CM, Jones KP, Quinn JD. Leiomyomatosis peritonealis disseminata treated with a gonadotropin-releasing hormone agonist. A case report. Am J Obstet Gynecol 1992;167:515-6.
303. Doyle MP, Li A, Villanueva CI, et al. Treatment of intravenous leiomyomatosis with cardiac extension following incomplete resection. Int J Vasc Med 2015;2015:756141.
304. Banner AS, Carrington CB, Emory WB, et al. Efficacy of oophorectomy in lymphangioleiomyomatosis and benign metastasizing leiomyoma. N Engl J Med 1981;305:204-9.
305. Abu-Rustum NR, Curtin JP, Burt M, Jones WB. Regression of uterine low-grade smooth-muscle tumors metastatic to the lung after oophorectomy. Obstet Gynecol 1997;89(Pt 2):850-2.
306. Lewis EI, Chason RJ, DeCherney AH, Armstrong A, Elkas J, Venkatesan AM. Novel hormone treatment of benign metastasizing leiomyoma: an analysis of five cases and literature review. Fertil Steril 2013;99:2017-24.
307. Stiller CA, Trama A, Serraino D, et al. Descriptive epidemiology of sarcomas in Europe: report from the RARECARE project. Eur J Cancer 2013;49:684-95.
308. Ferrari A, Sultan I, Huang TT, et al. Soft tissue sarcoma across the age spectrum: a population-based study from the Surveillance Epidemiology and End Results database. Pediatr Blood Cancer 2011;57:943-9.
309. Francis M, Dennis NL, Hirschowitz L, et al. Incidence and survival of gynecologic sarcomas in England. Int J Gynecol Cancer 2015;25:850-7.
310. Harlow BL, Weiss NS, Lofton S. The epidemiology of sarcomas of the uterus. J Natl Cancer Inst 1986;76:399-402.
311. Leibsohn S, d'Ablaing G, Mishell DR Jr, Schlaerth JB. Leiomyosarcoma in a series of hysterectomies performed for presumed uterine leiomyomas. Am J Obstet Gynecol 1990;162:968-74.
312. Hosh M, Antar S, Nazzal A, Warda M, Gibreel A, Refky B. Uterine sarcoma: analysis of 13,089 cases based on Surveillance, Epidemiology, and End Results Database. Int J Gynecol Cancer 2016;26:1098-104.
313. Silva EG, Tornos CS, Follen-Mitchell M. Malignant neoplasms of the uterine corpus in patients treated for breast carcinoma: the effects of tamoxifen. Int J Gynecol Pathol 1994;13:248-58.

314. Francis JH, Kleinerman RA, Seddon JM, Abramson DH. Increased risk of secondary uterine leiomyosarcoma in hereditary retinoblastoma. Gynecol Oncol 2012;124:254-9.
315. Gonzalez KD, Noltner KA, Buzin CH, et al. Beyond Li Fraumeni syndrome: clinical characteristics of families with p53 germline mutations. J Clin Oncol 2009;27:1250-6.
316. Ylisaukko-oja SK, Kiuru M, Lehtonen HJ, et al. Analysis of fumarate hydratase mutations in a population-based series of early onset uterine leiomyosarcoma patients. Int J Cancer 2006;119:283-7.
317. Barter JF, Smith EB, Szpak CA, Hinshaw W, Clarke-Pearson DL, Creasman WT. Leiomyosarcoma of the uterus: clinicopathologic study of 21 cases. Gynecol Oncol 1985;21:220-7.
318. Gadducci A, Landoni F, Sartori E, et al. Uterine leiomyosarcoma: analysis of treatment failures and survival. Gynecol Oncol 1996;62:25-32.
319. Major FJ, Blessing JA, Silverberg SG, et al. Prognostic factors in early-stage uterine sarcoma. A gynecologic oncology group study. Cancer 1993;71(4 Suppl):1702-9.
320. Schwartz Z, Dgani R, Lancet M, Kessler I. Uterine sarcoma in Israel: a study of 104 cases. Gynecol Oncol 1985;20:354-63.
321. Norris HJ, Taylor HB. Postirradiation sarcomas of the uterus. Obstet Gynecol 1965;26:689-94.
322. Botsis D, Koliopoulos C, Kondi-Pafitis A, Creatsas G. Myxoid leiomyosarcoma of the uterus in a patient receiving tamoxifen therapy: a case report. Int J Gynecol Pathol 2006;25:173-5.
323. Duk JM, Bouma J, Burger GT, Nap M, De Bruijn HW. CA 125 in serum and tumor from patients with uterine sarcoma. Int J Gynecol Cancer 1994;4:156-60.
324. Karti SS, Eren N, Sönmez M, et al. Leiomyosarcoma of the uterus presenting with thrombotic thrombocytopenic purpura. Turk J Haematol 2003;20:163-5.
325. Pal L, Parkash V, Chambers JT. Eosinophilia and uterine leiomyosarcoma. Obstet Gynecol 2003;101(Pt 2):1130-2.
326. Onishi S, Hojo N, Sakai I, et al. Secondary amyloidosis and eosinophilia in a patient with uterine leiomyosarcoma. Jpn J Clin Oncol 2005;35:617-21.
327. Bodon GR, Mijangos JA. Alkaline phosphatase-producing leiomyosarcoma of the uterus. Am J Surg 1972;124:673-5.
328. Tang SJ, Geevarghese S, Saab S, et al. A parathyroid hormone-related protein-secreting metastatic epithelioid leiomyosarcoma. A case report and review of the literature. Arch Pathol Lab Med 2003;127:e181-5.
329. Duff M, Dusenbery KE, Rodriguez FJ. Paraneoplastic encephalomyelitis: a case report and review of the literature. Gynecol Oncol 2006;102:593-5.
330. Roohi F, Smith PR, Bergman M, Baig MA, Sclar G. A diagnostic and management dilemma: combined paraneoplastic myasthenia gravis and Lambert-Eaton myasthenic syndrome presenting as acute respiratory failure. Neurologist 2006;12:322-6.
331. Abakka S, Elhalouat H, Khoummane N, et al. Uterine leiomyosarcoma and Leser-Trelat sign. Lancet 2013;381:88.
332. Liang S, Stone G, Chalas E, Pearl M, Callan F, Zheng W. A high-grade uterine leiomyosarcoma with human chorionic gonadotropin production. Int J Gynecol Pathol 2006;25:257-61.
333. Seidman MA, Oduyebo T, Muto MG, Crum CP, Nucci MR, Quade BJ. Peritoneal dissemination complicating morcellation of uterine mesenchymal neoplasms. PLoS One 2012;7:e50058.
334. Christopherson WM, Williamson EO, Gray LA. Leiomyosarcoma of the uterus. Cancer 1972;29:1512-7.
335. Friedrich M, Villena-Heinsen C, Mink D, Hell K, Schmidt W. Leiomyosarcomas of the female genital tract: a clinical and histopathological study. Eur J Gynaecol Oncol 1998;19:470-5.
336. Schwartz LB, Diamond MP, Schwartz PE. Leiomyosarcomas: clinical presentation. Am J Obstet Gynecol 1993;168(Pt 1):180-3.
337. Hsieh CH, Lin H, Huang CC, Huang EY, Chang SY, ChangChien CC. Leiomyosarcoma of the uterus: a clinicopathologic study of 21 cases. Acta Obstet Gynecol Scand 2003;82:74-81.
338. Nordal RR, Kristensen GB, Kaern J, Stenwig AE, Pettersen EO, Trope CG. The prognostic significance of stage, tumor size, cellular atypia and DNA ploidy in uterine leiomyosarcoma. Acta Oncol 1995;34:797-802.
339. Giuntoli RL 2nd, Metzinger DS, DiMarco CS, et al. Retrospective review of 208 patients with leiomyosarcoma of the uterus: prognostic indicators, surgical management, and adjuvant therapy. Gynecol Oncol 2003;89:460-9.
340. King ME, Dickersin GR, Scully RE. Myxoid leiomyosarcoma of the uterus. A report of six cases. Am J Surg Pathol 1982;6:589-98.
341. Burch DM, Tavassoli FA. Myxoid leiomyosarcoma of the uterus. Histopathology 2011;59:1144-55.
342. Mittal K, Popiolek D, Demopoulos RI. Uterine myxoid leiomyosarcoma within a leiomyoma. Hum Pathol 2000;31:398-400.
343. Yanai H, Wani Y, Notohara K, Takada S, Yoshino T. Uterine leiomyosarcoma arising in leiomyoma: clinicopathological study of four cases and literature review. Pathol Int 2010;60:506-9.

344. Coard KC, Fletcher HM. Leiomyosarcoma of the uterus with a florid intravascular component ("intravenous leiomyosarcomatosis"). Int J Gynecol Pathol 2002;21:182-5.
345. Mittal K, Joutovsky A. Areas with benign morphologic and immunohistochemical features are associated with some uterine leiomyosarcomas. Gynecol Oncol 2007;104:362-5.
346. Wang WL, Soslow R, Hensley M, et al. Histopathologic prognostic factors in stage I leiomyosarcoma of the uterus: a detailed analysis of 27 cases. Am J Surg Pathol 2011;35:522-9.
347. Lim D, Alvarez T, Nucci MR, et al. Interobserver variability in the interpretation of tumor cell necrosis in uterine leiomyosarcoma. Am J Surg Pathol 2013;37:650-8.
348. Yang EJ, Mutter GL. Biomarker resolution of uterine smooth muscle tumor necrosis as benign vs malignant. Mod Pathol 2015;28:830-5.
349. Taylor HB, Norris HJ. Mesenchymal tumors of the uterus. IV. Diagnosis and prognosis of leiomyosarcomas. Arch Pathol 1966;82:40-4.
350. Kempson RL, Bari W. Uterine sarcomas. Classification, diagnosis, and prognosis. Hum Pathol 1970;1:331-49.
351. Abeler VM, Royne O, Thoresen S, Danielsen HE, Nesland JM, Kristensen GB. Uterine sarcomas in Norway. A histopathological and prognostic survey of a total population from 1970 to 2000 including 419 patients. Histopathology 2009;54:355-64.
352. Chiang S, Oliva E. Recent developments in uterine mesenchymal neoplasms. Histopathology 2013;62:124-37.
353. Moinfar F, Azodi M, Tavassoli FA. Uterine sarcomas. Pathology 2007;39:55-71.
354. Veras E, Zivanovic O, Jacks L, Chiappetta D, Hensley M, Soslow R. "Low-grade leiomyosarcoma" and late-recurring smooth muscle tumors of the uterus: a heterogenous collection of frequently misdiagnosed tumors associated with an overall favorable prognosis relative to conventional uterine leiomyosarcomas. Am J Surg Pathol 2011;35:1626-37.
355. Burns B, Curry RH, Bell ME. Morphologic features of prognostic significance in uterine smooth muscle tumors: a review of eighty-four cases. Am J Obstet Gynecol 1979;135:109-14.
356. Clement PB. The pathology of uterine smooth muscle tumors and mixed endometrial stromal-smooth muscle tumors: a selective review with emphasis on recent advances. Int J Gynecol Pathol 2000;19:39-55.
357. Kyriazis AP, Kyriazis AA. Uterine leiomyoblastoma (epithelioid leiomyoma) neoplasm of low-grade malignancy. A histopathologic study. Arch Pathol Lab Med 1992;116:1189-91.
358. Lavin P, Hajdu SI, Foote FW Jr. Gastric and extragastric leiomyoblastomas: clinicopathologic study of 44 cases. Cancer 1972;29:305-11.
359. Tsukahara Y, Kotani T, Nakamura M, Fukuta T. Bizarre leiomyoblastoma (epithelioid leiomyosarcoma) of the uterus—a case with a malignant clinical course. Nihon Sanka Fujinka Gakkai Zasshi 1983;35:189-93.
360. Seidman JD, Yetter RA, Papadimitriou JC. Epithelioid component of uterine leiomyosarcoma simulating metastatic carcinoma. Arch Pathol Lab Med 1992;116:287-90.
361. Buscema J, Carpenter SE, Rosenshein NB, Woodruff JD. Epithelioid leiomyosarcoma of the uterus. Cancer 1986;57:1192-6.
362. Jones MW, Norris HJ. Clinicopathologic study of 28 uterine leiomyosarcomas with metastasis. Int J Gynecol Pathol 1995;14:243-9.
363. Silva EG, Tornos C, Ordoñez NG, Morris M. Uterine leiomyosarcoma with clear cell areas. Int J Gynecol Pathol 1995;14:174-8.
364. Levine PH, Mittal K. Rhabdoid epithelioid leiomyosarcoma of the uterine corpus: a case report and literature review. Int J Surg Pathol 2002;10:231-6.
365. Atkins K, Bell SW, Kempson RL. Myxoid smooth muscle tumors of the uterus. Mod Pathol. 2001;14:132A.
366. Shintaku M, Ashihara T, Koyama T. Myxoid leiomyosarcoma of the uterus with mature adipocytes and numerous bizarre multinucleated giant cells. Pathol Int 2015;65:205-7.
367. Pounder DJ, Iyer PV. Uterine leiomyosarcoma with myxoid stroma. Arch Pathol Lab Med 1985;109:762-4.
368. Salm R, Evans DJ. Myxoid leiomyosarcoma. Histopathology 1985;9:159-69.
369. Lu B, Shi H, Zhang X. Myxoid leiomyosarcoma of the uterus: a clinicopathological and immunohistochemical study of 10 cases. Hum Pathol 2017;59:139-46.
370. Chen E, O'Connell F, Fletcher CD. Dedifferentiated leiomyosarcoma: clinicopathological analysis of 18 cases. Histopathology 2011;59:1135-43.
371. Fukuda T, Ohnishi Y. Histological and immunohistochemical observations of dedifferentiated leiomyosarcoma of the uterus. Acta Pathol Jpn 1991;41:466-72.
372. Rawish KR, Fadare O. Dedifferentiated leiomyosarcoma of the uterus with heterologous elements: a potential diagnostic pitfall. Case Rep Obstet Gynecol 2012;2012:534634.
373. Bartosch C, Afonso M, Pires-Luis AS, et al. Distant metastases in uterine leiomyosarcomas: the wide variety of body sites and time intervals to metastatic relapse. Int J Gynecol Pathol 2017;36:31-41.

374. Darby AJ, Papadaki L, Beilby JO. An unusual leiomyosarcoma of the uterus containing osteoclast-like giant cells. Cancer 1975;36:495-504.
375. Marshall RJ, Braye SG, Jones DB. Leiomyosarcoma of the uterus with giant cells resembling osteoclasts. Int J Gynecol Pathol 1986;5:260-8.
376. Chen KT. Leiomyosarcoma with osteoclast-like giant cells. Am J Surg Pathol 1995;19:487-8.
377. Sieinski W. Malignant giant cell tumor associated with leiomyosarcoma of the uterus. Cancer 1990;65:1838-42.
378. Stout AP. Mesenchymoma, the mixed tumor of mesenchymal derivatives. Ann Surg 1948;127:278-90.
379. Shintaku M, Sekiyama K. Leiomyosarcoma of the uterus with focal rhabdomyosarcomatous differentiation. Int J Gynecol Pathol 2004;23:188-92.
380. Schoolmeester JK, Stamatakos MD, Moyer AM, Park KJ, Fairbairn M, Fader AN. Pleomorphic liposarcoma arising in a lipoleiomyosarcoma of the uterus: report of a case with genetic profiling by a next generation sequencing panel. Int J Gynecol Pathol 2016;35:321-6.
381. Verma M, Joseph G, McCluggage WG. Uterine composite tumor composed of leiomyosarcoma and embryonal rhabdomyosarcoma with immature cartilage. Int J Gynecol Pathol 2009;28:338-42.
382. Silverberg SG. Reproducibility of the mitosis count in the histologic diagnosis of smooth muscle tumors of the uterus. Hum Pathol 1976;7:451-4.
383. Kempson RL, Hendrickson MR. Pure mesenchymal neoplasms of the uterine corpus: selected problems. Semin Diagn Pathol 1988;5:172-98.
384. Mittal K, Demopoulos RI. MIB-1 (Ki-67), p53, estrogen receptor, and progesterone receptor expression in uterine smooth muscle tumors. Hum Pathol 2001;32:984-7.
385. Layfield LJ, Liu K, Dodge R, Barsky SH. Uterine smooth muscle tumors: utility of classification by proliferation, ploidy, and prognostic markers versus traditional histopathology. Arch Pathol Lab Med 2000;124:221-7.
386. D'Angelo E, Spagnoli LG, Prat J. Comparative clinicopathologic and immunohistochemical analysis of uterine sarcomas diagnosed using the World Health Organization classification system. Hum Pathol 2009;40:1571-85.
387. Liang Y, Zhang X, Chen X, Lu W. Diagnostic value of progesterone receptor, p16, p53 and pHH3 expression in uterine atypical leiomyoma. Int J Clin Exp Pathol 2015;8:7196-202.
388. Pang SJ, Li CC, Shen Y, Liu YZ, Shi YQ, Liu YX. Value of counting positive pHH3 cells in the diagnosis of uterine smooth muscle tumors. Int J Clin Exp Pathol 2015;8:4418-26.
389. Tapia C, Kutzner H, Mentzel T, Savic S, Baumhoer D, Glatz K. Two mitosis-specific antibodies, MPM-2 and phospho-histone H3 (Ser28), allow rapid and precise determination of mitotic activity. Am J Surg Pathol 2006;30:83-9.
390. Hisaoka M, Wei-Qi S, Jian W, Morio T, Hashimoto H. Specific but variable expression of h-caldesmon in leiomyosarcomas: an immunohistochemical reassessment of a novel myogenic marker. Appl Immunohistochem Mol Morphol 2001;9:302-8.
391. Abeler VM, Nenodovic M. Diagnostic immunohistochemistry in uterine sarcomas: a study of 397 cases. Int J Gynecol Pathol 2011;30:236-43.
392. Robin YM, Penel N, Perot G, et al. Transgelin is a novel marker of smooth muscle differentiation that improves diagnostic accuracy of leiomyosarcomas: a comparative immunohistochemical reappraisal of myogenic markers in 900 soft tissue tumors. Mod Pathol 2013;26:502-10.
393. Rubin BP, Fletcher CD. Myxoid leiomyosarcoma of soft tissue, an underrecognized variant. Am J Surg Pathol 2000;24:927-36.
394. McCluggage WG, Sumathi VP, Maxwell P. CD10 is a sensitive and diagnostically useful immunohistochemical marker of normal endometrial stroma and of endometrial stromal neoplasms. Histopathology 2001;39:273-8.
395. Toki T, Shimizu M, Takagi Y, Ashida T, Konishi I. CD10 is a marker for normal and neoplastic endometrial stromal cells. Int J Gynecol Pathol 2002;21:41-7.
396. Bodner K, Bodner-Adler B, Kimberger O, Czerwenka K, Leodolter S, Mayerhofer K. Estrogen and progesterone receptor expression in patients with uterine leiomyosarcoma and correlation with different clinicopathological parameters. Anticancer Res 2003;23:729-32.
397. Sutton GP, Stehman FB, Michael H, Young PC, Ehrlich CE. Estrogen and progesterone receptors in uterine sarcomas. Obstet Gynecol 1986;68:709-14.
398. Raspollini MR, Amunni G, Villanucci A, et al. Estrogen and progesterone receptors expression in uterine malignant smooth muscle tumors: correlation with clinical outcome. J Chemother 2003;15:596-602.
399. Zhai YL, Kobayashi Y, Mori A, et al. Expression of steroid receptors, Ki-67, and p53 in uterine leiomyosarcomas. Int J Gynecol Pathol 1999;18:20-8.
400. Wade K, Quinn MA, Hammond I, Williams K, Cauchi M. Uterine sarcoma: steroid receptors and response to hormonal therapy. Gynecol Oncol 1990;39:364-7.
401. Kelley TW, Borden EC, Goldblum JR. Estrogen and progesterone receptor expression in uterine and extrauterine leiomyosarcomas: an immunohistochemical study. Appl Immunohistochem Mol Morphol 2004;12:338-41.

402. Rao UN, Finkelstein SD, Jones MW. Comparative immunohistochemical and molecular analysis of uterine and extrauterine leiomyosarcomas. Mod Pathol 1999;12:1001-9.
403. Davidson B, Kjaereng ML, Forsund M, Danielsen HE, Kristensen GB, Abeler VM. Progesterone receptor expression is an independent prognosticator in FIGO stage I uterine leiomyosarcoma. Am J Clin Pathol 2016;145:449-58.
404. Silva EG, Deavers MT, Bodurka DC, Malpica A. Uterine epithelioid leiomyosarcomas with clear cells: reactivity with HMB-45 and the concept of PEComa. Am J Surg Pathol 2004;28:244-9.
405. Silva EG, Bodurka DC, Scouros MA, Ayala A. A uterine leiomyosarcoma that became positive for HMB45 in the metastasis. Ann Diagn Pathol 2005;9:43-5.
406. Zheng G, Martignoni G, Antonescu C, et al. A broad survey of cathepsin K immunoreactivity in human neoplasms. Am J Clin Pathol 2013;139:151-9.
407. Howitt BE, Schoolmeester JK, Quade BJ, Nucci MR. Immunohistochemical analysis of HMB-45, MelanA and Cathepsin K in a series of 35 uterine leiomyosarcoma. Mod Pathol 2013;26(suppl 2):279A.
408. Raspollini MR, Paglierani M, Taddei GL, Villanucci A, Amunni G, Taddei A. The protooncogene c-KIT is expressed in leiomyosarcomas of the uterus. Gynecol Oncol 2004;93:718.
409. Winter WE 3rd, Seidman JD, Krivak TC, et al. Clinicopathological analysis of c-kit expression in carcinosarcomas and leiomyosarcomas of the uterine corpus. Gynecol Oncol 2003;91:3-8.
410. Rushing RS, Shajahan S, Chendil D, et al. Uterine sarcomas express KIT protein but lack mutation(s) in exon 11 or 17 of c-KIT. Gynecol Oncol 2003;91:9-14.
411. Klein WM, Kurman RJ. Lack of expression of c-kit protein (CD117) in mesenchymal tumors of the uterus and ovary. Int J Gynecol Pathol 2003;22:181-4.
412. Atkins KA, Arronte N, Darus CJ, Rice LW. The use of p16 in enhancing the histologic classification of uterine smooth muscle tumors. Am J Surg Pathol 2008;32:98-102.
413. Schaefer IM, Hornick JL, Sholl LM, Quade BJ, Nucci MR, Parra-Herran C. Abnormal p53 and p16 staining patterns distinguish uterine leiomyosarcoma from inflammatory myofibroblastic tumour. Histopathology 2017;70:1138-46.
414. de Vos S, Wilczynski SP, Fleischhacker M, Koeffler P. p53 alterations in uterine leiomyosarcomas versus leiomyomas. Gynecol Oncol 1994;54:205-8.
415. Amada S, Nakano H, Tsuneyoshi M. Leiomyosarcoma versus bizarre and cellular leiomyomas of the uterus: a comparative study based on the MIB-1 and proliferating cell nuclear antigen indices, p53 expression, DNA flow cytometry, and muscle specific actins. Int J Gynecol Pathol 1995;14:134-42.
416. Hall KL, Teneriello MG, Taylor RR, et al. Analysis of Ki-ras, p53, and MDM2 genes in uterine leiomyomas and leiomyosarcomas. Gynecol Oncol 1997;65:330-5.
417. Blom R, Guerrieri C, Stal O, Malmstrom H, Simonsen E. Leiomyosarcoma of the uterus: A clinicopathologic, DNA flow cytometric, p53, and mdm-2 analysis of 49 cases. Gynecol Oncol 1998;68:54-61.
418. Croce S, Ribeiro A, Brulard C, et al. Uterine smooth muscle tumor analysis by comparative genomic hybridization: a useful diagnostic tool in challenging lesions. Mod Pathol 2015;28:1001-10.
419. Yang J, Du X, Chen K, et al. Genetic aberrations in soft tissue leiomyosarcoma. Cancer Lett 2009;275:1-8.
420. Kobayashi H, Uekuri C, Akasaka J, et al. The biology of uterine sarcomas: a review and update. Mol Clin Oncol 2013;1:599-609.
421. Fletcher JA, Morton CC, Pavelka K, Lage JM. Chromosome aberrations in uterine smooth muscle tumors: potential diagnostic relevance of cytogenetic instability. Cancer Res 1990;50:4092-7.
422. Sreekantaiah C, Davis JR, Sandberg AA. Chromosomal abnormalities in leiomyosarcomas. Am J Pathol 1993;142:293-305.
423. Hu J, Rao UN, Jasani S, Khanna V, Yaw K, Surti U. Loss of DNA copy number of 10q is associated with aggressive behavior of leiomyosarcomas: a comparative genomic hybridization study. Cancer Genet Cytogenet 2005;161:20-7.
424. Quade BJ, Pinto AP, Howard DR, Peters WA 3rd, Crum CP. Frequent loss of heterozygosity for chromosome 10 in uterine leiomyosarcoma in contrast to leiomyoma. Am J Pathol 1999;154:945-50.
425. Cho YL, Bae S, Koo MS, et al. Array comparative genomic hybridization analysis of uterine leiomyosarcoma. Gynecol Oncol 2005;99:545-51.
426. Raish M, Khurshid M, Ansari MA, et al. Analysis of molecular cytogenetic alterations in uterine leiomyosarcoma by array-based comparative genomic hybridization. J Cancer Res Clin Oncol 2012;138:1173-86.
427. Levy B, Mukherjee T, Hirschhorn K. Molecular cytogenetic analysis of uterine leiomyoma and leiomyosarcoma by comparative genomic hybridization. Cancer Genet Cytogenet 2000;121:1-8.
428. Croce S, Ducoulombier A, Ribeiro A, et al. Genome profiling is an efficient tool to avoid the STUMP classification of uterine smooth muscle lesions: a comprehensive array-genomic hybridization analysis of 77 tumors. Mod Pathol 2018;31:816-28.

429. Jeffers MD, Farquharson MA, Richmond JA, McNicol AM. p53 immunoreactivity and mutation of the p53 gene in smooth muscle tumours of the uterine corpus. J Pathol 1995;177:65-70.
430. Yang CY, Liau JY, Huang WJ, et al. Targeted next-generation sequencing of cancer genes identified frequent TP53 and ATRX mutations in leiomyosarcoma. Am J Transl Res 2015;7:2072-81.
431. Davidson B, Abeler VM, Hellesylt E, et al. Gene expression signatures differentiate uterine endometrial stromal sarcoma from leiomyosarcoma. Gynecol Oncol 2013;128:349-55.
432. Makinen N, Aavikko M, Heikkinen T, et al. Exome sequencing of uterine leiomyosarcomas identifies frequent mutations in TP53, ATRX, and MED12. PLoS Genet 2016;12:e1005850.
433. Liau JY, Tsai JH, Jeng YM, Lee JC, Hsu HH, Yang CY. Leiomyosarcoma with alternative lengthening of telomeres is associated with aggressive histologic features, loss of ATRX expression, and poor clinical outcome. Am J Surg Pathol 2015;39:236-44.
434. Kampjarvi K, Makinen N, Kilpivaara O, et al. Somatic MED12 mutations in uterine leiomyosarcoma and colorectal cancer. Br J Cancer 2012;107:1761-5.
435. Arias-Stella JA 3rd, Lewis N, Benayed R, et al. Novel PLAG1 gene rearrangement distinguishes a subset of uterine myxoid leiomyosarcoma from other uterine myxoid mesenchymal tumors. Am J Surg Pathol 2019;43:382-8.
436. Guo X, Jo VY, Mills AM, et al. Clinically relevant molecular subtypes in leiomyosarcoma. Clin Cancer Res 2015;21:3501-11.
437. Mills AM, Beck AH, Montgomery KD, et al. Expression of subtype-specific group 1 leiomyosarcoma markers in a wide variety of sarcomas by gene expression analysis and immunohistochemistry. Am J Surg Pathol 2011;35:583-9.
438. Miyata T, Sonoda K, Tomikawa J, et al. Genomic, epigenomic, and transcriptomic profiling towards identifying omics features and specific biomarkers that distinguish uterine leiomyosarcoma and leiomyoma at molecular levels. Sarcoma 2015;2015:412068.
439. Barlin JN, Zhou QC, Leitao MM, et al. Molecular subtypes of uterine leiomyosarcoma and correlation with clinical outcome. Neoplasia 2015;17:183-9.
440. Danielson LS, Menendez S, Attolini CS, et al. A differentiation-based microRNA signature identifies leiomyosarcoma as a mesenchymal stem cell-related malignancy. Am J Pathol 2010;177:908-17.
441. Davidson B, Abeler VM, Forsund M, et al. Gene expression signatures of primary and metastatic uterine leiomyosarcoma. Hum Pathol 2014;45:691-700.
442. Ravid Y, Formanski M, Smith Y, Reich R, Davidson B. Uterine leiomyosarcoma and endometrial stromal sarcoma have unique miRNA signatures. Gynecol Oncol 2016;140:512-7.
443. Vang R, Kempson RL. Perivascular epithelioid cell tumor ('PEComa') of the uterus: a subset of HMB-45-positive epithelioid mesenchymal neoplasms with an uncertain relationship to pure smooth muscle tumors. Am J Surg Pathol 2002;26:1-13.
444. Folpe AL, Mentzel T, Lehr HA, Fisher C, Balzer BL, Weiss SW. Perivascular epithelioid cell neoplasms of soft tissue and gynecologic origin: a clinicopathologic study of 26 cases and review of the literature. Am J Surg Pathol 2005;29:1558-75.
445. Schoolmeester JK, Howitt BE, Hirsch MS, Dal Cin P, Quade BJ, Nucci MR. Perivascular epithelioid cell neoplasm (PEComa) of the gynecologic tract: clinicopathologic and immunohistochemical characterization of 16 cases. Am J Surg Pathol 2014;38176-88.
446. Bennett JA, Braga AC, Pinto A, et al. Uterine PEComas: a morphological, immunohistochemical, and molecular analysis of 32 tumors. Am J Surg Pathol 2018;42:1370-83.
447. de Leval L, Lim GS, Waltregny D, Oliva E. Diverse phenotypic profile of uterine tumors resembling ovarian sex cord tumors: an immunohistochemical study of 12 cases. Am J Surg Pathol 2010;34:1749-61.
448. Shih IM, Kurman RJ. The pathology of intermediate trophoblastic tumors and tumor-like lesions. Int J Gynecol Pathol 2001;20:31-47.
449. Schoolmeester JK, Carlson J, Keeney GL, et al. Alveolar soft part sarcoma of the female genital tract: a morphologic, immunohistochemical, and molecular cytogenetic study of 10 cases with emphasis on its distinction from morphologic mimics. Am J Surg Pathol 2017;41:622-32.
450. Li XQ, Hisaoka M, Shi DR, Zhu XZ, Hashimoto H. Expression of anaplastic lymphoma kinase in soft tissue tumors: an immunohistochemical and molecular study of 249 cases. Hum Pathol 2004;35:711-21.
451. Lewis N, Soslow RA, Delair DF, et al. ZC3H7B-BCOR high-grade endometrial stromal sarcomas: a report of 17 cases of a newly defined entity. Mod Pathol 2018;31:674-84.
452. McCluggage WG, Young RH. Myxoid change of the myometrium and cervical stroma: description of a hitherto unreported non-neoplastic phenomenon with discussion of myxoid uterine lesions. Int J Gynecol Pathol 2010;29:351-7.
453. Pugh A, McCluggage WG, Hirschowitz L. Multifocal uterine myxoid change: a newly recognized association with neurofibromatosis type 1. Int J Gynecol Pathol 2012;31:580-3.

454. Veras E, Junkins-Hopkins JM, Marinis S, Vang R. Myometrial myxoidosis: a report of 2 cases of a distinctive type of secondary myometrial hypertrophy in patients with lupus erythematosus. Int J Gynecol Pathol 2009;28:164-71.
455. Bennett JA, Sanada S, Selig MK, Hariri LP, Nielsen GP, Oliva E. Giant cell tumor of the uterus: a report of 3 cases with a spectrum of morphologic features. Int J Gynecol Pathol 2015;34:340-50.
456. Giuntoli RL 2nd, Lessard-Anderson CR, Gerardi MA, et al. Comparison of current staging systems and a novel staging system for uterine leiomyosarcoma. Int J Gynecol Cancer 2013;23:869-76.
457. Leitao MM, Sonoda Y, Brennan MF, Barakat RR, Chi DS. Incidence of lymph node and ovarian metastases in leiomyosarcoma of the uterus. Gynecol Oncol 2003;91:209-12.
458. Giuntoli RL 2nd, Bristow RE. Uterine leiomyosarcoma: present management. Curr Opin Oncol 2004;16:324-7.
459. Gadducci A, Guerrieri ME. Pharmacological treatment for uterine leiomyosarcomas. Expert Opin Pharmacother 2015;16:335-46.
460. Mancari R, Signorelli M, Gadducci A, et al. Adjuvant chemotherapy in stage I-II uterine leiomyosarcoma: a multicentric retrospective study of 140 patients. Gynecol Oncol 2014;133:531-6.
461. Ricci S, Stone RL, Fader AN. Uterine leiomyosarcoma: epidemiology, contemporary treatment strategies and the impact of uterine morcellation. Gynecol Oncol 2017;145:208-16.
462. Altman AD, Nelson GS, Chu P, Nation J, Ghatage P. Uterine sarcoma and aromatase inhibitors: Tom Baker Cancer Centre experience and review of the literature. Int J Gynecol Cancer 2012;22:1006-12.
463. Babichev Y, Kabaroff L, Datti A, et al. PI3K/AKT/mTOR inhibition in combination with doxorubicin is an effective therapy for leiomyosarcoma. J Transl Med 2016;14:67.
464. Hyman DM, Sill MW, Lankes HA, et al. A phase 2 study of alisertib (MLN8237) in recurrent or persistent uterine leiomyosarcoma: an NRG oncology/gynecologic oncology group study 0231d. Gynecol Oncol 2017;144:96-100.
465. Larson B, Silfversward C, Nilsson B, Pettersson F. Prognostic factors in uterine leiomyosarcoma. A clinical and histopathological study of 143 cases. The Radiumhemmet series 1936-1981. Acta Oncol 1990;29:185-91.
466. Kapp DS, Shin JY, Chan JK. Prognostic factors and survival in 1396 patients with uterine leiomyosarcomas: emphasis on impact of lymphadenectomy and oophorectomy. Cancer 2008;112:820-30.
467. Pelmus M, Penault-Llorca F, Guillou L, et al. Prognostic factors in early-stage leiomyosarcoma of the uterus. Int J Gynecol Cancer 2009;19:385-90.
468. Bodner K, Bodner-Adler B, Kimberger O, Czerwenka K, Leodolter S, Mayerhofer K. Evaluating prognostic parameters in women with uterine leiomyosarcoma. A clinicopathologic study. J Reprod Med 2003;48:95-100.
469. Raut CP, Nucci MR, Wang Q, et al. Predictive value of FIGO and AJCC staging systems in patients with uterine leiomyosarcoma. Eur J Cancer 2009;45:2818-24.
470. Zivanovic O, Leitao MM, Iasonos A, et al. Stage-specific outcomes of patients with uterine leiomyosarcoma: a comparison of the international federation of gynecology and obstetrics and american joint committee on cancer staging systems. J Clin Oncol 2009;27:2066-72.
471. Prat J. FIGO staging for uterine sarcomas. Int J Gynaecol Obstet 2009;104:177-8.
472. Garg G, Shah JP, Liu JR, et al. Validation of tumor size as staging variable in the revised International Federation of Gynecology and Obstetrics stage I leiomyosarcoma: a population-based study. Int J Gynecol Cancer 2010;20:1201-6.
473. Lim D, Wang WL, Lee CH, Dodge T, Gilks B, Oliva E. Old versus new FIGO staging systems in predicting overall survival in patients with uterine leiomyosarcoma: a study of 86 cases. Gynecol Oncol 2013;128:322-6.
474. Zivanovic O, Jacks LM, Iasonos A, et al. A nomogram to predict postresection 5-year overall survival for patients with uterine leiomyosarcoma. Cancer 2012;118:660-9.
475. Rauh-Hain JA, Hinchcliff EM, Oduyebo T, et al. Clinical outcomes of women with recurrent or persistent uterine leiomyosarcoma. Int J Gynecol Cancer 2014;24:1434-40.
476. Tirumani SH, Deaver P, Shinagare AB, et al. Metastatic pattern of uterine leiomyosarcoma: retrospective analysis of the predictors and outcome in 113 patients. J Gynecol Oncol 2014;25:306-12.
477. Mayerhofer K, Obermair A, Windbichler G, et al. Leiomyosarcoma of the uterus: a clinicopathologic multicenter study of 71 cases. Gynecol Oncol 1999;74:196-201.
478. Bodner-Adler B, Bodner K, Kimberger O, Czerwenka K, Leodolter S, Mayerhofer K. MMP-1 and MMP-2 expression in uterine leiomyosarcoma and correlation with different clinicopathologic parameters. J Soc Gynecol Investig 2003;10:443-6.
479. Lennart K, Lennart B, Ulf S, Bernard T. Flow cytometric analysis of uterine sarcomas. Gynecol Oncol 1994;55(Pt 1):339-42.

480. Liu FS, Kohler MF, Marks JR, Bast RC Jr, Boyd J, Berchuck A. Mutation and overexpression of the p53 tumor suppressor gene frequently occurs in uterine and ovarian sarcomas. Obstet Gynecol 1994;83:118-24.
481. Leiser AL, Anderson SE, Nonaka D, et al. Apoptotic and cell cycle regulatory markers in uterine leiomyosarcoma. Gynecol Oncol 2006;101:86-91.
482. Kawaguchi K, Oda Y, Saito T, et al. Mechanisms of inactivation of the p16INK4a gene in leiomyosarcoma of soft tissue: decreased p16 expression correlates with promoter methylation and poor prognosis. J Pathol 2003;201:487-95.
483. Garcia C, Kubat JS, Fulton RS, et al. Clinical outcomes and prognostic markers in uterine leiomyosarcoma: a population-based cohort. Int J Gynecol Cancer 2015;25:622-8.
484. Espinosa I, Beck AH, Lee CH, et al. Coordinate expression of colony-stimulating factor-1 and colony-stimulating factor-1-related proteins is associated with poor prognosis in gynecological and nongynecological leiomyosarcoma. Am J Pathol 2009;174:2347-56.
485. Lee CH, Espinosa I, Vrijaldenhoven S, et al. Prognostic significance of macrophage infiltration in leiomyosarcomas. Clin Cancer Res 2008;14:1423-30.
486. Pritts EA, Vanness DJ, Berek JS, et al. The prevalence of occult leiomyosarcoma at surgery for presumed uterine fibroids: a meta-analysis. Gynecol Surg 2015;12:165-77.
487. Einstein MH, Barakat RR, Chi DS, et al. Management of uterine malignancy found incidentally after supracervical hysterectomy or uterine morcellation for presumed benign disease. Int J Gynecol Cancer 2008;18:1065-70.
488. Park JY, Park SK, Kim DY, et al. The impact of tumor morcellation during surgery on the prognosis of patients with apparently early uterine leiomyosarcoma. Gynecol Oncol 2011;122:255-9.
489. Slatter TL, Hsia H, Samaranayaka A, et al. Loss of ATRX and DAXX expression identifies poor prognosis for smooth muscle tumours of uncertain malignant potential and early stage uterine leiomyosarcoma. J Pathol Clin Res 2015;1:95-105.
490. Ha HI, Choi MC, Heo JH, et al. A clinicopathologic review and obstetric outcome of uterine smooth muscle tumor of uncertain malignant potential (STUMP) in a single institution. Eur J Obstet Gynecol Reprod Biol 2018;228:1-5.
491. Gupta M, Laury AL, Nucci MR, Quade BJ. Predictors of adverse outcome in uterine smooth muscle tumours of uncertain malignant potential (STUMP): a clinicopathological analysis of 22 cases with a proposal for the inclusion of additional histological parameters. Histopathology 2018;73:284-98.
492. Amant F, Moerman P, Vergote I. Report of an unusual problematic uterine smooth muscle neoplasm, emphasizing the prognostic importance of coagulative tumor cell necrosis. Int J Gynecol Cancer 2005;15:1210-2.
493. Peters WA 3rd, Howard DR, Andersen WA, Figge DC. Uterine smooth-muscle tumors of uncertain malignant potential. Obstet Gynecol 1994;83:1015-20.
494. Berretta R, Rolla M, Merisio C, Giordano G, Nardelli GB. Uterine smooth muscle tumor of uncertain malignant potential: a three-case report. Int J Gynecol Cancer 2008;18:1121-6.
495. Guntupalli SR, Ramirez PT, Anderson ML, Milam MR, Bodurka DC, Malpica A. Uterine smooth muscle tumor of uncertain malignant potential: a retrospective analysis. Gynecol Oncol 2009;113:324-6.
496. Shapiro A, Ferenczy A, Turcotte R, Bruchim I, Gotlieb WH. Uterine smooth-muscle tumor of uncertain malignant potential metastasizing to the humerus as a high-grade leiomyosarcoma. Gynecol Oncol 2004;94:818-20.
497. Ng JS, Han A, Chew SH, Low J. A clinicopathologic study of uterine smooth muscle tumours of uncertain malignant potential (STUMP). Ann Acad Med Singapore 2010;39:625-8.
498. Kempson RL. Sarcomas and related neoplasms. In: Norris HJ, Hertig AT, Abell MR, eds. The uterus. Baltimore: Williams & Wilkins; 1973:298-319.
499. Kempson RL, Hendrickson MR. Smooth muscle, endometrial stromal, and mixed Mullerian tumors of the uterus. Mod Pathol 2000;13:328-42.
500. Longacre TA, Hendrickson MR, Kempson RL. Predicting clinical outcome for uterine smooth muscle neoplasms with a reasonable degree of certainty. Adv Anat Pathol 1997;4:95-104.
501. Lee CH, Turbin DA, Sung YC, et al. A panel of antibodies to determine site of origin and malignancy in smooth muscle tumors. Mod Pathol 2009;22:1519-31.
502. Unver NU, Acikalin MF, Oner U, Ciftci E, Ozalp SS, Colak E. Differential expression of P16 and P21 in benign and malignant uterine smooth muscle tumors. Arch Gynecol Obstet 2011;284:483-90.
503. Devereaux KA, Kunder CA, Longacre TA. ALK-rearranged tumors are highly enriched in the STUMP subcategory of uterine tumors. Am J Surg Pathol 2018.
504. Ip PP, Cheung AN. Pathology of uterine leiomyosarcomas and smooth muscle tumours of uncertain malignant potential. Best Pract Res Clin Obstet Gynaecol 2011;25:691-704.

505. Bonetti F, Pea M, Martignoni G, Zamboni G. PEC and sugar. Am J Surg Pathol 1992;16:307-8.
506. Nese N, Martignoni G, Fletcher CD, et al. Pure epithelioid PEComas (so-called epithelioid angiomyolipoma) of the kidney: a clinicopathologic study of 41 cases: detailed assessment of morphology and risk stratification. Am J Surg Pathol 2011;35:161-76.
507. He W, Cheville JC, Sadow PM, et al. Epithelioid angiomyolipoma of the kidney: pathological features and clinical outcome in a series of consecutively resected tumors. Mod Pathol 2013;26:1355-64.
508. Tazelaar HD, Batts KP, Srigley JR. Primary extrapulmonary sugar tumor (PEST): a report of four cases. Mod Pathol 2001;14:615-22.
509. Zamboni G, Pea M, Martignoni G, et al. Clear cell "sugar" tumor of the pancreas. A novel member of the family of lesions characterized by the presence of perivascular epithelioid cells. Am J Surg Pathol 1996;20:722-30.
510. Mentzel T, Reisshauer S, Rutten A, Hantschke M, Soares de Almeida LM, Kutzner H. Cutaneous clear cell myomelanocytic tumour: a new member of the growing family of perivascular epithelioid cell tumours (PEComas). Clinicopathological and immunohistochemical analysis of seven cases. Histopathology 2005;46:498-504.
511. Bonetti F, Chiodera PL, Pea M, et al. Transbronchial biopsy in lymphangiomyomatosis of the lung. HMB45 for diagnosis. Am J Surg Pathol 1993;17:1092-102.
512. Matsui K, Tatsuguchi A, Valencia J, et al. Extrapulmonary lymphangioleiomyomatosis (LAM): clinicopathologic features in 22 cases. Hum Pathol 2000;31:1242-8.
513. Castro M, Shepherd CW, Gomez MR, Lie JT, Ryu JH. Pulmonary tuberous sclerosis. Chest 1995;107:189-95.
514. Longacre TA, Hendrickson MR, Kapp DS, Teng NN. Lymphangioleiomyomatosis of the uterus simulating high-stage endometrial stromal sarcoma. Gynecol Oncol 1996;63:404-10.
515. Folpe AL, Goodman ZD, Ishak KG, et al. Clear cell myomelanocytic tumor of the falciform ligament/ligamentum teres: a novel member of the perivascular epithelioid clear cell family of tumors with a predilection for children and young adults. Am J Surg Pathol 2000;24:1239-46.
516. Bonetti F, Martignoni G, Colato C, et al. Abdominopelvic sarcoma of perivascular epithelioid cells. Report of four cases in young women, one with tuberous sclerosis. Mod Pathol 2001;14:563-8.
517. Doyle LA, Hornick JL, Fletcher CD. PEComa of the gastrointestinal tract: clinicopathologic study of 35 cases with evaluation of prognostic parameters. Am J Surg Pathol 2013;37:1769-82.
518. Yamashita K, Fletcher CD. PEComa presenting in bone: clinicopathologic analysis of 6 cases and literature review. Am J Surg Pathol 2010;34:1622-9.
519. Liegl B, Hornick JL, Fletcher CD. Primary cutaneous PEComa: distinctive clear cell lesions of skin. Am J Surg Pathol 2008;32:608-14.
520. Sukov WR, Cheville JC, Amin MB, Gupta R, Folpe AL. Perivascular epithelioid cell tumor (PEComa) of the urinary bladder: report of 3 cases and review of the literature. Am J Surg Pathol 2009;33:304-8.
521. Martignoni G, Pea M, Zampini C, et al. PEComas of the kidney and of the genitourinary tract. Semin Diagn Pathol 2015;32:140-59.
522. Govender D, Sabaratnam RM, Essa AS. Clear cell 'sugar' tumor of the breast: another extrapulmonary site and review of the literature. Am J Surg Pathol 2002;26:670-5.
523. Bosincu L, Rocca PC, Martignoni G, et al. Perivascular epithelioid cell (PEC) tumors of the uterus: a clinicopathologic study of two cases with aggressive features. Mod Pathol 2005;18:1336-42.
524. Fadare O. Perivascular epithelioid cell tumor (PEComa) of the uterus: an outcome-based clinicopathologic analysis of 41 reported cases. Adv Anat Pathol 2008;15:63-75.
525. Fukunaga M. Perivascular epithelioid cell tumor of the uterus: report of four cases. Int J Gynecol Pathol 2005;24:341-6.
526. LeGallo RD, Stelow EB, Sukov WR, Duska LR, Alisanski SB, Folpe AL. Melanotic xp11.2 neoplasm of the ovary: report of a unique case. Am J Surg Pathol 2012;36:1410-4.
527. Lee SE, Choi YL, Cho J, Kim T, Song SY, Sung CO. Ovarian perivascular epithelioid cell tumor not otherwise specified with transcription factor E3 gene rearrangement: a case report and review of the literature. Hum Pathol 2012;43:1126-30.
528. Anderson AE, Yang X, Young RH. Epithelioid angiomyolipoma of the ovary: a case report and literature review. Int J Gynecol Pathol 2002;21:69-73.
529. Westaby JD, Magdy N, Fisher C, El-Bahrawy M. Primary ovarian malignant PEComa: a case report. Int J Gynecol Pathol 2017;36:400-4.
530. Fadare O, Parkash V, Yilmaz Y, et al. Perivascular epithelioid cell tumor (PEComa) of the uterine cervix associated with intraabdominal "PEComatosis": a clinicopathological study with comparative genomic hybridization analysis. World J Surg Oncol 2004;2:35.
531. Bradshaw MJ, Folpe AL, Croghan GA. Perivascular epithelioid cell neoplasm of the uterine cervix: an unusual tumor in an unusual location. Rare Tumors 2010;2:e56.

532. Yamada Y, Yamamoto H, Ohishi Y, et al. Sclerosing variant of perivascular epithelioid cell tumor in the female genital organs. Pathol Int 2011;61:768-72.
533. Kim HJ, Lim SJ, Choi H, Park K. Malignant clear-cell myomelanocytic tumor of broad ligament--a case report. Virchows Arch 2006;448:867-70.
534. Liang SX, Pearl M, Liu J, Hwang S, Tornos C. "Malignant" uterine perivascular epithelioid cell tumor, pelvic lymph node lymphangioleiomyomatosis, and gynecological pecomatosis in a patient with tuberous sclerosis: a case report and review of the literature. Int J Gynecol Pathol 2008;27:86-90.
535. Froio E, Piana S, Cavazza A, Valli R, Abrate M, Gardini G. Multifocal PEComa (PEComatosis) of the female genital tract associated with endometriosis, diffuse adenomyosis, and endometrial atypical hyperplasia. Int J Surg Pathol 2008;16:443-6.
536. Hornick JL, Fletcher CD. Sclerosing PEComa: clinicopathologic analysis of a distinctive variant with a predilection for the retroperitoneum. Am J Surg Pathol 2008;32:493-501.
537. Schoolmeester JK, Dao LN, Sukov WR, et al. TFE3 translocation-associated perivascular epithelioid cell neoplasm (PEComa) of the gynecologic tract: morphology, immunophenotype, differential diagnosis. Am J Surg Pathol 2015;39:394-404.
538. Ruco LP, Pilozzi E, Wedard BM, et al. Epithelioid lymphangioleiomyomatosis-like tumour of the uterus in a patient without tuberous sclerosis: a lesion mimicking epithelioid leiomyosarcoma. Histopathology 1998;33:91-3.
539. Gyure KA, Hart WR, Kennedy AW. Lymphangiomyomatosis of the uterus associated with tuberous sclerosis and malignant neoplasia of the female genital tract: a report of two cases. Int J Gynecol Pathol 1995;14:344-51.
540. Darai E, Bazot M, Barranger E, Detchev R, Cortez A. Epithelioid angiomyolipoma of the uterus: a case report. J Reprod Med 2004;49:578-81.
541. Cil AP, Haberal A, Hucumenoglu S, Kovalak EE, Gunes M. Angiomyolipoma of the uterus associated with tuberous sclerosis: case report and review of the literature. Gynecol Oncol 2004;94:593-6.
542. Yaegashi H, Moriya T, Soeda S, Yonemoto Y, Nagura H, Sasano H. Uterine angiomyolipoma: case report and review of the literature. Pathol Int 2001;51:896-901.
543. Sturtz CL, Dabbs DJ. Angiomyolipomas: the nature and expression of the HMB45 antigen. Mod Pathol 1994;7:842-5.
544. Rao Q, Cheng L, Xia QY, et al. Cathepsin K expression in a wide spectrum of perivascular epithelioid cell neoplasms (PEComas): a clinicopathological study emphasizing extrarenal PEComas. Histopathology 2013;62:642-50.
545. Martignoni G, Bonetti F, Chilosi M, et al. Cathepsin K expression in the spectrum of perivascular epithelioid cell (PEC) lesions of the kidney. Mod Pathol 2012;25:100-11.
546. Argani P, Aulmann S, Illei PB, et al. A distinctive subset of PEComas harbors TFE3 gene fusions. Am J Surg Pathol 2010;34:1395-406.
547. Agaram NP, Sung YS, Zhang L, et al. Dichotomy of genetic abnormalities in PEComas with therapeutic implications. Am J Surg Pathol 2015;39:813-25.
548. Miettinen M, McCue PA, Sarlomo-Rikala M, et al. Sox10—-a marker for not only schwannian and melanocytic neoplasms but also myoepithelial cell tumors of soft tissue: a systematic analysis of 5134 tumors. Am J Surg Pathol 2015;39:826-35.
549. Ahrens WA, Folpe AL. CD1a immunopositivity in perivascular epithelioid cell neoplasms: true expression or technical artifact? A streptavidin-biotin and polymer-based detection system immunohistochemical study of perivascular epithelioid cell neoplasms and their morphologic mimics. Hum Pathol 2011;42:369-74.
550. Pan CC, Jong YJ, Chai CY, Huang SH, Chen YJ. Comparative genomic hybridization study of perivascular epithelioid cell tumor: molecular genetic evidence of perivascular epithelioid cell tumor as a distinctive neoplasm. Hum Pathol 2006;37:606-12.
551. Simpson KW, Albores-Saavedra J. HMB-45 reactivity in conventional uterine leiomyosarcomas. Am J Surg Pathol 2007;31:95-8.
552. Albores-Saavedra J, Dorantes-Heredia R, Chable-Montero F, et al. Endometrial stromal sarcomas: immunoprofile with emphasis on HMB45 reactivity. Am J Clin Pathol 2014;141:850-5.
553. Chu P, Arber DA. Paraffin-section detection of CD10 in 505 nonhematopoietic neoplasms. Frequent expression in renal cell carcinoma and endometrial stromal sarcoma. Am J Clin Pathol 2000;113:374-82.
554. Ross H, Argani P. Xp11 translocation renal cell carcinoma. Pathology 2010;42:369-73.
555. Conlon N, Soslow RA, Murali R. Perivascular epithelioid tumours (PEComas) of the gynaecological tract. J Clin Pathol 2015;68:418-26.
556. Arndt CA, Donaldson SS, Anderson JR, et al. What constitutes optimal therapy for patients with rhabdomyosarcoma of the female genital tract? Cancer 2001;91:2454-68.
557. Ferguson SE, Gerald W, Barakat RR, Chi DS, Soslow RA. Clinicopathologic features of rhabdomyosarcoma of gynecologic origin in adults. Am J Surg Pathol 2007;31:382-9.

558. Li RF, Gupta M, McCluggage WG, Ronnett BM. Embryonal rhabdomyosarcoma (botryoid type) of the uterine corpus and cervix in adult women: report of a case series and review of the literature. Am J Surg Pathol 2013;37:344-55.
559. Garrett LA, Harmon DC, Schorge JO. Embryonal rhabdomyosarcoma of the uterine corpus. J Clin Oncol 2013;31:e48-50.
560. Fadare O, Bonvicino A, Martel M, Renshaw IL, Azodi M, Parkash V. Pleomorphic rhabdomyosarcoma of the uterine corpus: a clinicopathologic study of 4 cases and a review of the literature. Int J Gynecol Pathol 2010;29:122-34.
561. Montag TW, D'Ablaing G, Schlaerth JB, Gaddis O, Jr., Morrow CP. Embryonal rhabdomyosarcoma of the uterine corpus and cervix. Gynecol Oncol 1986;25:171-94.
562. Ordi J, Stamatakos MD, Tavassoli FA. Pure pleomorphic rhabdomyosarcomas of the uterus. Int J Gynecol Pathol 1997;16:369-77.
563. Hart WR, Craig JR. Rhabdomyosarcomas of the uterus. Am J Clin Pathol 1978;70:217-23.
564. Fadare O. Heterologous and rare homologous sarcomas of the uterine corpus: a clinicopathologic review. Adv Anat Pathol 2011;18:60-74.
565. Fukunaga M. Pure alveolar rhabdomyosarcoma of the uterine corpus. Pathol Int 2011;61:377-81.
566. Chiarle R, Godio L, Fusi D, Soldati T, Palestro G. Pure alveolar rhabdomyosarcoma of the corpus uteri: description of a case with increased serum level of CA-125. Gynecol Oncol 1997;66:320-3.
567. McCluggage WG, Lioe TF, McClelland HR, Lamki H. Rhabdomyosarcoma of the uterus: report of two cases, including one of the spindle cell variant. Int J Gynecol Cancer 2002;12:128-32.
568. Stolnicu S, Goyenaga P, Hincu M, Marian C, Murillo R, Nogales FF. Embryonal (botryoides) rhabdomyosarcoma of the uterus harboring a primitive neuroectodermal tumor component. Int J Gynecol Pathol 2012;31:387-9.
569. Cate F, Bridge JA, Crispens MA, et al. Composite uterine neoplasm with embryonal rhabdomyosarcoma and primitive neuroectodermal tumor components: rhabdomyosarcoma with divergent differentiation, variant of primitive neuroectodermal tumor, or unique entity? Hum Pathol 2013;44:656-63.
570. Folpe AL. MyoD1 and myogenin expression in human neoplasia: a review and update. Adv Anat Pathol 2002;9:198-203.
571. Riedlinger WF, Kozakewich HP, Vargas SO. Myogenic markers in the evaluation of embryonal botryoid rhabdomyosarcoma of the female genital tract. Pediatr Dev Pathol 2005;8:355-61.
572. Bahrami A, Gown AM, Baird GS, Hicks MJ, Folpe AL. Aberrant expression of epithelial and neuroendocrine markers in alveolar rhabdomyosarcoma: a potentially serious diagnostic pitfall. Mod Pathol 2008;21:795-806.
573. Harel M, Ferrer FA, Shapiro LH, Makari JH. Future directions in risk stratification and therapy for advanced pediatric genitourinary rhabdomyosarcoma. Urol Oncol 2016;34:103-15.
574. Clement PB, Scully RE. Mullerian adenosarcoma of the uterus: a clinicopathologic analysis of 100 cases with a review of the literature. Hum Pathol 1990;21:363-81.
575. Soslow RA, Ali A, Oliva E. Mullerian adenosarcomas: an immunophenotypic analysis of 35 cases. Am J Surg Pathol 2008;32:1013-21.
576. Kolin DL, Dong F, Baltay M, et al. SMARCA4-deficient undifferentiated uterine sarcoma (malignant rhabdoid tumor of the uterus): a clinicopathologic entity distinct from undifferentiated carcinoma. Mod Pathol 2018.
577. Cattani MG, Viale G, Santini D, Martinelli GN. Malignant rhabdoid tumour of the uterus: an immunohistochemical and ultrastructural study. Virchows Arch A Pathol Anat Histopathol 1992;420:459-62.
578. Cho KR, Rosenshein NB, Epstein JI. Malignant rhabdoid tumor of the uterus. Int J Gynecol Pathol 1989;8:381-7.
579. Hsueh S, Chang TC. Malignant rhabdoid tumor of the uterine corpus. Gynecol Oncol 1996;61:142-6.
580. Coffin CM, Watterson J, Priest JR, Dehner LP. Extrapulmonary inflammatory myofibroblastic tumor (inflammatory pseudotumor). A clinicopathologic and immunohistochemical study of 84 cases. Am J Surg Pathol 1995;19:859-72.
581. Rabban JT, Zaloudek CJ, Shekitka KM, Tavassoli FA. Inflammatory myofibroblastic tumor of the uterus: a clinicopathologic study of 6 cases emphasizing distinction from aggressive mesenchymal tumors. Am J Surg Pathol 2005;29:1348-55.
582. Gilks CB, Taylor GP, Clement PB. Inflammatory pseudotumor of the uterus. Int J Gynecol Pathol 1987;6:275-86.
583. Shintaku M, Fukushima A. Inflammatory myofibroblastic tumor of the uterus with prominent myxoid change. Pathol Int 2006;56:625-8.
584. Kargi HA, Ozer E, Gokden N. Inflammatory pseudotumor of the uterus: a case report. Tumori 1995;81:454-6.
585. Azuno Y, Yaga K, Suehiro Y, Ariyama S, Oga A. Inflammatory myoblastic tumor of the uterus and interleukin-6. Am J Obstet Gynecol 2003;189:890-1.
586. Olgan S, Saatli B, Okyay RE, Koyuncuoglu M, Dogan E. Hysteroscopic excision of inflammatory myofibroblastic tumor of the uterus: a case report and brief review. Eur J Obstet Gynecol Reprod Biol 2011;157:234-6.

587. Gupta N, Mittal S, Misra R. Inflammatory pseudotumor of uterus: an unusual pelvic mass. Eur J Obstet Gynecol Reprod Biol 2011;156:118-9.
588. Fuehrer NE, Keeney GL, Ketterling RP, Knudson RA, Bell DA. ALK-1 protein expression and ALK gene rearrangements aid in the diagnosis of inflammatory myofibroblastic tumors of the female genital tract. Arch Pathol Lab Med 2012;136:623-6.
589. Dehner LP. Inflammatory myofibroblastic tumor: the continued definition of one type of so-called inflammatory pseudotumor. Am J Surg Pathol 2004;28:1652-4.
590. Griffin CA, Hawkins AL, Dvorak C, Henkle C, Ellingham T, Perlman EJ. Recurrent involvement of 2p23 in inflammatory myofibroblastic tumors. Cancer Res 1999;59:2776-80.
591. Haimes JD, Stewart CJ, Kudlow BA, et al. Uterine inflammatory myofibroblastic tumors frequently harbor ALK fusions with IGFBP5 and THBS1. Am J Surg Pathol 2017;41:773-80.
592. Mariño-Enriquez A, Wang WL, Roy A, et al. Epithelioid inflammatory myofibroblastic sarcoma: an aggressive intra-abdominal variant of inflammatory myofibroblastic tumor with nuclear membrane or perinuclear ALK. Am J Surg Pathol 2011;35:135-44.
593. Antonescu CR, Suurmeijer AJ, Zhang L, et al. Molecular characterization of inflammatory myofibroblastic tumors with frequent ALK and ROS1 gene fusions and rare novel RET rearrangement. Am J Surg Pathol 2015;39:957-67.
594. Hornick JL, Sholl LM, Dal Cin P, Childress MA, Lovly CM. Expression of ROS1 predicts ROS1 gene rearrangement in inflammatory myofibroblastic tumors. Mod Pathol 2015;28:732-9.
595. Coffin CM, Hornick JL, Fletcher CD. Inflammatory myofibroblastic tumor: comparison of clinicopathologic, histologic, and immunohistochemical features including ALK expression in atypical and aggressive cases. Am J Surg Pathol 2007;31:509-20.
596. Keel SB, Clement PB, Prat J, Young RH. Malignant schwannoma of the uterine cervix: a study of three cases. Int J Gynecol Pathol 1998;17:223-30.
597. Gordon MD, Weilert M, Ireland K. Plexiform neurofibromatosis involving the uterine cervix, endometrium, myometrium, and ovary. Obstet Gynecol 1996;88(Pt 2):699-701.
598. Wei EX, Albores-Saavedra J, Fowler MR. Plexiform neurofibroma of the uterine cervix: a case report and review of the literature. Arch Pathol Lab Med 2005;129:783-6.
599. Miettinen M, Felisiak-Golabek A, Wang Z, Inaguma S, Lasota J. GIST manifesting as a retroperitoneal tumor: clinicopathologic immunohistochemical, and molecular genetic study of 112 cases. Am J Surg Pathol 2017;41:577-85.
600. Butrynski JE, D'Adamo DR, Hornick JL, et al. Crizotinib in ALK-rearranged inflammatory myofibroblastic tumor. N Engl J Med 2010;363:1727-33.
601. Vijayakumar A, Srinivas A, Chandrashekar BM. Uterine vascular lesions. Rev Obstet Gynecol 2013;6:69-79.
602. Bowers VM Jr, King JD. Benign hemangiomyoma of the uterus. Obstet Gynecol 1977;49(suppl 1):38-40.
603. Acevedo Gallegos S, Gallardo Gaona JM, Velazquez Torres B, Espino i Sosa S, Santarrosa Perez MA, Guzman Huerta ME. [Diffuse cavernous hemangioma of the uterus diagnosed during pregnancy. Case report]. Ginecol Obstet Mex 2011;79:447-51. [Spanish]
604. Kruse AJ, Sep S, Slangen BF, et al. Angiosarcomas of primary gynecologic origin: a clinicopathologic review and quantitative analysis of survival. Int J Gynecol Cancer 2014;24:4-12.
605. Morrel B, Mulder AF, Chadha S, Tjokrowardojo AJ, Wijnen JA. Angiosarcoma of the uterus following radiotherapy for squamous cell carcinoma of the cervix. Eur J Obstet Gynecol Reprod Biol 1993;49:193-7.
606. Prempree T, Tang CK, Hatef A, Forster S. Angiosarcoma of the vagina: a clinicopathologic report. A reappraisal of the radiation treatment of angiosarcomas of the female genital tract. Cancer 1983;51:618-22.
607. Olawaiye AB, Morgan JA, Goodman A, Fuller AF Jr, Penson RT. Epithelioid angiosarcoma of the uterus: a review of management. Arch Gynecol Obstet 2008;278:401-4.
608. Cardinale L, Mirra M, Galli C, Goldblum JR, Pizzolitto S, Falconieri G. Angiosarcoma of the uterus: report of 2 new cases with deviant clinicopathologic features and review of the literature. Ann Diagn Pathol 2008;12:217-21.
609. Schammel DP, Tavassoli FA. Uterine angiosarcomas: a morphologic and immunohistochemical study of four cases. Am Jo Surg Pathol 1998;22:246-50.
610. Drachenberg CB, Faust FJ, Borkowski A, Papadimitriou JC. Epithelioid angiosarcoma of the uterus arising in a leiomyoma with associated ovarian and tubal angiomatosis. Am J Clin Pathol 1994;102:388-9.
611. Lack EE, Bitterman P, Sundeen JT. Mullerian adenosarcoma of the uterus with pure angiosarcoma: case report. Hum Pathol 1991;22:1289-91.
612. Nielsen GP, Oliva E, Young RH, Rosenberg AE, Dickersin GR, Scully RE. Alveolar soft-part sarcoma of the female genital tract: a report of nine cases and review of the literature. Int J Gynecol Pathol 1995;14:283-92.

613. Kasashima S, Minato H, Kobayashi M, et al. Alveolar soft part sarcoma of the endometrium with expression of CD10 and hormone receptors. APMIS 2007;115:861-5.
614. Radig K, Buhtz P, Roessner A. Alveolar soft part sarcoma of the uterine corpus. Report of two cases and review of the literature. Pathol Res Pract 1998;194:59-63.
615. Burch DJ, Hitchcock A, Masson GM. Alveolar soft part sarcoma of the uterus: case report and review of the literature. Gynecol Oncol 1994;54:91-4.
616. Nolan NP, Gaffney EF. Alveolar soft part sarcoma of the uterus. Histopathology 1990;16:97-9.
617. Gray GF Jr, Glick AD, Kurtin PJ, Jones HW 3rd. Alveolar soft part sarcoma of the uterus. Hum Pathol 1986;17:297-300.
618. Zhang LL, Tang Q, Wang Z, Zhang XS. Alveolar soft part sarcoma of the uterine corpus with pelvic lymph node metastasis: case report and literature review. Int J Clin Exp Pathol 2012;5:715-9.
619. Ladanyi M, Antonescu CR, Drobnjak M, et al. The precrystalline cytoplasmic granules of alveolar soft part sarcoma contain monocarboxylate transporter 1 and CD147. Am J Pathol 2002;160:1215-21.
620. Wang H, Jacobson A, Harmon DC, et al. Prognostic factors in alveolar soft part sarcoma: a SEER analysis. J Surg Oncol 2016;113:581-6.
621. Pounder DJ. Fatty tumours of the uterus. J Clin Pathol 1982;35:1380-3.
622. Willen R, Gad A, Willen H. Lipomatous lesions of the uterus. Virchows Arch A Pathol Anat Histol 1978;377:351-61.
623. Fujimoto Y, Kasai K, Furuya M, et al. Pure uterine lipoma. J Obstet Gynaecol Res 2006;32:520-3.
624. Bapat K, Brustein S. Uterine sarcoma with liposarcomatous differentiation: report of a case and review of the literature. Int J Gynaecol Obstet 1989;28:71-5.
625. Sosnik H, Jelen M, Sosnik K, Pomorska M. Liposarcoma of the uterine corpus coexisting with preinvasive cervical cancer--a case report. Pol J Pathol 2006;57:171-3.
626. Mariño-Enriquez A, Nascimento AF, Ligon AH, Liang C, Fletcher CD. Atypical spindle cell lipomatous tumor: clinicopathologic characterization of 232 cases demonstrating a morphologic spectrum. Am J Surg Pathol 2017;41:234-44.
627. Lee HP, Tseng HH, Hsieh PP, Shih TF. Uterine lipoleiomyosarcoma: report of 2 cases and review of the literature. Int J Gynecol Pathol 2012;31:358-63.
628. Hong R, Lim SC, Jung H. A myxoid liposarcoma arising in a leiomyoma of the uterus: a case report. Arch Gynecol Obstet 2008;277:445-8.
629. Wakami K, Tateyama H, Kawashima H, et al. Solitary fibrous tumor of the uterus producing high-molecular-weight insulin-like growth factor II and associated with hypoglycemia. Int J Gynecol Pathol 2005;24:79-84.
630. Strickland KC, Nucci MR, Esselen KM, et al. A solitary fibrous tumor of the uterus presenting with lung metastases: a case report. Int J Gynecol Pathol 2016;35:25-9.
630a. Yang EJ, Howitt BE, Fletcher CDM, Nucci MR. Solitary fibrous tumour of the female genital tract: a clinicopathological analysis of 25 cases. Histopathology 2018;72:749-59.
631. Casanova J, Vizcaino JR, Pinto F, Cunha A, Madureira G. Abdominal mass mimicking a leiomyoma: malignant uterine solitary fibrous tumor. Gynecol Oncol Case Rep 2012;2:143-5.
632. Chu PW, Liu JY, Peng YJ, Yu MH. Solitary fibrous tumor of the uterus. Taiwan J Obstet Gynecol 2006;45:350-2.
633. Mohajeri A, Tayebwa J, Collin A, et al. Comprehensive genetic analysis identifies a pathognomonic NAB2/STAT6 fusion gene, nonrandom secondary genomic imbalances, and a characteristic gene expression profile in solitary fibrous tumor. Genes Chromosomes Cancer 2013;52:873-86.
634. Demicco EG, Park MS, Araujo DM, et al. Solitary fibrous tumor: a clinicopathological study of 110 cases and proposed risk assessment model. Mod Pathol 2012;25:1298-306.
635. Gomez-Laencina AM, Martinez Diaz F, Izquierdo Sanjuanes B, Vicente Sanchez EM, Fernandez Salmeron R, Meseguer Peña F. Localized neurofibromatosis of the female genital system: a case report and review of the literature. J Obstet Gynaecol Res 2012;38:953-6.
636. Clement PB. Chondrosarcoma of the uterus: report of a case and review of the literature. Hum Pathol 1978;9:726-32.
637. Zheng G, Richmond A, Liu C, et al. Clinicopathologic features and genetic alterations of a primary osteosarcoma of the uterine corpus. Int J Gynecol Pathol 2018.
638. Abraham C, O'Cearbhaill R, Soslow R. Primary osteosarcoma of the uterus with cardiac and pulmonary metastases. Gynecol Oncol Rep 2015;11:4-6.
639. Kostopoulou E, Dragoumis K, Zafrakas M, Myronidou Z, Agelidou S, Bontis I. Primary osteosarcoma of the uterus with immunohistochemical study. Acta Obstet Gynecol Scand 2002;81:678-80.

11 MIXED EPITHELIAL-STROMAL TUMORS

CARCINOSARCOMA

Definition. *Carcinosarcoma* is a biphasic malignant neoplasm composed of histologically high-grade epithelial and mesenchymal elements. Traditionally, carcinosarcoma was considered within the category of sarcomas. However, there is now widespread clinical, morphologic, and molecular evidence that carcinosarcomas are monoclonal neoplasms of epithelial derivation that secondarily undergo mesenchymal (sarcomatous) transformation (1–3). The term carcinosarcoma is preferred by the World Health Organization (WHO) (4), but the previous term, *malignant mixed müllerian tumor,* is still widely used by pathologists.

General Features. Carcinosarcomas constitute approximately 2 percent of all endometrial carcinomas, and almost all occur in a sporadic setting. Patients are most often in the 7th decade (range, 5th to 9th decades), but they have been reported in young patients. An association with breast carcinoma (5), tamoxifen therapy (6–11), and pelvic radiation (usually related to therapy of cervical or rectal carcinoma) (12–17) has been reported. African-Americans are at higher risk of developing carcinosarcoma compared to Caucasians, similar to patients with endometrial serous carcinomas. On rare occasion, carcinosarcomas are present in metastatic sites or in a recurrence following a diagnosis of primary endometrial serous carcinoma.

Clinical Features. Many patients present with vaginal bleeding and/or an enlarged uterus/mass associated with pelvic or abdominal pain or other related signs and symptoms. CA125 is frequently elevated (18). A large polypoid mass prolapsing through the cervical os is often seen on gynecologic exam (19–21). These tumors are frequently diagnosed at an advanced stage; thus, patients may present with signs/symptoms related to metastatic disease. Patients with carcinosarcomas share the same predisposing risk factors as those with endometrial carcinomas and tumors are staged like endometrial carcinomas, according to the 2009 revision to the International Federation of Gynecology and Obstetrics (FIGO) staging classification (22).

Gross Findings. Carcinosarcomas typically present as large, bulky polypoid tumors and occasionally fill the endometrial cavity and protrude through the cervical os, giving the impression of a primary cervical neoplasm (fig. 11-1). On sectioning, they have a soft, fleshy, heterogeneous surface with extensive areas of hemorrhage and necrosis. Deep infiltration of the myometrium or cervical stroma is often identified. On occasion, the tumor appears limited to an endometrial or endocervical polyp (19–21) and rarely, originates in the cervix (20), although the pathogenesis of cervical carcinosarcomas often differs from that of tumors arising in the corpus (23).

Microscopic Findings. With only rare exceptions, carcinosarcoma is composed of histologically high-grade carcinoma and high-grade sarcoma, with or without heterologous elements (figs. 11-2–11-6). Between 75 and 90 percent of carcinosarcomas contain serous or mixed high-grade endometrioid and serous carcinomas (fig. 11-3) (24). When present, the endometrioid carcinoma component may show tumor heterogeneity that includes admixtures of low- and high-grade carcinoma as well as undifferentiated carcinoma (25) and, not infrequently, a morphology that is a hybrid between endometrioid and serous carcinoma. Other components that have been reported include squamous, mucinous, or small cell neuroendocrine carcinoma (26).

The sarcoma component is typically high-grade spindle and/or pleomorphic, and often associated with intracytoplasmic hyaline globules (fig. 11-4). Although it has been stated that

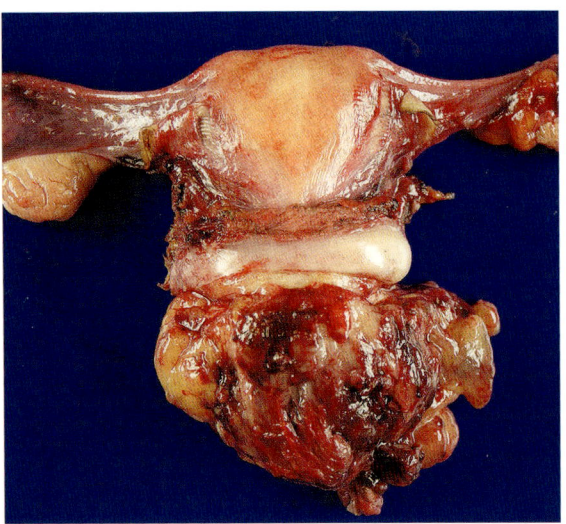
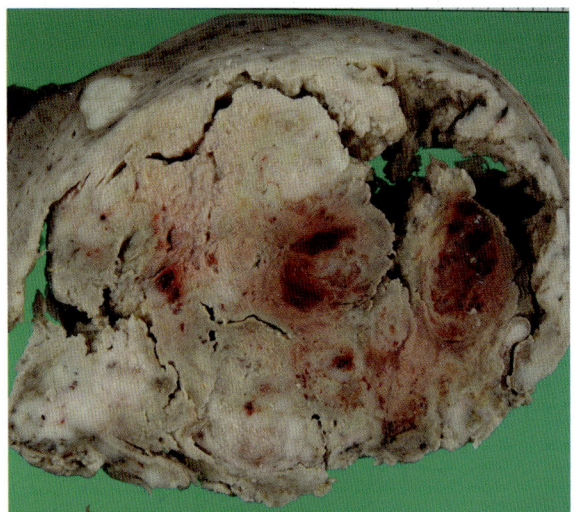

Figure 11-1

UTERINE CORPUS CARCINOSARCOMA

The tumor presents as a large, variegated polypoid mass that protrudes from the cervical os (left). They typically fill and distend the endometrial cavity and show extensive areas of necrosis and hemorrhage (right).

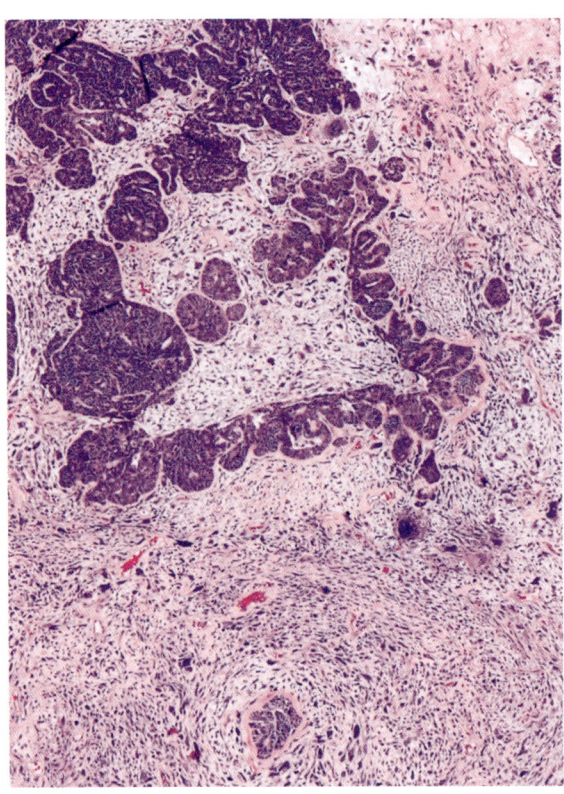
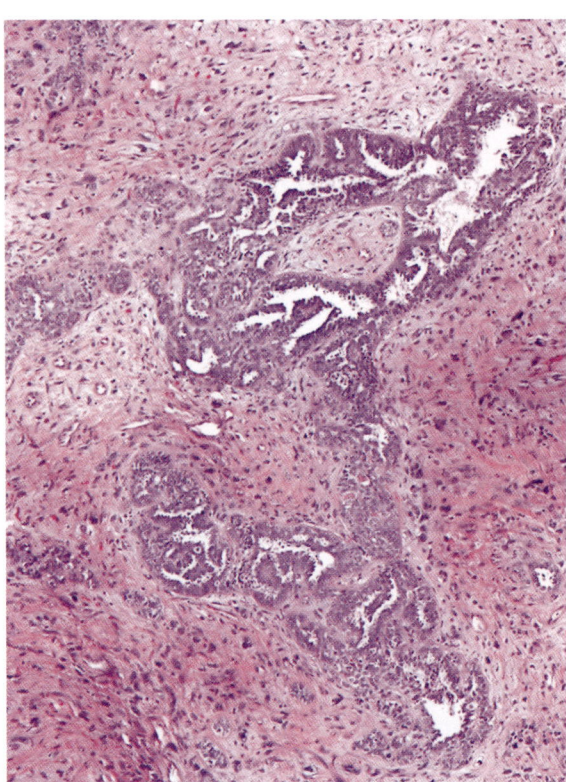

Figure 11-2

UTERINE CORPUS CARCINOSARCOMA

These biphasic, high-grade, malignant epithelial and mesenchymal neoplasms have a variable morphologic appearance of both carcinoma and sarcoma components.

Mixed Epithelial-Stromal Tumors

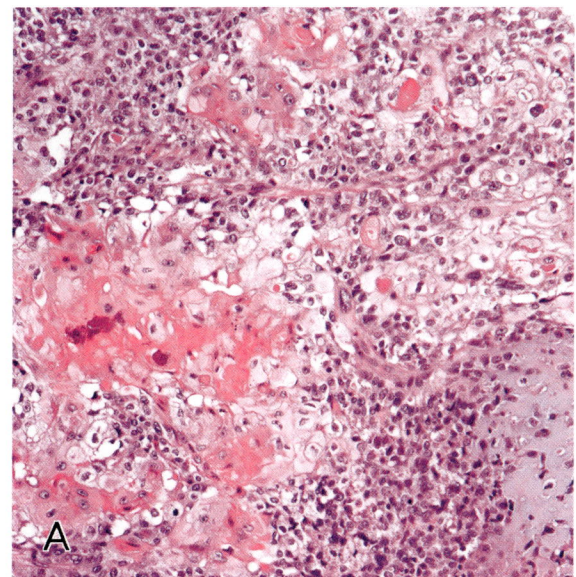

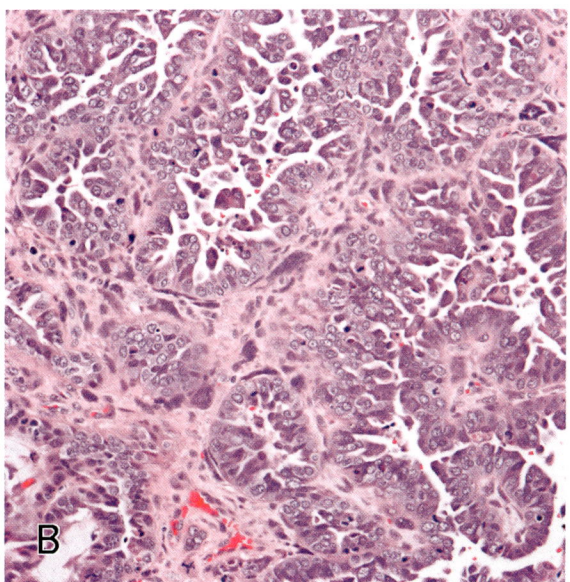

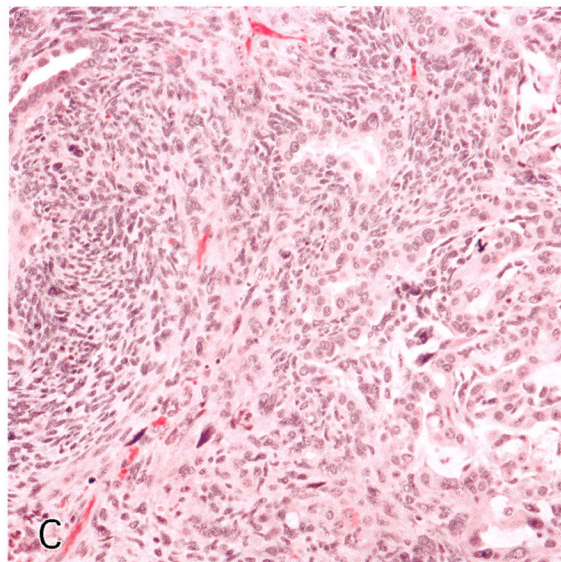

Figure 11-3

UTERINE CORPUS CARCINOSARCOMA: CARCINOMATOUS COMPONENTS

Squamous differentiation, indicative of endometrioid carcinoma (A). Serous carcinoma (B). High-grade carcinoma, not otherwise specified (C).

homologous-type sarcomatous components are represented by leiomyosarcoma or endometrial stromal sarcoma, most homologous carcinosarcomas do not contain such elements. A spindled sarcomatous component is more likely to be a spindle cell sarcoma, not otherwise specified, or a rhabdomyosarcoma with spindle cell morphology, while a component that resembles "high-grade endometrial stromal sarcoma" is more likely to be an undifferentiated carcinoma. In general, most homologous sarcomatous components of carcinosarcomas resemble what used to be diagnosed as "malignant fibrous histiocytoma" or high-grade "fibrosarcoma," and in the absence of the epithelial component, most tumors with homologous sarcomatous elements are currently diagnosed as undifferentiated uterine sarcomas of pleomorphic type (27).

Approximately half of carcinosarcomas contain heterologous elements (20,24), most commonly rhabdomyosarcoma and chondrosarcoma (figs. 11-5, 11-6) (24). When either element is present, a careful search often reveals the other component. Malignant osteoid is rare, and liposarcomatous and angiosarcomatous differentiation are even less common (20,28–30).

Figure 11-4

UTERINE CORPUS CARCINOSARCOMA WITH PLEOMORPHIC SARCOMATOUS ELEMENTS

The relationship between malignant glandular and pleomorphic sarcomatous elements is seen (A,B). Pleomorphic sarcomatous component with eosinophilic globules (C). The latter should not be misinterpreted as rhabdomyoblastic differentiation.

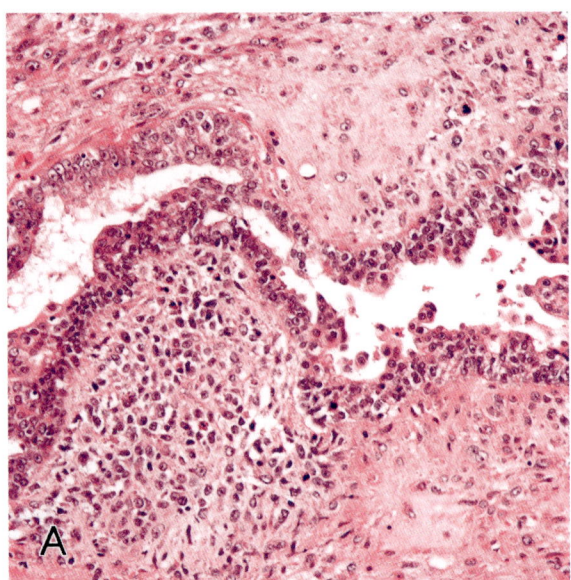

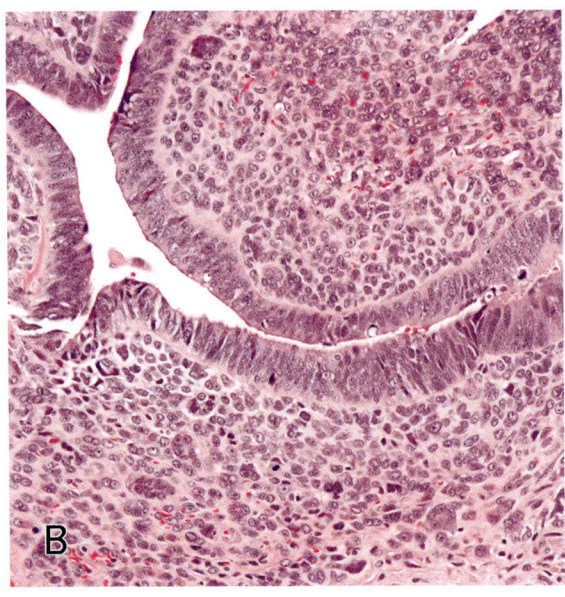

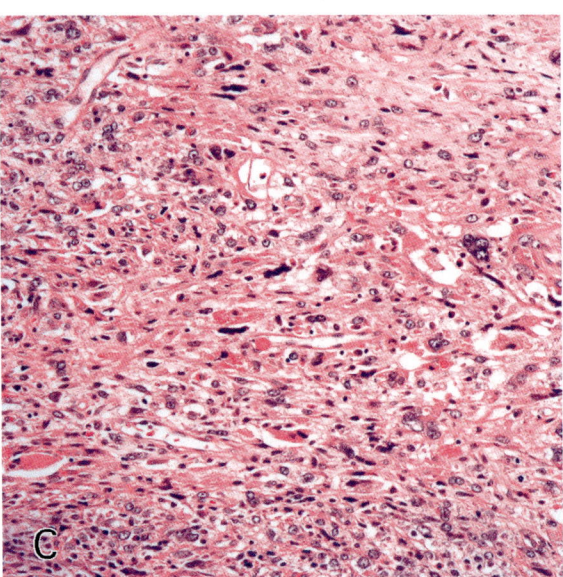

In addition to carcinomatous and sarcomatous elements, some carcinosarcomas contain components that resemble other tumor types, including central nervous system-type neuroectodermal differentiation (primitive neuroectodermal tumor [PNET] of central type), such as neuroblastoma, ependymoblastoma, and glioblastoma, and much less commonly, Wilms tumor and peripheral-type neuroectodermal tumor components (26,31–33). Rhabdoid or yolk sac tumor differentiation have been rarely reported (34,35).

The epithelial and mesenchymal elements are usually described as juxtaposed (fig. 11-7), without seamless transitions between the two. However, carcinosarcomas usually display both patterns, although the latter is usually much less apparent. Most carcinosarcomas have obvious representation of both epithelial and mesenchymal elements, but some are epithelial (fig. 11-8) or mesenchymal (fig. 11-9) predominant. The elements appear to be distributed randomly, but epithelial-predominant carcinosarcomas frequently display mesenchymal differentiation only in the most superficial areas of the tumor, which sometimes leads to diagnostic discrepancies between the original biopsy and subsequent hysterectomy. In

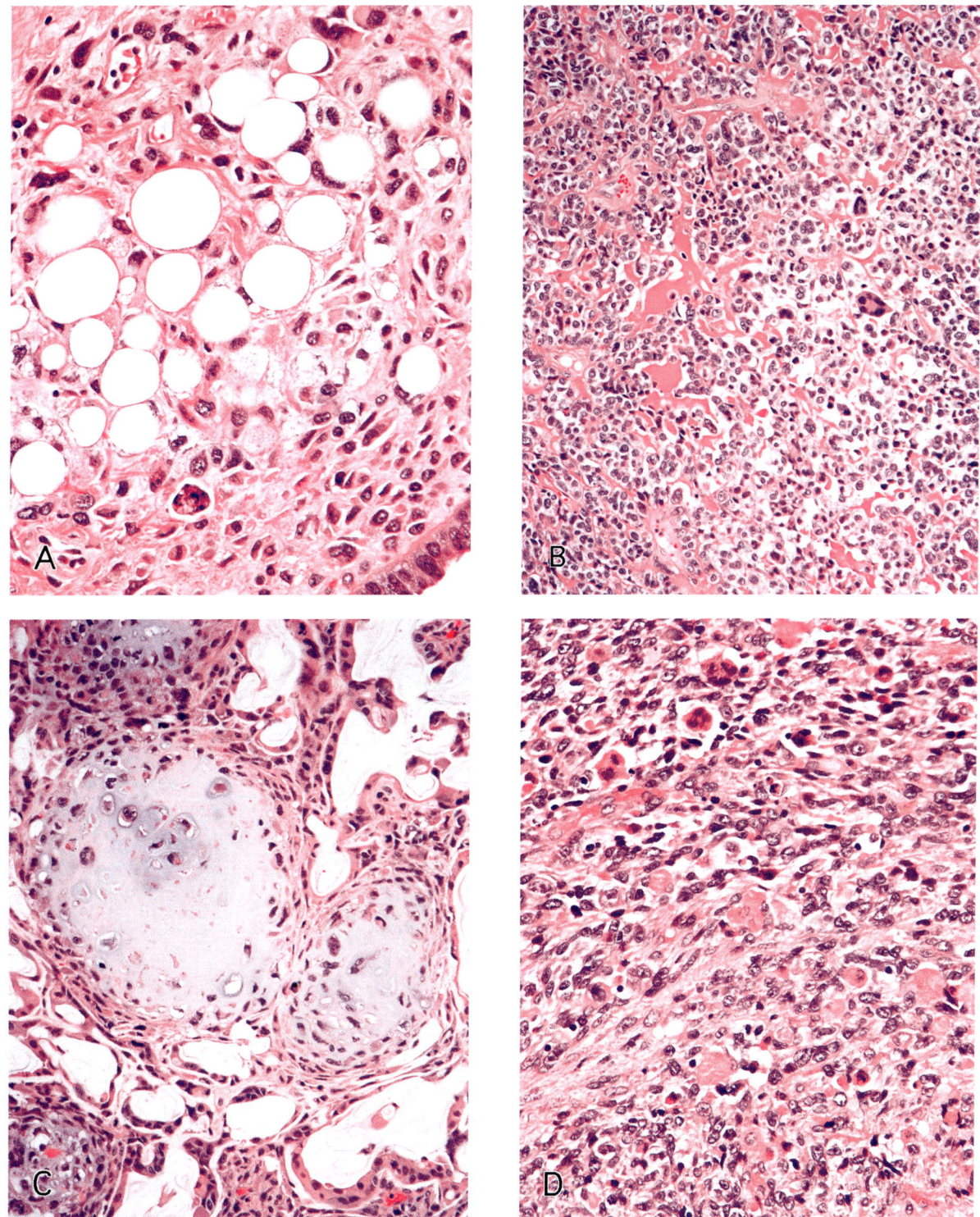

Figure 11-5

UTERINE CORPUS CARCINOSARCOMA WITH HETEROLOGOUS SARCOMATOUS ELEMENTS

Adipocytic (A), osteoid (B), cartilaginous (C), and skeletal muscle (D) differentiation. The latter two elements are more common.

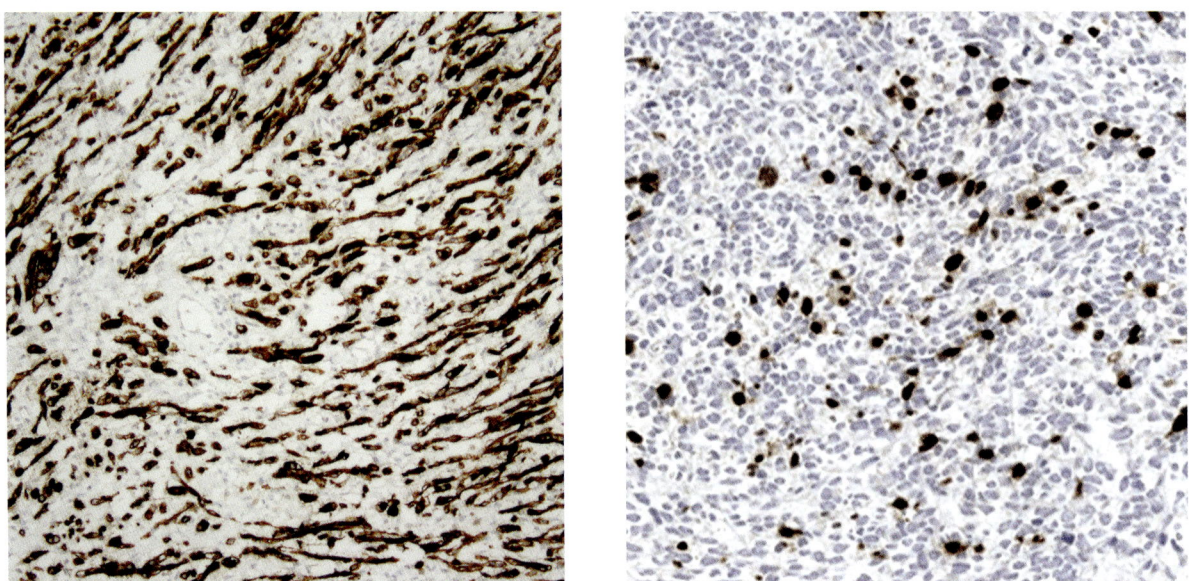

Figure 11-6

UTERINE CORPUS CARCINOSARCOMA WITH RHABDOMYOBLASTIC DIFFERENTIATION
Desmin (left) and myogenin (more specific) (right) confirm the presence of rhabdomyoblasts.

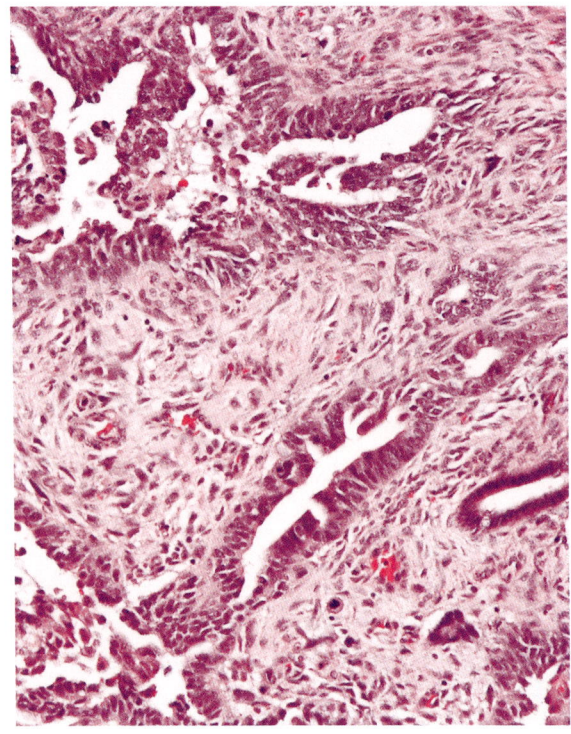

Figure 11-7

UTERINE CORPUS CARCINOSARCOMA
There is equal representation of epithelial and mesenchymal elements, which appear juxtaposed.

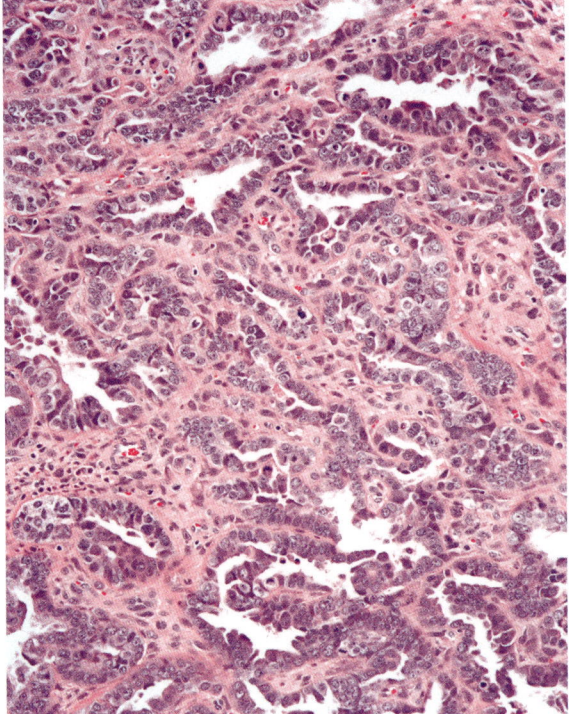

Figure 11-8

EPITHELIAL-PREDOMINANT UTERINE CORPUS CARCINOSARCOMA
The serous carcinoma comprises most of the tumor.

some other cases, extensive sampling is required to find a small component of carcinoma, thereby allowing for a diagnosis of carcinosarcoma.

In some carcinosarcomas, the epithelial component forms broad papillae or large irregular glands with a "phyllodes-type" morphology associated with condensation of the mesenchymal component under the epithelial component (figs. 11-10, 11-11). Such tumors have been described as having a low-power architecture resembling that of adenosarcoma, leading some authors to speculate as to whether some carcinosarcomas arise from adenosarcomas (36). On high-power examination, however, the epithelial and mesenchymal components are high grade, in contrast to the benign and low-grade malignant features of the epithelial and mesenchymal components in adenosarcoma (20,36–38).

Deep myometrial invasion as well as lymphovascular invasion are commonly seen. Tumor within vascular spaces is represented by carcinoma in over 95 percent of cases and only rarely by sarcoma or both (20,37). This finding correlates with the observation that metastases are most commonly composed of high-grade carcinoma (20,37).

Pathogenesis. Four theories have been postulated to explain the genesis of carcinosarcoma (2): 1) collision theory, in which carcinoma and sarcoma are two independent neoplasms; 2) combination theory, in which both components are derived from a single stem cell that undergoes divergent differentiation; 3) conversion theory, in which sarcomatous elements derive from the carcinoma; and 4) composition theory, in which the spindle cell component represents a pseudosarcomatous stromal reaction to the carcinoma. The recent Cancer Genomic Atlas Study provides data that strongly support the combination and conversion theories in the pathogenesis of carcinosarcomas (39). Some rare well-differentiated endometrioid adenocarcinomas that arise in the setting of mullerian adenosarcoma (considered by some to represent carcinosarcoma) may be explained by the collision theory (40). While spindle cell endometrioid carcinomas and related corded and hyalinized endometrioid carcinomas (41), (often misdiagnosed as carcinosarcoma) could be explained by the combination, conversion, or composition theories, a more modern ap-

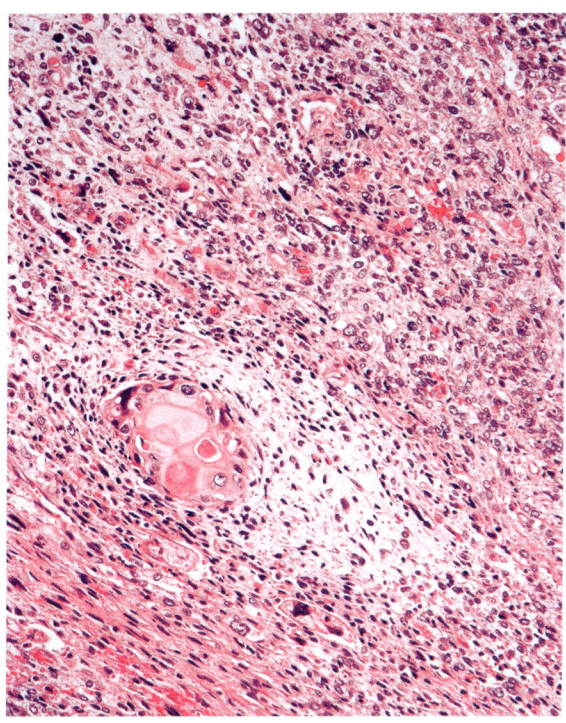

Figure 11-9

MESENCHYMAL-PREDOMINANT UTERINE CORPUS CARCINOSARCOMA

An undifferentiated pleomorphic sarcoma is the most extensive component and surrounds a nest of malignant squamous epithelium.

proach indicates that these tumors, as reported in carcinosarcomas, show evidence of epithelial to mesenchymal transition (39).

Immunohistochemical Findings. The immunophenotype of carcinosarcoma closely follows that of the individual elements present within the tumor. The epithelial component is often PAX8, epithelial membrane antigen (EMA), and keratin positive (42). Serous components show aberrant p53 expression while endometrioid components may show positivity for vimentin, CD10, and estrogen (ER) and progesterone (PR) receptors; variable PTEN and ARID1A loss of expression; and rarely, immunohistochemical loss of mismatch repair (MMR) proteins. Carcinosarcomas with an endometrioid component may also show aberrant expression of p53. Among heterologous elements, rhabdomyoblasts typically express desmin and myogenin (fig. 11-6) and S-100 protein may confirm a component of chondrosarcoma or liposarcoma.

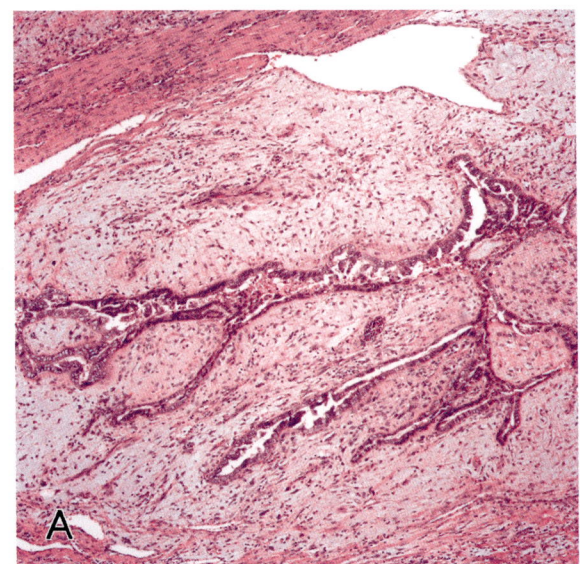

Figure 11-10

UTERINE CORPUS CARCINOSARCOMA WITH FEATURES OF ADENOSARCOMA

The low-power architecture suggests adenosarcoma (A). High-power magnification displays high-grade cytologic features of both epithelial and mesenchymal components (B,C).

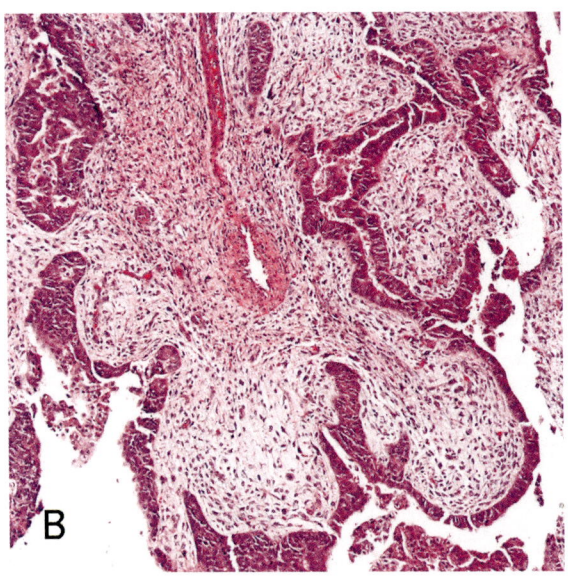

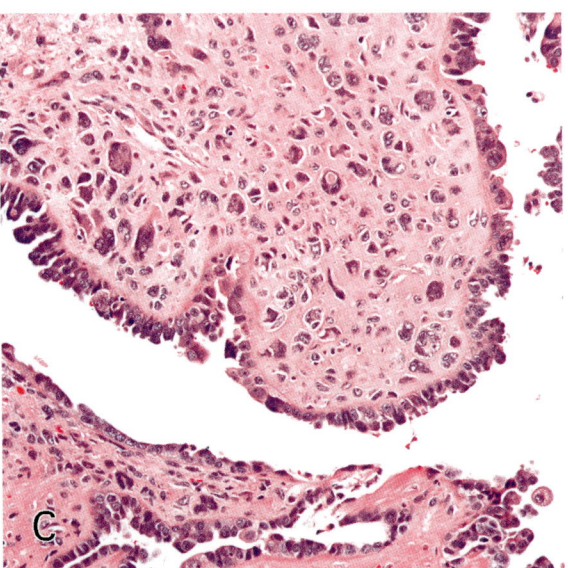

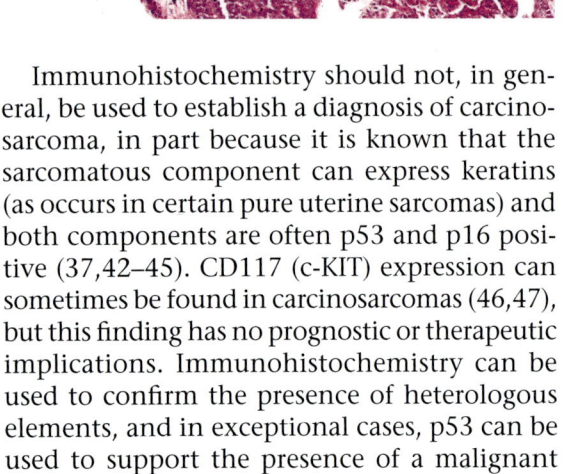

Immunohistochemistry should not, in general, be used to establish a diagnosis of carcinosarcoma, in part because it is known that the sarcomatous component can express keratins (as occurs in certain pure uterine sarcomas) and both components are often p53 and p16 positive (37,42–45). CD117 (c-KIT) expression can sometimes be found in carcinosarcomas (46,47), but this finding has no prognostic or therapeutic implications. Immunohistochemistry can be used to confirm the presence of heterologous elements, and in exceptional cases, p53 can be used to support the presence of a malignant epithelial component in a carcinosarcoma that may vaguely resemble an adenosarcoma (fig. 11-11).

Molecular Genetic Findings. Little is known about the genotype of carcinosarcomas (48,49). Tumors with serous and other high-grade carcinoma components have *TP53* and *PPP2R1A* mutations and those with an endometrioid component may have *PTEN, PIK3CA, KRAS, PPP2R1A, POLE, ARID1A,* and/or DNA MMR mutations (39). *p53* and *PTEN* mutations tend to be mutually exclusive.

As occurs with undifferentiated carcinomas, carcinosarcomas are thought to arise via epithelial to mesenchymal transition from an

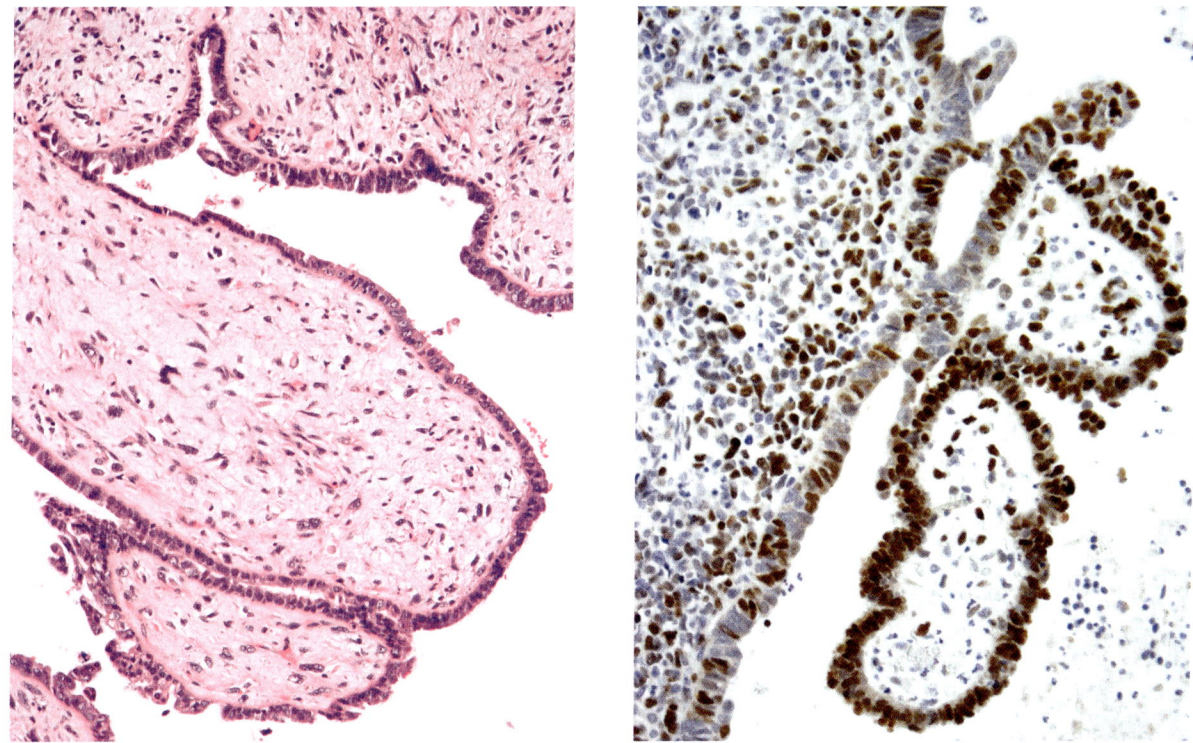

Figure 11-11

UTERINE CORPUS CARCINOSARCOMA

The tumor has an adenosarcomatous architecture and atypical, but not overtly malignant epithelium (left). p53 immunohistochemistry shows aberrant expression in atypical epithelium, as well as underlying stroma, supporting its malignant nature, and thus the diagnosis of carcinosarcoma (right).

epithelial substrate. Epithelial-mesenchymal transition is a process by which epithelial cells lose polarity and intercellular adhesion, while acquiring properties of mesenchymal cells. In uterine carcinosarcomas, epithelial-mesenchymal transition typically involves upregulation of the micro-RNA-200 series (39,50) with consequent upregulation of established EMT-related proteins such as ZEB-1 (51), SNAIL, and TWIST, and downregulation of E-cadherin as well as upregulation of *SLUG* gene by SOX4 and the beta-catenin/p300 complex (52).

Differential Diagnosis. *Endometrioid Adenocarcinoma with Corded and Hyalinized* or *Spindle Cell Elements*. The former is more often seen in the endometrium (41) while the latter is more frequently encountered in the ovary where it was first described (53). The presence of a "biphasic" pattern, myxohyaline change that mimics cartilage, and mitotically active, spindle cells may all contribute to diagnostic difficulties.

The endometrioid glands in the corded and hyalinized variant frequently show squamous metaplasia and transition to a corded growth associated with dense and often prominent stromal hyalinization. In endometrioid carcinomas with spindled cells, the glands also merge imperceptibly with the spindle component. In both, the cytologic features are low-grade in contrast to carcinosarcoma. Distinction between corded, hyalinized, or spindled endometrioid carcinoma and carcinosarcoma, however, may be challenging or impossible in some cases as some tumors may show a transition from low- to high-grade nuclear atypia in the corded or spindled components. The guiding principle remains that carcinosarcoma should be diagnosed when the spindle cell component of such tumors is pleomorphic or heterologous and high grade. Finally, some *FIGO Grade 3 endometrioid carcinomas* also display sex cord-like features, dense tromal hyalinization, and seamless fusion with spindled elements but no clearcut mesenchymal elements are present.

Endometrioid Adenocarcinoma with Metaplastic Osteoid Elements. These elements are histologically benign and occur in FIGO grades 1 and 2 endometrioid carcinomas, with conventional, spindle, or corded or hyalinized morphology. They are thought to behave clinically like typical low-grade endometrioid carcinomas (41).

Müllerian Adenosarcoma. As mentioned previously, some carcinosarcomas display an adenosarcoma-like architecture, however, they demonstrate high-grade carcinomatous components, frequently in the form of serous carcinoma, along with the high-grade sarcoma. In contrast, low-grade müllerian adenosarcomas show low-grade mesenchymal components and benign or atypical epithelial elements. If it is uncertain whether the epithelial component is neoplastic or metaplastic in nature, p53 immunostaining may be helpful in this differential diagnosis as aberrant expression is indicative of a serous or serous-like epithelial component, thereby excluding a diagnosis of adenosarcoma. If an adenosarcoma is associated with carcinoma, it is typically a FIGO grade 1 endometrioid carcinoma (40).

Undifferentiated and Dedifferentiated Carcinoma. The former might be mistakenly categorized as carcinosarcoma when patches of cytokeratin-immunoreactive cells are noted in a background of vimentin-positive but cytokeratin-negative cells. The presence of rhabdoid cells also may suggest a carcinosarcoma. Undifferentiated endometrial carcinoma, however, is not a biphasic tumor and immunohistochemistry should be avoided in this setting, as this may lead to the misinterpretation of the tumor as carcinosarcoma (54). Undifferentiated carcinomas may be associated with a low-grade endometrioid carcinoma ("dedifferentiated endometrial carcinoma" or "mixed endometrioid and undifferentiated carcinoma"), but do not meet the criteria for carcinosarcoma, as the epithelial component is typically FIGO grade 1 or 2. Distinction from carcinosarcoma can be problematic, however, when the dedifferentiated carcinoma contains a component of FIGO grade 3 endometrioid carcinoma. In this scenario, it is crucial to study the small, round blue cell component of the tumor; finding cellular dyshesion and uniform cytology supports a diagnosis of dedifferentiated carcinoma, in contrast to the pleomorphism typically seen in the sarcomatous components of a carcinosarcoma.

Combined Adenocarcinoma and Neuroendocrine Carcinoma. This can mimic carcinosarcoma since the glandular component may be similar in both entities and both have a biphasic appearance. However, areas with neuroendocrine differentiation histologically resemble their pulmonary counterparts, and are typically cytologically monomorphic (55–57). The recognition of a small cell carcinoma component is based on the presence of small cells with nuclear molding, salt and pepper chromatin, and abundant mitoses and apoptotic bodies. Immunohistochemistry should be used in conjunction with morphology in this differential diagnosis.

Mesonephric Carcinosarcomas. Although exceedingly rare when compared to mesonephric carcinomas, these tumors have been reported in the uterine cervix and corpus (58,59). The sarcomatous components may overlap significantly with müllerian carcinosarcomas since both can show heterologous rhabdomyoblastic and cartilaginous differentiation. The epithelial component should resemble mesonephric adenocarcinoma but may also contain a solid, poorly differentiated carcinoma, similarly to müllerian carcinosarcoma. The epithelial component may be PAX8, p16, CD10 and, rarely, ER positive (60), an immunohistochemical profile that overlaps with müllerian carcinosarcoma. Characteristic, but not necessarily diagnostic, is a glandular or tubular growth, with luminal eosinophilic colloid-like material. There is often an admixture of ductal, papillary, retiform, and glomeruloid architectures. Although no immunohistochemical data are reported for endometrial mesonephric carcinosarcoma, mesonephric carcinomas and mesonephric-like carcinomas may be GATA3 and TTF-1 positive, in contrast to most müllerian carcinomas (61) and have *K-RAS* mutations (62,63).

Rare tumors in the differential diagnosis include undifferentiated uterine sarcomas, heterologous sarcomas, Sertoli-Leydig cell tumor (64), teratoma (65), Wilms tumor (66-68), and PNETs of peripheral (Ewing) or central type (akin to medulloblastoma, for example) (31,32). The diagnosis of undifferentiated uterine sarcoma as well as heterologous sarcoma is one of exclusion and extensive sampling in such cases may be helpful in identifying a minor carcinoma component. Although Sertoli-Leydig cell tumors and teratomas are by far more common in the ovary, they are occasionally considered in the differential diagnosis of a müllerian carcinosarcoma since all may have heterologous elements including cartilage and rhabdomyoblastic differentiation. In contrast to carcinosarcoma, fetal-type cartilage is typical of Sertoli-Leydig cell tumors, Wilms tumors with heterologous elements, and teratoma, seen in association with other distinctive features of these tumors (65,69).

Rosettes and pseudorosettes of pure central-type PNET can be misinterpreted as epithelial elements, and thus, raise concern for a biphasic tumor such as a carcinosarcoma (31,32). In general, these epithelial-like elements are present in a background of central-type PNET, and typical areas of carcinosarcoma showing high-grade epithelial and mesenchymal components are lacking. Although keratin expression may be encountered in neuroectodermal tumors (31,32), strong expression of both cytokeratins and EMA is unusual; any such expression in a component of a biphasic tumor resembling a neuroectodermal tumor should prompt consideration of combined carcinoma and neuroectodermal tumor or combined carcinosarcoma and neuroectodermal tumor (when a sarcomatous component is also present). Carcinosarcomas with Ewing/PNET or central-type PNET components should contain areas of conventional malignant mixed mullerian tumor to establish a diagnosis of carcinosarcoma. The presence of carcinoma, sarcoma, and a neuroectodermal, Wilms or teratomatous component should suggest either carcinosarcoma with heterologous differentiation or so-called teratoid carcinosarcoma (34).

Treatment and Prognosis. The 5-year survival rate for patients with carcinosarcoma is approximately 30 percent while the 5-year survival rate for those with surgical stage I disease (confined to uterus) is approximately 50 percent (20,24,70–72). This very aggressive behavior contrasts with that of other high-grade endometrial carcinomas where the 5-year rate for stage I disease is 80 percent or higher (73,74). Stage is the most consistent independent predictor of outcome in these patients (75,76).

The wide range in 5-year survival rates, from 35 to 75 percent in women with early-stage disease has engendered several clinicopathologic studies to identify possible prognostic factors (20,24,37,70–72,76–79). The presence of deep myometrial invasion and lymphovascular invasion are important prognostic factors in patients with FIGO stage 1 and 2 carcinosarcomas that have not undergone comprehensive surgical staging, and can help to identify those women at highest risk of harboring occult metastases (20,77). As many as 60 percent of patients with seemingly organ-confined disease have occult extrauterine metastases, primarily in the abdomen and lymph nodes (20,71,77,78). These indices, however, have little prognostic value for women with comprehensively staged tumors confined to the uterine corpus (71).

It has been reported that the presence of heterologous elements is a poor prognostic factor in comprehensively staged, FIGO stage 1 tumors (24). In one study, 30 percent of patients with carcinosarcomas showing heterologous elements survived 5 years, compared to 80 percent of patients with homologous carcinosarcomas. Other prognostic factors studied include age, CA125 levels, tumor size, stage and grade of the carcinomatous and sarcomatous elements, percentage of tumor demonstrating sarcomatous differentiation, residual disease, and therapeutic modality (20,24,70–72,79). It is currently unclear whether the presence of heterologous elements has importance in the setting of advanced stage disease.

Following cytoreductive surgery (80), adjuvant therapy with chemotherapy alone or in combination with radiation therapy is now recommended for patients with carcinosarcoma (81). There are no data from prospective and randomized clinical trials to suggest that treating the predominant tumor component (i.e., rhabdomyosarcoma, when present) is preferable to standard therapy; however, a large, retrospective analysis (79) found platinum-based agents and anthracyclines to be beneficial for high-grade carcinoma with homologous sarcoma and high-grade carcinoma with heterologous sarcoma, respectively. That study also pointed out that the carcinomatous component tends to metastasize via lymphatics (involving lymph nodes), while the sarcomatous component tends to spread

Table 11-1

INTERNATIONAL FEDERATION OF GYNECOLOGY AND OBSTETRICS (FIGO) STAGING FOR MÜLLERIAN ADENOSARCOMA

IA	Tumor limited to endometrium/endocervix
IB	Myometrial invasion up to 50%
IC	Myometrial invasion >50%
IIA	Tumor extends to the pelvis, adnexal involvement
IIB	Tumor extends to extrauterine pelvic tissue
IIIA	Tumor invades abdominal tissues, one site
IIIB	Abdominal disease involving more than one site
IIIC	Metastasis to pelvic and/or para-aortic lymph nodes
IVA	Tumor invades bladder and/or rectum
IVB	Distant metastasis

locoregionally (vagina and cervical stroma). In line with the older literature, 74 percent of metastases were composed of carcinoma only, 18 percent were sarcoma only, and the remainder showed combinations of carcinoma and sarcoma. When comparing metastatic sites in carcinosarcoma and other high-grade endometrial carcinomas, carcinosarcomas appeared to more frequently metastasize to the lungs while rates of metastases to liver, peritoneum, lymph nodes, and vagina were not significantly different (75).

LOW-GRADE MÜLLERIAN ADENOSARCOMA

Definition. *Müllerian adenosarcoma* is a biphasic neoplasm composed of sarcoma, usually low-grade, associated with benign, metaplastic, or hyperplastic epithelium. The characteristic spatial organization of both elements distinguishes this tumor from other biphasic uterine neoplasms.

General Features. Adenosarcomas constitute less than 1 percent of endometrial malignancies and about 6 percent of uterine sarcomas, with the uterine corpus being the most common location within the female genital tract (cervical, adnexal, and peritoneal primary tumors are much less common) (82,83). Most patients are perimenopausal or postmenopausal, with a mean age at diagnosis of about 60 years (40, 84–86), but rare patients are premenopausal or even adolescents. An association with breast carcinoma, tamoxifen use, radiation therapy, and history of unopposed estrogens has been reported in some patients (87–89).

Clinical Features. Many patients present with vaginal bleeding or abdominal discomfort; a large polypoid mass prolapsing through the cervical os may be noted on gynecologic examination, and may give the false impression of a primary cervical tumor. Rarely, patients have a history of recurrent endometrial polyps (40, 90), but retrospective review has revealed a diagnostically challenging adenosarcoma. Uncommon presentations include symptoms related to prolapse, vaginal discharge, or an abnormal Pap smear. Some patients are asymptomatic.

Adenosarcomas are staged according to the 2009 FIGO classification (Table 11-1) (91). Almost all patients have a low-stage tumor at the time of initial diagnosis (confined to the uterus) in contrast to primary extrauterine adenosarcomas, which are more frequently high stage.

Gross Findings. Adenosarcomas typically present as large, bulky, polypoid tumors (fig. 11-12) with an average size of 5 cm, but both significantly smaller and larger tumors have been reported (range, 1 to 17 cm in largest study) (40). Occasionally, adenosarcomas fill the endometrial cavity. On sectioning, these tumors may display round and bulbous projections separated by clefts, set in a solid rubbery to fleshy and tan to grayish white background, with or without hemorrhage and necrosis. Multiple cysts, sometimes containing mucoid material or hemorrhage, may impart a spongy appearance. Less commonly, multiple small polyps or a diffuse growth is seen (40,92).

Most tumors are endometrial (corpus) based, with fewer arising in the lower uterine segment, cervix, and myometrium. The latter may be associated with adenomyosis or, rarely, an adenomyoma (40,87,93–95). Myometrial invasion can be detected on gross examination, but in most instances it is only superficial. If sarcomatous overgrowth is present, it displays a fleshy, gelatinous or encephaloid appearance, often gray-white color, sometimes with necrosis, hemorrhage, or both, and deep myometrial invasion is frequently found (40,96). Tumors associated with sex cord-like overgrowth may display discrete masses that have well-circumscribed margins and homogeneous, soft, tan to yellow cut surfaces (96–98). Synchronous

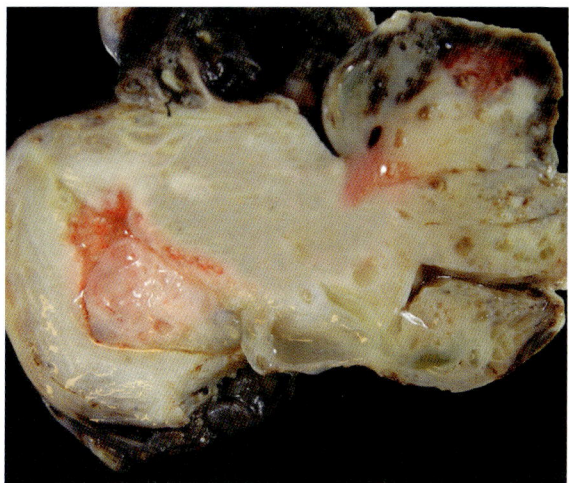 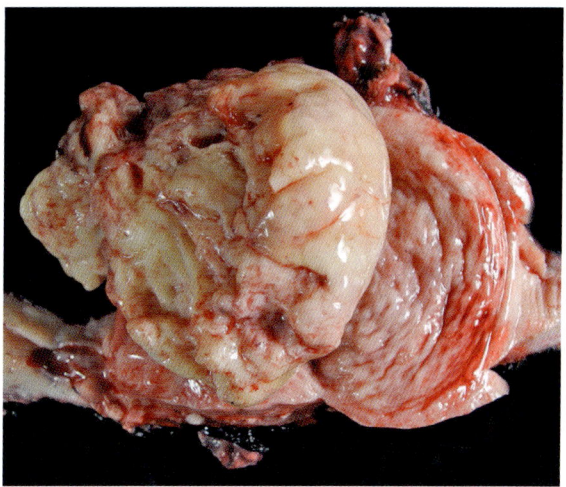

Figure 11-12

MÜLLERIAN ADENOSARCOMA

The tumor is polypoid and protrudes through the cervical canal. The cut surface is homogenous, showing multiple cysts containing mucus and lacks necrosis in contrast to carcinosarcomas (left). Sarcomatous overgrowth shows a fleshy cut surface (right).

uterine and extrauterine adenosarcomas have been reported (40,93).

Microscopic Findings. At scanning magnification, adenosarcomas typically exhibit homogeneously distributed glands and cysts containing stromal papillae and leaf-like formations associated with subepithelial stromal condensation (collaring) and less cellular interglandular stroma (figs. 11-13–11-15), an overall appearance often reminiscent of an intracanalicular fibroadenoma or phyllodes tumor of the breast. Club-like stromal papillae may protrude onto the endometrial surface (fig. 11-14). Some cysts have a round and "rigid" appearance, without intraglandular stromal projections (fig. 11-15), while glands distorted by stromal projections can display slit-like outlines. This very ordered epithelial-stromal spatial relationship is maintained throughout the tumor if stromal overgrowth is absent.

The epithelial component of adenosarcoma is typically composed of glands, cysts, clefts, and fronds lined by endometrioid-type cells often reminiscent of the proliferative-phase endometrium, less commonly inactive or atrophic, and almost always benign in appearance. Metaplastic changes as encountered in non-neoplastic endometrium are also noted (fig. 11-16), most commonly squamous (typically nonkeratinizing), tubal, and, less commonly, eosinophilic, mucinous, secretory, papillary, or hobnail (99). In rare instances, the epithelium may be hyperplastic or even show architectural features of a well-differentiated endometrioid adenocarcinoma (40), such as cribriform and back-to-back glands; epithelial cytologic atypia may also be encountered. In the largest series published in the literature, these changes were reported in 10 percent and one-third of tumors, respectively, although importantly they were typically focal (40). In that series, six adenosarcomas had a component of atypical hyperplasia, one showed a well-differentiated endometrioid adenocarcinoma, and another had a synchronous, well-differentiated endometrioid adenocarcinoma secondarily involving the adenosarcoma. One intraepithelial clear cell carcinoma has been reported, although in an ovarian adenosarcoma (100). The finding of focal well-differentiated endometrioid adenocarcinoma should not lead to a reflexive diagnosis of carcinosarcoma; it is preferred to report these as carcinoma present or arising in a background of adenosarcoma (40).

The stromal component is hypercellular and low grade, typically condensing around the epithelium (periglandular cuffing) or forming intraluminal polypoid projections. In tumors lacking stromal overgrowth, the stroma intervening between glands is hypocellular, thereby

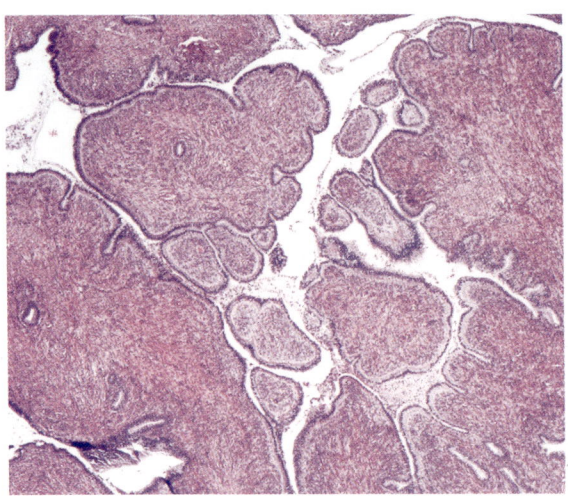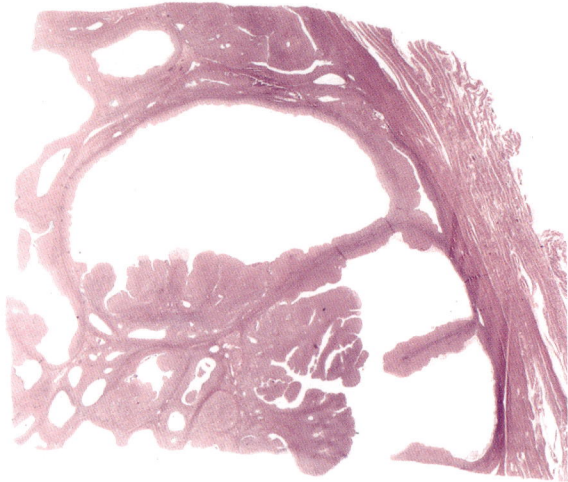

Figure 11-13

LOW-GRADE MÜLLERIAN ADENOSARCOMA

Typical bulbous fronds and subtle subepithelial stromal condensation are seen (left). Even within the cysts, bulbous projections are appreciated (right).

Figure 11-14

LOW-GRADE MÜLLERIAN ADENOSARCOMA WITH PHYLLODES-LIKE ARCHITECTURE

Club-like (A), phyllodes-like (B), and intraglandular stromal papillary (C) architectural patterns are seen.

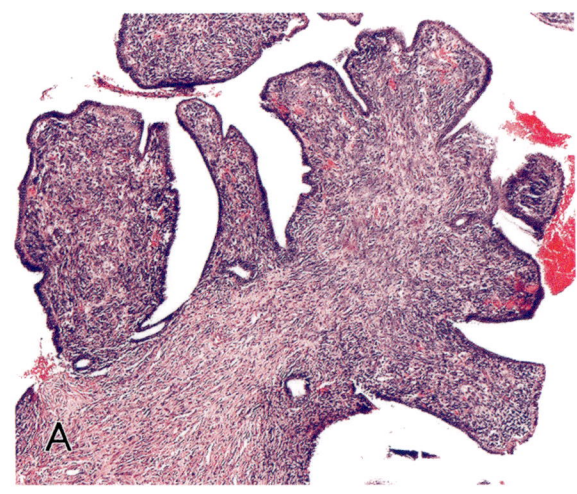
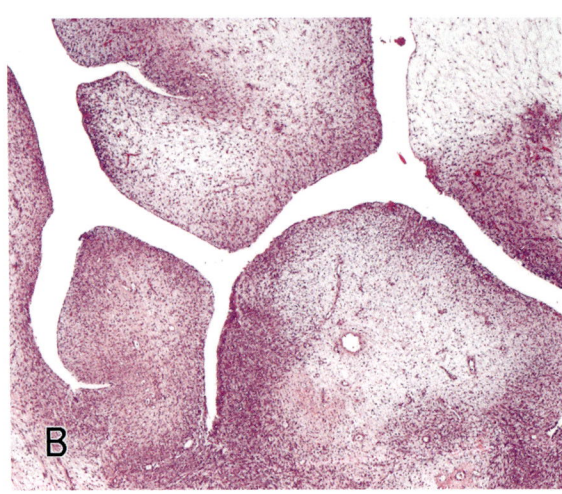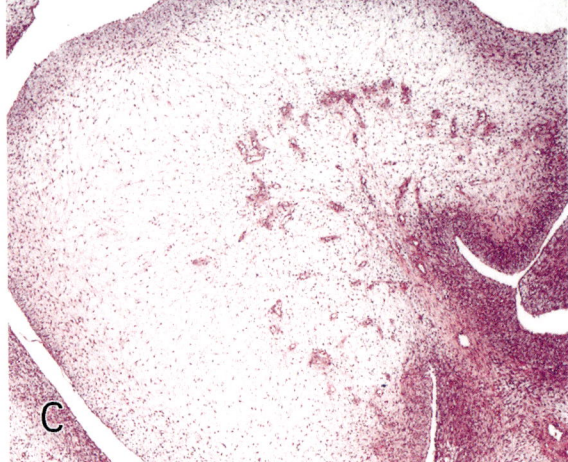

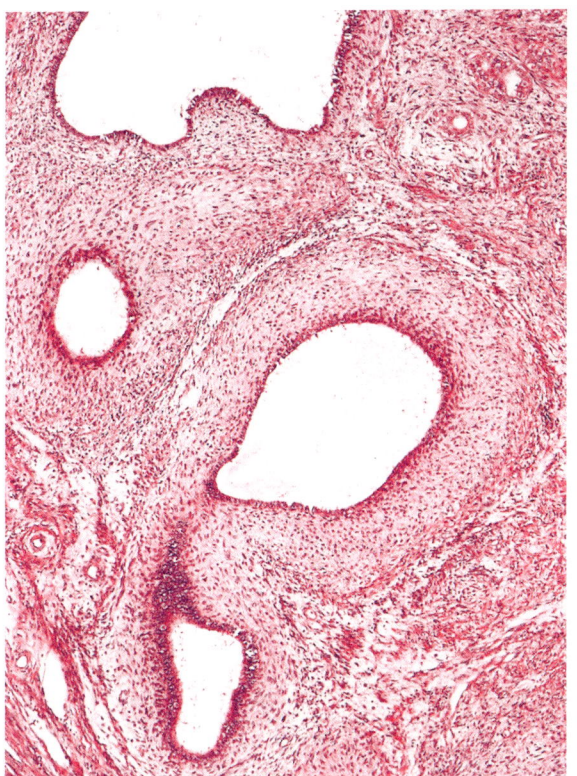 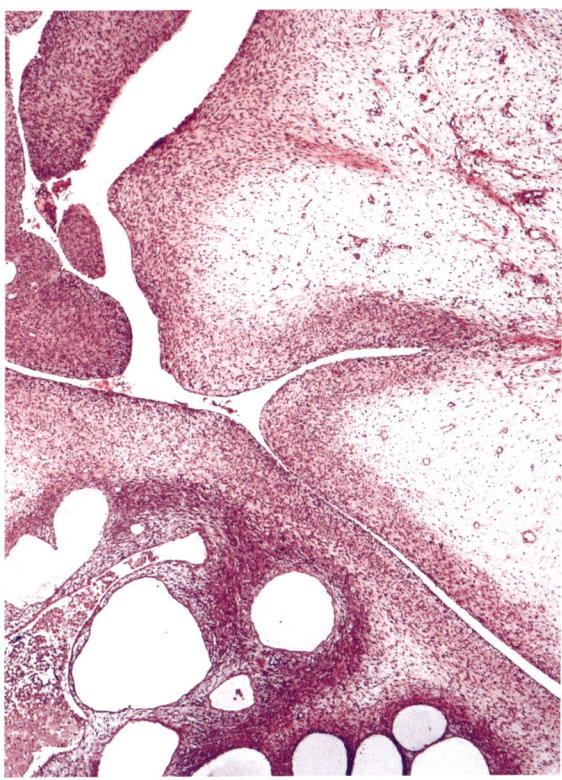

Figure 11-15

LOW-GRADE MÜLLERIAN ADENOSARCOMA

"Rigid" cysts (left) and elongated glands (right) are surrounded by a variably thickened hypercellular stromal cuff.

contrasting with the appearance of the periglandular stromal cuffs. The band of stromal condensation around glands, however, may be thin or attenuated and rarely the stroma may be uniformly cellular. The hypercellular areas exhibit a proliferation of small, nondescript, ovoid to spindled cells with scant cytoplasm and plump nuclei with variable mitotic activity, most often resembling the morphology of an endometrial stromal sarcoma (about 60 percent), sometimes with pseudodecidual change (fig. 11-17).

The stromal nuclear features are usually mildly to moderately atypical, although rare tumors display severe cytologic atypia, which should prompt additional sampling to detect stromal overgrowth. The hypercellular areas may also have a histologic appearance similar to a low-grade fibroblastic or myofibroblastic sarcoma (about 10 percent) or show other types of differentiation including smooth muscle differentiation (fig. 11-18) (40). The latter may have a spindle or epithelioid morphology, and when found in a periglandular location, the typical condensation of stroma may not be apparent (88,101).

Approximately 20 percent of adenosarcomas contain heterologous elements, usually only focally. Fetal-type cartilage and scattered rhabdomyoblasts are most common; less commonly, adipose or even neuroectodermal tissue can be present (40,85). Some adenosarcomas contain sex cord-like elements in the form of nests, trabeculae, cords, hollow or solid tubules, and nests or sheets of cells with eosinophilic, pale or finely vacuolated cytoplasm and round to oval nuclei, sometimes with grooves or small nucleoli. These features impart an overall appearance similar to granulosa, Sertoli, or Sertoli-Leydig cell tumors of the ovary (fig. 11-19) (96–98,102). Sex cord-like elements may represent more than 50 percent of the total tumor, and in such cases (sex cord overgrowth), the microscopic appearance correlates with a well-demarcated mass on gross examination (96–98,102).

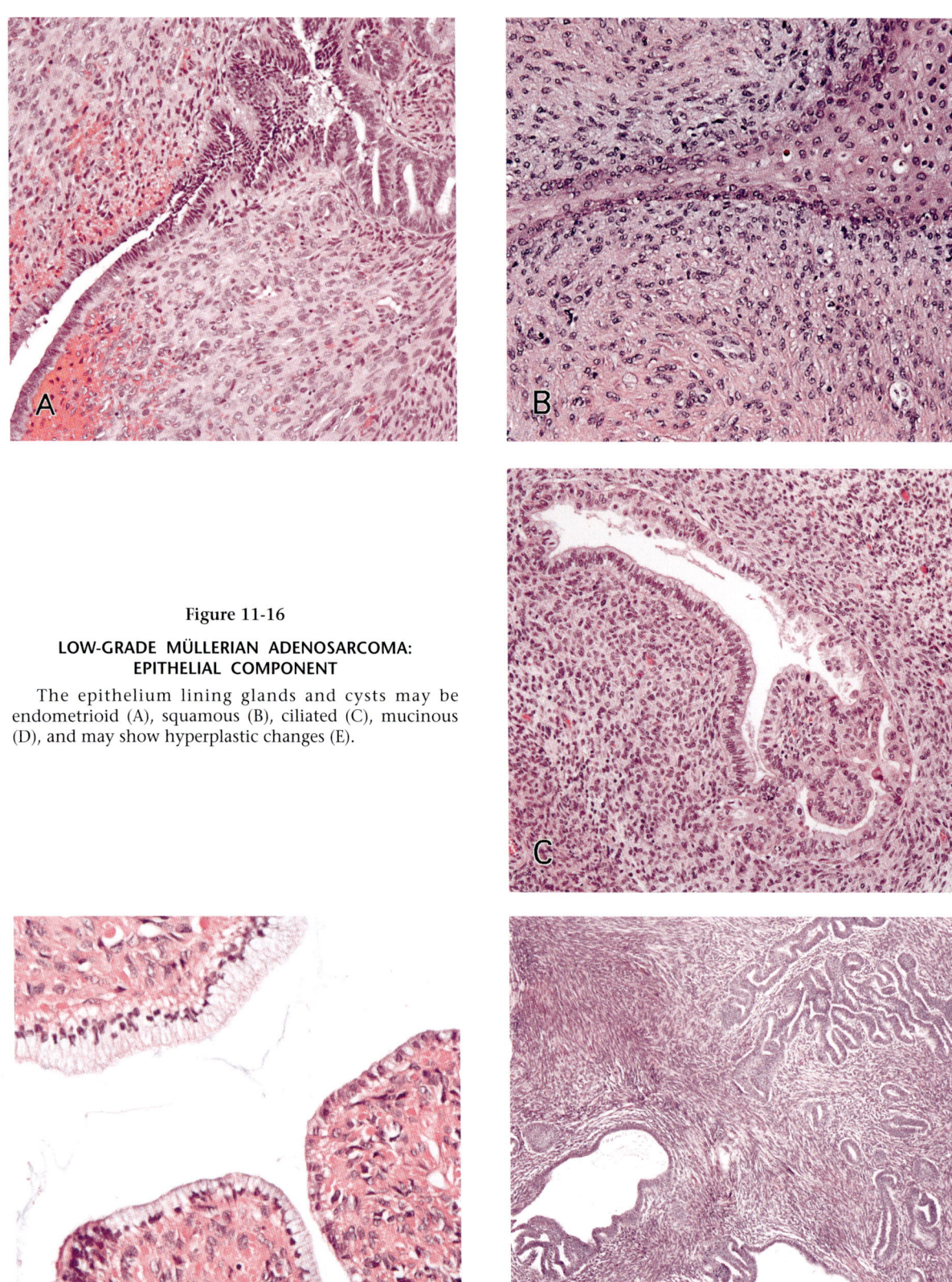

Figure 11-16

LOW-GRADE MÜLLERIAN ADENOSARCOMA: EPITHELIAL COMPONENT

The epithelium lining glands and cysts may be endometrioid (A), squamous (B), ciliated (C), mucinous (D), and may show hyperplastic changes (E).

Mixed Epithelial-Stromal Tumors

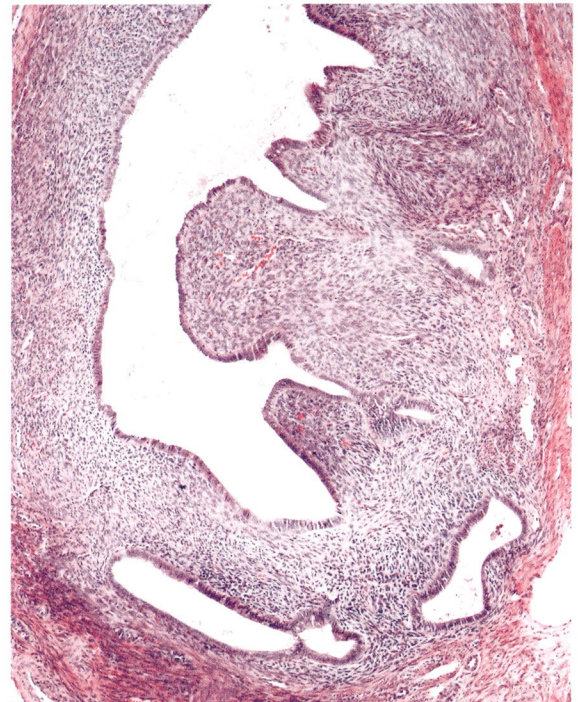
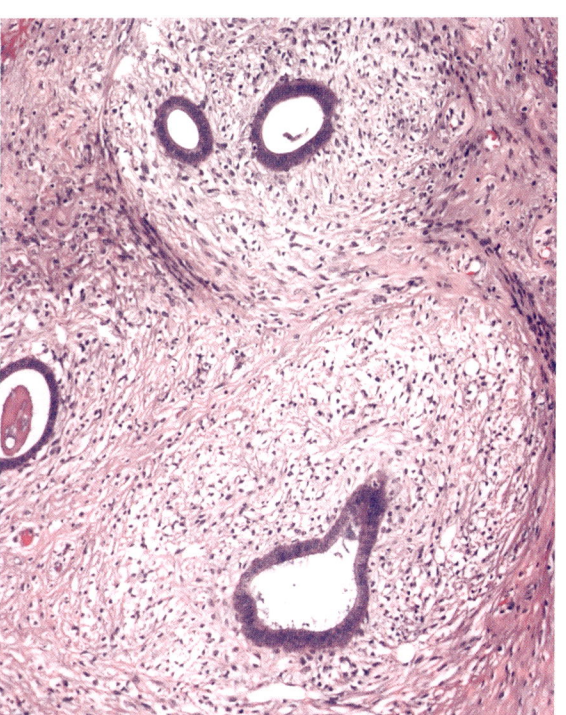

Figure 11-17

STROMA IN LOW-GRADE MÜLLERIAN ADENOSARCOMA

The stroma often resembles endometrial stroma (left) which may be myxoid (right).

Nonspecific changes often seen within the neoplastic stroma include edema, myxoid change (fig. 11-17), fibrosis, and hyalinization and, less commonly, abundant foamy histiocytes, multinucleated giant cells, chronic inflammatory infiltrate, and hemosiderin-laden macrophages (99). A uterine adenosarcoma with a predominant histiocytic (xanthomatous) stroma has been reported (103). The interglandular stroma is, as mentioned earlier, hypocellular and usually cytologically less "atypical" than stroma in the subepithelial cuffs.

In the past, the finding of at least 4 mitoses per 10 high-power fields in the stromal component was required for the diagnosis of adenosarcoma (86), but this rule no longer appears to be uniformly followed. Tumor architecture takes diagnostic precedence over mitotic index since rare tumors with low mitotic counts can have an aggressive clinical course. In the largest study to date (40), the mean mitotic index in the sarcomatous component was 9 mitoses per 10 high-power fields, but rare tumors with fewer than 2 mitoses per 10 high-power fields have

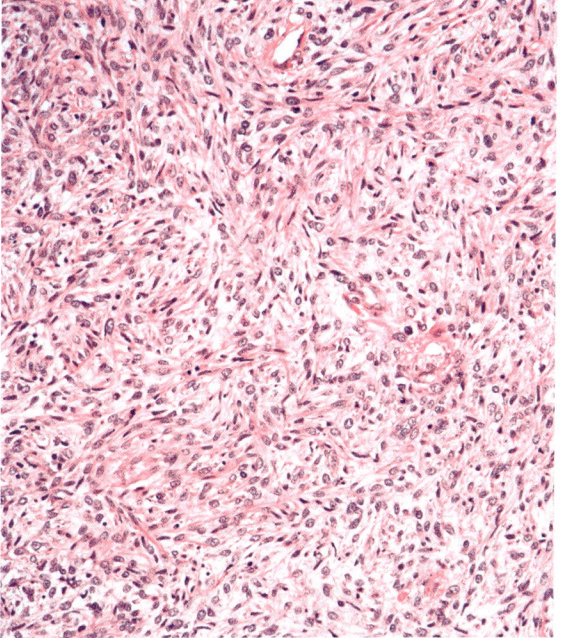

Figure 11-18

STROMA IN LOW-GRADE MÜLLERIAN ADENOSARCOMA

The stroma resembles that of fibrosarcoma.

Figure 11-19
LOW-GRADE MÜLLERIAN ADENOSARCOMA WITH SEX CORD-LIKE DIFFERENTIATION

Clusters and nests of lipidized cells are noted within the neoplastic endometrial-like stroma (A). Overgrowth of sex cord-like elements is juxtaposed to typical adenosarcoma (B). Inhibin stains areas of sex cord-like differentiation (C). (A and C courtesy of Dr. S. Stonilcu, Targu Mures, Romania).

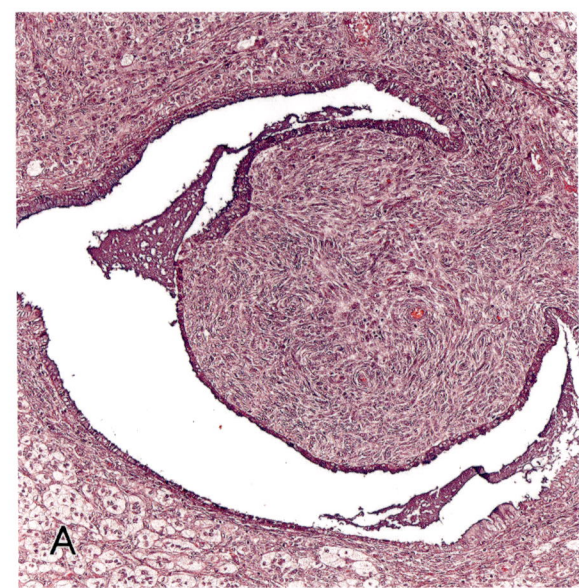
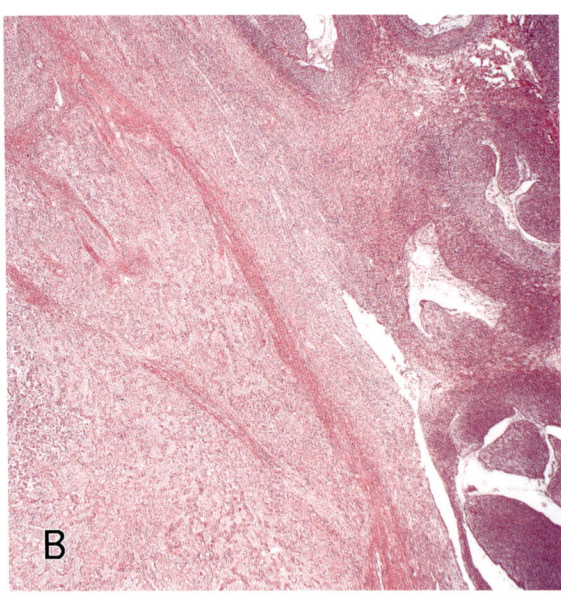
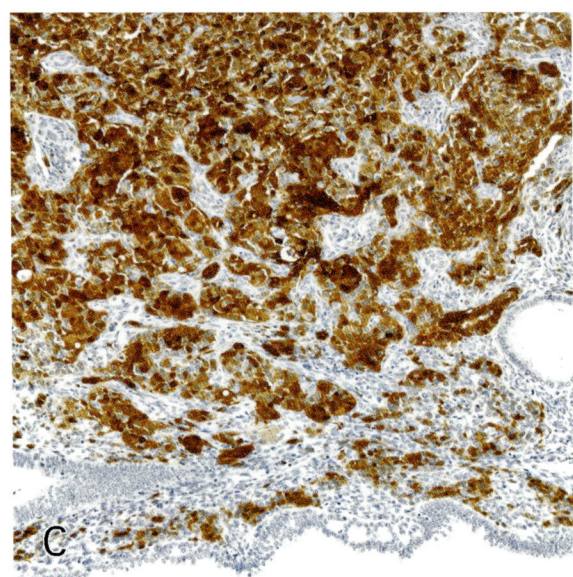

recurred even in the absence of stromal overgrowth. Tumors with lower mitotic rates have been reported in more contemporary studies, indicating the diagnostic importance of architectural features for the diagnosis of low-grade adenosarcoma (40,92,104,105). It is important to keep in mind that there may be interobserver variation in counting mitoses, and progesterone may influence mitotic rates.

In about 10 percent of adenosarcomas, there is sarcomatous overgrowth (fig. 11-20). Originally, sarcomatous overgrowth was defined as sarcoma, without associated epithelium, that constituted at least 25 percent of the tumor (105a), but this definition was recently amended in the 2014 WHO classification to indicate that the sarcoma should be histologically high grade (4). The term "low-grade sarcomatous overgrowth" has been used for adenosarcomas associated with overgrowth of a low-grade homologous sarcoma, but this phenomenon is exceedingly rare, and although associated with recurrences, these tumors have an indolent behavior (106). Compared to typical müllerian adenosarcomas, those with sarcomatous overgrowth more commonly invade deeply into

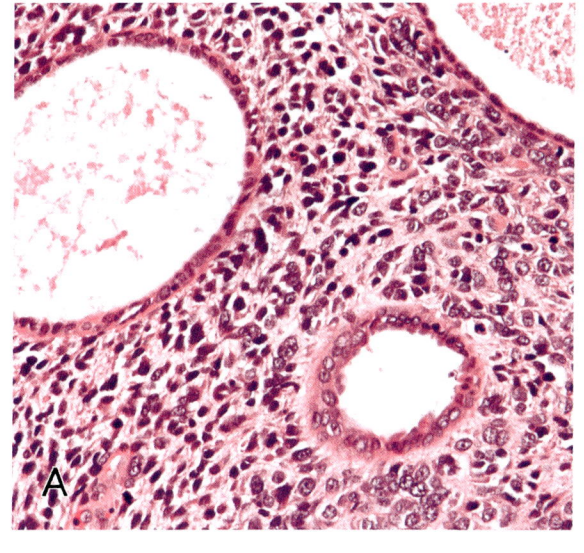
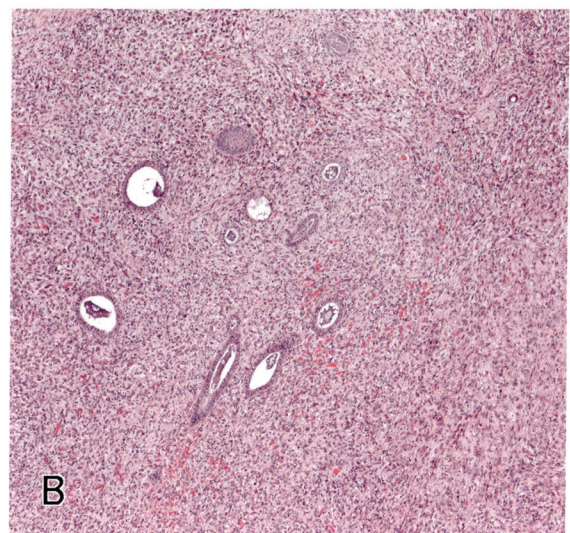
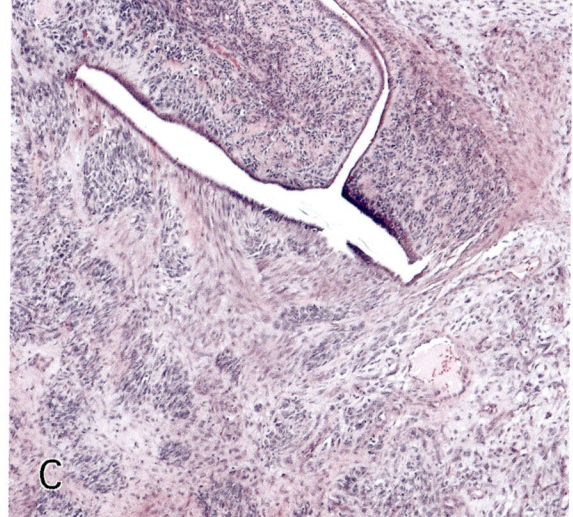

Figure 11-20

HIGH-RISK MORPHOLOGIC FEATURES IN MÜLLERIAN ADENOSARCOMA

Epitheliotropic rhabdomyosarcoma originating in adenosarcoma (latter not shown) (A). Abundant malignant stroma to suggest the presence of sarcomatous overgrowth (B). Overt sarcomatous overgrowth (C). Myometrial invasion that shows both glandular and stromal elements (D). Myometrial invasion consisting only of sarcoma (E).

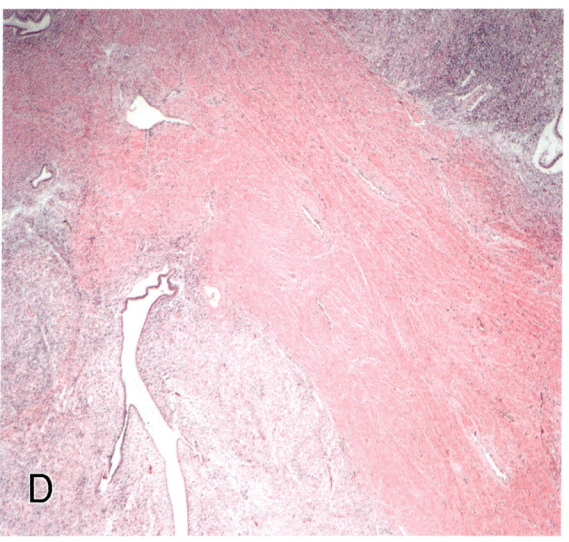
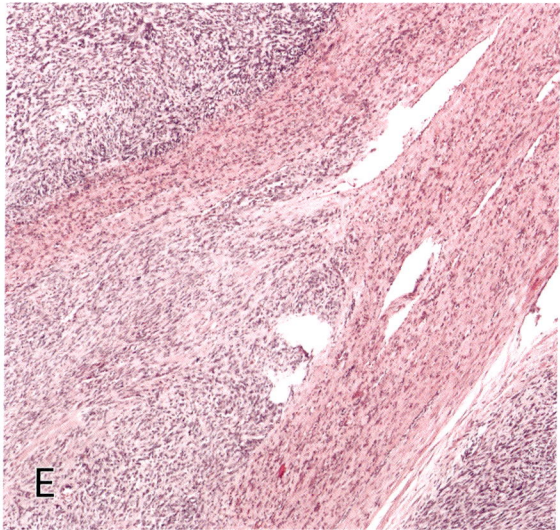

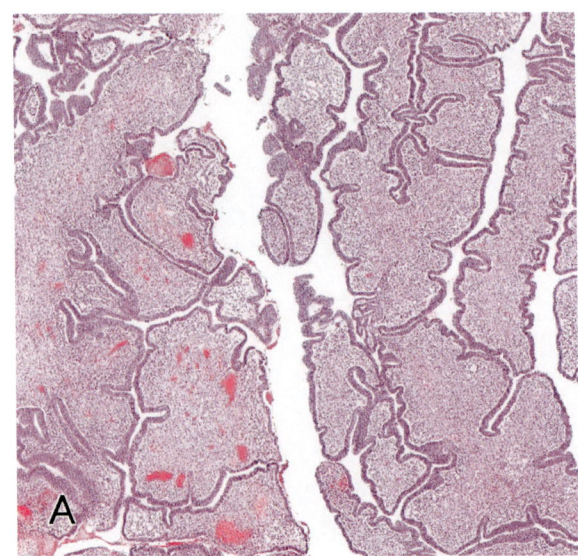

Figure 11-21

HIGH-GRADE MÜLLERIAN ADENOSARCOMA

At low (A) and high (B) power, the stromal component is high-grade but the overall architecture of typical adenosarcoma is preserved and no stromal overgrowth is seen. Aberrant p53 staining in the high-grade stromal compartment (C). (Courtesy of Dr. C. Parra-Herran, Toronto, Canada.)

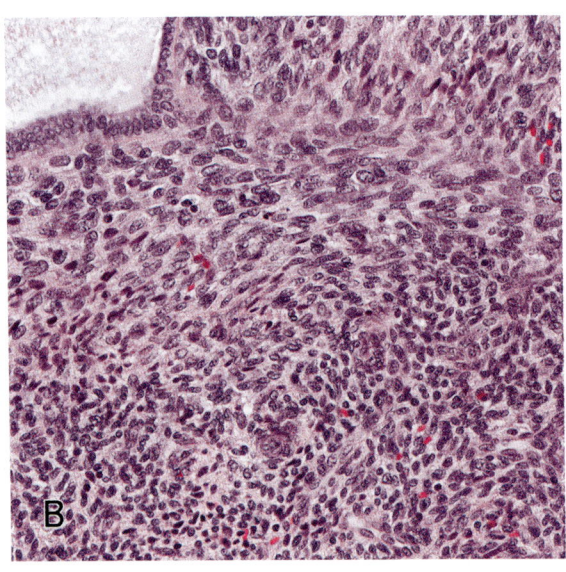

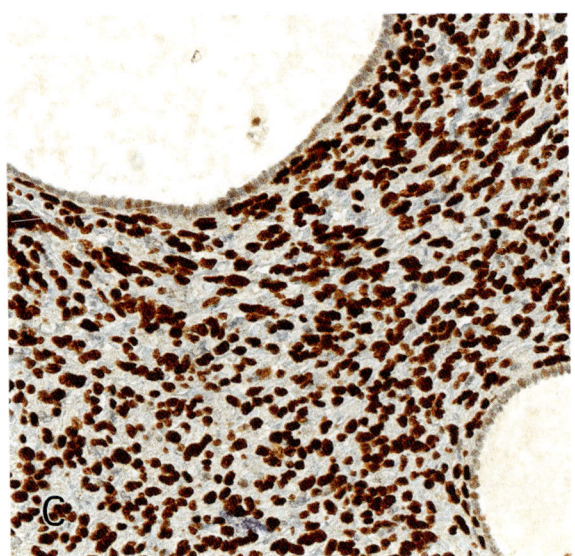

myometrium (fig. 11-20D), are more frequently high grade (105a), and contain heterologous elements, such as rhabdomyosarcoma (99). High-grade homologous sarcomatous components may resemble high-grade fibrosarcoma, malignant fibrous histiocytoma, pleomorphic undifferentiated uterine sarcoma, or an anaplastic small round cell tumor. The latter should suggest rhabdomyosarcoma, which can be confirmed either by finding strap cells and rhabdomyoblasts with cross striations or by immunohistochemical expression of myogenin or myoD-1. Aside from rhabdomyosarcoma, the most common type of heterologous differentiation (fig. 11-20A), rare types of sarcomatous overgrowth have been reported, including primitive neuroectodermal tumor (32,107) and angiosarcoma (108). A high-grade sarcoma occupying less than 25 percent of the tumor is not currently classified as sarcomatous overgrowth (fig. 11-20B,C), but it is still a good practice to report (figs. 11-20E). The finding of high-grade malignant stroma in a tumor with typical architecture should also be reported (high-grade müllerian adenosarcoma) (fig. 11-21) (109).

Myometrial invasion is found in approximately 15 percent of adenosarcomas (fig. 11-20D), usually with a destructive pattern. In the absence of stromal overgrowth, the invasive component

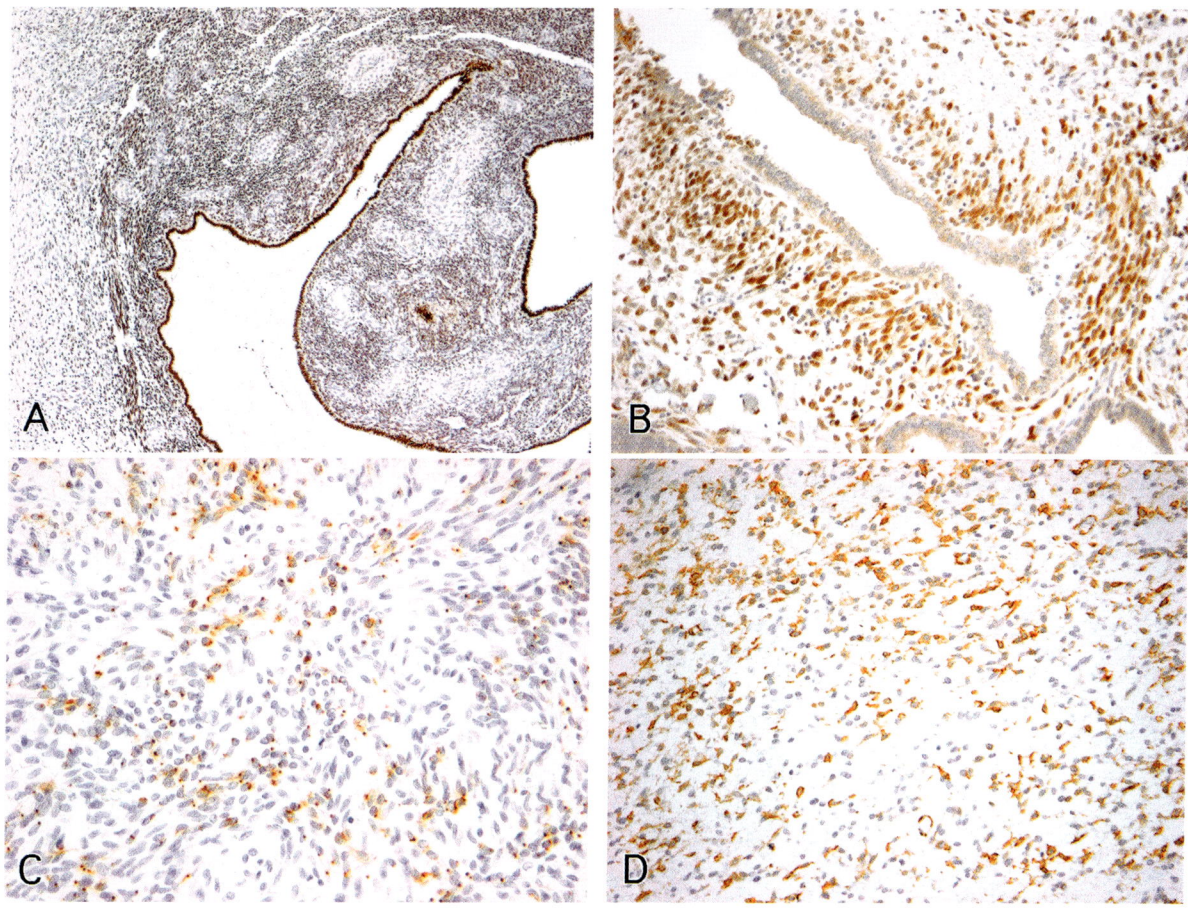

Figure 11-22

LOW-GRADE MÜLLERIAN ADENOSARCOMA: IMMUNOPHENOTYPE

ER expression is best seen in the periglandular cuff (A) as is WT1 (B). Rare adenosarcomas show punctate cytokeratin expression (C) and diffuse expression of smooth muscle actin (D). (Figure 2 from Soslow RA, Ali A, Oliva E. Mullerian adenosarcomas: an immunophenotypic analysis of 35 cases. Am J Surg Pathol 2008;32:1013-21.)

often shows both epithelial and stromal components, whereas in tumors with stromal overgrowth, high-grade sarcomatous components usually predominate. Lymphovascular invasion is uncommon (40).

Immunohistochemical Findings. The immunophenotype of the stromal component of low-grade adenosarcoma lacking sarcomatous overgrowth and heterologous elements is similar to that observed in low-grade endometrial stromal tumors with nearly universal expression of CD10, WT1, ER, and PR (fig. 11-22) (92,105, 110,111). Many tumors also express AE1/3 cytokeratin, CD34, and calretinin, although the latter two are often typically patchy and weak. ER, PR, and CD10 expression is typically lost in areas of sarcomatous overgrowth relative to the conventional low-grade stromal component, likely indicative of stromal dedifferentiation, while WT1 expression appears to be preserved (fig. 11-23) (105). Smooth muscle actin and desmin are positive if smooth muscle differentiation is noted, while myogenin and myo-D1 are positive when rhabdomyoblastic differentiation exists. Areas of sex cord-like differentiation are variably positive for inhibin, calretinin, CD99, and melan A (97,102,105). The mean Ki-67 labeling index may range markedly within the low-grade malignant stromal component of adenosarcoma (less than 5 to 40 percent; mean, 12 to 20 percent) but when sarcomatous overgrowth is present, the proliferative rates are

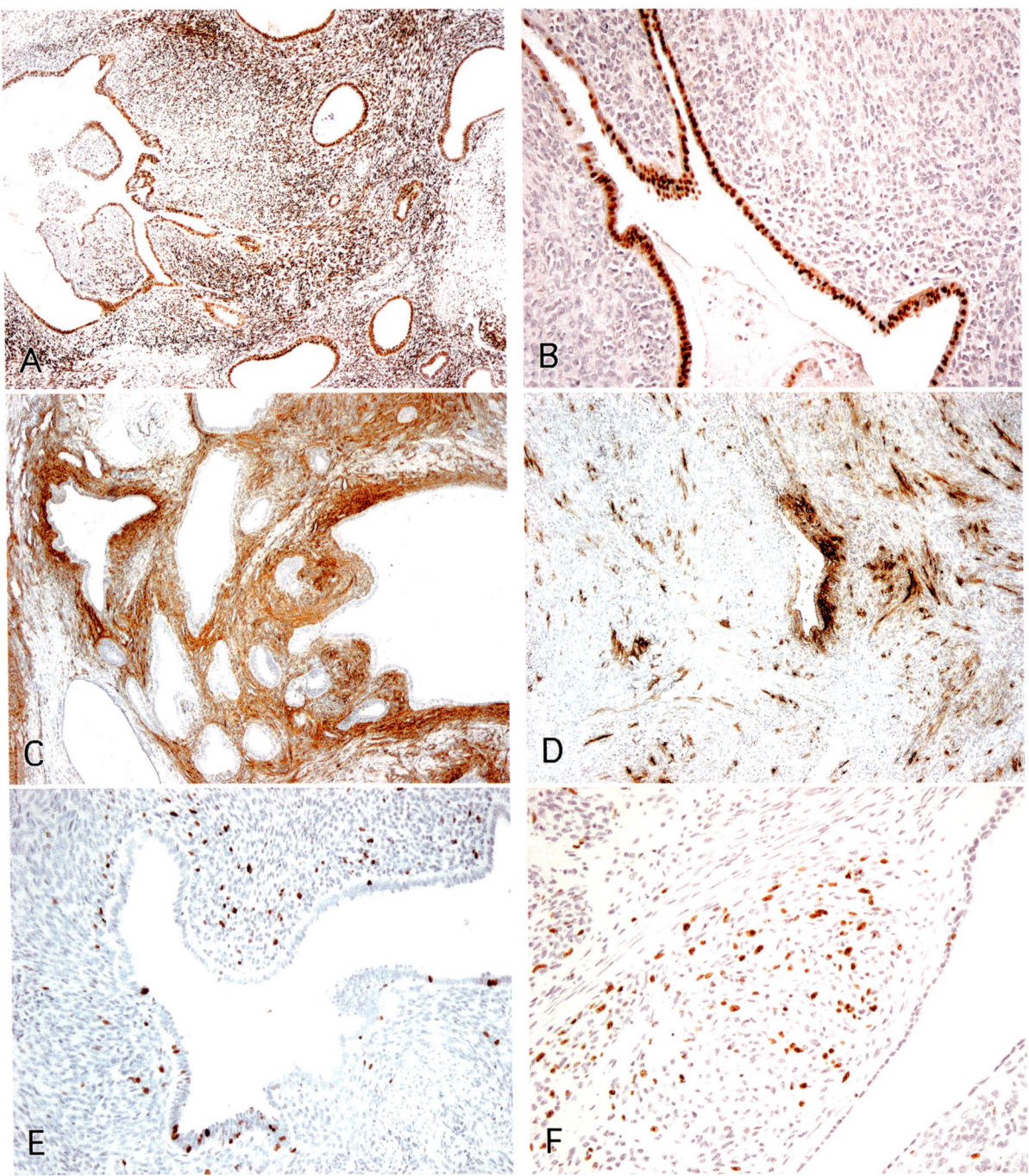

Figure 11-23

LOW-GRADE MÜLLERIAN ADENOSARCOMA WITH AND WITHOUT STROMAL OVERGROWTH: IMMUNOPHENOTYPE

Expression of PR (A,B) and CD10 (C,D) is significantly more diffuse in adenosarcomas without stromal overgrowth (A,C) than adenosarcomas with stromal overgrowth (B,D). Note that epithelial expression of PR is retained in this adenosarcoma with stromal overgrowth (B). Most adenosarcomas without stromal overgrowth show a proliferative index with mib-1 or less than 5 percent overall, but the proliferative index is also generally elevated in periglandular cuffs (E). The proliferative index in adenosarcomas with stromal overgrowth almost always exceeds 5 percent. (Figure 2 from Soslow RA, Ali A, Oliva E. Mullerian adenosarcomas: an immunophenotypic analysis of 35 cases. Am J Surg Pathol 2008;32:1017.)

much higher (92,105,112). The epithelial compartment is often positive for ER, PR, and AE1/3 cytokeratin, and rarely expresses CD10 or AR.

Molecular Genetic Findings. It has recently been reported that adenosarcomas are mesenchymal neoplasms that contain a nonclonal epithelial proliferation (113). Despite some histologic and immunohistochemical similarities between low-grade müllerian adenosarcoma and endometrial stromal sarcoma, there are significant cytogenetic and genomic differences. None of the translocations that have been reported in endometrial stromal sarcomas have been detected in müllerian adenosarcomas (114). In a recent study (115), the most frequent genomic abnormality was an amplification involving *MDM2* and *CDK4* (5 of 18 cases), accompanied by diffuse expression of HMGA2 and, focally, CDK4 and MDM2. Alterations in PIK3CA/AKT/PTEN pathway constituents were seen in 72 percent of the 18 tumors. Adenosarcomas with stromal overgrowth more often showed high copy number changes, including *MYBL1* amplification, while overall, *TP53* mutations were uncommon, present in only 2 tumors with stromal overgrowth. *Tp53* mutations and aberrant p53 staining can also be encountered in the histologically high-grade sarcomatous components of tumors with or without stromal overgrowth (fig. 11-21) (109). Three of the 18 tumors (17 percent) had mutations in *ATRX* (as seen in uterine leiomyosarcomas), and, interestingly, all were associated with stromal overgrowth (115).

Another recent study of 19 adenosarcomas reported 2 with fusion genes involving *NCOA* family members as well as recurrent *FGFR2*, *KMT2C*, and *DICER1* mutations (2 cases each) (113). Twenty-six percent and 21 percent of müllerian adenosarcomas harbored *MDM2/CDK4/HMGA2* and *TERT* gene amplifications, respectively, while only one adenosarcoma with heterologous rhabdomyoblastic differentiation had a *DICER1* mutation. Mitochondrial DNA sequencing has revealed that epithelial and mesenchymal components of adenosarcomas are clonally unrelated, consistent with the principle that these tumors are primarily mesenchymal in nature (113). Frequent abnormalities involving chromosome 8 also have been reported (116).

Differential Diagnosis. *Adenofibroma.* This tumor is so uncommon that its existence has been questioned by some investigators. Extraordinarily rare examples conforming to historical diagnostic criteria do, indeed, exist. Since adenosarcomas may have very subtle periglandular collaring and less than 1 mitoses per 10 high-power fields, and both tumors display bulbous fronds and phyllodes-like architecture, a diagnosis of adenofibroma should only be made in the absence of stromal cellularity, periglandular cuffing, stromal nuclear atypia, and stromal mitotic activity. The tumor should be well sampled before establishing a diagnosis of adenofibroma. Some tumors originally diagnosed as "adenofibromas" have recurred and have been associated with adverse outcome, and in retrospect, likely represented low-grade müllerian adenosarcomas (86,92).

Adenomyoma. Adenomyoma may be in the differential diagnosis of adenosarcoma since it is also a biphasic tumor. Although adenosarcomas may contain benign smooth muscle and endometrioid-type adenomyomas may show a rim of endometrial-type stroma, there are significant differences between these tumors. On gross examination, endometrioid adenomyomas may be submucosal, but they typically have a cut surface that closely overlaps with that of a leiomyoma except for the occasional presence of cysts. On microscopic examination, this tumor lacks the phyllodes-like architecture or polypoid projections of stroma into glands. Although a periglandular component of endometrial stroma may be seen, it does not show condensation around the glands or cytologic atypia (117,118). A rare adenosarcoma has been reported to arise in a background of an adenomyoma, but in these instances, the two components are clearly demarcated (87,94).

Atypical Endometrial Polyp. This lesion resembles adenosarcoma in three situations: 1) when the polyp is highly cellular; 2) when it shows focal and subtle stromal condensation around glands or focal and subtle adenosarcoma-like architecture (fig. 11-24); or 3) when it contains bizarre stromal cells. In the first scenario, stromal cellularity is homogenous throughout the polyp and the stroma is atrophic and compacted. The glands have an inactive or atrophic appearance and lack the phyllodes-type architecture seen in adenosarcomas. Endometrial polyps may show focally phyllodes-type architecture, periglandular stromal condensation, and increased

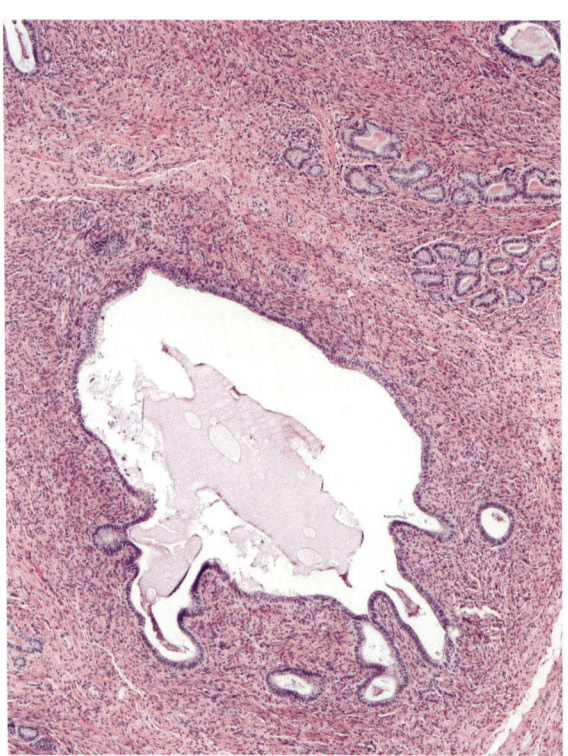 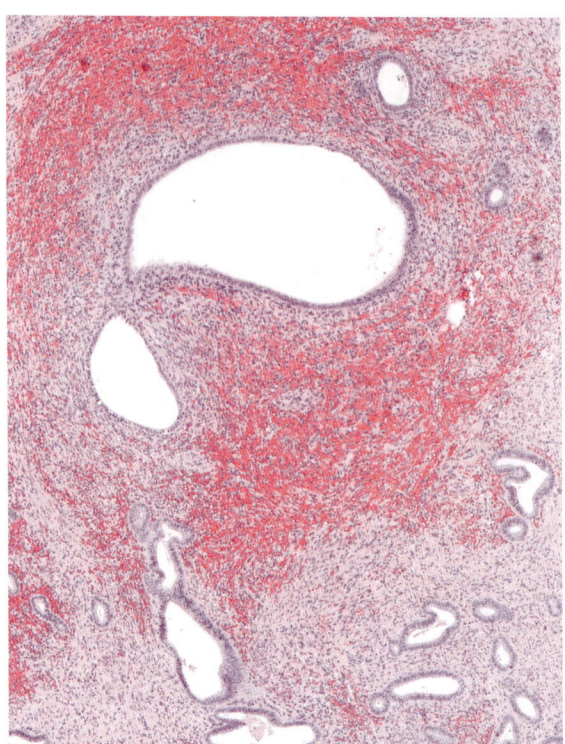

Figure 11-24

ATYPICAL ENDOMETRIAL POLYP

Incompletely developed features of adenosarcoma are seen as focal and subtle stromal hypercellularity around the endometrial glands, some of which are enlarged.

mitoses, however, such atypical polyps tend to measure less than 3 cm, the periglandular condensation tends to be subtle, and stromal cytologic atypia is typically absent. Follow-up in these patients, although relatively short, has been uneventful (62). It is important to note that there is no consensus about where to draw the line between atypical endometrial polyp and adenosarcoma, and in some instances, the distinction is arbitrary. In the setting of fertility preservation, it is important to convey that the polyp must be entirely excised with a negative curetting, myometrial invasion excluded on imaging, and close clinical follow-up maintained to detect any early recurrence. The third type of endometrial polyp described above resembles a typical endometrial polyp except for the presence of atypical stromal cells, many of which resemble floret cells and those encountered in vaginal polyps (119). These polyps lack typical adenosarcoma architecture, stromal condensation, and mitotic activity.

Carcinosarcoma. In contrast to adenosarcoma, carcinosarcoma contains histologically high-grade epithelial and mesenchymal components. Some carcinosarcomas have adenosarcoma-like areas at low-power examination, including high-grade sarcoma juxtaposed to seemingly bland-appearing epithelium (20,36,37). At high power, however, both carcinomatous and sarcomatous components are high grade, at least focally, in contrast to adenosarcoma. Low-grade adenosarcomas may have a component of carcinoma or an adenocarcinoma may secondarily involve an adenosarcoma. In the former scenario, the carcinomas are typically small, low grade, and endometrioid, in contrast to the high-grade cytologic features in carcinosarcoma. These tumors should be diagnosed as adenosarcoma with a second diagnosis of carcinoma.

Rhabdomyosarcomas. Among rhabdomyosarcomas, embryonal rhabdomyosarcoma may resemble müllerian adenosarcoma as both may feature periglandular condensation and contain fetal-type cartilage. However, there are several important differentiating features. At low power, the epithelium of adenosarcoma grows in concert with the sarcomatous components and is distributed within the tumor in an orderly fashion, while in rhabdomyosarcoma, endometrial-type glands are entrapped, typically much less numerous, and lack phyllodes-type growth, fronds, or intraluminal polypoid projections. In gland-poor areas, rhabdomyosarcoma frequently displays hypocellular and hypercellular areas, and at high-power magnification, the cells are primitive and hyperchromatic in appearance when compared to the low-grade endometrial-type stroma seen in most adenosarcomas. Metaplastic changes within the epithelial component of adenosarcomas are not a feature of rhabdomyosarcoma (120).

Pleomorphic rhabdomyosarcoma enters in the differential diagnosis of adenosarcoma with high-grade sarcomatous overgrowth. Thus, extensive sampling should be undertaken in order to identify even a small component of conventional adenosarcoma (or carcinosarcoma).

Currently, it is not certain whether there are important prognostic differences between adult patients with rhabdomyosarcoma or adenosarcoma with extensive heterologous differentiation in the form of rhabdomyosarcoma. Rhabdomyosarcomas in adults are usually treated with surgery, with or without adjuvant chemotherapy or radiotherapy, in contrast to adenosarcoma, which should be treated with surgery primarily.

Endometrial Stromal Sarcoma. This tumor may rarely contain endometrioid glands. The glands tend to be round, with or without cyst formation, haphazardly distributed, and they lack extensive metaplastic changes and phyllodes-like architecture (121). In contrast to adenosarcoma, these tumors have a prominent myometrial component in most instances, with or without an endometrial component. Myometrial invasion shows a permeative pattern (tongue-like) in contrast to the destructive invasion seen in adenosarcomas. Since many myometrial-invasive adenosarcomas also feature high-grade stromal overgrowth, the myoinvasive component of such tumors is of higher grade when compared to low-grade endometrial stromal sarcoma.

Uterine Tumor Resembling Ovarian Sex Cord Tumor (UTROSCT). This tumor is sometimes difficult to distinguish from adenosarcoma with sex cord-stromal elements, especially when the latter component is extensive or the tumor is incompletely sampled. The finding of sex cord-like differentiation in a curettage should invoke a differential diagnoses of endometrial stromal tumor, adenosarcoma with sex cord-like differentiation, endometrioid adenocarcinoma with sex cord-like features, and UTROSCT. Hysterectomy should be performed in order to provide a definitive diagnosis. Immunohistochemistry is not diagnostically helpful as significant overlap exists between most of these entities (122).

Treatment and Prognosis. Müllerian adenosarcoma of the uterus is a tumor with a favorable clinical outcome, with an overall survival rate of 75 to 90 percent (92). In the largest study in the literature, Clement and Scully (40) noted that only 26 percent of patients with müllerian adenosarcoma experienced recurrence(s), with myometrial invasion being among the most important adverse risk factors (46 percent rate of recurrence compared to 12 percent in patients with no myometrial invasion). Fifty percent of patients experiencing recurrence succumbed to disease (40), a finding that has been corroborated in other studies (86,123–125). Overall, myometrial invasion, sarcomatous overgrowth, and high-grade cytology or heterologous stromal elements (high-risk histologic features), are associated with diminished survival (40,92,99). As many as 70 percent of patients whose tumors have sarcomatous overgrowth experience recurrence, and overall survival is reduced to approximately 50 percent.

Patients with organ-confined adenosarcoma without high-risk histologic features are probably best treated with hysterectomy alone (83). Patients who present at advanced stages or have tumors with high-risk histologic features are commonly treated with pelvic radiation, with the goal of decreasing local recurrence, even though this intervention is not strongly evidence-based. The role of chemotherapy in this setting is not well defined. Treatment with progestational agents is sometimes considered, as most tumors lacking stromal overgrowth contain mesenchymal components that express ER and PR (105).

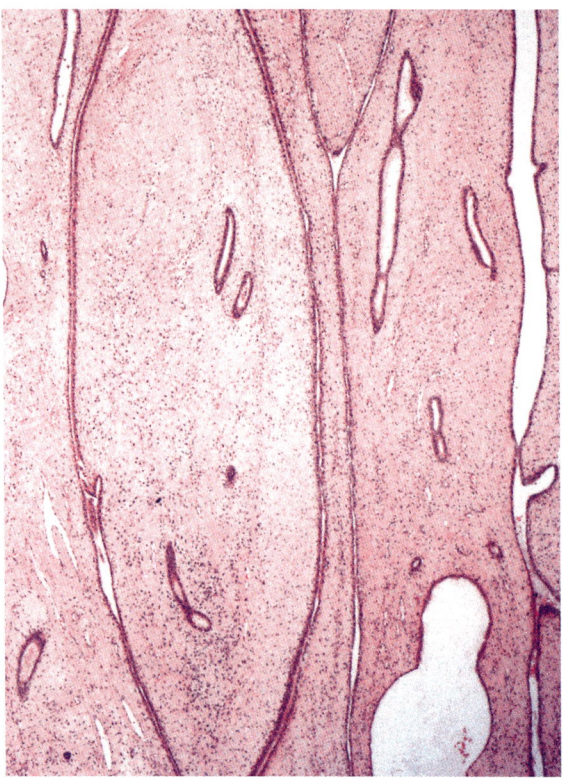

Figure 11-25

MULLERIAN ADENOFIBROMA

Although the low-power architectural features display some similarity to adenosarcoma, there is no stromal cuffing, stromal cellularity, atypia, or mitotic activity.

The mean time to recurrence is about 3 to 4 years, but tumors may recur a decade after the original diagnosis. Sites of recurrence include vagina, pelvis, and abdomen, in both peritoneal and retroperitoneal locations (40). Hematogenous metastases are rare (40) as are lymph node metastases (126). Recurrences and metastases following a diagnosis of adenosarcoma can be solely sarcomatous, biphasic, or rarely, as carcinosarcoma (40). It is not unusual for the mesenchymal component in either biphasic or monophasic recurrences to display a higher grade than that present in the primary tumor but infrequently contains heterologous elements. Sarcomatous overgrowth is often associated with hematogenous spread and pulmonary or bone metastases. These patients have a higher mortality rate that is similar to those with other high-grade sarcomas or carcinosarcomas of the uterus (38,105a,127,128).

MÜLLERIAN ADENOFIBROMA

Endometrial and *cervical adenofibromas* are rare (40,86,129,130). A description of their gross appearance may not be accurate as some tumors diagnosed as adenofibromas in the past likely represent low-grade adenosarcomas, especially when using current criteria that emphasize tumor architecture over mitotic index. In the series reported by Clement and Scully (40) as well as Zaloudek and Norris (86), the tumors were described as broad-based polypoid masses with a villous surface, a spongy appearance on sectioning, and cystic spaces surrounded by firm white-tan tissue.

Adenofibromas may resemble adenosarcomas on low-power magnification, but they lack subepithelial stromal condensation, stromal cytologic atypia, and any stromal mitotic activity (fig. 11-25). They have fibromatous and uniform background stroma throughout.

As endometrial and cervical tumors demonstrating the above specific features are exceptionally rare, it is best to reserve a diagnosis of adenofibroma for well-sampled tumors in hysterectomy specimens. In the series of 10 cases reported by Zaloudek and Norris (86), all patients underwent hysterectomy and 8 out of 10 with follow-up were apparently cured, although only 3 patients were followed for more than 5 years (86). In contrast, in the series reported by Gallardo and Prat (92), one patient with a diagnosis of cervical adenofibroma with less than 1 mitoses per 10 high-power fields and treated by polypectomy, developed a low-grade myoinvasive adenosarcoma of the uterine corpus 7 years later followed by two pelvic recurrences and pulmonary metastases, dying 11 year after the initial diagnosis. This case illustrates the very high threshold needed before making a diagnosis of müllerian adenofibroma. A case of an adenomyofibroma containing skeletal muscle and a lipoadenofibroma have been reported in the literature as variant forms of adenofibroma (131,132).

ADENOMYOMA

Definition. *Adenomyoma* is a biphasic tumor composed of benign endometrioid-type epithelium plus or minus endometrial stroma in a predominant background of benign smooth muscle.

Clinical Features. The median age of patients is 40 years. They most commonly present with vaginal bleeding followed by pelvic pain and are often thought to have symptomatic uterine fibroids.

Gross Findings. The most common type of adenomyoma, endometrioid adenomyoma, usually occurs within the uterine corpus and may involve the endometrium, myometrium, or serosa (fig. 11-26). Endocervical and broad ligament adenomyomas (117,118,133–135) as well as those associated with endometriosis (136) have also been described. In the largest series (117), approximately 80 percent were polypoid and protruded into the endometrial cavity or were exophytic and subserosal; the remainder were centered in the myometrium. A smaller series (118), however, reported a substantially larger proportion of tumors centered in the myometrium.

The median size of an adenomyoma is approximately 4 cm, although wide variation has been reported (less than 5 mm to 17 cm) (117). Adenomyomas are smooth surfaced when polypoid, although erosion and ulceration are common. They are typically well circumscribed and most are solid, but they may be solid and cystic or predominantly cystic on occasion. When polypoid, they may be confused with endometrial polyps or considered to be adenomyomatous polyps; if mural, they are often misconstrued as leiomyomas. On sectioning, they are variably firm, often whorled or trabeculated with a variable number of cysts that on occasion may be large and filled with hemorrhagic contents. Many patients also have leiomyomas and adenomyosis.

Microscopic Findings. Although this is a biphasic tumor, the epithelial component is typically minor compared to the smooth muscle component. The endometrioid-type glands are generally well spaced and have simple outlines, although occasional small glandular aggregates and cystically dilated glands are also present (fig. 11-27). The endometrioid glands, usually with a proliferative appearance, may show tubal, mucinous endocervical, squamous, or rarely clear cell metaplasia (117). The cells are cytologically bland, with low mitotic activity.

Smooth muscle is the predominant mesenchymal component, typically located around the endometrioid components and spindle in morphology. This component varies from hypocellular and edematous or hyalinized to hypercellular, a histologic appearance that closely overlaps with

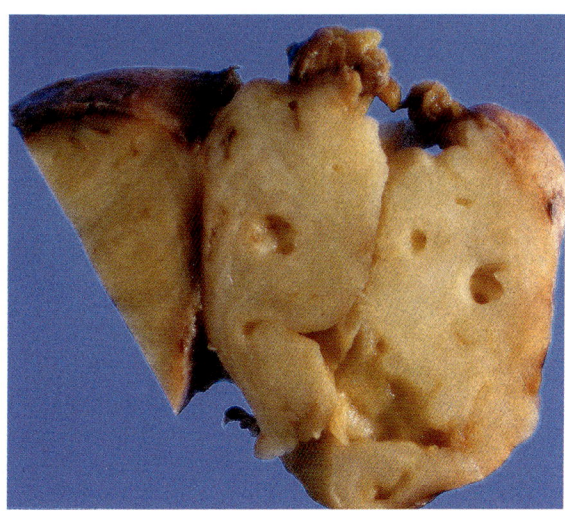

Figure 11-26

ENDOMETRIOID ADENOMYOMA

The overall appearance is similar to that seen in leiomyoma, with a white to tan, firm cut surface. However, in contrast to the latter, small cysts, some filled with blood, are noted.

that seen in leiomyomas. Smooth muscle cells with bizarre nuclei can be found, but the muscle component is cytologically bland (117,118).

The endometrial stroma located around the glands is variably prominent, sometimes difficult to discern, and usually resembles proliferative endometrial stroma. Rarely, it has a myofibroblastic appearance or contains sex cord-like elements. Mature adipose tissue has been reported (137). Mitoses, when present within the mesenchymal compartment, are more common within the endometrial stromal areas but typically are fewer than 5 per 10 high-power fields (117).

Adenomyomatosis, a diffuse/multifocal process (138), and intravenous adenomyomatosis (139) have been rarely reported. The latter is considered by some to be a form of intravenous leiomyomatosis.

Differential Diagnosis. *Leiomyoma.* On gross examination, leiomyoma may have an appearance and consistency identical to adenomyoma. If glands are present on microscopic examination, however, they are typically at the periphery of the leiomyoma. Submucosal examples can have entrapped endometrial glands, subserosal leiomyomas may entrap endometriosis at their periphery, and intramural examples

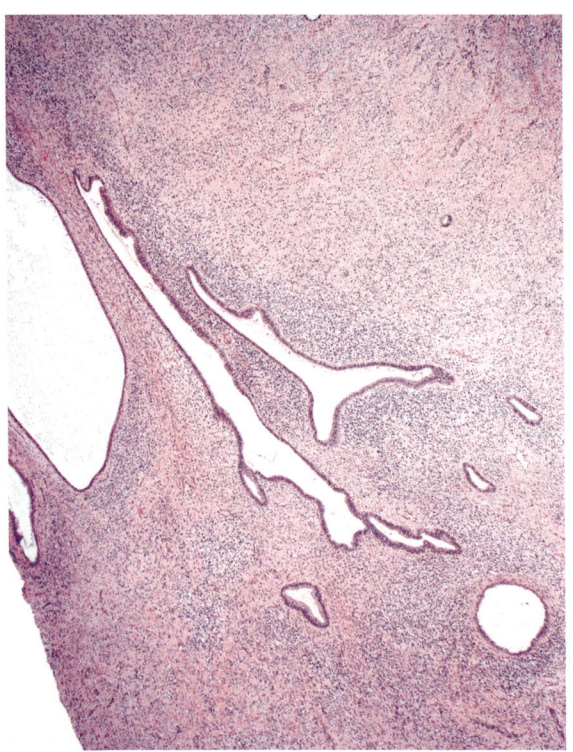 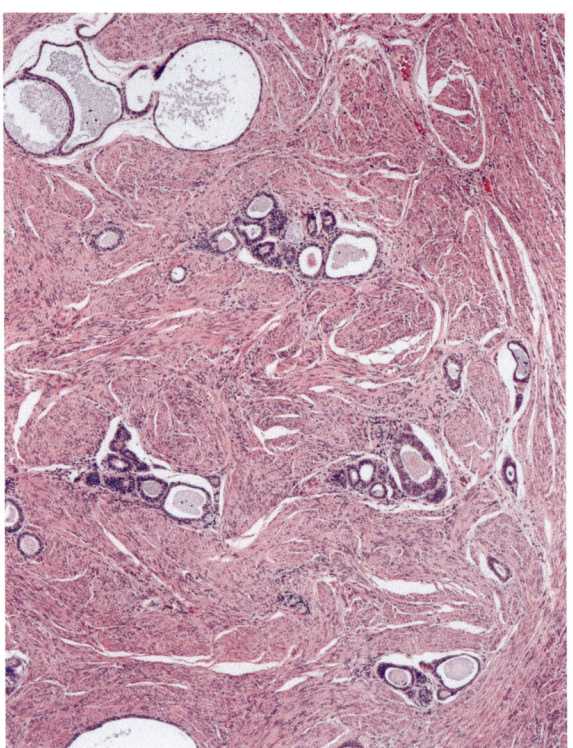

Figure 11-27

UTERINE (ENDOMETRIOID) ADENOMYOMA

The glands are surrounded by a small rim of endometrial stroma invested in hyperplastic smooth muscle (left). (Courtesy of Dr. G. Turashvili, Toronto, Canada.) Some tumors lack the endometrial stromal component. Glands may be small and form clusters (right).

may be juxtaposed against adenomyosis, thus correlation with gross appearance is helpful.

Endometrial Polyp with a Prominent Muscular Component. Endometrial glands are located at the periphery of the polyp, in contrast to adenomyomas.

Adenomyosis. This is characterized by a trabeculated appearance on gross examination secondary to the presence of small cysts surrounded by a rim of firmer, hyperplastic myometrium, but it rarely forms a sizable, circumscribed mass and is instead a diffuse microscopic finding. When foci of adenomyosis are circumscribed and mass-forming (i.e., nodular) and have a predominant muscular component, the term "nodular adenomyosis" is used.

Atypical Polypoid Adenomyoma. This is probably the most important entity in the differential diagnosis. In contrast to typical adenomyoma, atypical polypoid adenomyoma is more frequently located in the lower uterine segment, often measures under 2 cm, and contains an epithelial component with a vaguely nodular architecture that predominates over the myoid stroma. Although the smooth muscle component is benign, the glands may be crowded and sometimes complex, with squamous morules. This contrasts with the limited and simple epithelial component of typical adenomyoma (140–142).

Adenosarcoma. This is also a biphasic tumor and may show smooth muscle differentiation within the stromal component. Both the epithelial and mesenchymal elements differ from adenomyoma. Mullerian adenosarcoma displays phyllodes-like architecture with low-grade sarcomatous stroma that cuffs around benign endometrioid epithelium. Regardless of the presence of smooth muscle differentiation, the orderly relationship between epithelium and neoplastic stroma is maintained in nearly every case (101,105).

Treatment and Prognosis. Endometrioid adenomyomas are benign tumors treated surgically by excision or hysterectomy. No recurrences have been reported when polypectomy was performed without hysterectomy (117).

ATYPICAL POLYPOID ADENOMYOMA

Definition. *Atypical polypoid adenoma* is a biphasic tumor, typically polypoid, containing a proliferation of often complex and atypical endometrioid glands, characteristically with squamous morules, set in a myoid or myofibromatous stroma (143).

Clinical Features. Atypical polypoid adenomyomas disproportionately affect women in their 4th and 5th decades, with an average age of 38 to 40 years, although they may occur in other age groups. They have a predilection for the lower uterine segment, where approximately 35 to 57 percent of atypical polypoid adenomyomas are centered (140–142). They are occasionally located in the endocervix (140,144). Patients are typically premenopausal and nulligravid (55 to 76 percent), and present with vaginal bleeding. An additional 20 to 40 percent of patients are known to be infertile or are diagnosed with atypical polypoid adenomyoma during evaluation for infertility (140–142). Association with Turner (142) or Cowden syndrome (145) has been reported.

Gross Findings. Most atypical polypoid adenomyomas form sessile or pedunculated polyps, usually attached to the endometrium by a broad base (fig. 11-28). The average size is 2 cm, although they may be considerably larger. They are generally described as bulging, lobulated or bosselated, with a firm or rubbery, yellow to gray to white cut surface. When sessile, they are well circumscribed and the interface between their base and myometrium can be easily discerned (140,142). Although some atypical polypoid adenomyomas contain foci of adenocarcinoma, this is rarely grossly appreciable.

Microscopic Findings. In hysterectomy specimens, the circumscribed base of the lesion is bounded by non-neoplastic basalis or directly abuts the myometrium (fig. 11-29). Rarely, the interface is irregular (140,142). At low-power magnification, atypical polypoid adenomyomas have two components: endometrioid glands and myoid or myofibromatous stroma (fig. 11-

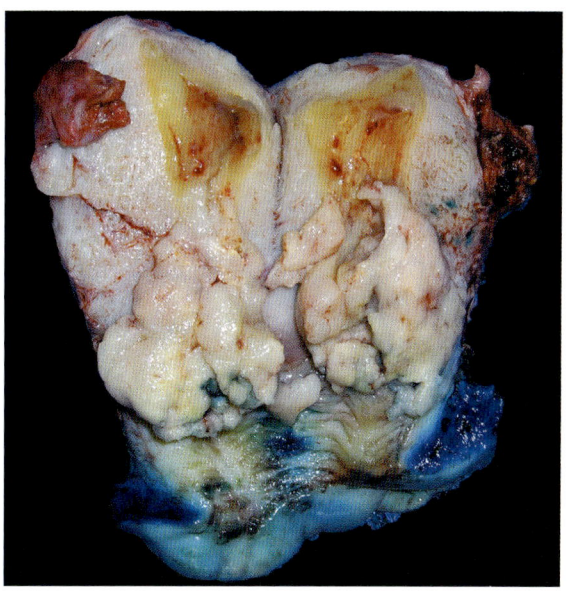

Figure 11-28

ATYPICAL POLYPOID ADENOMYOMA

The polypoid tumor is to be centered in the lower uterine segment and has a multinodular but homogeneous appearance. (Courtesy of Dr. N. Abu-Rustum, New York, NY.)

29). The glands may be haphazardly arranged, but vague lobulation is typical. In up to 50 percent of tumors, glands vary in size and cluster irregularly, resembling complex hyperplasia (fig. 11-30) (140). A true glandular cribriform pattern is unusual but a "pseudocribriform" appearance is often noted due to the presence of squamous morules, a common finding (fig. 11-29) (140). Squamous morules may obliterate gland lumina in large areas and central comedo-like necrosis may be present (142). Small foci of keratinizing squamous differentiation and tubal and mucinous metaplasia have also been reported (140,142). The cells lining the glands are cuboidal to columnar and often show nuclear pseudostratification. Cytologic atypia is usually mild, but moderate atypia may be seen. Mitoses are absent to rare in about 30 percent of tumors, but they can be found easily during a dedicated search at high-power magnification (usually with 2 or fewer mitoses per 10 high-power fields).

The myoid stroma of atypical polypoid adenomyomas demonstrates intersecting fascicles of smooth muscle cells, the appearance of which

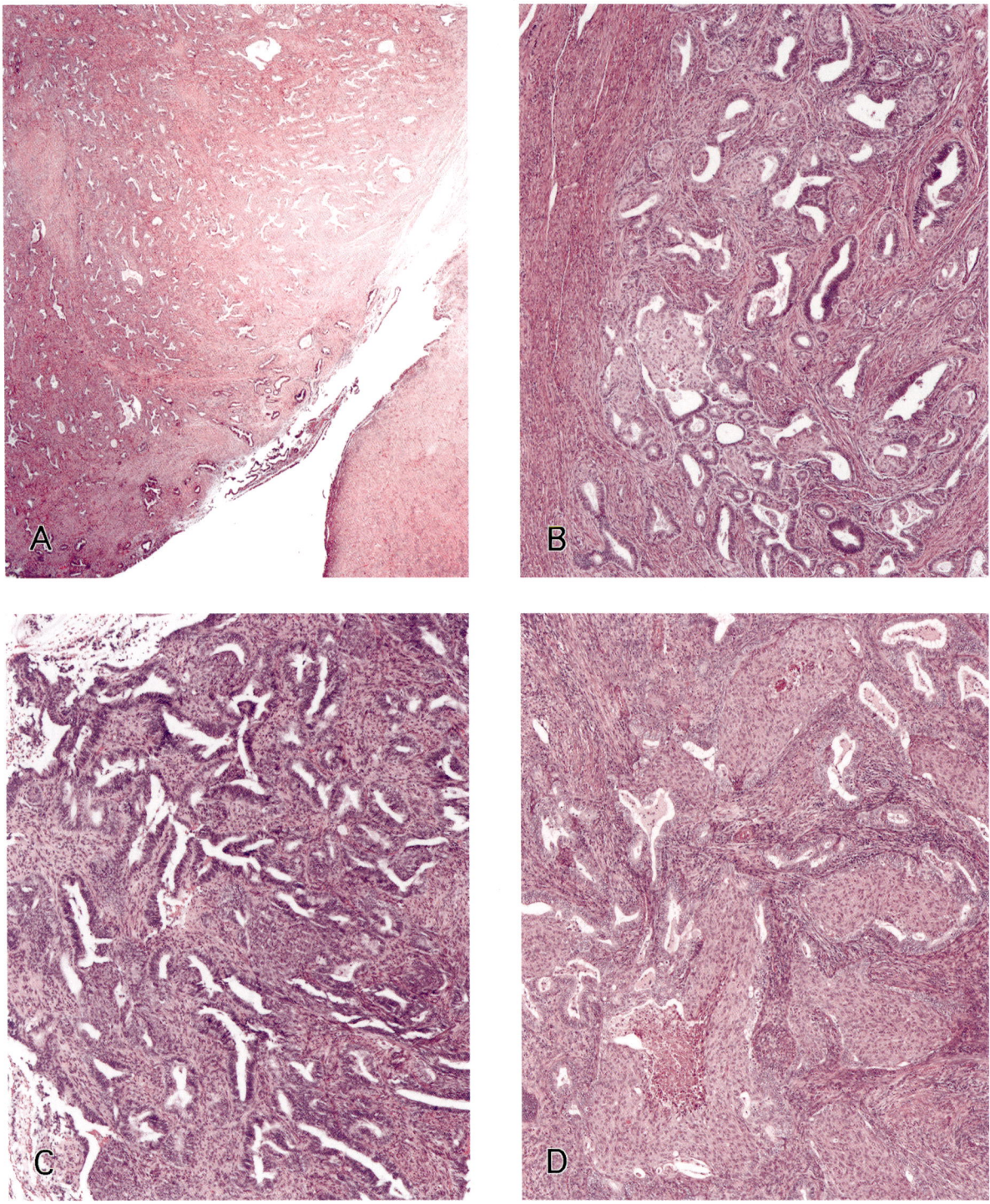

Figure 11-29

ATYPICAL POLYPOID ADENOMYOMA

The tumor has a well-circumscribed margin and displays a vaguely nodular configuration (A). Simple (B) and crowded (C) endometrioid glands are embedded in a myofibromatous stroma. There is good demarcation between tumor and adjacent myometrium (B). Squamous morules are a characteristic feature. They may be confluent and have central necrosis, neither of which is diagnostically informative (B and D).

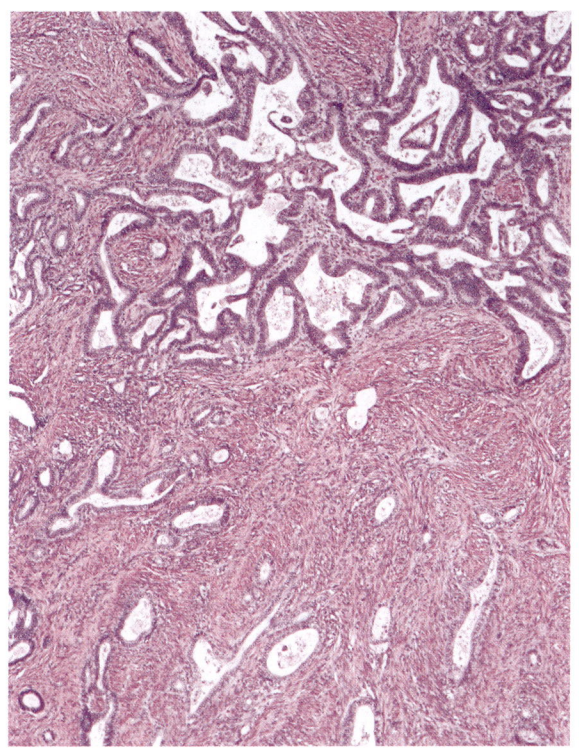

Figure 11-30
ATYPICAL POLYPOID ADENOMYOMA
Overt gland crowding is seen.

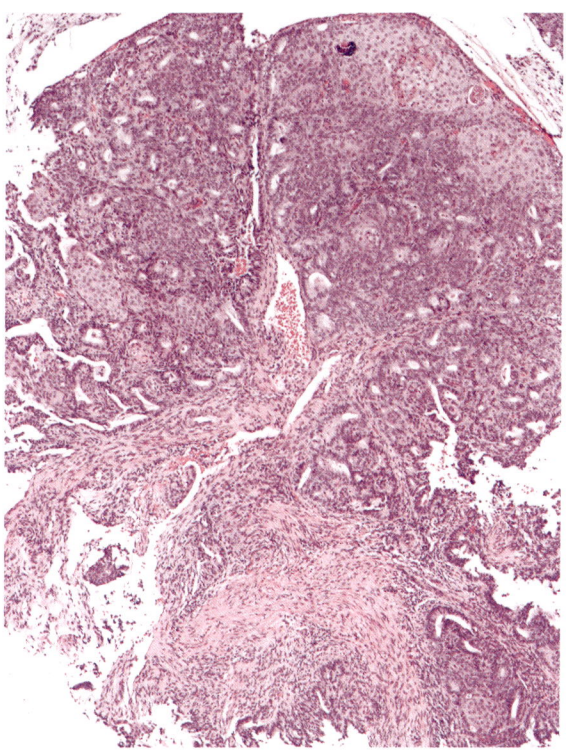

Figure 11-31
WELL-DIFFERENTIATED ENDOMETRIOID ADENOCARCINOMA ARISING IN ATYPICAL POLYPOID ADENOMYOMA

This lesion has been referred to as "atypical polypoid adenomyofibroma of low malignant potential" because of rare associated myometrial invasion.

tends to differ from that of myometrium, and rarely, is highly cellular, similar to leiomyomas. The smooth muscle component may be variably admixed with fibromatous stroma, with areas of hyalinization, patches of endometrial stroma, clusters of chronic inflammatory cells, and stromal calcifications (140,142). No periglandular condensation is noted. Nuclear atypia is uncommon.

The glands may be architecturally complex (crowded, branching, cribriforming) with minimal intervening stroma and may be indistinguishable from atypical hyperplasia or well-differentiated endometrioid adenocarcinoma (fig. 11-31) (140,141). Seventeen percent of atypical polypoid adenomyomas were reported to contain foci of adenocarcinoma in one study (141) while in another, 45 percent of tumors were reported to have a high architectural index (30 percent or more of complex glandular architecture). Despite this finding, myometrial invasion is not found at hysterectomy in most cases. In the series reported by Longacre et al.

(140), 19 of 48 patients underwent hysterectomy following biopsy, curettage, or polypectomy diagnosis; only 2 patients had superficial foci of myometrial invasive endometrioid adenocarcinoma, and all had an uneventful outcome. Interestingly, one of the patients had a synchronous, histologically similar lesion in one ovary.

In approximately 10 percent of hysterectomy specimens, foci of atypical hyperplasia are found adjacent to or noncontiguous to the atypical polypoid adenomyoma (140). In practice, a few atypical polypoid adenomyomas have atypical hyperplasia at biopsy or curettage of nonpolypoid endometrium, which illustrates the importance of evaluating the nonpolypoid endometrium.

Immunohistochemical and Molecular Genetic Findings. The myoid component of atypical polypoid adenomyoma universally expresses smooth muscle actin, and at least half of tumors display desmin expression as well. Expression of ER and PR is typically found in both the epithelial and myoid components (148).

Little is known about the immunophenotype and genomics of atypical polypoid adenomyoma. The epithelial component displays aberrant nuclear expression of β-catenin in morules in approximately three fourths of tumors and a similar proportion displays hepatocyte nuclear factor 1-β expression; loss of PTEN expression is noted in approximately one third, with wild-type p53 expression.

Abnormalities in DNA MMR have been rarely reported, but none in association with Lynch syndrome (146,147). In a study of six atypical polypoid adenomyomas, two exhibited *MLH1* promoter hypermethylation with only geographic loss of MLH1 immunostaining in the absence of microsatellite instability (147). Occasional *PTEN* gene deletions have been reported as well as frequent *KRAS* mutations (146).

Differential Diagnosis. *Myometrial-Invasive Adenocarcinoma.* With rare exceptions, a diagnosis of myometrial-invasive adenocarcinoma should be avoided in biopsies or curettings, as atypical polypoid adenomyomas and adenocarcinomas that invade polyp stroma may simulate myometrial-invasive adenocarcinoma. A lobulated growth is suggestive of atypical polypoid adenomyoma. In hysterectomy specimens, in contrast to myoinvasive carcinomas, the former lacks myometrial invasion with a well delineated margin with myometrium.

Polypoid Adenomyoma. Polypoid adenomyomas contain fewer glands than atypical polypoid adenomyomas and usually do not show gland crowding, as the glandular component is minor in most instances. One specific feature that is seen in most adenomyomas and is rare or nonexistent in atypical polypoid adenomyoma is the presence of endometrial stroma around the endometrioid glands (117).

Müllerian Adenosarcoma. Only occasional müllerian adenosarcomas contain myoid stroma. Features typically present in adenosarcomas with myoid stroma that are not found in atypical polypoid adenomyomas are stromal cuffing of glands and phyllodes-like architecture.

Treatment and Prognosis. As these lesions rarely harbor an endometrioid adenocarcinoma that invades the myometrium, it is considered safe to manage premenopausal patients conservatively. This usually includes hysteroscopic polypectomy and endometrial curettage, followed by administration of progestational agents. Even though these tumors are prone to recur, with rates ranging from 24 percent (141) to 45 percent (140), and some patients experience more than one recurrence, conservative management still appears appropriate.

The mean time to recurrence is about 1 year, although the range extends to almost 5 years. There is one case report of a patient who developed a FIGO grade 2 endometrioid adenocarcinoma with cervical and lymphovascular invasion after having been managed conservatively for atypical polypoid adenomyoma 8 years previously (149). The goal of conservative therapy, obviously, is maintenance of fertility. In the series of 55 patients reported by Longacre et al. (140), 5 patients with recurrent or persistent atypical polypoid adenomyoma became pregnant and delivered at full-term. Hysterectomy remains a curative option in patients who fail conservative therapy or do not desire fertility.

The morphology, immunophenotype, genotype, and clinical biology of these tumors lead to the conclusion that atypical polypoid adenomyoma is a type of complex hyperplasia, usually with a *CTNNB1* (beta-catenin) mutation in a myomatous polyp (146). If the atypical polypoid adenomyoma contains atypical hyperplasia or even adenocarcinoma, it should behave similarly to atypical hyperplasia or adenocarcinoma confined to an endometrial polyp, with low rates of myometrial invasion (150).

Since myometrial invasion is only a rare occurrence, and no patient has ever reportedly died of adenocarcinoma associated with atypical polypoid adenomyoma, Longacre et al. (140) proposed the term "atypical polypoid adenomyofibroma of low malignant potential" for atypical polypoid adenomyoma containing foci of adenocarcinoma comprising more than 30 percent of the lesion. It is reasonable to use this term, provided the gynecologist is familiar with it and understands its significance. A more prevalent practice is to report "atypical polypoid adenomyoma with a focus of well-differentiated endometrioid adenocarcinoma" and explain the significance and expected clinical outcome in a note.

REFERENCES

1. McCluggage WG. Uterine carcinosarcomas (malignant mixed mullerian tumors) are metaplastic carcinomas. Int J Gynecol Cancer 2002;12:687-90.
2. McCluggage WG. Malignant biphasic uterine tumours: carcinosarcomas or metaplastic carcinomas? J Clin Pathol 2002;55:321-5.
3. McCluggage WG. A practical approach to the diagnosis of mixed epithelial and mesenchymal tumours of the uterus. Mod Pathol 2016;29(Suppl1):S78-91.
4. Kurman RJ, Carcangiu ML, Herrington CS, Young RH, eds. WHO classification of tumours of female reproductive organs, 4th ed. Lyon IARC Press; 2014:6.
5. Wilson BT, Cordell HJ. Uterine carcinosarcoma/malignant mixed Mullerian tumor incidence is increased in women with breast cancer, but independent of hormone therapy. J Gynecol Oncol 2015;26:249-51.
6. Bland AE, Calingaert B, Secord AA, et al. Relationship between tamoxifen use and high risk endometrial cancer histologic types. Gynecol Oncol 2009;112:150-4.
7. Brinton LA, Felix AS, McMeekin DS, et al. Etiologic heterogeneity in endometrial cancer: evidence from a Gynecologic Oncology Group trial. Gynecol Oncol 2013;129:277-84.
8. Ferguson SE, Soslow RA, Amsterdam A, Barakat RR. Comparison of uterine malignancies that develop during and following tamoxifen therapy. Gynecol Oncol 2006;101:322-6.
9. Hoogendoorn WE, Hollema H, van Boven HH, et al. Prognosis of uterine corpus cancer after tamoxifen treatment for breast cancer. Breast Cancer Res Treat 2008;112:99-108.
10. Magriples U, Naftolin F, Schwartz PE, Carcangiu ML. High-grade endometrial carcinoma in tamoxifen-treated breast cancer patients. J Clin Oncol 1993;11:485-90.
11. Silva EG, Tornos C, Malpica A, Mitchell MF. Uterine neoplasms in patients treated with tamoxifen. J Cell Biochem Suppl 1995;23:179-83.
12. Fehr PE, Prem KA. Malignancy of the uterine corpus following irradiation therapy for squamous cell carcinoma of the cervix. Am J Obstet Gynecol 1974;119:685-92.
13. Gallion HH, van Nagell JR Jr, Donaldson ES, Powell DE. Endometrial cancer following radiation therapy for cervical cancer. Gynecol Oncol 1987;27:76-83.
14. Parkash V, Carcangiu ML. Uterine papillary serous carcinoma after radiation therapy for carcinoma of the cervix. Cancer 1992;69:496-501.
15. Pothuri B, Ramondetta L, Eifel P, et al. Radiation-associated endometrial cancers are prognostically unfavorable tumors: a clinicopathologic comparison with 527 sporadic endometrial cancers. Gynecol Oncol 2006;103:948-51.
16. Pothuri B, Ramondetta L, Martino M, et al. Development of endometrial cancer after radiation treatment for cervical carcinoma. Obstet Gynecol 2003;101(Pt 1):941-5.
17. Rodriguez J, Hart WR. Endometrial cancers occurring 10 or more years after pelvic irradiation for carcinoma. Int J Gynecol Pathol 1982;1:135-44.
18. Harano K, Hirakawa A, Yunokawa M, et al. Prognostic factors in patients with uterine carcinosarcoma: a multi-institutional retrospective study from the Japanese Gynecologic Oncology Group. Int J Clin Oncol 2016;21:168-76.
19. Barwick KW, LiVolsi VA. Malignant mixed mullerian tumors of the uterus. A clinicopathologic assessment of 34 cases. Am J Surg Pathol 1979;3:125-35.
20. Silverberg SG, Major FJ, Blessing JA, et al. Carcinosarcoma (malignant mixed mesodermal tumor) of the uterus. A Gynecologic Oncology Group pathologic study of 203 cases. Int J Gynecol Pathol 1990;9:1-19.
21. Spanos WJ Jr, Wharton JT, Gomez L, Fletcher GH, Oswald MJ. Malignant mixed mullerian tumors of the uterus. Cancer 1984;53:311-6.
22. Pecorelli S. Revised FIGO staging for carcinoma of the vulva, cervix, and endometrium. Int J Gynaecol Obstet 2009;105:103-4.
23. Grayson W, Taylor LF, Cooper K. Carcinosarcoma of the uterine cervix: a report of eight cases with immunohistochemical analysis and evaluation of human papillomavirus status. Am J Surg Pathol 2001;25:338-47.
24. Ferguson SE, Tornos C, Hummer A, Barakat RR, Soslow RA. Prognostic features of surgical stage I uterine carcinosarcoma. Am J Surg Pathol 2007;31:1653-61.
25. Tafe LJ, Garg K, Chew I, Tornos C, Soslow RA. Endometrial and ovarian carcinomas with undifferentiated components: clinically aggressive and frequently underrecognized neoplasms. Mod Pathol 2010;23:781-9.
26. Fukunaga M, Nomura K, Endo Y, Ushigome S, Aizawa S. Carcinosarcoma of the uterus with extensive neuroectodermal differentiation. Histopathology 1996;29:565-70.

27. Kurihara S, Oda Y, Ohishi Y, et al. Endometrial stromal sarcomas and related high-grade sarcomas: immunohistochemical and molecular genetic study of 31 cases. Am J Surg Pathol 2008;32:1228-38.
28. Clement PB, Scully RE. Uterine tumors with mixed epithelial and mesenchymal elements. Semin Diagn Pathol 1988;5:199-222.
29. Costa MJ, Khan R, Judd R. Carcinoma (malignant mixed mullerian [mesodermal] tumor) of the uterus and ovary. Correlation of clinical, pathologic, and immunohistochemical features in 29 cases. Arch Pathol Lab Med 1991;115:583-90.
30. Sangoi AR, Kshirsagar M, Horvai AE, Roma AA. SATB2 expression is sensitive but not specific for osteosarcomatous components of gynecologic tract carcinosarcomas: a clinicopathologic study of 60 cases. Int J Gynecol Pathol 2017;36:140-5.
31. Chiang S, Snuderl M, Kojiro-Sanada S, et al. Primitive neuroectodermal tumors of the female genital tract: a morphologic, immunohistochemical, and molecular study of 19 cases. Am J Surg Path 2017;41:761-72.
32. Euscher ED, Deavers MT, Lopez-Terrada D, Lazar AJ, Silva EG, Malpica A. Uterine tumors with neuroectodermal differentiation: a series of 17 cases and review of the literature. Am J Surg Pathol 2008;32:219-28.
33. Gersell DJ, Duncan DA, Fulling KH. Malignant mixed mullerian tumor of the uterus with neuroectodermal differentiation. Int J Gynecol Pathol 1989;8:169-78.
34. Garcia-Galvis OF, Cabrera-Ozoria C, Fernandez JA, Stolnicu S, Nogales FF. Malignant mullerian mixed tumor of the ovary associated with yolk sac tumor, neuroepithelial and trophoblastic differentiation (teratoid carcinosarcoma). Int J Gynecol Pathol 2008;27:515-20.
35. Mount SL, Lee KR, Taatjes DJ. Carcinosarcoma (malignant mixed mullerian tumor) of the uterus with a rhabdoid tumor component. An immunohistochemical, ultrastructural, and immunoelectron microscopic case study. Am J Clin Pathol 1995;103:235-9.
36. Seidman JD, Chauhan S. Evaluation of the relationship between adenosarcoma and carcinosarcoma and a hypothesis of the histogenesis of uterine sarcomas. Int J Gynecol Pathol 2003;22:75-82.
37. Bitterman P, Chun B, Kurman RJ. The significance of epithelial differentiation in mixed mesodermal tumors of the uterus. A clinicopathologic and immunohistochemical study. Am J Surg Pathol 1990;14:317-28.
38. Krivak TC, Seidman JD, McBroom JW, MacKoul PJ, Aye LM, Rose GS. Uterine adenosarcoma with sarcomatous overgrowth versus uterine carcinosarcoma: comparison of treatment and survival. Gynecol Oncol 2001;83:89-94.
39. Cherniack AD, Shen H, Walter V, et al. Integrated molecular characterization of uterine carcinosarcoma. Cancer Cell 2017;31:411-23.
40. Clement PB, Scully RE. Mullerian adenosarcoma of the uterus: a clinicopathologic analysis of 100 cases with a review of the literature. Hum Pathol 1990;21:363-81.
41. Murray SK, Clement PB, Young RH. Endometrioid carcinomas of the uterine corpus with sex cord-like formations, hyalinization, and other unusual morphologic features: a report of 31 cases of a neoplasm that may be confused with carcinosarcoma and other uterine neoplasms. Am J Surg Pathol 2005;29:157-66.
42. Chen X, Arend R, Hamele-Bena D, et al. Uterine carcinosarcomas: clinical, histopathologic and immunohistochemical characteristics. Int J Gynecol Pathol 2017;36:412-9.
43. Buza N, Tavassoli FA. Comparative analysis of P16 and P53 expression in uterine malignant mixed mullerian tumors. Int J Gynecol Pathol 2009;28:514-21.
44. George E, Manivel JC, Dehner LP, Wick MR. Malignant mixed mullerian tumors: an immunohistochemical study of 47 cases, with histogenetic considerations and clinical correlation. Hum Pathol 1991;22:215-23.
45. Sreenan JJ, Hart WR. Carcinosarcomas of the female genital tract. A pathologic study of 29 metastatic tumors: further evidence for the dominant role of the epithelial component and the conversion theory of histogenesis. Am J Surg Pathol 1995;19:666-74.
46. Menczer J, Kravtsov V, Levy T, Berger E, Glezerman M, Avinoach I. Expression of c-kit in uterine carcinosarcoma. Gynecol Oncol 2005;96:210-5.
47. Raspollini MR, Susini T, Amunni G, et al. COX-2, c-KIT and HER-2/neu expression in uterine carcinosarcomas: prognostic factors or potential markers for targeted therapies? Gynecol Oncol 2005;96:159-67.
48. Jones S, Stransky N, McCord CL, et al. Genomic analyses of gynaecologic carcinosarcomas reveal frequent mutations in chromatin remodelling genes. Nat Commun 2014;19:5006.
49. McConechy MK, Ding J, Cheang MC, et al. Use of mutation profiles to refine the classification of endometrial carcinomas. J Pathol 2012;228:20-30.
50. Castilla MA, Moreno-Bueno G, Romero-Perez L, et al. Micro-RNA signature of the epithelial-mesenchymal transition in endometrial carcinosarcoma. J Pathol 2011;223:72-80.
51. Singh M, Spoelstra NS, Jean A, et al. ZEB1 expression in type I vs type II endometrial cancers: a marker of aggressive disease. Mod Pathol 2008;21:912-23.

52. Inoue H, Takahashi H, Hashimura M, et al. Cooperation of Sox4 with beta-catenin/p300 complex in transcriptional regulation of the Slug gene during divergent sarcomatous differentiation in uterine carcinosarcoma. BMC Cancer 2015;16:53.
53. Tornos C, Silva EG, Ordoñez NG, Gershenson DM, Young RH, Scully RE. Endometrioid carcinoma of the ovary with a prominent spindle-cell component, a source of diagnostic confusion. A report of 14 cases. Am J Surg Pathol 1995;19:1343-53.
54. Soslow RA. Mixed Mullerian tumors of the female genital tract. Surg Pathol Clin 2009;2:707-30.
55. Manivel C, Wick MR, Sibley RK. Neuroendocrine differentiation in mullerian neoplasms. An immunohistochemical study of a "pure" endometrial small-cell carcinoma and a mixed mullerian tumor containing small-cell carcinoma. Am J Clin Pathol 1986;86:438-43.
56. Posligua L MA, Liu J, Brown J, Deavers MT. Combined large cell neuroendocrine carcinoma and papillary serous carcinoma of the endometrium with pagetoid spread. Arch Pathol Lab Med 2008;132:1821-4.
57. Shaco-Levy R, Manor E, Piura B, Ariel I. An unusual composite endometrial tumor combining papillary serous carcinoma and small cell carcinoma. Am J Surg Pathol 2004;28:1103-6.
58. Bague S, Rodriguez IM, Prat J. Malignant mesonephric tumors of the female genital tract: a clinicopathologic study of 9 cases. Am J Surg Pathol 2004;28:601-7.
59. Clement PB, Young RH, Keh P, Ostor AG, Scully RE. Malignant mesonephric neoplasms of the uterine cervix. A report of eight cases, including four with a malignant spindle cell component. Am J Surg Pathol 1995;19:1158-71.
60. Kenny SL, McBride HA, Jamison J, McCluggage WG. Mesonephric adenocarcinomas of the uterine cervix and corpus: HPV-negative neoplasms that are commonly PAX8, CA125, and HMGA2 positive and that may be immunoreactive with TTF1 and hepatocyte nuclear factor 1-beta. Am J Surg Pathol 2012;36:799-807.
61. McFarland M, Quick CM, McCluggage WG. Hormone receptor-negative, thyroid transcription factor 1-positive uterine and ovarian adenocarcinomas: report of a series of mesonephric-like adenocarcinomas. Histopathology 2016;68:1013-20.
62. Howitt BE, Quade BJ, Nucci MR. Uterine polyps with features overlapping with those of Mullerian adenosarcoma: a clinicopathologic analysis of 29 cases emphasizing their likely benign nature. Am J Surg Pathol 2015;39:116-26.
63. Mirkovic J, McFarland M, Garcia E, et al. Targeted genomic profiling reveals recurrent KRAS mutations in mesonephric-like adenocarcinomas of the female genital tract. Am J Surg Pathol 2017. [Epub ahead of print]
64. Czernobilsky B, Mamet Y, David MB, Atlas I, Gitstein G, Lifschitz-Mercer B. Uterine retiform sertoli-leydig cell tumor: report of a case providing additional evidence that uterine tumors resembling ovarian sex cord tumors have a histologic and immunohistochemical phenotype of genuine sex cord tumors. Int J Gynecol Pathol 2005;24:335-40.
65. Stolnicu S, Szekely E, Molnar C, et al. Mature and immature solid teratomas involving uterine corpus, cervix, and ovary. Int J Gynecol Pathol 2017;36:222-7.
66. Bittencourt AL, Britto JF, Fonseca LE Jr. Wilms' tumor of the uterus: the first report of the literature. Cancer 1981;47:2496-9.
67. Garcia-Galvis OF, Stolnicu S, Muñoz E, Aneiros-Fernandez J, Alaggio R, Nogales FF. Adult extrarenal Wilms tumor of the uterus with teratoid features. Hum Pathol 2009;40:418-24.
68. McAlpine J, Azodi M, O'Malley D, et al. Extrarenal Wilms' tumor of the uterine corpus. Gynecologic oncology 2005;96:892-6.
69. Prat J, Young RH, Scully RE. Ovarian Sertoli-Leydig cell tumors with heterologous elements. II. Cartilage and skeletal muscle: a clinicopathologic analysis of twelve cases. Cancer 1982;50:2465-75.
70. George E, Lillemoe TJ, Twiggs LB, Perrone T. Malignant mixed mullerian tumor versus high-grade endometrial carcinoma and aggressive variants of endometrial carcinoma: a comparative analysis of survival. Int J Gynecol Pathol 1995;14:39-44.
71. Major FJ, Blessing JA, Silverberg SG, et al. Prognostic factors in early-stage uterine sarcoma. A Gynecologic Oncology Group study. Cancer 1993;71(Suppl):1702-9.
72. Yamada SD, Burger RA, Brewster WR, Anton D, Kohler MF, Monk BJ. Pathologic variables and adjuvant therapy as predictors of recurrence and survival for patients with surgically evaluated carcinosarcoma of the uterus. Cancer 2000;88:2782-6.
73. Alektiar KM, McKee A, Lin O, et al. Is there a difference in outcome between stage I-II endometrial cancer of papillary serous/clear cell and endometrioid FIGO Grade 3 cancer? Int J Radiat Oncol Biol Phys 2002;54:79-85.
74. Soslow RA, Bissonnette JP, Wilton A, et al. Clinicopathologic analysis of 187 high-grade endometrial carcinomas of different histologic subtypes: similar outcomes belie distinctive biologic differences. Am J Surg Pathol 2007;31:979-87.
75. Amant F, Cadron I, Fuso L, et al. Endometrial carcinosarcomas have a different prognosis and pattern of spread compared to high-risk epithelial endometrial cancer. Gynecol Oncol 2005;98:274-80.

76. Sartori E, Bazzurini L, Gadducci A, et al. Carcinosarcoma of the uterus: a clinicopathological multicenter CTF study. Gynecol Oncol 1997;67:70-5.
77. Dinh TV, Slavin RE, Bhagavan BS, Hannigan EV, Tiamson EM, Yandell RB. Mixed mullerian tumors of the uterus: a clinicopathologic study. Obstet Gynecol 1989;74(Pt 1):388-92.
78. Iwasa Y, Haga H, Konishi I, et al. Prognostic factors in uterine carcinosarcoma: a clinicopathologic study of 25 patients. Cancer 1998;82:512-9.
79. Matsuo K, Takazawa Y, Ross MS, et al. Significance of histologic pattern of carcinoma and sarcoma components on survival outcomes of uterine carcinosarcoma. Ann Oncol 2016;27:1257-66.
80. Berton-Rigaud D, Devouassoux-Shisheboran M, Ledermann JA, et al. Gynecologic Cancer InterGroup (GCIG) consensus review for uterine and ovarian carcinosarcoma. Int J Gynecol Cancer 2014;24(Suppl 3):S55-60.
81. Makker V, Kravetz SJ, Gallagher J, et al. Treatment outcomes in completely resected stage I to stage IV uterine carcinosarcoma with rhabdomyosarcoma differentiation. Int J Gynecol Cancer 2013;23:1635-41.
82. Abeler VM, Royne O, Thoresen S, Danielsen HE, Nesland JM, Kristensen GB. Uterine sarcomas in Norway. A histopathological and prognostic survey of a total population from 1970 to 2000 including 419 patients. Histopathology 2009;54:355-64.
83. Seagle BL, Kanis M, Strohl AE, Shahabi S. Survival of women with mullerian adenosarcoma: a National Cancer Data Base study. Gynecol Oncol 2016;143:636-41.
84. Clement PB, Scully RE. Mullerian adenosarcoma of the uterus. A clinicopathologic analysis of ten cases of a distinctive type of mullerian mixed tumor. Cancer 1974;34:1138-49.
85. Fox H, Harilal KR, Youell A. Mullerian adenocoma of the uterine body: a report of nine cases. Histopathology 1979;3:167-80.
86. Zaloudek CJ, Norris HJ. Adenofibroma and adenosarcoma of the uterus: a clinicopathologic study of 35 cases. Cancer 1981;48:354-66.
87. Bocklage T, Lee KR, Belinson JL. Uterine mullerian adenosarcoma following adenomyoma in a woman on tamoxifen therapy. Gynecol Oncol 1992;44:104-9.
88. Clement PB, Oliva E, Young RH. Mullerian adenosarcoma of the uterine corpus associated with tamoxifen therapy: a report of six cases and a review of tamoxifen-associated endometrial lesions. Int J Gynecol Pathol 1996;15:222-9.
89. Press MF, Scully RE. Endometrial "sarcomas" complicating ovarian thecoma, polycystic ovarian disease and estrogen therapy. Gynecol Oncol 1985;21:135-54.
90. Kerner H, Lichtig C. Mullerian adenosarcoma presenting as cervical polyps: a report of seven cases and review of the literature. Obstet Gynecol 1993;81(Pt 1):655-9.
91. Pecorelli S. Revised FIGO staging for carcinoma of the vulva, cervix, and endometrium. Int J Gynecol Obstet 2009;105:103-4.
92. Gallardo A, Prat J. Mullerian adenosarcoma: a clinicopathologic and immunohistochemical study of 55 cases challenging the existence of adenofibroma. Am J Surg Pathol 2009;33:278-88.
93. Clarke BA, Mulligan AM, Irving JA, McCluggage WG, Oliva E. Mullerian adenosarcomas with unusual growth patterns: staging issues. Int J Gynecol Pathol 2011;30:340-7.
94. Elshafie M, Rahimi S, Ganesan R, Hirschowitz L. Mullerian adenosarcoma arising in a subserosal adenomyoma. Int J Surg Pathol 2013;21:186-9.
95. Gollard R, Kosty M, Bordin G, Wax A, Lacey C. Two unusual presentations of mullerian adenosarcoma: case reports, literature review, and treatment considerations. Gynecol Oncol 1995;59:412-22.
96. Clement PB, Scully RE. Mullerian adenosarcomas of the uterus with sex cord-like elements. A clinicopathologic analysis of eight cases. Am J Clin Pathol 1989;91:664-72.
97. Mohammadizadeh F, Rajabi P, Behnamfar F, Hani M, Bagheri M. Extensive overgrowth of sex cord-like differentiation in uterine mullerian adenosarcoma: a rare and challenging entity. Int J Gynecol Pathol 2016;35:153-61.
98. Stolnicu S, Balachandran K, Aleykutty MA, et al. Uterine adenosarcomas overgrown by sex-cord-like tumour: report of two cases. J Clin Pathol 2009;62:942-4.
99. Kaku T, Silverberg SG, Major FJ, Miller A, Fetter B, Brady MF. Adenosarcoma of the uterus: a Gynecologic Oncology Group clinicopathologic study of 31 cases. Int J Gynecol Pathol 1992;11:75-88.
100. Eichhorn JH, Young RH, Clement PB, Scully RE. Mesodermal (mullerian) adenosarcoma of the ovary: a clinicopathologic analysis of 40 cases and a review of the literature. Am J Surg Pathol 2002;26:1243-58.
101. Fehmian C, Jones J, Kress Y, Abadi M. Adenosarcoma of the uterus with extensive smooth muscle differentiation: ultrastructural study and review of the literature. Ultrastruct Pathol 1997;21:73-9.
102. Stolnicu S, Molnar C, Barsan I, Boros M, Nogales FF, Soslow RA. The impact on survival of an extensive sex cord-like component in mullerian adenosarcomas: a study comprising 6 cases. Int J Gynecol Pathol 2016;35:147-52.

103. Garcia CR, Toro Rojas M, Morales Jimenez C, Lopez Beltran A, Nogales Ortiz F, Nogales Fernandez F. Uterine mullerian adenosarcoma with histiocytic (xanthomatous) mesenchymal component. Histol Histopathol 1991;6:363-7.

104. Czernobilsky B, Hohlweg-Majert P, Dallenbach-Hellweg G. Uterine adenosarcoma: a clinicopathologic study of 11 cases with a re-evaluation of histologic criteria. Arch Gynecol 1983;233:281-94.

105. Soslow RA, Ali A, Oliva E. Mullerian adenosarcomas: an immunophenotypic analysis of 35 cases. Am J Surg Pathol 2008;32:1013-21.

105a. Clement PB. Mullerian adenosarcomas of the uterus with sarcomatous overgrowth. A clinicopathological analysis of 10 cases. Am J Surg Pathol 1989;13:28-38.

106. Wu RI, Schorge JO, Dal Cin P, Young RH, Oliva E. Mullerian adenosarcoma of the uterus with low-grade sarcomatous overgrowth characterized by prominent hydropic change resulting in mimicry of a smooth muscle tumor. Int J Gynecol Pathol 2014;33:573-80.

107. Hodgson A, Amemiya Y, Seth A, Djordjevic B, Parra-Herran C. high-grade mullerian adenosarcoma: genomic and clinicopathologic characterization of a distinct neoplasm with prevalent TP53 Pathway alterations and aggressive behavior. Am J Surg Pathol 2017;41:1513-22.

108. Bhardwaj M, Batrani M, Chawla I, Malik R. Uterine primitive neuroectodermal tumor with adenosarcoma: a case report. J Med Case Rep 2010;4:195.

109. Lack EE, Bitterman P, Sundeen JT. Mullerian adenosarcoma of the uterus with pure angiosarcoma: case report. Hum Pathol 1991;22:1289-91.

110. Amant F, Schurmans K, Steenkiste E, et al. Immunohistochemical determination of estrogen and progesterone receptor positivity in uterine adenosarcoma. Gynecol Oncol 2004;93:680-5.

111. Amant F, Steenkiste E, Schurmans K, et al. Immunohistochemical expression of CD10 antigen in uterine adenosarcoma. Int J Gynecol Cancer 2004;14:1118-21.

112. Aggarwal N, Bhargava R, Elishaev E. Uterine adenosarcomas: diagnostic use of the proliferation marker Ki-67 as an adjunct to morphologic diagnosis. Int J Gynecol Pathol 2012;31:447-52.

113. Piscuoglio S, Burke KA, Ng CK, et al. Uterine adenosarcomas are mesenchymal neoplasms. J Pathol 2016;238:381-8.

114. Chiang S, Oliva E. Cytogenetic and molecular aberrations in endometrial stromal tumors. Hum Pathol 2011;42:609-17.

115. Howitt BE, Sholl LM, Dal Cin P, et al. Targeted genomic analysis of Mullerian adenosarcoma. J Pathol 2015;235:37-49.

116. Howitt BE, Dal Cin P, Nucci MR, Quade BJ. Involvement of chromosome 8 in mullerian adenosarcoma. Int J Gynecol Pathol 2017;36:24-30.

117. Gilks CB, Clement PB, Hart WR, Young RH. Uterine adenomyomas excluding atypical polypoid adenomyomas and adenomyomas of endocervical type: a clinicopathologic study of 30 cases of an underemphasized lesion that may cause diagnostic problems with brief consideration of adenomyomas of other female genital tract sites. Int J Gynecol Pathol 2000;19:195-205.

118. Tahlan A, Nanda A, Mohan H. Uterine adenomyoma: a clinicopathologic review of 26 cases and a review of the literature. Int J Gynecol Pathol 2006;25:361-5.

119. Tai LH, Tavassoli FA. Endometrial polyps with atypical (bizarre) stromal cells. Am J Surg Pathol 2002;26:505-9.

120. Li RF, Gupta M, McCluggage WG, Ronnett BM. Embryonal rhabdomyosarcoma (botryoid type) of the uterine corpus and cervix in adult women: report of a case series and review of the literature. Am J Surg Pathol 2013;37:344-55.

121. Oliva E, Clement PB, Young RH. Endometrial stromal tumors: an update on a group of tumors with a protean phenotype. Adv Anat Pathol 2000;7:257-81.

122. de Leval L, Lim GS, Waltregny D, Oliva E. Diverse phenotypic profile of uterine tumors resembling ovarian sex cord tumors: an immunohistochemical study of 12 cases. Am J Surg Pathol 2010;34:1749-61.

123. Bernard B, Clarke BA, Malowany JI, et al. Uterine adenosarcomas: a dual-institution update on staging, prognosis and survival. Gynecol Oncol 2013;131:634-9.

124. Blom R, Guerrieri C. Adenosarcoma of the uterus: a clinicopathologic, DNA flow cytometric, p53 and mdm-2 analysis of 11 cases. Int J Gynecol Cancer 1999;9:37-43.

125. Carroll A, Ramirez PT, Westin SN, et al. Uterine adenosarcoma: an analysis on management, outcomes, and risk factors for recurrence. Gynecol Oncol 2014;135:455-61.

126. Machida H, Nathenson MJ, Takiuchi T, Adams CL, Garcia-Sayre J, Matsuo K. Significance of lymph node metastasis on survival of women with uterine adenosarcoma. Gynecol Oncol 2017;144:524-30.

127. Mbatani N, Olawaiye AB, Prat J. Uterine sarcomas. Int J Gynaecol Obstet 2018;143(Suppl 2):51-8.

128. Verschraegen CF, Vasuratna A, Edwards C, et al. Clinicopathologic analysis of mullerian adenosarcoma: the M.D. Anderson Cancer Center experience. Oncol Rep 1998;5:939-44.

129. Vellios F. Papillary adenofibroma-adenosarcoma: the uterine phyllodes. Prog Surg Pathol 1980;1:205-19.
130. Ostor AG, Fortune DW. Benign and low grade variants of mixed Mullerian tumour of the uterus. Histopathology 1980;4:369-82.
131. Horie Y, Ikawa S, Kadowaki K, Minagawa Y, Kigawa J, Terakawa N. Lipoadenofibroma of the uterine corpus. Report of a new variant of adenofibroma (benign mullerian mixed tumor). Arch Pathol Lab Med 1995;119:274-6.
132. Sinkre P, Miller DS, Milchgrub S, Hameed A. Adenomyofibroma of the endometrium with skeletal muscle differentiation. Int J Gynecol Pathol 2000;19:280-3.
133. Cullen TS. Adenomyomas of the Uterus. Philadelphia: Saunders; 1908.
134. Breen JL, Lukeman JM, Neubecker RD. Nodular fasciitis of the round ligament. Report of a case. Obstet Gynecol 1962;19:397-400.
135. Redman R, Wilkinson EJ, Massoll NA. Uterine-like mass with features of an extrauterine adenomyoma presenting 22 years after total abdominal hysterectomy-bilateral salpingo-oophorectomy: a case report and review of the literature. Arch Pathol Lab Med 2005;129:1041-3.
136. Tandon N, Showalter J, Sultana S, Zhao B, Zhang S. Extrauterine Adenomyoma of the liver in a 50 year old female with pelvic endometriosis. Ann Clin Lab Sci 2017;47:208-12.
137. Payne F, Rollason TP, Sivridis E. Adenomyolipoma of the endometrium—a hamartoma? Histopathology 1992;20:357-9.
138. Silverberg SG. Adenomyomatosis of endometrium and endocervix—a hamartoma. Am J Clin Pathol 1975;64:192-9.
139. Hirschowitz L, Mayall FG, Ganesan R, McCluggage WG. Intravascular adenomyomatosis: expanding the morphologic spectrum of intravascular leiomyomatosis. Am J Surg Pathol 2013;37:1395-400.
140. Longacre TA, Chung MH, Rouse RV, Hendrickson MR. Atypical polypoid adenomyofibromas (atypical polypoid adenomyomas) of the uterus. A clinicopathologic study of 55 cases. Am J Surg Pathol 1996;20:1-20.
141. Matsumoto T, Hiura M, Baba T, et al. Clinical management of atypical polypoid adenomyoma of the uterus. A clinicopathological review of 29 cases. Gynecol Oncol 2013;129:54-7.
142. Young RH, Treger T, Scully RE. Atypical polypoid adenomyoma of the uterus. A report of 27 cases. Am J Clin Pathol 1986;86:139-45.
143. Mazur MT. Atypical polypoid adenomyomas of the endometrium. Am J Surg Pathol 1981;5:473-82.
144. Ramos P, Valenzuela P, Santana A, Ruiz A, Solano J. Atypical polypoid adenomyoma of the uterine cervix: a diagnostic problem. J Obstet Gynaecol 2003;23:319-21.
145. Edwards JM, Alsop S, Modesitt SC. Coexisting atypical polypoid adenomyoma and endometrioid endometrial carcinoma in a young woman with Cowden syndrome: case report and implications for screening and prevention. Gynecol Oncol Case Rep 2012;2:29-31.
146. Nemejcova K, Kenny SL, Laco J, et al. Atypical polypoid adenomyoma of the uterus: an immunohistochemical and molecular study of 21 cases. Am J Surg Pathol 2015;39:1148-55.
147. Ota S, Catasus L, Matias-Guiu X, et al. Molecular pathology of atypical polypoid adenomyoma of the uterus. Hum Pathol 2003;34:784-8.
148. Soslow RA, Chung MH, Rouse RV, Hendrickson MR, Longacre TA. Atypical polypoid adenomyofibroma (APA) versus well-differentiated endometrial carcinoma with prominent stromal matrix: an immunohistochemical study. Int J Gynecol Pathol 1996;15:209-16.
149. Inoue K, Tsubamoto H, Hori M, Ogasawara T, Takemura T. A case of endometrioid adenocarcinoma developing 8 years after conservative management for atypical polypoid adenomyoma. Gynecol Oncol Case Rep 2014;8:21-3.
150. Leitao MM Jr, Han G, Lee LX, et al. Complex atypical hyperplasia of the uterus: characteristics and prediction of underlying carcinoma risk. Am J Obstet Gynecol 2010;203:349.e1-6.

12 MISCELLANEOUS AND METASTATIC MALIGNANCIES

Although most tumors within the uterine corpus are categorized as endometrial carcinomas, smooth muscle, stromal, or mixed müllerian tumors, neoplasms that are more commonly diagnosed outside the uterine corpus and metastases can also occur.

NEUROENDOCRINE CARCINOMAS

General Features. Three large series have reported 10, 16, and 25 patients, respectively, with *neuroendocrine carcinomas* or *endometrial tumors with neuroendocrine differentiation* (1–3). These patients ranged in age from 30 to 87 (median, 57) years and although they typically presented with uterine bleeding, paraneoplastic syndromes such as paraneoplastic retinopathy (4–7) and Cushing syndrome (8) occasionally were reported.

Neuroendocrine carcinomas are typically bulky and polypoid, and often invade the myometrium. More than two thirds of patients present with high-stage disease at the time of initial diagnosis and have a poor prognosis despite aggressive treatment, except in one series, where about 30 percent of patients (including those with stage 3 disease) survived more than 5 years (2). In the largest series to date, 60 percent of tumors were admixed with an endometrial adenocarcinoma (fig. 12-1A), most often endometrioid (1–3), and, rarely, serous carcinoma (2) or carcinosarcoma (malignant mixed müllerian tumor) (3). The neuroendocrine component may be represented by a small cell or large cell neuroendocrine carcinoma, or both.

Microscopic and Immunohistochemical Findings. A diagnosis of small cell neuroendocrine carcinoma starts with an appreciation of the classic cytologic features. The cells are small, oval to slightly spindled, with scant cytoplasm (high nuclear to cytoplasmic [N/C] ratio), nuclear molding, and crush artifact. Nuclei show finely dispersed chromatin (salt and pepper) or are hyperchromatic with apoptosis and brisk mitotic activity (fig. 12-1B). Cells often grow in diffuse or trabecular patterns. If needed, immunohistochemistry for neuroendocrine markers can be performed, but it is not required for the diagnosis of small cell carcinoma. Furthermore, not every small cell carcinoma has extensive expression of neuroendocrine markers, and cytokeratin expression may be attenuated or absent, particularly in small samples (9–11).

Large cell neuroendocrine carcinomas often show insular (organoid/nesting) growth, with or without solid components, while trabecular or ribbon-like patterns are less common. The cells are typically polygonal and medium to large, with considerable amounts of amphophilic or eosinophilic cytoplasm (fig. 12-1C). The nuclei are large and vesicular, and have prominent nucleoli. Large bizarre nuclei may be observed, geographic necrosis is common, and mitotic rate is very high. In order to establish a diagnosis of large cell neuroendocrine carcinoma, more than 10 percent of tumor cells should show positivity for one neuroendocrine marker in the appropriate histologic context (fig. 12-1D).

In the largest series to date (2), all neuroendocrine carcinomas expressed at least one neuroendocrine marker, such as chromogranin, synaptophysin, or CD56, and most expressed more than one. Pancytokeratin was typically positive and p16 was overexpressed in some, while high-risk human papillomavirus (HPV) in situ hybridization was negative in all tumors tested. Only one third of large cell neuroendocrine carcinomas showed PAX8 expression and about 50 percent had loss of expression of at least one DNA mismatch repair (MMR) protein, almost exclusively MLH1/PMS2 (2).

Differential Diagnosis. The differential diagnosis of these tumors varies depending upon the presence of small or large cells. Once a diagnosis of small cell carcinoma has been established, the possibility of small cell carcinoma of cervix should be considered, which, in contrast to small cell carcinoma of the endometrium, is

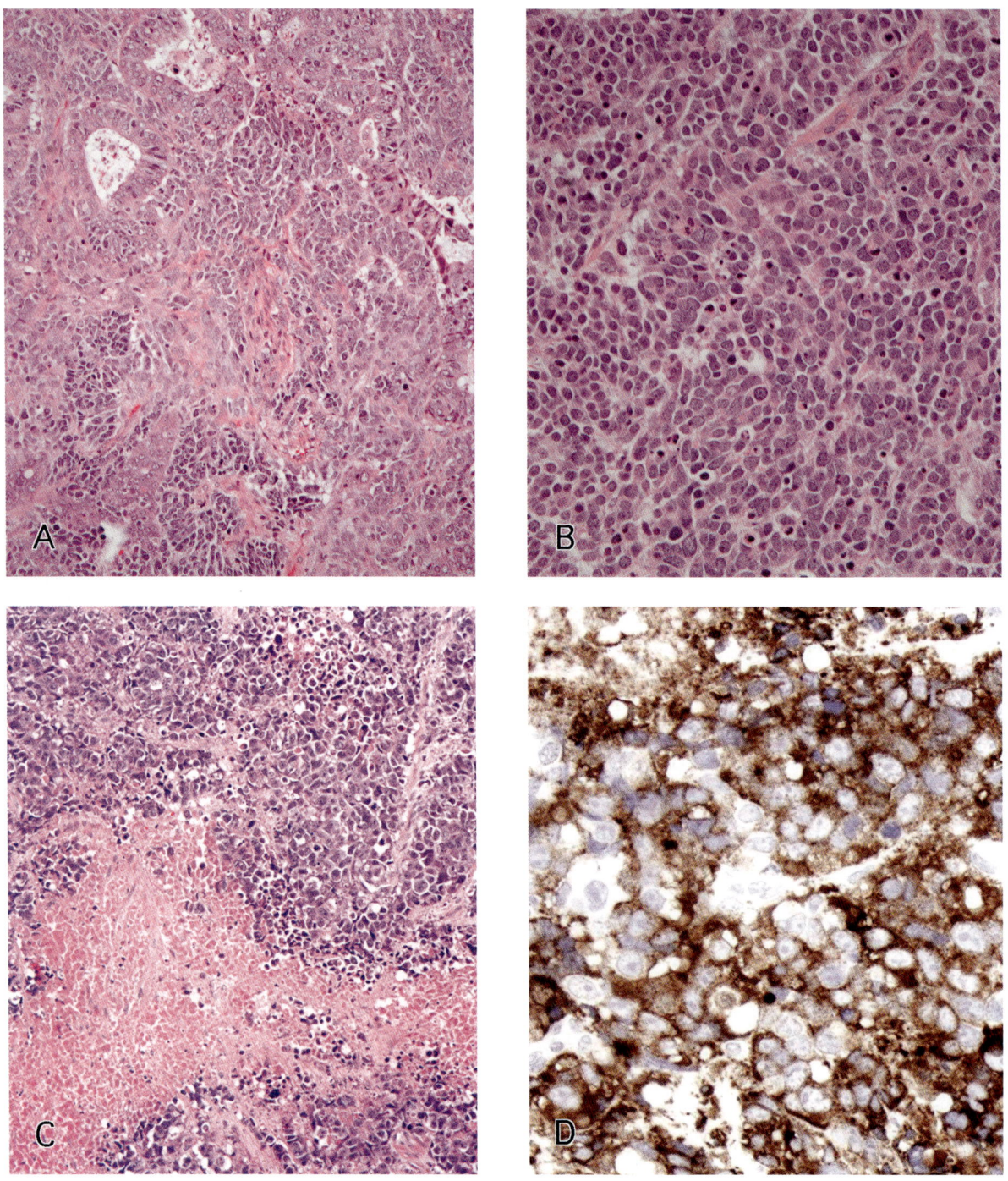

Figure 12-1

NEUROENDOCRINE CARCINOMAS OF ENDOMETRIUM

Small cell carcinoma shows nests of small blue cells juxtaposed to well-developed endometrioid glands (A). Small cell carcinoma is characterized by cells with a high nuclear to cytoplasmic ratio, nuclear molding, common apoptoses, and mitoses (B). Large cell neuroendocrine carcinoma displays cords and nests of cells with abundant cytoplasm. These tumors are often associated with geographic necrosis (C). (Courtesy of Dr. A. Malpica, Houston, TX). Chromogranin positivity confirms the diagnosis of large cell neuroendocrine carcinoma. In contrast to small cell carcinoma, positivity for one neuroendocrine marker in more than 10 percent of cells is necessary to establish this diagnosis (D). (Courtesy of Dr. A. Malpica, Houston, TX).

frequently etiologically associated with HPV infection, and thus, HPV positive.

The possibility of central- or peripheral-type primitive neuroectodermal tumor (PNET), lymphoma, and leukemia should also be considered. Central-type PNET may show glial, ependymal, or medulloepithelial differentiation, while the peripheral type is typically associated with t(11,22). These tumors lack the mitotic activity, nuclear molding, and frequent apoptoses seen in small cell carcinoma. Keratin positivity without glial fibrillary acidic protein (GFAP) expression favors neuroendocrine carcinoma over PNET. Involvement by leukemia or lymphoma is typically part of a systemic disease and the tumor cells are typically negative for neuroendocrine and epithelial markers.

Recognition of a pure or mixed neuroendocrine carcinoma is often problematic, as evidenced by frequent diagnostic discrepancies reported in one series (2). Both large and small cell carcinoma may simulate the appearance of a high-grade endometrioid carcinoma due to shared solid architecture. Furthermore, endometrioid carcinomas may show neuroendocrine differentiation by immunohistochemistry but this finding does not classify the tumor as a neuroendocrine carcinoma.

Undifferentiated endometrial carcinoma differs from small cell carcinoma not only by the cytologic features, but also by the immunophenotype. By definition, undifferentiated carcinoma does not show more than weak, focal expression of neuroendocrine markers, however, distinction based only on immunohistochemistry may be misleading (12).

SQUAMOUS CELL CARCINOMA

General Features. *Squamous cell carcinoma* is an uncommon tumor, with fewer than 100 cases reported in the literature. The diagnosis can only be established when a primary cervical squamous cell carcinoma has been excluded and no endometrioid glandular differentiation is present (13–15).

Patients are typically postmenopausal at the time of diagnosis (average age, about 60 years). The most frequent presenting symptom is vaginal bleeding. Chronic pyometra secondary to cervical stenosis, nulliparity, and prior radiation are known predisposing factors. The uterus is

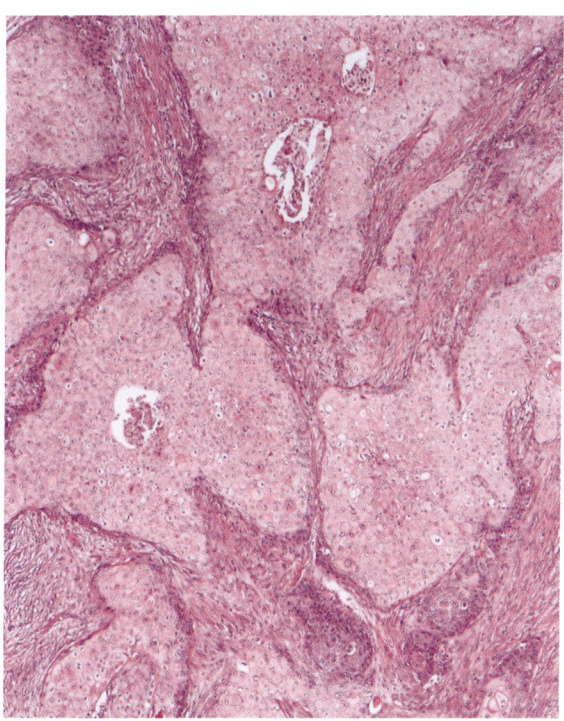

Figure 12-2

SQUAMOUS CELL CARCINOMA OF ENDOMETRIUM

Cervical squamous carcinoma and endometrioid carcinoma with squamous differentiation should be excluded before making this diagnosis.

often enlarged and the endometrium may show granular excrescences, papillary fronds that on occasion have a condylomatous or verrucous appearance, and purulent material.

Microscopic Findings. Tumors may be highly differentiated (fig. 12-2), often resembling benign, reactive, or mildly atypical mature squamous epithelium of the cervix in cytologic preparations, biopsies, and curettings; nevertheless, poorly differentiated, including sarcomatoid, tumors can occur. Variable degrees of keratinization are present. The pattern of myometrial infiltration can vary from "pushing" in well-differentiated tumors, with some characterized by a burrowing growth within the myometrium that is noted grossly as central cysts with white material, or may show destructive invasion, particularly in high-grade carcinomas.

These tumors are typically HPV unrelated (16) and show no or minimal p16 nuclear expression (14,17). Associated findings include pyometria, chronic endometritis, and squamous metaplasia.

Differential Diagnosis. The differential diagnosis includes cervical squamous carcinoma and high-grade squamous intraepithelial lesion extending to endometrium, endometrioid adenocarcinoma with extensive squamous differentiation, transitional cell carcinoma, and ichthyosis uteri (i.e., extensive, plaque-like squamous metaplasia of endometrium) (14,18,19). To establish a diagnosis of primary uterine corpus squamous cell carcinoma, extension from a concurrent or preexistent cervical primary tumor should be excluded and no connection with the cervical squamous epithelium should be noted. Squamous cell carcinoma of the cervix may extend to the endometrium, replacing surface epithelium and glands, and it has been rarely reported to extend along the surface of the fallopian tube and involve the ovary (20). The location of the mass, prior clinical history, and different p16 results are helpful in difficult settings (14,17).

Some endometrioid carcinomas have a prominent squamous cell component that resembles pure squamous cell carcinoma of the endometrium. As immunohistochemistry results also overlap, extensive sampling is required in order to identify endometrioid glands or morular squamous metaplasia.

Transitional cell carcinoma of the endometrium may have prominent papillary growth and histologically may be difficult to distinguish from squamous cell carcinoma. Distinction between these two entities may be subjective and not clinically relevant (21). On gross examination, transitional cell carcinomas are typically polypoid and most importantly almost never seen in a pure form but associated with squamous differentiation (squamotransitional carcinomas) or another component, usually endometroid carcinoma. The immunohistochemical profile is similar to that of primary endometrial carcinomas since they are CK7 positive and CK20 negative.

Squamous cell carcinoma can be distinguished from ichthyosis uteri in the presence of moderate or severe nuclear atypia and/or myometrial invasion. Rare squamous carcinomas arising in ichthyosis have been reported (22,23). The finding of abundant benign-appearing or mildly atypical squamous cells in an endometrial curetting from a postmenopausal patient should prompt clinical workup.

Treatment and Prognosis. Although 80 percent of patients in one study had stage 1 disease, deep myometrial invasion is common. Survival is stage dependent and possibly associated with the presence of lymphovascular invasion. In one study, none of the patients who experienced recurrence survived. Both local and distant recurrences, including peritoneal carcinomatosis, have been reported (15).

MESONEPHRIC-LIKE CARCINOMA

Recent studies indicate the rare existence of *mesonephric-like carcinomas* of the uterine corpus, although with a much lower frequency than in the cervix (24). They may be centered in the outer half of the myometrium.

As seen in the cervix, mesonephric-like carcinomas of the uterine corpus show a combination of architectural patterns, most commonly small glands and tubules with eosinophilic secretions, glomeruloid structures, and sieve-like spaces (fig. 12-3A–C). Papillary (fig. 12-3D), solid, or spindled growth patterns are less frequently noted. The cells display vesicular or grooved, often overlapping nuclei with variable amounts of clear to more commonly eosinophilic cytoplasm. These tumors are frequently positive for nuclear thyroid transcription factor 1 (TTF1); variably positive with CD10, calretinin, and GATA-3; and consistently negative for ER and PR, with wild-type p53 expression (24,25).

The architectural patterns of mesonephric-like carcinoma may simulate an endometrioid, clear cell, or serous carcinoma. Clues to an accurate diagnosis include a mixture of characteristic patterns as described above, and lack of squamous or mucinous differentiation (seen in endometrioid carcinoma), and dyshesive cells with pleomorphic nuclei (seen in serous carcinoma). Endometrioid carcinomas are typically ER/PR positive, but most are GATA-3 negative and only occasionally express TTF1 (26,27) while serous carcinomas show mutation-type p53 staining (28–33). Clear cell carcinoma rarely enters in this differential diagnosis, and it is important to note that two examples of mesonephric-like carcinoma were reported to be HNF1-beta and napsin A positive (24). Although the clinical behavior of these tumors is not well established, mesonephric carcinomas may behave more aggressively than differentiated endometrioid

Miscellaneous and Metastatic Malignancies

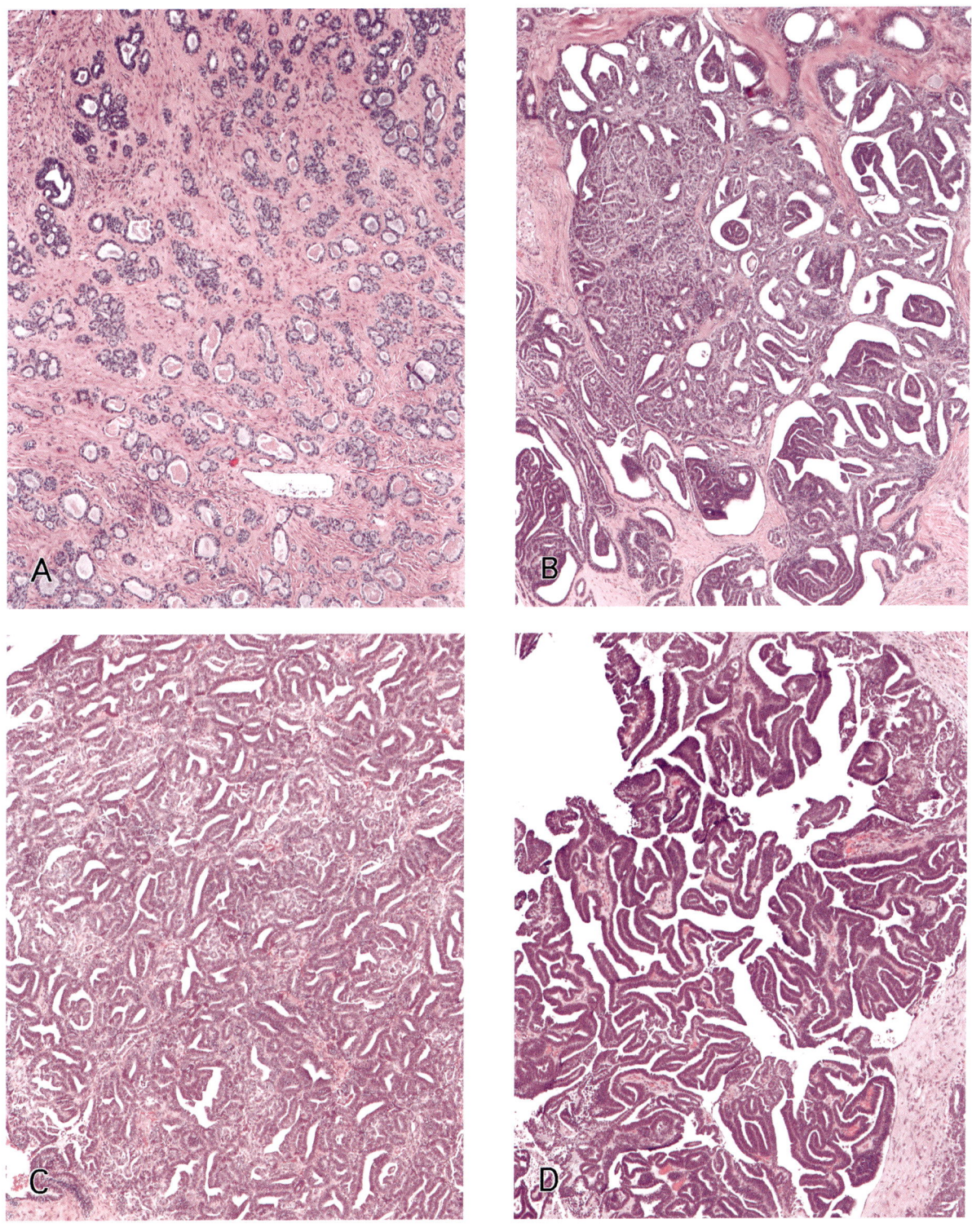

Figure 12-3

MESONEPHRIC-LIKE ADENOCARCINOMA

Typical tubular pattern (A); glomeruloid architecture (B); glandular morphology resembling endometrioid adenocarcinoma (C); and papillary growth resembling papillary endometrioid, and, less frequently, serous carcinoma (D).

carcinomas, with a potential propensity for pulmonary metastases (personal observation).

PRIMITIVE NEUROECTODERMAL TUMORS

Since the seminal publication by Daya et al. (34), only two large clinicopathologic series of *primitive neuroectodermal tumors* (PNETs) have been reported in the literature, one on uterine tumors associated with primitive neuroectodermal differentiation (17 cases) (35) and another on PNETs of the female genital tract (19 cases) including 8 uterine examples (36). Patients ranged in age from 26 to 81 (median, 57) years, but were often postmenopausal. Vaginal bleeding was the most common presentation and most patients had advanced stage disease at diagnosis. Eighteen out of 25 tumors were pure PNETs, while in 10, the primitive neuroectodermal component was associated with a variety of uterine neoplasms, including endometrioid carcinoma, unclassified sarcoma, rhabdomyosarcoma, adenosarcoma, and carcinosarcoma. Almost all tumors contained a component of fibrillary, neuropil-like background, albeit not necessarily extensive (fig. 12-4A,B). Ganglion-like cells were noted in one (35). When these tumors are of "central-type" (central nervous system [CNS] type) they may contain neuropil and Homer-Wright rosettes, an appearance similar to neuroblastoma, or ependymal-type rosettes and perivascular pseudorosettes recapitulating the appearance of ependymoblastoma (fig. 12-4C,D). Tumors with a morphology resembling medulloblastoma and even glioblastoma have also been encountered (34). The majority of these tumors are negative for cytokeratins, while most are positive with at least two of the following: synaptophysin, neurofilaments, CD99, Fli-1, and GFAP (fig. 12-4E), the latter in about 50 percent of cases in one series (36). None of the "central-type" tumors harbors the t(11;22) and *EWSR1* gene rearrangement.

The possibility of a peripheral-type PNET/Ewing sarcoma should be considered when the tumor shows a diffuse growth of small cells lacking astrocytic, glial, or neuronal differentiation (fig. 12-5A,B). Peripheral-type PNETs are typically positive for CD99 (fig. 12-5C) and Fli-1 but are GFAP negative, and show t(11;22) and *EWSR1* gene rearrangements. There appears to be fewer than 15 published cases with molecular confirmation, making this type of PNET less common than its central-type counterpart. If a peripheral-type PNET (i.e., Ewing sarcoma) is suspected, the diagnosis should be confirmed with molecular testing or fluorescence in situ hybridization (FISH) for detection of the *EWSR1* rearrangement. Rare tumors that have the morphologic and immunophenotypic features of peripheral PNET/Ewing sarcoma, but lack *EWSR1* rearrangement may harbor less common alterations (*FUS, BCOR, CCNB3, CIC,* or *DUX4*) which are reported in the Ewing family of tumors involving bone and soft tissues (36).

A pure PNET or a component of neuroectodermal tumor in a uterine tumor with heterogeneous morphology may be overlooked if undue emphasis is placed on equating solid architecture with FIGO grade 3 endometrioid carcinoma. Furthermore, PNETs with obvious rosettes can be misinterpreted as gland-forming endometrioid carcinomas (fig. 12-4C–D). The correct diagnosis includes the presence of fibrillary stroma, rosettes, or pseudorosettes rather than glands, a primitive appearance of the nuclei, and the absence of confirmatory endometrioid features. Helpful immunostains in the diagnosis of central-type PNETs include neurofilaments and GFAP in the absence of strong pancytokeratin expression as carcinomas may very rarely be GFAP positive (37).

Undifferentiated carcinoma also enters in the differential diagnosis of PNET as there is substantial morphologic and immunohistochemical overlap. Both tumors often display a diffuse growth of monotonous, dyshesive cells with limited or absent expression of epithelial markers and positivity for neuroendocrine markers. By definition, however, the latter are only focally expressed in undifferentiated carcinoma (12), in contrast to PNET. Diffuse and strong membranous CD99 and nuclear Fli-1 positivity with at least one neuroendocrine marker and minimal to absent keratin positivity supports the diagnosis of PNET over undifferentiated carcinoma. In contrast, undifferentiated carcinomas may show loss of BRG1, BRM, and INI1 expression (38,39). DNA MMR protein deficiency favors endometrioid and undifferentiated carcinomas over PNET. Rarely, other primary or metastatic tumors, such as Wilms tumor, malignant melanoma, lymphoma, small cell carcinoma, and

Miscellaneous and Metastatic Malignancies

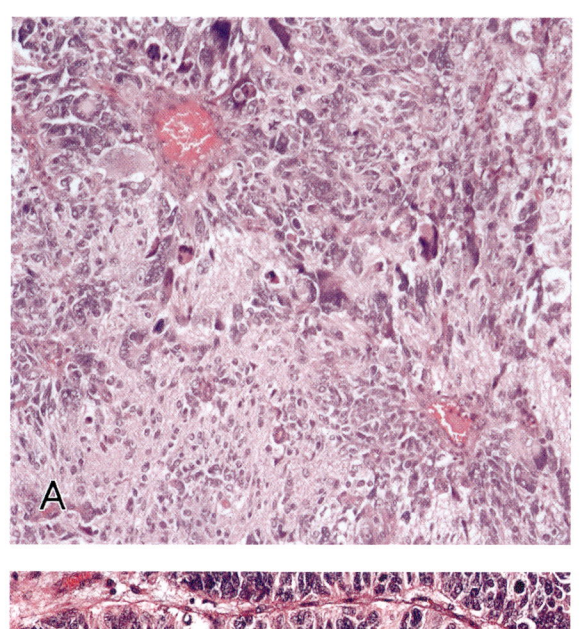
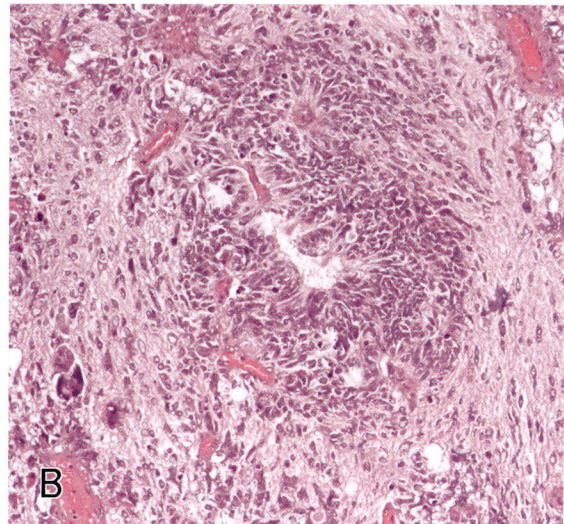
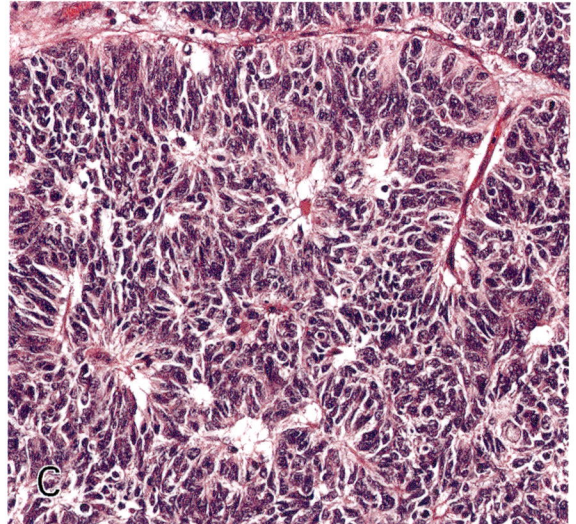
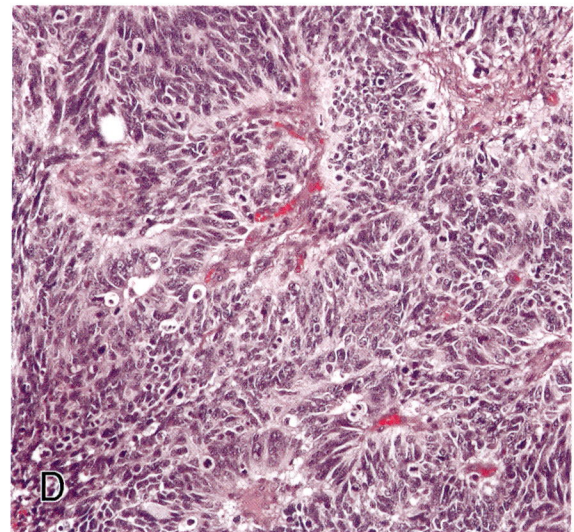
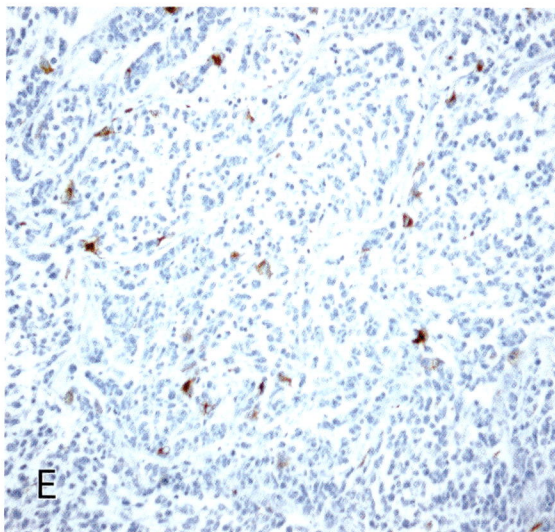

Figure 12-4

CENTRAL-TYPE PRIMITIVE NEUROECTODERMAL TUMOR

The finding of glial fibrillary stroma is helpful in establishing the correct diagnosis (A,B). Rosettes and perivascular pseudorosettes in a primitive tumor may raise suspicion for high-grade endometrioid adenocarcinoma (C,D). Glial fibrillary acidic protein (GFAP) is positive in up to 50 percent of central-type peripheral neuroectodermal tumors, although may be focal, but not their peripheral counterpart (E).

Figure 12-5

PERIPHERAL-TYPE PRIMITIVE NEUROECTODERMAL TUMOR

The tumor cells have a diffuse growth pattern (A). They have scant cytoplasm and round to oval nuclei with small nucleoli and fine chromatin (B). CD99 shows diffuse membranous positivity (C).

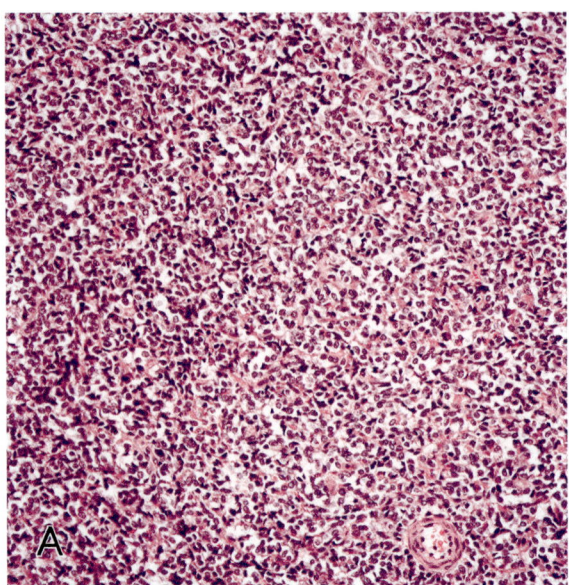
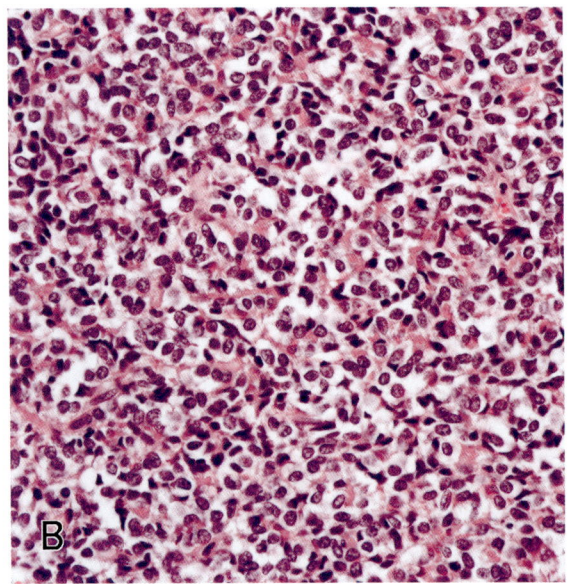
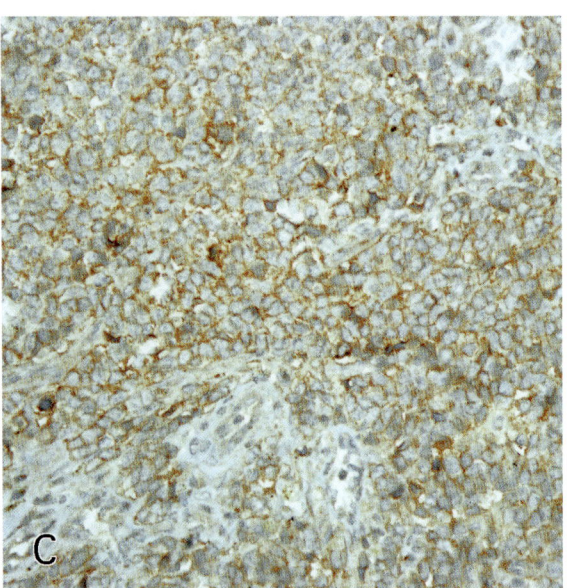

other round cell sarcomas, may enter in the differential diagnosis of PNET.

WILMS TUMOR

Extrarenal *Wilms tumor* is a highly unusual neoplasm that may occur in the uterus. Even though fewer than 20 cases have been reported in the literature (40–42), the uterus is the most common location in the female genital tract, with involvement of the corpus being more common than the cervix. These tumors show a slight predominance in children over adults. Although most tumors are pure, occasionally they occur within müllerian adenosarcomas (43), carcinosarcomas, and teratoid carcinosarcomas (carcinosarcoma with epithelial, mesenchymal, neuroectodermal, and endodermal differentiation) (41).

Wilms tumors typically present as bulky polypoid masses. They are characterized by a variable admixture of three components: blastema, simple epithelial tubules and glomeruloid structures, and immature mesenchyme (fig. 12-6). The mesenchymal component may show smooth muscle, rhabdomyoblastic, and rarely, cartilaginous differentiation, while the background stroma may be myxoid. The cytologic

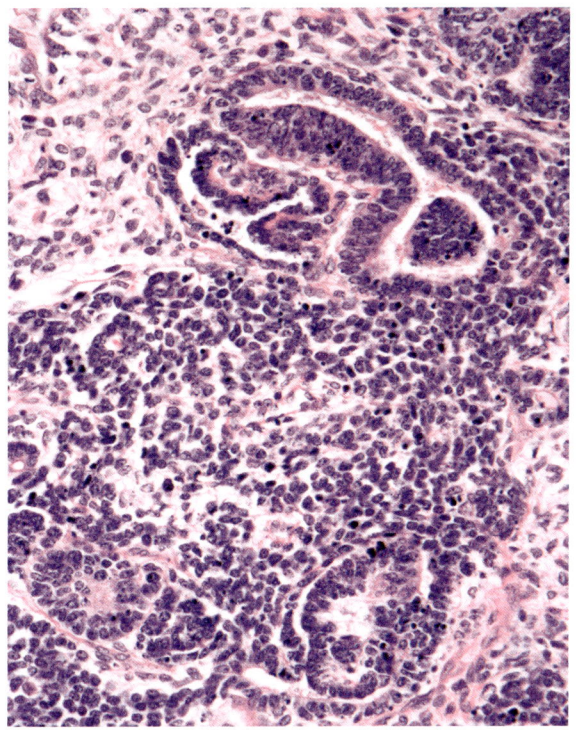

Figure 12-6

EXTRARENAL WILMS TUMOR

Primitive tubules and glomeruli as well as blastema are seen.

features are primitive with a high N/C ratio and brisk mitotic activity in the blastomatous component. These tumors are typically WT1 positive but also express CD56, CD99, and neuron-specific enolase (NSE) (44–47). The rhabdomyoblastic component is positive for Myo-D1 and myogenin.

The differential diagnosis of pure extrarenal Wilms tumor includes carcinosarcoma, especially when it has rhabdomyoblastic differentiation, and less commonly, adenosarcoma with sarcomatous overgrowth. The former is characterized by high-grade cytologic atypia in both the epithelial and stromal components while adenosarcoma with stromal overgrowth typically shows at least focal condensation of stroma around glands, the latter lined by müllerian-type epithelium, while the overgrowth of the sarcomatous component is typically high grade. Resemblance to an endometrioid carcinoma with tubular and spindle cell features may occur, especially in biopsy specimens when the epithelial component of the Wilms tumor is overrepresented. A diagnosis of endometrioid carcinoma requires confirmatory endometrioid features including squamous or mucinous differentiation and lack of primitive nuclei that are typical of blastema. The newly described mesonephric-like carcinoma of the uterine corpus (24) may resemble Wilms tumor to a significant degree when glomeruloid structures that sometimes merge with spindle cells are noted, however, all reported mesonephric-like tumors of the uterine corpus have been WT1 negative (24).

The origin of extrarenal Wilms tumors is unclear. It has been postulated that the close proximity of the genital and urinary structures during embryologic development may promote displacement of the latter to müllerian structures, with subsequent malignant transformation. Pure Wilms tumor is associated with a good prognosis when confined to the uterus.

PURE GERM CELL TUMORS AND CARCINOMAS WITH GERM CELL DIFFERENTIATION

Yolk Sac Tumors

Both pure *yolk sac tumors* and *endometrial carcinomas with yolk sac differentiation* have been reported (48–50). Pure yolk sac tumors more commonly occur in young women, with a mean age of 33 (range, 24 to 49) years (48). Preoperative serum alpha-fetoprotein (AFP) levels range from 1,762 to 18,530 ng/mL. Patients tend to present with disease confined to the uterine corpus, and have a favorable prognosis when treated with chemotherapy.

Yolk sac tumors in older patients are much more likely to be associated with an endometrioid carcinoma and much less commonly clear cell carcinoma (51) or represent a component of a carcinosarcoma (52), and a subset displays hepatoid differentiation (51). These tumors tend to present at high stage and are associated with poor prognosis. Given the clinical and histologic characteristics of these tumors, including presentation at older age and poor response to chemotherapy, as well as frequent coexistence with a müllerian-type carcinoma, it has been suggested that yolk sac tumors occurring in this setting represent *carcinomas with divergent differentiation* (53).

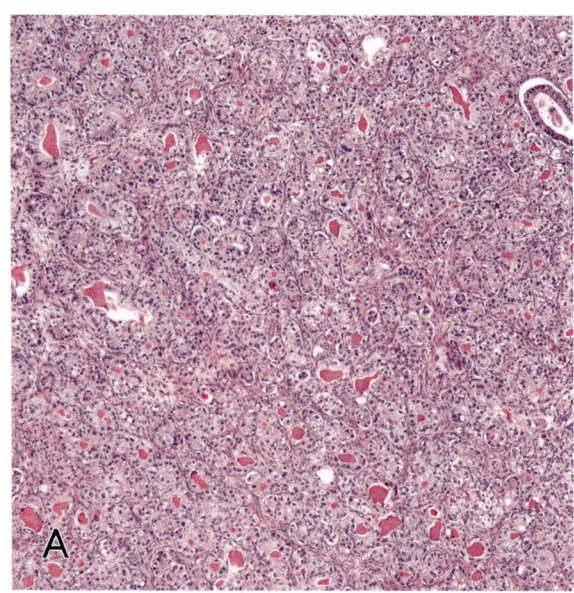

Figure 12-7

YOLK SAC TUMOR

These tumors may feature small, round tubules (A), glands lined by cells resembling secretory endometrium (B), and primitive epithelium surrounded by stromal mucin (C).

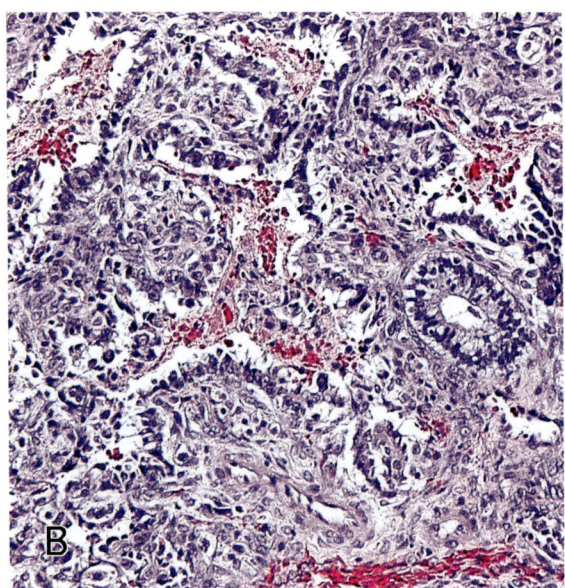

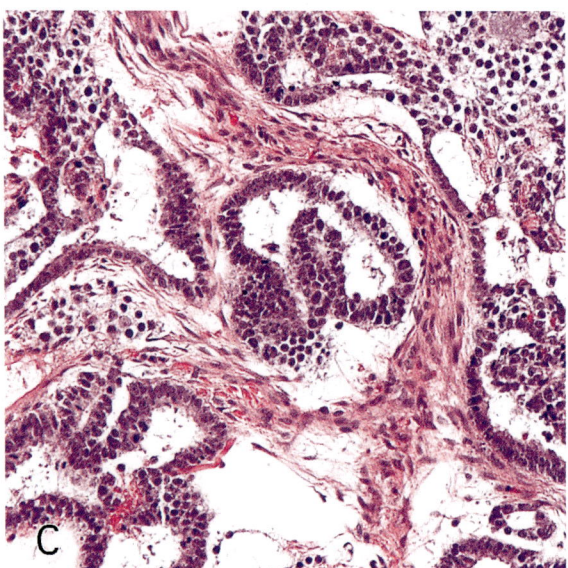

The most helpful histologic features suggesting a component of yolk sac tumor is a reticular (most common), microcystic, macrocystic, papillary, glandular, or polyvesicular vitelline patterns present in a loose myxoid background (fig. 12-7). The cells have a primitive appearance consisting of large vesicular nuclei with nucleoli and pale to clear cytoplasm that may contain hyaline globules. Schiller-Duval bodies may be seen (54,55). Mitotic activity is brisk and necrosis common.

Yolk sac differentiation in the context of an associated endometrial adenocarcinoma can be difficult to recognize when the yolk sac component displays clear cells arranged in papillary, glandular, and solid patterns that simulate endometrioid carcinoma with secretory features, or rarely, an adenocarcinoma with intestinal differentiation (56). Therefore, tumors with primitive-appearing cells such as high-grade adenocarcinoma with a component resembling endometrioid carcinoma with secretory changes; adenocarcinoma with solid and trabecular arrangements of polygonal eosinophilic cells resembling hepatocytes (fig. 12-8A); and adenocarcinoma with features suggesting a colorectal adenocarcinoma should be evaluated by extensive sampling and/or immunohistochemistry, in an effort to disclose yolk sac differentiation.

The yolk sac component shows SALL-4 and glypican-3 expression in the absence of EMA, CK7, and PAX8, with exceptions since some yolk sac tumors express CK7 and up to 25 percent express PAX8 (51,57,58). HepPar-1, albumin, and arginase may highlight glandular and hepatoid yolk sac components (fig. 12-8B) (59). The immunophenotype of primitive yolk sac tumors and differentiating or "somatic glandular" yolk sac tumors differs, the latter demonstrating evidence of enteric differentiation. Primitive yolk sac tumors are more easily recognized than the differentiating examples. Primitive yolk sac tumors exhibit the characteristic yolk sac growth patterns and the classic immunophenotype: SALL-4, AFP, villin (56,60), and GATA-3 (61) positive, typically without EMA or CK7 expression. Differentiating yolk sac tumors that mimic endometrioid carcinomas and primitive enteric carcinomas, as described above, are less likely to express AFP, glypican-3 3, and GATA-3 (60), and more likely to express CK20, CK7, and even PAX8 (56). CK7 and PAX8, when expressed, are focal in distribution.

Clear cell carcinoma is another entity in the differential diagnosis of yolk sac tumor and some clear cell carcinomas may display a yolk sac component (51). Clear cell carcinomas show focal glypican-3 positivity (62) and glandular yolk sac tumors, particularly, express CK7, EMA, and even PAX8 (63,64), as mentioned above. HNF1β is often positive in both tumors, but napsin-A and racemase are typically negative in yolk sac tumors (51,65); therefore, applying a panel of antibodies is preferred given this differential diagnosis. It is best to avoid AFP immunohistochemistry as some clear cell carcinomas are positive and immunohistochemical results with this marker are frequently equivocal due to high background staining.

Hepatoid Tumors

Hepatoid tumors occur in the endometrium, typically in association with an endometrial adenocarcinoma (fig. 12-8C) (66–68), more often mixed with serous carcinoma, and anecdotally, endometrioid carcinoma. Although not proven, it is likely that such tumors represent somatically-derived yolk sac tumors with hepatoid differentiation. Hepatoid tumors typically express the full spectrum of yolk sac-associated markers, including HepPar-1 and SALL4 (fig. 12-8D) (49,60). It is expected that these tumors also contain albumin and express arginase as do yolk sac tumors with hepatoid differentiation (69).

Uterine Teratomas

Fewer than a dozen *uterine teratomas* have been reported to involve the endometrium, cervix, or both. Most are solid teratomas, with a subset of immature teratomas. The gross and histologic appearance is similar to their ovarian counterparts. They are often polypoid, with a solid and cystic cut surface; the latter may contain keratin debris (fig. 12-9, left). On microscopic examination, there is a variable admixture of the three embryonic layers (fig. 12-9, right), with the presence of immature neural tissue being the determinant feature for the diagnosis of immature teratoma (55,70–72).

Differentiating high-grade immature teratoma from central-type PNET should be accomplished in the same manner as in the ovary. The finding of geographic, tumor-like outgrowth of solely immature neuroectoderm confirms a diagnosis of central-type PNET, whereas an admixture of immature and mature elements is diagnostic of high-grade immature teratoma. A case of high-grade immature teratoma followed by relapse in the form of central-type PNET has been reported (73). Although it was previously suggested that uterine teratomas were gestationally derived, a recent case report suggests that they are more likely of nongestational origin (55).

Nongestational Tumors with Trophoblastic Differentiation

These are rare tumors with only about 20 cases reported (48,74–76). Patients are typically perimenopausal or postmenopausal (over 50 years) with preoperative serum β-human chorionic gonadotropin (hCG) levels over 1,000,000 mIU/mL. Associated carcinomas range from endometrioid, most commonly, to serous and clear cell carcinomas and carcinosarcomas (61,77–79). Choriocarcinoma is probably the most common type of somatically-derived trophoblastic neoplasm, but some tumors only display syncytiotrophoblastic cells (fig. 12-10,

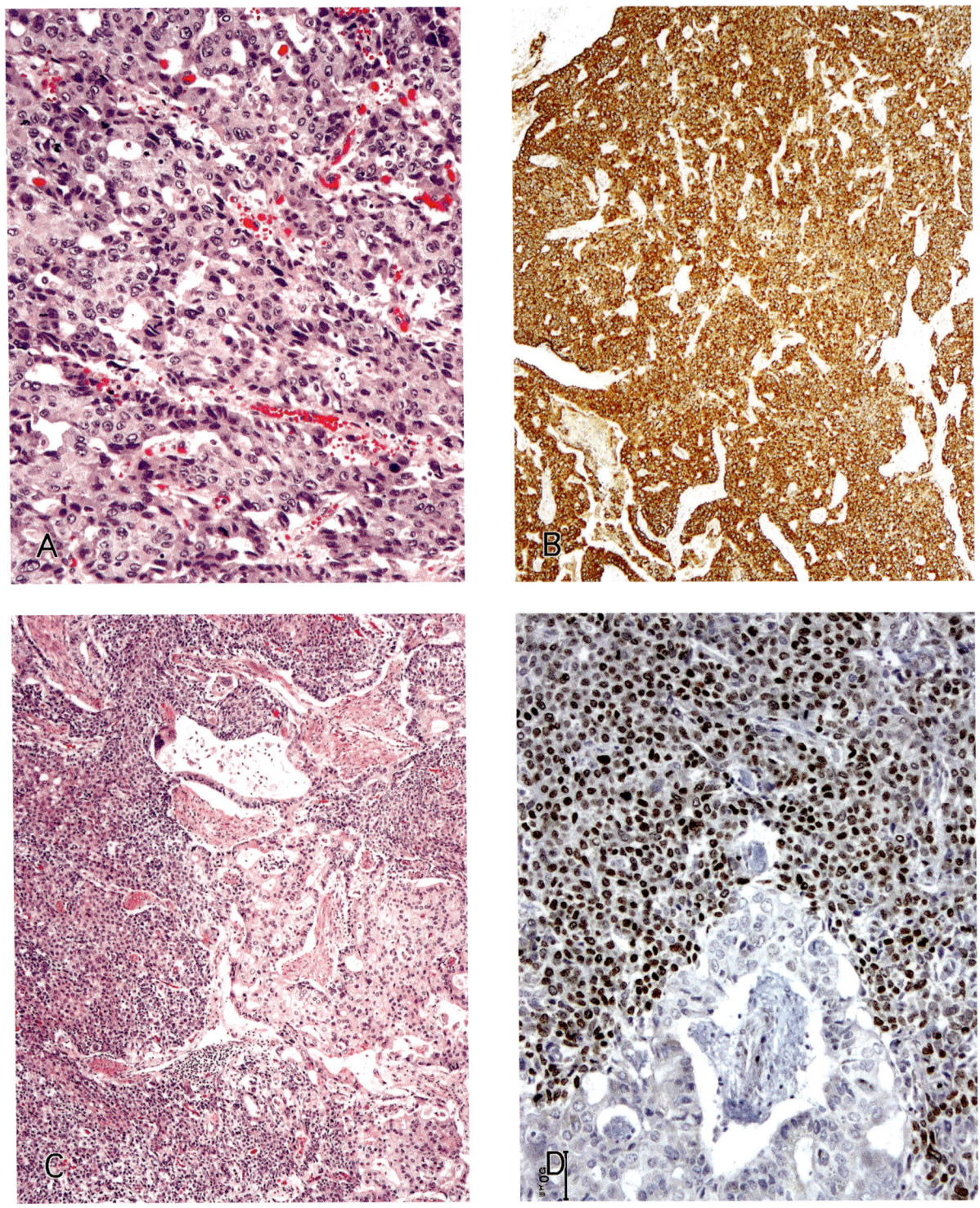

Figure 12-8

CARCINOMA WITH YOLK SAC HEPATOID DIFFERENTIATION AND HEPATOID CARCINOMA

The cells have abundant eosinophilic cytoplasm and round nuclei with nucleoli (A). Hepar1 immunostain highlights tumor cells with hepatoid differentiation (B). Mixed endometrioid adenocarcinoma and hepatoid carcinoma (C). SALL4 stains the hepatoid component (D).

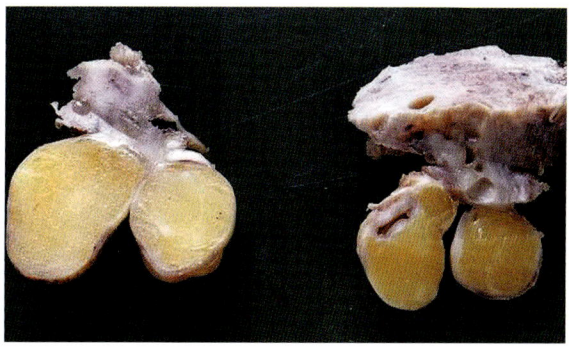
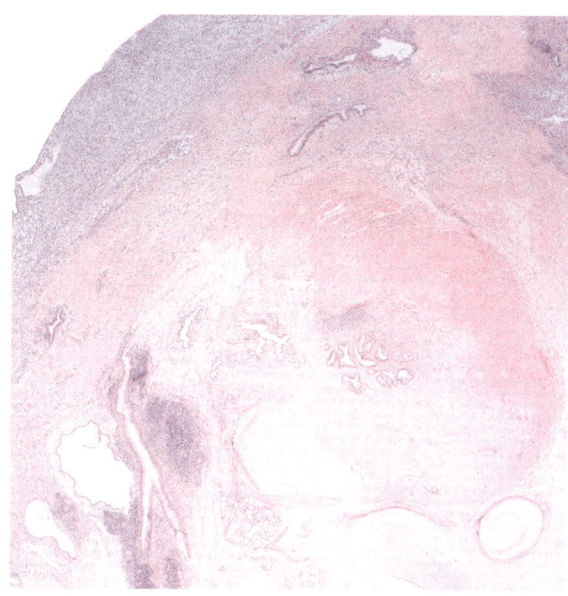

Figure 12-9

SECONDARY UTERINE SEROSAL AND CERVICAL INVOLVEMENT OF CORPUS TERATOMA

Notice yellow cut surface due to adipose tissue (above). (Courtesy of Dr. S. Stolnicu, Targu Mures, Romania). Squamous and respiratory epithelium as well as fetal cartilage and a nodule of glial tissue are seen (right).

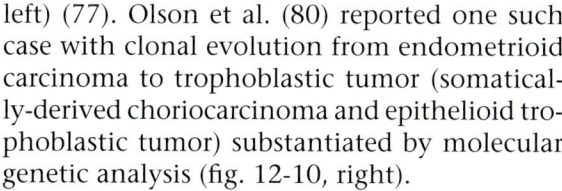

left) (77). Olson et al. (80) reported one such case with clonal evolution from endometrioid carcinoma to trophoblastic tumor (somatically-derived choriocarcinoma and epithelioid trophoblastic tumor) substantiated by molecular genetic analysis (fig. 12-10, right).

Regardless of the context, cells demonstrating trophoblastic differentiation express pantrophoblastic markers such as CD10, GATA-3, and inhibin (the latter except for cytotrophoblast) (81–83). Syncytiotrophoblast expresses hCG and chorionic-type intermediate trophoblast preferentially expresses p63 (84) and p40 (85) over human placental lactogen (hPL). The presence of rare, scattered hCG-positive cells without an intimate admixture of mononuclear trophoblast supports a diagnosis of carcinoma with syncytiotrophoblastic giant cells, whereas numerous hCG-positive cells that surround aggregates of mononuclear trophoblast is diagnostic of a choriocarcinomatous component.

Nongestational tumors with trophoblastic differentiation are highly likely to represent divergent differentiation from a carcinomatous substrate, as occurs with yolk sac tumors and primitive neuroectodermal tumors in adults. Tumors with a choriocarcinomatous component and markedly elevated serum β-hCG levels are thought to be highly aggressive, whereas tumors containing scattered syncytiotrophoblast cells are thought to behave similarly to adenocarcinomas lacking fully developed trophoblastic differentiation (77). This parallels the distinction of seminoma with syncytiotrophoblastic cells from a malignant mixed germ cell tumor with seminoma and choriocarcinoma in the testis.

SEX CORD-STROMAL TUMORS

Only one *Sertoli-Leydig cell tumor* originating in the uterine corpus has been reported (86). Although it was suggested that this tumor represented an unusual variant of a uterine tumor resembling an ovarian sex cord tumor (UTROSCT), a cornual example shown to be indistinguishable from an ovarian Sertoli-Leydig cell tumor has been recently seen by one author (fig. 12-11).

METASTASES AND DIRECT EXTENSION TO UTERINE CORPUS FROM ADJACENT GYNECOLOGIC ORGANS

Although a comprehensive review of metastases to the uterine corpus has not been published, adnexa and uterine cervix are the most common origins (87) based on anecdotal experience, and carcinomas are by far more common. Metastases to the uterine corpus represent less than 10 percent of all metastases to the female genital tract, with the uterine serosa and subadjacent myometrium, (typical of metastatic ovarian carcinoma) being more commonly involved than the endometrium.

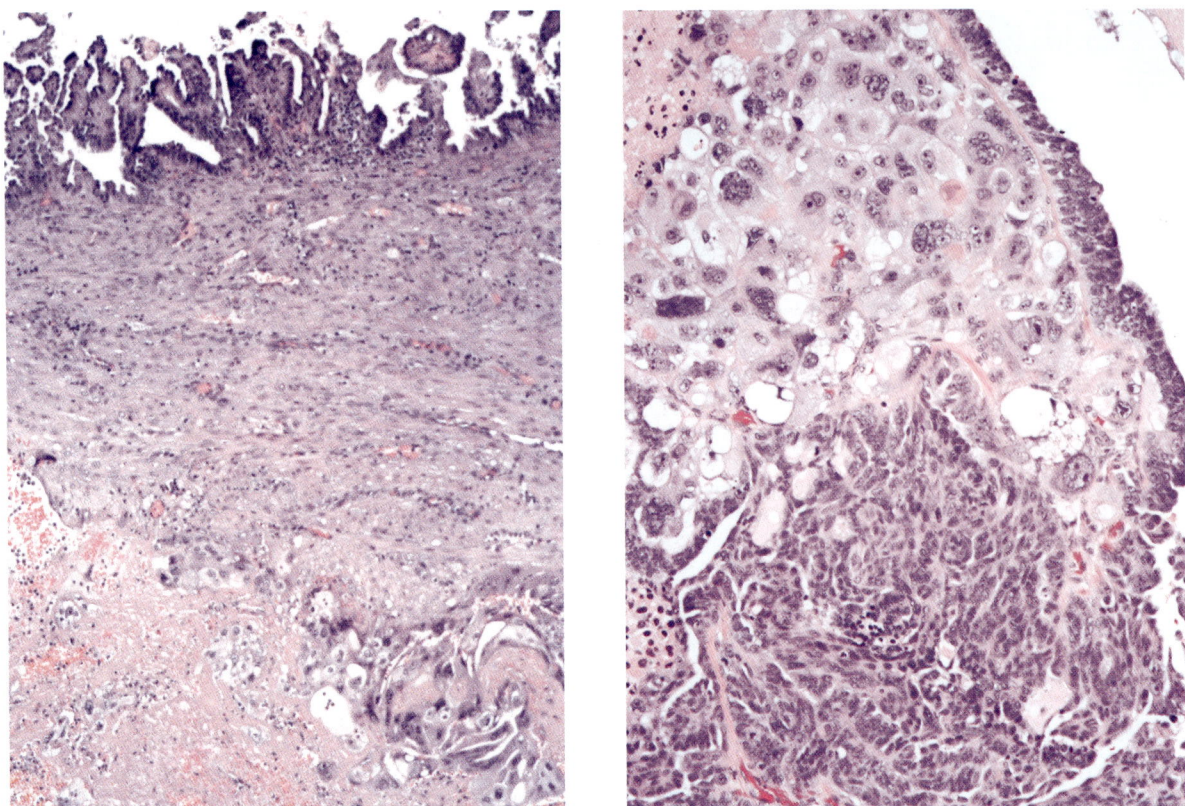

Figure 12-10

CHORIOCARCINOMA JUXTAPOSED TO AN ENDOMETRIOID CARCINOMA

The choriocarcinoma shows a biphasic population of mononucleated and multinucleated cells (left). (Courtesy of Dr. M. F. Lerwill, Boston, MA.) Endometrial serous carcinoma with intermediate chorionic-type trophoblastic differentiation (right).

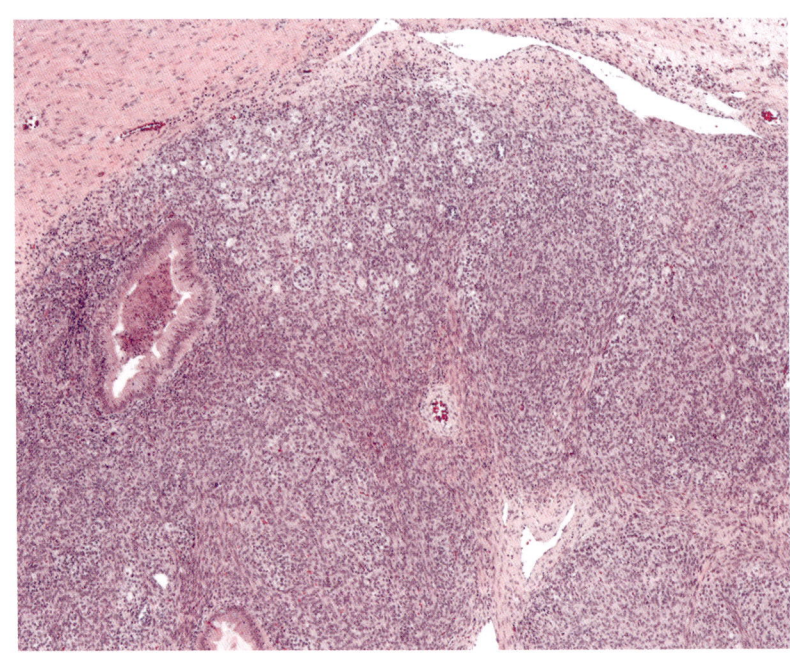

Figure 12-11

SERTOLI-LEYDIG CELL TUMOR OF THE UTERINE CORNU

Intermediate differentiation and intestinal (heterologous) elements are present.

Primary Adnexal/Peritoneal Carcinomas

Although there are no data-driven criteria that allow reproducible recognition of "drop metastasis" from the ovary, fallopian tube, and peritoneum to the endometrium, there are some characteristic findings that can suggest this diagnosis (fig. 12-12; fig. 6-16, chapter 6). Rarely, ovarian endometrioid, serous, or clear cell carcinomas invade through the myometrium to involve the endometrium by direct extension, but almost all drop metastases from the adnexa are serous carcinomas.

In an endometrial biopsy or curettage specimen, drop metastasis is suggested in the presence of the following: age younger than 60 years, low-grade serous carcinoma, and small and dissociated serous carcinoma fragments in a background of non-neoplastic endometrium, especially when an endometrial polyp is not present (88). In a hysterectomy specimen with serous carcinoma in the adnexa and endometrium, drop metastasis is favored when extensive serous tubal intraepithelial carcinoma and diffuse WT1 positivity are found in a patient younger than 60 years, particularly when carcinoma is unassociated with an endometrial polyp (88).

Most serous carcinomas with the above characteristics are confined to the endometrium or show limited myometrial invasion, with some demonstrating apparent multifocality within the endometrium. It can be difficult or impossible to ascertain the primary site when there is extensive involvement of both adnexa and endomyometrium. Diffuse WT1 positivity in endometrium and adnexa may provide some support for drop metastasis to endometrium.

Primary Cervical Carcinomas

Primary cervical tumors, including high-grade squamous intraepithelial lesion, endocervical adenocarcinoma in situ, invasive squamous cell carcinoma (fig. 12-13A), and endocervical adenocarcinoma (including endocervical mucinous [fig. 12-13A,C], gastric-type mucinous [fig. 12-13D], mesonephric, and clear cell carcinomas) can colonize the endometrium and invade the myometrium. The latter occurs either by direct extension or by invasion from foci of endometrial colonization (89,90).

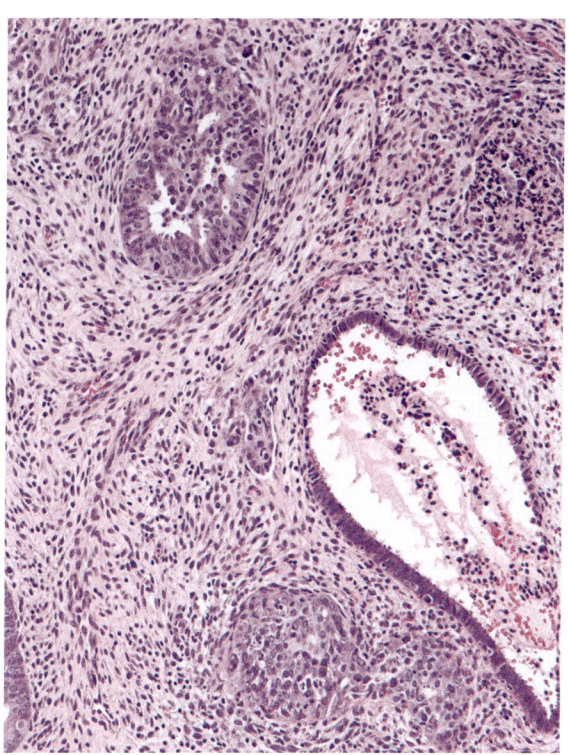

Figure 12-12

DROP METASTASIS OF HIGH-GRADE SEROUS CARCINOMA TO ENDOMETRIUM

The tumor is often an incidental microscopic finding.

Primary cervical squamous carcinomas that involve the endometrium are typically large (over 4 cm) and deeply invasive into cervical stroma. In some cases, the tumor invades endometrial stroma and myometrium without endometrial glandular involvement, but in others, endometrial glandular involvement is also present. "Carpet-like" replacement of the endometrium, fallopian tube mucosa, and even ovaries has been reported on occasion (20,91).

Several different patterns of involvement of the uterine corpus are seen with endocervical adenocarcinoma: endometrial colonization by adenocarcinoma in situ resembling atypical hyperplasia when the architecture is simple or endometrioid adenocarcinoma in the presence of complex architecture; colonization of adenomyosis; and myometrial invasion, typically associated with large and deeply invasive endocervical adenocarcinoma (89). As occurs with squamous cell carcinoma, in most instances there is a mass centered in the endocervix.

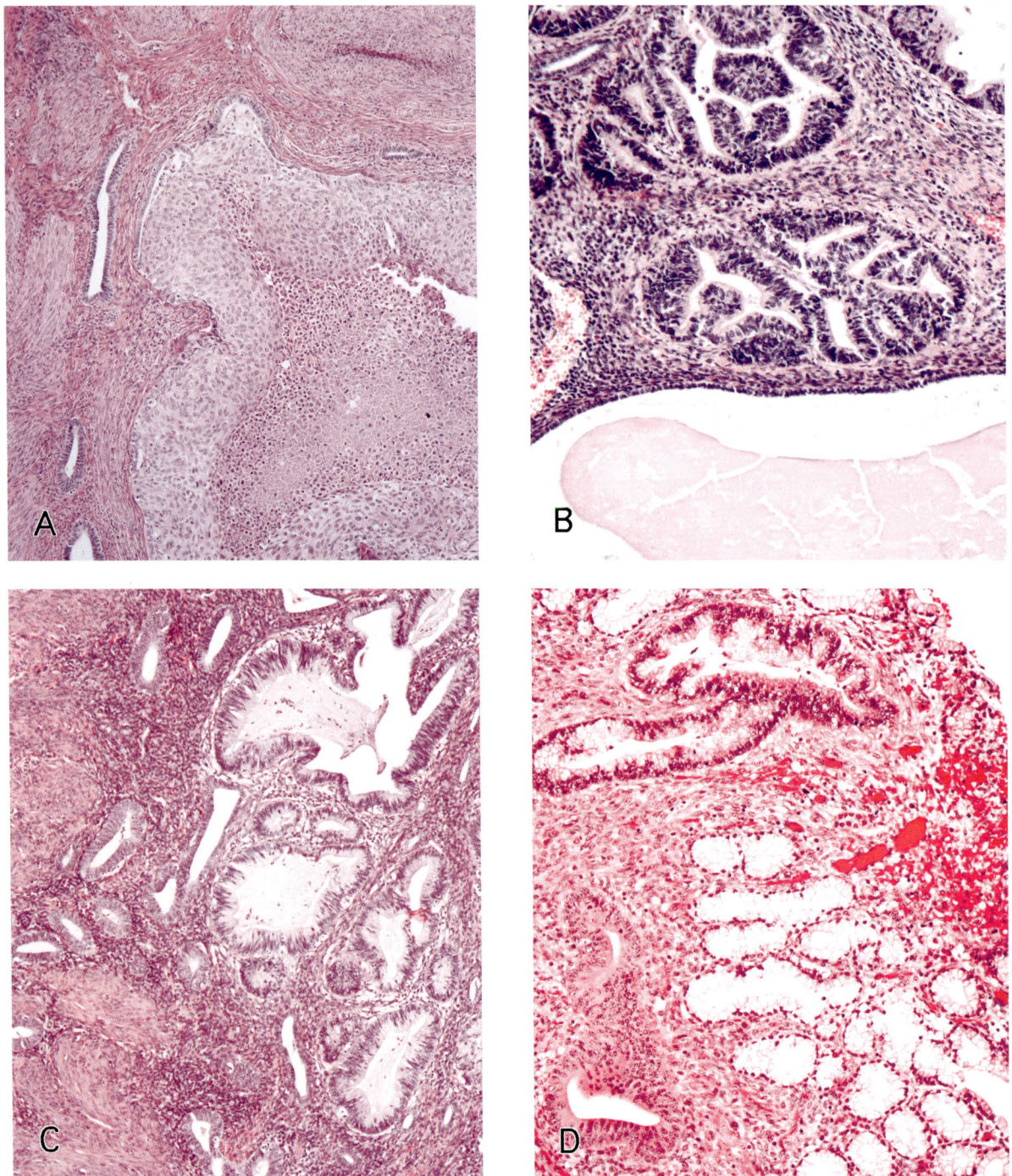

Figure 12-13

CERVICAL CARCINOMAS INVOLVING UTERINE CORPUS

Squamous cell carcinoma of the cervix. The tumor replaces preexisting glandular epithelium of the lower uterine segment and is focally associated with desmoplastic reaction (A). Secondary involvement of endometrium by cervical adenocarcinoma, usual type, with typical cytologic characteristics including nuclear pseudostratification, hyperchromasia, and apical mitoses (B). The cytologic features of the usual cervical adenocarcinoma may be subtle (C) (courtesy of Dr. K. Park, New York, NY). Gastric-type adenocarcinoma is found at the top, while lobular pyloric metaplasia is seen at right overlying the proliferative endometrial glands at left (D) (courtesy of Dr. K. Park, New York, NY).

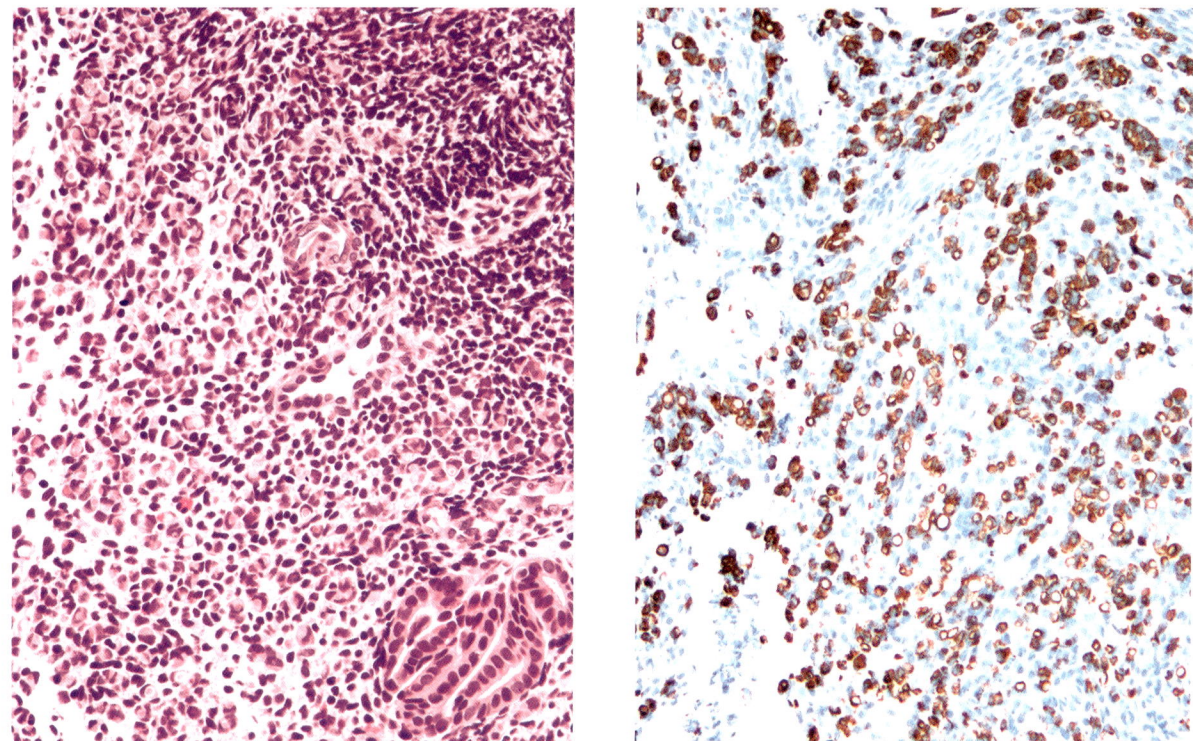

Figure 12-14

METASTATIC LOBULAR CARCINOMA

The tumor cells have a noncohesive appearance and some show intracytoplasmic vacuoles (left). CK7 immunostain highlights a larger number of neoplastic cells within the stroma (right).

METASTASES FROM EXTRAGYNECOLOGIC SITES

A PubMed literature search from 2010 to present revealed only about 20 case reports describing secondary uterine involvement from extragynecologic tumors. In a review of genital tract metastases, 7 involved the endometrium (out of a total of 149 reviewed) (87). Typically, metastatic carcinoma from extragynecologic sites is an incidental finding, but the uterus may be enlarged or the uterine serosa studded by tumor. Occasionally, metastases are limited to a leiomyoma (92).

Breast carcinomas, usually lobular (substantially more common) and ductal types metastasize to the uterus, particularly to endometrial stroma. In curettage specimens, a lobular carcinoma may be overlooked as evidence may be minimal and only isolated cells or small groups of tumor cells may be present (fig. 12-14). It is important to carefully examine all endometrial fragments and polyps especially in patients treated with tamoxifen in order to exclude metastases.

Other tumors reported to metastasize to the uterine corpus include colorectal (fig. 12-15), gastric, mucinous appendiceal, and renal clear cell carcinomas, pulmonary adenocarcinoma, melanoma, cholangiocarcinoma, and squamous cell carcinoma originating in an ovarian teratoma (93–96). Colorectal and, less commonly, gastric carcinoma may mimic the appearance of endometrioid carcinoma, but finding simple or cribriform glands with luminal "dirty necrosis" and high-grade nuclear features suggests metastasis and should prompt further workup. PAX8, estrogen receptor (ER), progesterone receptor (PR), CK20, CDX2, and SATB2 are helpful in this differential diagnosis as is a confirmatory history.

Mucinous appendiceal tumors may colonize the endometrium, with a banal appearance similar to that seen in mucinous metaplasia (97). Mucin dissection within the endometrial stroma ("pseudomyxoma endometrii") has also

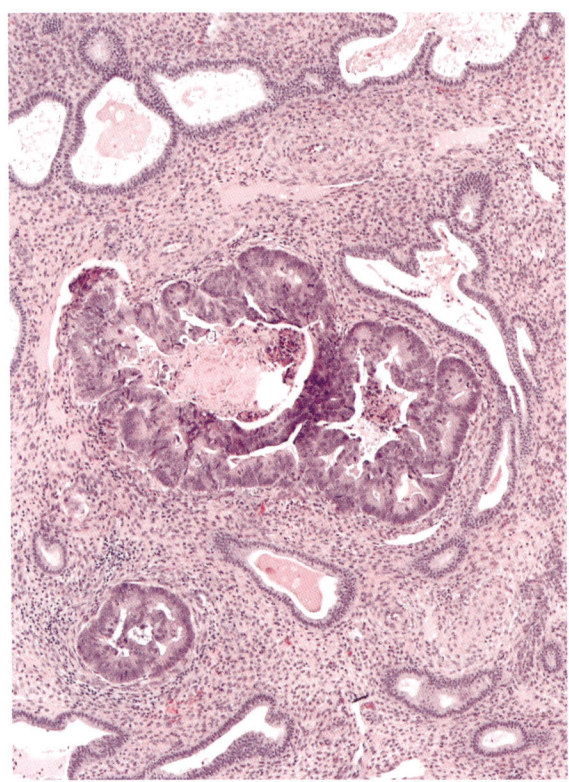 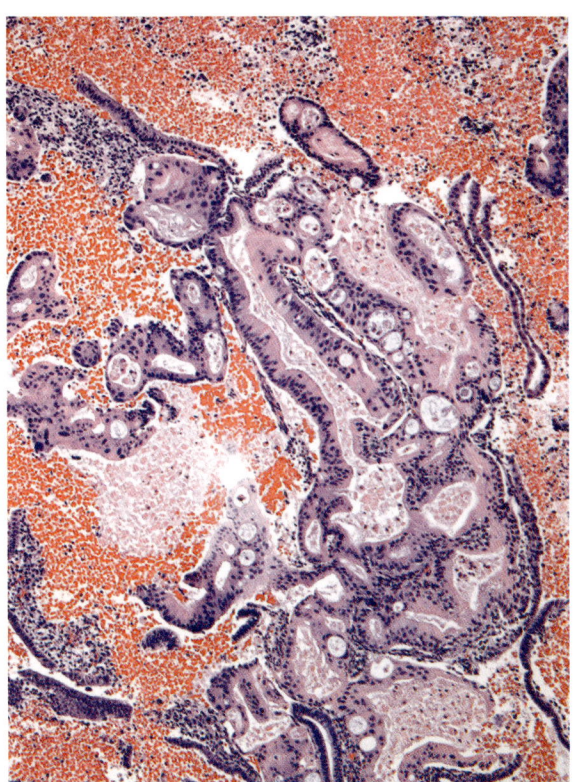

Figure 12-15

COLORECTAL ADENOCARCINOMA METASTATIC TO ENDOMETRIUM

The neoplastic glands show luminal dirty necrosis (left). An endometrial curettage specimen shows metastatic colorectal carcinoma that resembles an endometrial adenocarcinoma. Focal segmental necrosis of glands and "dirty" necrosis are seen in the background (right).

been reported (fig. 2-10, chapter 2) (97a). Metastases to the uterine corpus reflects disseminated disease and is associated with a poor prognosis.

HEMATOLYMPHOID MALIGNANCIES

Hematolymphoid malignancies only rarely present in the gynecologic tract, although gynecologic involvement by leukemia in autopsy series is not uncommon (98). In an extensive literature search from 2000 to the present, nine cases of acute myeloid malignancies have been documented to involve the uterus, including cervix, mostly in the form of extramedullary myeloid tumor/myeloid sarcoma (99–103), as myeloid leukemias are more common than lymphoblastic leukemias (104).

There are three series reporting involvement of the uterine corpus by lymphoma (105-108). The only study reporting both primary and secondary involvement by lymphoma suggests that primary lymphoma may be more common than secondary involvement (16 of 23 cases), at least in surgical resection specimens (106). In the most recent review of 697 primary lymphomas of the female genital tract, 16.5 percent involved the uterine corpus: diffuse large B-cell lymphoma (76.5 percent), mucosa-associated lymphoid tissue (MALT) lymphomas (i.e., extranodal marginal zone lymphomas) (11.2 percent) (fig. 12-16), follicular lymphoma (9.2 percent), and Burkitt lymphoma (3.1 percent). In this series of gynecologic lymphomas, localized disease, premenopausal status, and follicular histology were prognostically favorable parameters, but excisional surgery usually performed for carcinomas and sarcomas did not confer any clinical benefit (107).

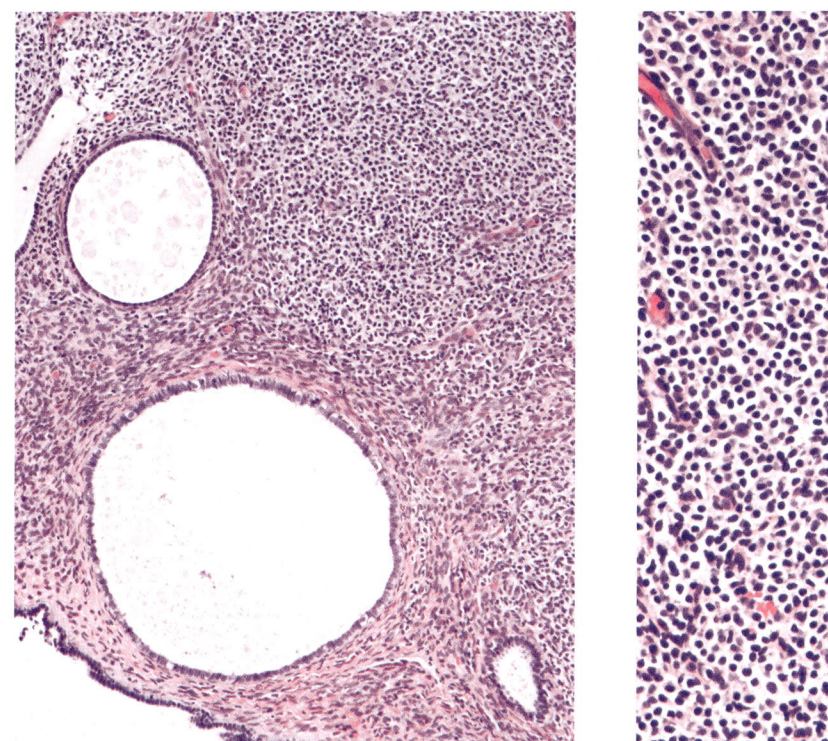 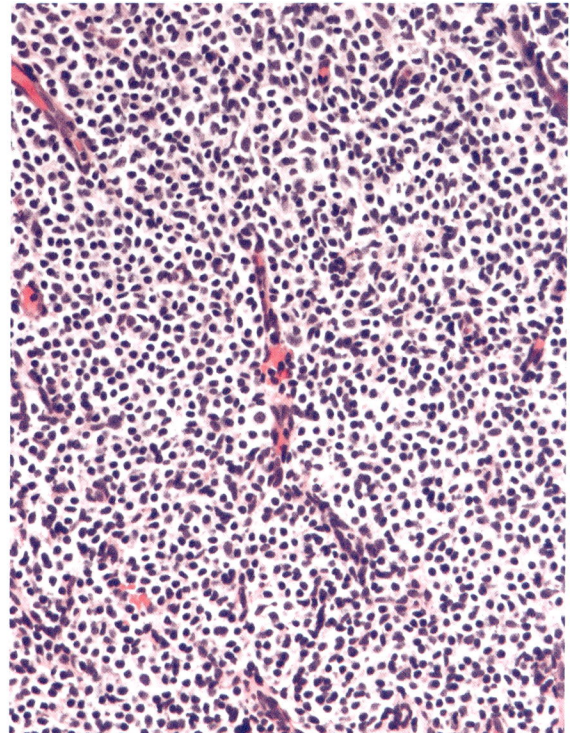

Figure 12-16

MARGINAL ZONE LYMPHOMA INVOLVING THE ENDOMETRIUM

The tumor cells grow diffusely between the residual endometrial glands (left). The cells are homogeneously small with pale cytoplasm and round nuclei (right).

REFERENCES

1. Huntsman DG, Clement PB, Gilks CB, Scully RE. Small-cell carcinoma of the endometrium. A clinicopathological study of sixteen cases. Am J Surg Pathol 1994;18:364-75.
2. Pocrnich CE, Ramalingam P, Euscher ED, Malpica A. Neuroendocrine carcinoma of the endometrium: a clinicopathologic study of 25 cases. Am J Surg Pathol 2016;40:577-86.
3. van Hoeven KH, Hudock JA, Woodruff JM, Suhrland MJ. Small cell neuroendocrine carcinoma of the endometrium. Int J Gynecol Pathol 1995;14:21-9.
4. Campo E, Brunier MN, Merino MJ. Small cell carcinoma of the endometrium with associated ocular paraneoplastic syndrome. Cancer 1992;69:2283-8.
5. Crofts JW, Bachynski BN, Odel JG. Visual paraneoplastic syndrome associated with undifferentiated endometrial carcinoma. Can J Ophthalmol 1988;23:128-32.
6. Ju W, Park IA, Kim SH, Lee SE, Kim SC. Small cell carcinoma of the uterine corpus manifesting with visual dysfunction. Gynecol Oncol 2005;99:504-6.
7. Sekiguchi I, Suzuki M, Sato I, Ohkawa T, Kawashima H, Tsuchida S. Rare case of small-cell carcinoma arising from the endometrium with paraneoplastic retinopathy. Gynecol Oncol 1998;71:454-7.
8. Sato H, Kanai G, Kajiwara H, Itoh J, Osamura RY. Small-cell carcinoma of the endometrium presenting as Cushing's syndrome. Endocr J 2010;57:31-8.
9. Kontogianni K, Nicholson AG, Butcher D, Sheppard MN. CD56: a useful tool for the diagnosis of small cell lung carcinomas on biopsies with extensive crush artefact. J Clin Pathol 2005;58:978-80.
10. Lyda MH, Weiss LM. Immunoreactivity for epithelial and neuroendocrine antibodies are useful in the differential diagnosis of lung carcinomas. Hum Pathol 2000;31:980-7.

11. Rekhtman N. Neuroendocrine tumors of the lung: an update. Arch Pathol Lab Med 2010;134:1628-38.
12. Altrabulsi B, Malpica A, Deavers MT, Bodurka DC, Broaddus R, Silva EG. Undifferentiated carcinoma of the endometrium. Am J Surg Pathol 2005;29:1316-21.
13. Fluhmann CF. Squamous epithelium in the endometrium in benign and malignant conditions. Surg Gynecol Obstet 1928;46:209-316.
14. Chew I, Post MD, Carinelli SG, et al. p16 expression in squamous and trophoblastic lesions of the upper female genital tract. Int J Gynecol Pathol 2010;29:513-22.
15. Goodman A, Zukerberg LR, Rice LW, Fuller AF, Young RH, Scully RE. Squamous cell carcinoma of the endometrium: a report of eight cases and a review of the literature. Gynecol Oncol 1996;61:54-60.
16. Horn LC, Richter CE, Einenkel J, Tannapfel A, Liebert UG, Leo C. p16, p14, p53, cyclin D1, and steroid hormone receptor expression and human papillomaviruses analysis in primary squamous cell carcinoma of the endometrium. Ann Diagn Pathol 2006;10:193-6.
17. Yoo SH, Son EM, Sung CO, Kim KR. Primary squamous cell carcinoma of the upper genital tract: utility of p16(INK4a) expression and HPV DNA status in its differential diagnosis from extended cervical squamous cell carcinoma. Korean J Pathol 2013;47:549-56.
18. Bewtra C, Xie QM, Hunter WJ, Jurgensen W. Ichthyosis uteri: a case report and review of the literature. Arch Pathol Lab Med 2005;129:e124-5.
19. Brown D Jr, Spjut HJ. Extensive squamous metaplasia of the endometrium (ichthyosis uteri). South Med J 1982;75:593-5.
20. Pins MR, Young RH, Crum CP, Leach IH, Scully RE. Cervical squamous cell carcinoma in situ with intraepithelial extension to the upper genital tract and invasion of tubes and ovaries: report of a case with human papilloma virus analysis. Int J Gynecol Pathol 1997;16:272-8.
21. Lininger RA, Ashfaq R, Albores-Saavedra J, Tavassoli FA. Transitional cell carcinoma of the endometrium and endometrial carcinoma with transitional cell differentiation. Cancer 1997;79:1933-43.
22. Murhekar K, Majhi U, Sridevi V, Rajkumar T. Does "ichthyosis uteri" have malignant potential? A case report of squamous cell carcinoma of endometrium associated with extensive ichthyosis uteri. Diagn Pathol 2008;3:4.
23. Takeuchi K, Tsujino T, Yabuta M, Kitazawa S. A case of primary squamous cell carcinoma of the endometrium associated with extensive "ichthyosis uteri." Eur J Gynaecol Oncol 2012;33:552-4.
24. McFarland M, Quick CM, McCluggage WG. Hormone receptor-negative, thyroid transcription factor 1-positive uterine and ovarian adenocarcinomas: report of a series of mesonephric-like adenocarcinomas. Histopathology 2016;68:1013-20.
25. Kenny SL, McBride HA, Jamison J, McCluggage WG. Mesonephric adenocarcinomas of the uterine cervix and corpus: HPV-negative neoplasms that are commonly PAX8, CA125, and HMGA2 positive and that may be immunoreactive with TTF1 and hepatocyte nuclear factor 1-beta. Am J Surg Pathol 2012;36:799-807.
26. Howitt BE, Emori MM, Drapkin R, et al. GATA3 is a sensitive and specific marker of benign and malignant mesonephric lesions in the lower female genital tract. Am J Surg Pathol 2015;39:1411-9.
27. Roma AA, Goyal A, Yang B. Differential expression patterns of gata3 in uterine mesonephric and nonmesonephric lesions. Int J Gynecol Pathol 2015;34:480-6.
28. Lax SF, Kendall B, Tashiro H, Slebos RJ, Hedrick L. The frequency of p53, K-ras mutations, and microsatellite instability differs in uterine endometrioid and serous carcinoma: evidence of distinct molecular genetic pathways. Cancer 2000;88:814-24.
29. Prat J, Oliva E, Lerma E, Vaquero M, Matias-Guiu X. Uterine papillary serous adenocarcinoma. A 10-case study of p53 and c-erbB-2 expression and DNA content. Cancer 1994;74:1778-83.
30. Sherman ME, Bur ME, Kurman RJ. p53 in endometrial cancer and its putative precursors: evidence for diverse pathways of tumorigenesis. Hum Pathol 1995;26:1268-74.
31. Soslow RA, Shen PU, Chung MH, Isacson C. Distinctive p53 and mdm2 immunohistochemical expression profiles suggest different pathogenetic pathways in poorly differentiated endometrial carcinoma. Int J Gynecol Pathol 1998;17:129-34.
32. Tashiro H, Isacson C, Levine R, Kurman RJ, Cho KR, Hedrick L. p53 gene mutations are common in uterine serous carcinoma and occur early in their pathogenesis. Am J Pathol 1997;150:177-85.
33. Zheng W, Khurana R, Farahmand S, Wang Y, Zhang ZF, Felix JC. p53 immunostaining as a significant adjunct diagnostic method for uterine surface carcinoma: precursor of uterine papillary serous carcinoma. Am J Surg Pathol 1998;22:1463-73.
34. Daya D, Lukka H, Clement PB. Primitive neuroectodermal tumors of the uterus: a report of four cases. Hum Pathol 1992;23:1120-9.
35. Euscher ED, Deavers MT, Lopez-Terrada D, Lazar AJ, Silva EG, Malpica A. Uterine tumors with neuroectodermal differentiation: a series of 17 cases and review of the literature. Am J Surg Pathol 2008;32:219-28.

36. Chiang S, Snuderl M, Kojiro-Sanada S, et al. Primitive neuroectodermal tumors of the female genital tract: a morphologic, immunohistochemical, and molecular study of 19 cases. Am J Surg Pathol 2017;41:761-72.
37. Moll R, Pitz S, Levy R, Weikel W, Franke WW, Czernobilsky B. Complexity of expression of intermediate filament proteins, including glial filament protein, in endometrial and ovarian adenocarcinomas. Hum Pathol 1991;22:989-1001.
38. Ramalingam P, Croce S, McCluggage WG. Loss of expression of SMARCA4 (BRG1), SMARCA2 (BRM) and SMARCB1 (INI1) in undifferentiated carcinoma of the endometrium is not uncommon and is not always associated with rhabdoid morphology. Histopathology 2017;70:359-66.
39. Rosa-Rosa JM, Leskela S, Cristobal-Lana E, et al. Molecular genetic heterogeneity in undifferentiated endometrial carcinomas. Mod Pathol 2016;29:1390-8.
40. Bittencourt AL, Britto JF, Fonseca LE, Jr. Wilms' tumor of the uterus: the first report of the literature. Cancer 1981;47:2496-9.
41. Garcia-Galvis OF, Stolnicu S, Muñoz E, Aneiros-Fernandez J, Alaggio R, Nogales FF. Adult extrarenal Wilms tumor of the uterus with teratoid features. Hum Pathol 2009;40:418-24.
42. McAlpine J, Azodi M, O'Malley D, et al. Extrarenal Wilms' tumor of the uterine corpus. Gynecol Oncol 2005;96:892-6.
43. Clement PB. Müllerian adenosarcomas of the uterus with sarcomatous overgrowth. A clinicopathological analysis of 10 cases. Am J Surg Pathol 1989;13:28-38.
44. Barnoud R, Sabourin JC, Pasquier D, et al. Immunohistochemical expression of WT1 by desmoplastic small round cell tumor: a comparative study with other small round cell tumors. Am J Surg Pathol 2000;24:830-6.
45. Ghanem MA, Van der Kwast TH, Den Hollander JC, et al. Expression and prognostic value of Wilms' tumor 1 and early growth response 1 proteins in nephroblastoma. Clin Cancer Res 2000;6:4265-71.
46. Hussong JW, Perkins SL, Huff V, et al. Familial Wilms' tumor with neural elements: characterization by histology, immunohistochemistry, and genetic analysis. Pediatr Dev Pathol 2000;3:561-7.
47. Vasei M, Moch H, Mousavi A, Kajbafzadeh AM, Sauter G. Immunohistochemical profiling of Wilms tumor: a tissue microarray study. Appl Immunohistochem Mol Morph 2008;16:128-34.
48. Ji M, Lu Y, Guo L, Feng F, Wan X, Xiang Y. Endometrial carcinoma with yolk sac tumor-like differentiation and elevated serum beta-hCG: a case report and literature review. Onco Targets Ther 2013;6:1515-22.
49. McNamee T, Damato S, McCluggage WG. Yolk sac tumours of the female genital tract in older adults derive commonly from somatic epithelial neoplasms: somatically derived yolk sac tumours. Histopathology 2016;69:739-51.
50. Shokeir MO, Noel SM, Clement PB. Malignant mullerian mixed tumor of the uterus with a prominent alpha-fetoprotein-producing component of yolk sac tumor. Mod Pathol 1996;9:647-51.
51. Nogales FF, Prat J, Schuldt M, et al. Germ cell tumor growth patterns originating from clear cell carcinomas of the ovary and endometrium: a comparative immunohistochemical study favouring their origin from somatic stem cells. Histopathology 2018;72:634-47.
52. Oguri H, Sumitomo R, Maeda N, Fukaya T, Moriki T. Primary yolk sac tumor concomitant with carcinosarcoma originating from the endometrium: case report. Gynecol Oncol 2006;103:368-71.
53. Damato S, Haldar K, McCluggage WG. Primary endometrial yolk sac tumor with endodermal-intestinal differentiation masquerading as metastatic colorectal adenocarcinoma. Int J Gynecol Pathol 2016;35:316-20.
54. Clement PB, Young RH, Scully RE. Extraovarian pelvic yolk sac tumors. Cancer 1988;62:620-6.
55. Wang WC, Lee MS, Ko JL, Lai YC. Origin of uterine teratoma differs from that of ovarian teratoma: a case of uterine mature cystic teratoma. Int J Gynecol Pathol 2011;30:544-8.
56. Ravishankar S, Malpica A, Ramalingam P, Euscher ED. Yolk Sac tumor in extragonadal pelvic sites: still a diagnostic challenge. Am J Surg Pathol 2017;41:1-11.
57. Laury AR, Perets R, Piao H, et al. A comprehensive analysis of PAX8 expression in human epithelial tumors. Am J Surg Pathol 2011;35:816-26.
58. Ramalingam P, Malpica A, Silva EG, Gershenson DM, Liu JL, Deavers MT. The use of cytokeratin 7 and EMA in differentiating ovarian yolk sac tumors from endometrioid and clear cell carcinomas. Am J Surg Pathol 2004;28:1499-505.
59. Arora K, Bal M, Shih A, et al. Fetal-type gastrointestinal adenocarcinoma: a morphologically distinct entity with unfavourable prognosis. J Clin Pathol 2017. [Epub ahead of print]
60. Nogales FF, Quinonez E, Lopez-Marin L, Dulcey I, Preda O. A diagnostic immunohistochemical panel for yolk sac (primitive endodermal) tumours based on an immunohistochemical comparison with the human yolk sac. Histopathology 2014;65:51-9.
61. Schuldt M, Rubio A, Preda O, Nogales FF. GATA binding protein 3 expression is present in primitive patterns of yolk sac tumours but is not expressed by differentiated variants. Histopathology 2016;68:613-5.

62. Maeda D, Ota S, Takazawa Y, et al. Glypican-3 expression in clear cell adenocarcinoma of the ovary. Mod Pathol 2009;22:824-32.
63. Nogales FF, Preda O, Nicolae A. Yolk sac tumours revisited. A review of their many faces and names. Histopathology 2012;60:1023-33.
64. Sangoi AR, McKenney JK, Brooks JD, Bonventre JV, Higgins JP. Evaluation of putative renal cell carcinoma markers PAX-2, PAX-8, and hKIM-1 in germ cell tumors: a tissue microarray study of 100 cases. Applied immunohistochem Mole Morphol 2012;20:451-3.
65. Fadare O, Zhao C, Khabele D, et al. Comparative analysis of Napsin A, alpha-methylacyl-coenzyme A racemase (AMACR, P504S), and hepatocyte nuclear factor 1 beta as diagnostic markers of ovarian clear cell carcinoma: an immunohistochemical study of 279 ovarian tumours. Pathology 2015;47:105-11.
66. Ishibashi K, Kishimoto T, Yonemori Y, Hirashiki K, Hiroshima K, Nakatani Y. Primary hepatoid adenocarcinoma of the uterine corpus: a case report with immunohistochemical study for expression of liver-enriched nuclear factors. Pathol Res Pract 2011;207:332-6.
67. Takano M, Shibasaki T, Sato K, Aida S, Kikuchi Y. Malignant mixed Mullerian tumor of the uterine corpus with alpha-fetoprotein-producing hepatoid adenocarcinoma component. Gynecol Oncol 2003;91:444-8.
68. Yamamoto R, Ishikura H, Azuma M, et al. Alpha-fetoprotein production by a hepatoid adenocarcinoma of the uterus. J Clin Pathol 1996;49:420-2.
69. Shih AR, Liu XL, Silva A, et al. Refined characterization of hepatoid differentiation in gynecologic tract neoplasms. Mod Pathol 2016;29(Suppl 2):309A.
70. Kamgobe E, Massinde A, Matovelo D, Ndaboine E, Rambau P, Chaula T. Uterine myometrial mature teratoma presenting as a uterine mass: a review of literature. BMC Clin Pathol 2016;16:5.
71. Papadia A, Rutigliani M, Gerbaldo D, Fulcheri E, Ragni N. Mature cystic teratoma of the uterus presenting as an endometrial polyp. Ultrasound Obstet Gynecol 2007;29:477-8.
72. Stolnicu S, Szekely E, Molnar C, et al. Mature and immature solid teratomas involving uterine corpus, cervix, and ovary. Int J Gynecol Pathol 2017;36:222-7.
73. Ben Ameur El Youbi M, Mohtaram A, Kharmoum J, et al. Primary immature teratoma of the uterus relapsing as malignant neuroepithelioma: case report and review of the literature. Case Rep Oncol Med 2013;2013:971803.
74. Kalir T, Seijo L, Deligdisch L, Cohen C. Endometrial adenocarcinoma with choriocarcinomatous differentiation in an elderly virginal woman. Int J Gynecol Pathol 1995;14:266-9.
75. Pesce C, Merino MJ, Chambers JT, Nogales F. Endometrial carcinoma with trophoblastic differentiation. An aggressive form of uterine cancer. Cancer 1991;68:1799-802.
76. Savage J, Subby W, Okagaki T. Adenocarcinoma of the endometrium with trophoblastic differentiation and metastases as choriocarcinoma: a case report. Gynecol Oncol 1987;26:257-62.
77. Horn LC, Hanel C, Bartholdt E, Dietel J. Serous carcinoma of the endometrium with choriocarcinomatous differentiation: a case report and review of the literature indicate the existence of 2 prognostically relevant tumor types. Int J Gynecol Pathol 2006;25:247-51.
78. Gao HJ, Zhou W, Zhang XF, Zhou CY, Qian JH. Coexistent gestational choriocarcinoma and mixed adenocarcinoma of the uterus. Eur J Gynaecol Oncol 2013;34:362-7.
79. Rawish KR, Buza N, Zheng W, Fadare O. Endometrial carcinoma with trophoblastic components: clinicopathologic analysis of a rare entity. Int J Gynecol Pathol 2017. [Epub ahead of print]
80. Olson MT, Gocke CD, Giuntoli RL 2nd, Shih IeM. Evolution of a trophoblastic tumor from an endometrioid carcinoma—a morphological and molecular analysis. Int J Gynecol Pathol 2011;30:117-20.
81. Shih IM, Seidman JD, Kurman RJ. Placental site nodule and characterization of distinctive types of intermediate trophoblast. Hum Pathol 1999;30:687-94.
82. Shih IM, Kurman RJ. Immunohistochemical localization of inhibin-alpha in the placenta and gestational trophoblastic lesions. Int J Gynecol Pathol 1999;18:144-50.
83. Banet N, Gown AM, Shih IeM, et al. GATA-3 expression in trophoblastic tissues: an immunohistochemical study of 445 cases, including diagnostic utility. Am J Surg Pathol 2015;39:101-8.
84. Shih IM, Kurman RJ. p63 expression is useful in the distinction of epithelioid trophoblastic and placental site trophoblastic tumors by profiling trophoblastic subpopulations. Am J Surg Pathol 2004;28:1177-83.
85. Zhang HJ, Xue WC, Siu MK, Liao XY, Ngan HY, Cheung AN. P63 expression in gestational trophoblastic disease: correlation with proliferation and apoptotic dynamics. Int J Gynecol Pathol 2009;28:172-8.
86. Czernobilsky B, Mamet Y, David MB, Atlas I, Gitstein G, Lifschitz-Mercer B. Uterine retiform sertoli-leydig cell tumor: report of a case providing additional evidence that uterine tumors resembling ovarian sex cord tumors have a histologic and immunohistochemical phenotype of genuine sex cord tumors. Int K Gynecol Pathol 2005;24:335-40.

87. Mazur MT, Hsueh S, Gersell DJ. Metastases to the female genital tract. Analysis of 325 cases. Cancer 1984;53:1978-84.
88. Soslow RA. Practical issues related to uterine pathology: staging, frozen section, artifacts, and Lynch syndrome. Mod Pathol 2016;29(Suppl 1):S59-77.
89. Reyes C, Murali R, Park KJ. Secondary involvement of the adnexa and uterine corpus by carcinomas of the uterine cervix: a detailed morphologic description. Int J Gynecol Pathol 2015;34:551-63.
90. Yemelyanova A, Vang R, Seidman JD, Gravitt PE, Ronnett BM. Endocervical adenocarcinomas with prominent endometrial or endomyometrial involvement simulating primary endometrial carcinomas: utility of HPV DNA detection and immunohistochemical expression of p16 and hormone receptors to confirm the cervical origin of the corpus tumor. Am J Surg Pathol 2009;33:914-24.
91. Gungor T, Altinkaya SO, Ozat M, Akbay S, Mollamahmutoglu L. Unusual form of superficial spreading squamous cell carcinoma of cervix involving the endometrium, bilateral tubes and ovaries: a case report with literature review. Arch Gynecol Obstet 2011;283:323-7.
92. Kiyokoba R, Yagi H, Yahata H, et al. Tumor-to-tumor metastasis of poorly differentiated gastric carcinoma to uterine lipoleiomyoma. Case Rep Obstet Gynecol 2015;2015:352369.
93. Dendas W, Cappelle L, Verguts J, Orye G. Cholangiocarcinoma presenting as uterine metastasis. Case Rep Obstet Gynecol 2014;2014:204915.
94. Giordano G, Gnetti L, Ricci R, Merisio C, Melpignano M. Metastatic extragenital neoplasms to the uterus: a clinicopathologic study of four cases. Int J Gynecol Cancer 2006;16(Suppl 1):433-8.
95. Kumar NB, Hart WR. Metastases to the uterine corpus from extragenital cancers. A clinicopathologic study of 63 cases. Cancer 1982;50:2163-9.
96. Singh K, DiSilvestro PA, Lawrence WD, Quddus MR. An isolated metastasis from clear cell renal cell carcinoma to the uterus: a case report and review of literature. Int J Gynecol Pathol 2016;35:419-22.
97. McVeigh G, Shah V, Longacre TA, McCluggage W. Endometrial involvement in pseudomyxoma peritonei secondary to low-grade appendiceal mucinous neoplasm: report of 2 cases. Int J Gynecol Pathol 2015;34:232-8.
97a. Shaw K, Kokh D, Ioffe OB, Staats PN. "Pseudomyxoma endometrii": endometrial deposition of acellular mucin from a low-grade appendiceal mucinous neoplasm as a rare mimic of myxoid uterine tumors. Int J Gynecol Pathol 2015;34:351-6.
98. Barcos M, Lane W, Gomez GA, et al. An autopsy study of 1206 acute and chronic leukemias (1958 to 1982). Cancer 1987;60:827-37.
99. Gregor M, Tomsova M, Siroky O. Granulocytic sarcoma of the uterus. Int J Gynaecol Obstet 2008;103:73-4.
100. Kilic G, Boruban MC, Bueco-Ramos C, Konoplev SN. Granulocytic sarcoma involving the uterus and right fallopian tube with negative endometrial biopsy. Eur J Gynaecol Oncol 2007;28:270-2.
101. Ko SW, Kim YK, Jin GY, Lee SY, Kim CS. Granulocytic sarcoma manifested as a parametrial mass mimicking a haemorrhagic abscess: a case report with CT and MR findings. Br J Radiol 2007;80:e128-30.
102. Lambein K, Janssens A, Weyers S, Praet M, De Paepe P. Presence of myeloid precursor cells in the endometrium of an AML patient: a diagnostic challenge! Virchows Arch 2007;451:1097-8.
103. Oliva E, Ferry JA, Young RH, Prat J, Srigley JR, Scully RE. Granulocytic sarcoma of the female genital tract: a clinicopathologic study of 11 cases. Am J Surg Pathol 1997;21:1156-65.
104. Garcia MG, Deavers MT, Knoblock RJ, et al. Myeloid sarcoma involving the gynecologic tract: a report of 11 cases and review of the literature. Am J Clin Pathol 2006;125:783-90.
105. Bennett JA, Oliva E, Nardi V, Lindeman N, Ferry JA, Louissaint A, Jr. Primary endometrial marginal zone lymphoma (MALT lymphoma): a unique clinicopathologic entity. Am J Surg Pathol 2016;40:1217-23.
106. Kosari F, Daneshbod Y, Parwaresch R, Krams M, Wacker HH. Lymphomas of the female genital tract: a study of 186 cases and review of the literature. Am J Surg Pathol 2005;29:1512-20.
107. Nasioudis D, Kampaktsis PN, Frey M, Witkin SS, Holcomb K. Primary lymphoma of the female genital tract: an analysis of 697 cases. Gynecol Oncol 2017;145:305-9.
108. Vang R, Medeiros LJ, Ha CS, Deavers M. Non-Hodgkin's lymphomas involving the uterus: a clinicopathologic analysis of 26 cases. Mod Pathol 2000;13:19-28.

13 GESTATIONAL TROPHOBLASTIC DISEASE

The trophoblast is a unique and specialized epithelium associated with the placenta, and therefore normally present during pregnancy. It is predominantly in an intrauterine location, either within the placenta proper, surrounding chorionic villi mainly as cytotrophoblast and syncytiotrophoblast, as extravillous trophoblast between chorionic villi, or within the decidua and myometrium. *Gestational trophoblastic disease* (GTD) is a broad term that encompasses a range of clinical conditions associated with abnormal proliferation and/or persistence of gestationally derived trophoblast outside of normal pregnancy.

Since gestational trophoblast is derived from the conceptus, which is genetically distinct from maternal tissue and has a paternal genetic contribution, GTD can be conceptually thought of as an unusual form of a potentially malignant "allograft." As GTD is composed of abnormal trophoblastic tissue, many entities within this category are characterized by the production of pregnancy-associated hormones such as human chorionic gonadotrophin (hCG), which can be useful biomarkers to diagnose and monitor response to therapy.

GTD is generally subclassified into two main categories: *hydatidiform moles* (HM), which are genetically abnormal conceptions with associated abnormal proliferation of chorionic villous trophoblast, and *gestational trophoblastic tumors* (GTTs), characterized by abnormal proliferation of villous (*choriocarcinoma*) or extravillous (*placental-site trophoblastic tumor* and *epithelioid trophoblastic tumor*) trophoblast, usually not associated with a conceptus or chorionic villi. Other non-neoplastic trophoblastic lesions are sometimes included within the spectrum of GTD, such as exaggerated placental-site reaction and placental site nodule/plaque (Table 13-1) (1).

Patients with HMs most often present with vaginal bleeding or early pregnancy failure. Although most HMs are not malignant, they are associated with an increased risk of development of subsequent malignant disease requiring chemotherapy (*persistent gestational trophoblastic disease* [pGTD]). All HMs share the finding of excessive proliferation of villous trophoblast, although there are two morphologic and genetic types: *complete hydatidiform mole* (CHM), a diploid, hyperdiploid, or tetraploid conception in which the nuclear genome is only paternally derived in most cases, and *partial hydatidiform mole* (PHM), a triploid conception with at least two sets of paternal and one set of maternal chromosomes (Table 13-2).

The term CHM was originally based on the diffuse hydropic appearance of the abnormally large chorionic villi of fully developed examples, historically diagnosed in the second trimester of pregnancy, which could be observed on gross examination. In contrast, in PHM, such hydropic change was characteristically focal, and thus, the term "partial." However, since most HMs are now evacuated and examined at an early stage of pregnancy (first trimester), these macroscopic features are no longer apparent, but the terms

Table 13-1

WORLD HEALTH ORGANIZATION (WHO) CLASSIFICATION OF GESTATIONAL TROPHOBLASTIC DISEASE

Hydatidiform Mole
  Complete hydatidiform mole
  Partial hydatidiform mole
  Invasive hydatidiform mole

(Abnormal Nonmolar Villous Lesions)[a]

Non-Neoplastic Trophoblastic Lesions[a]
  Exaggerated placental-site reaction
  Placental site nodule(s) and plaque(s)

Neoplasms (Gestational Trophoblastic Tumors)
  Choriocarcinoma
  Placental-site trophoblastic tumor
  Epithelioid trophoblastic tumor

[a]These lesions are not strictly GTDs but are included in the WHO classification and also included here.

Table 13-2

DIFFERENTIAL DIAGNOSIS OF SUSPECTED MOLAR PRODUCTS OF CONCEPTION

	Nonmolar Miscarriage	PHM[a]	CHM[a]
Clinical features[b]	PV[a] bleeding, incidental finding of pregnancy failure on routine ultrasound scan	PV bleeding, incidental finding of pregnancy failure on routine ultrasound scan	PV bleeding, incidental finding of pregnancy failure on routine ultrasound scan
Villous hydrops[c]	Mild to marked	Mild to marked	Mild to marked
Villous morphology	Round and ovoid villous outlines, hypocellular stroma, no abnormal trophoblast hyperplasia	Irregular villous outlines with pseudoinclusions, angiomatoid vessels with nucleated red blood cells, focal abnormal trophoblast hyperplasia	Budding villous outlines, hypercellular stroma with karyorrhectic debris, prominent abnormal trophoblast hyperplasia, abnormal implantation site
Villous p57 immunostaining	Positive	Positive	Negative
Genetic findings	Diploid/aneuploid	Triploid	Diploid androgenetic[d]

[a]PHM = partial hydatidiform mole; CHM = complete hydatidiform mole; PV = per vaginum.
[b]PHM and CHM are rarely symptomatic in current clinical practice in developed nations.
[c]Extent of hydrops is not a useful diagnostic feature in products of conception evacuated in the first trimester.
[d]See section on biparental CHM.

CHM and PHM remain in use, primarily relating to the distinct underlying genetic abnormalities that characterize these two entities. Most HMs (approximately 85 percent of CHMs and over 99 percent of PHMs) are associated with no significant clinical consequences and resolve completely following uterine evacuation; a minority progresses to pGTD and these patients require chemotherapy.

Invasive mole is an aggressive form of HM defined by molar chorionic villi, usually after a previously diagnosed complete, but occasionally partial, HM, that invade the myometrium with or without associated invasion of adjacent structures. Its frequency has decreased in developed countries due to contemporary obstetric practices.

GTTs represent a wide spectrum of neoplasms that originate from the extravillous trophoblast, have variable malignant potential, and typically originate in the uterus, although can be encountered at other locations, both within the female genital tract and at other sites (e.g., lung). Patients generally have a favorable prognosis and better response to specific chemotherapeutic regimens than those with nongestational malignant genital tract neoplasms, and thus their recognition is important.

Typically, choriocarcinoma is predominantly composed of cells resembling villous cytotrophoblast and syncytiotrophoblast but, in contrast to HM, no chorionic villi are present (except in the rare setting of intraplacental choriocarcinoma). It is frequently associated with metastases and fatal without treatment, but highly responsive to current chemotherapy and, thus, associated with overall good outcome.

Placental-site and epithelioid trophoblastic tumors (PSTT and ETT), are less common, and almost always arise in the uterus. They are more chemoresistant than choriocarcinoma, and surgical intervention is the most important initial treatment modality (Table 13-3).

GTD represents a spectrum of conditions associated with abnormal trophoblast proliferation, with the specific features depending on genotype and trophoblast phenotype. Further discussion broadly focuses on HM and GTTs as separate subgroups, although some overlap exists.

NORMAL TROPHOBLAST DEVELOPMENT

Trophoblast is one of the earliest differentiated cell types to develop after fertilization. It is formed from the outer cell mass of the blastocyst and involved in implantation of the embryo and subsequent placental development (2,3). In addition to its role in implantation, with adhesion of the blastocyst to the uterine wall, one of the important early functions of trophoblast is production of hCG which, by having effects on maternal tissues, supports the

Table 13-3

DIFFERENTIAL DIAGNOSIS OF GESTATIONAL TROPHOBLASTIC TUMORS

	Choriocarcinoma	PSTT[a]	ETT[a]
Clinical features[b]	Abnormal PV[a] bleeding or unusual symptoms postpartum	Abnormal PV bleeding	Abnormal PV bleeding
Macroscopic features	Hemorrhagic uterine mass	Hemorrhagic and solid uterine mass	Hemorrhagic and solid uterine mass
Microscopic features	Necrosis with viable areas of abnormal pleomorphic trophoblast showing a biphasic pattern	Nests and sheets of relatively bland mononuclear trophoblasts with local infiltration	Hyalinized nodules containing nests of bland mononuclear trophoblast around vessels
Immunostaining	High proliferation index, diffuse hCG expression, inhibin expression in syncytotrophoblast, HLAG positive	Moderate proliferation index, focal hCG expression, inhibin and hPL positive, p63 negative, HLAG positive	Moderate proliferation index, focal hCG expression, inhibin and p63 positive, HPL negative, HLAG positive

[a]PSTT = placental-site trophoblastic tumor; ETT = epithelioid trophoblastic tumor; PV = per vaginum.
[b]A wide range of clinical features have been described depending on metastatic site and hormone production but most cases present as noted.

production of progesterone by the corpus luteum until the trophoblast can produce adequate amounts of steroid hormones (4).

The normal placenta includes villous and extravillous trophoblast. The villous trophoblast covers chorionic villi and consists of cytotrophoblast and syncytiotrophoblast, the former representing the presumed trophoblastic stem cell compartment (fig. 13-1A–C). Cytotrophoblast cells are mononuclear cells that form the inner layer of trophoblast overlying the chorionic villi. They are prominent in the first trimester of pregnancy but much less conspicuous in mature placentas. They display clear to granular cytoplasm (probably reflecting a paucity of cellular organelles) with prominent cell borders and large and round nuclei. They are associated with a high mitotic rate, especially in early gestation. They are metabolically and endocrinologically inactive, producing few hormones compared to syncytiotrophoblast cells. They express cytokeratin, CD10, p57, and p63 but not hCG or human placental lactogen (HPL) and do not express α-inhibin throughout gestation (5).

Syncytiotrophoblast cells are formed by the fusion of cytotrophoblasts and cannot proliferate directly. This true syncytium presents as an outer layer within the chorionic villi. The cells have abundant basophilic to amphophilic dense cytoplasm with vacuoles or lacunae, dense brush borders, and multinucleation with nuclei that are smaller without associated mitotic activity when compared to cytotrophoblast cells. Syncytiotrophoblast cells are responsible for the exchange of oxygen and nutrients with maternal blood and act as the major metabolic and endocrine component of the placenta, secreting many hormones including hCG, HPL, placental alkaline phosphatase (PLAP), SP-1, and a wide range of other pregnancy-associated factors. Syncytiotrophoblast also has an important role in producing steroid hormones, such as estrogen and progesterone. As pregnancy progresses, hCG production decreases while HPL and PLAP production increase (6,7). Alpha-inhibin is consistently expressed by syncytiotrophoblast cells, especially in the first trimester (5). Syncytiotrophoblast cells also express low- and high-molecular weight keratins and CD10 but not p57 or p63 (8).

The extravillous trophoblast is composed of intermediate trophoblast, although the latter is also present within trophoblastic columns of anchoring villi. Intermediate trophoblast cells have features intermediate between proliferating cytotrophoblast and terminal syncytiotrophoblast. Intermediate trophoblast is divided into three subtypes (fig. 13-2): 1) villous, located in the villous columns acting as a source for the other subtypes of intermediate trophoblast; 2) implantation site, responsible for establishing effective maternal-fetal circulation by infiltrating decidua, spiral arteries (causing

Tumors of the Uterine Corpus and Gestational Trophoblastic Diseases

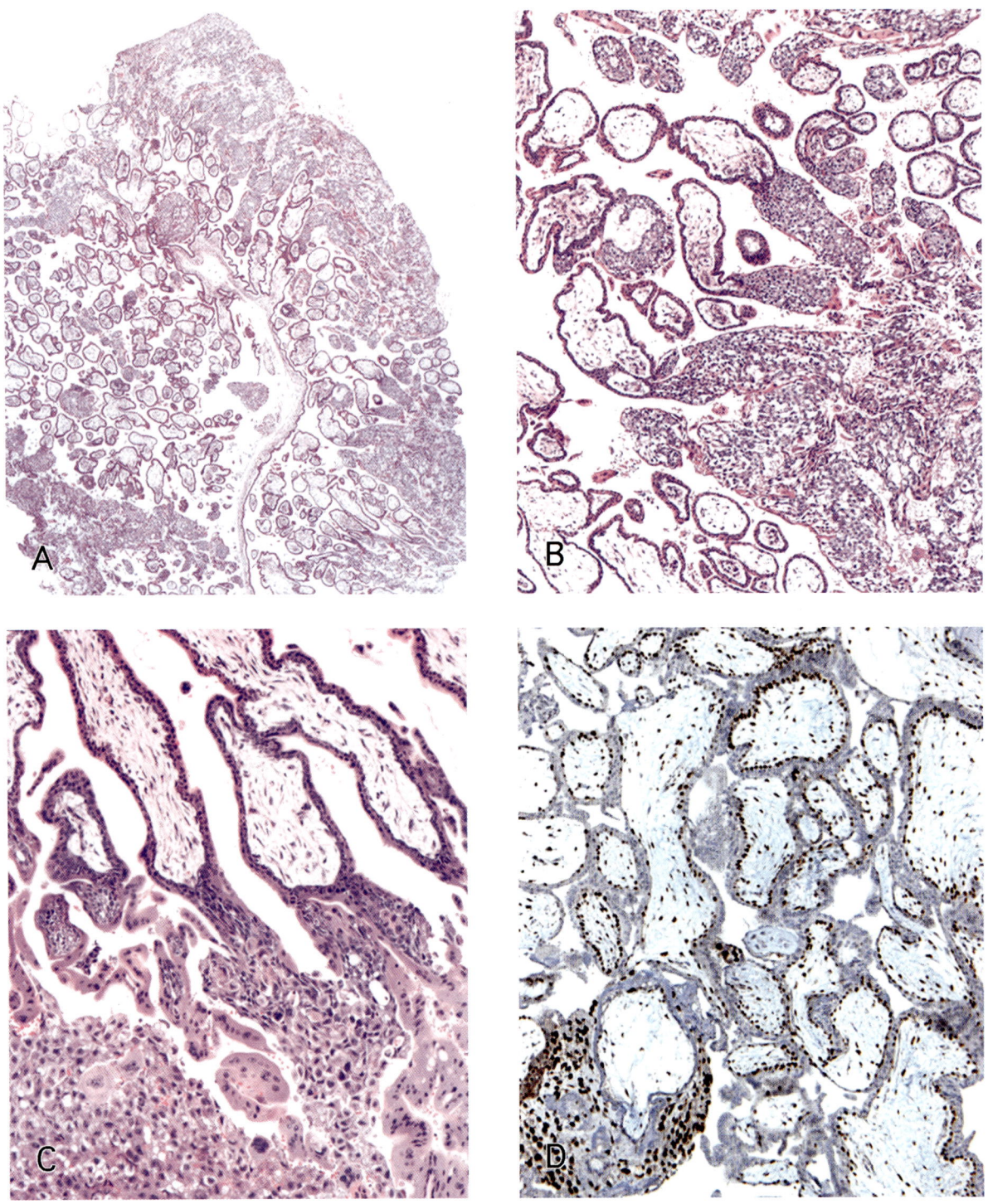

Figure 13-1

NONMOLAR CONCEPTION

Normal early conception with organized and regular chorionic villi and florid trophoblast shell formation (A). Trophoblast is streaming from one pole of the chorionic villi in contrast to the circumferential distribution in established hydatidiform mole (B,C). Diffuse nuclear expression of p57^{KIP2} is present in villous stroma and cytotrophoblast but absent in syncytiotrophoblast (D).

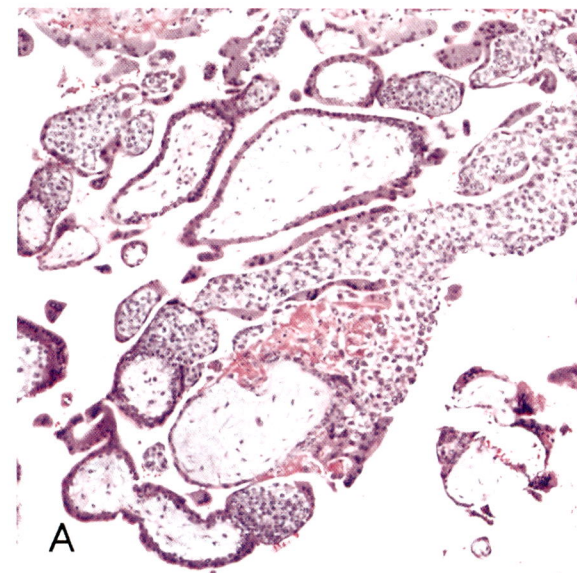

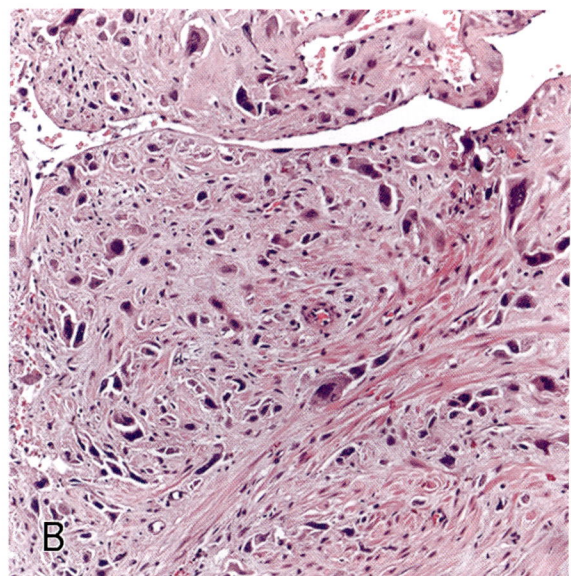
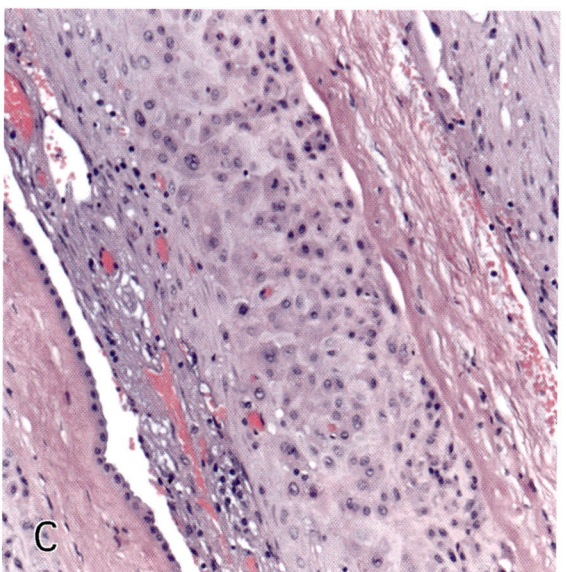

Figure 13-2

EXTRAVILLOUS TROPHOBLAST

Villous trophoblast is located within the villous columns and is a source for the other subtypes of intermediate trophoblast (A). Implantation trophoblast is seen between the maternal tissues (decidua and myometrium) (B). Chorionic-type trophoblast is located in the chorionic laeve (C).

fibrinoid necrosis but leaving the vascular outline intact), and myometrium (9); and 3) chorionic, located in the chorionic laeve of the fetal membranes. The latter potentially acts as a maternal immune mechanical barrier and may also have a function in fetal allograft survival, besides helping to maintain the tensile strength of the fetal membranes by synthesis of extracellular matrix components (9).

Intermediate trophoblast cells within the trophoblastic columns are cohesive and have larger nuclei than cytotrophoblasts but smaller than implantation intermediate trophoblasts with polygonal clear cytoplasm. Intermediate trophoblast cells from the implantation site tend to have abundant eosinophilic to amphophilic cytoplasm and frequently are difficult to distinguish from decidual cells. In contrast to the latter, they have irregular and frequently hyperchromatic nuclei. The chorionic-type extravillous trophoblast is typically composed of a uniform population of cells with clear or eosinophilic cytoplasm. The cells are larger than cytotrophoblast but smaller than the implantation trophoblast cells as occurs with the villous extravillous trophoblasts. Extravillous

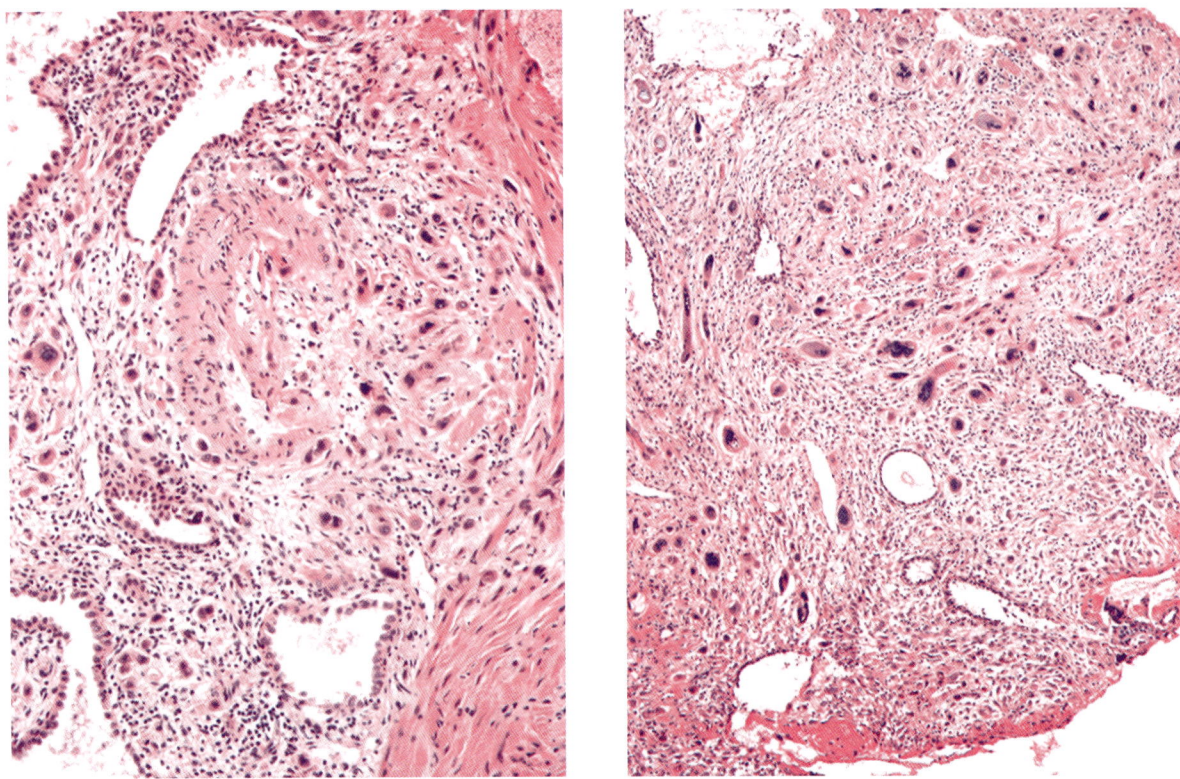

Figure 13-3

IMPLANTATION SITE

The intermediate trophoblast in early implantation invades vessels (left) as well as endomyometrium (right).

trophoblast cells are predominantly mononuclear but may be binucleated and are rarely multinucleated, especially within the implantation site and chorionic laeve. They coexpress HPL and cytokeratins with minimal hCG and PLAP expression (5,10). They also express epithelial membrane antigen (EMA), inhibin, CD10, and human leukocyte antigen (HLA)-G.

The functions of extravillous trophoblast, especially that of the implantation site, probably include production of proteolytic enzymes to facilitate tissue invasion, production of thromboplastin and plasminogen activator to control fibrin formation, control of vascular conversion and patency, expression of HLA types, which may be important in immunologic function, and endocrine/paracrine roles (11).

Trophoblast Stem Cells and Early Development

Trophoblast develops from the outer layer of the blastocyst and has important roles mediating maternal-fetal interaction, including endocrine functions in early implantation and covering chorionic villi in the placenta. The process of early implantation and development of the placenta involves invasion of maternal tissues (endometrium/decidua and myometrium) by the trophoblast and complex remodelling of the maternal vasculature in order to appropriately supply the placenta with oxygen and nutrients (fig. 13-3).

Although there have been significant advances in understanding the overall genetic and cellular control of the process of implantation, the precise mechanisms that control the extent of trophoblast infiltration remain uncertain in humans (12–14). There is also interest in knowing how trophoblast manages to evade immune detection and secondary destruction by maternal response, given that trophoblast is genetically distinct from maternal tissue, and the conceptus essentially acts as a graft. Although, this remains an area of intense research, it is recognized that the invading interstitial trophoblast expresses unique patterns of HLA molecules, which have a significant role in trophoblast-host interaction, in addition to the production of a range of biologically active compounds that likely influence the local immune response (15,16).

There has been increased understanding of the intrinsic role of trophoblast infiltration in modifying the maternal vascular supply to the developing placenta, a process that is more complex than initially suggested (17–19). Compared to the nonpregnant state, in the late stages of pregnancy, branches of the uterine spiral arteries are converted from normal muscular arteries into poorly muscularized, dilated, low-resistance uteroplacental vessels. It is now recognized that in the early stages of pregnancy, infiltration by intermediate trophoblast at the implantation site involves both invasion into decidua/endometrium and myometrium as well as invasion of the maternal vasculature by a specific subtype of extravillous trophoblast (endovascular trophoblast) (20–22).

Subsequent conversion of the spiral arteries into low-resistance uteroplacental vessels appears to be a coordinated process involving both endovascular trophoblast and surrounding interstitial extravillous trophoblast, resulting in the remodelling of these vessels. Furthermore, the endovascular trophoblast probably plays an important role in early pregnancy by forming solid intravascular "plugs" to minimize oxygenated arterial blood flow to the early implanting embryo. As pregnancy proceeds through the late first trimester, these endovascular plugs dissolve, allowing increased blood flow to reach the intervillous space as required for subsequent fetal growth (23,24).

Because gestational trophoblastic disease represents abnormal trophoblast development, there has been much interest in understanding trophoblast stem cells (TSCs). In mammals, trophoblast is the first established lineage during development. In mice, TSCs are derived from blastocyst and can differentiate into a full range of trophoblast lineages (25). In mice, a wide range of transcriptional networks and signalling pathways are required for normal placental development, which determine the fate of TSCs (26). In humans, the identification of TSCs has remained elusive, particularly as they appear to be derived from, or differentiate toward, different trophoblast populations (25,27,28). Further understanding has been gained in trophoblast research with the discovery that human embryonic stem cells (ES cells) differentiate toward trophoblast lineages. BMP4 (bone morphogenic protein 4, a member of the transforming growth factor-beta superfamily) (27,29,30), or other such factors, identify ES cells, although whether the end cells represent true trophoblast identical to normal early human trophoblast remains controversial (31).

The phenomenon of imprinting, which is defined by differential expression of genes depending on whether they are inherited from the maternal or paternal genome, appears to be important in trophoblast development. Several studies have demonstrated that androgenetic conceptions, in both mice and humans, exhibit marked preferential trophoblast development while conceptions only derived from the maternal genome show poor trophoblast development. A range of imprinted genes, such as insulin-like growth factor, have been implicated in trophoblast development but their precise role remains uncertain (32,33).

Although knowledge of the embryologic basis and functions of trophoblast is not required for adequate histologic diagnosis of gestational trophoblastic diseases/tumors, such information provides a framework to better understand diseases of the trophoblast, especially of gestational trophoblastic tumors, as well as an appreciation of the patterns of differentiation and invasion of trophoblast. Specifically, the dominant phenotype in different gestational trophoblastic tumors closely resembles specific types of trophoblast present during normal placentation. Awareness of these different trophoblast populations enhances their detection and also conceptually may explain the finding of differing trophoblast phenotypes in the same tumor. For example, choriocarcinoma demonstrates abnormal villous-type trophoblast differentiation, including cytotrophoblast and syncytiotrophoblast-like components, with the proliferation of syncytiotrophoblast explaining the rapid growth, prominent hCG production, and marked response to chemotherapy, analogous to the behavior of normal placental trophoblast. Placental-site and epithelioid trophoblastic tumors conversely demonstrate an extravillous implantation site or chorionic-type intermediate trophoblast phenotype with relative lack of hCG production and predominant local invasion (mostly PSTT) requiring surgical intervention (1). There remains uncertainty however, whether these tumors are derived from partially differentiated cells within these anatomic populations or from common TSCs with differentiation along different pathways (34). In some cases, especially following chemotherapy, more than one trophoblast morphologic phenotype is identified in the same tumor, suggesting some degree of plasticity.

GESTATIONAL TROPHOBLASTIC DISEASE

Staging

Both the TNM (35) and International Federation of Gynecology and Obstetrics (FIGO) (36) staging systems are used for GTD classification, based on the extent of local invasion and presence or absence of metastatic disease (Table 13-4) (34,37,38). Most specialized centers currently use the revised FIGO staging system, which includes anatomic staging and other prognostic indicators for stages I to IV in addition to risk stratification scores (Table 13-5) (36).

The optimal management of gestational trophoblastic neoplasia requires a thorough assessment of the extent of disease and risk factors prior to the initiation of treatment. Patients undergo physical examination, hCG evaluation, and metastatic imaging screening for complete FIGO staging. Prognostic scoring is based on sites of metastases, tumor burden, duration of disease, and prior chemotherapy exposure and resistance. Patients with low risk of persistent GTD have extremely high cure rates with chemotherapy regardless of protocol (single agent, methotrexate or actinomycin D in most cases). Five to 15 percent of low-risk patients may not be cured with first line chemotherapy and require multiagent chemotherapy (39–41). For placental-site and epithelioid trophoblastic tumors, hysterectomy is the main treatment with further therapy directed by stage. Choriocarcinoma is usually treated initially with chemotherapy (42–44).

Epidemiology

The overall incidence of GTD is 0.5 to 1.0/1,000 live births/pregnancies in most countries, including those in Western countries and China (34,45,46). Higher rates are reported in some areas, such as Japan (around 2/1,000 pregnancies) (47,48) compared to Europe (0.6

Table 13-4

REVISED INTERNATIONAL FEDERATION OF GYNECOLOGY AND OBSTETRICS (FIGO) STAGING SYSTEM

Stage I	Disease confined to the uterus
Stage II	Extension outside the uterus but limited to genital structures (adnexa, vagina, broad ligament)
Stage III	Extension to the lungs with or without genital tract involvement
Stage IV	All other metastatic sites

Table 13-5

FIGO RISK FACTOR SCORING VALUES[a]

FIGO Scoring	0	1	2	4
Age	<40	≥40	–	–
Antecedent pregnancy	Mole	Abortion	Term	–
Interval months from index pregnancy	<4	4 – <7	7 – <13	≥13
Pretreatment serum hCG (IU/L)	$<10^3$	$10^3 - <10^4$	$10^4 - <10^5$	$\geq 10^5$
Largest tumor size (including uterus) in cm	<3	3 – <5	≥5	–
Site of metastases	Lung	Spleen, kidney	Gastrointestinal	Liver, brain
Number of metastases	–	1 – 4	5 – 8	>8
Previous failed chemotherapy	–	–	Single drug	2 or more drugs

[a]Identification of an individual patient's stage and risk score is expressed by allotting a Roman numeral to the stage and an Arabic numeral to the risk score separated by a colon.

to 1.1/1,000 pregnancies) (49,50). Early studies suggested that GTD may be more common in American Indians and Eskimos (51) and Asian populations (52) and several reasons for possible geographic differences have been suggested, including differences in maternal age, diet, ethnicity, and gravidity, poor social-economic conditions, and infection, but none have been proven. No specific environmental factors have been identified that can be linked with certainty to an increased risk for GTD, while the demographic risk factors are broadly similar for PHM and CHM (49). The incidence rates of GTD in the United States and Europe have remained fairly constant in recent decades (49).

The age-specific incidence of GTD demonstrates a typical J-shaped curve, with HM (both PHM and CHM, although more marked for CHM) more frequent at the extremes of reproductive age, with rates greater if patients are under 15 years of age, and especially for those over 40 years (53–55). Most pregnancies are not in women at these extremes, even though the relative risks are greater, most patients affected by GTD are women between 18 and 40 years, which represents the normal reproductive age range.

There are several issues with the data derived from these epidemiologic studies. The true number of affected patients and the denominator used (for example, clinical pregnancies, live births) to calculate incidence are difficult to determine. There are inconsistencies when comparing historical population data to contemporary data from specialized centers using molecular genetic testing. Identification of persistent GTD is even more problematic, since it is based on monitoring hCG with surveillance programs in some countries, with variation in cut-off values, and based only on clinical features in others. In addition, it is likely that all hospital-based studies tend to have falsely elevated incidence rates, whereas populations with poor medical services likely under report these diseases.

GTD is mainly represented by HMs. The risk of pGTD and choriocarcinoma varies greatly: approximately 1 in 40 to 50,000 following a normal term pregnancy to 1 in 40 following an HM (56,57). Epidemiologic studies have reported varying ratios of CHM and PHM, likely due to differences in ascertainment, especially with underdetection of PHM. Data obtained from large tertiary centers suggest a 1- to 2-fold excess of PHM when compared to CHM with complete ascertainment (58).

A history of a previous HM is associated with increased risk of subsequent ones (59,60): 1 to 2 percent following one previous HM, 10- to 20-fold greater than the baseline risk, particularly for patients with CHM. Those patients with a history of multiple prior HMs have a greater risk of subsequent HM, probably due to inclusion of a subgroup of patients with biparental familial recurrent HM (BiFRHM). Other than an increased risk of recurrence of HM, the outcome of future pregnancies appears unaffected in these patients (61).

Since choriocarcinoma often develops from a CHM, many epidemiologic risk factors are shared. With the introduction of screening following the detection of HM, fully developed symptoms/signs of choriocarcinoma (as opposed to biochemical pGTD following HM) have become less common. The relative proportion of clinically apparent choriocarcinoma occurring following term nonmolar pregnancies has increased (34).

The largest and most comprehensive dataset on the incidence of GTD was undertaken at the national trophoblastic disease service in England and Wales, based on centralized national recruitment with high ascertainment of cases (58). Of 8,242,511 pregnant women, there were 5,793 CHMs and 7,790 PHMs, with an overall incidence of around 1/600 HMs (1/1,400 for CHM and 1/1,000 for PHM, with a slight excess of PHM). The overall risk of developing pGTD requiring chemotherapy was 14 percent and 1 percent following CHM and PHM, respectively. The previously reported significant association with maternal age extremes was confirmed, especially for CHM. Following a previous HM, the risk of a subsequent one was 1 in 70; women with CHM had a 1 in 100 and 1 in 4 risk of further CHM after one or two consecutive CHM, respectively. Women with PHM had only a small increase in risk for further HM (60).

Genetics

It has long been recognized that HMs represent the phenotypic correlates of distinct genetically abnormal conceptions. Before recognition of the different subtypes, it had been reported that HMs typically demonstrated a 46,XX female karyotype (62,63), with a few being triploid (64). Differences in the genetic background as well as clinical and morphologic differences led to the concept that genetically and phenotypically distinct subgroups of HMs exist, namely, CHM and PHM (65–67). It was proposed, and is now accepted, that CHMs are diploid, with a 46,XX karyotype while PHMs are triploid. Although CHMs appeared to have a normal chromosome number, further insight was gained from the finding that their genetic material was all derived from the paternal genome (androgenetic) (68–73), mostly from duplication of a normal haploid sperm at fertilization (71,73). In addition, it is now recognized that some CHMs result from fertilization of an anucleate egg by two different haploid sperms (74,75), and modern molecular genotyping has shown that this mechanism is responsible for around 20 percent of them (76,77). CHMs with a 46,YY karyotype have not yet been reported, suggesting that are nonviable. While it is now accepted that CHMs occur by fusion of one or two sperm with an anucleate oocyte, the mechanism of formation of the anucleate egg remains uncertain. Finally, it has been suggested that postzygotic diploidization of a triploid conceptus may be an alternative mechanism for the development of a CHM, but, if it occurs, it is exceedingly rare (78).

In contrast to CHM, PHMs are almost always triploid (69,XXX, 69,XXY, or 69,XYY) (68,79,80), being the result of fertilization of an ovum by two sperms (common) or by a diploid sperm (rare) (81,82). PHMs, therefore, contain one copy of the maternally derived genome and an extra set of paternally derived chromosomes with overexpression of associated genes (83). The "diploid" PHMs described in early studies likely represent either nonmolar miscarriages or early CHMs, based on data from the application of modern molecular techniques (84,85). Although PHMs are triploid, not all triploid pregnancies are PHM; 70 to 80 percent of triploid conceptions are paternally derived PHMs, the remainder are nonmolar digynic triploid conceptions (84,86).

Data on the genetics of HMs has become more complex in recent years with the widespread routine use of molecular genotyping in clinical practice. Although most are classified either as androgenetic diploid or diandric triploid, occasional HMs do not demonstrate these typical patterns, including rare tetraploid cases (87,88), although these still demonstrate an excess of paternally derived material. The genetic etiology of HMs is further complicated since mosaicism, placental mosaicism or chimera formation (89,90), with both androgenetic and biparental cell lines admixed, has been reported in CHMs. Examples of biparental/androgenetic mosaicism (all derived from the same sperm) or biparental/androgenetic chimerism (fusion of genetically different lines) have now been described (91–95). The placental phenotype in these cases appears to be related to the distribution of cell lines: fully androgenetic areas exhibit placental mosaicism for CHM (92), and if androgenetic cells are restricted to mesenchymal components, the phenotype is that of placental mesenchymal dysplasia (PMD) (93). Finally, a well-characterized group of biparental CHMs is now recognized (see section below).

Imprinting

The development of HM is associated with the overexpression of paternally-derived genes, a feature of genetic imprinting in which gene activity or function is dependent on whether the allele is maternally or paternally inherited. In HM, there is either complete or relative overexpression of paternal genes resulting in trophoblastic overgrowth and defective or absent embryonic development. When only paternal material is present, CHM develops, while presence of maternal genome is associated with some degree of fetal development and PHM. These findings have been confirmed in mouse models (96,97), demonstrating that both maternal and paternal contributions to the genome are required for normal development.

This phenomenon is used in diagnostic pathology practice since immunohistochemical staining for p57^{KIP2}, the product of the imprinted gene *CDKN1C* (a cyclin dependent kinase inhibitor, which acts as a tumor suppressor gene), can be used to confirm a diagnosis of CHM. p57 is only expressed in villous tissue (mesenchyme and cytotrophoblast) when derived from the maternal genome (fig. 13-1D) (94,98–103). Villous p57^{KIP2} expression is, therefore, absent in CHM, but expressed in all other pregnancies (normal and abnormal) and is a reliable immunohistochemical marker of defective imprinting (see below).

Familial Recurrent (Biparental) Hydatidiform Moles

Most CHMs are sporadic with increased, but still low, recurrence risk. There are some families, however, in which affected women have most of their conceptions affected by CHM, with few or no livebirths (61,104–108). It is now recognized that they are affected by a rare diploid form of HM that is biparental, with a normal genotype, known as *familial recurrent biparental HM* (FR-BHM) (105,109,110). In such cases, CHMs are diploid, as with sporadic forms, but the chromosomal constitution of the HM is biparental rather than androgenetic (111,112).

Inheritance patterns suggest a maternal autosomal recessive defect at 19q13.3-13.4 (111) subsequently identified as *NLRP7* (*NALP7*), with different mutations affecting around 80 percent of these women (112–116). *NLRP7* is involved in immunologic and inflammatory pathways, but the precise mechanisms by which the mutations cause CHM remain uncertain. It appears to involve disruption of imprinting with a number of genes that normally carry a maternal methylation imprint, having been shown to assume a paternal epigenetic pattern on the maternal allele. Mutations on the *C6ORF221* gene have been detected in 5 percent of women with BFRHM syndrome but no other specific mutations have been seen in the remaining 15 percent (117,118). These mutations do not appear to be involved in other pregnancy complications of nonfamilial HMs or recurrent miscarriages (119).

FRBHMs are generally histopathologically indistinguishable from typical androgenetic CHMs and also show an abnormal p57^{KIP2} expression pattern (101). This suggests that the phenotype is a consequence of abnormal imprinting control, possibly with variable penetrance to account for the varied pregnancy outcomes. In one large review of published series of recurrent HMs including over 150 pregnancies from 37 affected women from 14 families, 113 of the conceptions (74 percent) were CHMs, 26 (17 percent) nonmolar miscarriages, 6 (4 percent) PHMs, and 7 (5 percent) phenotypically normal pregnancies (61). Despite the occurrence of non-CHM in patients from these families, most (more than 70 percent) pregnancies in affected women were CHMs, a figure that may be even higher since some may be missed when miscarriage tissue is not available for histologic examination.

Women with FRBHM syndrome should be made aware of the low (less than 5 percent) chance that they will have a normal pregnancy resulting in livebirth with no treatment. The risk of progression to pGTD appears to be similar to that seen in usual CHM. In the above study, 11 percent of CHMs failed to resolve spontaneously, similar to what is reported in sporadic CHM (61). Recent data support that there is no significant difference in the risk of developing pGTD in sporadic CHM when compared to FRBHM (60).

Genetic Testing of Hydatidiform Moles

The distinction of a HM from a nonmolar miscarriage is important for future patient management. hCG screening to detect pGTD and counselling regarding recurrent risk of persistent GTD are necessary. A correct diagnosis of HM based on morphology alone is possible in approximately 90 percent of cases in specialized referral centers (120,121). In some instances, however, due to sampling issues, degenerative changes secondary to tissue retention, or histologic overlap with other chromosomal abnormalities, a definite diagnosis is not possible on routine sections and ancillary techniques are required (99,122–126).

Genetic testing aims to assess ploidy, and, more recently, direct molecular genetic analysis aims to determine parental origin of the conceptus, using a range of specific markers. Ploidy can theoretically be assessed using karyotype, flow cytometry, and in situ hybridization with chromosome specific probes (a technique applicable to routinely processed formalin-fixed paraffin-embedded tissue) (87,127–134). Although ploidy may be useful to distinguish PHM from CHM and nonmolar miscarriages, it cannot distinguish between molar and nonmolar triploid or diploid pregnancies or determine the causative pregnancy in gestational trophoblastic tumors.

Most modern molecular genetic approaches use polymerase chain reaction (PCR)-based techniques to identify specific variations in DNA sequences, such as restriction fragment length polymorphisms, DNA fingerprinting, minisatellite probes, and microsatellite polymorphisms (135–137). Many of these techniques are also used with formalin-fixed paraffin-embedded material including that derived from histologic sections (138,139). These approaches can reliably identify androgenetic CHM, including distinguishing monospermic from dispermic CHM, and diandric triploid PHM (124,126). Molecular testing combined with histologic examination is mandatory to identify FRBHM (including specific assessment for mutations in known regions such as *NLRP7*) (112) and for reliable diagnosis of GTT versus nongestational hCG-producing tumors (140).

Genetic Features Influencing Outcome

Prediction of the biological behavior of HMs remains a major clinical challenge since, despite the markedly increased risk of pGTD compared to nonmolar pregnancies, most patients with CHM (85 percent) and PHM (over 99 percent) do not require chemotherapy (141). Women having such diagnoses undergo registration and follow-up in countries where surveillance is performed. Genetic approaches have been suggested but to date have been unsuccessful. It was initially suggested that the risk of pGTD could be greater with dispermic CHM (141), however, the frequency of invasive mole and metastatic disease following monospermic and dispermic CHM was not different in other studies (142). Similarly, there is no significant difference in the risk of developing pGTD in sporadic CHM compared to FRBHM (60).

Genetic Testing of Gestational Trophoblastic Tumors

Genetic testing based on molecular genotyping is primarily performed to distinguish gestational from nongestational GTTs when unusual clinical or pathologic findings are noted. There are no distinctive or clinically prognostic genetic markers in GTTs and their genetic background depends on the type of pregnancy from which they are derived. In general, choriocarcinomas are aneuploid (143–145), with chromosomal gains, losses, and rearrangements, but with no consistent findings. Some genes, such as *NECC1* (4q11-q12), are expressed in normal placenta but absent in choriocarcinoma, although the clinical significance of such findings remains to be determined (146). PSTTs show similar nonconsistent chromosomal findings, but most are genetically "female," suggesting that the presence of a Y chromosome might be less compatible with their development (147,148).

Although GTTs, as their name implies, show trophoblast differentiation and express hCG, occasional nongestational nontrophoblastic tumors display overlapping features and the differential diagnosis may be difficult, especially if the tumor is associated with an unusual presentation (140,149,150). The distinction between GTTs and nongestational tumors is important since the former respond better to chemotherapy. The genetic origin of such tumors is now easily determined based on molecular genotyping approaches, with GTTs containing paternal and maternal DNA (or only paternal if arising from a CHM) compared to nongestational tumors which show a genotype similar to the surrounding nontumor tissue, but with no paternal component from another individual (151,152).

GTTs develop from both molar and nonmolar conceptions. Histologic examination cannot determine the causative pregnancy based on either morphologic examination or $p57^{KIP2}$ expression (100). Origin can be determined, however, using molecular genotyping, which has demonstrated that the pregnancy immediately preceding the clinical presentation of the GTT may not always be the one from which the tumor is genetically derived (153–155). For some tumors, the causative pregnancy may even be from a previous HM, with intervening nonmolar pregnancies.

The risk of developing a GTT following a definite nonmolar hydropic miscarriage is low, probably less than 1 in 50,000. Most examples previously described are likely misdiagnosed early CHMs or nonmolar miscarriages preceding the GTT, but not the genetically causative pregnancy (154,155). Molecular studies suggest that approximately one quarter of GTTs are not derived from the immediately antecedent pregnancy (153). Such knowledge allows improved understanding of the development of these tumors and may in the future facilitate targeted therapies.

Human Chorionic Gonadotrophin as a Biomarker of Gestational Trophoblastic Disease

hCG is a glycoprotein hormone composed of two subunits, alpha and beta, with variable side chain modifications (156). In GTD, as in normal pregnancy, trophoblast produces hCG, which may, in the setting of GTT, be detected as intact hCG molecules, free subunits, degraded fragments, and hyperglycosylated variants in serum or urine (150,157). hCG is only normally detected during pregnancy and, therefore, it is a reliable, sensitive, and specific marker of the presence of hCG-producing tissue, usually containing trophoblast. Depending on laboratory protocols and assays used, blood levels reported may represent intact hCG, free β-hCG, nicked hCG, and hyperglycosylated hCG, with a degradation product, β-core fragment, also detectable in urine (158).

Many commercial hCG assays are available but almost all are primarily designed for uncomplicated pregnancies and are based on standard "sandwich type" detection methods (using antibodies against various hCG subunits). Different assays preferentially detect different types of hCG-related molecules, which is not a clinically significant issue in normal pregnancy, since in this setting intact hCG is the main molecule expressed. For the detection and monitoring of GTD, however, this may cause issues since a range of hCG variants are produced by different tumors (159). For example, hyperglycosylated hCG is the most prevalent subtype in choriocarcinoma, possibly with an autocrine function (160–162), whereas PSTT is generally associated with increased levels of free β-hCG (163). Cleaved forms of hCG are more common following treatment of GTTs (164). For these reasons, recurrence of invasive disease may be missed and false negative results occur if assays are used which do not detect the full spectrum of hCG subtypes (158) and false positives may also occur from interfering antibodies rather than hCG (165–167).

It has been suggested that hCG findings may have diagnostic and management implications beyond confirmation of GTD. For example, increased levels of hyperglycosylated hCG may be useful to discriminate GTD requiring no therapy from those that need treatment (168). PSTT is generally associated with significantly lower hCG levels than choriocarcinoma, the latter characteristically associated with hyperglycosylated hCG, and the former typically having greater serum levels of free β-hCG and urine β-core fragment (164,168).

Gestational Trophoblastic Disease Subtypes

There are several specific practical issues to consider regarding GTD diagnosis. First, a main function of normal pregnancy-associated trophoblast is to invade the endomyometrium and gain access to maternal circulation. Normal trophoblast, therefore, also invades vessels and is hematogenously transported to lungs and other sites, a behavior which in most other settings would be regarded as evidence of malignancy (169–171). Thus, tissue invasion and "metastases" are poor criteria to diagnose malignancy or predict behavior in GTD.

Second, GTD, and GTT in particular, are rare and, therefore, often unfamiliar to both physicians and pathologists in nonspecialized centers. This, coupled with frequent technical difficulties and risks in obtaining adequate samples from deeply invasive and/or hemorrhagic lesions, make pathologic diagnosis difficult or impossible. Patients may be treated, and many cured, based on clinical and serologic findings without histologic confirmation of the underlying disease process, especially in the setting of postmolar surveillance; hence, the use of nonspecific terms such as GTD and pGTD (34,46).

Third, widespread use of routine ultrasound examination in detection, diagnosis, and management of early pregnancy complications has resulted in much earlier evacuation of HMs and prompt chemotherapy for those on hCG surveillance programs (172,173). Such approaches have resulted in a marked reduction in the proportion of patients with HM presenting with typical clinical features such as enlarged uterine size, hyperemesis, toxemia, or hyperthyroidism (174,175). Most patients with HM now present with vaginal bleeding or early pregnancy failure toward the end of the first trimester. At this stage, pathologic criteria used to establish the diagnosis of late second trimester HM are no longer valid and revised criteria are required (see below) (176).

For patients with HM, 5 to 10 percent require chemotherapy following uterine evacuation. Patients on surveillance programs who develop pGTD posthydatidiform mole have cure rates approaching 100 percent; patients presenting with clinical complications, choriocarcinoma, or PSTT often require more extensive therapy, although with current regimes, there is still a high likelihood of cure.

The histopathologic diagnosis of GTT may be difficult in nonspecialized centers since the success of modern chemotherapeutic regimens has resulted in reduction in the number of viable choriocarcinoma specimens available for examination. Specific classification of some gestational trophoblastic tumors may be difficult as histologic features may be altered by treatment, and some lesions have a mixed phenotypic morphology (177,178).

HYDATIDIFORM MOLES

In contemporary clinical practice in developed countries, patients with HMs typically present with non-specific symptoms/signs such as vaginal bleeding or abdominal pain, or are asymptomatic and the HM is detected as early pregnancy failure on routine first trimester ultrasound examination. Although maternal serum hCG levels are generally elevated in HM compared to normal pregnancy, hCG alone cannot reliably distinguish HM from non-molar pregnancies due to significant overlap, especially in the context of pregnancy failure, although presence of free β-hCG provides improved detection of CHM.

The classic findings of HM, excessive uterine enlargement, hyperemesis, and pre-eclampsia, are now rarely encountered in countries where ultrasound scan evaluation is available, either routinely or for investigation of pregnancy associated vaginal bleeding (174). Heavy bleeding, anemia, and lung metastases are, however, still recorded in areas where routine ultrasound remains unavailable. Ultrasound examination correctly identifies approximately 80 percent CHMs and 30 percent of PHMs in the first and early second trimesters, with the remainder sonographically diagnosed as otherwise unremarkable early pregnancy failures. In the latter scenario, the diagnosis of HM is made following routine histologic evaluation of evacuated products of conception. In settings with widely available first trimester ultrasound assessment, HM is evacuated at an average of 8 to 9 weeks of gestation (179).

Following evacuation, approximately 15 percent of patients with CHM and 1 percent with PHM on hCG surveillance programs develop pGTD and thus, require chemotherapy (180). Early identification of patients that require treatment remains currently impossible, hence all patients should undergo hCG surveillance following a diagnosis of HM. Regardless of the cut-offs used in specific programmes, general indications for treatment include plateauing or rising hCG levels, persistently elevated hCG levels, evidence of metastatic disease, heavy vaginal bleeding, and a histologic diagnosis of GTT.

Patients who present with symptomatic pGTD but have not been part of an hCG surveillance program have more severe clinical symptoms/signs, including hemorrhage, anemia and metastatic disease and require more intensive therapy compared to those identified via surveillance programs (181). Some patients with vaginal bleeding and persistent molar tissue in the uterine cavity after initial evacuation undergo further surgical evacuation, although, this approach is normally contraindicated since many such patients still require chemotherapy and the second evacuation is associated with increased risk of uterine perforation (182). Earlier diagnosis and management of HM have not resulted in significant reduction of postmolar pGTD rates (172). Indeed, data from a large series indicate that the risk of pGTD is unrelated to the duration of pregnancy/gestational age at evacuation (183).

Traditional descriptions of the pathologic features of HM are based on examples with well-developed, macroscopically identifiable, villous hydrops since they were detected during the mid-second trimester (figs. 13-4–13-6). In contemporary practice, with almost universal availability of ultrasound examination, the average gestational age at which products of conception undergo histologic evaluation for possible HM is now in the first trimester. The morphologic descriptions below are primarily focused on findings described in early HM from contemporary practice. Currently, in well-developed countries, the characteristic features of CHM are most commonly encountered in the setting of a dichorionic twin pregnancy with a co-existent HM that was managed expectantly.

Despite differences between the groups, both CHMs and PHMs are characterized by two

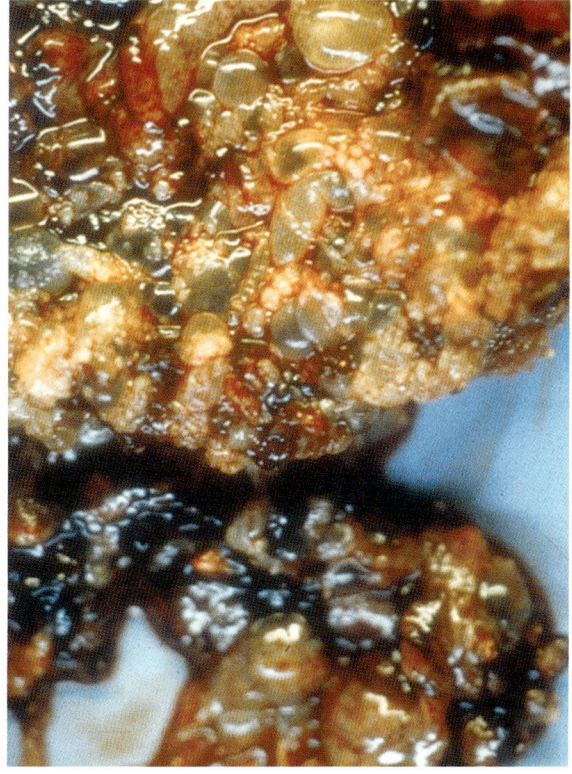

Figure 13-4

MIDGESTATION COMPLETE HYDATIDIFORM MOLE

Numerous chorionic villi display vesicle formation identifiable by the naked eye. Such changes are uncommon if evacuated in the first trimester where the diagnosis is suspected on histologic examination only.

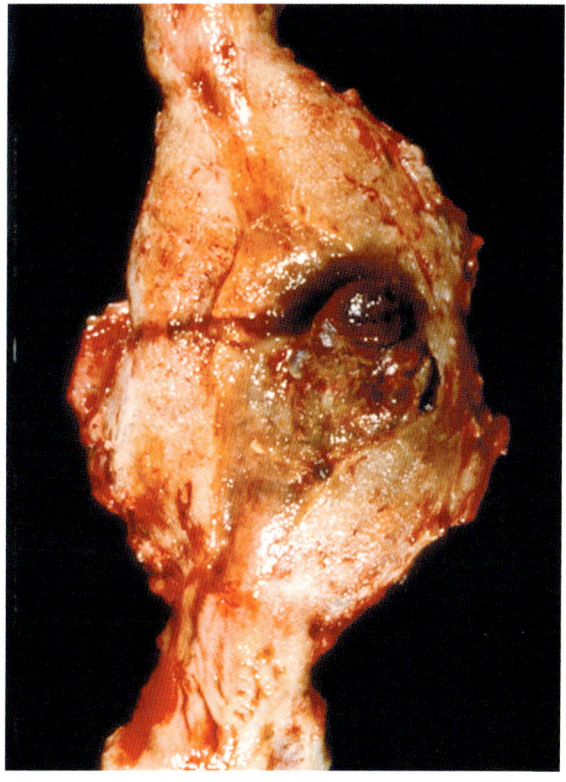

Figure 13-5

COMPLETE HYDATIDIFORM MOLE IN HYSTERECTOMY SPECIMEN

The tissue is bloody but grape-like vesicles are seen.

major pathologic features compared to normal pregnancies: presence of abnormal villous morphology (villous dysmorphism) and abnormal villous trophoblast hyperplasia. The histologic features described below expand these features and illustrate how specific findings allow distinction between them (123,185–187).

The gross (macroscopic) findings are of limited use in assessing early gestational age products of conception for possible HM. In some cases, scattered hydropic vesicles may be identified in CHM, PHM, and even nonmolar hydropic miscarriage, but conversely, many early HMs do not demonstrate macroscopically identifiable hydropic change. In the rare HM presenting in later pregnancy, or HM in association with planned pregnancy continuation such as HM with co-twin, the classic macroscopic "bunch of grapes" appearance may still occur and the amount of tissue procured in HM is often more abundant than that of an uncomplicated miscarriage.

Complete Hydatidiform Mole

Traditionally, histologic examination of CHM demonstrated markedly enlarged and hydropic chorionic villi, many of which were surrounded by an abnormal and excessive circumferential villous trophoblast proliferation. Fluid accumulated and formed "cisterns" in the central portion of the chorionic villi. No fetal blood vessels or nucleated red blood cells were noted. Villous trophoblast showed marked nuclear pleomorphism while extravillous trophoblast often also showed hyperplasia and striking cytologic atypia. This description is characteristic for CHMs evacuated in the mid-late second trimester but CHMs are now evacuated at a much earlier stage (173,175,180) and the most

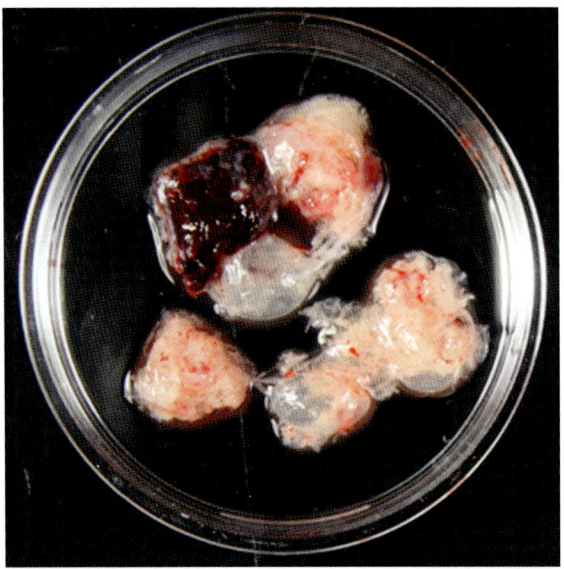 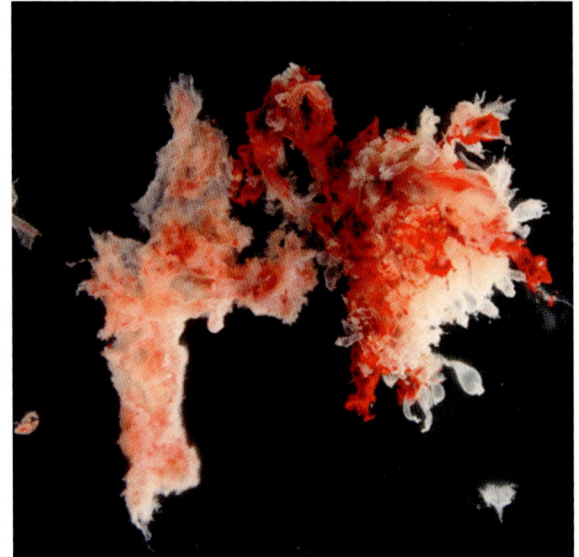

Figure 13-6

PARTIAL HYDATIDIFORM MOLE

Gross examination of evacuated products of conception demonstrate patchy villous hydrops, seen as small to medium-sized transparent "grapes." There is also increased amount of tissue evacuated in contrast to a normal abortion.

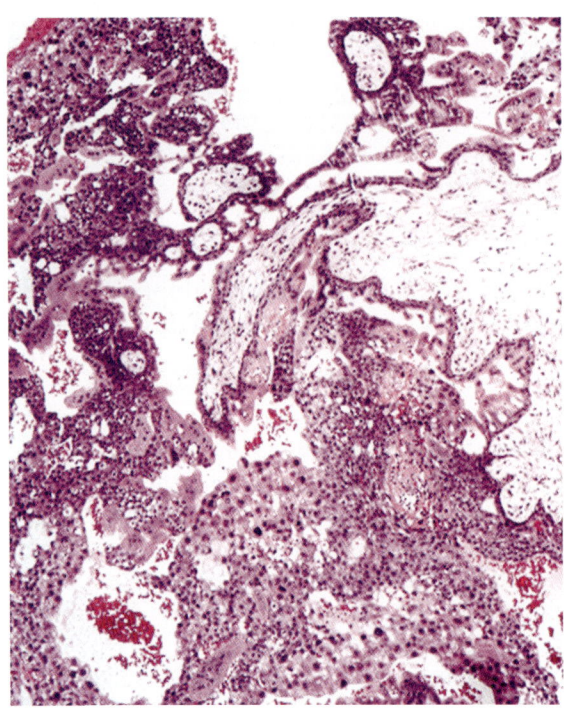

Figure 13-7

COMPLETE HYDATIDIFORM MOLE

The complex outlines of the chorionic villi and the striking biphasic circumferential proliferation of cytotrophoblast and syncytiotrophoblast-like are seen.

useful histopathologic features of earlier CHMs are described below (99,121,188).

Abnormal Circumferential Trophoblast Hyperplasia. Abnormal trophoblast hyperplasia is a constant feature in CHM. It is defined by the presence of more than two layers of trophoblast forming sprouts and more extensive circumferential masses at multiple points around the villous circumference, rather than the normal polar trophoblast columns associated with chorionic villi (figs. 13-7, 13-8). Trophoblast is typically associated with varying degrees of nuclear pleomorphism. No consistent morphologic differences have been reported between XX and XY CHMs. Most CHMs are diploid, but examination of large numbers of cells from CHMs has demonstrated that hyperdiploid and tetraploid fractions are seen in about 40 percent and this finding has been reported with the increased presence of pleomorphic nuclei in molar trophoblast. Biparental CHM have subtle differences from typical androgenetic CHM, with slightly less marked trophoblast hyperplasia and hydrops, but the genetic background is essentially indistinguishable for an individual case on a morphologic basis (189).

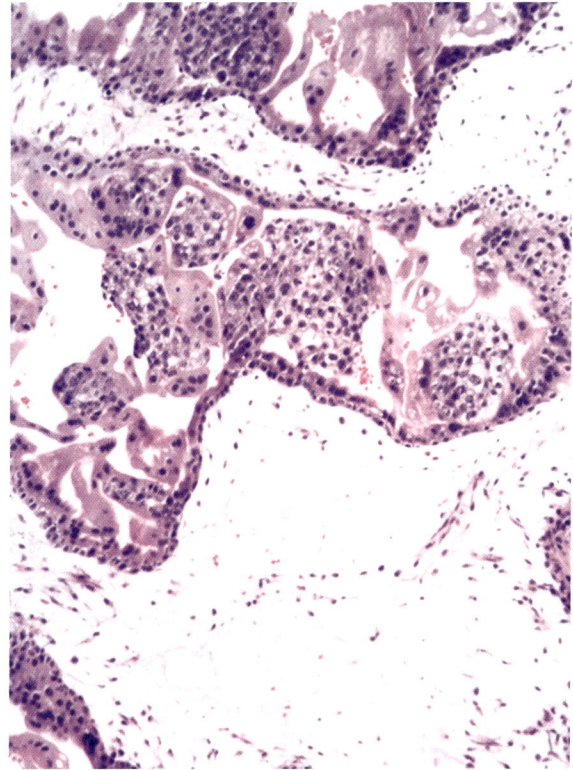

Figure 13-8

COMPLETE HYDATIDIFORM MOLE

Nests of cytotrophoblast-like cells are surrounded by syncytiotrophoblast without striking cytologic atypia. There is a large edematous villus.

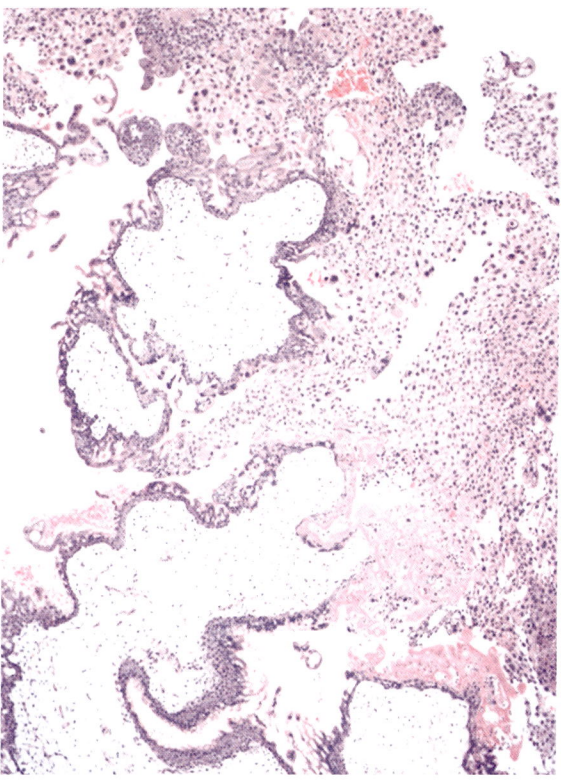

Figure 13-9

EARLY COMPLETE HYDATIDIFORM MOLE

The abnormal villous architecture is associated with prominent trophoblast proliferation.

Although a relationship is suggested between the finding of more abundant and pleomorphic trophoblast and worse prognosis, this finding has not been confirmed (190). This may be explained by the fact that excess trophoblast is only loosely attached to chorionic villi and the amount of trophoblast seen in histologic sections is not representative of the total. In some cases, excess villous trophoblast (fig. 13-9) is easier to detect in earlier gestational age CHMs since fully developed hydrops in well-developed moles may be associated with attenuation of villous trophoblast. This is presumably due to trophoblast detachment, as evidenced by features of third trimester CHM associated with normal co-twin. The extent and distribution of trophoblast hyperplasia is, however, variable among CHMs, especially in early gestation forms, where the stromal and architectural changes may be prominent with only focal abnormal trophoblast hyperplasia (fig. 13-10). In a morphometric study of early CHMs, only 30 percent of chorionic villi demonstrated unequivocal abnormal trophoblast hyperplasia (191).

Abnormal Villous Architecture. In early gestation CHM, low-power architectural features often provide useful diagnostic information. In normal early placentation, secondary chorionic villi form from primary chorionic villi, and are regular in size, with well-organized polar trophoblast proliferation (190,192,193). In contrast, in early CHM, the architecture demonstrates a characteristic "budding" or "branching" phenotype (fig. 13-11). Chorionic villi are also irregular in size and distribution, with abnormal nonpolar trophoblast "circumferential" proliferation (fig. 13-12). This abnormal budding architecture may result in the appearance of oval trophoblastic pseudoinclusions due to the sectioning plane. These are morphologically different than the inclusions associated with PHM (see below) (121).

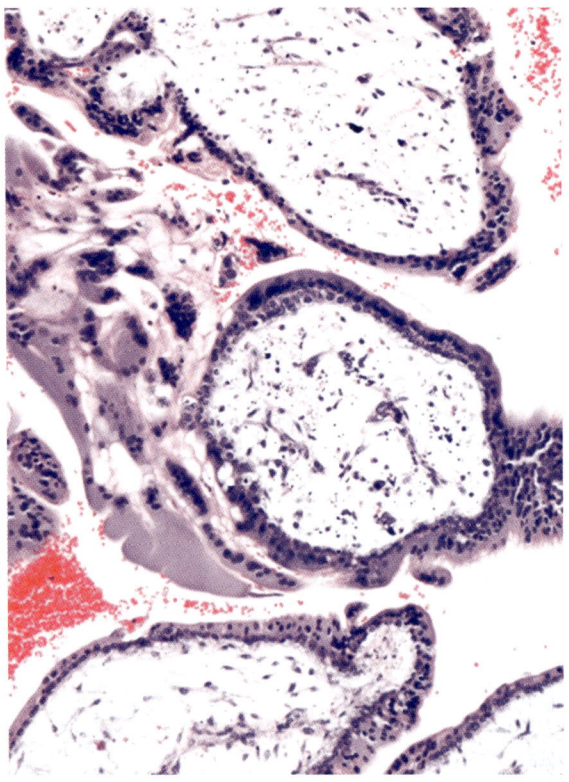

Figure 13-10

EARLY GESTATION COMPLETE HYDATIDIFORM MOLE

There is minimal trophoblast proliferation. Thin and collapsed stromal blood vessels and stromal karyorrhexis are present.

In addition to the budding phenotype, early gestation CHMs often demonstrate basophilic and myxoid villous stroma (fig. 13-11C), with only small amounts of reticulin (194,195). With the development of hydrops, collagen may be seen in the condensed stroma at the periphery of cisterns but fibrosis is not a major feature of the villous stroma in CHM even with prolonged intrauterine retention. In early gestation CHMs, the combination of budding architecture, basophilic stroma, and invaginations of the trophoblast result in a characteristic "lobulated" appearance, which has been suggested as superficially resembling a fibroadenoma (196).

Villous Hydrops. The extensive villous hydrops resulting in the well-described "grape-like" macroscopic appearance of classic CHM is only present from the mid-second trimester. Hydropic change in the late first or early second trimester does occur but is less marked and more focal, while well-formed cistern formation is absent or only focal in early gestations (fig. 13-13). The extent and distribution of hydropic change/cistern formation alone should, therefore, not be used to identify or classify HM at early gestational age, especially since marked hydropic change may also be seen in nonmolar miscarriages.

Villous Vascular and Stromal Changes. In classic descriptions of CHM in the late second trimester, fetal blood vessels were not identified. However, several publications have since described the frequent presence of stromal blood vessels in CHMs evacuated at early gestational ages (190,196). In fact, most CHMs examined before the end of the first trimester contain stromal blood vessels. These vessels are collapsed and empty (figs. 13-10, 13-14), since there is no fetus or fetal circulation, although in a few, even nucleated red blood cells are present (109,197). In such cases, the intravascular contents are karyorrhectic. However, intravascular karyorrhexis is also identified in PHM and nonmolar pregnancies following fetal death, and it should not be confused with stromal karyorrhexis in CHM, which is usually marked and characteristic, although the underlying mechanism remains undetermined.

The finding of villous vessels in CHM may be explained by the fact that normal early villous vascular development occurs independently of fetal development, with subsequent fusion to form the fetoplacental circulation. Therefore, in early CHM, the presence of some stromal blood vessel development is common, with presumed involution with increasing gestational age in the absence of fetal vasculature.

Extensive stromal karyorrhexis (nuclear debris) in otherwise well-preserved (nondegenerated) chorionic villi is present in almost all early gestation CHMs and is one of the most useful diagnostic features. It is more striking beneath the villous surface and it is typically accompanied by myxoid stroma as well scattered primitive stellate cells (fig. 13-10) (122,198,199).

Abnormal Implantation Site. Normal implantation involves the organized and sequential controlled invasion of maternal endomyometrium and vessels by extavillous trophoblast. This process is defective in CHM and the implantation site lacks normal endovascular

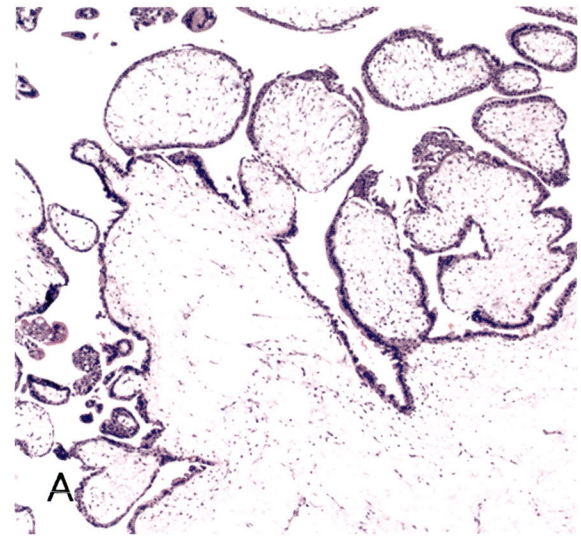
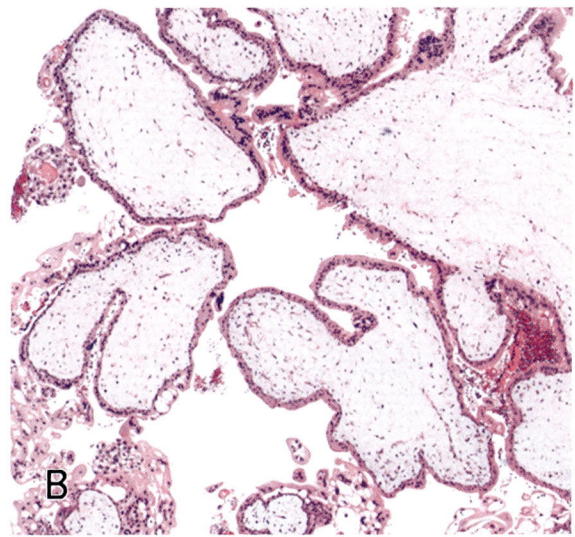
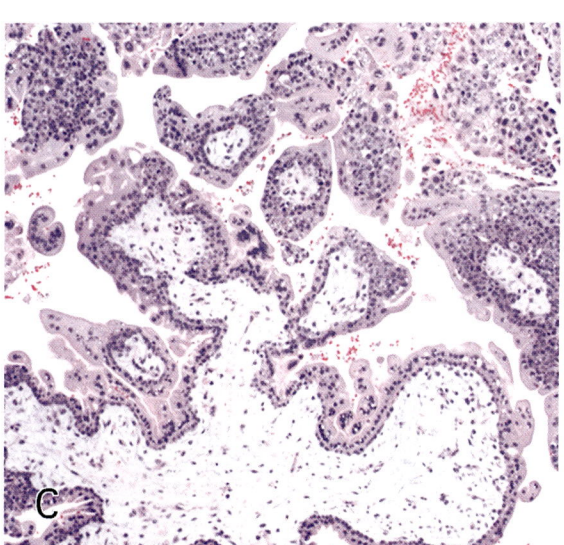

Figure 13-11

EARLY COMPLETE HYDATIDIFORM MOLE

The outer contour of the chorionic villi impart a characteristic low-power appearance "clubbing" (A–C). During the first trimester, many of the villi may not show any abnormal trophoblastic proliferation. The villous stroma is typically myxoid (C).

Figure 13-12

EARLY COMPLETE HYDATIDIFORM MOLE

There is abnormal villous architecture with exuberant abnormal trophoblast proliferation.

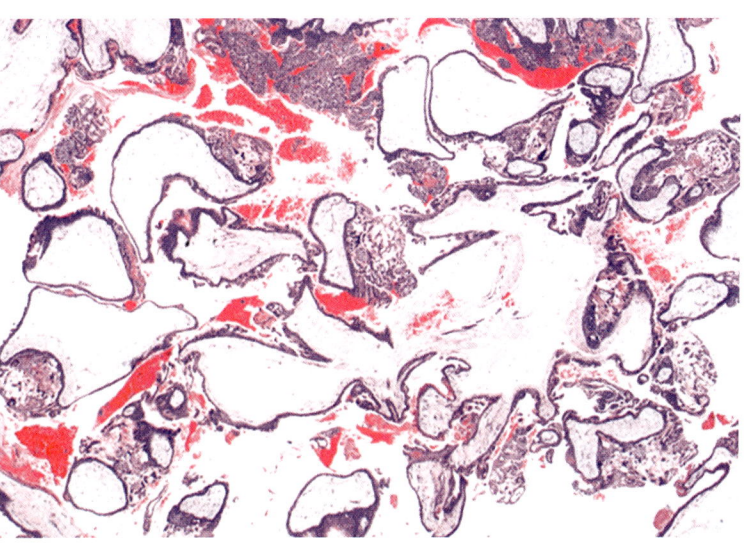

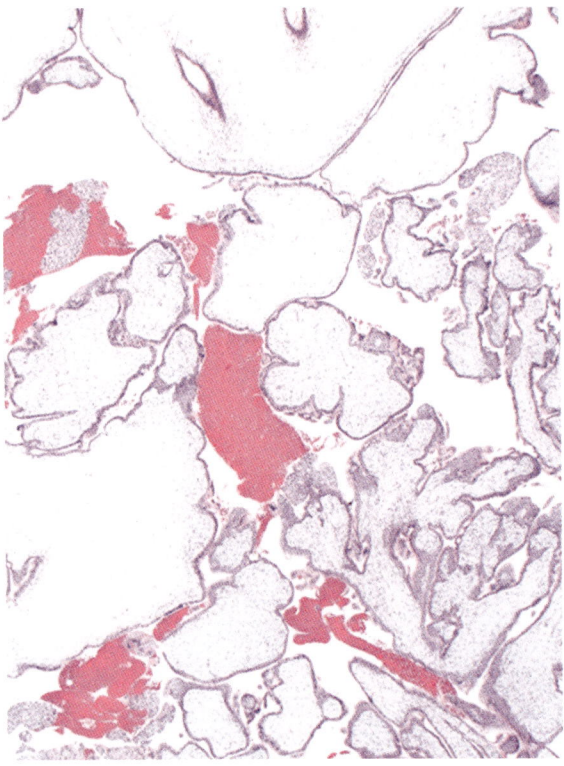

Figure 13-13

EARLY COMPLETE HYDATIDIFORM MOLE

Some chorionic villi are enlarged due to marked edema but are unassociated with any trophoblastic proliferation (top). A large cistern is present.

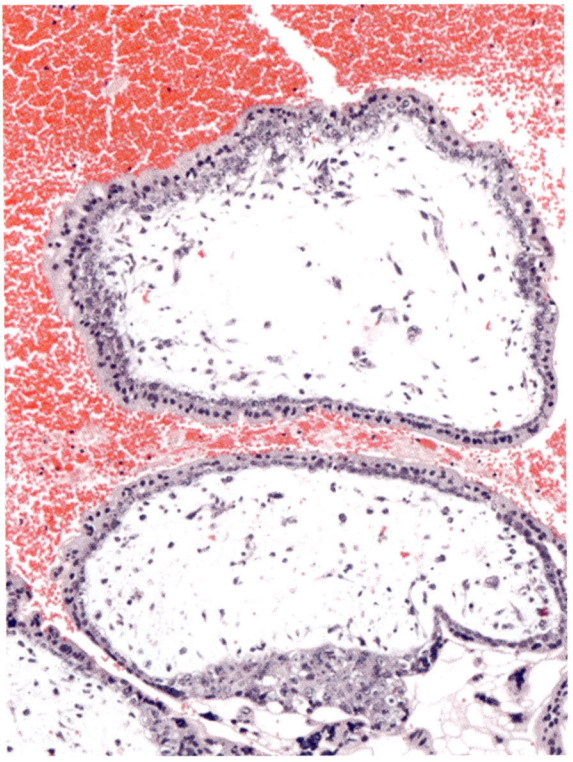

Figure 13-14

EARLY COMPLETE HYDATIDIFORM MOLE

Relatively normal-looking chorionic villi are present in this field. In early gestation in CHM, not every villus exhibits the diagnostic features.

trophoblastic plugging, instead demonstrating florid interstitial infiltration of trophoblast, with or without cytologic atypia (fig. 13-15) (200–202). These features have no clinical or prognostic significance but can provide additional diagnostic clues if presented with limited material and may provide an explanation for the common presentation of vaginal bleeding and early pregnancy failure in CHM.

Embryonic Development. Due to their androgenetic nature and the impact of imprinting on fetal and placental development, most CHMs are not associated with evidence of embryonic development. However, in rare cases of confirmed early singleton CHM, the presence of nucleated fetal red blood cells, fragments of amnion, or other embryonic tissues has been well described (109,197,198). The mechanism for the presence of fetal red cells in molar villi remains unexplained and the possibility that some early embryonic development may occur in CHM cannot be excluded. In usual clinical practice, however, the presence of significant embryonic tissue in CHM is highly unlikely and in the presence of otherwise typical CHM features, should raise the possibility of twin pregnancy or mosaicism.

Ideally, the morphologic diagnosis of CHM should be confirmed by genetic studies for completeness, and certainly may be required for research studies. In clinical practice, however, this is rarely necessary since in most cases the morphologic findings in CHM are distinctive and diagnostic. If required, other additional ancillary studies may confirm the diagnosis, including flow cytometry, immunostaining, and molecular studies.

Partial Hydatidiform Mole

Historical descriptions of PHM included hydropic chorionic villi in triploid conceptions with typically focal changes, often in association with a malformed fetus. Abnormal

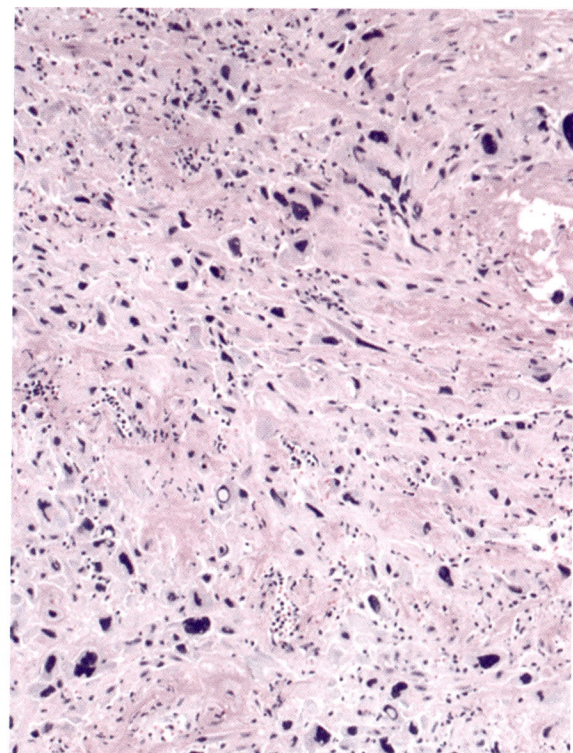

Figure 13-15

ABNORMAL IMPLANTATION SITE IN COMPLETE HYDATIDIFORM MOLE

The implantation-site trophoblast is exuberant and markedly atypical. This finding in isolation is not diagnostic but should suggest CHM.

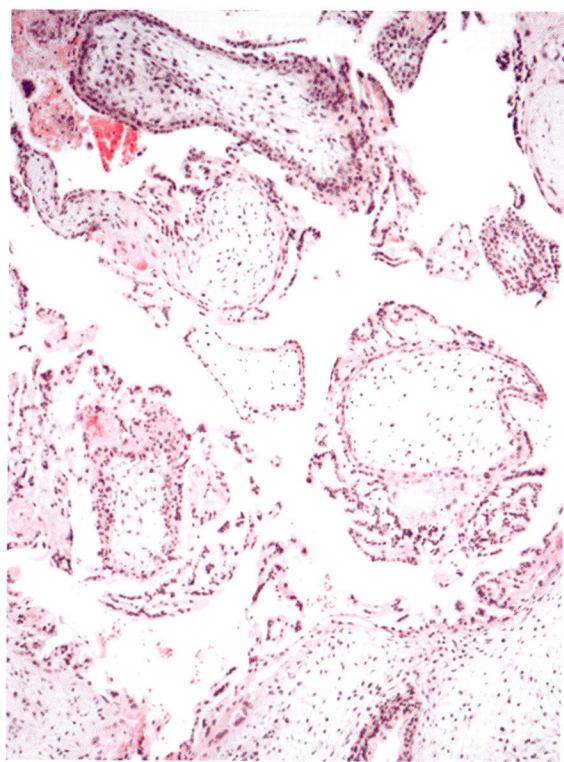

Figure 13-16

PARTIAL HYDATIDIFORM MOLE

Prominent syncytiotrophoblast hyperplasia in a "lacy" configuration and prominent cytoplasmic vacuolization of the cells are seen. There is a morphologically normal villus (center).

and excessive trophoblastic proliferation was reported to be focal, affecting a minority of villi (fig. 13-16) (79,64,81,203–206). Analogous to CHMs, PHMs are also now evacuated at earlier gestational ages, most being unsuspected on sonographic examination and presenting as either vaginal bleeding or early pregnancy failure (173,180).

Dealing with evacuation of HM within the first trimester, diagnostic issues may arise when differentiating PHM from CHM if only historical histologic criteria are applied and features of early CHM are not taken into consideration. For example, the diagnosis of PHM based only on the presence of stromal blood vessels, fetal nucleated red blood cells, or focal hydrops may be incorrect (see above) as these features may also be seen in early CHM. Similarly, a diagnosis of PHM based on the presence of fetal tissues such amnion may be incorrect, since CHM may occur as part of a twin pregnancy or with mosaicism. Nevertheless, several histologic features allow reliable distinction between CHM and PHM even at early gestational age, especially when ancillary techniques such as immunohistochemistry or molecular studies are used. The distinction is important as the risk of development of pGTD in PHM, although greater than the background risk in the general population, is much lower than that observed in CHM. Chemotherapy is required following 1 in 100 to 200 PHMs (60), and rarely, PHM precedes the development of choriocarcinoma (34,181,207–209).

In daily clinical practice, the much more frequent and difficult scenario is the morphologic distinction between PHM and nonmolar miscarriage specimens, especially when the latter are associated with other nonandrogenic chromosomal abnormalities and sampling is limited. Nonmolar miscarriages with morphologic features similar to

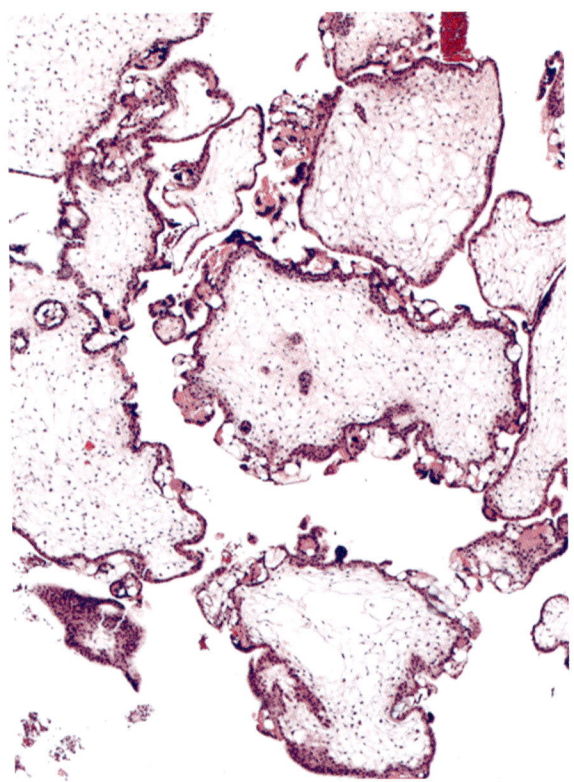

Figure 13-17

PARTIAL HYDATIDIFORM MOLE

Villous dysmorphism with irregular outlines, trophoblastic pseudoinclusions including intravillous trophoblast (single cells or groups of cells), and focal abnormal trophoblast hyperplasia are characteristic.

PHM include trisomies, monosomies, chromosomal translocations, and maternally derived triploid pregnancies (210–215). They represented approximately 10 to 20 percent of gestations initially suspected to be PHMs at one regional center in the United Kingdom and in contrast to PHM do not have increased risk of pGTD (155).

The main morphologic features useful in the diagnosis of PHMs at earlier gestation ages are described below (83,121,127,185,187,216):

Abnormal Trophoblast Hyperplasia. Abnormal trophoblast hyperplasia is required for the morphologic diagnosis of PHM in the absence of genetic confirmation, but the trophoblast excess is often focal in early PHM, much less marked than in CHM, and may not be identified if only limited material is available. There may be obvious circumferential trophoblast hyperplasia affecting a variable proportion of chorionic villi, both hydropic and nonhydropic. In one study, the number of chorionic villi with abnormal trophoblast hyperplasia was over 10 percent (190). Since the extent of villous trophoblast hyperplasia is generally less in PHM than CHM, extravillous trophoblast fragments are also less commonly seen.

The villous trophoblast proliferation in PHM is limited to the syncytiotrophoblast, which often demonstrates a "lacy" and "vacuolated" appearance, with only a mild degree of nuclear pleomorphism (fig. 13-16). The amount of abnormal trophoblast and its proliferative activity are significantly less than those seen in CHM (190).

Villous Architecture. Dysmorphic chorionic villi with abnormal architecture are a characteristic feature of PHM. These villi have been described as "scalloped" in appearance compared to the normal round chorionic villi in cross section (figs. 13-17–13-19). This irregular architecture results in invaginations of villous syncytiotrophoblast, which on histologic sections are evident as irregular pseudoinclusions (fig. 13-17). Unlike the abnormal budding architecture of early CHM, PHM villi appear more angulated. Irregular villous outlines and pseudoinclusions may also be present in nonmolar miscarriages, especially when chromosomally abnormal, as seen with trisomies or monosomy X, and should not be used a sole diagnostic criterium for PHM. Additional features of abnormal excess trophoblast are required for a definitive diagnosis of PHM (83,121,185).

Villous Hydrops. Hydrops and cistern formation characteristically involve only some of the chorionic villi in PHM (fig. 13-18), and focal hydrops may also be seen in early CHMs. Cistern formation is often minimal in first trimester PHM, therefore, this feature in isolation is a poor morphologic marker of PHM. In contrast to CHM, PHM often demonstrates extensive stromal fibrosis of chorionic villi rather than marked hydrops (fig. 13-20), possibly related to early fetal demise.

A well-recognized diagnostic pitfall is the erroneous interpretation of folded fragments of gestational sac in nonmolar specimens as representing an enlarged chorionic villous with cistern formation. In this scenario, the finding of more collagen within the "hydropic villous" than in the surrounding chorionic villi should

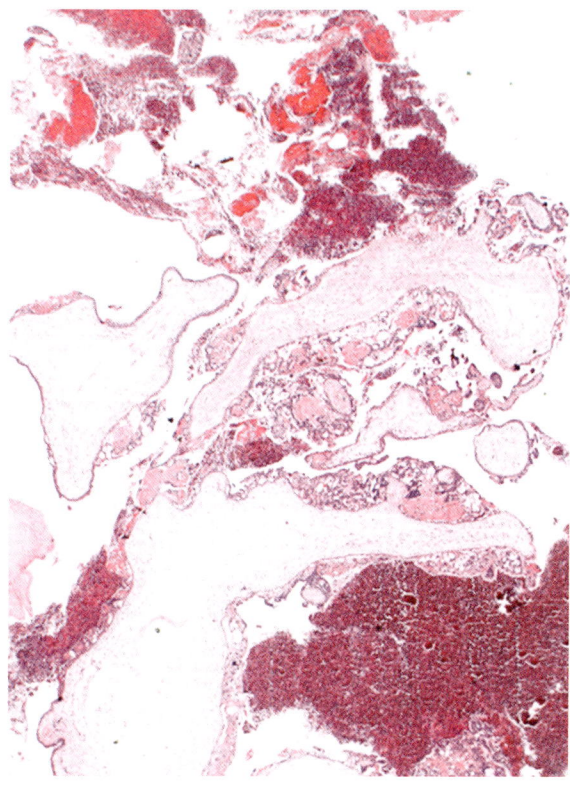

Figure 13-18

PARTIAL HYDATIDIFORM MOLE

There are large, abnormally shaped chorionic villi; marked edema; and focal cistern formation. The proliferation of syncytiotrophoblast-like cells is only focal.

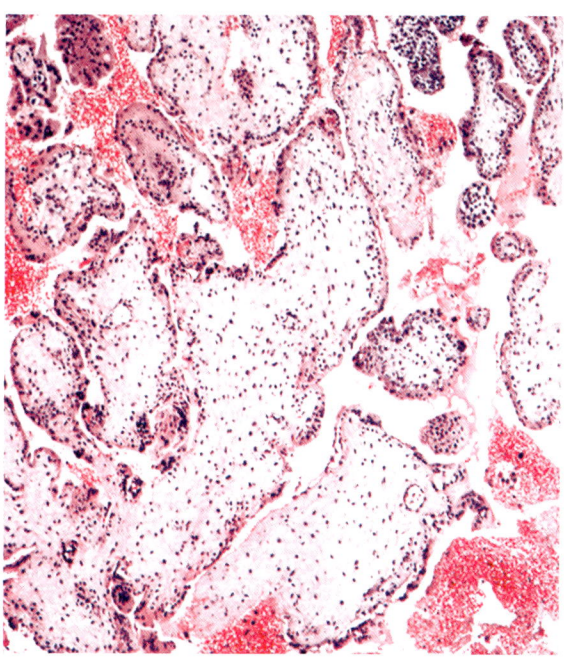

Figure 13-19

GENETICALLY CONFIRMED PARTIAL HYDATIDIFORM MOLE WITH FOCAL ABNORMAL TROPHOBLAST HYPERPLASIA

There are two types of chorionic villi: normal and abnormal; the latter show scalloped outlines.

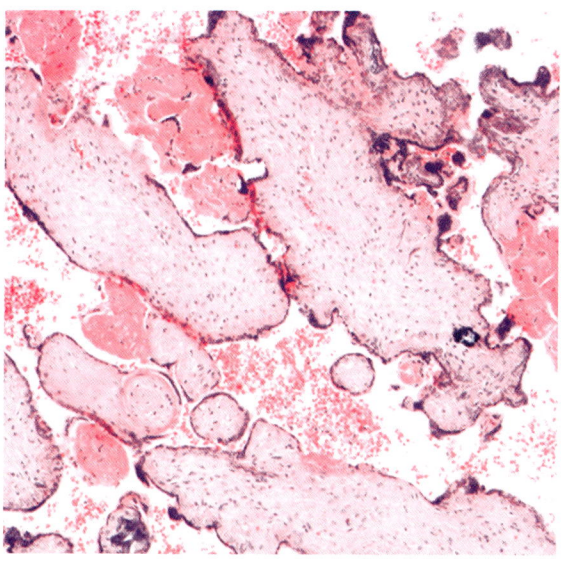

Figure 13-20

PARTIAL HYDATIDIFORM MOLE

There is villous dysmorphism and striking stromal sclerosis but no diagnostically abnormal trophoblast hyperplasia. In such cases, definitive diagnosis may require molecular testing.

suggest the diagnosis of gestational sac, and this possibility should always be considered when apparent huge cisterns are rare and surrounded by smaller, nonmolar chorionic villi.

Distinguishing hydropic nonmolar products of conception from PHM is straightforward in most instances since nonmolar gestations generally demonstrate uniform hydropic villous change, with round villous outlines on cross section, with few or absent trophoblastic inclusions and lack of stromal cellularity (fig. 13-21). Despite awareness of the described features, however, this distinction may be difficult or impossible in some cases, especially with limited sampling, and ancillary molecular testing may be required for definitive diagnosis.

Villous Vascular and Stromal Changes. The stromal components of early PHM differ from those of early CHM. Specifically, villous stromal blood vessels, usually containing nucleated fetal

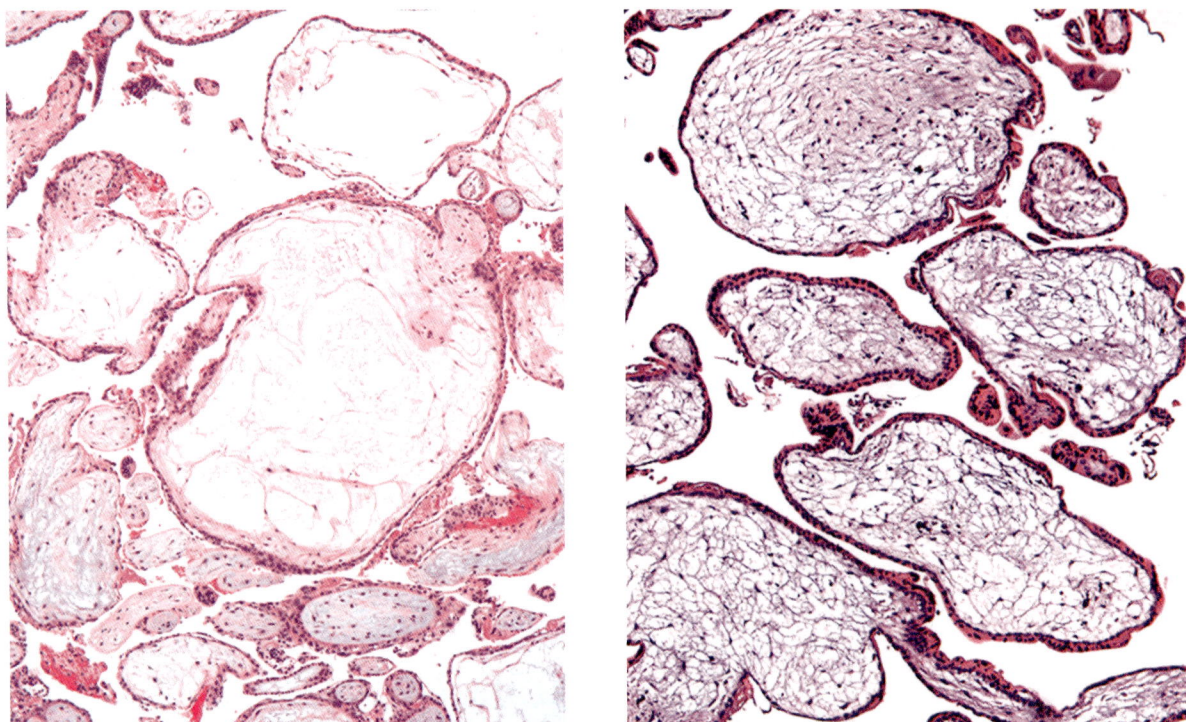

Figure 13-21

HYDROPIC NONMOLAR MISCARRIAGE

There is marked but variable villous hydrops (left). Many of the villi have a round configuration with paucicellular stroma, but more importantly, lack villous hyperplasia. In some chorionic villi (right), the stroma may be myxoid causing concern for an early complete hydatidiform mole. However, there is no "clubbing" or abnormal villous hyperplasia.

red blood cells, are common and well-formed, with patent vessels compared to the collapsed, empty vessels of early CHM. If evacuated in the later second trimester, the apparent villous vascularity decreases, likely as a consequence of fetal demise, absent fetal circulation, and secondary changes.

Pseudoangiomatoid vascular change, defined as abnormal, dilated and irregular vessels throughout the villous stroma, is a rare but striking and characteristic feature present in 10 to 15 percent of PHMs (fig. 13-22) (218,219). In contrast to CHM, stromal karyorrhexis is rare and the nuclear debris present within stromal vascular walls and lumens should not be confused with true stromal karyorrhexis, since it represents secondary changes due to fetal demise.

The villous stroma of PHM often contains abundant collagen, which increases with gestational age, and apparent stromal fibrosis may be a prominent feature of retained PHM. If evacuated at earlier gestational age, a network of reticulin fibers may be present. Additionally, stromal condensation may be seen surrounding cisterns within hydropic villi.

Embryonic Development. Evidence of an embryo or fetus is common in PHM, but the fetus is almost always malformed and often dies during early pregnancy, hence, the absence of fetal tissue in histologic material is of no diagnostic value. Definite fetal tissue has been identified in around 20 percent of histologic sections of PHM, with fetal nucleated red blood cells and fetal membranes present in 50 and 40 percent of cases, respectively (108,176). Although the presence of fetal tissues coexisting with molar villi is supportive of PHM, CHM as part of a twin pregnancy or mosaic is a diagnostic possibility and the final diagnosis should be based on villous features and ancillary tests, rather than presence or absence of fetal tissue.

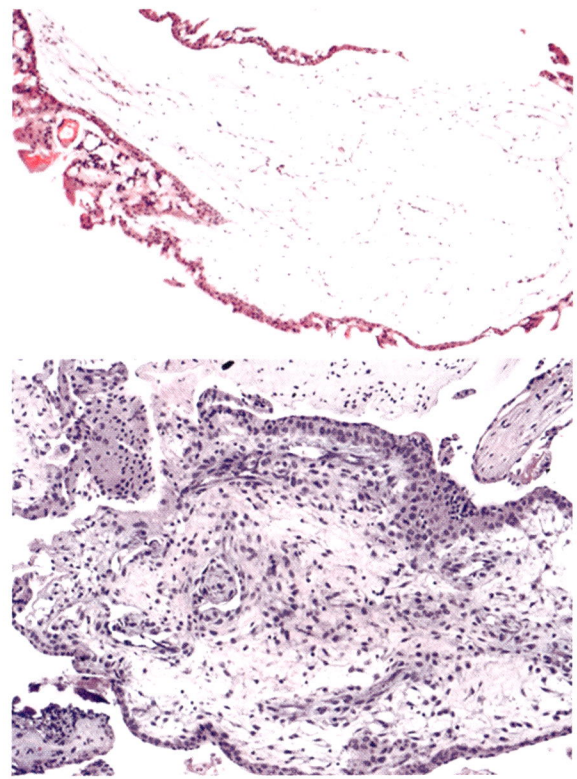

Figure 13-22

PARTIAL HYDATIDIFORM MOLE

Pseudoangiomatoid stromal vascular change is not common but may be striking.

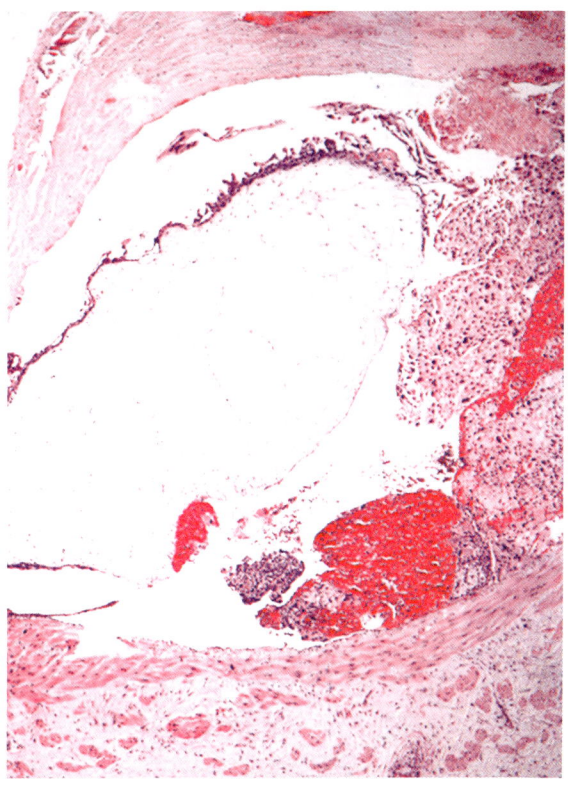

Figure 13-23

INVASIVE COMPLETE HYDATIDIFORM MOLE

An enlarged chorionic villus associated with prominent trophoblastic proliferation is noted within a vascular space in the myometrium.

Invasive Hydatidiform Mole

Invasive mole does not represent a specific disease entity but rather the presentation of a HM with histologic evidence of myometrial invasion (220). Although most HMs are confined to the uterine cavity with superficial "implantation," some degree of myometrial invasion by molar villi does occur and may result in complications such as uterine perforation or extension to adjacent organs. The frequency of myometrial invasion remains unknown since, in most instances, evacuation (rather than hysterectomy) is the standard diagnostic procedure followed by hCG surveillance, therefore, myometrial invasion cannot be assessed. Vascular invasion by chorionic villi is also described (fig. 13-23).

It has been suggested that invasive moles represent approximately 5 percent of CHMs, but due to the issues noted above, in addition to selection bias of published cases, its true frequency remains unknown (143). Based on clinical presentation, it is clear that invasive mole represents a rare complication of molar pregnancy, since most of the latter are confined to the uterine cavity and resolve spontaneously.

The histologic appearance of an invasive mole is identical to that of CHM or PHM, but with chorionic villi found deeply in, or beyond, the myometrial wall. The diagnosis of HM type is based on the type of excessive trophoblastic proliferation and villous dysmorphism, but hydropic change may be limited in the deeply invasive chorionic villi.

Although no standard nomenclature exits, the terminology used for invasive HM is generally analogous to that for abnormally invasive placenta according to the depth of myometrial invasion, namely accreta, increta, and percreta for superficial, deep, and transmural invasion, respectively. As hysterectomy

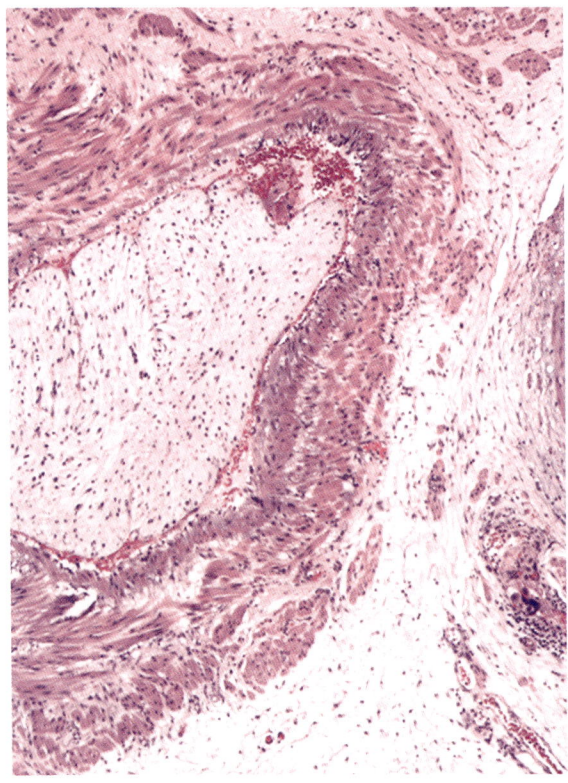

Figure 13-24

METASTATIC COMPLETE HYDATIDIFORM MOLE

Metastatic villi may not be associated with marked trophoblastic proliferation.

is rarely required with current management of HM, only unsuspected pregnancies presenting as an acute abdomen due to uterine perforation show hemorrhage and molar chorionic villi implanted in a pelvic organ (220–222). Most invasive HMs confirmed in hysterectomy specimens correspond to CHM, but rare confirmed invasive triploid PHMs requiring hysterectomy as well as PHM with deeply implanted myometrial villi in curettage specimens have been reported (223).

Metastatic Molar Disease

HM, especially CHM, may spread locally to involve cervix, vagina, and vulva, but with current chemotherapeutic regimens this finding does not necessarily confer a worse prognosis. Early series suggested that up to 10 percent of patients presenting clinically with a CHM had radiologically detected pulmonary lesions, interpreted as metastases (fig. 13-24).

In contemporary practice, with much earlier gestational age at diagnosis and evacuation, and commencement of chemotherapy based on abnormal serum hCG levels, clinically detectable metastatic disease is rare. The finding of metastases long after evacuation of a CHM may indicate pGTD or choriocarcinoma (224).

Ectopic Hydatidiform Mole

As seen in nonmolar ectopic pregnancies, HM, although rare, also occurs at ectopic sites, with the fallopian tube being the most common location. Tubal ectopic HMs are frequently overdiagnosed, since nonmolar ectopic pregnancies often show hydropic villous change, extensive extravillous trophoblast proliferation associated with early trophoblast shell, and an apparently "invasive" implantation site in the absence of decidua. Data from regional specialized centers suggest that fewer than 10 percent of cases initially diagnosed as tubal HM are confirmed as molar following review (225,226). Persistent pGTD and choriocarcinoma have been reported following tubal HM (227,228).

Twin Pregnancy with Hydatidiform Mole

HM may be part of a dizygotic, dichorionic twin pregnancy consisting of an HM and nonmolar co-twin. The coexistence of molar and nonmolar pregnancy affects 1 in 200 pregnancies with histologically confirmed CHM (229). The combination of a PHM and normal gestation appears to be much rarer, probably since the distinction of nonmolar villi from PHM alone may be difficult, particularly in early miscarriages. The coexistence of a CHM and a normal gestation may cause diagnostic confusion with PHM, both on antenatal ultrasonographic examination and histologic evaluation of the products of conception, unless the diagnostic criteria described above are recognized (fig. 13-25).

Placentas or products of conception from pregnancies affected by CHM with a coexisting normal co-twin exhibit geographically distinct areas with histologically normal chorionic villi and other chorionic villi with typical diagnostic features of CHM. Histologically confirmed CHM and co-twin pregnancies were initially thought to be associated with poor outcome (230). Recent data based on complete ascertainment of unselected cases have demonstrated that the risk of pGTD is similar to that following a singleton CHM, and is not significantly different for patients managed by early elective termination of pregnancy versus those that continue pregnancy. With continuation of pregnancy, however, several complications may develop including fetal loss before 24 weeks' gestation in approximately 50 percent, late intrauterine death in about 25 percent, and early preterm delivery in 40 percent. Other complications of pregnancy continuation include vaginal bleeding/antepartum hemorrhage and severe pre-eclampsia (229).

Immunohistochemical Findings

Histologic diagnosis of CHM and PHM, even at early gestational age, is primarily dependent on the recognition of the distinctive morphologic features. Special stains highlight certain histologic features, as for example, trichrome stain for collagen, but overall, these do not provide useful additional diagnostic information. A wide range of potential immunohistochemical markers have been reported but, with one major exception, these markers generally have minimal diagnostic value in HM (in contrast to numerous markers used in the diagnosis of GTTs). Markers of cell proliferation, such as PCNA and Ki-67, have been studied and reported to be of little practical use in the distinction between hydropic abortus, CHM, and PHM. A review of the literature compiling findings from 88 studies reported that there is an association between p53, EGFR, HER2, c-erbB-2, and telomerase, and increased risk of progression to pGTD (231). However, methodologic issues complicating interpretation, including small datasets and uncertainty of classification of HM, were also noted, thus, the clinical significance of the reported results was uncertain. A subsequent prospective blind study based on assessment of these immunohistochemical markers (along with other quantitative morphologic features) reported no significant association with outcome, defined as development of pGTD (190). There are, therefore, currently no histopathologic or immunohistochemical features to reliably predict biologic behavior and requirement for chemotherapy (190,232).

$P57^{KIP2}$ is the exception to the general lack of diagnostic utility of immunomarkers in this setting. Since molar pregnancies represent

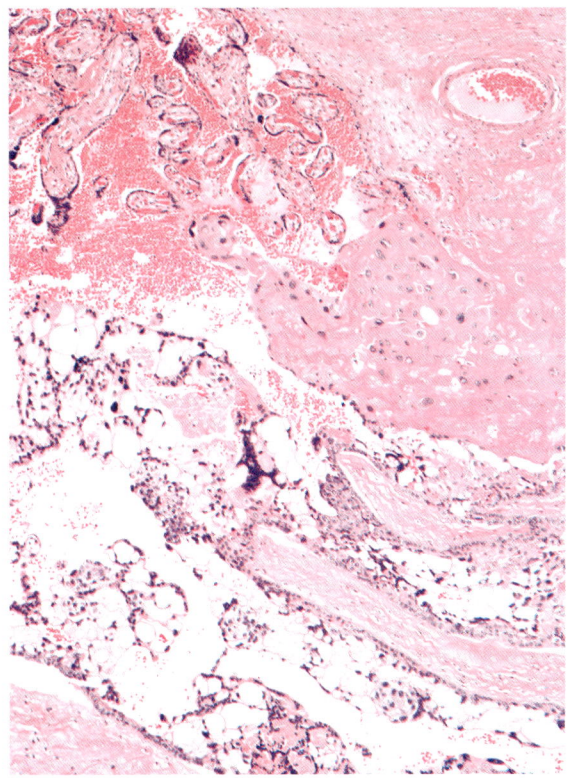

Figure 13-25

TWIN GESTATION WITH A COMPLETE HYDATIDIFORM MOLE

Normal-appearing villi (top left) are juxtaposed to enlarged and abnormal chorionic villi of the complete mole (bottom). This biphasic appearance should not be confused with a partial hydatidiform mole.

abnormalities in imprinting, with relative or absolute overexpression of paternally derived genes, it is logical that abnormal expression of imprinted gene products is diagnostically useful. Although the distinction between CHM and PHM is usually possible based on morphologic features, in some cases, especially very early gestations or when only limited material is available, this may be difficult. $P57^{KIP2}$ is a cell cycle inhibitor that is strongly paternally imprinted, therefore expressed predominantly from the maternal allele. Nuclear $p57^{KIP2}$ expression is normally detected in cytotrophoblast and villous mesenchymal cells in all pregnancies that have the maternal allele, including PHM and nonmolar miscarriages, whereas expression is absent in CHM since it lacks maternal alleles (fig. 13-26, left). $P57^{KIP2}$ immunostaining confirms

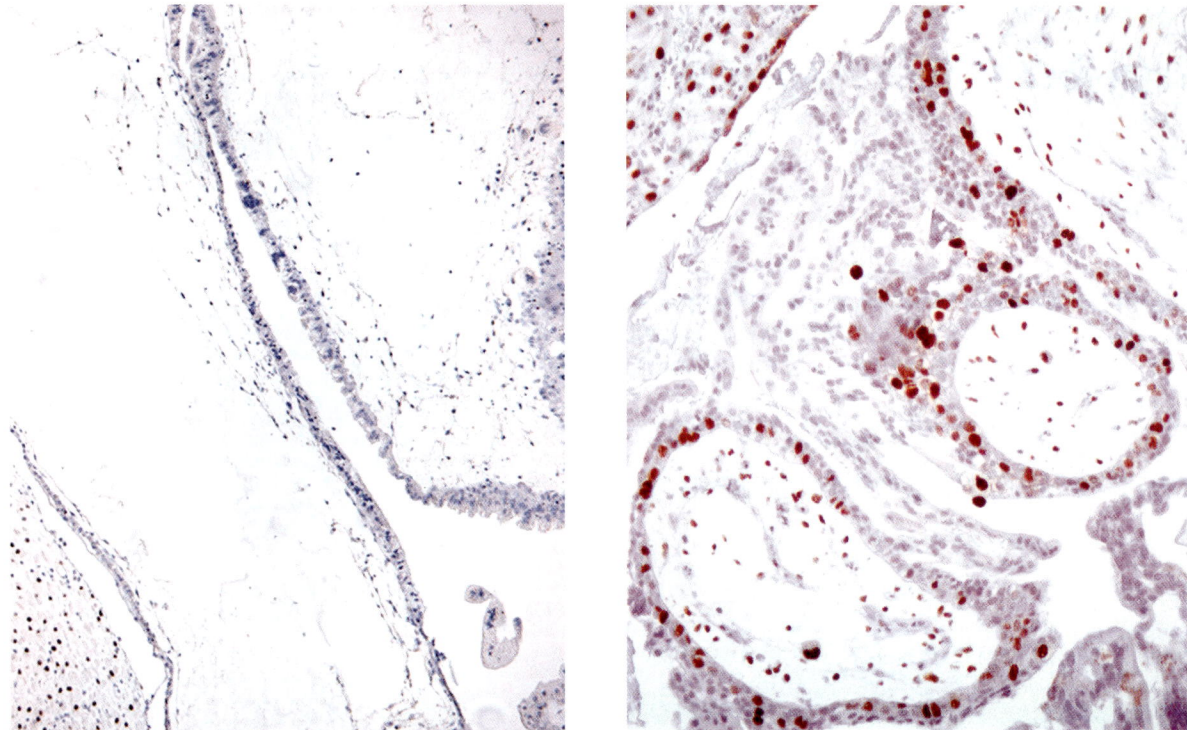

Figure 13-26

COMPLETE HYDATIDIFORM MOLE

P57 is absent in cytotrophoblast and villous mesenchyme (in contrast to partial hydatidiform mole) (left). A rare exception occurs when there is preservation of maternal chromosome 11. In such instances p57 expression is noted even in CHM (right).

a CHM but cannot separate PHM from a nonmolar miscarriage (233,234). Even in CHM with absent chorionic villi, p57^{KIP2} expression is seen in extravillous trophoblast for reasons that remain unclear in conjunction with normal maternal tissue, providing a useful internal positive control (101). Thus, for diagnostic purposes, only villous expression should be assessed for p57 expression.

In the setting of mosaic CHM, p57^{KIP2} stains unaffected chorionic villi but not the affected molar villi. In biparental CHM, although a maternal genome is present, due to imprinting defects, the maternal genes are not expressed and hence p57^{KIP2} expression is lost as it occurs in typical androgenetic CHM (188). Although useful in establishing a diagnosis of CHM, p57^{KIP2} expression cannot determine the origin of the GTT, since variable expression is seen in different tumors regardless of their origin (CHM or nonmolar conceptions) (99).

With the combination of molecular genetic testing and p57^{KIP2} immunostaining, cases of androgenetic/biparental mosaicism have been increasingly described, including those affecting villous stroma or trophoblast populations (234). Atypical p57^{KIP2} staining may occur (less than 1 percent), including p57^{KIP2} positivity in CHM with retained maternal chromosome 11 (fig. 13-26, right) and p57-negative PHM or nonmolar miscarriages with loss of maternal chromosome 11. The findings indicate that p57 expression strongly relates to genotype but in unusual or apparently discordant cases, molecular studies are also required for correct interpretation (fig. 13-27) (123,185,235).

Differential Diagnosis

Pleomorphic Trophoblast in the Absence of Chorionic Villi. Pleomorphic trophoblast, either villous, extravillous, or within the implantation site, is a common feature of CHM and lacks prognostic significance (190). It has been suggested that extensive trophoblast pleomorphism might represent coexistence of CHM and

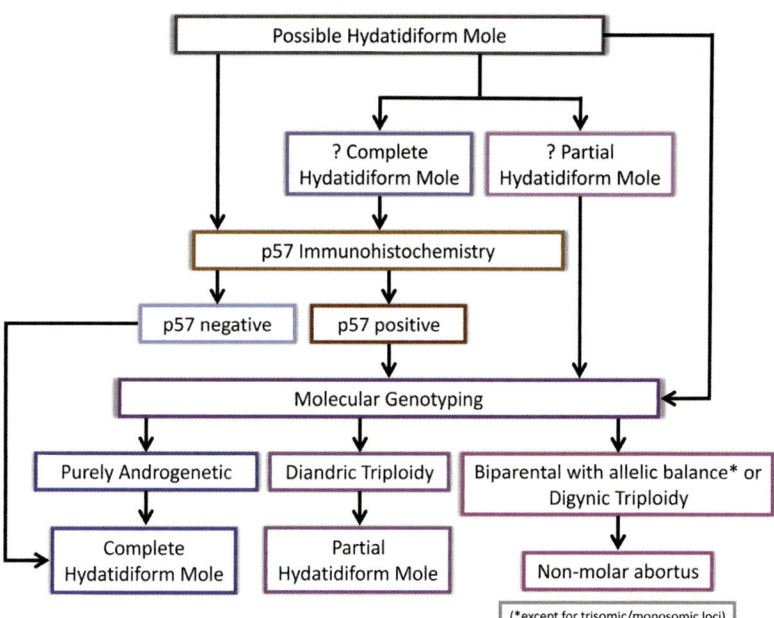

Figure 13-27

ALGORITHMIC APPROACH TO DIAGNOSIS OF HYDATIDIFORM MOLES

Per one approach, potentially molar specimens are universally subjected to immunohistochemical analysis of p57 expression, with triage to genotyping based on this result. The p57 negative cases are diagnosed as complete hydatidiform mole, and p57 positive cases are genotyped to distinguish partial hydatidiform moles from nonmolar specimens. In another approach, potentially molar specimens are universally subjected to genotyping. In yet another approach, some triage to p57 immunohistochemistry versus genotyping is performed based on morphologic assessment as favoring complete hydatidiform mole versus partial hydatidiform mole, respectively. (Fig. 13 from Ronnett BM. Hydatidiform moles: ancillary techniques to refine diagnosis. Arch Pathol Lab Med 2018;142:1500.)

choriocarcinoma (237). However, until further data are available, the consensus is that choriocarcinoma should not be diagnosed regardless of the degree of trophoblast pleomorphism in a background of a CHM with chorionic villi. Accordingly, CHM with choriocarcinoma is not included as a category in the most recent World Health Organization (WHO) classification (1).

The most problematic scenario is the finding of blood clot and fragments of pleomorphic trophoblast without associated chorionic villi, or other specific features, in a curettage specimen. In such cases, it is most likely that such trophoblast derives from a CHM or, sometimes, trophoblast shell from an early gestation, although definitive exclusion of choriocarcinoma on such limited material is not possible. Such specimens should be reported as "atypical trophoblast" after complete assessment of material, with further clinical and biochemical surveillance being indicated. For practical purposes, in early pregnancy specimens, the presence of chorionic villi in curettings excludes the diagnosis of choriocarcinoma (fig. 13-28). The diagnosis of choriocarcinoma should be reserved for cases in which there is a proliferation of biphasic, highly atypical trophoblast in the absence of chorionic villi, in conjunction with other abnormal clinical (invasion, mass lesion, metastases) and biochemical (highly elevated serum hCG levels) features.

The only exception to this approach is the finding of choriocarcinoma in a third trimester nonmolar placenta (intraplacental choriocarcinoma). In this scenario, the gross appearance is usually nonspecific, but may overlap with that of a placental thrombus. Choriocarcinoma, however, is commonly central, an unusual location for thrombi, which are typically peripheral within the placenta. On microscopic examination, there are normally developed third trimester chorionic villi juxtaposed to an area with clusters of abnormal chorionic villi surrounded by a proliferation of biphasic atypical trophoblasts associated with fibrin deposition.

Mosaic CHM. Rarely, the placental tissue, both sonographically and histologically, demonstrates an admixture of normal and molar chorionic villi, representing genetically a mosaic CHM. These cases have been detected since the introduction of genetic testing, and represent around 2 percent of CHMs. They are associated with abnormal molar villi which are scattered throughout the placental parenchyma (in contrast to the geographic distribution of chorionic villi in a CHM within co-twin) (238). The affected chorionic villi have the typical morphology of CHM, but they are admixed with a larger population of normal, nonmolar chorionic villi. Such gestations have been described in the second and third trimesters,

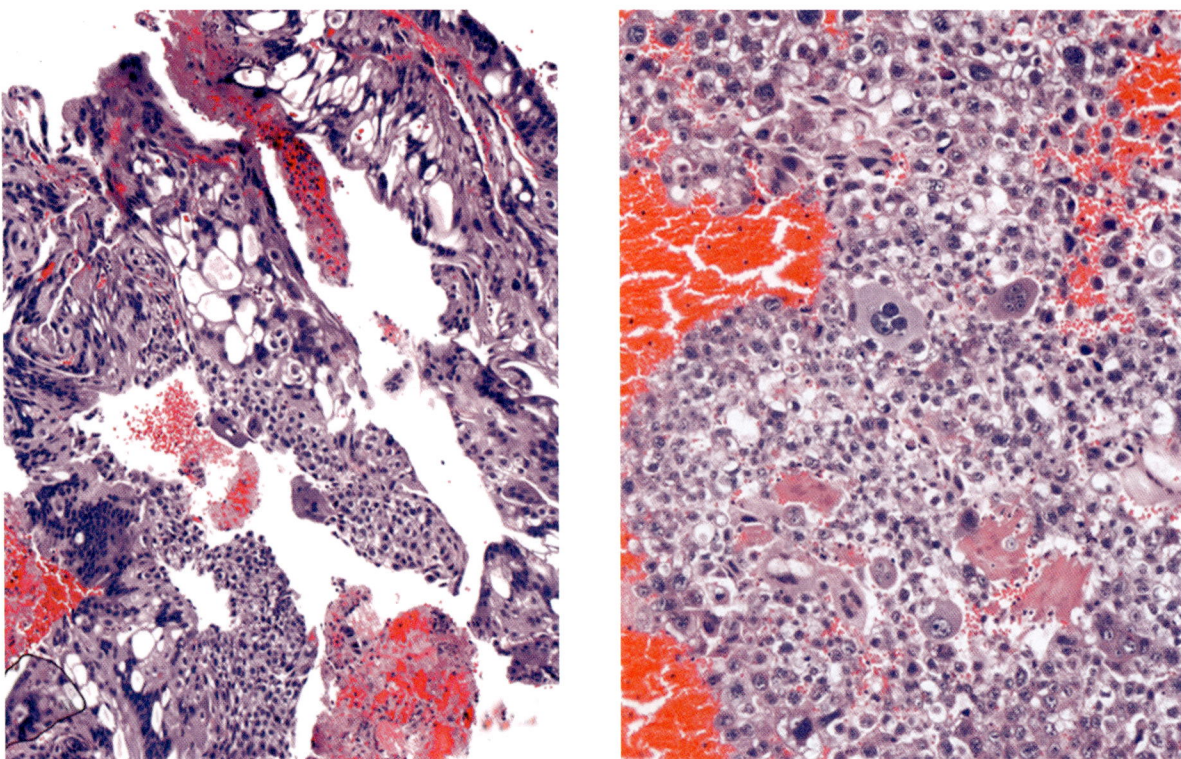

Figure 13-28

EARLY COMPLETE HYDATIDIFORM MOLE WITH PLEOMORPHIC TROPHOBLAST

Although highly atypical and exuberant, a diagnosis of choriocarcinoma should not be rendered in this setting. Atypical trophoblast with no chorionic villi in curettage specimen should suggest further levels and inclusion of all material in order to disclose normal (very early gestation) or abnormal (molar) chorionic villi.

with abnormal sonographic features, usually in association with a structurally normal fetus (92,120). This may be impossible to distinguish from a twin pregnancy with CHM in curettage specimens, especially if material is limited. In such instances, ancillary tests are useful to highlight the distribution of affected villi and to genetically confirm the diagnosis.

Placental Mesenchymal Dysplasia. Diffuse but scattered "molar" change in the placenta detected sonographically in the mid and late trimesters in association with an anatomically normal fetus has been described in association with the condition of *placental mesenchymal dysplasia* (PMD) which does not fall within the family of GTD, but rather represents an associated mosaic disorder of imprinting. In contrast to HMs, which are characterized by overexpression of paternal genes in both villous stroma and trophoblast, PMD is associated with normal biparental trophoblast but with overexpression of paternal genes within the stromal component (93–95,239). As an imprinting disorder, it may also be associated with underlying conditions such as Beckwith-Wiedemann syndrome (238).

Characteristically, there is no trophoblast hyperplasia but rather marked hydrops of stem chorionic villi, with associated normal-appearing terminal villi (fig. 13-29A). Although these features are easily identified in full-term placentas, they may not be detected in a curettage specimen where the overall architecture of the chorionic villi is more difficult to visualize and diagnostic features of early PMD are not described. Chorionic vascular anomalies and angiomatoid villous stromal changes may also be present (239,240). It is important to distinguish PMD from mosaic CHM and PHM, since PMD does not appear to be associated with the increased risk of pGTD and hence maternal hCG

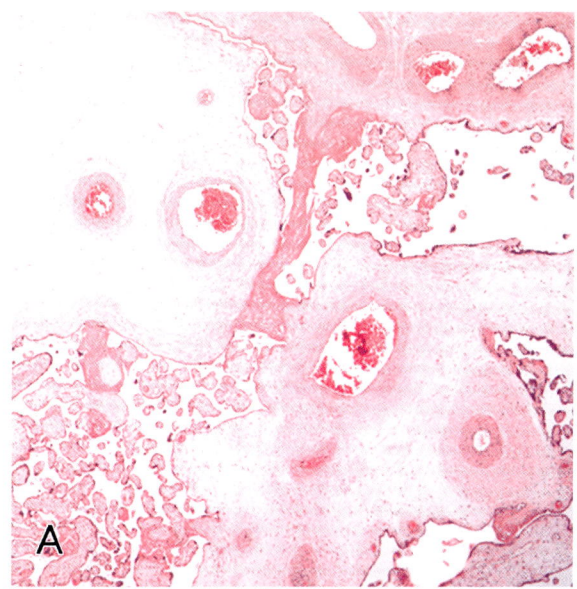
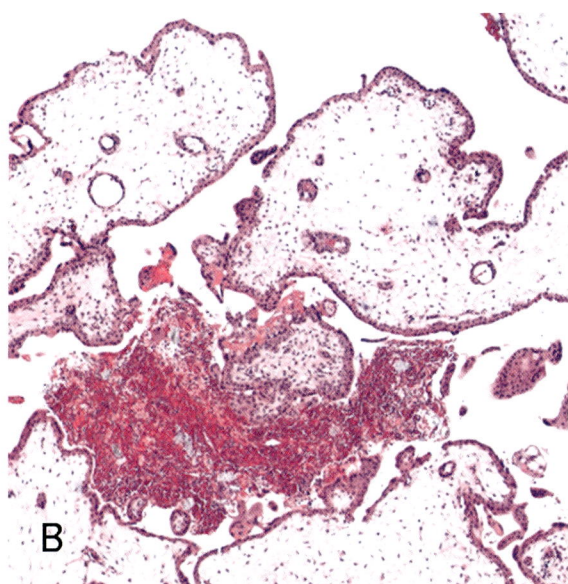
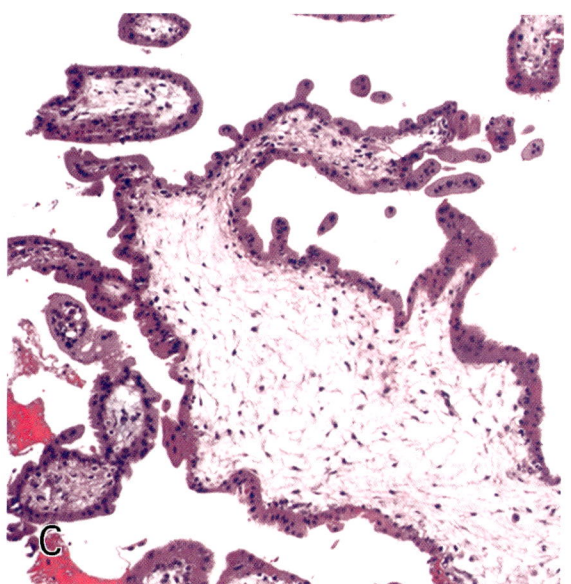

Figure 13-29

MIMICKERS OF PARTIAL HYDATIDIFORM MOLE

Placental mesenchymal dysplasia shows marked hydrops of stem villi, but normal distal villi and absence of trophoblast hyperplasia (A). Triploid nonmolar gestation with prominent villous dysmorphism with irregular outlines and trophoblastic pseudoinclusions (B). Associated syncytiotrophoblast hyperplasia is lacking (C).

surveillance is not required. The potential infant associations remain to be fully determined.

Triploid Nonmolar Pregnancies or Other Aneuploidy. These may be difficult to distinguish from PHM by morphology alone. In such cases, proliferation of syncytiotrophoblast is more limited and does not show the characteristic "lacy" circumferential growth seen in PHM (fig. 13-29B,C). A definitive diagnosis requires ancillary genetic studies.

Nonmolar Hydropic Miscarriage. This entity is characterized by marked hydropic change with round or ovoid villous cross sections without abnormal proliferation of trophoblast. Some of the villi normally show typical polar columns of trophoblast, a feature that is lacking in HM.

Treatment and Prognosis

With early detection and current treatment regimens, low-risk GTD has a cure rate of almost 100 percent; high-risk GTD, however, is associated with a 40 to 50 percent mortality rate. The important impact of chemotherapy can be seen in patients with choriocarcinoma, with an increased 5-year survival rate of 20 to 30 percent in the 1960s to over 90 percent in the 1990s and over 95 percent currently (241–243). This risk is not related to the gestational age at evacuation (183). Over 95 percent of pGTN post-HMs develop within 6 months of evacuation, either presenting as ongoing vaginal bleeding or, more commonly, rising/plateauing serum hCG levels on surveillance.

The reported incidence of CHMs needing treatment varies according to criteria used for the diagnosis of pGTD and whether PHMs and nonmolar miscarriages have been reliably excluded. For example, in the United Kingdom, around 8 percent of all HMs require treatment including approximately 15 percent and 0.5 to1.0 percent following CHM and PHM, respectively (59,60). Figures of up to 30 percent reported from the United States are a consequence of different criteria used for the diagnosis of pGTN (244).

No immortalized cell lines have been obtained from molar trophoblast whereas choriocarcinoma cell lines are well described, suggesting that first, molar trophoblast and pGTN/choriocarcinomas are probably phenotypically distinct, and second, that early molecular prognostication might be possible. At present, no successful stratification strategies have been described and all patients currently require surveillance post HM. A greater frequency of pGTD was initially suggested in heterozygous (dispermic) HM but this has not been supported by more recent studies (74,141,245).

Historically, the greater frequencies of pGTD post PHM almost certainly were due to the inclusion of many "diploid PHMs" which likely represented unrecognized early CHMs (84). The specific incidence of choriocarcinoma after PHM is not known but occasional histologically and genetically confirmed cases are reported. The factors that control the differences in behavior from HM to pGTD remain unknown and there is no relationship between any histologic feature and development of pGTN (190).

GESTATIONAL TROPHOBLASTIC TUMORS

Choriocarcinoma

Definition. Since *choriocarcinoma* represents the malignant counterpart of villous trophoblast, it is histologically characterized by a biphasic growth of cytotrophoblast-like and syncytiotrophoblast-like components, with prominent hCG production. It has been recognized that choriocarcinoma essentially represents malignant transformation of villous trophoblast which may show a range of differentiation patterns. It behaves aggressively if untreated but is highly chemosensitive.

Clinical Features. Choriocarcinoma follows any type of conception, including CHM, PHM, and normal nonmolar pregnancies. The true incidence of choriocarcinoma after CHM remains undetermined but is estimated to be approximately 2 to 3 percent while it is much lower following a PHM (less than 0.5 percent). The risk of choriocarcinoma developing from a normal nonmolar pregnancy is estimated to be 1 in 50,000, implying that the development of choriocarcinoma is 1,000-fold more likely following a CHM than a nonmolar conception. In the era prior to hCG surveillance following a diagnosis of HM, half of choriocarcinomas arose in that setting. With contemporary approaches in which most patients with pGTD are diagnosed early and treated without histologic confirmation of disease subtype, a greater number of choriocarcinomas are recognized following nonmolar term pregnancies. The frequency of choriocarcinomas that are preceded by HM varies between 40 and 80 percent, although this frequency may be underestimated due to historical misclassification of early gestation CHM as nonmolar miscarriage. Furthermore, since molecular genetic testing has established that the immediate antecedent pregnancy may not be the genetic origin of a choriocarcinoma, these numbers may be even less reliable (154,246–248). Geographic variations in frequency similar to those noted in CHM occur in choriocarcinoma, as both conditions are strongly related (49,56,131,207,246,249).

Abnormal vaginal bleeding is the most common clinical presentation (250). However, because choriocarcinoma may be associated with early metastases, a variety of clinical presentations have been described ranging from cervical or vaginal nodules to pulmonary, central nervous system, and liver metastases with secondary cor-pulmonale or intracerebral hemorrhage (34,251,252). Any unusual clinical symptoms/signs in a woman of childbearing age should raise the possibility of choriocarcinoma (253,254). Failure to recognize these findings has resulted in the development of

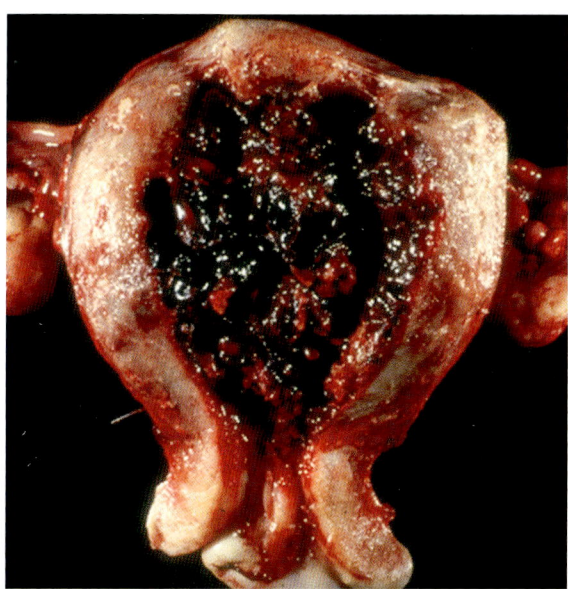

Figure 13-30

CHORIOCARCINOMA

An extensively hemorrhagic and necrotic polypoid mass fills and distends the endometrial cavity.

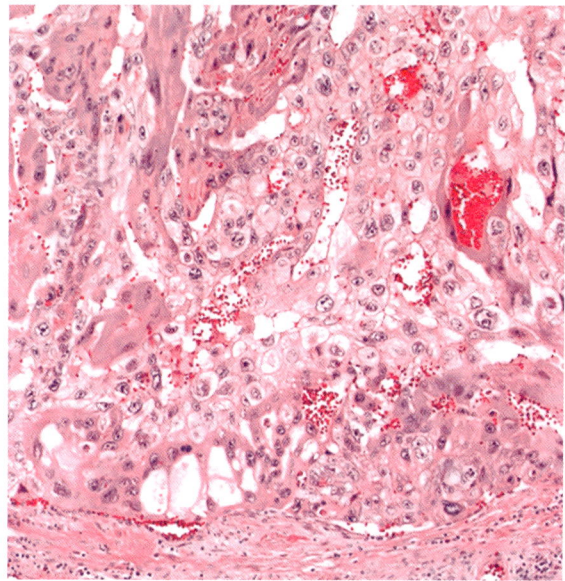

Figure 13-31

CHORIOCARCINOMA

The typical biphasic growth of syncytiotrophoblast and cytotrophoblast-like abnormal trophoblast is striking, with the syncytiotrophoblast stretching and surrounding cytotrophoblast in the absence of chorionic villi.

choriocarcinoma in immunosuppressed organ recipients (255). Melena or hematuria secondary to involvement of gastrointestinal or renal tract has been reported, and metastases to other even more unusual sites have been described (256–262). Since lymph node involvement is unusual, the finding of nodal involvement by a tumor with apparent trophoblastic differentiation, without definite evidence of a gestational disease, should raise the possibility of a nongestational neoplasm with trophoblastic differentiation such as germ cell tumor or carcinoma.

Choriocarcinoma is typically associated with very high hCG serum levels, since synthesis of hCG occurs mainly in villous syncytiotrophoblast, although some tumors may secrete lower amounts, especially if they are predominantly composed of cytotrophoblast-like cells. hCG is a sensitive marker of choriocarcinoma, although a wide range of hCG types may be secreted and appropriate assays are required. Ovarian luteal cysts that occur secondary to the high hCG levels are often multiple and bilateral and should not be mistaken for metastases (263–265).

Gross Findings. Choriocarcinomas most typically appear as variably sized, friable, hemorrhagic nodules with varying degrees of necrosis. They are centered in the endomyometrium and associated with irregular margins (fig. 13-30). Given the response to chemotherapy, this tumor is rarely treated by hysterectomy and samples obtained for pathologic examination often consist of curettings, biopsy of metastatic lesions, or postchemotherapy hysterectomy specimens in which the macroscopic and histologic features may be significantly altered.

Microscopic Findings. Histologically, choriocarcinoma typically demonstrates a biphasic growth of mononuclear cytotrophoblast-like and syncytiotrophoblast-like cells recapitulating villous type trophoblast, usually growing in sheets without intervening stroma (figs. 13-31, 13-32). Cytotrophoblast-like cells typically appear in the center and are surrounded by syncytiotrophoblast cells, the latter often showing vacuolated cytoplasm. Marked nuclear pleomorphism is common, especially if there is prominent syncytiotrophoblast-like differentiation (fig. 13-32). No chorionic villi are present (with the exception of choriocarcinoma arising in a term placenta (intraplacental choriocarcinoma) (fig. 13-33).

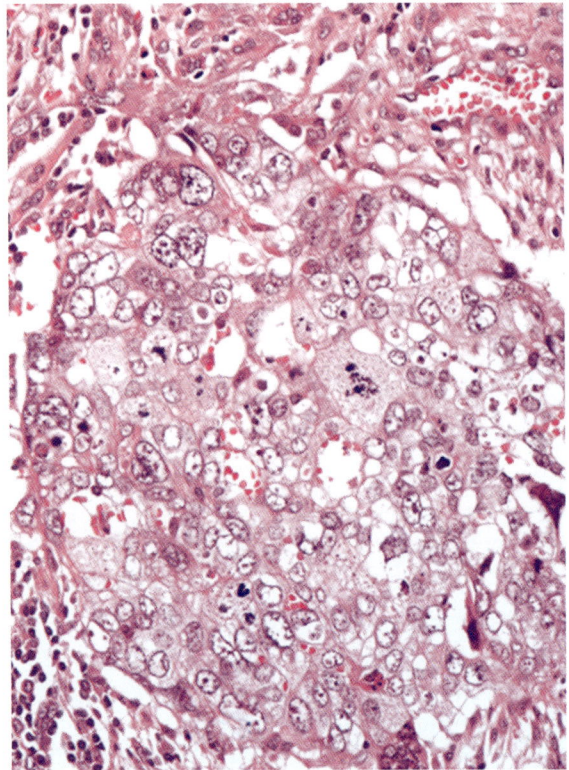

Figure 13-32

CHORIOCARCINOMA

Choriocarcinoma cells show marked cytologic atypia as well as mitotic figures.

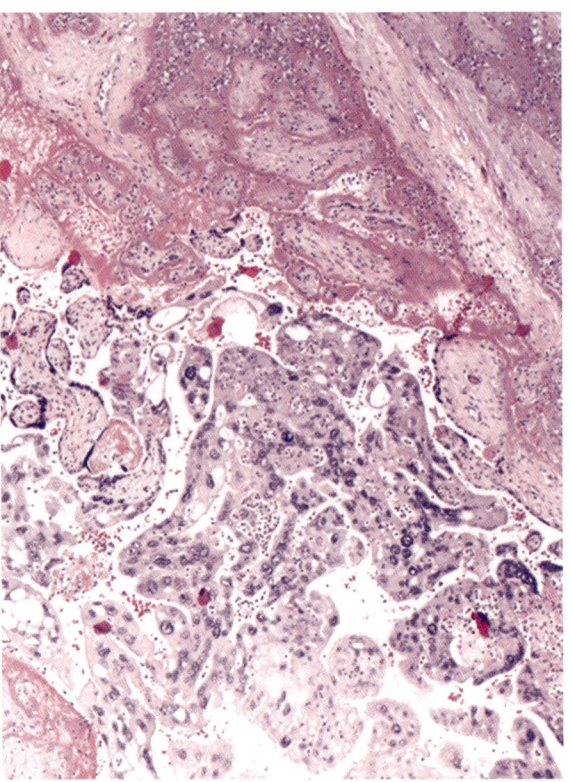

Figure 13-33

INTRAPLACENTAL CHORIOCARCINOMA

Third trimester mature chorionic villi are juxtaposed to a biphasic growth of cytotrophoblast-like and syncytiotrophoblast-like cells as seen in choriocarcinoma.

Extensive sampling may be necessary due to areas of hemorrhage and necrosis, especially in postchemotherapy hysterectomy specimens, with viable tumor often present only at the periphery (fig. 13-34). Residual viable tumor may exhibit extensive mononuclear, cytotrophoblast-like and intermediate trophoblast-like differentiation with marked pleomorphism, which may lead to diagnostic difficulty, especially if the previous clinical circumstances are not documented.

Choriocarcinoma may be associated with a marked lymphocytic inflammatory infiltrate. Prior to effective chemotherapeutic regimens, a correlation had been reported between intensity of the infiltrate and favorable prognosis, although this association has not been corroborated by other studies (266). Vascular invasion may be prominent since the tumor does not have its own vascular supply (267).

As noted earlier, the diagnosis of choriocarcinoma in limited samples may be difficult, particularly the distinction between choriocarcinoma and atypical trophoblast associated with CHM in the absence of chorionic villi. Curettage specimens may also sometimes demonstrate sheets and groups of pleomorphic trophoblast with mitotic activity in early nonmolar miscarriage, usually representing the trophoblastic shell of the early gestational sac. For practical purposes, the presence of chorionic villi in curettings in early pregnancy specimens excludes the diagnosis of choriocarcinoma and suggests either nonmolar pregnancy failure or CHM. In the setting of CHM, although highly pleomorphic trophoblast is occasionally seen in the absence of chorionic villi, it does not usually demonstrate the biphasic growth of cytotrophoblast and syncytiotrophoblast as seen in choriocarcinoma. A diagnosis of "atypical trophoblast" should be suggested if a

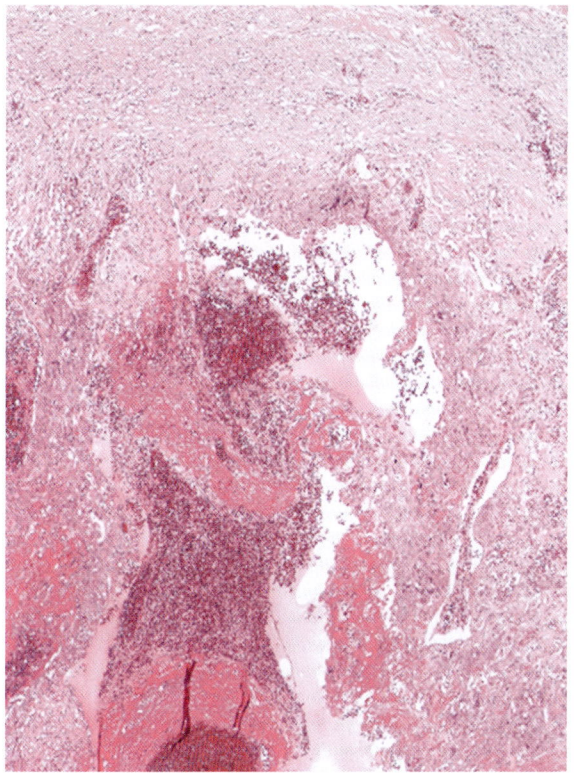

Figure 13-34

CHORIOCARCINOMA

Marked necrosis and hemorrhage are often noted. Close scrutiny at the periphery of these areas discloses typical areas of choriocarcinoma.

final diagnosis cannot be reached, indicating that the patient requires further clinical, imaging, and biochemical follow-up studies (268).

It is well-recognized that choriocarcinoma may follow, and be genetically derived from, nonmolar pregnancies, and when occurring in the third trimester placenta is termed intraplacental choriocarcinoma. In this setting, an atypical trophoblast proliferation develops within an otherwise normally developed placenta, surrounding clusters of chorionic villi, with trophoblast shedding into the maternal intervillous space and hence to the maternal circulation (fig. 13-33). The placental tumor may not be macroscopically visible or identified, since extensive pathologic examination of placentas from normal pregnancies is not performed. If a lesion is noted, however, the appearance may be nonspecific, usually initially presumed to be placental infarcts or intervillous thrombi at an unusual location. Thus, any lesion that grossly resembles a placental infarct and has a central location should be sampled in order to exclude an intraplacental choriocarcinoma. On histologic examination, apparently normal chorionic villi are surrounded by a highly pleomorphic, bilaminar trophoblast proliferation, which often locally fills the intervillous space and is associated with fibrin deposition (fig. 13-33) (269).

Molecular genetic testing has confirmed that both maternal and fetal metastatic diseases are derived from intraplacental choriocarcinoma, presenting as typical post-term pregnancy choriocarcinoma in the mother and choriocarcinoma of the liver in infants (270,271). Molecular studies have also confirmed that intraplacental choriocarcinomas are genetically derived from the placenta from which they are found, hence from term nonmolar villi rather than retained trophoblast from previous molar pregnancies (272). Although, intraplacental choriocarcinoma may be initially asymptomatic or missed, the diagnosis is made following pathologic placental examination in the setting of clinical maternal or infant choriocarcinoma or in the setting of other complications such as intrauterine death or fetal distress which complicate around 35 percent of these tumors. In approximately 50 percent of reported intraplacental choriocarcinomas, maternal choriocarcinoma/pGTD is also present (269,273–275).

Choriocarcinoma also develops outside the uterus and indeed, primary choriocarcinoma of the fallopian tube is rare but well described (276–282). Approximately two thirds of these patients present with symptoms of vaginal bleeding and abdominal pain, with a positive pregnancy test, clinically identical to a routine ectopic pregnancy. Others present with an apparent ovarian mass, suggesting an ovarian tumor, or with metastatic disease (fig. 13-35). Tubal choriocarcinoma has been described following fertility treatment (283). The prognosis of patients with tubal choriocarcinoma is similar to its uterine counterpart, with most patients now surviving following chemotherapy. In contrast to ectopic tubal choriocarcinoma, primary choriocarcinoma in other organs including lung, breast, stomach, intestine, liver, adrenal gland, pancreas, bladder, and kidney represent nongestational carcinomas with aberrant trophoblastic

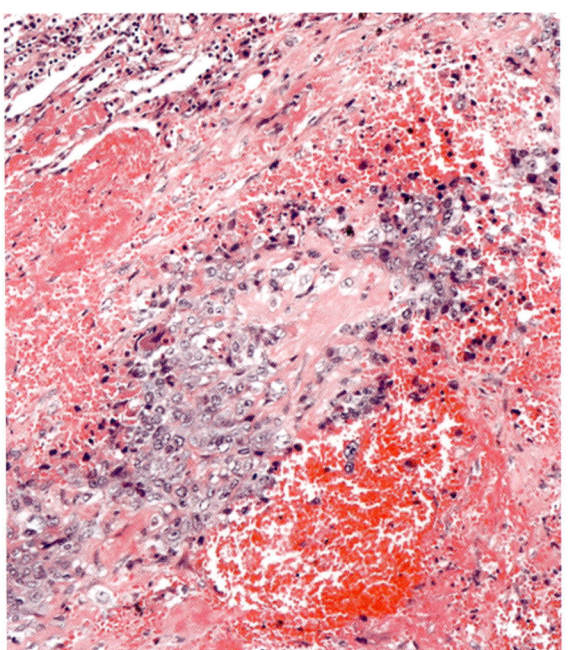 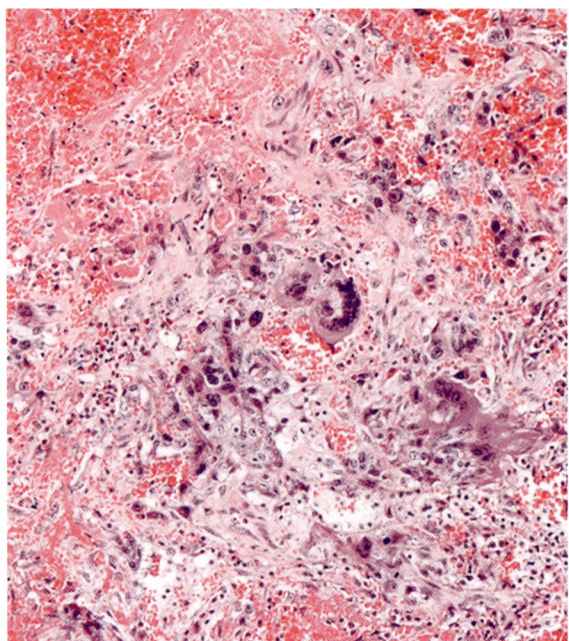

Figure 13-35

PULMONARY METASTASES OF CHORIOCARCINOMA

Tumor at metastatic sites may be composed only of highly atypical mononuclear cells (left) or display a biphasic growth of mononucleated and multinucleated cells (right). The associated hemorrhage is prominent.

differentiation, which can now be confirmed by molecular genotyping (140,284).

Immunohistochemical and Molecular Genetic Findings. Although there are clinical, biochemical, and morphologic features that are characteristic in choriocarcinoma, they may not be obvious, especially when postchemotherapy material is limited in atypical clinical circumstances. Also, trophoblastic differentiation is observed in nongestational tumors. Thus, immunohistochemistry may be diagnostically useful, but definitive distinction between gestational and nongestational tumors requires molecular genotyping.

Choriocarcinomas show strong and uniform cytokeratin expression, including AE1/3 but are typically negative for CK5/6 and CK18. They also typically express CD10 and inhibin but are negative for p63, HPL (with rare exceptions), and CEA (285). HLAG expression confirms gestational trophoblastic origin and may be useful in the distinction from nongestational tumors (285). hCG expression is seen in all tumors and is almost always present within syncytiotrophoblast-like cells, but may be patchy (fig. 13-36, left). HPL expression is usually present in syncytiotrophoblast-like cells but seen in less than 50 percent of the neoplasms. The Ki-67 proliferation index is high (over 70 percent) in most tumors (fig. 13-36, right) (286).

Although choriocarcinoma predominantly shows differentiation toward bilaminar villous type trophoblast, a mononuclear subpopulation of cells showed diffuse membranous and cytoplasmic MUC4 expression with variable HLAG and mel-CAM expression in a recent study (287). These markers are typically associated with trophoblast column and implantation site-type intermediate trophoblast. These data suggest that the spectrum of differentiation in choriocarcinoma may be wider than originally suggested. Only a few mononuclear cells expressed nuclear β-catenin, a marker of cytotrophoblast, thus suggesting that potentially choriocarcinoma is composed of intermediate trophoblast and syncytiotrophoblast. The authors hypothesized that cytotrophoblastic cells may potentially represent cancer stem cells in these tumors.

Although a range of molecular findings has been described in choriocarcinoma, no distinctive diagnostically or prognostically useful

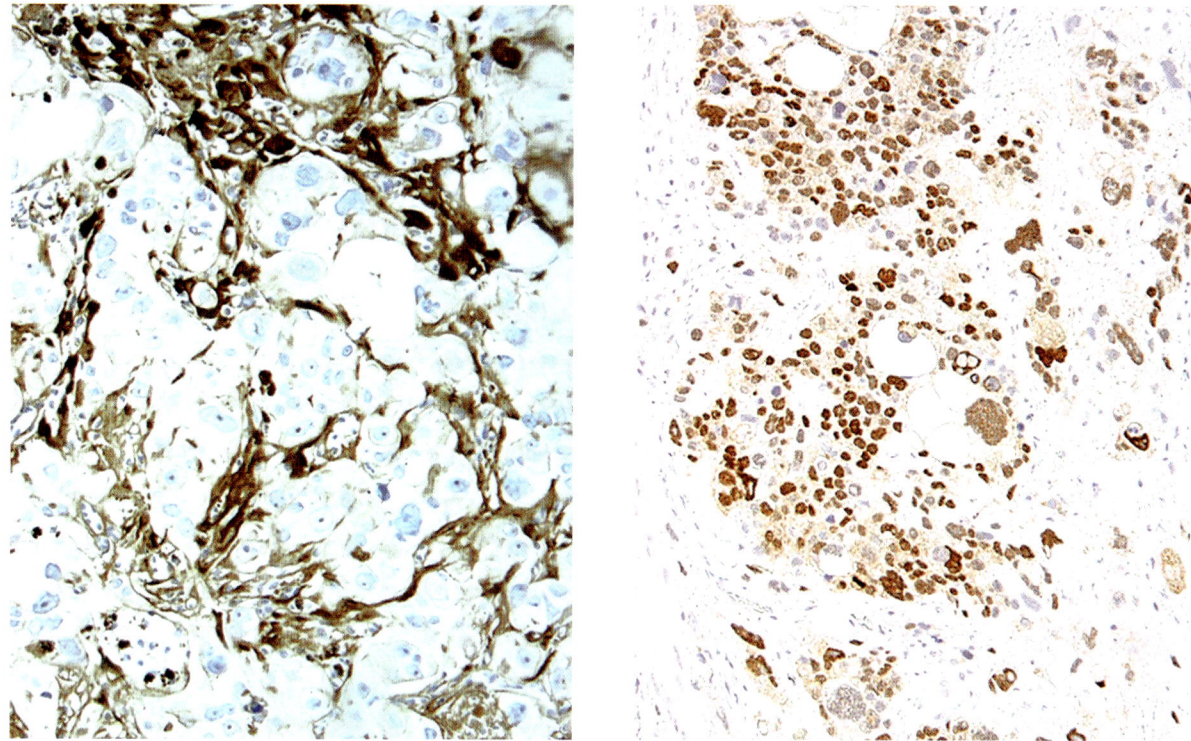

Figure 13-36

CHORIOCARCINOMA

hCG shows strong positivity within the syncytiotrophoblast-like cells (left) while Ki-67 shows a high proliferation rate (right).

molecular signature exists. Studies have often been performed in choriocarcinoma cell lines (288–291) and overexpression of VEGF292 and downregulation of ASPP2 (a p53 binding protein) (292) have been reported, but at present no consistent or reliable alterations have been identified for clinical use.

Treatment and Prognosis. Chemotherapy is the mainstay of treatment for choriocarcinoma, with overall cure rates of over 90 percent since these are highly chemosensitive tumors. Prognosis depends on risk group, which is based on factors such as tumor stage, interval from preceding pregnancy, antecedent term pregnancy, hCG levels, location and number of metastases, and history of failed treatment. In contemporary practice, however, major morbidity and mortality associated with choriocarcinoma predominantly occur in patients exhibiting extensive metastatic disease at presentation, especially central nervous system involvement, which may result in both severe complications and difficulties in treatment (293).

Intermediate Trophoblastic Lesions

Intermediate trophoblast is derived predominantly from nonvillous trophoblast and is mainly associated with normal placental implantation site and chorionic membranes. A range of lesions arise from intermediate trophoblast: *exaggerated placental-site reaction* (EPSR), *placental-site nodule/plaque* (PSN), *placental-site trophoblastic tumor* (PSTT), and *epithelioid trophoblastic tumor* (ETT). EPSR and PSTT most closely recapitulate implantation site trophoblast whereas PSN and ETT more closely resemble chorionic-type intermediate trophoblast. Conceptually, EPSR and PSN can be thought of as the non-neoplastic counterparts of PSTT and ETT, respectively. The latter two are subtypes of malignant GTT, and although phenotypically and immunohistochemically distinct, there is overlap in their clinical and pathologic features (294).

Placental-Site Trophoblastic Tumor. The term trophoblastic pseudotumor was initially suggested for these tumors because it was

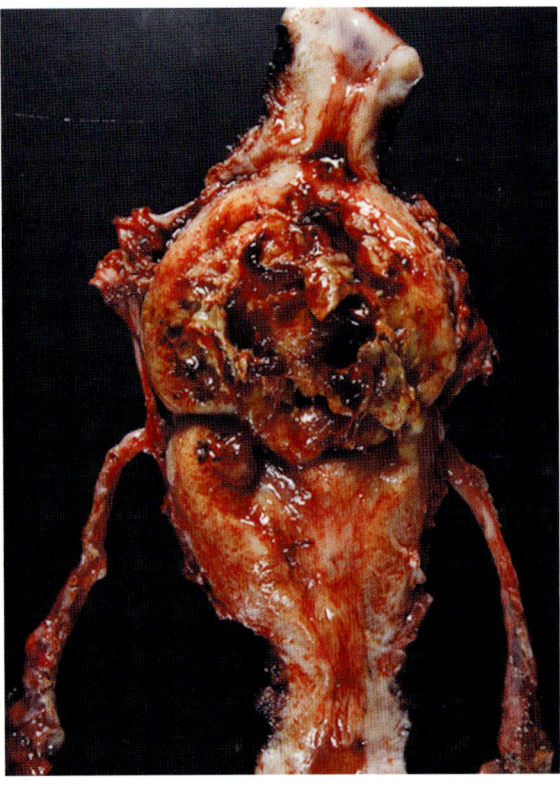

Figure 13-37

PLACENTAL-SITE TROPHOBLASTIC TUMOR

A large, focally necrotic, polypoid tumor is present within the endometrial cavity and extensively infiltrates the myometrial wall.

originally thought that they were associated with a favorable prognosis (295). Further evidence has shown that PSTT can behave aggressively, exhibiting local invasion and even metastatic spread. The term PSTT was introduced based on its clinical behavior and phenotypic similarity to the implantation site associated with normal placentation (9,296–299).

Clinical Features. Most patients are of child-bearing age and less commonly, peri/postmenopausal (300,301). They present with vaginal bleeding or amenorrhea (296,300–303). Local extension may be noted on initial physical examination, but patients also present with metastatic disease involving lungs, peritoneum, liver, pancreas, and brain. The interval between the last known antecedent pregnancy and clinical presentation ranges from months to years (average, 3 years), in contrast to the usually short interval period in choriocarcinoma (44).

PSTT genetically arises from both molar and nonmolar conceptions, with an unexplained but striking predominance of female conceptions (148,302,304,305). Serum hCG levels are almost always increased, but, consistent with its extravillous trophoblast phenotype, hCG concentrations are usually far less elevated than in choriocarcinoma, and may include specific hCG subtypes, particularly the free-β fraction (306,307). Rarely, PSTT is associated with paraneoplastic syndromes or secondary manifestations, including nephrotic syndrome due to glomerular intracapillary deposits of immunoglobulin and fibrin, and virilization due to hormonal stimulation (308,309).

Gross Findings. PSTTs typically form a mass, which may be small (1 to 2 cm) or may replace most of the uterus. They are well or poorly circumscribed, with a soft, white to tan to yellow cut surface often associated with patchy areas of necrosis and hemorrhage (fig. 13-37). Deep myometrial invasion, including extension to adjacent organs, is noted in 60 percent of tumors.

Microscopic Findings. PSTTs are characterized by a diffuse growth of monomorphic intermediate trophoblast-like cells that show an irregular infiltrating pattern into the myometrium, typically separating myometrial fibers ("splitting") (fig. 13-38). Replacement of uterine blood vessel walls, with preservation of vessel lumens, and associated with extensive fibrinoid deposition, is another characteristic feature, similar to the appearance of normal implantation site (fig. 13-39). Destructive vascular invasion with hemorrhage is less frequent than seen in choriocarcinoma.

Most cells are mononuclear and polygonal with abundant amphophilic or eosinophilic cytoplasm, but cells with clear cytoplasm and large cytoplasmic pseudoinclusions are seen. Most cells have a single, irregular, hyperchromatic nucleus but binucleated and rarely, multinucleated cells may be present (fig. 13-40A,B). Syncytiotrophoblast-like giant cells are not usually seen. Eosinophilic fibrinoid-like material may be seen in a patchy distribution throughout the tumor (fig. 13-40C). The mitotic rate is typically low in most tumors but atypical mitotic figures may be seen.

In longstanding or postchemotherapy tumors, secondary dystrophic calcification is identified,

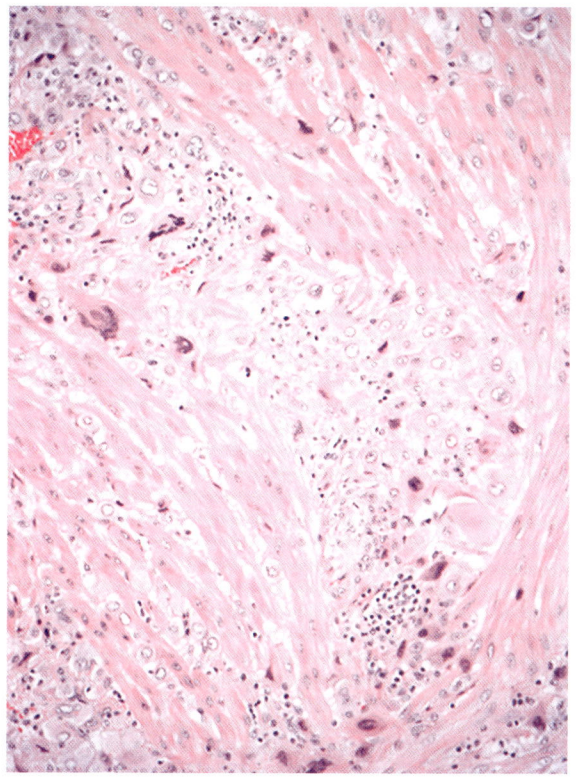

Figure 13-38

PLACENTAL-SITE TROPHOBLASTIC TUMOR

The neoplastic cells typically split the muscle fibers at the periphery since these tumors are characterized by an infiltrative border.

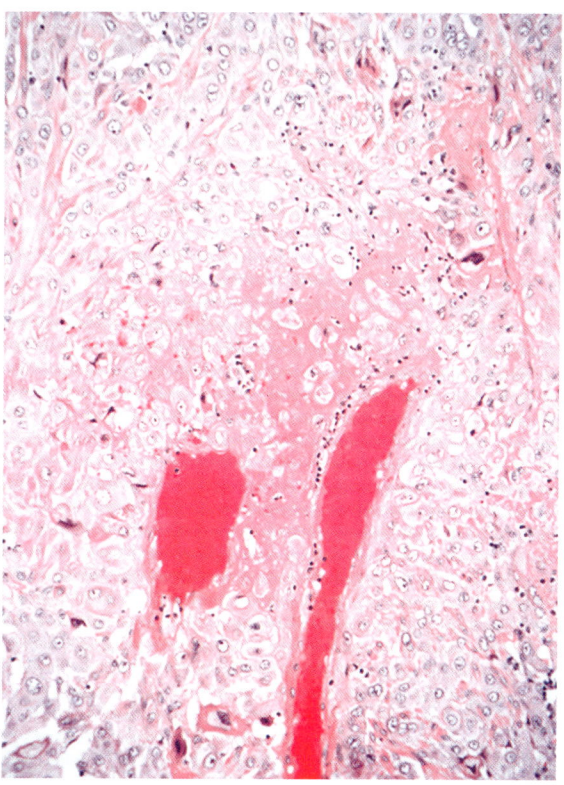

Figure 13-39

PLACENTAL-SITE TROPHOBLASTIC TUMOR

The cells typically infiltrate and destroy vessel walls and are associated with fibrinoid necrosis as tumor recapitulates the normal implantation site.

with viable tumor cells only identified at the periphery close to vessels (298). Since PSTTs are gestational in origin, they may occur at extrauterine sites as occurs in choriocarcinoma, including fallopian tube and ovary (310–312).

Immunohistochemical and Molecular Genetic Findings. In contrast to HM and choriocarcinoma, immunohistochemical stains often provide useful diagnostic information. There is widespread expression of cytokeratin (fig. 13-41A), in keeping with trophoblast lineage, greater expression of HPL than PLAP or hCG (fig. 13-41B), and expression of cyclin E, HLAG, inhibin (fig. 13-41C), and CD146 (mel CAM) (9,313–317). HLAG is only normally expressed by intermediate trophoblast and is, therefore, a useful marker for all intermediate-type trophoblastic lesions, but does not further discriminate among them; choriocarcinoma also expresses HLAG despite not morphologically recapitulating intermediate trophoblast. p63 expression is typically absent in PSTT and thus, is useful in distinguishing PSTT from ETT, which typically shows strong p63 expression (285,313,318). Immunohistochemical panels provide a useful and practical approach to the classification of trophoblastic lesions and appropriate algorithms are well described (313).

The electron microscopic features of GTTs are similar to trophoblast of normal pregnancy. This technique does not currently have a role in clinical diagnosis (319–321).

Most PSTTs are diploid (322,323). There is a confirmed and marked female predominance of these gestational tumor cells, which remains unexplained (148,324). Genetic studies have otherwise demonstrated no consistent chromosomal loss or gains and molecular testing currently does not provide useful diagnostic or prognostic information (177,325).

Figure 13-40
PLACENTAL-SITE TROPHOBLASTIC TUMOR

Cells are typically mononuclear and polygonal, with abundant amphophilic or eosinophilic cytoplasm, and may show large cytoplasmic pseudoinclusions (A). Most cells have a single irregular hyperchromatic nucleus but binucleated and rarely multinucleated cells are present (B). Fibrinoid material is present between the tumor cells (C).

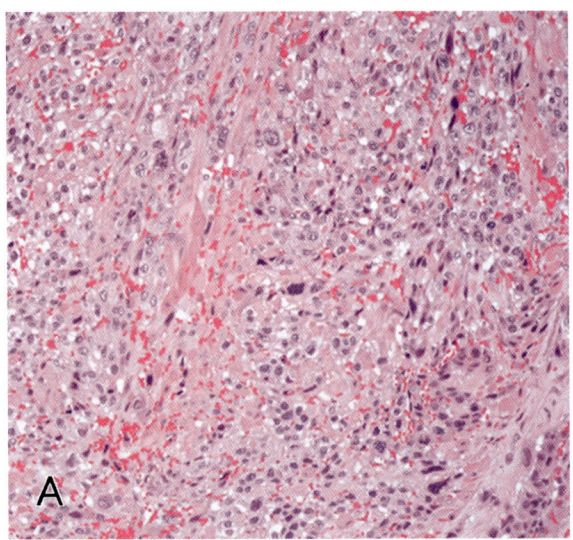
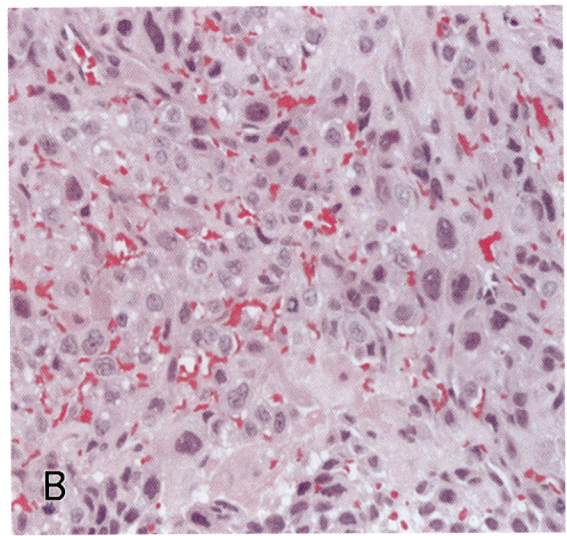
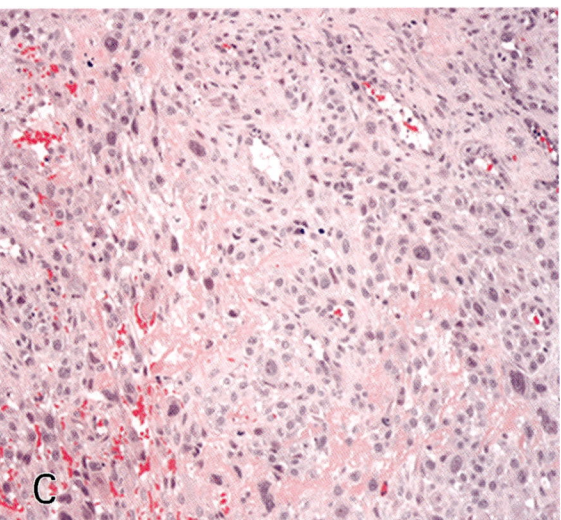

Treatment and Prognosis. Predictive factors for outcome in these tumors have been difficult to assess, mainly due to their rarity even in specialized centers. The largest study, based on multicenter registry data, reported overall survival rates of 70 percent at 10 years, dropping from 90 percent in patients with stage I disease to 50 percent in those with stage III or IV disease (301). Multivariate analysis, including a range of clinical and histologic features, demonstrated that the only significant predictor of survival was time from antecedent pregnancy, with intervals of over 48 months associated with a marked increase in risk of adverse outcome (44,298,301,326). Among other factors that have been implicated in the prognosis of PSTT, only stage and clear cytoplasm were suggested as predictors of overall survival in a review (298). Currently, no definitive molecular findings or histologic features (in addition to extent of disease) have been described to allow reliable risk stratification among these patients.

When compared to choriocarcinoma, PSTTs are relatively unresponsive to chemotherapy, and, therefore, surgery is the treatment of choice (301,327), although local pelvic extension in particular may be difficult to manage (44). Sites of metastases in order of frequency include lungs, liver, vagina, gastrointestinal tract, pelvis, bladder, and brain. Brain metastases tend to be fatal due to associated hemorrhage. Recent data have demonstrated that although less

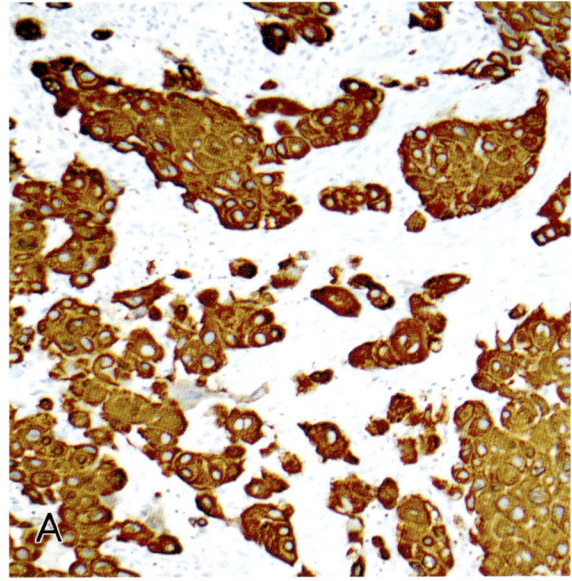
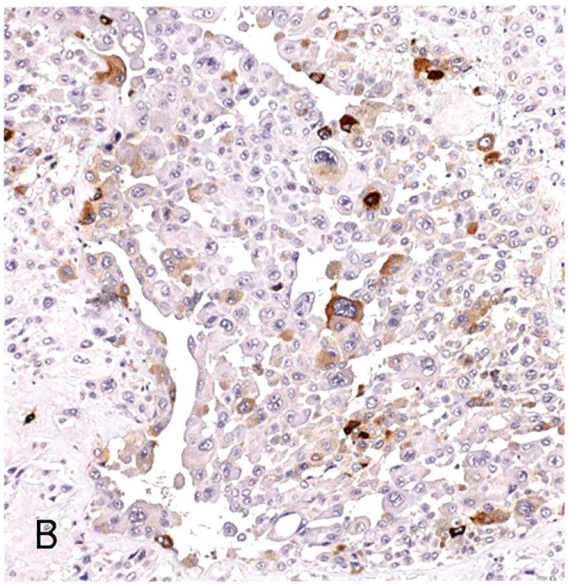
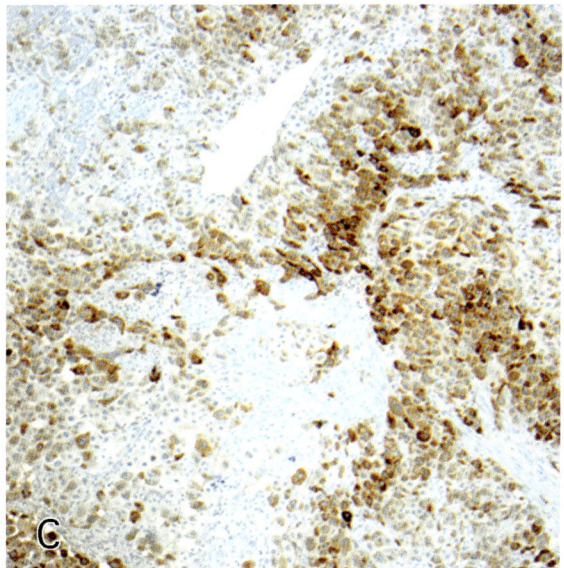

Figure 13-41

PLACENTAL-SITE TROPHOBLASTIC TUMOR

Cytokeratin is frequently diffusely and strongly positive (A). Some cells stain for hCG (B) while inhibin is typically positive in the implantation-site intermediate trophoblast (C).

responsive than pGTD, not otherwise specified, and choriocarcinoma, PSTTs respond to some extent to chemotherapy with a variety of multiagent protocols (302,328–330).

Epithelioid Trophoblastic Tumor. This subtype of trophoblastic tumor was initially described and termed "atypical choriocarcinoma," and subsequently recognized as a distinct entity (314).

Clinical Features. Patients are usually in their reproductive years with a history that includes a full term delivery (70 percent) followed by spontaneous miscarriage (15 percent) and HM (15 percent). The interval between previous gestation and diagnosis may be long (average, 6.2 years) and is slightly longer than that seen in PSTT (331,332). The most common presenting complaint is vaginal bleeding, but patients also present with metastases (333). As with PSTT, serum hCG is almost always elevated at the time of diagnosis, but levels are low when compared to those seen in patients with choriocarcinoma.

Gross Findings. Epithelioid trophoblastic tumors are usually solid, hemorrhagic, polypoid uterine masses with an expansile growth (fig. 13-42). They may be located in the uterine corpus, lower uterine segment, or cervix. They have a solid and cystic brown cut surface with frequent areas of necrosis and hemorrhage.

Microscopic Findings. On microscopic examination, the tumors often appear well circumscribed, although focal infiltration may be seen at the periphery. The most striking morphologic feature is the presence of a nodular architecture, which contrasts with the prominent infiltrative growth of PSTT (fig. 13-43, left). There is a monotonous population of mononucleated intermediate trophoblast cells that resemble the chorionic leave-type intermediate trophoblast. They are arranged in nests, cords, and islands, sometimes distributed around vessels and are intimately associated with hyalinized material (331, 334,335), imparting a "geographic" appearance.

The tumor blood vessels are preserved, with focal deposition of amorphous fibrinoid material, but vascular wall infiltration is not a striking feature (fig. 13-44). A peritumoral lymphocytic infiltrate is seen in approximately half of cases. The tumor cells have eosinophilic or clear cytoplasm, well-defined cell membranes, and round uniform

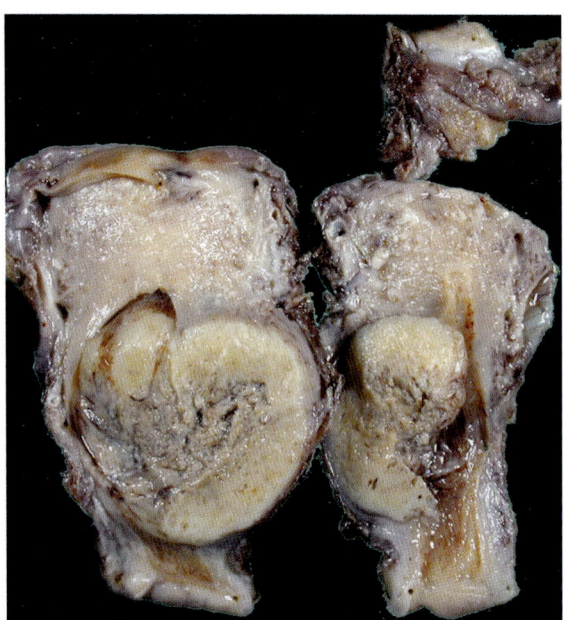

Figure 13-42

EPITHELIOID TROPHOBLASTIC TUMOR

The mass is solid, polypoid, and well demarcated.

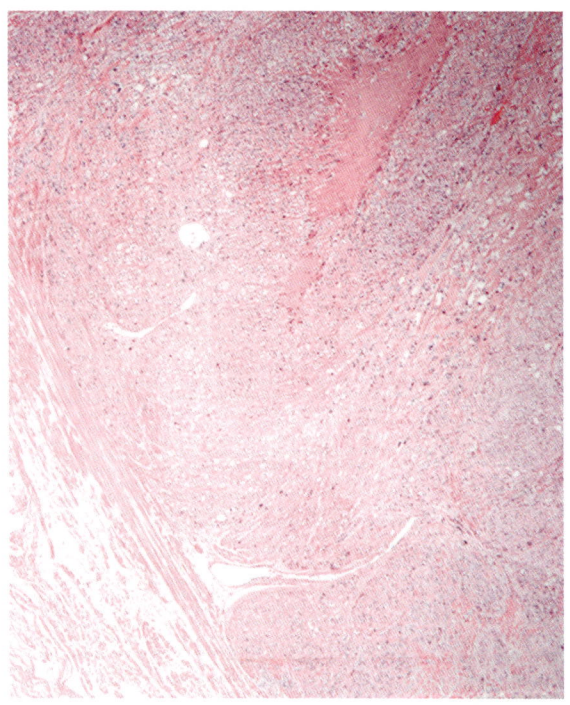
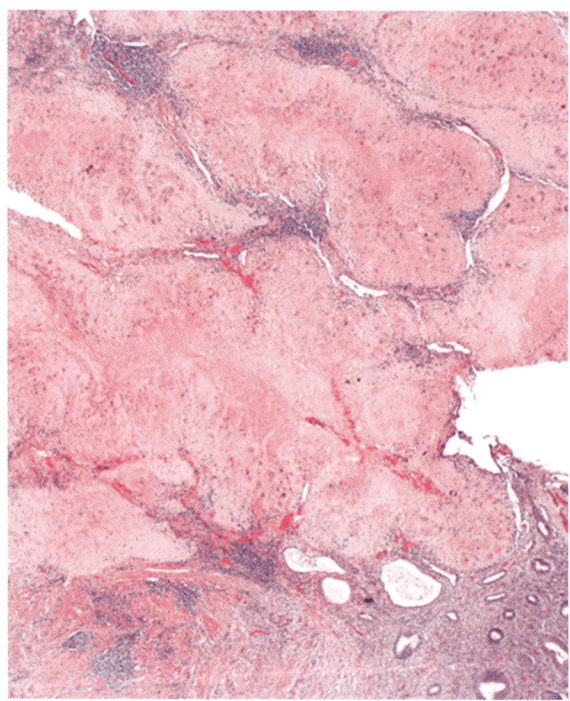

Figure 13-43

EPITHELIOID TROPHOBLASTIC TUMOR

The tumor is circumscribed (left), with extensive hyalinized areas and a nodular architecture (right). This is in contrast to the destructive infiltration and diffuse growth seen in placental-site trophoblastic tumor.

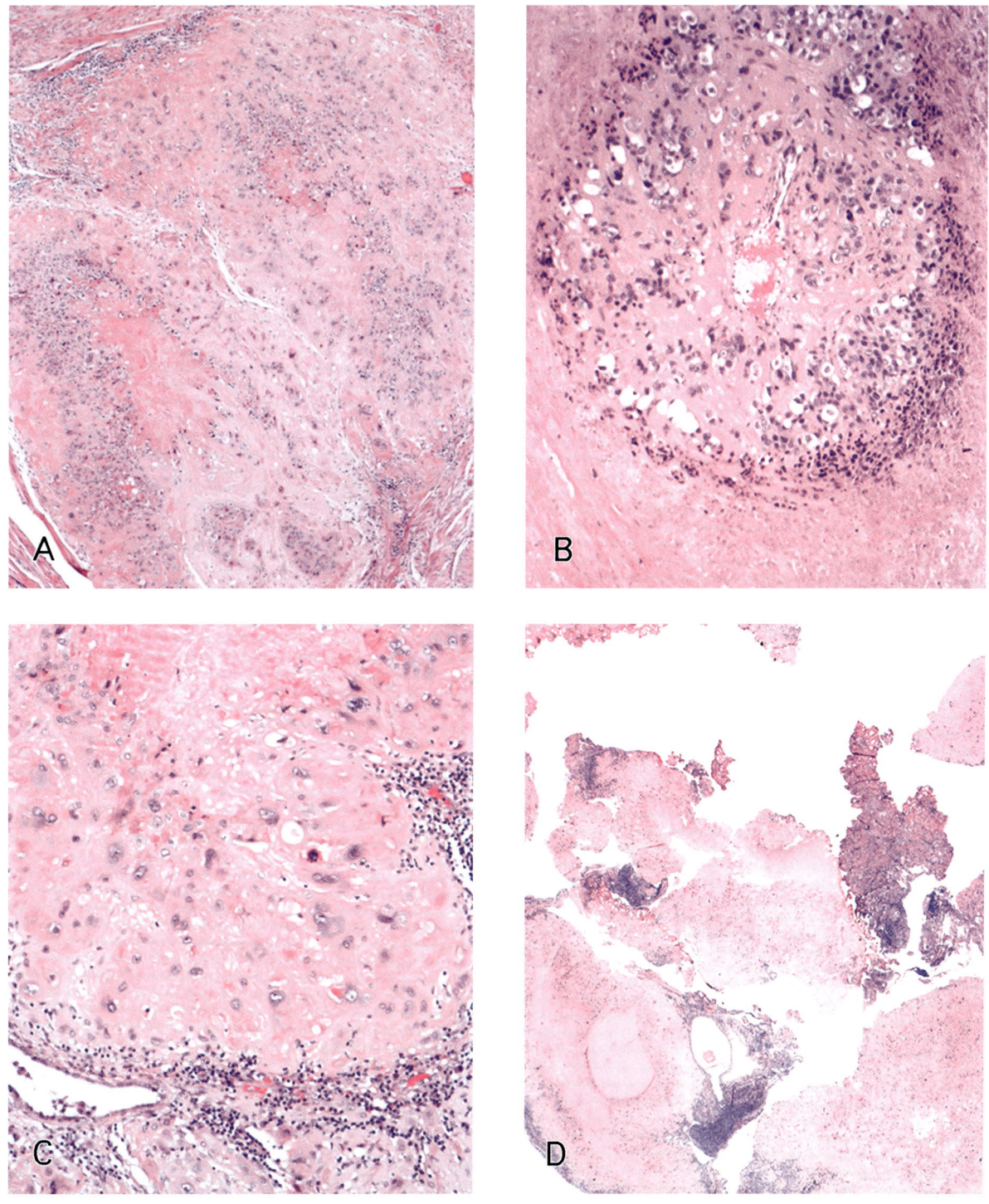

Figure 13-44

EPITHELIOID TROPHOBLASTIC TUMOR

Individual nodules have an appearance that is reminiscent of placental-site nodule (A). The tumor cells are arranged in nests, cords, and islands, sometimes distributed around vessels and intimately associated with hyalinized material, imparting a "geographic" appearance (B). The cells are fairly monotonous but may show variation in nuclear size (C). In a curettage specimen, the presence of large nodules suggest this entity since placental nodules are typically small in this setting (D).

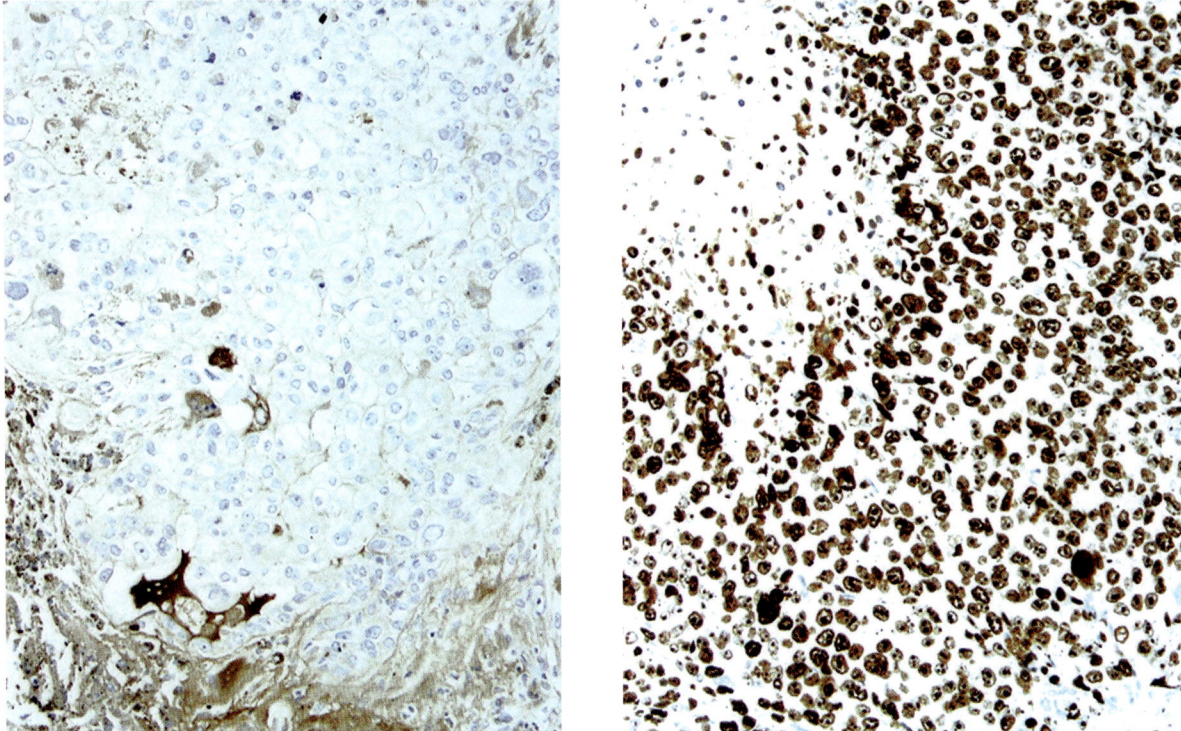

Figure 13-45

EPITHELIOID TROPHOBLASTIC TUMOR

Rare neoplastic cells are positive for β-HCG (left) and most are strongly and diffusely positive for p63 (right) in contrast to lesions derived from the implantation-site intermediate trophoblast.

nuclei and are smaller and show less nuclear pleomorphism than PSTT cells. Mitotic counts average of 2 mitoses per 10 high-power fields but can be higher, and the Ki-67 proliferation index is about 20 percent (335). Other types of GTTs when examined postchemotherapy may have a morphologic phenotype that overlaps with ETT, often showing extensive necrosis with only scanty viable peripheral mononuclear tumor cells, low Ki-67 index, and p63 positivity (336).

Immunohistochemical Findings. The tumor cells express pancytokeratin, EMA, and inhibin and usually demonstrate diffuse PLAP positivity; expression of hCG (fig. 13-45, left) and HPL is weak and focal (313–315,337). P63 is reliably positive in ETT and is a useful marker in the differential diagnosis with other malignant trophoblastic tumors (fig. 13-45, right) (310,314,318,331,335,338–341). There is increased expression of cyclin E when compared to PSN, but PSTT also shows cyclin E positivity.

Immunohistochemical algorithms have been suggested to aid in the differential diagnosis of GTT and are useful in clinical practice. Specifically, HLAG reliably identifies intermediate trophoblast and p63 separates ETT (strong expression) from PSTT (absent expression) (313). CD146 (mel-CAM) is expressed by intermediate trophoblast during normal implantation and is a useful marker for both ETT and PSTT, while ETT usually shows stronger positivity for PLAP and weaker staining for HPL, with the opposite profile being characteristic of PSTT (314,331,335,339).

Molecular Genetic Findings. There are no characteristic molecular genetic findings, although gestational origin and female preponderance have been confirmed (304,342).

Treatment and Prognosis. Patients often undergo hysterectomy, with or without adjuvant chemotherapy. Determinants of prognosis are not well characterized due to the rarity and recent recognition of this subset of malignant trophoblastic tumors. Data from pooled cases suggest that the main factor relating to outcome is FIGO stage, with a recent small series suggesting that interval from prior pregnancy of greater than 4 years is associated with adverse outcome, similar to what has been reported in PSTT (333,343).

Curettage Specimens of Trophoblastic Tissue. In a curettage specimen, fragments of myometrium infiltrated by trophoblastic cells from PSTT with dense eosinophilic cytoplasm and moderately pleomorphic nuclei may be difficult to distinguish from a placental-site reaction, since there may be scanty material and both infiltrate the myometrium. Confluent growth of monomorphic cells with mitoses and elevated Ki-67 index (over 1 percent) are suggestive of PSTT even in limited material (286,344).

Issues arise in the differential diagnosis between placental-site nodule and ETT for similar reasons (9,344). The finding of an irregular border, mitotic activity, and Ki-67 index of over 10 percent should favor a diagnosis of ETT over placental-site nodule. Interpretation of the histologic findings in these scenarios must always be in the appropriate clinical, imaging, and biochemical context, ideally as part of a multidisciplinary team approach.

Exaggerated Placental-Site Reaction. *Exaggerated placental-site reaction* (EPSR) does not represent a trophoblast neoplasm but rather is the residual morphologic expression of the implantation site reaction following a recent gestation. EPSR is usually diagnosed following curettage when evaluating postconception vaginal bleeding.

On microscopic examination, fragments of endomyometrium are infiltrated by individual and nests of intermediate trophoblast, with organization and morphologic characteristics of normal implantation site (fig. 13-46). There is no confluent growth or destruction of the underlying myometrial architecture. The presence of admixed implantation site-type multinucleated trophoblast giant cells is a useful diagnostic feature (9,286,345–347).

In some cases the diagnosis of PSTT is suggested in a postconception curettage specimen in which retained chorionic villi are also present in association with a florid implantation-site reaction. In such cases, the presence of villi largely excludes the diagnosis of PSTT. Distinction of EPSR from

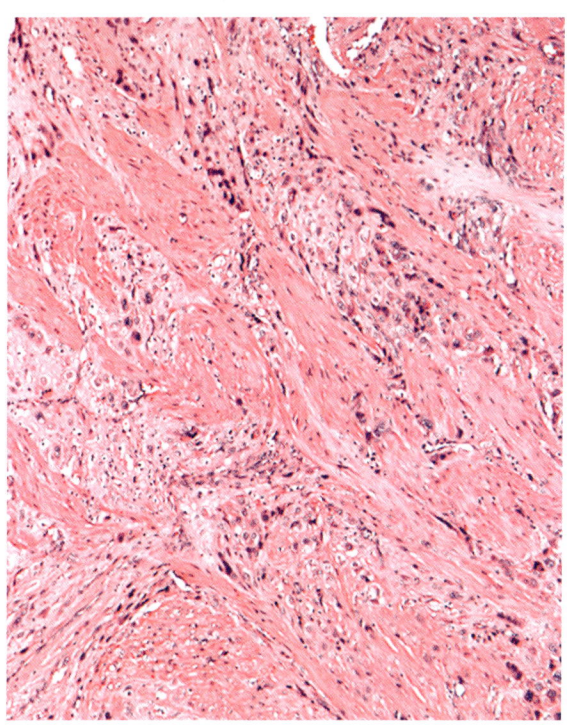

Figure 13-46

EXAGGERATED PLACENTAL-SITE REACTION

There is striking infiltration of the myometrium by numerous intermediate trophoblast cells. The cells do not form a mass.

PSTT is based on both clinical and morphologic findings and the immunohistochemical profile. EPSR demonstrates no mitotic activity and an extremely low (less than 1 percent) or zero proliferation index (286). Although not required in clinical practice, EPSRs are genetically different from PSTTs, with a normal expected ratio of male and female trophoblast-derived cells in EPSR versus the documented female predominance in PSTT (347).

Florid implantation-site reaction is well-described in association with CHM. It should not in this context be regarded as EPSR or PSTT (200).

Placental-Site Nodule/Atypical PSN. *Placental site nodule* (PSN) is a non-neoplastic proliferation derived from the intermediate chorionic laeve trophoblast occurring in women of child-bearing age (348). PSN is not a proliferative lesion and thus is not associated with elevated hCG levels (348–350). It is most often identified incidentally in endometrial curettings performed for menstrual disorders or other indications. A pregnancy may be documented more than 10 years prior to diagnosis. As occurs with ETT, it can occur anywhere within the uterus but often is centered in the cervix/low-uterine segment. Rarely, PSN is documented in the fallopian tube including in tubal ligation specimens (350a).

PSNs correspond to one or more typically small (less than 10 mm), well-circumscribed nodules rarely grossly visible. On microscopic examination, they are often seen as lobulated nodules or plaques in which intermediate trophoblast cells are embedded in a hypocellular and hyalinized background. Central cavitation may be seen. The periphery of the nodules sometimes show small pseudopods that mimic invasion, thus causing concern for a malignant trophoblastic tumor or even squamous cell carcinoma if located in the cervix of a young woman. Small groups, nests, or single cells may be seen within the hyalinized nodule and may show degenerative-type cytologic atypia including nuclear pseudoinclusions (fig. 13-47). In contrast to ETT, they are less cellular and have an absent or low proliferation index (less than 10 and likely less than 5 percent) (348–350,351).

Trophoblast origin is confirmed by expression of PLAP, cytokeratin, CD10 (fig. 13-48A), inhibin (fig. 13-48B), and EMA. PSN cells also express p63, as seen in ETT, but they lack cyclin E expression (348,349,351). p63 positivity may help if PSTT is in the differential diagnosis since PSTT is typically negative. As occurs with ETT, rare cells may be HPL positive (fig. 13-48C).

In a curettage specimen, PSNs often maintain the lobular architecture and the diagnosis is often straightforward. If cellular or with unusual features, a diagnosis of PSN in curettage specimens should be interpreted in light of the clinical/radiologic findings, since in the presence of a image-identifiable lesion, sampling at the periphery of an ETT, or less often, a PSTT may erroneously suggest a PSN (352).

Although patients with typical PSNs do not require further follow-up, recently, a subgroup of tumors was identified with features of PSN but also showing larger size, cellular atypia, or increased mitotic rate. Such lesions are categorized as *atypical PSN* (aPSN) (fig. 13-49) (348,353). Data regarding this group of tumors is limited but in the largest available series to date, 15 percent were associated with a malignant GTT, either concurrently or developing within 16 months of the aPSN diagnosis (353). Examples of PSTT/ETT in hysterectomy specimens in which morphologic areas of both PSN and PSTT/ETT are present have also been reported (352), as well as PSN transforming into a malignant ETT with pelvic lymph node and lung metastases (354).

Mixed Gestational Trophoblastic Tumors. Although GTTs are generally described as clinically and pathologically distinct entities, it is increasingly recognized that examination of hysterectomy specimens occasionally demonstrates tumors in which there are areas morphologically suggestive of choriocarcinoma and/or PSTT/ETT (178).

Distinction of choriocarcinoma from PSTT/ETT is usually straightforward based on clinical features and serum hCG concentrations. If prechemotherapy specimens are sampled, histologic examination demonstrates their distinctive features. Choriocarcinomas examined postchemotherapy may demonstrate extensive necrosis, with only small peripheral areas of mononuclear viable cells, which may be confused with PSTT/ETT (178). In such cases, interpretation should rely on clinical findings since both immunostaining and molecular studies may be nondiagnostic.

In some cases, histologic findings are iatrogenic and represent residual PSTT/ETT-like mononuclear areas of choriocarcinoma following chemotherapy (336,355). Other tumors may, however, have genuine mixed PSTT/ETT and choriocarcinoma morphology in the uterus but choriocarcinoma-like appearance in distant metastases. Other tumors have areas of PSTT juxtaposed with areas of choriocarcinoma (331,335,339). Such cases may also demonstrate variable immunostaining in the different areas with markers such as SALL4 (356).

Distinguishing PSTT and ETT may not be possible, and in one of the seminal publications describing ETT, some illustrated cases had areas of apparent PSTT-like morphology (314). It is possible that choriocarcinoma and PSTT/ETT arise from similar progenitor cells, with differentiation pathways dependent on environmental or other factors, including chemotherapy which may select chemoresistant clones.

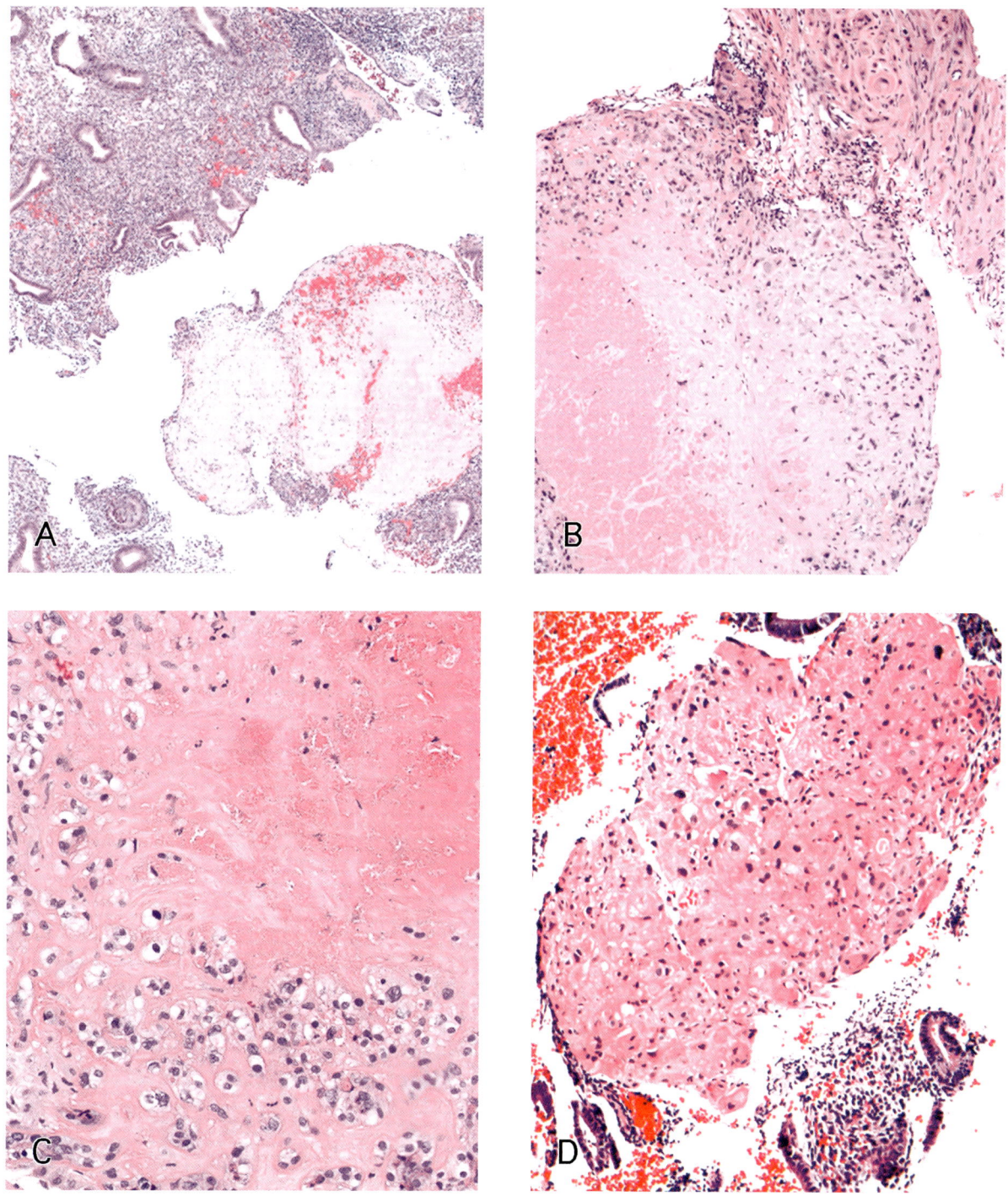

Figure 13-47

PLACENTAL-SITE NODULE

A well-demarcated, extensively hyalinized nodule with a slightly peripheral cellular rim is embedded within the endometrium (A). On higher magnification, the peripheral cellular areas are composed of intermediate trophoblast cells. The small irregular pseudopod at the periphery of the nodule (top right) should not be misconstrued as invasion (B). Nodules often have a central hyalinization or fibrinoid deposit (C). The intermediate trophoblast cells are either single or form small nests with pale of eosinophilic cytoplasm and variably sized nuclei that may be hyperchromatic (D).

Figure 13-48

PLACENTAL-SITE NODULE

The intermediate trophoblast cells in a placental-site nodule are typically CD10 positive (A). Inhibin shows extensive positivity (B) while HPL displays only minimal positivity as the cells are derived from chorionic laeve (C) (in contrast to implantation-site intermediate trophoblast).

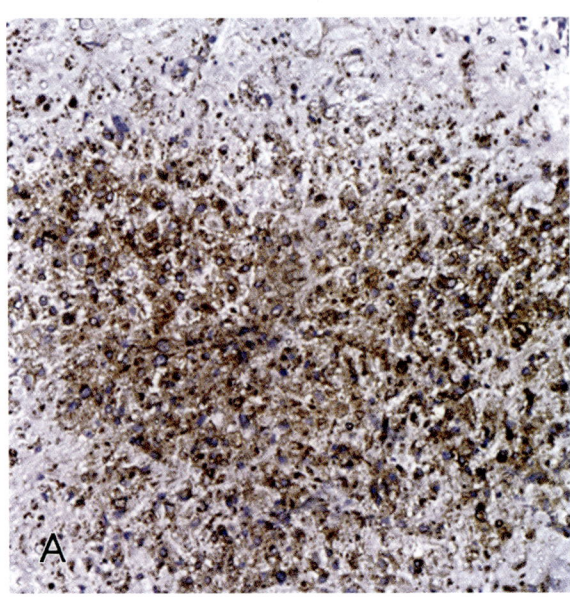
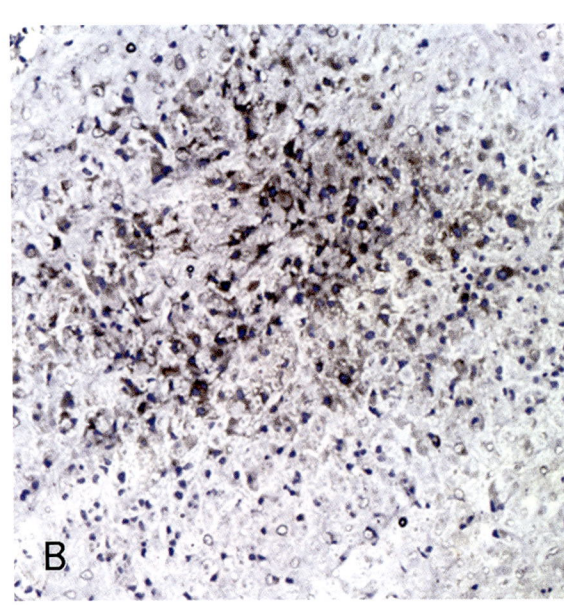
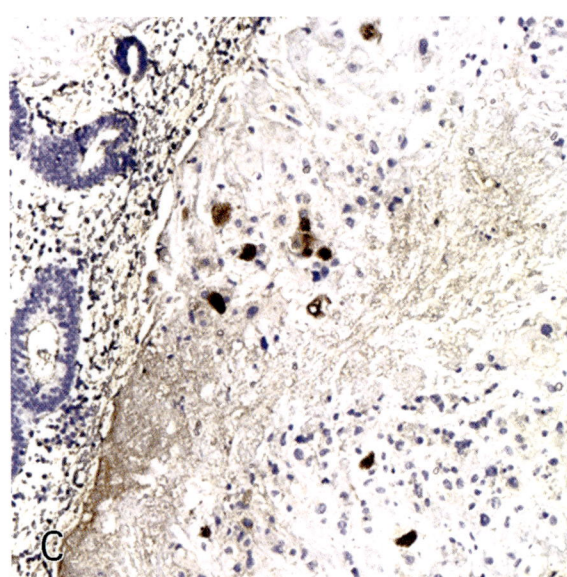

NONGESTATIONAL TUMORS WITH TROPHOBLASTIC PHENOTYPE

A range of poorly differentiated carcinomas have been reported that clinically and morphologically overlap with GTT, including expression of hCG (141,357). Definitive diagnosis is achieved using molecular methods as described above, but often immunostains and generous sampling are helpful in establishing the final diagnosis. Specifically, epithelioid leiomyosarcoma may be confused with PSTT/ETT but finding spindle morphology as well as positivity for smooth muscle markers but negative staining for trophoblast markers aid in the diagnosis (358). Rarely, squamous cell carcinoma may mimic PSTT or ETT. Although p16 is used as a surrogate marker of high-risk human papillomavirus in cervical squamous neoplasia, trophoblastic proliferations may stain, although not diffusely and strongly, for this marker. It is also important to note that squamous cell carcinomas are p63 positive. Thus, a panel of antibodies should be used in this differential diagnosis including inhibin, hPL, HLAG, and different keratins (359).

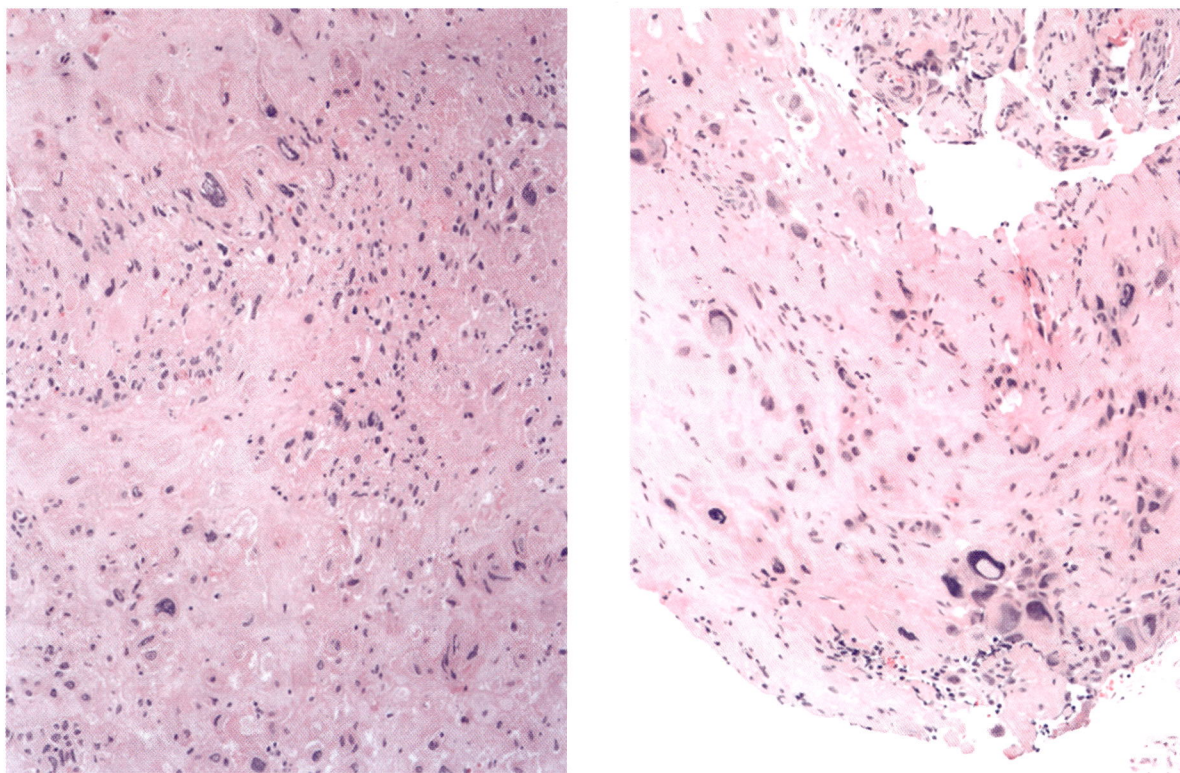

Figure 13-49

ATYPICAL PLACENTAL-SITE NODULE

Intermediate trophoblast cells are larger and have more cellular atypia than typical placental-site nodule.

REFERENCES

1. Kurman RJ, Carcangiu ML, Herrington ML, Young RH, eds. WHO classification of tumours of female reproductive organs, 4th ed. Lyon: IARC Press; 2014:6.
2. Pfeffer PL, Pearton DJ. Trophoblast development. Reproduction 2012;143:231-46.
3. Senner CE, Hemberger M. Regulation of early trophoblast differentiation—lessons from the mouse. Placenta 2010;31:944-50.
4. Lunghi L, Ferretti ME, Medici S, Biondi C, Vesce F. Control of human trophoblast function. Reprod Biol Endocrinol 2007;5:6.
5. Shih IM, Kurman RJ. Immunohistochemical localization of inhibin-alpha in the placenta and gestational trophoblastic lesions. Int J Gynecol Pathol 1999;18:144-50.
6. Hamilton WJ, Boyd JD. Development of the human placenta in the first three months of gestation. J Anat 1960;94(Pt 3):297-328.
7. Kurman RJ, Young RH, Norris HJ, Main CS, Lawerence WD, Scully RE. Immunocytochemical localization of placental lactogen and chorionic gonadotropin in the normal placenta and trophoblastic tumors, with emphasis on intermediate trophoblast and the placental site trophoblastic tumor. Int J Gynecol Pathol 1984;3:101-21.
8. Ino K, Suzuki T, Uehara C, et al. The expression and localization of neutral endopeptidase 24.11/CD10 in human gestational trophoblastic diseases. Lab Invest 2000;80:1729-38.
9. Shih IM, Kurman RJ. The pathology of intermediate trophoblastic tumors and tumor-like lesions. Int J Gynecol Pathol 2001;20:31-47.

10. Yeh IT, O'Connor DM, Kurman RJ. Intermediate trophoblast: further immunocytochemical characterization. Mod Pathol 1990;3:282-7.
11. Wells M, Bulmer JN. The human placental bed: histology, immunohistochemistry and pathology. Histopathology 1988;13:483-98.
12. Rashid NA, Lalitkumar S, Lalitkumar PG, Gemzell-Danielsson K. Endometrial receptivity and human embryo implantation. Am J Reprod Immunol 2011;66(suppl 1):23-30.
13. Diedrich K, Fauser BC, Devroey P, Griesinger G. The role of the endometrium and embryo in human implantation. Hum Reprod Update 2007;13:365-77.
14. Staun-Ram E, Shalev E. Human trophoblast function during the implantation process. Reprod Biol Endocrinol 2005;3:56.
15. Huppertz B. The feto-maternal interface: setting the stage for potential immune interactions. Semin Immunopathol 2007;29:83-94.
16. Erlebacher A. Immunology of the maternal-fetal interface. Annu Rev Immunol 2013;31:387-411.
17. Kam EP, Gardner L, Loke YW, King A. The role of trophoblast in the physiological change in decidual spiral arteries. Hum Reprod 1999;14:2131-8.
18. Chen JZ, Sheehan PM, Brennecke SP, Keogh RJ. Vessel remodelling, pregnancy hormones and extravillous trophoblast function. Mol Cell Endocrinol 2012;349:138-44.
19. Wallace AE, Fraser R, Cartwright JE. Extravillous trophoblast and decidual natural killer cells: a remodelling partnership. Hum Reprod Update 2012;18:458-71.
20. Cross JC, Hemberger M, Lu Y, et al. Trophoblast functions, angiogenesis and remodeling of the maternal vasculature in the placenta. Molecular Cell Endocrinol 2002;187:207-12.
21. Soares MJ, Chakraborty D, Renaud SJ, et al. Regulatory pathways controlling the endovascular invasive trophoblast cell lineage. J Reprod Dev 2012;58:283-7.
22. Huppertz B, Weiss G, Moser G. Trophoblast invasion and oxygenation of the placenta: measurements versus presumptions. J Reprod Immunol 2014;101-102:74-9.
23. Burton GJ, Jauniaux E. Placental oxidative stress: from miscarriage to preeclampsia. J Soc Gynecol Investig 2004;11:342-52.
24. Johns J, Jauniaux E, Burton G. Factors affecting the early embryonic environment. Rev Gynaecol Perinat Pract 2006;6:199-210.
25. Quinn J, Kunath T, Rossant J. Mouse trophoblast stem cells. Methods Mol Med 2006;121:125-48.
26. Roberts RM, Fisher SJ. Trophoblast stem cells. Biol Reprod 2011;84:412-21.
27. Xu RH, Chen X, Li DS, et al. BMP4 initiates human embryonic stem cell differentiation to trophoblast. Nat Biotechnol 2002;20:1261-4.
28. Kunath T, Strumpf D, Rossant J. Early trophoblast determination and stem cell maintenance in the mouse—a review. Placenta 2004;25(suppl A):S32-8.
29. Golos TG, Giakoumopoulos M, Gerami-Naini B. Review: trophoblast differentiation from human embryonic stem cells. Placenta 2013;34(suppl 1):s56-61.
30. Amita M, Adachi K, Alexenko AP, et al. Complete and unidirectional conversion of human embryonic stem cells to trophoblast by BMP4. Proc Natl Acad Sci U S A 2013;110:E1212-21.
31. Roberts RM, Loh KM, Amita M, et al. Differentiation of trophoblast cells from human embryonic stem cells: To be or not to be? Reproduction 2014;147:D1-12.
32. Wilkins JF, Haig D. What good is genomic imprinting: the function of parent-specific gene expression. Nat Rev Genet 2003;4:359-68.
33. Ferguson-Smith AC, Moore T, Detmar J, et al. Epigenetics and imprinting of the trophoblast —a workshop report. Placenta 2006;27(suppl a):122-6.
34. Seckl MJ, Sebire NJ, Berkowitz RS. Gestational trophoblastic disease. Lancet 2010;376:717-29.
35. Chen LM, Olawaiye B, Bhosale PR, et al. Gestational trophoblastic neoplasms. In: Amin MB, Edge SB, Green FL, eds. AJCC cancer staging manual, 8th ed. New York: Springer; 2018:691-7.
36. FIGO Committee on Gynecologic Oncology. Current FIGO staging for cancer of the vagina, fallopian tube, ovary, and gestational trophoblastic neoplasia. Int J Gynaecol Obstet 2009;105:3-4.
37. Hancock BW. Staging and classification of gestational trophoblastic disease. Best Pract Res Clin Obstet Gynaecol 2003;17:869-83.
38. Gardner E. Gestational trophoblastic neoplasia: staging and treatment. UpToDate. http://www.uptodate.com/contents/gestational-trophoblastic-neoplasia-staging-and-treatment?-source=related_link#H52. Published 2013.
39. Homesley HD. Single-agent therapy for nonmetastatic and low-risk gestational trophoblastic disease. J Reprod Med 1998;43:69-74.
40. Roberts JP, Lurain JR. Treatment of low-risk metastatic gestational trophoblastic tumors with single-agent chemotherapy. Am J Obstet Gynecol 1996;174:1917-24.
41. Foulmann K, Guastalla JP, Caminet N, et al. What is the best protocol of single-agent methotrexate chemotherapy in nonmetastatic or low-risk metastatic gestational trophoblastic tumors? A review of the evidence. Gynecol Oncol 2006;102:103-10.

42. Feltmate CM, Genest DR, Wise L, Bernstein MR, Goldstein DP, Berkowitz RS. Placental site trophoblastic tumor: a 17-year experience at the New England Trophoblastic Disease Center. Gynecol Oncol 2001;82:415-9.
43. Lathrop JC, Lauchlan S, Nayak R, Ambler M. Clinical characteristics of placental site trophoblastic tumor (PSTT). Gynecol Oncol 1988;31:32-42.
44. Papadopoulos AJ, Foskett M, Seckl MJ, et al. Twenty-five years' clinical experience with placental site trophoblastic tumors. J Reprod Med 2002;47:460-4.
45. Berkowitz RS, Goldstein DP. Clinical practice. Molar pregnancy. N Engl J Med 2009;360:1639-45.
46. Sebire NJ, Seckl MJ. Gestational trophoblastic disease: current management of hydatidiform mole. BMJ 2008;337:453-8.
47. Takeuchi S. Incidence of gestational trophoblastic disease by regional registration in Japan. Hum Reprod 1987;2:729-34.
48. Hando T, Ohno M, Kurose T. Recent aspects of gestational trophoblastic disease in Japan. Int J Gynaecol Obstet 1998;60(Suppl 1):S71-6.
49. Altieri A, Franceschi S, Ferlay J, Smith J, La Vecchia C. Epidemiology and aetiology of gestational trophoblastic diseases. Lancet Oncol 2003;4:670-8.
50. Palmer JR. Advances in the epidemiology of gestational trophoblastic disease. J Reprod Med 1994;39:155-62.
51. Martin PM. High frequency of hydatidiform mole in native Alaskans. Int J Gynaecol Obstet 1978;15:395-6.
52. Kim SJ, Bae SN, Kim JH, et al. Epidemiology and time trends of gestational trophoblastic disease in Korea. Int J Gynaecol Obstet 1998;60(Suppl 1):S33-8.
53. Sebire NJ, Foskett M, Fisher RA, Rees H, Seckl M, Newlands E. Risk of partial and complete hydatidiform molar pregnancy in relation to maternal age. BJOG 2002;109:99–102.
54. Altman AD, Bentley B, Murray S, Bentley JR. Maternal age-related rates of gestational trophoblastic disease. Obstet Gynecol 2008;112(Pt 1):244-50.
55. Parazzini F, La Vecchia C, Pampallona S. Parental age and risk of complete and partial hydatidiform mole. Br J Obstet Gynaecol 1986;93:582-5.
56. Brinton LA, Bracken MB, Connelly RR. Choriocarcinoma incidence in the United States. Am J Epidemiol 1986;123:1094-100.
57. Smith HO, Qualls CR, Prairie BA, Padilla LA, Rayburn WF, Key CR. Trends in gestational choriocarcinoma: a 27-year perspective. Obstet Gynecol 2003;102:978-87.
58. Savage PM, Sita-Lumsden A, Dickson S, et al. The relationship of maternal age to molar pregnancy incidence, risks for chemotherapy and subsequent pregnancy outcome. J Obstet Gynaecol 2013;33:406-11.
59. Sebire NJ, Fisher RA, Foskett M, Rees H, Seckl MJ, Newlands ES. Risk of recurrent hydatidiform mole and subsequent pregnancy outcome following complete or partial hydatidiform molar pregnancy. BJOG 2003;110:22-6.
60. Eagles N, Sebire NJ, Short D, Savage PM, Seckl MJ, Fisher RA. Risk of recurrent molar pregnancies following complete and partial hydatidiform moles. Hum Reprod 2015;30:2055-63.
61. Fisher RA, Hodges MD, Newlands ES. Familial recurrent hydatidiform mole: a review. J Reprod Med 2004;49:595-601.
62. Sasaki M, Fukuschima T, Makino S. Some aspects of the chromosome constitution of hydatidiform moles and normal chorionic villi. Gan 1962;53:101-6.
63. Makino S, Sasaki MS, Fukuschima T. Cytological studies of tumors. XLI. Chromosal instiability in human chorionic. Okajimas Folia Anat Jpn 1965;40:439-65.
64. Makino S, Sasaki MS, Fukuschima T. Triploid chromosome constitution in human chorionic lesions. Lancet 1964;2:1273-5.
65. Vassilakos P, Kajii T. Letter: hydatidiform mole: two entities. Lancet 1976;1:259.
66. Vassilakos P, Riotton G, Kajii T. Hydatidiform mole: two entities. A morphologic and cytogenetic study with some clinical consideration. Am J Obstet Gynecol 1977;127:167-70.
67. Lawler SD, Pickthall VJ, Fisher RA, Povey S, Evans MW, Szulman AE. Genetic studies of complete and partial hydatidiform moles. Lancet 1979;2:580.
68. Kajii T, Ohama K. Androgenetic origin of hydatidiform mole. Nature 1977;268:633-4.
69. Wake N, Takagi N, Sasaki M. Androgenesis as a cause of hydatidiform mole. J Natl Cancer Inst 1978;60:51-7.
70. Jacobs PA, Wilson CM, Sprenkle JA, Rosenshein NB, Migeon BR. Mechanism of origin of complete hydatidiform moles. Nature 1980;286:714-6.
71. Jacobs PA, Hassold TJ, Matsuyama AM, Newlands IM. Chromosome constitution of gestational trophoblastic disease. Lancet 1978;2:49.
72. Lawler SD, Povey S, Fisher RA, Pickthall VJ. Genetic studies on hydatidiform moles. II. The origin of complete moles. Ann Hum Genet 1982;46(Pt 3):209-22.
73. Ohama K, Kajii T, Okamoto E, et al. Dispermic origin of xy hydatidiform moles. Nature 1981;292:551-2.
74. Surti U, Szulman AE, O'Brien S. Dispermic origin and clinical outcome of three complete hydatidiform moles with 46,xy karyotype. Am J Obstet Gynecol 1982;144:84-7.

75. Kovacs BW, Shahbahrami B, Tast DE, Curtin JP. Molecular genetic analysis of complete hydatidiform moles. Cancer Genet Cytogenet 1991;54:143-52.
76. Fisher RA, Povey S, Jeffreys AJ, Martin CA, Patel I, Lawler SD. Frequency of heterozygous complete hydatidiform moles, estimated by locus-specific minisatellite and y chromosome-specific probes. Hum Genet 1989;82:259-63.
77. Golubovsky MD. Postzygotic diploidization of triploids as a source of unusual cases of mosaicism, chimerism and twinning. Hum Reprod 2003;18:236-42.
78. Szulman AE, Surti U. The syndromes of hydatidiform mole. I. Cytogenetic and morphologic correlations. Am J Obstet Gynecol 1978;131:665-71.
79. Jacobs PA, Hunt PA, Matsuura JS, Wilson CC, Szulman AE. Complete and partial hydatidiform mole in Hawaii: cytogenetics, morphology and epidemiology. Br J Obstet Gynaecol 1982;89:258-66.
80. Jacobs PA, Angell RR, Buchanan IM, Hassold TJ, Matsuyama AM, Manuel B. The origin of human triploids. Ann Hum Genet 1978;42:49-57.
81. Kajii T, Niikawa N. Origin of triploidy and tetraploidy in man: 11 cases with chromosomes markers. Cytogenet Cell Genet 1977;18:109-25.
82. Lawler SD, Fisher RA, Pickthall VJ, Povey S, Evans MW. Genetic studies on hydatidiform moles. I. The origin of partial moles. Cancer Genet Cytogenet 1982;5:309-20.
83. Genest DR. Partial hydatidiform mole: clinicopathological features, differential diagnosis, ploidy and molecular studies, and gold standards for diagnosis. Int J Gynecol Pathol 2001;20:315-22.
84. Genest DR, Ruiz RE, Weremowicz S, Berkowitz RS, Goldstein DP, Dorfman DM. Do nontriploid partial hydatidiform moles exist? A histologic and flow cytometric reevaluation of nontriploid specimens. J Reprod Med 2002;47:363-8.
85. Zaragoza MV, Surti U, Redline RW, Millie E, Chakravarti A, Hassold TJ. Parental origin and phenotype of triploidy in spontaneous abortions: predominance of diandry and association with the partial hydatidiform mole. Am J Hum Genet 2000;66:1807-20.
86. Lawler SD, Fisher RA, Dent J. A prospective genetic study of complete and partial hydatidiform moles. Am J Obstet Gynecol 1991;164(5 Pt 1):1270-7.
87. Vejerslev LO, Fisher RA, Surti U, Walke N. Hydatidiform mole: cytogenetically unusual cases and their implications for the present classification. Am J Obstet Gynecol 1987;157:180-4.
88. Sarno AP Jr, Moorman AJ, Kalousek DK. Partial molar pregnancy with fetal survival: an unusual example of confined placental mosaicism. Obstet Gynecol 1993;82(4 Pt 2 Suppl):716-9.
89. Zhang P, McGinniss MJ, Sawai S, Benirschke K. Diploid/triploid mosaic placenta with fetus. Towards a better understanding of "partial moles." Early Hum Dev 2000;60:1-11.
90. Ford JH, Brown JK, Lew WY, Peters GB. Diploid complete hydatidiform mole, mosaic for normally fertilized cells and androgenetic homozygous cells. Case report. Br J Obstet Gynaecol 1986;93:1181-6.
91. Makrydimas G, Sebire NJ, Thornton SE, Zagorianakou N, Lolis D, Fisher RA. Complete hydatidiform mole and normal live birth: a novel case of confined placental mosaicism: case report. Hum Reprod 2002;17:2459-63.
92. Kaiser-Rogers KA, McFadden DE, Livasy CA, et al. Androgenetic/biparental mosaicism causes placental mesenchymal dysplasia. J Med Genet 2006;43:187-92.
93. Hoffner L, Dunn J, Esposito N, Macpherson T, Surti U. P57KIP2 immunostaining and molecular cytogenetics: combined approach aids in diagnosis of morphologically challenging cases with molar phenotype and in detecting androgenetic cell lines in mosaic/chimeric conceptions. Hum Pathol 2008;39:63-72.
94. Robinson WP, Lauzon JL, Innes AM, Lim K, Arsovska S, McFadden DE. Origin and outcome of pregnancies affected by androgenetic/biparental chimerism. Hum Reprod 2007;22:1114-22.
95. Surani MA, Barton SC, Norris ML. Development of reconstituted mouse eggs suggests imprinting of the genome during gametogenesis. Nature 1984;308:548-50.
96. Barton SC, Surani MA, Norris ML. Role of paternal and maternal genomes in mouse development. Nature. 1984;311:374-6.
97. Castrillon DH, Sun D, Weremowicz S, Fisher RA, Crum CP, Genest DR. Discrimination of complete hydatidiform mole from its mimics by immunohistochemistry of the paternally imprinted gene product p57KIP2. Am J Surg Pathol 2001;25:1225-30.
98. McConnell TG, Murphy KM, Hafez M, Vang R, Ronnett BM. Diagnosis and subclassification of hydatidiform moles using p57 immunohistochemistry and molecular genotyping: validation and prospective analysis in routine and consultation practice settings with development of an algorithmic approach. Am J Surg Pathol 2009;33:805-17.
99. Sebire NJ, Rees HC, Peston D, Seckl MJ, Newlands ES, Fisher RA. P57(KIP2) immunohistochemical staining of gestational trophoblastic tumours does not identify the type of the causative pregnancy. Histopathology 2004;45:135-41.

100. Fisher RA, Hodges MD, Rees HC, et al. The maternally transcribed gene p57(KIP2) (CDNK1C) is abnormally expressed in both androgenetic and biparental complete hydatidiform moles. Hum Mol Genet 2002;11:3267-72.
101. Sebire NJ, Lindsay I. P57KIP2 immunostaining in the diagnosis of complete versus partial hydatidiform moles. Histopathology 2006;48:873-4.
102. Fukunaga M. Immunohistochemical characterization of p57(KIP2) expression in early hydatidiform moles. Hum Pathol 2002;33:1188-92.
103. Xiong Y, Cao Y, Li H. Low and maternal-specific expression of p57KIP2 in hydatidiform mole and its clinical implication. J Huazhong Univ Sci Technol Med Sci 2002;22:121-2, 157.
104. Helwani MN, Seoud M, Zahed L, Zaatari G, Khalil A, Slim R. A familial case of recurrent hydatidiform molar pregnancies with biparental genomic contribution. Hum Genet 1999; 105:112-5.
105. Fallahian M, Foroughi F, Vasei M, et al. Outcome of subsequent pregnancies in familial molar pregnancy. Int J Fertil Steril 2013;7:63-6.
106. Fallahian M. Familial gestational trophoblastic disease. Placenta 2003;24:797-9.
107. Parazzini F, La Vecchia C, Franceschi S, Mangili G. Familial trophoblastic disease: case report. Am J Obstet Gynecol 1984;149:382-3.
108. Fisher RA, Paradinas FJ, Soteriou BA, Foskett M, Newlands ES. Diploid hydatidiform moles with fetal red blood cells in molar villi. 2 - genetics. J Pathol 1997;181:189-95.
109. Fisher RA, Khatoon R, Paradinas FJ, Roberts AP, Newlands ES. Repetitive complete hydatidiform mole can be biparental in origin and either male or female. Hum Reprod 2000;15:594-8.
110. Moglabey YB, Kircheisen R, Seoud M, El Mogharbel N, Van den Veyver I, Slim R. Genetic mapping of a maternal locus responsible for familial hydatidiform moles. Hum Mol Genet 1999;8:667-71.
111. Nguyen NM, Slim R. Genetics and epigenetics of recurrent hydatidiform moles: basic science and genetic counselling. Curr Obstet Gynecol Rep 2014;3:55-64.
112. Murdoch S, Djuric U, Mazhar B, et al. Mutations in NALP7 cause recurrent hydatidiform moles and reproductive wastage in humans. Nat Genet 2006;38:300-2.
113. Qian J, Deveault C, Bagga R, Xie X, Slim R. Women heterozygous for NALP7/NLRP7 mutations are at risk for reproductive wastage: report of two novel mutations. Hum Mutat 2007;28:741.
114. Wang CM, Dixon PH, Decordova S, et al. Identification of 13 novel NLRP7 mutations in 20 families with recurrent hydatidiform mole; missense mutations cluster in the leucine-rich region. J Med Genet 2009;46:569-75.
115. Dixon PH, Trongwongsa P, Abu-Hayyah S, et al. Mutations in NLRP7 are associated with diploid biparental hydatidiform moles, but not androgenetic complete moles. J Med Genet 2012;49:206-11.
116. Fallahian M, Sebire NJ, Savage PM, Seckl MJ, Fisher RA. Mutations in NLRP7 and KHDC3L confer a complete hydatidiform mole phenotype on digynic triploid conceptions. Hum Mutat 2013;34:301-8.
117. Parry DA, Logan CV., Hayward BE, et al. Mutations causing familial biparental hydatidiform mole implicate C6orf221 as a possible regulator of genomic imprinting in the human oocyte. Am J Hum Genet 2011;89:451-8.
118. Manokhina I, Hanna CW, Stephenson MD, McFadden DE, Robinson WP. Maternal NLRP7 and C6orf221 variants are not a common risk factor for androgenetic moles, triploidy and recurrent miscarriage. Mol Hum Reprod 2013;19:539-44.
119. Andreasen L, Bolund L, Niemann I, Hansen ES, Sunde L. Mosaic moles and non-familial biparental moles are not caused by mutations in NLRP7, NLRP2 or C6orf221. Mol Hum Reprod 2012;18:593-8.
120. Fisher RA, Tommasi A, Short D, Kaur B, Seckl MJ, Sebire NJ. Clinical utility of selective molecular genotyping for diagnosis of partial hydatidiform mole; a retrospective study from a regional trophoblastic disease unit. J Clin Pathol 2014;67:980-4.
121. Sebire NJ. Histopathological diagnosis of hydatidiform mole: contemporary features and clinical implications. Fetal Pediatr Pathol 2010;29:1-16.
122. Murphy KM, Ronnett BM. Molecular analysis of hydatidiform moles: Utilizing p57 immunohistochemistry and molecular genotyping to refine morphologic diagnosis. Pathol Case Rev 2010;15:126-34.
123. Hui P, Buza N, Murphy KM, Ronnett BM. Hydatidiform moles: genetic basis and precision diagnosis. Annu Rev Pathol 2017;12:449-85.
124. Ronnett BM, DeScipio C, Murphy KM. Hydatidiform moles: ancillary techniques to refine diagnosis. Int J Gynecol Pathol 2011;30:101-16.
125. Murphy KM, McConnell TG, Hafez MJ, Vang R, Ronnett BM. Molecular genotyping of hydatidiform moles: analytic validation of a multiplex short tandem repeat assay. J Mol Diagn 2009;11:598-605.
126. Jeffers MD, Michie BA, Oakes SJ, Gillan JE. Comparison of ploidy analysis by flow cytometry and image analysis in hydatidiform mole and non-molar abortion. Histopathology 1995;27:415-21.

127. Genest DR, Dorfman DM, Castrillon DH. Ploidy and imprinting in hydatidiform moles. Complementary use of flow cytometry and immunohistochemistry of the imprinted gene product p57KIP2 to assist molar classification. J Reprod Med 2002;47:342-6.

128. Lage JM, Driscoll SG, Yavner DL, Olivier AP, Mark SD, Weinberg DS. Hydatidiform moles. Application of flow cytometry in diagnosis. Am J Clin Pathol 1988;89:596-600.

129. Lage JM, Popek EJ. The role of DNA flow cytometry in evaluation of partial and complete hydatidiform moles and hydropic abortions. Semin Diagn Pathol 1993;10:267-74.

130. Topalovski M, Hankin RC, Michael C, Hunter SV, Edwards AM, Chen JC. Ploidy analysis of products of conception by image and flow cytometry with cytogenetic correlation. Am J Clin Pathol 1995;103:409-14.

131. Fukunaga M, Endo Y, Ushigome S. Flow cytometric and clinicopathologic study of 197 hydatidiform moles with special reference to the significance of cytometric aneuploidy and literature review. Cytometry 1995;22:135-8.

132. Yver M, Carles D, Bloch B, Bioulac-Sage P, Martin Negrier ML. Determination of DNA ploidy by fluorescence in situ hybridization (FISH) in hydatidiform moles: evaluation of FISH on isolated nuclei. Hum Pathol 2004;35:752-8.

133. Sumithran E, Cheah PL, Susil BJ, Looi LM. Problems in the histological assessment of hydatidiform moles: a study on consensus diagnosis and ploidy status by fluorescent in situ hybridisation. Pathology 1996;28:311-5.

134. Saji F, Tokugawa Y, Kimura T, et al. A new approach using DNA fingerprinting for the determination of androgenesis as a cause of hydatidiform mole. Placenta 10:399-405.

135. Takahashi H, Kanazawa K, Ikarashi T, Sudo N, Tanaka K. Discrepancy in the diagnoses of hydatidiform mole by macroscopic and microscopic findings and the deoxyribonucleic acid fingerprint method. Am J Obstet Gynecol 1990;163(Pt 1):112-3.

136. Ko TM, Hsieh CY, Ho HN, Hsieh FJ, Lee TY. Restriction fragment length polymorphism analysis to study the genetic origin of complete hydatidiform mole. Am J Obstet Gynecol 1991;164:901-6.

137. Bell KA, van Deerlin V, Addya K, Clevenger CV, Van Deerlin PG, Leonard DG. Molecular genetic testing from paraffin-embedded tissue distinguishes nonmolar hydropic abortion from hydatidiform mole. Mol Diagn 1999;4:11-9.

138. Lane SA, Taylor GR, Ozols B, Quirke P. Diagnosis of complete molar pregnancy by microsatellites in archival material. J Clin Pathol 1993;46:346-8.

139. Vang R, Gupta M, Wu LS, et al. Diagnostic reproducibility of hydatidiform moles: ancillary techniques (p57 immunohistochemistry and molecular genotyping) improve morphologic diagnosis. Am J Surg Pathol 2012;36:443-53.

140. Fisher RA, Savage PM, MacDermott C, et al. The impact of molecular genetic diagnosis on the management of women with hcg-producing malignancies. Gynecol Oncol 2007;107:413-9.

141. Baasanjav B, Usui H, Kihara M, et al. The risk of post-molar gestational trophoblastic neoplasia is higher in heterozygous than in homozygous complete hydatidiform moles. Hum Reprod 2010;25:1183-91.

142. Bynum J, Murphy KM, DeScipio C, et al. Invasive complete hydatidiform moles: analysis of a case series with genotyping. Int J Gynecol Pathol 2016;35:134-41.

143. Wake N, Tanaka K, Chapman V, Matsui S, Sandberg AA. Chromosome and cellular origin of choriocarcinoma. Cancer Res 1981;41:3137-43.

144. Sasaki S, Katayama PK, Roesler M, Pattillo RA, Mattingly RF, Ohkawa K. Cytogenetic analysis of choriocarcinoma cell lines. Nihon Sanka Fujinka Gakkai Zasshi 1982;34:2253-6.

145. Sheppard DM, Fisher RA, Lawler SD. Karyotypic analysis and chromosome polymorphisms in four choriocarcinoma cell lines. Cancer Genet Cytogenet 1985;16:251-8.

146. Asanoma K, Kato H, Inoue T, Matsuda T, Wake N. Analysis of a candidate gene associated with growth suppression of choriocarcinoma and differentiation of trophoblasts. J Reprod Med 2004;49:617-26.

147. Hui P, Wang HL, Chu P, et al. Absence of Y chromosome in human placental site trophoblastic tumor. Mod Pathol 2007;20:1055-60.

148. Zhao S, Sebire NJ, Kaur B, Seckl MJ, Fisher RA. Molecular genotyping of placental site and epithelioid trophoblastic tumours; female predominance. Gynecol Oncol 2016;142:501-7.

149. Braunstein GD, Vaitukaitis JL, Carbone PP, Ross GT. Ectopic production of human chorionic gonadotrophin by neoplasms. Ann Intern Med 1973;78:39-45.

150. Stenman UH, Alfthan H, Hotakainen K. Human chorionic gonadotropin in cancer. Clin Biochem 2004;37:549-61.

151. Fisher RA, Newlands ES, Jeffreys AJ, et al. Gestational and nongestational trophoblastic tumors distinguished by DNA analysis. Cancer 1992;69:839-45.

152. Arima T, Imamura T, Sakuragi N, et al. Malignant trophoblastic neoplasms with different modes of origin. Cancer Genet Cytogenet 1995;85:5-15.

153. Suzuki T, Goto S, Nawa A, Kurauchi O, Saito M, Tomoda Y. Identification of the pregnancy responsible for gestational trophoblastic disease by DNA analysis. Obstet Gynecol 1993;82(Pt 1):629-34.
154. Fisher RA, Soteriou BA, Meredith L, Paradinas FJ, Newlands ES. Previous hydatidiform mole identified as the causative pregnancy of choriocarcinoma following birth of normal twins. Int J Gynecol Cancer 1995;5:64-70.
155. Sebire NJ, Foskett M, Fisher RA, Lindsay I, Seckl MJ. Persistent gestational trophoblastic disease is rarely, if ever, derived from non-molar first-trimester miscarriage. Med Hypotheses 2005;64:689-93.
156. Cole LA. HCG, five independent molecules. Clin Chim Acta 2012;413:48-65.
157. Cole LA. New discoveries on the biology and detection of human chorionic gonadotropin. Reprod Biol Endocrinol 2009;7:8.
158. Cole LA, Sutton JM, Higgins TN, Cembrowski GS. Between-method variation in human chorionic gonadotropin test results. Clin Chem 2004;50:874-82.
159. Burler SA, Khanlian SA, Cole LA. Detection of early pregnancy forms of human chorionic gonadotropin by home pregnancy test devices. Clin Chem 2001;47:2131-6.
160. Cole LA. HCG and hyperglycosylated hCG in the establishment and evolution of hemochorial placentation. J Reprod Immunol 2009;82:112-8.
161. Cole LA. Proportion hyperglycosylated hCG: a new test for discriminating gestational trophoblastic diseases. Int J Gynecol Cancer 2014;24:1709-14.
162. Cole LA, Muller CY. Hyperglycosylated hCG in the management of quiescent and chemorefractory gestational trophoblastic diseases. Gynecol Oncol 2010;116:3-9.
163. Cole LA, Khanlian SA, Muller CY, Giddings A, Kohorn E, Berkowitz R. Gestational trophoblastic diseases: 3. Human chorionic gonadotropin-free beta-subunit, a reliable marker of placental site trophoblastic tumors. Gynecol Oncol 2006;102:160-4.
164. Kardana A, Cole LA. Human chorionic gonadotropin beta-subunit nicking enzymes in pregnancy and cancer patient serum. J Clin Endocrinol Metab 1994;79:761-7.
165. Cole LA, Khanlian SA. Inappropriate management of women with persistent low hCG results. J Reprod Med 2004;49:423-32.
166. Cole LA, Khanlian SA, Giddings A, et al. Gestational trophoblastic diseases: 4. Presentation with persistent low positive human chorionic gonadotropin test results. Gynecol Oncol 2006;102:165-72.
167. Kohorn EI. Persistent low-level "real" human chorionic gonadotropin: a clinical challenge and a therapeutic dilemma. Gynecol Oncol 2002;85:315-20.
168. Rinne K, Shahabi S, Cole L. Following metastatic placental site trophoblastic tumor with urine beta-core fragment. Gynecol Oncol 1999;74:302-3.
169. Mueller UW, Hawes CS, Wright AE, et al. Isolation of fetal trophoblast cells from peripheral blood of pregnant women. Lancet 1990;336:197-200.
170. Covone AE, Mutton D, Johnson PM, Adinolfi M. Trophoblast cells in peripheral blood from pregnant women. Lancet 1984;2:841-3.
171. Hawes CS, Suskin HA, Petropoulos A, Latham SE, Mueller UW. A morphologic study of trophoblast isolated from peripheral blood of pregnant women. Am J Obstet Gynecol 1994;170(Pt 1):1297-300.
172. Sun SY, Melamed A, Goldstein DP, et al. Changing presentation of complete hydatidiform mole at the New England Trophoblastic Disease Center over the past three decades: does early diagnosis alter risk for gestational trophoblastic neoplasia? Gynecol Oncol 2015;138:46-9.
173. Sun SY, Melamed A, Joseph NT, et al. Clinical presentation of complete hydatidiform mole and partial hydatidiform mole at a Regional Trophoblastic Disease Center in the United States over the past 2 decades. Int J Gynecol Cancer 2016;26:367-70.
174. Soto-Wright V, Bernstein M, Goldstein DP, Berkowitz RS. The changing clinical presentation of complete molar pregnancy. Obstet Gynecol 1995;86:775-9.
175. Mangili G, Garavaglia E, Cavoretto P, Gentile C, Scarfone G, Rabaiotti E. Clinical presentation of hydatidiform mole in northern Italy: has it changed in the last 20 years? Am J Obstet Gynecol 2008;198:302.
176. Paradinas FJ, Browne P, Fisher RA, Foskett M, Bagshawe KD, Newlands E. A clinical, histopathological and flow cytometric study of 149 complete moles, 146 partial moles and 107 non-molar hydropic abortions. Histopathology 1996;28:101-10.
177. Xue WC, Guan XY, Ngan HY, Shen DH, Khoo US, Cheung AN. Malignant placental site trophoblastic tumor: a cytogenetic study using comparative genomic hybridization and chromosome in situ hybridization. Cancer 2002;94:2288-94.
178. Shen DH, Khoo US, Ngan HYS, et al. Coexisting epithelioid trophoblastic tumor and choriocarcinoma of the uterus following a chemoresistant hydatidiform mole. Arch Pathol Lab Med 2003;127:291-3.

179. Fowler DJ, Lindsay I, Seckl MJ, Sebire NJ. Routine pre-evacuation ultrasound diagnosis of hydatidiform mole: experience of more than 1000 cases from a regional referral center. Ultrasound Obstet Gynecol 2006;27:56-60.

180. Seckl MJ, Fisher RA, Salerno G, et al. Choriocarcinoma and partial hydatidiform moles. Lancet 2000;356:36-9.

181. Seckl MJ, Gillmore R, Foskett M, Sebire NJ, Rees H, Newlands ES. Routine terminations of pregnancy—should we screen for gestational trophoblastic neoplasia? Lancet 2004;364:705-7.

182. Pezeshki M, Hancock BW, Silcocks P, et al. The role of repeat uterine evacuation in the management of persistent gestational trophoblastic disease. Gynecol Oncol 2004;95:423-9.

183. Seckl MJ, Dhillon T, Dancey G, et al. Increased gestational age at evacuation of a complete hydatidiform mole: does it correlate with increased risk of requiring chemotherapy? J Reprod Med 2004;49:527-30.

184. Banet N, DeScipio C, Murphy KM, et al. Characteristics of hydatidiform moles: analysis of a prospective series with p57 immunohistochemistry and molecular genotyping. Mod Pathol 2014;27:238-54.

185. Ronnett BM. Hydatidiform moles: ancillary techniques to refine diagnosis. Arch Pathol Lab Med 2018;142:1485-502.

186. Sebire NJ, Makrydimas G, Agnantis NJ, Zagorianakou N, Rees H, Fisher RA. Updated diagnostic criteria for partial and complete hydatidiform moles in early pregnancy. Anticancer Res 2003;23:1723-8.

187. Sebire NJ, Fisher RA, Rees HC. Histopathological diagnosis of partial and complete hydatidiform mole in the first trimester of pregnancy. Pediatr Dev Pathol 2002;6:69-77.

188. Sebire NJ, Savage PM, Seckl MJ, Fisher RA. Histopathological features of biparental complete hydatidiform moles in women with NLRP7 mutations. Placenta 2013;34:50-6.

189. Genest DR, Laborde O, Berkowitz RS, Goldstein DP, Bernstein MR, Lage J. A clinicopathologic study of 153 cases of complete hydatidiform mole (1980-1990): histologic grade lacks prognostic significance. Obstet Gynecol 1991;78(Pt 1):402-9.

190. Petts G, Fisher RA, Short D, Lindsay I, Seckl MJ, Sebire NJ. Histopathological and immunohistochemical features of early hydatidiform mole in relation to subsequent development of persistent gestational trophoblastic disease. J Reprod Med 2014;59:213-20.

191. Hoffner L, Surti U. The genetics of gestational trophoblastic disease: a rare complication of pregnancy. Cancer Genet 2012;205:63-77.

192. Szulman AE, Surti U. The syndromes of hydatidiform mole. II. Morphologic evolution of the complete and partial mole. Am J Obstet Gynecol 1978;132:20-7.

193. Kim K, Park BH, Hong YO, Kwon HC, Robboy SJ. The villous stromal constituents of complete hydatidiform mole differ histologically in very early pregnancy from the normally developing placenta. Am J Surg Pathol 2009;33:176-85.

194. Paradinas FJ, Fisher RA. Pathology and molecular genetics of trophoblastic disease. Cur Obstet Gynaecol Rep 1995;5:6-12.

195. Dickson-González SM, García de Barriola V, Barbella-Aponte RA, Figueira L, Cortés-Charry R, Naranjo de Gómez M. Histopathologic and immunohistochemical evaluation of blood vessels in complete and partial hydatidiform mole. J Reprod Med 2006;51:933-7.

196. Zaragoza MV, Keep D, Genest DR, Hassold T, Redline RW. Early complete hydatidiform moles contain inner cell mass derivatives. Am J Med Genet 1997;70:273-7.

197. Sebire NJ, Rees H. Diagnosis of gestational trophoblastic disease in early pregnancy. Curr Diagn Pathol 2002;8:430-40.

198. Kim KR, Park BH, Hong YO, Kwon HC, Robboy SJ. The villous stromal constituents of complete hydatidiform mole differ histologically in very early pregnancy from the normally developing placenta. Am J Surg Pathol 2009;33:176-85.

199. Kim MJ, Kim KR, Ro JY, Lage JM, Lee HI. Diagnostic and pathogenetic significance of increased stromal apoptosis and incomplete vasculogenesis in complete hydatidiform moles in very early pregnancy periods. Am J Surg Pathol 2006;30:362-9.

200. Sebire NJ, Rees H, Paradinas F, et al. Extravillus endovascular implantation site trophoblast invasion is abnormal in complete versus partial molar pregnancies. Placenta 2001;22:725-8.

201. Wells M. The pathology of gestational trophoblastic disease: recent advances. Pathology 2007;39:88-96.

202. Sebire NJ, Lindsay I. Current issues in the histopathology of gestational trophoblastic tumors. Fetal Pediatr Pathol 2010;29:30-44.

203. Philipp T, Grillenberger K, Separovic ER, Philipp K, Kalousek DK. Effects of triploidy on early human development. Prenat Diagn 2004;24:276-81.

204. Doshi N, Surti U, Szulman AE. Morphologic anomalies in triploid liveborn fetuses. Hum Pathol 1983;14:716-23.

205. Leisti JT, Raivio KO, Rapola MH, Saksela EJ, Aula PP. The phenotype of human triploidy. Birth Defects Orig Artic Ser 1974;10:248-53.

206. Mittal TK, Vujanic GM, Morrissey BM, Jones A. Triploidy: antenatal sonographic features with post-mortem correlation. Prenat Diagn 1998;18:1253-62.
207. Bracken MB, Brinton LA, Hayashi K. Epidemiology of hydatidiform mole and choriocarcinoma. Epidemiol Rev 1984;6:52-75.
208. Medeiros F, Callahan MJ, Elvin JA, Dorfman DM, Berkowitz RS, Quade BJ. Intraplacental choriocarcinoma arising in a second trimester placenta with partial hydatidiform mole. Int J Gynecol Pathol 2008;27:247-51.
209. Heifetz SA, Czaja J. In situ choriocarcinoma arising in partial hydatidiform mole: implications for the risk of persistent trophoblastic disease. Pediatr Pathol 1992;12:601-11.
210. Kajii T, Ohama K, Mikamo K. Anatomic and chromosomal anomalies in 944 induced abortuses. Hum Genet 1978;43:247-58.
211. Dhadial RK, Machin AM, Tait SM. Chromosomal anomalies in spontaneously aborted human fetuses. Lancet 1970;2:20-1.
212. Choi TY, Lee HM, Park WK, Jeong SY, Moon HS. Spontaneous abortion and recurrent miscarriage: a comparison of cytogenetic diagnosis in 250 cases. Obstet Gynecol Sci 2014;57:518-25.
213. Novak R, Agamanolis D, Dasu S, et al. Histologic analysis of placental tissue in first trimester abortions. Pediatr Pathol 1988;8:477-82.
214. Honoré LH, Dill FJ, Poland BJ. Placental morphology in spontaneous human abortuses with normal and abnormal karyotypes. Teratology 1976;14:151-66.
215. Eiben B, Borgmann S, Schübbe I, Hansmann I. A cytogenetic study directly from chorionic villi of 140 spontaneous abortions. Hum Genet 1987;77:137-41.
216. Ishikawa N, Harada Y, Tokuyasu Y, Nagasaki M, Maruyama R. Re-evaluation of the histological criteria for complete hydatidiform mole: comparison with the immunohistochemical diagnosis using p57KIP2 and CD34. Biomed Res 2009;30:141-7.
217. Lage JM, Mark SD, Roberts DJ, Goldstein DP, Bernstein MR, Berkowitz RS. A flow cytometric study of 137 fresh hydropic placentas: correlation between types of hydatidiform moles and nuclear DNA ploidy. Obstet Gynecol 1992;79:403-10.
218. Carles D, Pelluard F, André G, Naudion S, Saura R. [Maze-like vascular anomaly in partial mole. Interest for the pathological diagnosis of partial mole on chorionic villous sampling]. Ann Pathol 2009;29:424-7.
219. Feist H, Caliebe A, Oates J, Sarioglu N, Hussein K. Partial hydatidiform mole with extensive angiomatoid vessel configuration in a first trimester miscarriage. Int J Gynecol Pathol 2015;34:253-6.
220. Nair K, Al-Khawari H. Invasive mole of the uterus-a rare case diagnosed by ultrasound:a case report. Med Ultrason 2014;16:175-8.
221. Okumura M, Fushida K, Pulcineli Vieira Francisco R, Schultz R, Zugaib M. Sonographic appearance of an advanced invasive mole and associated metastatic thrombus in the inferior vena cava. J Clin Ultrasound 2013;41:113-5.
222. Tanizaki Y, Nanjo S, Mizoguchi M, et al. Three cases of invasive mole arising from complete mole within very short periods. Placenta 2012;33:A109.
223. Zhou X, Chen Y, Li Y, Duan Z. Partial hydatidiform mole progression into invasive mole with lung metastasis following in vitro fertilization. Oncol Lett 2012;3:659-61.
224. Agarwal R, Alifrangis C, Everard J, et al. Management and survival of patients with FIGO high-risk gestational trophoblastic neoplasia: the U.K. experience, 1995-2010. J Reprod Med 2014;59:7-12.
225. Burton JL, Lidbury EA, Gillespie AM, et al. Over-diagnosis of hydatidiform mole in early tubal ectopic pregnancy. Histopathology 2001;38:409-17.
226. Sebire NJ, Lindsay I, Fisher RA, Savage P, Seckl MJ. Overdiagnosis of complete and partial hydatidiform mole in tubal ectopic pregnancies. Int J Gynecol Pathol 2005;24:260-4.
227. Siozos A, Sriemevan A. A case of true tubal hydatidiform mole and literature review. BMJ Case Rep 2010;2010.
228. Beena D, Teerthanath S, Jose V, Shetty J. Molar pregnancy presents as tubal ectopic pregnancy: a rare case report. J Clin Diagn Res 2016;10:ED10-1.
229. Sebire NJ, Foskett M, Paradinas FJ, et al. Outcome of twin pregnancies with complete hydatidiform mole and healthy co-twin. Lancet 2002;359:2165-6.
230. Steller MA, Genest DR, Bernstein MR, Lage JM, Goldstein DP, Berkowitz RS. Natural history of twin pregnancy with complete hydatidiform mole and coexisting fetus. Obstet Gynecol 1994;83:35-42.
231. Sebire NJ, Seckl MJ. Immunohistochemical staining for diagnosis and prognostic assessment of hydatidiform moles: current evidence and future directions. J Reprod Med 2010;55:236-46.
232. Rice LW, Genest DR, Berkowitz RS, Goldstein DP, Bernstein MR, Redline RW. Pathologic features of sharp curettings in complete hydatidiform mole. Predictors of persistent gestational trophoblastic disease. J Reprod Med 1991;36:17-20.
233. Sarmadi S, Izadi-Mood N, Abbasi A, Sanii S. P57KIP2 immunohistochemical expression: a useful diagnostic tool in discrimination between complete hydatidiform mole and its mimics. Arch Gynecol Obstet 2011;283:743-8.

234. Banet N, DeScipio C, Murphy KM, et al. Characteristics of hydatidiform moles: analysis of a prospective series with p57 immunohistochemistry and molecular genotyping. Mod Pathol 2014;27:238-54.
235. Lewis GH, DeScipio C, Murphy KM, et al. Characterization of androgenetic/biparental mosaic/chimeric conceptions, including those with a molar component: morphology, p57 immnohistochemistry, molecular genotyping, and risk of persistent gestational trophoblastic disease. Int J Gynecol Pathol 2013;32:199-214.
236. Gupta M, Vang R, Yemelyanova AV, et al. Diagnostic reproducibility of hydatidiform moles: ancillary techniques (p57 immunohistochemistry and molecular genotyping) improve morphologic diagnosis for both recently trained and experienced gynecologic pathologists. Am J Surg Pathol 2012;36:1747-60.
237. Shih IM, Mazur MT, Kurman RJ. Gestational trophoblastic tumors and related tumor-like lesions. In: Kurman RJ, Ellenson LH, Ronnett BM, eds. Blaustein's pathology of the female genital tract, 6th ed. New York: Springer; 2010:1075-135.
238. Paradinas FJ, Sebire NJ, Fisher RA, et al. Pseudo-partial moles: placental stem vessel hydrops and the association with Beckwith-Wiedemann syndrome and complete moles. Histopathology 2001;39:447-54.
239. Cohen MC, Roper EC, Sebire NJ, Stanek J, Anumba DO. Placental mesenchymal dysplasia associated with fetal aneuploidy. Prenat Diagn 2005;25:187-92.
240. Moscoso G, Jauniaux E, Hustin J. Placental vascular anomaly with diffuse mesenchymal stem villous hyperplasia. A new clinico-pathological entity? Pathol Res Pract 1991;187:324-8.
241. Ngan HY, Seckl MJ, Berkowitz RS, et al. Update on the diagnosis and management of gestational trophoblastic disease. Int J Gynaecol Obstet 2018;143(Suppl 2):79-85
242. Alifrangis C, Agarwal R, Short D, et al. EMA/CO for high-risk gestational trophoblastic neoplasia: good outcomes with induction low-dose etoposide-cisplatin and genetic analysis. J Clin Oncol 2013;31:280-6.
243. Sita-Lumsden A, Short D, Lindsay I, et al. Treatment outcomes for 618 women with gestational trophoblastic tumours following a molar pregnancy at the Charing Cross Hospital, 2000-2009. Br J Cancer 2012;107:1810-4.
244. Lurain JR, Brewer JI, Torok EE, Halpern B. Natural history of hydatidiform mole after primary evacuation. Am J Obstet Gynecol 1983;145:591-5.
245. Lipata F, Parkash V, Talmor M, et al. Precise DNA genotyping diagnosis of hydatidiform mole. Obstet Gynecol 2010;115:784-94.
246. Buckley JD. The epidemiology of molar pregnancy and choriocarcinoma. Clin Obstet Gynecol 1984;27:153-9.
247. Zhao J, Xiang Y, Wan XR, Feng FZ, Cui QC, Yang XY. Molecular genetic analyses of choriocarcinoma. Placenta 2009;30:816-20.
248. Zhao J, Xiang Y, Wan X, Feng FZ, Cui QC, Yang XY. [Genetic genesis of choriocarcinoma.] Zhonghua Fu Chan Ke Za Zhi 2010;45:35-40. [Chinese]
249. Loukovaara M, Pukkala E, Lehtovirta P, Leminen A. Epidemiology of choriocarcinoma in Finland, 1953 to 1999. Gynecol Oncol 2004;92:252-5.
250. Ryu N, Ogawa M, Matsui H, Usui H, Shozu M. The clinical characteristics and early detection of postpartum choriocarcinoma. Int J Gynecol Cancer 2015;25:926-30.
251. Tidy JA, Rustin GJ, Newlands ES, et al. Presentation and management of choriocarcinoma after nonmolar pregnancy. Br J Obstet Gynaecol 1995;102:715-9.
252. Nugent D, Hassadia A, Everard J, Hancock BW, Tidy JA. Postpartum choriocarcinoma presentation, management and survival. J Reprod Med 2006;51:819-24.
253. Bonnet L, Raposo N, Blot-Souletie N, et al. Stroke caused by a pulmonary vein thrombosis revealing a metastatic choriocarcinoma. Circulation 2015;131:2093-4.
254. Dadlani R, Furtado SV, Ghosal N, Prasanna KV, Hegde AS. Unusual clinical and radiological presentation of metastatic choriocarcinoma to the brain and long-term remission following emergency craniotomy and adjuvant EMA-CO chemotherapy. J Cancer Res Ther 2010;6:552-6.
255. Braun-Parvez L, Charlin E, Caillard S, et al. Gestational choriocarcinoma transmission following multiorgan donation. Am J Transplant 2010;10:2541-6.
256. Arora A, Thawrani A, Kirnake V, et al. An unusual cause of lower GI bleeding in a young woman: metastatic gestational choriocarcinoma. Gastrointest Endosc 2013;77:152-4.
257. Cho EB, Byun JM, Jeong DH, et al. Metastatic choriocarcinoma as initial presentation of small bowel perforation in absence of primary uterine lesion: a case report. Tumori 2016;102:(suppl 2).
258. Dhrami-Gavazi E, Lo C, Patel P, Galic V, Pareja F, Kazim M. Gestational choriocarcinoma metastasis to the extraocular muscle: a case report. Ophthalmic Plast Reconstr Surg 2014;30:e75-7.

259. Hazan A, Katz MS, Leder H, Blace N, Szlechter M. Choroidal metastases of choriocarcinoma. Retin Cases Brief Rep 2014;8:95-6.
260. Heil R, Tran T, Stawick L, Herschman B. Metastatic choriocarcinoma of the small intestine presenting as refractory anemia and melena. ACG Case Rep J 2015;2:131-2.
261. Mukherjee S, Nagarsenkar A, Chandra S, Sahasrabhojanee M. Primary choriocarcinoma metastasizing to skeletal muscles, presenting as an abdominal wall mass: a rare presentation. J Nat Sci Biol Med 2013;4:497-9.
262. Yazgan Y, Öncü K, Kaplan M, et al. Upper gastrointestinal bleeding as an initial manifestation of metastasis secondary to choriocarcinoma. Turk J Gastroenterol 2013;24:565-7.
263. Osathanondh R, Berkowitz RS, de Cholnoky C, Smith BS, Goldstein DP, Tyson JE. Hormonal measurements in patients with theca lutein cysts and gestational trophoblastic disease. J Reprod Med 1986;31:179-83.
264. Montz FJ, Schlaerth JB, Morrow CP. The natural history of theca lutein cysts. Obstet Gynecol 1988;72:247-51.
265. Requard CK, Mettler FA Jr. The use of ultrasound in the evaluation of trophoblastic disease and its response to therapy. Radiology 1980;135:419-222.
266. Deligdisch L, Driscoll SG, Goldstein DP. Gestational trophoblastic neoplasms: morphologic correlates of therapeutic response. Am J Obstet Gynecol 1978;130:801-6.
267. Shih IeM. Trophoblastic vasculogenic mimicry in gestational choriocarcinoma. Mod Pathol 2011;24:646-52.
268. Elston CW, Bagshawe KD. The diagnosis of trophoblastic tumours from uterine curettings. J Clin Pathol 1972;25:111-8.
269. Sebire NJ, Lindsay I, Fisher RA, Seckl MJ. Intraplacental choriocarcinoma: experience from a tertiary referral center and relationship with infantile choriocarcinoma. Fetal Pediatr Pathol 2005;24:21-9.
270. Jacques SM, Qureshi F. Intraplacental choriocarcinoma without associated maternal or fetal metastases. Int J Gynecol Pathol 2011;30:364-5.
271. Bolze PA, Weber B, Fisher RA, Seckl MJ, Golfier F. First confirmation by genotyping of transplacental choriocarcinoma transmission. Am J Obstet Gynecol 2013;209:e4-6.
272. Kanehira K, Starostik P, Kasznica J, Khoury T. Primary intraplacental gestational choriocarcinoma: histologic and genetic analyses. Int J Gynecol Pathol 2013;32:71-5.
273. Brudie LA, Ahmad S, Radi MJ, Finkler NJ. Metastatic choriocarcinoma in a viable intrauterine pregnancy treated with EMA-CO in the third trimester: a case report. J Reprod Med 56:359-63.
274. Liu J, Guo L. Intraplacental choriocarcinoma in a term placenta with both maternal and infantile metastases: a case report and review of the literature. Gynecol Oncol 2006;103:1147-51.
275. Jiao L, Ghorani E, Sebire NJ, Seckl MJ. Intraplacental choriocarcinoma: systematic review and management guidance. Gynecol Oncol 2016;141:624-31.
276. Boynukalin FK, Erol Z, Aral AI, Boyar IH. Gestational choriocarcinoma arising in a tubal ectopic pregnancy: case report. Eur J Gynaecol Oncol 2011;32:592-3.
277. Karaman E, Çetin O, Kolusari A, Bayram I. Primary tubal choriocarcinoma presented as ruptured ectopic pregnancy. J Clin Diagn Res 2015;9:QD17-8.
278. Mehrotra S, Singh U, Goel M, Chauhan S. Ectopic tubal choriocarcinoma: a rarity. BMJ Case Rep 2012;2012.
279. Nakayama M, Namba A, Yasuda M, Hara M, Ishihara O, Itakura A. Gestational choriocarcinoma of Fallopian tube diagnosed with a combination of p57KIP2 immunostaining and short tandem repeat analysis: case report. J Obstet Gynaecol Res 2011;37:1493-6.
280. Petre I, Bernad E, Muresan A, et al. Choriocarcinoma developed in a tubal pregnancy - a case report. Rom J Morphol Embryol 2015;56(Suppl 2):871-4.
281. Rettenmaier MA, Khan HJ, Epstein HD, Nguyen D, Abaid LN, Goldstein BH. Gestational choriocarcinoma in the fallopian tube. J Obstet Gynaecol 2013;33:912-4.
282. Wan J, Li XM, Gu J. Primary choriocarcinoma of the fallopian tube: a case report and literature review. Eur J Gynaecol Oncol 2014;35:604-7.
283. Ober WB, Maier RC. Gestational choriocarcinoma of the fallopian tube. Diagn Gynecol Obstet 1981;3:213-31.
284. Brunner J, Högberg T, Malmström H, Simonsen E. Postmenopausal extragenital choriocarcinoma. A case report and review of the literature. Eur J Gynaecol Oncol 1991;12:395-8.
285. Kalhor N, Ramirez PT, Deavers MT, Malpica A, Silva EG. Immunohistochemical studies of trophoblastic tumors. Am J Surg Pathol 2009;33:633-8.
286. Shih IM, Kurman RJ. Ki-67 labeling index in the differential diagnosis of exaggerated placental site, placental site trophoblastic tumor, and choriocarcinoma: a double immunohistochemical staining technique using Ki-67 and Mel-CAM antibodies. Hum Pathol 1998;29:27-33.
287. Mao TL, Kurman RJ, Huang CC, Lin MC, Shih IeM. Immunohistochemistry of choriocarcinoma: an aid in differential diagnosis and in elucidating pathogenesis. Am J Surg Pathol 2007;31:1726-32.

288. Liu X, Li X, Yin L, Ding J, Jin H, Feng Y. Genistein inhibits placental choriocarcinoma cell line JAR invasion through ERβ/MTA3/Snail/E-cadherin pathway. Oncol Lett 2011;2:891-7.
289. Al-Shami R, Sorensen ES, Ek-Rylander B, Andersson G, Carson DD, Farach-Carson MC. Phosphorylated osteopontin promotes migration of human choriocarcinoma cells via a p70 S6 kinase-dependent pathway. J Cell Biochem 2005;94:1218-33.
290. Thang NM, Kumasawa K, Tsutsui T, et al. Overexpression of endogenous TIMP-2 increases the proliferation of BeWo choriocarcinoma cells through the MAPK-signaling pathway. Reprod Sci 2013;20:1184-92.
291. Huining L, Jingting C, Keren H. Metastasis gene expression analyses of choriocarcinoma and the effect of silencing metastasis-associated genes on metastatic ability of choriocarcinoma cells. Eur J Gynaecol Oncol 2011;32:264-8.
292. Mak VC, Lee L, Siu MK, et al. Downregulation of ASPP2 in choriocarcinoma contributes to increased migratory potential through Src signaling pathway activation. Carcinogenesis 2013;34:2170-7.
293. Cagayan MS, Lu-Lasala LR. Management of gestational trophoblastic neoplasia with metastasis to the central nervous system: a 12-year review at the Philippine General Hospital. J Reprod Med 2006;51:785-92.
294. Kurman RJ, Shih IeM. Discovery of a cell: reflections on the checkered history of intermediate trophoblast and update on its nature and pathologic manifestations. Int J Gynecol Pathol 2014;33:339-47.
295. Kurman RJ, Scully RE, Norris HJ. Trophoblastic pseudotumor of the uterus: an exaggerated form of "syncytial endometritis" simulating a malignant tumor. Cancer 1976;38:1214-26.
296. Behtash N, Karimi Zarchi M. Placental site trophoblastic tumor. J Cancer Res Clin Oncol. 2008;134:1-6.
297. Feltmate CM, Genest DR, Goldstein DP, Berkowitz RS. Advances in the understanding of placental site trophoblastic tumor. J Reprod Med 2002;47:337-41.
298. Baergen RN, Rutgers JL, Young RH, Osann K, Scully RE. Placental site trophoblastic tumor: a study of 55 cases and review of the literature emphasizing factors of prognostic significance. Gynecol Oncol 2006;100:511-20.
299. Piura B. Placental site trophoblastic tumor - a challenging rare entity. Eur J Gynaecol Oncol 2006;27:545-51.
300. Bower M, Paradinas FJ, Fisher RA, et al. Placental site trophoblastic tumor: molecular analysis and clinical experience. Clin Cancer Res 1996;2:897-902.
301. Schmid P, Nagai Y, Agarwal R, et al. Prognostic markers and long-term outcome of placental-site trophoblastic tumours: a retrospective observational study. Lancet 2009;374:48-55.
302. Hassadia A, Gillespie A, Tidy J, et al. Placental site trophoblastic tumour: clinical features and management. Gynecol Oncol 2005;99:603-7.
303. Hyman DM, Bakios L, Gualtiere G, et al. Placental site trophoblastic tumor: analysis of presentation, treatment, and outcome. Gynecol Oncol 2013;129:58-62.
304. Oldt RJ 3rd, Kurman RJ, Shih IeM. Molecular genetic analysis of placental site trophoblastic tumors and epithelioid trophoblastic tumors confirms their trophoblastic origin. Am J Pathol 2002;161:1033-7.
305. Fisher RA, Paradinas FJ, Newlands ES, Boxer GM. Genetic evidence that placental site trophoblastic tumours can originate from a hydatidiform mole or a normal conceptus. Br J Cancer 1992;65:355-8.
306. Cole LA, Khanlian SA, Muller CY. Blood test for placental site trophoblastic tumor and nontrophoblastic malignancy for evaluating patients with low positive human chorionic gonadotropin results. J Reprod Med 2008;53:457-64.
307. Harvey RA, Pursglove HD, Schmid P, Savage PM, Mitchell HD, Seckl MJ. Human chorionic gonadotropin free beta-subunit measurement as a marker of placental site trophoblastic tumors. J Reprod Med 2008;53:643-8.
308. Nagelberg SB, Rosen SW. Clinical and laboratory investigation of a virilized woman with placental-site trophoblastic tumor. Obstet Gynecol 1985;65:527-34.
309. Young RH, Scully RE, McCluskey RT. A distinctive glomerular lesion complicating placental site trophoblastic tumor: report of two cases. Hum Pathol 1985;16:35-42.
310. Gupta N, Mittal S, Misra R, Vimala N, Das AK. Placental site trophoblastic tumor originating in a tubal ectopic pregnancy. Eur J Obstet Gynecol Reprod Biol 2006;129:92-4.
311. Su YN, Cheng WF, Chen CA, et al. Pregnancy with primary tubal placental site trophoblastic tumor—a case report and literature review. Gynecol Oncol 1999;73:322-5.
312. Palmieri C, Fisher RA, Sebire NJ, Smith JR, Newlands ES. Placental-site trophoblastic tumour: an unusual presentation with bilateral ovarian involvement. Lancet Oncol 2005;6:59-61.
313. Shih IM, Kurman RJ. P63 expression is useful in the distinction of epithelioid trophoblastic and placental site trophoblastic tumors by profiling trophoblastic subpopulations. Am J Surg Pathol 2004;28:1177-83.

314. Shih IM, Kurman RJ. Epithelioid trophoblastic tumor: a neoplasm distinct from choriocarcinoma and placental site trophoblastic tumor simulating carcinoma. Am J Surg Pathol 1998;22:1393-403.
315. Mao TL, Seidman JD, Kurman RJ, Shih IeM. Cyclin E and p16 immunoreactivity in epithelioid trophoblastic tumor--an aid in differential diagnosis. Am J Surg Pathol 2006;30:1105-10.
316. Singer G, Kurman RJ, McMaster MT, Shih IeM. HLA-G immunoreactivity is specific for intermediate trophoblast in gestational trophoblastic disease and can serve as a useful marker in differential diagnosis. Am J Surg Pathol 2002;26:914-20.
317. Shih IM. The role of CD146 (Mel-CAM) in biology and pathology. J Pathol 1999;189:4-11.
318. Sung WJ, Shin HC, Kim MK, Kim MJ. Epithelioid trophoblastic tumor: clinicopathologic and immunohistochemical analysis of three cases. Korean J Pathol 2013;47:67-73.
319. Gloor E, Hürlimann J. Trophoblastic pseudotumor of the uterus: clinicopathologic report with immunohistochemical and ultrastructural studies. Am J Surg Pathol 1981;5:5-13.
320. Kodama S, Kase H, Aoki Y, et al. Recurrent placental site trophoblastic tumor of the uterus: clinical, pathologic, ultrastructural, and DNA fingerprint study. Gynecol Oncol 1996;60:89-93.
321. Soma H, Osawa H, Oguro T, et al. P57kip2 immunohistochemical expression and ultrastructural findings of gestational trophoblastic disease and related disorders. Med Mol Morphol 2007;40:95-102.
322. Sugimori H, Kashimura Y, Kashimura M, Taki I. Nuclear DNA content of trophoblastic tumors. Acta Cytol 1978;22:542-5.
323. Fukunaga M, Ushigome S. Malignant trophoblastic tumors: immunohistochemical and flow cytometric comparison of choriocarcinoma and placental site trophoblastic tumors. Hum Pathol 1993;24:1098-106.
324. Hui P, Parkash V, Perkins AS, Carcangiu ML. Pathogenesis of placental site trophoblastic tumor may require the presence of a paternally derived X chromosome. Lab Invest 2000;80:965-72.
325. Hui P, Riba A, Pejovic T, Johnson T, Baergen RN, Ward D. Comparative genomic hybridization study of placental site trophoblastic tumour: a report of four cases. Mod Pathol 2004;17:248-51.
326. Finkler NJ, Berkowitz RS, Driscoll SG, Goldstein DP, Bernstein MR. Clinical experience with placental site trophoblastic tumors at the New England Trophoblastic Disease Center. Obstet Gynecol 1988;71(Pt 1):854-7.
327. Brewer CA, Adelson MD, Elder RC. Erythrocytosis associated with a placental-site trophoblastic tumor. Obstet Gynecol 1992;79(Pt 2):846-9.
328. Dessau R, Rustin GJ, Dent J, Paradinas FJ, Bagshawe KD. Surgery and chemotherapy in the management of placental site tumor. Gynecol Oncol 1990;39:56-9.
329. Mangili G, Garavaglia E, De Marzi P, Zanetto F, Taccagni G. Metastatic placental site trophoblastic tumor. Report of a case with complete response to chemotherapy. J Reprod Med 2001;46:259-62.
330. Randall TC, Coukos G, Wheeler JE, Rubin SC. Prolonged remission of recurrent, metastatic placental site trophoblastic tumor after chemotherapy. Gynecol Oncol 2000;76:115-7.
331. Palmer JE, Macdonald M, Wells M, Hancock BW, Tidy JA. Epithelioid trophoblastic tumor: a review of the literature. J Reprod Med 2008;53:465-75.
332. Moutte A, Doret M, Hajri T, et al. Placental site and epithelioid trophoblastic tumours: diagnostic pitfalls. Gynecol Oncol 2013;128:568-72.
333. Davis MR, Howitt BE, Quade BJ, et al. Epithelioid trophoblastic tumor: a single institution case series at the New England Trophoblastic Disease Center. Gynecol Oncol 2015;137:456-61.
334. Zavadil M, Feyereisl J, Safar P, Pán M. [Undifferentiated choriocarcinomas—epithelioid trophoblastic tumors treated at the Center for Trophoblastic Diseases in the Czech Republic 1955-2003.] Ceska Gynekol 2003;68:420-6. [Czech]
335. Li J, Shi Y, Wan X, Qian H, Zhou C, Chen X. Epithelioid trophoblastic tumor: a clinicopathological and immunohistochemical study of seven cases. Med Oncol 2011;28:294-9.
336. Lu B, Zhang X, Liang Y. Clinicopathologic analysis of postchemotherapy gestational trophoblastic neoplasia: an entity overlapping with epithelioid trophoblastic tumor. Int J Gynecol Pathol 2016;35:516-24.
337. Kamoi S, Ohaki Y, Mori O, et al. Epithelioid trophoblastic tumor of the uterus: cytological and immunohistochemical observation of a case. Pathol Int 2002;52:75-81.
338. Bouchet-Mishellany F, Ledoux-Pilon A, Darcha C, Déchelotte P. [Trophoblastic gestational disease: a placental site trophoblastic tumor and an epithelioid trophoblastic tumor.] Ann Pathol 2004;24:167-71. [French]
339. Allison KH, Love JE, Garcia RL. Epithelioid trophoblastic tumor: review of a rare neoplasm of the chorionic-type intermediate trophoblast. Arch Pathol Lab Med 2006;130:1875-7.
340. Fadare O, Parkash V, Carcangiu ML, Hui P. Epithelioid trophoblastic tumor: clinicopathological features with an emphasis on uterine cervical involvement. Mod Pathol 2006;19:75-82.
341. Scott EM, Smith AL, Desouki MM, Olawaiye AB. Epithelioid trophoblastic tumor: a case report and review of the literature. Case Rep Obstet Gynecol 2012;2012:862472.

342. Zhao J, Xiang Y, Wan XR, Cui QC, Yang XY. Clinical and pathologic characteristics and prognosis of placental site trophoblastic tumor. J Reprod Med 2006;51:939-44.
343. Zhang X, Lü W, Lü B. Epithelioid trophoblastic tumor: an outcome-based literature review of 78 reported cases. Int J Gynecol Cancer 2013;23:1334-8.
344. Collins RJ, Ngan HY, Wong LC. Placental site trophoblastic tumor: with features between an exaggerated placental site reaction and a placental site trophoblastic tumor. Int J Gynecol 1990;9:170-7.
345. Yeasmin S, Nakayama K, Katagiri A, et al. Exaggerated placental site mimicking placental site trophoblastic tumor: case report and literature review. Eur J Gynaecol Oncol 2010;31:586-9.
346. Menczer J, Livoff A, Malinger G, Girtler O, Zakut H. Exaggerated placental site erroneously diagnosed as non-metastatic trophoblastic disease. A case report. Eur J Gynaecol Oncol 1999;20:115-6.
347. Dotto J, Jorge D, Hui P. Lack of genetic association between exaggerated placental site reaction and placental site trophoblastic tumor. Int J Gynecol Pathol 2008;27:562-7.
348. Shih IM, Seidman JD, Kurman RJ. Placental site nodule and characterization of distinctive types of intermediate trophoblast. Hum Pathol 1999;30:687-94.
349. Jacob S, Mohapatra D. Placental site nodule: a tumor-like trophoblastic lesion. Indian J Pathol Microbiol 2009;52:240-1.
350. Huettner PC, Gersell DJ. Placental site nodule: a clinicopathologic study of 38 cases. Int J Gynecol Pathol 1994;13:191-8.
350a. Nayar R, Snell J, Silverberg SG, Lage JM. Placental site nodule occurring in a fallopian tube. Hum Pathol 1996;27:1243-5.
351. Shitabata PK, Rutgers JL. The placental site nodule: an immunohistochemical study. Hum Pathol 1994;25:1295-301.
352. Chen BJ, Cheng CJ, Chen WY. Transformation of a post-cesarean section placental site nodule into a coexisting epithelioid trophoblastic tumor and placental site trophoblastic tumor: a case report. Diagn Pathol 2013;8:85.
353. Kaur B, Short D, Fisher RA, Savage PM, Seckl MJ, Sebire NJ. Atypical placental site nodule (APSN) and association with malignant gestational trophoblastic disease; a clinicopathologic study of 21 cases. Int J Gynecol Pathol 2015;34:152-8.
354. Tsai HW, Lin CP, Chou CY, et al. Placental site nodule transformed into a malignant epithelioid trophoblastic tumour with pelvic lymph node and lung metastasis. Histopathology 2008;53:601-4.
355. Shen DH, Khoo US, Ngan HY, et al. Coexisting epithelioid trophoblastic tumor and choriocarcinoma of the uterus following a chemoresistant hydatidiform mole. Arch Pathol Lab Med 2003;127:e291-3.
356. Stichelbout M, Devisme L, Franquet-Ansart H, et al. SALL4 expression in gestational trophoblastic tumors: a useful tool to distinguish choriocarcinoma from placental site trophoblastic tumor and epithelioid trophoblastic tumor. Hum Pathol 2016;54:121-6.
357. Hirata Y, Yanaihara N, Yanagida S, et al. Molecular genetic analysis of nongestational choriocarcinoma in a postmenopausal woman: a case report and literature review. Int J Gynecol Pathol 2012;31:364-8.
358. Fukuda T, Ohnishi Y. Histological and immunohistochemical observations of dedifferentiated leiomyosarcoma of the uterus. Acta Pathol Jpn 1991;41:466-72.
359. Chew I, Post MD, Carinelli SG, et al. P16 expression in squamous and trophoblastic lesions of the upper female genital tract. Int J Gynecol Pathol 2010;29:513-22.

Index*

A

Actinomyces endometritis, 46
Adenoacanthosis, 28
Adenocarcinoma, *see* Endometrioid adenocarcinoma
Adenofibroma, 405, **408**
    Differentiation from low-grade mullerian sarcoma, 405
    Mullerian adenofibroma, 408
Adenoma malignum-like endometrial invasion, 122
Adenomyoma, 252, 405, **408**
    Diagnostic features, 408
Differentiation from endometrial stromal tumor, 252; from low-grade mullerian sarcoma, 405
Adenomyomatosis, intravascular, 255
Adenomyosis, 52, 255
    Florid, differentiation from endometrial stromal tumor, 255
Alveolar soft part sarcoma, 347, **356**
    Differentiation from PEComa, 347
Amsterdam criteria for Lynch syndrome, 211
Amyloidosis, 54
Anatomy, normal uterus, 2
Angioleiomyoma, 296
Angioma, 356
Angiomyolipoma, 345
Angiosarcoma, 356
Apoplectic leiomyoma, 290
Arias-Stella reaction, 33, 200
    Differentiation from clear cell carcinoma, 200
Arteriovenous malformation, 356
Atypical hyperplasia, differentiation from endometrial carcinoma, 137
Atypical leiomyoma, *see* Smooth muscle tumors of uncertain malignant potential
Atypical polypoid adenomyoma, 139, **411**
    Diagnostic features, 411
    Differentiation from endometrial carcinoma, 139
Atypical stromal cells, endometrium, 49

B

Benign metastasizing leiomyoma, 295, **315**
Bethesda criteria for Lynch syndrome, 211
Blue nevus, 54
BRCA syndromes, 224

C

Carcinoma, *see* Endometrioid carcinoma
Carcinoma with yolk sac differentiation, differentiation from endometrial carcinoma, 148
Carcinosarcoma, 177, **383,** 406
    Clinical features, 383
    Differential diagnosis, 391; differentiation from low-grade mullerian sarcoma, 406
    General features, 383
    Immunohistochemical findings, 389
    Microscopic findings, 383
    Molecular genetic findings, 390
    Pathogenesis, 389
Cartilaginous metaplasia, 38
Cellular endometrial polyps, differentiation from endometrial stromal tumors, 250
Cellular intravenous leiomyomatosis, differentiation from endometrial stromal tumor, 254
Cellular leiomyoma, 301
Chemotherapy-induced endometrial changes, 45
Chondrosarcoma, 359
Choriocarcinoma, 476
    Clinical features, 476
    Gross findings, 477
    Immunohistochemical and molecular genetic findings, 480
    Microscopic findings, 477
    Treatment and prognosis, 481
Ciliated carcinoma, 111
Ciliated metaplasia, *see* Tubal metaplasia
Clear cell carcinoma, 144, 176, **187**
    Anaplastic clear cell carcinoma, 192
    Clinical features, 187
Differential diagnosis, 197; differentiation from endometrial adenocarcinoma, 144, 197; from serous carcinoma, 176
    General features, 187
    Gross findings, 187
    Immunohistochemical findings, 195
    Microscopic findings, 188
    Molecular genetic findings, 196
    Precursors, 195
    Treatment and prognosis, 202
        Clear cell changes, 33

*In a series of numbers, those in boldface indicate the main discussion of the entity.

Complete hydatidiform mole, 459
　Abnormal circumferential trophoblast hyper-
　　plasia, 460
　Abnormal implantation site, 462
　Abnormal villous architecture, 461
　Mosaic complete hydatidiform mole, 473
　Embryonic development, 464
　Villous hydrops, 462
　Villous vascular and stromal changes, 462
Cotyledonoid leiomyoma, 293, **304**
Cowden syndrome, 223
Cowden-like syndrome, 224
Cytomegalovirus endometritis, 46

D

Dedifferentiated endometrial carcinoma, **112**, 146
　Differentiation from endometrial adenocarcin-
　　oma, 146
Dedifferentiated (pleomorphic) leiomyosarcoma, 333
Diffuse leiomyomatosis, 290, **311,** 347
　Differentiation from lymphangiomyomatosis, 347
Diffuse leiomyomatosis peritonealis (diffuse perito-
　neal leiomyomatosis), 293, **312**
Dissecting leiomyoma, 293, **304**
Dissecting noncotyledonoid leiomyoma, 293

E

Embryology, normal uterus, 1
Endocervical adenocarcinoma, 139, 178
Differentiation from endometrial carcinoma, 139; from serous carcinoma, 178; from clear cell carcinoma, 200
Endocervical-type metaplasia, *see* Mucinous meta-
　plasia
Endometrial carcinoma, *see* Endometrioid carcinoma
Endometrial cycle, normal, 5
Endometrial hyperplasia, 75, *see also* Precancerous
　neoplasia
Endometrial intraepithelial neoplasia, 75, 137
　Differentiation from endometrial carcinoma, 137
Endometrial intraepithelial carcinoma, 173
Endometrial metaplasia, 9, **19**
　Epithelial metaplasias, 19
　　Arias-Stella reaction, 33
　　Clear cell changes, 33
　　Eosinophilic metaplasia, 32
　　Hobnail changes, 33
　　Mucinous metaplasia, 21
　　Mucinous metaplasia of intestinal type, 21
　　Mucinous metaplasia of pyloric type, 21
　　Papillary proliferations, 24
　　Papillary syncytial metaplasia, 10, **30**
　　Pregnancy-related changes, 33
　　Squamous metaplasia, 10, **28**
　　Tubal metaplasia, 10, **19**
　Stromal metaplasias, 37
　　Cartilaginous metaplasia, 38
　　Extramedullary hematopoiesis, 39
　　Fatty metaplasia, 38
　　Glial heterotopia, 38
　　Osseous metaplasia, 37
　　Smooth muscle metaplasia, 37
Endometrial neoplasia, 108
　Bethesda classification, 108
Endometrial polyp, **63**, 405
　Atypical, 405
　Clinical features, 63
　Differential diagnosis, 68
　Gross findings, 63
　Microscopic findings, 64
　Pathogenesis, 63
Endometrial serous carcinoma, differentiation
　　from endometrial adenocarcinoma, 142
Endometrial stromal nodule, 229
　Clinical features, 229
　Differential diagnosis, 250
　Gross findings, 229
　Immunohistochemical findings, 244
　Microscopic findings, 231
　Molecular genetic findings, 247
　Treatment and prognosis, 256
Endometrial stromal sarcoma, **229**, 347, 407
　Clinical features, 229
　Differential diagnosis, 250; differentiation from
　　PEComa, 347; from low-grade mullerian
　　sarcoma, 407
　Gross findings, 230
　High-grade sarcomas, 258, *see also* High-grade
　　endometrial stromal sarcomas
　Immunohistochemical findings, 244
　Microscopic findings, 231
　Molecular genetic findings, 247
　Treatment and prognosis, 256
　With variant morphology, 231, 236
Endometrial stromal tumors, 229, *see also under*
　individual entities
　Endometrial stromal nodule, 229
　Endometrial stromal sarcoma, 229
　High-grade endometrial stromal sarcomas, 258
　Undifferentiated uterine sarcomas, 268

Uterine tumors resembling ovarian sex cord tumors, 270
Endometritis, 40
　Acute, 40
　Chronic, 40
　Cytomegalovirus, 46
　Herpes, 46
　Lymphoma-like lesions, 43
　Necrotizing, 43
Endometrioid carcinomas, **89**, 174, 212, 429
　Adenocarcinoma, 91
　Binary grading system for endometrioid carcinomas, 106
　Ciliated carcinoma, 111
　Clinical features, 91
　Differential diagnosis, 137; differentiation from serous carcinoma, 174; from clear cell carcinoma, 197
　Endometrial neoplasia, 108
　Epidemiology, 89
　General features, 89
　Grading, 90, **103**
　　FIGO system, 103
　　Non-FIGO grading, 106
　Gross findings, 91
　Immunohistochemical findings, 131
　International Federation of Gynecology and Obstetrics (FIGO), 90, 103, 119
　　Grades, 90, 103
　　Stage, 119
　Lynch syndrome association, 212
　Markers of carcinoma, 131
　Microscopic findings, 91
　　Architectural features, 91
　　Cellular features, 93
　　　Cytologic, 93
　　　Nuclear, 97
　　Stromal features, 99
　　Treatment-related changes, 101
　Molecular genetic findings, 133
　Mucinous adenocarcinoma, 111
　Mucinous carcinoma, 111
　Secretory carcinoma, 111
　Staging, 119
　　Adenoma malignum-like invasion, 122
　　Cervical involvement, 125
　　FIGO stage, 119
　　Lymph node metastases, 129
　　Lymphovascular invasion, 124
　　MELF (microcystic, elongated, and fragmented) invasion, 121
　　Myometrial invasion, 119
　　Synchronous endometrial and ovarian carcinomas, 128
　Treatment and prognosis, 149
　Undifferentiated/dedifferentiated carcinoma, 112
　Villoglandular carcinoma, 111
　With yolk sac-like differentiation, 429
Endometrium, normal, 4
　Cytology, 13
Eosinophilic metaplasia, 32
Eosinophilic syncytial change, 30
Epithelial metaplasias, 19, *see also under individual entities*
Epithelioid leiomyoma, 309
Epithelioid leiomyosarcoma, 330
Epithelioid plexiform tumorlets, 309
Epithelioid trophoblastic tumor, 485
Exaggerated placental-site reaction, 489
Extramedullary hematopoiesis, 39

F

Familial cancer syndromes, 209, *see also under individual entities*
　BRCA syndromes, 224
　Cowden syndrome, 223
　Lynch syndrome, 209
　Lynch-like syndrome, 209
　Other mutations, 224
　POLE mutations, 223
Familial recurrent hydatidiform moles, 455
Fatty metaplasia, 38
FIGO grading of endometrial carcinoma, *see* Internation Federation of Gynecology and Obstetrics (FIGO) classification
Fumerate hydratase (FH)-deficient leiomyoma, 300

G

Genes and endometrial carcinoma, 133
Gestational trophoblastic diseases, 445, *see also under individual entities*
　Choriocarcinoma, 476
　Epidemiology, 452
　Epithelioid trophoblastic tumor, 485
　Exaggerated placental-site reaction, 489
　Familial recurrent hydatidiform moles, 455
　Genetics, 453
　Genetic testing, 456
　Human chorionic gonadotropin, 457
　Hydatidiform moles, 458
　Imprinting, 454

Mixed gestational trophoblastic tumors, 490
Placental-site nodule, 489
Placental-site trophoblastic tumor, 481
Staging, 452
Trophoblast development, 446
Trophoblast stem cells, 450
World Health Organization (WHO) classification, 445
Gland poor/intravascular adenomyosis, differentiation from endometrial stromal tumors, 251
Glial heterotopia, 38
Gonadotropin-releasing hormone reactive changes, 36
Granulomas, endometrial, 48

H

Hematolymphoid metastatic malignancies, 438
Hemorrhagic cellular (apoplectic) leiomyoma, 290, **306**
Hepatoid carcinoma, differentiation from endometrial carcinoma, 148
Hepatoid tumors, 431
Hereditary breast and ovarian cancer syndromes, 224
Hereditary nonpolyposis colorectal carcinoma, see Lynch syndrome
Herpes endometritis, 46
High-grade endometrial stromal sarcomas, 258
    YWHAE-FAM22 (*YWHAE-NUTM2*) sarcomas, 258
    ZC3H7B-BCOR sarcomas, 262
    With low-grade endometrial stromal sarcomas, 267
Histology, normal uterus, 3
Hobnail changes, 33
Hydatidiform moles, 455, **458**
    Complete hydatidiform mole, 459, see also Complete hydatidiform mole
    Ectopic hydatidiform mole, 470 add
    Familial recurrent, 455
    Genetic testing, 455
    Invasive hydatidiform mole, 469
    Metastatic disease, 470
    Partial hydatidiform mole, 464, see also Partial hydatidiform mole
    With twin pregnancy, 470
Hyperplasia, see Endometrial hyperplasia

I

Immunohistochemical carcinoma markers, 131
Inflammatory myofibroblastic tumor, 351
    Differentiation from smooth muscle tumors, 355

Intermediate-type trophoblastic tumor, 202
International Federation of Gynecology and Obstetrics (FIGO) classification, 90, 103, 119, 452
    Grading system for endometrial carcinoma, 90, 103
    Staging system for endometrial carcinoma, 119
    Trophoblastic diseases, 452
Intraepithelial clear cell carcinoma, 195
Intraepithelial serous carcinoma, 168, 173
Intrauterine device-related endometrial changes, 46
Intravascular adenomyomatosis, 255
Intravenous leiomyomatosis, 294, **313**, 347
    Diagnostic features, 313
    Differentiation from lymphangiomyomatosis, 347
Intravenous leiomyosarcomatosis, 325
Invasive hydatidiform mole, 469

L

Lehman and Hart endometrial proliferations, see Papillary metaplasia
Leiomyohybernoma, 310
Leiomyoma, 252, **289**, 335
    Angioleiomyoma, 296
    Benign metastasizing leiomyoma, 295, **315**
    Cellular leiomyoma, 301
    Clinical features, 290
    Differential diagnosis, 319; differentiation from endometrial stromal tumor, 252; from leiomyosarcomas, 335
Diffuse leiomyomatosis, 290, **311**
Diffuse leiomyomatosis peritonealis (diffuse peritoneal leiomyomatosis), 293, **312**
Dissecting leiomyoma, 293, **304**
Dissecting noncotyledonoid leiomyoma, 293
Drug-related changes, 308
Epidemiology, 289
Epithelioid leiomyoma, 309
    Gross findings, 291
    FH-deficient leiomyoma, 300
    FH germline mutations, 289
    General features, 289
    Hemorrhagic cellular (apoplectic) leiomyoma, 290, **306**
    Immunohistochemical findings, 315
    Intravenous leiomyomatosis, 294, **313**
Leiomyohybernoma, 310
Lipoleiomyoma, 310
    Microscopic findings, 295
    Mitotically active leiomyoma, 302
    Molecular genetic findings, 317

Myxoid leiomyoma, 310
Parasitic leiomyoma, 291, **311**
Perinodular hydropic leiomyoma, 293
Pyomyoma, 296
Seedling leiomyoma, 296
Treatment and prognosis, 323
With bizarre nuclei, 297
With heterologous elements, 310
With hydropic change, 304
With vascular invasion, 312
Leiomyosarcoma, **324**, 347
    Clinical features, 325
    Dedifferentiated (pleomorphic) leiomyosarcoma, 333
    Differential diagnosis, 335; differentiation from PEComa, 347
    Epidemiology, 324
    Epithelioid leiomyosarcoma, 330
    General features, 324
    Gross findings, 325
    Immunohistochemical findings, 333
    Intravenous leiomyosarcomatosis, 325
    Microscopic findings, 326
    Molecular genetic findings, 334
    Myxoid leiomyosarcoma, 331
    Spindle cell leiomyosarcoma, 326
    Treatment and prognosis, 337
Ligneous endometritis, 54
Lipoma, 358
Lipoleiomyoma, 310
Liposarcoma, 358
Lymphangiomyomatosis, and PEComa, 344
Lymphoma, metastatic, 438
Lymphoma-like lesions, 43
Lynch syndrome, 209
    Associated endometrioid carcinomas, 212
    General features, 209
    Genetics, 209
        Mismatch repair genes, 209, 216
    Gross findings, 212
    Immunohistochemical findings, 216
    Microsatellite instability (MSI), 212
    Microscopic findings, 212
    Screening and diagnosis, 210, 220
        Amsterdam criteria, 211
        Bethesda criteria, 211
    Treatment and prognosis, 220
Lynch-like syndrome, 222
    Mismatch repair genes, 222

M

Malakoplakia, endometrium, 48
Malignant rhabdoid tumor/*SMARCA-4* deficient uterine sarcoma, 359
MELF (microcystic, elongated and fragmented) invasion, 119
Mesenchymal tumors, 340
    Alveolar soft part tumor, 356
    Inflammatory myofibroblastic tumor, 351
    Lipoma, 358
    Liposarcoma, 358
    PEComa, 340
    Rhabdomyosarcoma, 348
    Solitary fibrous tumor, 358
Mesonephric-like carcinoma, 200, **424**
Metaplasia, *see* Endometrial metaplasia
Metastases, to uterine corpus, 433
    From extragynecologic sites, 437
    Hematolymphoid malignancies, 438
    Primary adnexal/peritoneal carcinomas, 435
    Primary cervical carcinomas, 435
Metastatic adenocarcinoma, 148
    Differentiation from endometrial adenocarcinoma, 148
Metastatic molar disease, 470
Mismatch repair genes, 209, 216, 222
Mixed carcinomas with a serous component, 176
Mixed endometrioid and clear cell carcinoma, 198
Mixed epithelial-stromal tumors, 383
MLH genes, 209, 222
Molar pregnancy, *see* Gestational trophoblastic diseases
Mucinous metaplasia, 10, **21**
    Differential diagnosis, 22
    Of intestinal type, 21
    Of pyloric type, 21
Mullerian adenofibroma, 408
Mullerian adenosarcoma, low-grade, 394
    Clinical features, 394
    Differential diagnosis, 305
    General features, 394
    Gross findings, 394
    Immunohistochemical findings, 403
    Microscopic findings, 395
    Molecular genetic findings, 405
    Treatment and prognosis, 407
Myxoid change, endometrium, 50
Myxoid leiomyoma, 310
Myxoid leiomyosarcoma, 331

N

Necrotizing endometritis, 43
Nerve sheath tumors, 359
Neuroendocrine carcinomas, 421
Nongestational tumors with trophoblastic differentiation, 431, 492

O

Osseous metaplasia, 37
Osteosarcoma, 359
Ovulation, 5

P

Papillary proliferations, 24
Papillary syncytial metaplasia, 10, **30**
Parasitic leiomyoma, 291, **311**
Partial hydatidiform mole, 464
    Abnormal trophoblast hyperplasia, 466
    Embryonic development, 468
    Villous architecture, 466
    Villous hydrops, 466
    Villous vascular and stromal changes, 467
PEComa, 340
    Angiomyolipomas, 345
    Association with lymphangiomyomatosis, 344
    Clinical features, 341
    Differential diagnosis, 346
    Epidemiology, 341
    Immunohistochemical findings, 345
    Microscopic findings, 341
    PEComatosis, 341
    Treatment and prognosis, 347
PEComatosis, 344
Perinodular hydropic leiomyoma, 293
Perivascular epithelioid cell tumor (PEComa), 201
Placental mesenchymal dysplasia, 474
Placental site nodule/plaque, 489
Placental site trophoblastic tumor, 346, **481**
    Diagnostic features, 481
differentiation from PEComa, 346
Pleomorphic undifferentiated carcinoma, 178
Plexiform tumorlets, 309
POLD1 genes and mutations, 222, **223**
POLE genes and mutations, 222, **223**
Precancerous neoplasia, endometrial, 75
    Atypical hyperplasia, 75, 80
    Clinical features, 76
    Diagnostic criteria, 77
    Differential diagnosis, 82

Endometrial intraepithelial neoplasia, 75, 80
    Epidemiology, 75
    Gross findings, 76
    Molecular genetic findings, 76
Nonatypical hyperplasia, 75, 80
Secretory hyperplasia, 83
Pregnancy-related endometrial changes, 33
Primitive neuroectodermal tumor, 148, 359, **426**
    Diagnostic features, 426
    Differentiation from endometrial carcinoma, 148
Progesterone-related reactive changes, 35
Pseudomyxoma endometrii, 51
Pyomyoma, 296

R

Radiation-induced endometrial changes, 45
Reactive changes, 179
Rhabdomyosarcoma, **348**, 405
    Alveolar, 348
    Botryoid, 348
    Embryonal, 348
    Pleomorphic, 348

S

Sarcoidosis, endometrial, 48
Secretory carcinoma, 111
Seedling leiomyoma, 296
Serous carcinoma, **165,** 199
    Clinical features, 165
    Differential diagnosis, 174; differentiation from clear cell carcinoma, 199
    General features, 165
    Gross findings, 166
    Immunohistochemical findings, 174
    Intraepithelial serous carcinoma, 168
    Microscopic findings, 166
    Minimal serous carcinoma, 168
    Molecular genetic findings, 174
    Precursors, 173
    Treatment and prognosis, 179
Serous endometrial intraepithelial carcinoma, 173
Sex cord-stromal tumors, 433
Small cell neuroendocrine carcinoma, differentiation from endometrial carcinoma, 146
Smooth muscle metaplasia, 37
Smooth muscle tumors, **289,** 346, *see also under individual entities*
    Differentiation from PEComa, 346
    Leiomyoma, 289
    Leiomyosarcoma, 324

Smooth muscle tumors of uncertain malignant potential, 339
Solitary fibrous tumor, 358
Spindle cell leiomyosarcoma, 326
Squamous cell carcinoma, 146, **423**
    Differentiation from endometrial carcinoma, 146
Squamous metaplasia, 10, **28**
Squamous morules, 28
Staging endometrial carcinoma, 119
    Cervical involvement, 125
    FIGO stage, 119
    Lymphovascular invasion, 124
    Myometrial invasion, 119
    Synchronous endometrial and ovarian involvement, 128
Sternberg tumor, 304
Stromal endometrial metaplasias, 37
Surface papillary syncytial change, *see* Papillary syncytial metaplasia
Symplastic leiomyoma, 297

T

Tamoxifen-related endometrial changes, 36
Teratoma, 431
Thermal ablation changes, 43
Trophoblast, 446
    Development, 446
    Differential diagnosis of tumors, 447
    Stem cells, 450
Tubal metaplasia, 10, **19**

U

Undifferentiated endometrial carcinoma, **112**, 145
    Differentiation from endometrial adenocarcinoma, 145
    Monomorphic, 112
    Pleomorphic, 112
Undifferentiated uterine sarcoma, 268
Uterine tumor resembling ovarian sex cord tumor (UTROSCT), 147, 254, **270,** 407
    differentiation from endometrial carcinoma, 147; from endometrial stromal tumors, 254; from low-grade mullerian sarcoma, 407

V

Vascular tumors, 356
    Angiomas, 356
    Angiosarcomas, 356
    Arteriovenous malformation, 356
Vasculature, normal uterus, 3
Vasculitis, 54
Villoglandular carcinoma, 111
Viral infections, 46

W

Wilms tumor, 148, **428**
    Diagnostic features, 428
    Differentiation from endometrial carcinoma, 148
Wnt genes, 1

X

Xanthogranulomatous endometritis, 47

Y

Yolk sac tumor, 202, **429**
YWHAE-FAM22 (YWHAE-NUTM2) high-grade endometrial stromal sarcoma, 255, **258**

Z

ZC3H7B-BCOR high-grade endometrial stromal sarcoma, 262